CLINICAL NURSING:

Pathophysiological and Psychosocial Approaches

Contributors:

ESTHER H. READ, A.B., M.Ed., R.N.

Associate Professor of Nursing, College of Nursing
Wayne State University, Detroit, Michigan

JANE FRANCES RONAN, B.S., A.M., R.N.

Assistant Professor of Nursing, College of Nursing
Wayne State University, Detroit, Michigan

NANCY MARTIN, B.S., M.A., R.N.

Assistant Professor, College of Nursing
University of Illinois, Chicago, Illinois

JOYCE PASSOS, B.S., M.S., R.N.

Assistant Professor of Nursing, College of Nursing
Wayne State University, Detroit, Michigan

CLINICAL NURSING:

Pathophysiological and Psychosocial Approaches

IRENE L. BELAND, B.S., M.S., R.N.
Professor of Nursing, College of Nursing
Wayne State University, Detroit, Michigan

THE MACMILLAN COMPANY
COLLIER-MACMILLAN LIMITED, LONDON

Ninth Printing, 1969

Library of Congress catalog card number: 65-15589

THE MACMILLAN COMPANY
COLLIER-MACMILLAN CANADA, LTD., TORONTO, ONTARIO

Printed in the United States of America

Preface

This book is written for the nursing student who is studying medical-surgical nursing for the first time. The approach that is used has been developed in the teaching of medical-surgical nursing over a period of many years. An attempt has been made to organize a vast quantity of material into a meaningful whole and to present the person who is ill as a total individual, not as a sick arm, leg, or heart. To further this objective the content of one chapter is related to and built upon earlier chapters and anticipates the content of later ones. Content is selected from the biological, physical, and social sciences. Emphasis is on normal as well as pathological physiology. Throughout the text the relationship of the function of one part to that of other parts of the body has been stressed. Since derangement in the function of one part is likely to affect other functions, including psychological and emotional functioning, these relationships are included. Further, an attempt has been made to organize all aspects of a function so that the interrelationships of different bodily functions are shown. As an example, one vital function is the maintenance of nutrition. All elements entering into the nutritional status from those affecting food supply and the ingestion, digestion, and absorption of food, to its utilization by cells, are presented. Through this approach, it is hoped that the student will have a broader base from which to evaluate the needs of each patient. A conscientious effort has been made to show how a variety of elements such as age, hereditary background, cultural background, state of nutrition, causative agent or agents, and the organs affected influence the effects of illness and the behavior manifested by the patient and his nursing requirements.

Surgery is regarded by the writer as a form of treatment. Recognition is given to the fact that the person experiencing surgical therapy has some special requirements. However, because he is a human being who has an illness, many of his needs are similar to those of other sick persons.

In the selection of content, three criteria have been given priority: first, that the information act as a basis for answering the question "Why?"; second, that it have broad rather than limited applicability; and third, that it have relevance to the practice of nursing as defined by the writer. Though nurses perform many activities, including acting as the physician's assistant, and as the protector and custodian of machines, their function in ministering to and in behalf of the patient has been emphasized.

Extensive footnoting and bibliographies have been used. It is hoped that sufficient content has been included to provide the student with a base to which she can continue to add. No effort has been made to be encyclopedic.

With the rapid expansion of knowledge and techniques, it is essential that the nurse be prepared to continue her own learning. Hopefully, the content of the book will also help to prepare the student for change and to make changes. If nursing is to survive, the members of the profession must be prepared to accept and effect change. The maintenance of the *status quo* is no longer adequate.

In the development of the content a number of concepts[1] have been presented and discussed. They include:

1. Adaptation is basic to survival.
   a. The human organism is flexible and permits adaptations at all levels of activity (physiological, psychological, social).
   b. As an organism increases in complexity, specialized structures are required to facilitate adaptive functions.
   c. In health, physiological and psychological changes are regulated within limits.
   d. Some of the effects observed in disease result from the utilization of adaptive mechanisms.
   e. In disease, adaptation may be deficient, excessive, disorganized, or initiated by inappropriate stimuli.
   f. The physiological and psychological changes occurring in disease have a cause or causes, and within limits, some of them serve a useful purpose.
2. Heredity and environment interact to create individual potentials and differences.
3. Patient needs determine patient care.
4. Organization facilitates the utilization of resources to meet human needs.
5. Optimum health is a desirable goal.
6. The value of an observation depends on the integrity and detachment with which it is made and on its specificity.
7. Perceptions of reality vary with the perceiver.
8. The interaction of multiple factors determines the outcome of a situation.
9. Progress from disease toward health involves an increase in the capacity of the patient to cope with stress. During illness and recovery, the patient's needs shift from dependence, to independence, to interdependence.
10. Manifestations of disease and behavior during illness result from:
    a. An attempt on the part of the organism to adapt to or to compensate for disturbed function.
    b. The mobilization of defense mechanisms.
    c. The effect of injury on cells comprising a tissue or organ.
    d. The meaning that a disease and its treatment has for a person.

[1] Many of these concepts were developed by a group of the faculty of Wayne State University College of Nursing.

11. What a person does when he is ill depends on what he believes to be the cause of his illness and how he thinks it should be treated.
12. Therapy in disease includes one or more of the following: neutralizing the cause, encouraging compensatory mechanisms, and providing rest to the diseased organ so that healing can take place.
13. Respect for the rights and dignity of man is fundamental in a democratic society. This is just as essential to the sick as to the well.
14. Mutual trust is basic to the establishment of constructive nurse-patient relationships.
15. Acceptance of the patient involves considering the meaning of his behavior and recognizing that it has a cause and serves a purpose. It does not require the nurse to compromise her own system of values.
16. The behavior of a person is affected by and affects all persons and events with which he is involved.
17. Rehabilitation is a continuous process which begins with the first contact with the patient.
18. The patient has a right to participate in plans concerning his welfare.
19. The nurse has a responsibility to assist the patient and his family to utilize his resources constructively.
20. Nurses have an obligation to explore interests and aptitudes with the patient to increase his skills in living.
21. Nursing procedures can be used to facilitate communication.
22. There are limits to what can be accomplished by medical science.
23. Birth, growth, health, disease, and death are all phenomena of life.

For some readers, too much content may be provided in some areas and too little in others. Certain specialized areas of the body now included in medical-surgical nursing texts have not been included. No attempt has been made to include a wide variety of procedures. For the most part, procedures are included for the purpose of illustrating or emphasizing a point or points. Although the nurse does have a responsibility for using machines properly and for knowing whether or not they are operating properly, little attention has been given to the operation and care of machines employed in the treatment of disease. When directions provided by the manufacturer are inadequate, technicians from the factory are usually available to instruct in the use and care of complicated machines.

The writer would like to express her appreciation to the many persons who assisted in countless ways in the preparation of the manuscript. First are the students, who, over the years, asked the question, "When are you going to write a medical-surgical nursing book based on physiology?" or made statements such as, "Nursing makes more sense and is more fun when you are encouraged to seek answers to the question 'Why?' " Finally, the graduates of the class of 1962 provided concrete assistance by trying out and making constructive suggestions used in the revision of the "Guide for Assessing the Needs of Patients."

Certainly, the manuscript would have never been started or completed had it not been for the cooperation, patience, and prodding of Dean Katharine Faville of the College of Nursing of Wayne State University. Among others who provided encouragement are Miss Sylvia Peabody, R.N., Dean Mary Kelly Mullane, R.N., and Dean Rozella Schlotfeldt, R.N.

Those who read parts of the manuscript and assisted with the library research that went into its preparation and writing include the following: Mrs. Mary Ann Gray, R.N., Mrs. Joyce Passos, R.N., Miss Nancy Couture, R.N., Miss Milenca Herc, R.N. (deceased), Mrs. Lorene Fischer, R.N., Mrs. Mildred Konlande, Miss Kathlene Monahan, R.N., Mrs. Charlotte Pickering, R.N., Mrs. Claudia Watson, R.N., and Mrs. Dawn Zagornik, R.N. Special thanks go to Mr. Theodore Draves, who typed and retyped the manuscript in all of its revisions. I am greatly indebted to Dr. Gordon Doty, who, with the exception of the chapters on the special requirements of patients treated surgically and neural integration, read the entire manuscript. Dr. Raymond C. Read took time from a busy schedule to read the chapter on the special requirements of surgical patients. Dr. John Sterling Meyer read and commented on the chapter on neural integration. My gratitude also goes to my colleagues who cheerfully assumed some of my responsibilities when the manuscript was in preparation and to those who participated in the identification of nursing concepts.

Finally, the writer wishes to express sincere appreciation to the staff of the Macmillan Company, and especially to Mr. Henry Van Swearingen, for their help and cooperation during the preparation and production of this book.

Irene L. Beland

Contents

1 : Introduction

> She opened her hands to the needy and stretched out her hands to the poor. . . . Strength and honesty are her clothing. . . . She rendered good, not evil, all the days of her life. . . . The law of clemency is on her tongue. . . . Many daughters have gathered together riches but the valiant woman has surpassed them all.
>
> The Book of Proverbs

The purpose of this chapter is to introduce the reader to: (1) the writer's views about nursing as a profession, (2) how other nurses, the sociologist, and the patient view the role of the nurse, (3) some factors that should be considered in assessing patients' needs, (4) a suggested guide for assessing the needs of the patient, (5) methods used by the nurse in the practice of nursing, (6) a definition of medical-surgical nursing, and (7) a preview of future chapters.

PROFESSIONAL STATUS OF NURSING

The two questions "What is nursing?" and "Is nursing a profession?" have been the subject of both thought and disagreement. Neither have been answered to the satisfaction of everyone. Henderson,[1] while recognizing the difficulty in defining nursing, states: "Nursing is primarily assisting the individual (sick or well) in the performance of those activities contributing to health, or to its recovery (or to a peaceful death) that he would perform unaided if he had the necessary strength, will, or knowledge. It is likewise the. unique contribution of nursing to help the individual to be independent of such assistance as soon as possible."

The question "Is nursing a profession?" raises two further questions. What are the characteristics of a professional person? And what are the characteristics of a profession? Darley[2] describes the characteristics of a professional person as follows: "The truly professional person is one, who, by virtue of intellectual capacity, education and moral outlook, is capable of the exercise of intellectual and moral judgment at a high level of responsibility." In his discussion of the professional person, Darley emphasizes the importance of

---

[1] Bertha Harmer, revised by Virginia Henderson, *Textbook of Principles and Practice of Nursing*, 5th ed., The Macmillan Company, New York, 1955, p. 4.
[2] Ward Darley, "The Professions and Professional People," *Nursing Forum*, I, Winter 1961, p. 83.

judgment based on "broad knowledge, penetrating wisdom and great moral certitude."

Nursing, as it is practiced today, is not always on a professional level. The writer believes, however, that nursing can and should qualify as a profession. This belief is supported by Towle,[3] who has included nursing in her list of professions.

In order to examine the possibility of nursing's being a profession, the principal characteristics of a profession and of professional practice that are suggested by Towle will be considered. They are: (1) a profession has attitudes toward the recipients of its service which are essential to the giving of service in ways that are helpful to the recipients, (2) a profession has something to give which is unique and which other members of the community do not have to offer to the same degree, and (3) a profession demands of its members competence, in both knowledge and skill, in its practice.

ATTITUDES ABOUT NURSING

What are some of the attitudes of a profession toward recipients of its service which are essential to the giving of service in ways that are helpful?

The attitude that is fundamental to the practice of professions that have as their purpose helping people is respect for every person as an individual human being with dignity and rights. Every person has and retains his dignity and rights whatever his state in life, his religion, color, national origin, economic status, age, state of health, or personal habits. True respect for the dignity and rights of the individual is demonstrated in many ways. The person is treated with kindness, thoughtfulness, and courtesy. Service, whether it be for, to, or with the individual, is given in a way that meets the needs of the individual. Moreover, service is continued as long but only as long as it is required. The person who is sick is allowed to be sick, but as soon as he is able to resume the management of his own affairs he is encouragd to do so. Emphasis is on helping the individual to identify his strengths and resources and on assisting him in utilizing them rather than taking over and acting for him. When the latter is necessary, as it sometimes is, the reason should be to meet a need of the patient and not to meet a need of the nurse. An important objective is to identify and meet the needs of the patient in ways that are appropriate to the person and his situation. The behavior of the patient is recognized to have a cause and to serve a purpose. Respect for him as an individual demands that an effort be made to consider the meaning of his behavior and to act accordingly.

Another attitude that the truly professional person has is acceptance that the recipient has needs, physiological, psychological, social, intellectual, and

[3] Charlotte Towle, *The Learner in Education for the Professions*, University of Chicago Press, Chicago, 1954, p. 3.

spiritual, which must be met if he is to survive and be productive. At times one need may take precedence over others; however, when the nurse is attending to a dominant need, other needs should not be ignored. It is the responsibility of the profession to try to identify what needs it is prepared to meet and how it can go about meeting them. Moreover, the member of the profession provides service without expecting the recipient to express his gratitude or otherwise directly reward the professional for his efforts. The professional person gives service because the person needs it rather than for selfish reasons.

RECAPITULATION

To recapitulate, nursing as a profession is concerned with the welfare of the individual as an individual. It professes to respect the rights and dignity of each and every patient. It recognizes that each patient has needs some of which can be met through the practice of nursing. It accepts the premise that each patient has the right to participate to the degree that he can in plans for his welfare. Although practice of nursing involves doing to, for, and with the patient, it further involves assisting him to become independent of the services of nursing as soon as he is able to do so. The profession has as a general objective the meeting of the needs of the patient, in distinction to meeting its own needs—that is, either those of the individual nurse or those of the profession. The above list of attitudes characteristic of a profession is not exhaustive nor is it meant to be. Rather the intention has been to examine some of the attitudes fundamental to a profession. To the extent that these attitudes influence positively the practice of nursing, nursing can be said to be a profession.

NURSING CARE IS UNIQUE

The second characteristic of a profession is that it has some services or skills which are unique to that profession and which other members of the community do not have to the same degree. Despite some investigation and discussion, nurses are not agreed about what the skills are that are unique to nursing.

What skills or services does professional nursing have that other members of the community do not have to the same degree?

One view is that the area which is uniquely nursing is the giving of physical care. Those who espouse this view do not mean, nor do they intend to mean, that nursing is limited to the physical care of the patient. When it is, it is a mechanical or technical procedure, just as any service to people may be. Physical care is made professional by the manner in which it is provided and by the degree to which the nurse identifies and meets other needs of the patient. Nurses too often fail to respect the importance of physical care to the patient, both to his immediate welfare and as a means of establishing a helping relationship with him. Nurses, like other members of the American culture, tend to look at the part away from the whole and to want a single answer to each question or problem. Perhaps this pitfall could be avoided if the needs of the patient were identified and priorities established for what is important in the care of a patient at a particular time. Care would then be planned in terms of the needs of the patient. Those needs for which the professional nurse possesses competence would be met by the practice of nursing. Those for which she lacked competence would be referred to or performed by others, such as the physician, social worker, occupational therapist, or clergyman.

Kreuter, although not attempting to state what is unique about nursing, defines nursing care as ". . . acting and interacting with the patient through physical and personal contact for his welfare, and intervening in his behalf between him and those stresses in the physical environment and in the social climate that impinge on him."[4]

COMPONENTS OF NURSING PRACTICE

In an attempt to delineate the components of nursing practice, Kreuter[5] lists the following: (1) providing nursing care; (2) coordinating the care given not only by nurses, but by the members of other professions; (3) planning for the continuity of care not only within the hospital or agency, but with other community agencies; (4) evaluating the care of the patient; and (5) directing others in the care of the patient, including members of the family. Kreuter further emphasizes that nursing care includes the activities performed directly with the patient and those performed away from the patient, but in his behalf.

COMPETENCE

The third characteristic of a profession is that it demands a high degree of competence, both in knowledge and in skill, in its practice. No one denies that nursing requires a high degree of skill. There is less agreement as to how much or even what knowledge is required. Towle[6] quotes Tyler as emphasizing: ". . . that it is in the nature of a profession that it bases its techniques of operation upon principles rather than upon rule-of-thumb procedures or simple routine tasks, . . . "Nursing faces the task of identifying the principles on which the practice of nursing is based. Because this has not been done very

---

[4] Frances Kreuter, "What Is Good Nursing Care?" *Nursing Outlook*, V, May, 1957, p. 302.
[5] *Ibid.*, p. 302.
[6] *Op. cit.*, p. 5.

well, this is an area where the status of nursing as a profession is weak. There is little doubt that the welfare of the patient often depends on the exercise of considerable judgment on the part of the nurse. Basic to making valid judgments is a body of knowledge of the principles on which judgment is based. Studies presently underway as well as those of the future will in time lead to the identification of these principles.

In the preceding paragraphs nursing as a profession has been examined in reference to three of the characteristics of a profession. While the discussion has not exhausted the possibilities, perhaps the reader will be stimulated to think about what being professional means and what nursing must do to be, or to become, a profession. Sometimes insight can be gained into what one does or ought to do by examining the views of persons who are not of the profession.

THE ROLE OF THE NURSE IN PATIENT CARE

Recently sociologists have developed an interest in the role of the nurse in patient care. They suggest that the actions taken by nurses in the care of patients can be classified under two roles. One, the therapeutic role, includes all those actions directed toward the prevention and treatment of disease. The other is called the expressive role by some and the mother-substitute role by others. It includes all those activities directed toward creating an environment in which the patient feels comforted, accepted, protected, cared for, and supported. The emphasis in the performance of the expressive role is not on cure, but on the manner in which care is provided. Johnson and Martin[7] and Schulman[8] emphasize that the physical care of the patient is an important vehicle for communicating to the patient the concern of the nurse for his welfare.

Since the therapeutic role of the nurse has as its goal the prevention and cure of disease, discussion of the details of this role will be included in later chapters. Inasmuch as all patients experience the manner in which they are nursed, the expressive role of the nurse will be considered in some detail here. Johnson and Martin[9] state that the objective of the expressive role is the relief of tension in the group. The group referred to here is composed of the doctor, nurse, and patient. Though they do not so state, the group actually consists of all those who have some relationship to the patient including the members of his family and his friends. They further state that, in any social system, certain problems must be solved if the system is to maintain itself. That is, it must move forward toward the accomplishment of a common goal and it must

[7] Miriam M. Johnson and Henry W. Martin, "A Sociological Analysis of the Nurses Role," *American Journal of Nursing*, LVIII, March, 1958, pp. 373-77.
[8] Sam Schulman, "Basic Functional Roles in Nursing: Mother Surrogate and Healer" in *Patients, Physicians and Illness*, ed. E. Gartley Jaco, The Free Press, Glencoe, Illinois, 1958, pp. 528-37.
[9] *Loc. cit.*, p. 373.

maintain internal equilibrium. They explain by stating ". . . relationships between the social system members must be harmonious and integrated and each member must feel good both within himself and toward other group members." They emphasize the importance of the nurse in this role by suggesting that it is here she is the expert and as such should give leadership. She stands as an intermediary between the patient and the doctor and what he does for and to the patient. If this view is accepted, the nurse also stands between the patient and the other persons who participate in his care. To fulfill this role she must know what the common goal or objective is and give leadership to those working toward its achievement. She does this by utilizing her skills in such a manner that each person feels "good within himself and toward other members of the group." Martin and Johnson[10] emphasize that the physical care of the patient is important because it gives the nurse an opportunity to reduce the tension of the patient and to promote good feeling.

Schulman[11] compares the feeling that the nurse should have for her patient as being similar to the feeling that a mother has for her child. The early phase of the mother-child relationship is largely physical and marked by tenderness and compassion. The mother tends her child and stands between him and harm. She comforts him and soothes his hurts. As the child grows and develops in his ability to care for himself, she encourages him to become independent of her. The mother gives of herself and of her material resources to meet his needs, because he is her child.

Johnson and Martin[12] state that the expressive role of the nurse can be carried too far and that the needs and wants of a patient can be so gratified that he prefers sickness to health. As in other situations, multiple factors contribute to the preference of the patient for sickness to health. The nurse should not assume that she is necessarily the one who is responsible when a patient prefers sickness to health. She should, of course, examine her behavior to be sure that she is not contributing to the situation. The physician usually is responsible for indicating to the patient that he is not trying to get well and that his behavior is not acceptable. The nurse has the responsibility for recognizing the signs indicating that the patient is finding the secondary gains of illness preferable to returning to the healthy state and for supporting the physician and the patient when the physician decides the time has come to help the patient move toward recovery.

A second problem in the practice of the expressive role concerns the nurse. She must have and convey to the patient a very real concern for his welfare and at the same time develop in herself the ability to evaluate objectively both his behavior and the effect of her own behavior on him. She may find that in one instance she was too supporting and in another she withdrew her support too soon, or that she was too permissive or too limiting. She may also find

[10] *Ibid.*, p. 373.
[11] *Loc. cit.*, p. 530.
[12] *Loc cit.*, p. 376.

that she felt so strongly with the patient that she was unable to give him the support he needed to consider his alternatives or to do what he knew he had to do. Psychologists emphasize that the more the person is concerned with himself, the less he is able to be concerned with others. The nurse contributes to the welfare of the patient when she not only is able to communicate to him her interest in and concern for his welfare, but also maintains enough objectivity to evaluate his needs and act in the manner that is best suited to meet them.

What do patients want from nursing?

A study performed by Abdellah and Levine[13] to determine what patients want from nursing provides some answers to the above question. In summarizing their study, they say that a patient wants:

1. To be treated as an individual, that is, he wants his care to be personalized rather than depersonalized
2. An explanation of his care
3. To be considered as a partner in his care
4. To have his behavior as a sick person accepted as a part of his illness
5. To be treated with thoughtfulness, kindness, and firmness

THE PATIENT AS A PERSON

How can the care of the patient be personalized or individualized?

Basic to the treatment of each patient as an individual is respect for him as a person. This respect is demonstrated in many ways. The treatment of each patient with the same courtesy that one expects from one's associates goes a long way toward establishing the fact that the patient is an individual. This courtesy should be extended to the patient's family and friends. They do have a right to be concerned about the patient and his welfare as well as a role to play in his recovery. An effort should be made to allow the family to express their feelings and to interpret their behavior in the light of its meanings. The effect of their behavior on the patient should also be evaluated. When some change is necessary, explanations should be in terms of the needs of the patient and recognition should be given to the interest of the family in the welfare of the patient. If the nurse accepts the fact that she has a responsibility for the welfare of the patient, she will intervene when the quality or quantity of visiting is likely to be detrimental to his interests.

A recent exaggerated, but nevertheless true, example of the abdication by

[13] Faye Abdellah and Eugene Levine, "What Patients Say About Their Nursing Care," *Hospitals,* XXXI, No. 1, 1957, pp. 44-48.

the nurse of her responsibility to protect the patient from harm is illustrated by the following anecdote. Mary Lively, age 17, was hospitalized on Friday night. She had been in an automobile accident and had two crushed lumbar vertebrae. She also had some superficial scalp wounds. On the following Sunday, she and her roommate had 84 visitors. When Mary's mother visited her in the evening, she found Mary in a state of near collapse. When Mrs. Lively complained, she was told that it was the responsibility of the family to regulate visitors. Though Mrs. Lively had visited Mary in the morning, she had not been in the hospital at the time when most of the visitors arrived. She had asked that a sign be placed on the door indicating that not more than two visitors be admitted at a time. The visitors cooperated. They lined up and entered the room two at a time until the room was full. The conclusion that the nurse in this situation had lost sight of her responsibility to protect the patient and that she failed to exercise reasonable judgment is an understatement. Moreover, patients other than those immediately involved must have suffered.

One of the really unique characteristics of each person is his name. If this premise is accepted, a way to show respect for an individual is to call him by his name and title. Despite a trend toward informality, an adult should be called by his surname preceded by the appropriate title, that is Mr., Mrs., or Miss. Unless there is a specific and identified reason, an adult should not be addressed by his first name. Certainly first names should not be used to indicate that the social or economic status of the patient is less than that of those who care for him. Calling an elderly person "Grandma" or "Grandpa" may express affection, but it may also be interpreted by the patient to indicate a lack of respect for him and his potential. Some elderly persons bitterly resent being called "Grandpa" or "Grandma" by anyone except their grandchildren. A patient who is addressed by his first name or who is nameless does not always express his resentment openly, but this does not mean that he fails to feel resentment.

Respect for the individual is expressed by the nurse when she greets the patient when entering his presence and includes him in any conversation carried on in his presence. Other courtesies too often neglected include asking the permission of the patient when it is necessary to interrupt his activities or his care. That his care should not be interrupted unless it is absolutely necessary is obvious. Respect for the patient as an individual also includes sensitivity to his feelings. This is expressed when the nurse tries to modify her behavior so that the patient knows that she appreciates how he feels. She tries to avoid being excessively cheerful in the presence of a downcast or gloomy patient. On the other hand, she also avoids being gloomy herself.

Respect for the patient is evidenced when his suggestions, opinions, and concerns are treated with courtesy and thoughtfulness. It is also evidenced when the nurse protects him from unnecessary embarrassment by protecting his modesty and by helping him prepare for the visit of his doctor or family.

Respect for the patient as a human being is demonstrated by trying to create an environment in which the patient is able to express his feelings, and when the nurse interprets his behavior as an expression of an unmet need or needs and then acts appropriately. Sometimes a patient is demanding and aggressive because he feels depersonalized. He fights to be recognized as a human being. The patient may relax when he is certain that he can depend on the nursing staff to meet his needs as an individual human being.

The nurse is likely to find individualization of each patient's care easier if she has some awareness of her own values as well as of her biases and prejudices. No one is completely free of prejudice. When an individual knows what he values and what his biases and prejudices are, he may be able to limit their effect on the care he provides the patient. For example, Mrs. Laura, a public health nurse, took pride in being unprejudiced. One day as she was thinking about how unsuccessful she had been with the Hill family, she thought, "How could anyone be successful with those hillbillies?" As she talked about her experience later, she said that she was shocked to learn that she too had prejudices and thought of people not as individuals, but as stereotypes. After she recognized what she had been feeling, she was better able to manage her feelings and as a result to enlist the cooperation of Mrs. Hill.

Although numerous situations in which care of a patient was or was not individualized could be cited, only three will be presented. In the first situation failure to meet an obvious or overt need of the patient contributed to the feeling on the part of the patient of depersonalization and to a failure of the nursing personnel to experience satisfaction. In the second situation, the nurse recognized and met a covert need of a patient. The last illustrates why it is impossible to individualize care by rule.

The first patient, Mrs. Devoted Family, had undergone major surgery several days previous to the incident cited below. Following her operation, both she and her family expressed their concern about her progress openly and volubly. One of her less serious complaints, from the point of view of the personnel, was that her feet were cold. Though she complained to everyone who participated in her care, nothing was done to relieve her discomfort. Her family, however, took their mother's discomfort seriously and bought her a lovely white wool shawl, which they placed over her feet. A few days later the shawl was discarded with the bed linen. Naturally, Mrs. Family and her children were upset. The nursing staff responded by saying that they had no responsibility for the personal belongings of the patient; nothing could be done to recover the shawl. In this instance, the simple procedure of placing a bath blanket over Mrs. Family's feet might have been sufficient to relieve her discomfort. Mrs. Family might well have had her feelings of importance enhanced had the nurse placed a blanket over her feet in such a manner that the patient knew that the nurse wanted her to be comfortable. Moreover, the manner of the nurse might also have suggested that if the blanket did not accomplish the objective, there were other things that she could and would do.

She could give Mrs. Family a hot-water bottle or ask her daughter to bring her some bed or ankle socks. In any event the patient's feeling of depersonalization might have been reduced by any one of several simple acts. As it was, both the patient and her family felt that Mrs. Family was neglected. She had suffered a double injury—cold feet and a lack of appropriate action to correct her discomfort as well as the loss of a valued possession. These feelings were strengthened by the loss of the shawl and failure of the nursing staff to appear to make any effort to retrieve it. The nursing staff was also deprived because they failed to achieve any sense of satisfaction in the care of Mrs. Family.

The next patient is Mr. Johnson. In the care of Mr. Johnson the nurse recognized and responded to a need that the patient was unable to express directly. Mr. Johnson was a middle-aged, obese man with a diagnosis of far-advanced carcinoma of the lung. He was allowed bathroom privileges and permitted to sit in a chair as he desired. In this hospital, patients who were up and about were expected to take their own sponge baths. Showers and bath-tubs were not available. One busy morning just before noon, Miss Team Leader stopped to check with Mr. Johnson to see whether or not he had taken his bath. In response to Miss Team Leader's inquiry, he said, "I did the best I could." Now Miss Team Leader might have said, "I'll make your bed, or send Mrs. Aide in to do it." She, however, interpreted Mr. Johnson's statement as saying, "I was not able to take a very good bath and I'd like to be given one." She thought a moment about his reply and realized that although he was up and about, even a small amount of exertion caused Mr. Johnson to be short of breath. She got a basin of warm water and *gave* him a bath. As she was bathing him, he lay back against his pillows, sighed, and relaxed, saying "This is the first bath that I've had since I came here."

The third patient is Mrs. Willow. Mrs. Willow was a young middle-aged woman who some months earlier had had a radical mastectomy for cancer of the breast. The cancer had since metastasized to her spine and now impinged upon her spinal cord. She was unable to control the movements of her lower extremities. Slight movement or jarring of her body resulted in muscular spasms that were accompanied by severe pain. Mrs. Willow was in the hospital for the purpose of determining the amount of a curarizing drug that would control the muscular spasms without paralyzing the muscles of respiration. After spending three days in a ten-bed ward, she was moved to a double room and was placed in the bed next to the door. She spent her days sitting in bed and guarding herself each time someone came into the room. Her general expression was that of a frightened fawn. In this instance, the head nurse at the daily nursing care conference talked with the group about Mrs. Willow. Together the members of the group worked out ways to protect Mrs. Willow from avoidable suffering. A sign was placed on the door to warn those who were entering to be especially careful not to jar her bed. The dietary aide was asked to call a nurse when Mrs. Willow's tray was ready rather than to deliver it to the room. As soon as the patient in the bed away from the door was discharged, Mrs. Willow's bed was moved. A special procedure was planned with Mrs. Willow, so that her bed linen could be changed without causing her unnecessary discomfort. Other procedures were also modified. Suggestions were recorded on the "Nursing Care Record" so that the information about Mrs. Willow's special needs could be communicated to all members of the staff.

Though there was no possibility of cure in the instance either of Mr. Johnson or of Mrs. Willow, both these patients benefited from thoughtful and creative nursing. In both these instances, the nurses also experienced satisfaction, inasmuch as they concentrated on and were able to improve the situation of the patient. In the care of Mr. Johnson and Mrs. Willow, nurses demonstrated their concern for the welfare of the patient largely through physical care, and they exercised judgment in the realm that is nursing. In neither instance was the amount of time involved great. In fact, time was probably saved in the care of Mrs. Willow.

PREPARING THE PATIENT FOR WHAT TO EXPECT

How may nurses prepare patients for what to expect?

In addition to the wish of the patient to be treated as an individual, Abdellah and Levine[14] found that he wants an explanation of his care. Another way this may be said is that he wants to know what to expect and what is expected of him. Wertham[15] a psychiatrist, in discussing his own experience as a patient, made the following comments: "Medical and surgical patients need psychological advice about how they should act, what their experiences mean; they need psychological preparation for what to expect; they need guidance, so that they can make the best of their possibilities."

Preparing the patient for what to expect includes acquainting him with such hospital routines as when meals are served and medicines administered, when his friends may visit or telephone him, and how to call the nurse. He should be informed about those aspects of his care requiring some change in his behavior. For example, he is to stay in bed until seen by his physician, or he is free to move about and go to the solarium, or he should stay in his room. Most persons who are ill are more or less anxious; they frequently need to have instructions repeated a number of times as high levels of anxiety interfere with the ability to learn. Since the patient often has questions about his illness and the plan of therapy, the nurse will find it helpful to know what information the physician has given the patient. Even when the physician has given the patient a careful explanation of his disease and of what is required

---

[14] *Loc cit.*, p. 48.
[15] Fredric Wertham, "A Psychosomatic Study of Myself," *When Doctors Are Patients*, ed. Max Pinner and Benjamin Miller, W. W. Norton & Co., Inc., New York, 1952, pp. 102-18.

in its treatment, he may have failed to comprehend what was said. When the nurse knows what the patient has been told, she can answer his questions, or refer them to his physician with the expectation that she is relieving rather than creating further tension.

Part of preparing the patient for what to expect is to determine what the patient expects and wants to know. Patients are frequently subjected to un-necessary anxiety, unless time has been taken to determine what their expec-tations are. To illustrate, Mrs. Fox, who had had a mitral commissurotomy two weeks previously, was found lying on a cart in the hall outside the room where cardiac catheterizations were performed. The nurse who stopped to greet her learned that she had "been waiting for hours," and that she expected "to be stabbed in the back" without benefit of anesthesia. The fact that the catheter was to be introduced through an arm vein made her suffering quite unnecessary, had someone taken the time to determine her understanding of the procedure and to correct her misinformation. Moreover, she might have been less apprehensive if someone had stayed with her.

Determination of what the patient expects and wants to know helps to prevent giving him information that suggests problems or difficulties he has not anticipated. Wertham[16] makes this point in regard to his own situation. A surgeon made the comment to him that phlebitis seldom affects the arms. Previous to this time, the possibility that his arms might be involved had not occurred to him and it became a source of worry. He found himself trying to detect pain first in one arm and then in the other.

PARTICIPATION OF THE PATIENT IN HIS CARE

How can a patient participate as a partner in his care?

The fact that a patient wants to be a partner in his care is partly taken care of by preparing him for what to expect and for what is expected of him. When he is prepared to help himself by such activities as exercising, deep breathing, and coughing, he knows that he has a part in his recovery. Moreover, ap-praisal of how long a painful procedure will take and comments indicating progress help to keep the patient informed about how long he has to continue to brace himself. Further, both types of comments assure him that the person who is performing the procedure is aware of his needs. He is then better able to follow instructions relative to his part in the procedure.

Patients are often asked to assume responsibility for aspects of their own care. When this is done, the patient should understand that he is encouraged to take this responsibility because it furthers his recovery. Too often patients gain the impression that they are asked to bathe themselves or ambulate because the nurses are too busy, or do not want to care for them, rather than because activity is part of their therapeutic regime.

At other times, patients wish to retain certain responsibilities or privileges.

[16] *Ibid.*

These are sometimes denied them without adequate thought being given to the reason for the refusal or to the value that the responsibility has to them. To illustrate, Mrs. Lottie Gamely had disseminated cancer of the breast which had metastasized to the cervical spine. She was in more or less constant pain and was very fearful lest any activity increase it. Her husband brought her some tablets of Empirin[17] compound, which she planned to take as needed. In the course of giving Mrs. Gamely care, the nurse discovered the Empirin compound in Mrs. Gamely's bedside table. Before removing the medication, she talked with Mrs. Gamely's physician. The decision was made to leave the Empirin compound at the bedside because it gave Mrs. Gamely the feeling that she had some control over her pain. The possibility of any harm resulting was negligible. Later, this patient expressed her feeling that she was a partner in her care. This was revealed when the nurse told Mrs. Gamely that she was going on vacation and that she had enjoyed working with her. Mrs. Gamely responded by saying, "I've enjoyed working with you, too."

The satisfaction of the wish of the patient to be considered a partner in his care depends on the belief that each individual, sick or well, has a right to participate in plans concerning his welfare. The nurse has a responsibility to provide the individual with the information he needs in order to consider his alternatives, and with support to carry out his decision once it is made, or to change his mind. Sometimes a patient is pressed to make decisions that he is unable or unprepared to make. If he feels that he is censured or blamed for failing to make the "right" decision, he may be unable to change his mind. Physicians and nurses sometimes forget that a patient may be asked to adjust to or make a decision about a procedure that may affect the entire course of his life and to do it quickly. Human beings tend to react to change with anxiety. Excessive anxiety makes the objective evaluation of his situation by the patient difficult, if not impossible.

In the practice of nursing, the nurse will see persons whose diseases require prompt action, and yet who refuse to have treatment. Mrs. Youthful Thirty-Five was such an individual. She was found to have an ulcer on the left labia majora, which on examination proved to be cancer. Her physician explained why she should have a resection of the labia, and she entered the hospital to be prepared for surgery. On the morning of her operation she told Miss Noll, the nurse who was preparing her for surgery, that she had changed her mind. She would not have the operation. Miss Noll related the information to the surgeon. He came to see Mrs. Thirty-Five and calmly reassured her that she was free to decide whether or not she would have the operation. He tried to convey to her that he understood her feelings and that should she change her mind the operation could be performed at a later time. He encouraged her to remain in the hospital for a few days, so that the ulcer could be treated medically.

He left orders for sitz baths and dressings, as the lesion was draining. A

[17] Trade name for tablets containing phenacetin 0.15 gm (gr. 2½); acetylsalicylic acid 0.23 gm (gr. 3½); caffeine 30 mgm (gr. ½).

plan was made to encourage Mrs. Thirty-Five to talk about her fears, but not to force her to do so. Careful attention was given to her physical care. Her doctor saw her regularly. About a week later she decided to have the operation. It was not easy even then. She had had, however, an opportunity to consider her alternatives and to come to the decision that the operation was preferable to allowing the disease to progress.

In addition to the patient wanting to be treated as an individual, to have an explanation of his care, and to be considered as a partner in his care, Abdellah and Levine found that he wants to have his behavior as a sick person accepted as part of his illness and to be treated with thoughtfulness, kindness, and firmness. Mr. Tenny, a young man who had suffered a cervical cord injury when struck by a car, expressed this desire when he said, "I've been difficult, I know. But then doctors and nurses ought to understand how difficult this whole experience has been for me."

MEETING THE PATIENT'S NEEDS

Though not stated explicitly in Abdellah and Levine's study, the patient wants to feel he can trust those who are responsible for his care. The confidence of the patient is built on his being accepted as an individual and on the confidence of the nurse in her ability to meet his needs. It is facilitated by the way his care is provided, its timing, and by attention to details of his care, especially those that are important to him. It is strengthened by keeping promises and by keeping the patient informed about the status of those that take time to fulfill. For example, Mr. Samuel was promised a "high-low bed." When the nurse called the storeroom, she learned that one would not be available for several hours. She relayed this information to Mr. Samuel. Later, when it had not arrived at the expected time, she called the storeroom and told Mr. Samuel that the bed was on its way. The fact that the nurse kept Mr. Samuel informed helped to develop his confidence that she was concerned with his welfare.

The nurse may not always be able to fulfill all of the expectations of the patient, nor is she always responsible for the fact that they are not met. She is responsible for trying to determine what they are and for considering them in his care. Most persons who are sick enough to require medical and nursing care suffer some degree of anxiety. When they are hospitalized, the environment is strange and frightening. A sick person should not be expected to be at his best. Despite his illness, he remains a human being and should be treated with courtesy and thoughtfulness. Interest in him as a person, concern for his welfare, kindness, and a desire to be helpful—all should contribute to his confidence that his needs will be met.

On what should the patient's nursing care be based?

The nursing care of each patient should be based on his individual needs. Briefly stated, patient needs determine patient care. This implies that the needs of the patient be assessed and those with which he requires assistance identified. From the data collected a nursing diagnosis can be established. The nursing diagnosis serves as a basis for the formulation of a nursing care plan that is directed toward the accomplishment of both long-term and immediate goals. Since needs of the patient are seldom static, regular re-evaluation of the plan is essential if his needs are to continue to be met.

In the chapters that follow, content basic to understanding each of the needs of the patient will be discussed in some detail. As the various needs are discussed, the fact that a human being functions as a whole should not be lost from sight. A disturbance in the capacity of an individual to meet one or more needs affects the whole person, not just a part of him. Moreover, a disturbance in the capacity of the individual to meet one need may interfere with his ability to meet other needs. Except in the terminal stages of an illness, however, the patient can be expected to be able to meet some of his needs without the aid of others.

If nursing care is to be based on the needs of the patient, it is obvious that the nurse must be able to assess or identify what they are. In order to assess the needs of the patient that can be met through the practice of nursing, understanding of what is meant by the term "need," as well as what the needs of the human being are, is essential. Moreover, to understand how needs are affected by illness, and how to assist the patient in meeting his needs, some knowledge of the mechanisms used to defend and protect himself against changes in the environment is necessary. Knowledge of the mechanisms utilized to limit injury and to repair any injury or disturbance is also essential. Finally, assessment of the success of the patient in meeting his own needs depends on knowledge of the behavior that indicates he is or is not successful.

What are some of the understandings that are essential to fulfilling the concept "Patient needs determine patient care"?

Murray's[18] definition of need is paraphrased by King[19] as follows: "A concept that stands for a force of some nature in the brain region, an organizing force that affects thinking, knowing, perceiving in such a way as to change an existing unsatisfying situation in certain directions. Each need is accompanied by a particular feeling or emotion, and even though sometimes weak or momentary, it usually persists and gives rise to overt behavior or fantasy, which may change the external circumstances sufficiently to appease or satisfy the organism and still the need."

Needs must be satisfied if the organism is to carry on one or more of the activities of life. These activities may be classified as: (1) use of food and oxygen with the release of energy, (2) response to the environment, (3) growth, (4) reproduction, and (5) productivity. Needs may arise from, or be

[18] Henry A. Murray, *Explorations in Personality*, Oxford University Press, New York, 1938, pp. 123-24.
[19] Stanley H. King, *Perceptions of Illness and Medical Practice*, Russell Sage Foundation, New York, 1962, p. 43.

met at, any of the levels of organization of the human being—biochemical, cellular, organ, psychological, interpersonal, and social.

According to Gordon, four basic phenomena of the nervous system make it possible for man to adapt, to survive, and to satisfy his needs in an ever-changing environment. They are: pain, hunger, fear, and rage.[20]

Though needs may be listed in endless detail, they will be considered in five broad categories. They are the physiological, safety, psychological, social, and spiritual needs. All living beings have needs. On the cellular level they are similar for all organisms. Man differs from other living beings in his psychological, social, and spiritual needs. The needs common to all species are sometimes referred to as basic or survival needs. These are the requirements that must be met to maintain life. Basic needs are prepotent, or take precedence, over others. Another way this concept can be stated is that needs are organized in a hierarchy with lower needs demanding satisfaction first. They must be satisfied before other needs are manifested and given attention. For example, physiological needs must be met to some degree before psychological needs can be expressed. Even among the basic needs some are more urgent than others. Some physiological needs, such as the need for oxygen, take precedence over the need for food or water. Knowledge of the fact that some needs are more important to survival than others has implications to the practice of nursing. For example, the patient who is acutely short of oxygen is unlikely to be interested in food, much less in conversation or other intellectual activities. Even more significant, his survival may well depend on correction of his oxygen deficit. Most students have at some time tried to study when they were cold, hungry, or angry and found that they were unsuccessful until they put on a sweater, had something to eat, or recovered from their anger.

What factors alter the capacity of the individual to tolerate the frustration of a need?

The capacity of the individual to tolerate frustration of one or more needs depends on a number of factors. One factor is the adequacy of his structures and processes for meeting the need and for adapting to change. This is exemplified by the brain-damaged individual, such as one who has had a stroke, who may have very little tolerance for frustration. He may become excited or upset when faced with minor difficulties. A general anaesthetic reduces the ability of the person to adapt the caliber of his blood vessels to changes in position. The child who is born with a defect in the structure of his heart may be unable to meet the need of his tissues for oxygen during exercise. In general the individual can tolerate the frustration of a need better if the condition that is responsible develops slowly rather than rapidly. Time allows

[20] Gerald Gordon, "To Live or Not to Live with Your Job," *Nursing Forum*, I, Winter 1961-62, p. 38.

the organism an opportunity to adapt to the change both by altering its requirements and by initiating mechanisms that increase the effectiveness with which it utilizes its supplies. The capacity to tolerate frustration, particularly of psychological needs, depends also on the degree to which the need has been met in the past, especially in early life. Since illness involves the failure to meet one or more needs, the capacity of the sick person to tolerate frustration of his needs is often limited. For example, the patient who is in the period immediately following a major operation is unable to anticipate and adapt to changes in his environment. Changes such as moving him from the stretcher to the bed, or loud noises, may be followed by a fall in blood pressure. Until he fully recovers from the anesthetic, he must be protected from falling out of bed. Until he is up and about, procedures to maintain the patency of his airway are required. Until his alimentary canal can tolerate food and fluids, they must be administered parenterally.

The meeting of needs also depends on the availability of supplies or materials. For example, the requirement for oxygen cannot be met unless there is oxygen in the atmosphere. The need to be loved and to give love cannot be met unless love is available.

As has been previously implied, the capacity of an individual to meet his needs depends on processes and mechanisms which in health are regulated so that their action is appropriate, effective, and constructive. Structures and processes are required for the regulation of intake, distribution, use, storage, output, and elimination of excesses of supply or of waste products resulting from activity. Not only are individual processes regulated so that a need is met, but each process is regulated so that it is integrated into the activities of the total individual. In man many structures and functions may be involved in satisfying one need. To illustrate, the physiological need for water involves structures and processes whereby a deficit of water is recognized and is translated into the sensation of thirst. Further, coordinated activity is required to obtain, drink, and absorb water into the blood stream. Many more processes are involved in the distribution of water to the cells, in its temporary storage, and in the elimination of an excess by the kidney.

To assist the nurse in assessing the needs of each patient, an outline that may be used as a guide has been prepared (see pages 21-29). The purpose of this guide is to provide a basis for the organized collection of data required to make a nursing diagnosis. Not all the information suggested is available for every patient, nor is it always necessary. Some of it may be obtained from the patient's hospital chart and medical history. Moreover, continuous assessment is essential. As the patient recovers or fails, his needs change. As a consequence, his nursing care requirements also change.

To collect the information required to make a nursing diagnosis, knowledge and skill in the field of interpersonal relationships, as well as in the observation and interpretation of the signs and symptoms indicating deviations from normal functioning and behavior, are essential. After the data are collected, they should be analyzed and the problems which can be met through the practice of nursing identified. Problems outside the province of nursing or that are shared with other disciplines should be referred to the appropriate persons. The welfare of the patient often depends on the coordination of the activities of all who have a part in his care. In fact, the patient's care cannot be said to be truly comprehensive without it.

For example, to meet the food requirements of a patient, persons from a number of disciplines combine their efforts to make the proper food available to the patient. The physician prescribes the diet. The dietitian translates the prescription into food and is responsible for its preparation and serving. When the patient requires formal dietary instruction, this is frequently the responsibility of the dietitian. The nurse prepares the patient for his meal and feeds him, when necessary. She answers his questions about his nutritional needs, or his diet, or refers them to the physican or dietitian. The nutritional needs of many patients are met by each individual nurse, physician, and dietitian, performing his functions. When problems arise, however, their solution may depend on the combined efforts of the nurse, dietitian, physician, patient, and even the members of the family.

To illustrate, Mary Ellen Cliff was a young woman with a diagnosis of rheumatoid arthritis. She ate very little and consequently was weak, lacking in energy, thin, and frail-looking. She was cared for at home by her mother and a visiting nurse who visited her twice a week. In the course of her visits Miss Visiting Nurse learned that Mary Ellen ate poorly. She discussed this problem with Mary Ellen's physician, who said that her weakness and lack of energy were directly related to inadequate food intake. He prescribed a high-calorie diet and said that he would again talk to Mary Ellen about the importance of eating. In order to evaluate Mary Ellen's food pattern, the nurse asked her to keep a record of her food intake for three days. Miss V. Nurse gave Mary Ellen and her mother instructions about how to make the study as well as how the information was to be used. As a result of the study, Miss V. Nurse's previous suspicion that Mrs. Cliff was an indifferent and unimaginative cook was borne out. Part of the problem stemmed from poorly prepared and unattractively served food. Miss V. Nurse arranged for a consultation with the agency dietitian. Miss Dietitian talked with the physician, and then she planned a diet that included foods Mary Ellen liked and, if eaten, would be adequate to her needs. She also suggested that Miss V. Nurse take some recipes with her that Mrs. Cliff might try to use. Mary Ellen was encouraged to try to eat even when she did not feel like it. After six months of continued effort Mary Ellen had gained 10 lb. and her appetite had improved considerably. She was able to be out of bed and was beginning to think about seeking employment. Mrs. Cliff's cooking, though not in the gourmet class, was much improved. In this particular instance the nurse carried more of the responsibility for the instruction and the management of the patient and her mother than she might have in the hospital. The solution of the problem, however, depended on the cooperative efforts of the members of several disciplines.

SAFETY OF THE PATIENT

In assessing the needs of the patient for nursing, one of the factors to be evaluated is safety. Since safety is a factor in all aspects of patient care, the content relating to safety will be integrated throughout. There are, however, a few general points that bear emphasis. The first of these is that safety has two aspects. One is the actual danger or threat to the welfare of the patient. The other is the feeling that the person has of being safe or in danger. Conditions endangering the patient may have their origin in either his internal or external environment. For example, the life of the patient is threatened by any condition that deprives him of some substance required by his cells or by failure to remove excesses of supply or products of metabolism. The life of the patient may also be endangered by conditions in the external environment such as extremes in temperature or radioactive active substances or rays. What the person regards as being unsafe depends on his past experience and the unknown elements in his situation.

A second point is that the safety of the patient depends on all those who participate in his care. They must assume responsibility for the identification of threats to his well-being and for the institution of appropriate measures to anticipate, forestall, and control harmful agents or conditions. This is both a legal and a moral responsibility. Since one of the goals in the practice of nursing is to prevent and relieve suffering, appropriate measures should also be taken to help the patient feel safe and protected. Actual safety and a feeling of safety require not only that the physical environment of the patient be made safe, but that his social and emotional climate be safe as well. In identification of threats to the emotional well-being of the patient, the point that man learns to fear harmless things should not be neglected. This means that what each person fears is an individual matter. To prevent unnecessary fear requires some knowledge of the expectations of the patient and how he perceives his situation. The feeling of being safe and protected depends on the belief that conditions that may cause harm are under control, either by the individual himself or by someone in his environment whom he trusts.

Though all patients should be protected from unnecessary risks, the need is greatest in those who are unable to identify or control dangers to themselves. Some patients, by virtue of their age or condition, are completely vulnerable. An example is the unconscious patient who is unable to satisfy his needs or protect himself. He has to be protected from the effects of heat, cold, and pressure and even from his own body secretions. Dangers to which the fully conscious, as well as the unconscious, patient may be exposed include infection, falling, incorrect drugs, and the failure to identify and report significant signs and symptoms. The patient may suffer insults to his dignity and self-esteem and to his feeling that his welfare is important to those who are responsible for his care. These may lead to doubt on the part of the patient that he can really trust the members of the nursing staff to be there when they are needed.

A third general point about safety is what Chapman[21] calls the unsafe act. In discussing the causes of accidents, Chapman emphasizes that they all have their origin in an unsafe act. Knowledge of certain facts about unsafe acts contributes to their control. Few unsafe acts result in injury and still fewer result in death. The person who is responsible for an accident is not always the one who is injured. Sometimes the relationship between the unsafe act and the accident is not immediate or direct. Moreover, an accident may result from a series of unsafe acts. The latter is illustrated by the instance of the man who was killed by an iron bar falling from an open window. The first unsafe act was the construction of an apartment or other building with windows opening directly over the street. The second was the use of an iron bar to prop a window open. The third was failure to remove the bar from the window sill preparatory to opening the window. When the effect of an unsafe act is delayed, as it was in the above anecdote, until the bar fell from the window, the identification of the cause may be difficult, if not impossible.

A similar example, though less serious in outcome, occurred in General Hospital. The physician wrote the following order: "phenobarbital 30 mg tid to be administered by subcutaneous injection." The order was transferred to a medicine card and written on the Kardex by a ward clerk. The head nurse initialed the medicine card. The nurse caring for the patient administered Phenobarbital tablets U.S.P. instead of the more soluble form, Phenobarbital sodium U.S.P. Although no harm came to the patient, his safety was threatened by a series of unsafe acts. The one person in the series who was not negligent was the ward clerk.

Finally, the control of accidents depends on knowledge of the potential dangers and of the human factors entering into the performance of unsafe acts. Accident prevention takes planning, preparation, and instruction so that people learn what the dangers are and develop the attitude that accidents can and should be prevented. Their prevention is the responsibility of everyone. In terms of the latter example, each person had a responsibility to assure the patient's getting the correct drug in the correct form.

What tool or tools are available for use in identifying the needs of patients?

Observation is an essential tool in assessing the needs of the patient. Because the process of observation may be confused with that of interpretation, it is essential to distinguish between them. Observation is defined as the act of noting some *fact* or *occurrence*. In contrast, interpretation is the act of *explaining* or *translating* an event or occurrence. An observation is what is. Interpretation is why it is. A man's blood pressure is 90/60, an observation of a fact or occurrence. The interpretation of what a blood pressure of 90/60

[21] Albert L. Chapman, "The Anatomy of an Accident," *Public Health Reports*, LXXV, July, 1960, p. 630.

means in this man depends not only on an actual level, but on other facts as well. A blood pressure of 90 systolic and 60 diastolic may be his usual blood pressure or it may indicate that he is in severe shock. The kinds of questions that are answered by observation include: What do I see? Hear? Feel? Smell? What amount or quantity? What quality? Interpretation answers the questions: What do these data mean? Why? Both observation and interpretation are useful tools when appropriately used. The value of an observation depends on the integrity and detachment with which it is made and on its specificity. The value of an interpretation depends on the adequacy of the facts and the knowledge of the interpreter of all the factors that contribute to the situation. It also depends on the ability to appropriately relate what is known.

Accurate observation is essential to the correct interpretation of a situation. Florence Nightingale acknowledged the importance of astute observation to effective nursing when she wrote: "It may safely be said, not that the habit of ready and correct observation will by itself make us useful nurses, but that without it we shall be useless with all our devotion."[22]

To illustrate, Mrs. Smart is lying quietly in bed. Her hair is neat and she has polish on her fingernails. On her bedside table is a picture of a little boy. These are observations or facts. What interpretations can be made from these facts? Are there enough facts to conclude that the little boy is her son? He may not be; he may be her nephew or grandson or the child of a friend. What are her feelings toward him? What other *facts* must be known before these questions can be answered? To emphasize, through observations, the *facts* in a situation are determined. These facts have value inasmuch as they are accurately and clearly described. The facts are used to explain an occurrence or event.

Sometimes the data available are inadequate to explain the event; then an educated guess, or hypothesis, may be made. For example, the man whose blood pressure is 90/60 had just arrived in a hospital emergency room following an automobile collision. There is a large wound in his right arm from which he has been bleeding. Though his normal blood pressure is not known, from the known facts, the assumption that he is in shock is reasonable. What is fact and what is assumed to be fact, however, should be kept clearly in mind. As new evidence is uncovered, new or different interpretations may be required.

Facts about the individual patient, and how he interprets his situation, what his expectations are for himself and for others can be obtained by purposeful conversation with him and with the members of his family. Purposeful conversation as a tool in nursing care of the patient is discussed in Chapter 6. For students who wish to read further in this area, references have been included in the References for Chapter 6.

[22] Florence Nightingale, *Notes on Nursing; What It Is, and What It Is Not*, Harrison and Sons, London, 1860, p. 160.

The guide for assessing the patient's needs and the nursing skills required to meet these needs follows.

Assessing the Needs of the Patient for Nursing

1. The general objectives toward which the nursing care of each patient is planned
   1.1 To personalize the care of each patient
   1.2 To support and maintain his capacity for meeting his physiological, psychological, social, and spiritual needs
   1.3 To protect the patient from the threats to his safety, comfort, and well-being
   1.4 To support, comfort, sustain the patient, and to ease his suffering during all phases of illness
   1.5 To assist in the restoration of the patient to the fullest capacity of which he is capable
   1.6 To consider the members of the family of the patient and his friends as persons who have a legitimate interest in and a role to play in his well-being

Guide For Assessing The Needs of The Patient

1. Personal information
   1.1 General impression
   1.2 Apparent degree of illness
       1.21 Acutely ill, seriously ill, critically ill, improving, convalescent, failing to improve
   1.3 Cerebral activity[23]
       1.31 Mental status[24]
           1.311 Oriented
           1.312 Disoriented
       1.32 Level of consciousness[24]
           1.321 Fully conscious
           1.322 Inattentive
           1.323 Drowsy
           1.324 Confused
           1.325 Stuporous
           1.326 Comatose
   1.4 Previous experience with illness in hospital _____
       Previous experience with illness at home   _____
   1.5 Age _____ Sex _____

[23] Although the following characteristics of cerebral activity might appropriately be included under the "Physical and Physiological Status" heading of this guide, they are elaborated here because of their essentiality to the nurse in assessing the priority of needs of the patient.
[24] For definition of these terms, the reader is referred to glossaries of neurological and psychiatric terms.

1.6 Problems with communication
    1.61 Language
        1.611 Does not speak English _____
        1.612 Inability to speak   _____
        1.613 Impediment in speech   _____
        1.614 Hearing impairment   _____
        1.615 Other _____
    1.62 Manner in which patient communicates satisfaction or dissatisfaction _____
    1.63 How does he seem to relate to others? _____
1.7 Cultural differences that may affect his attitudes, food preferences, expectations, or modesty pattern   _____
1.8 Religion _____
    1.81 Does he wish to see minister, priest, rabbi?   _____
    1.82 Religious practices with which he desires assistance   _____
1.9 Education and intellectual level
    1.91 Level of schooling   _____
    1.92 Interest in learning   _____
    1.93 Hobbies and recreational interests   _____
    1.94 What does the patient like to talk about?   _____
    1.95 Prejudices   _____
    1.96 Aspirations   _____
1.10 Role and place in family
    1.101 Position in family   _____
    1.102 Position in community   _____
    1.103 Apparent image of himself. How does he answer the questions Where am I? What am I? Who am I?   _____
    1.104 How does his family appear to regard him?   _____
    1.105 Is there anything in the family relationship that may have an effect on the patient?
        1.1051 Favorable   _____
        1.1052 Unfavorable   _____
    1.106 Is there a relative or friend who may be helpful in meeting patient's needs?   _____
    1.107 If he has no family, what resources are available as a substitute?   _____
    1.108 Who is the head of the family?   _____
2. Social and economic status
    2.1 Occupation and position   _____
    2.2 Insurance
        2.21 Hospital   _____
        2.22 Medical   _____
        2.23 Income   _____
    2.3 Adequacy of income to meet needs   _____

2.4 Adequacy of housing   _____

3. Emotional status[25]

   3.1   Apprehensive   _____

   3.2   Anxious   _____

   3.3   Agitated   _____

   3.4   Restless   _____

   3.5   Irritable   _____

   3.6   Shy, timid   _____

   3.7   Withdrawn   _____

   3.8   Depressed   _____

   3.9   Discouraged   _____

   3.10 Happy   _____

   3.11 Demanding   _____

4. Patient's expectations

   4.1 How does he view his role as a sick person?   _____

   4.2 What does he expect of those who care for him?

     4.21 Nurses   _____

     4.22 Doctors   _____

     4.23 Others   _____

   4.3 How does he expect his family to behave?   _____

   4.4 How does he think his illness should be treated?   _____

   4.5 What does he want to know and do?   _____

5. Previous experience and background that may be factors in his reactions and his expectations

   5.1 Previous hospitalizations   _____

   5.2 Previous care by nurses   _____

   5.3 Life experiences   _____

6. Personal habits (which of these is the patient able to perform for himself, with which does he require assistance, which must be performed for him?)

   6.1 Mouth care

     6.11 Dentures   _____

     6.12 Brushing teeth   _____

   6.2 Bathing

     6.21 Modifications   _____

   6.3 Hair (clean, dirty, tangled, matted)

     6.31 Shampoo   _____

     6.32 Combing   _____

   6.4 Nails (clean, dirty, long, short)   _____

   6.5 Beard   _____

---

[25] See Footnote 24. These terms are intended to assist the nurse in identifying the nature of the emotional needs of the patient, to enable her to formulate the most effective plan, or approach, possible. Their purpose is not to label, or categorize, the patient, but rather to help the nurse better understand and describe his behavior as a necessary first step to assisting him in coping with his illness.

6.6 Bowel or defecation habits
    6.61 Usual time   _____
    6.62 Time of last defecation   _____
    6.63 Abnormalities   _____
        6.631 Constipation   _____
        6.632 Diarrhea   _____
        6.633 Incontinence
    6.64 Dependent drainage   _____
        6.641 Colostomy   _____
        6.642 Ileostomy   _____
        6.643 Fistula   _____
        6.644 Draining wound   _____

6.7 Sleep and resting habits
    6.71 Rest periods   _____
    6.72 Sleep   _____
        6.721 Usual time for retiring   _____
        6.722 Usual hour for arising   _____
        6.723 Any assistance or modifications that he requires to get adequate sleep   _____

6.8 Food habits and pattern   _____
    6.81 Likes, dislikes, preferences   _____
    6.82 Timing of meals when at home   _____
    6.83 Any ideas about food that may have a bearing on patient's food intake   _____

7. Exercise
    7.1 Active or sedentary habits   _____
    7.2 Usual forms of exercise   _____
    7.3 Limits of exercise   _____
        7.31 Paralysis   _____
        7.32 Weakness   _____
        7.33 Prostheses   _____

8. With what daily activities of living does the patient require help?
    8.1 Eating   _____
    8.2 Bathing   _____
    8.3 Dressing   _____
    8.4 Getting out of bed   _____
    8.5 Walking   _____
    8.6 Bathroom   _____
    8.7 Uses crutches, braces, wheelchair, walker, etc.   _____

9. Physical and physiological status
    9.1 Height_____Weight_____
        (lean, normal, overweight)
    9.2 Vital signs: Temperature_____Pulse_____Respiration_____
    9.3 Blood pressure   _____

  9.4 Condition of skin   _____
      9.41 Intact   _____
      9.42 Breaks or wounds   _____
      9.43 Dry   _____
      9.44 Moist   _____
      9.45 Wrinkled   _____
      9.46 Tense   _____
      9.47 Bruised   _____
      9.48 Rash   _____
      9.49 Flushed   _____
      9.50 Pale   _____
      9.51 Jaundiced   _____
      9.52 Ulcers or sores   _____
      9.53 Edematous areas   _____
  9.5 Teeth
      9.51 Own teeth   _____
      9.52 Edentulous   _____
      9.53 Dentures   _____
  9.6 Vision
      9.61 Good   _____
      9.62 Defective   _____
      9.63 Blind   _____
      9.64 Prosthesis   _____
  9.7 Eyes
      9.71 Conjunctiva   _____
      9.72 Lids   _____
  9.8 Hearing
      9.81 Good   _____
      9.82 Impaired   _____
  9.9 Body alignment   _____
  9.10 Position   _____
  9.11 General sensation   _____
      9.111 Sensory deficit   _____
      9.112 Inability to detect changes in temperature   _____
10. Needs with which the patient requires assistance
  10.1 Maintenance of oxygen supply   _____
      10.11 Clear airway   _____
      10.12 Assistance with breathing   _____
      10.13 Additional supply of oxygen   _____
          10.131 Mask or catheter in proper position   _____
          10.132 Mask comfortable   _____
          10.133 Tent tucked in   _____
      10.14 Evidence of general oxygen deficit   _____
      10.15 Difficulty in breathing   _____
      10.16 Signs or symptoms indicating deficit of oxygen   _____

10.2 Maintenance of water balance _____
    10.21 Intake _____
    10.22 Output _____
    10.23 Weight _____
    10.24 Condition of skin and mucous membranes _____
    10.25 Thirst _____
10.3 Nutritional needs _____
    10.31 Interference with capacity to eat _____
        10.311 Anorexia, nausea, vomiting _____
    10.32 Condition preventing absorption of food
        10.321 Diarrhea _____
10.4 Capacity to maintain excretory function
    10.41 Urine _____
        10.411 Voids _____
        10.412 Indwelling catheter _____
        10.413 Color, odor, appearance of urine _____
    10.42 Bowel _____
10.5 Special observation of urine
    10.51 Glucose _____
    10.52 Acetone _____
    10.53 Specific gravity _____
11. Capacity to maintain motor function
    11.1 Difficulty in swallowing _____
    11.2 Difficulty in walking _____
    11.3 Difficulty with grasping _____
    11.4 Motor incoordination _____
    11.5 Motor instability _____
    11.6 Motor weakness _____
12. Ability to maintain appropriate position and body alignment _____
13. Therapeutic measures and devices
    13.1 Blood transfusions _____
    13.2 Indwelling catheter _____
    13.3 Cast _____
    13.4 Nasogastric or gastric suction _____
    13.5 Surgical procedure _____
    13.6 Barron pump _____
    13.7 Tracheostomy _____
    13.8 Other _____
14. Signs and symptoms associated with a disease state
    14.1 Pain { Location / Quality / Severity } _____
    14.2 Fever _____
    14.3 Abdominal distention _____
15. Medical diagnosis _____

16. Condition of physical environment
    16.1 Equipment used in the care of the patient   ————
    16.2 Furnishings   ————
    16.3 Floors—clean and dry   ————
    16.4 Room temperature and ventilation   ————
    16.5 Lights   ————
17. Safety precautions
    17.1 Side rails   ————
    17.2 Low bed   ————
    17.3 Other   ————
18. What instruction does he require?
19. What problems does he have in accepting the goals that are possible for him?
20. What aspects of the medical care plan have a bearing on the patient's needs for nursing?
    20.1 Diagnostic measures
    20.2 Therapy
21. Which aspects of the patient's care require assistance from members of other disciplines?
22. What care and service is he likely to require following his discharge from hospital? Need for continuing care?
23. What nursing skills are necessary to meeting the patient's needs?[26]
    23.1 Observation of health status of the patient
    23.2 Skills of communication
        Verbal
        Nonverbal
        Written
    23.3 Application of knowledge
        Physical sciences
        Biological sciences
        Social sciences
        Nursing sciences
    23.4 Teaching of patients and families
        Spontaneous teaching
        Planned individual instruction
        Spontaneous group teaching
        Planned group teaching
    23.5 Planning and organization of work
        Individual patient care
        Group care of patient

[26] Modified from Faye G. Abdellah, Almeda Martin, Irene L. Beland, and Ruth V. Matheny, *Patient-Centered Approaches to Nursing*, The Macmillan Company, New York, 1960, pp. 17-19.

Inhalation
Removal
Applications
Diagnostic procedures
Comfort and support
Safety

Abdellah[27] summarizes the elements in the practice of nursing as follows:

The first element is the continuous mastery of human relations, including the mastery of technical and of managerial skills needed to take care of patients.

The second element is the ability to observe and report with clarity the signs and symptoms, and deviation from normal behavior, which a patient presents. This element would include the mastery of basic communication skills.

The third element is the ability to interpret the signs and symptoms which comprise the deviation from health and constitute nursing problems. The deviations from health usually are identified from one or more signs and symptoms which the nurse has observed. They involve nursing problems. Thus a nursing problem exists in a situation involving patient care, a possible solution to which is found through the services which are the functions of nursing.

The fourth element requires the analysis of nursing problems which will guide the nurse in carrying out nursing functions, and the selection of the necessary course of action which will help the patient attain a goal that is realistic for him, as she plans for total patient care.

The fifth element is the organization of her efforts to assure the desired outcome. Effective patient care would thus result when the nurse is able to help the patient to return to health or what can be approximate normal health for him. This process may be referred to as nursing diagnosis and treatment.

To this point nursing as a profession and some of the elements in the practice of professional nursing have been considered. The next question is "How does medical and surgical nursing fit into this framework?" "What is medical-surgical nursing?"

The definition of medical-surgical nursing that follows is based on the philosophy that every person is an individual human being with dignity and rights. A person does not, or should not, lose his dignity and rights as an individual because he is sick or well, old or young, clean or unclean, rich or poor. Further, he has needs, physiological, psychological, social, and spiritual, which must be met if he is to survive, grow, and be productive. In health he is able to meet his needs through his own efforts. When he is ill he requires assistance in meeting one or more of his needs.

The definition is also based on the conviction that the practice of professional nursing requires a body of knowledge of facts, theories, principles, and concepts. This body of knowledge is derived from the humanities, the biological, physical, and behavioral sciences and is necessary to the understanding of (1) the role of the nurse, (2) the needs of people, (3) the importance of the ability to adapt physiologically, emotionally, and socially to changes in

[27] Abdellah, *et al., Op. cit.,* p. 26.

the environment, (4) some failures of man to adapt, and (5) how, through nursing, the nurse may be of service to him.

Last, the definition is based on the belief that professional nursing has a real contribution to make in the promotion of health, in the prevention of disease, and in the care of those who are sick, those who will be cured, and those for whom cure is unlikely and/or for whom this is the last illness. The term "to give nursing care" has real meaning when it expresses the attitude of the nurse as she bestows on her patient her concern for his welfare, freely and without the expectation that he will reward her directly. The nurse expresses this concern for the patient both by doing and by her manner of doing.

The practice of medical-surgical nursing is defined as the branch of nursing concerned with people whose presenting problem is primarily physiological. Like many definitions this one is not too helpful for it tells how, but not why, the person is ill. Whatever its nature, any illness is the consequence of the interaction of multiple factors. Moreover, disturbances at any level of organization—biochemical, cellular, organ, psychological, interpersonal, or social—are likely to result in disturbances at other levels. For example, Mr. Quick is angry with his wife. He not only feels and looks angry, but he manifests his anger by changes in behavior. On the physiological level, his muscles contract, he loses his appetite, and his blood vessels constrict. On the interpersonal level he shouts at his wife, is sharp with his son, and is rude to the neighbor next door. He gets into his car and backs out of the driveway, narrowly missing a two-year-old child playing in the street. In other words, Mr. Quick is angry as a whole individual and he manifests his anger as a unit, not as a part.

The practice of medical-surgical nursing requires a body of knowledge and skills that enable the practitioner to:

1. Assess the needs of the patient for nursing
2. Collect information from appropriate sources—patient, family, patient's record, community, literature, physician, and others who have some responsibility for the patient—so that essential information is at hand
3. Make a plan of care
   a. State the patient's needs as nursing problems and translate them into objectives of care
   b. Establish priorities
   c. Select appropriate nursing methods
   d. Make an appropriate time plan
   e. Coordinate or dovetail plan with plans for other patients in group
   f. Coordinate and integrate all the activities that enter into the overall plan of therapy
   g. Anticipate needs for future care
4. Inform the patient of the details of the plan that help him to know what to expect and what is expected of him
5. Carry out the plan

6. Record observations and care given so that necessary information is available for future reference

7. Evaluate and modify plan, in light of its effectiveness and changes in the patient's condition

None of the above is unique to the practice of medical-surgical nursing; it is part of all nursing.

In this chapter an attempt has been made to review nursing as a profession and the broad role of the nurse. Since the writer believes that nursing has the responsibility for assisting the patient to meet needs that he is unable to meet by himself, a concept of need has been briefly explored. A nursing guide for assessing the needs of patients has been outlined. By meeting the needs of the patient for nursing, the nurse contributes to the welfare of the patient by what she does, and by how she cares for him.

REFERENCES

Books

Brown, Esther Lucille, *Newer Dimensions of Patient Care. Part I*, Russell Sage Foundation, New York, 1961.

Blauch, Lloyd E. (ed.), *Education for the Professions*, Government Printing Office, Washington, D.C., 1955.

King, Stanley H., *Perceptions of Illness and Medical Practice*, Russell Sage Foundation, New York, 1962.

Maslow, A. H., *Motivation and Personality*, Harper and Brothers, New York, 1954.

Nightingale, Florence, *Notes on Nursing: What It Is and What It Is Not.* D. Appleton and Co., New York, 1938.

Osler, Sir William, *The Evolution of Modern Medicine*, Yale University Press, New Haven, Conn., 1921.

Roueché, Berton, *Eleven Blue Men*, Berkley Publishing Company, New York, 1955.

Towle, Charlotte, *The Learner in Education for the Professions*, The University of Chicago Press, Chicago, 1954.

Articles

Aberg, Harriet L., "Nurse's Role in Hospital Safety," *Nursing Outlook*, V, March, 1957, pp. 160-62.

"ANA Board Approves a Definition of Nursing Practice Act," *American Journal of Nursing*, LV, December, 1955, p. 1474.

Anderson, Odin W., "Medical Care: Its Social and Organizational Aspects," *New England Journal of Medicine*, CCLXIX, October 17, 1963, pp. 839-43.

Austin, Catherine L., "The Basic Six Needs of the Aging," *Nursing Outlook*, VII, March, 1959, pp. 138-41.

Becker, Howard S., "The Nature of a Profession," *National Society for the Study of Education Sixty-first Yearbook*, Part II, 1962, Chapter 2.

Benne, Kenneth D., and Warren Bennis, "Role Confusion and Conflict in Nursing, What Is Real Nursing?" *American Journal of Nursing*, LIX, March, 1959, pp. 380-83.

Benne, Kenneth D., and Warren Bennis, "What Is Real Nursing?" *Canadian Nurse*, LVII, February, 1961, pp. 122-27.

Bixler, Genevieve K., and Roy M. Bixler, "The Professional Status of Nursing," *American Journal of Nursing*, LIX, August, 1959, pp. 1142-46.

Cameron, Charles, and Agnes F. Campbell, "Accident Prevention for Older People," *Nursing Outlook,* IV, June, 1956, pp. 332-34.

"The Expert Nurse Practitioner," *American Journal of Nursing,* LVIII, February, 1958, pp. 199.

Flores, F., "Role of the Graduate Nurse Today," *New England Journal of Medicine,* CCLXVII, September 6, 1962, pp. 487-91.

Girdwood, R. H., "Patient Care in the Age of Science," *British Medical Journal,* I, No. 5331, March 9, 1963, pp. 631-36.

Henderson, Virginia, "The Nature of Nursing," *American Journal of Nursing,* LXIV, August 1964, pp. 62-68.

"Hospital Manners," *British Medical Journal,* II, No. 5352, August 3, 1963, pp. 265-66.

Jahoda, Marie, "A Social Psychologist Views Nursing as a Profession," *American Journal of Nursing,* LXI, July 1961, pp. 52-56.

Johnson, Dorothy E., "A Philosophy of Nursing," *Nursing Outlook,* VII, April 1959, pp. 198-200.

Johnson, Dorothy E., "The Nature of a Science of Nursing," *Nursing Outlook,* VII, May 1959, pp. 291-94.

Johnson, Miriam M., and Henry W. Martin, "A Sociological Analysis of the Nurse Role," *American Journal of Nursing,* LVIII, March 1958, pp. 373-77.

Jourard, Sidney M., "To Whom Can a Nurse Give Personalized Care," *American Journal of Nursing,* LXI, March, 1961, pp. 86-88.

Keeler, Hazel, "The Nurses' Grail—Good Nursing," *Canadian Nurse,* LVII, February 1961, pp. 127-31.

Komorita, Nori I., "Nursing Diagnosis," *American Journal of Nursing,* LXIII, December 1963, pp. 83-86.

Kreuter, Frances, "What Is Good Nursing Care?" *Nursing Outlook,* V, May, 1957, p. 302.

Kyle, Irma M., "From Handmaid to Partner," *American Journal of Nursing,* LXI, January 1961, pp. 84-86.

Larsen, Virginia L., "What Hospitalization Means to Patients," *American Journal of Nursing,* LXI, May 1961, pp. 44-47.

Lauterstein, R. H., and L. F. Mustoe, "Accidents Involve People," *Nursing Outlook,* VIII, February 1960, pp. 96-98.

Litwack, Janice, and Lawrence Litwack, "Four Stages of Nursing Care," *American Journal of Nursing,* LXII, January 1962, pp. 95-96.

Meyer, Genevieve Rogge, *Tenderness and Technique: Nursing Values in Transition,* Institute of Industrial Relations, University of California, Los Angeles, 1960.

National Society for the Study of Education, "Education for the Professions," *Sixty-first Yearbook,* Part II, 1962.

Newton, Mildred E., "As Nursing Research Comes of Age," *American Journal of Nursing,* LXII, August 1962, pp. 46-50.

Parrish, H. M., *et al.,* "Accidents to Patients Can be Prevented," *American Journal of Nursing,* LVIII, May 1958, pp. 679-82.

Price, Alice W., "The Nurse as a Teacher," *Nursing Outlook,* VII, February, 1959, pp. 98-99.

Saunders, Lyle, "Permanence and Change," *American Journal of Nursing,* LVIII, July 1958, pp. 969-72.

Schulman, Sam, "Basic Functional Roles in Nursing: Mother Surrogate and Healer," *Patients, Physicians and Illness.* ed., E. Gartley Jaco. The Free Press, Glencoe, Illinois, 1958.

Simmons, Leo W., "Past and Potential Images of the Nurse," *Nursing Forum,* I, Summer 1962, pp. 16-33.

Stevens, Leonard, "What Makes a Ward Climate Therapeutic?" *American Journal of Nursing,* LXI, March 1961, pp. 95-96.

Taylor, Carol Dickinson, "Sociological Sheepsheering," *Nursing Forum,* I, No. 2, Spring 1962, pp. 78-89.

"Twenty-One Nursing Problems," *American Journal of Nursing,* LX, October 1960, p. 1473.

Tyler, Ralph W., "Distinctive Attributes of Education for the Professions," *Social Work Journal,* XXIII, 1952, pp. 52-62.

Webb, Marvin W., "The Nurse and the Challenge of the Sixties," *American Journal of Nursing,* LXI, August 1961, pp. 48-50.

Whitaker, Judith G., "The Changing Role of the Professional Nurse in the Hospital," *American Journal of Nursing,* LXII, February 1962, pp. 65-69.

Whiting, Leila, and Joseph F. Whiting, "Finding the Core of Hospital Nursing," *American Journal of Nursing,* LXII, August, 1962, pp. 80-83.

2 : Elements in Health and Disease

All theories have a life history. They start tentatively, grow piece-meal, and slowly mature. Then they can successfully handle new facts and also have considerable predictive value. But sooner or later a discrepancy appears between fact and theory. Then the theory will become modified, and perhaps will entirely disintegrate, to be succeeded by something new.[1]

Fade far away, dissolve, and quite forget
What thou among the leaves hast never known,
The weariness, the fever, and the fret
Here, where men sit and. hear each other groan.
"Ode to a Nightingale": John Keats

'Tis a little thing
To give a cup of water; yet its draught
Of cool refreshment, drained by fevered lips,
May give a shock of pleasure to the frame
More exquisite than when nectarean juice
Renews the life of joy in happiest hours.
Ion (1835), Act I, Scene 2:
Sir Thomas Noon Talfourd (1795-1854)

Nursing is concerned not only with the individual as a person, but with the problems arising from the fact that disease is one of the realities of life. Because nurses spend their professional lives in the care of the sick and in activities that are for the purpose of preventing and curing sickness, they may come to view the world as being inhabited by sick people. This is far from the truth. For most people, during most of their lives, health is the rule. A vague hope of many is that disease will be eliminated, but this is not likely to happen. In a paper in which he considers the possibility of eradicating tuber-culosis, Perkins[2] states that to date man has never eradicated a communi-cable disease. There is, however, sufficient knowledge and experience to elim-inate "smallpox (almost certainly); tuberculosis, syphilis, typhoid fever,

---

[1] Lester S. King, *The Growth of Medical Thought*, The University of Chicago Press, Chicago, 1963, p. 232.
[2] James E. Perkins, "Can Tuberculosis Be Eradicated," *Public Health Reports*, LXXVIII, May, 1963, p. 419.

cholera (probably); malaria (perhaps)." He further indicates that man will never be free of all communicable disease, as new etiological agents pathogenic for man evolve that are not subject to eradication. As future discussion

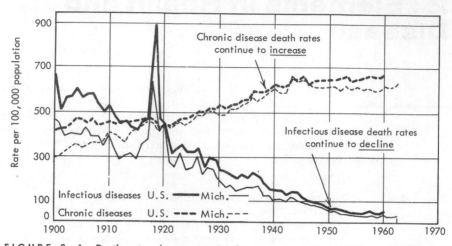

FIGURE 2—1. Death rates due to certain chronic and infectious diseases, Michigan and United States, 1900–1962, which clearly illustrates both the decrease in the incidence of infectious diseases, and the increase in the incidence of chronic disease. Includes following diseases indicated by International Classification Seventh Revision Detailed List Numbers in parenthesis: *Chronic Diseases*—Cancer (140–205), Diabetes (260), Vascular lesions affecting central nervous system (330–334), Diseases of heart (400–443), Chronic and unspecified nephritis (592–594), Ulcer of stomach or duodenum (540–541), and Cirrhosis of liver (581). *Infectious Diseases*—Typhoid fever (40), Scarlet fever (50), Whooping cough (56), Diphtheria (55), Tuberculosis (1–19), Dysentery (45–48), Malaria (110–117), Syphilis (20–29), Measles (85), Pneumonia and Influenza (480–493), Diarrhea, enteritis, and ulceration of intestines (543, 571, 572). (Source of United States data: Building America's Health, Vol. III, Table 36, and Vital Statistics of United States, Vol. I, II. U.S. data for 1961 and 1962 not available.) (Adapted. Courtesy of Statistical Methods Section, Michigan Department of Health.)

will show, infectious diseases remain under control[3] only as long as procedures for their control are effectively applied.

As the incidence of infectious diseases have been lessened, the diseases of middle and later life have increased.

The onset of these diseases can be delayed and their progress slowed by the application of present-day knowledge. Whether these diseases can be entirely eliminated is open to question. As a consequence of the increase in the average life span and the industrialization of our society, new health problems relating to health have been created. Some of the most pressing of these are: How can emphasis in the health professions and society be shifted from a concern for diseases and death to that of health and its fulfillment? How can these years be rendered meaningful that have been gained by life as a result of the control of infectious diseases? How can the new hazards to

[3] By control is meant that the disease is kept from attaining epidemic proportions. There continue to be occasional cases of the disease, but it does not spread rapidly to a large number of persons. It is endemic or sporadic rather than epidemic.

health such as those arising out of the use of radioactive materials and air and water pollution be controlled? None of these problems are the exclusive concern of the members of the health professions. They are problems of the entire nation and world, nor are these the only problems relating to health which face our society.

How is health defined?

Because health is the norm and is the objective toward which the efforts of the health professions are directed, health will be defined and some of the factors in its maintenance will be presented as a background for the general discussion of disease. Beyond general agreement that health is more than a lack of disease, definitions of health do not go very far toward establishing the specific nature of health. There are undoubtedly many reasons for this. One is that health is not easily measured. A disease may be well established or even far advanced before a person has signs or symptoms indicating that he is ill.[4]

Perkins[5] defines health as "a state of relative equilibrium of body form and function which results from its successful dynamic adjustment to forces tending to disturb it. It is not a passive interplay between the body substance and forces impinging on it, but an active response of body forces working toward adjustment." Francis[6] extends the concept of adequate structure and function by adding "adequate reserve." Adding the phrase "adequate reserve" to the definition, an individual can be presumed to be in a state of health as long as he is able to adapt to changes in his environment in such a manner that structure, function, and reserve capacity are preserved. In fact, he is likely to appear to be healthy as long as his reserve capacity is sufficient for him to carry on his usual activities.

Define Adaptation.

One of the outstanding characteristics of the healthy individual is his capacity to adapt to a constantly changing environment. Through appropriate adjustments in behavior, the individual maintains the nutrition of his cells and responds to his environment in such ways that injury is prevented. Adaptation occurs at all levels of organization. In unicellular organisms, the cell carries on all life processes. In multicellular organisms, some cells specialize, and with specialization, some of the capacity of these cells to adapt is lost. For example, the growth potential of nerve and muscle cells is so small that it is of little practical significance. Cellular specialization, however, is to the over-all

[4] Since most students are undoubtedly familiar with the World Health Organization's definition of health, it will not be quoted here. See *Everyman's United Nations*, United Nations Department of Information, New York, 1959, p. 386.

[5] W. H. Perkins, *Cause and Prevention of Disease*, Lea & Febiger, Philadelphia, 1938, p. 21.

[6] Thomas Francis, "Research in Preventive Medicine," *Journal of the American Medical Association*, CLXXII, March 5, 1960, pp. 993-99.

advantage of the individual. It makes him better able to find food and water, escape his enemies, and modify the environment so that it meets his needs. All cells retain one common characteristic—they carry on the biochemical activities essential to metabolism. Although all cells are capable of adapting to changes in the supply of food, those with a high rate of metabolism are quickly injured by marked deprivation.

In addition to the capacity to adapt the rate of metabolism to the supply of nutrients, some cells can respond to a change in the environment by undergoing cell division. For example, following a small injury to the skin or mucous membrane, the epithelial cells multiply and repair the damage. More extensive breaks are repaired by fibrous connective tissue. Exposure to low oxygen tension, such as occurs at high altitudes, results in an increase in the number of erythrocytes in the blood. Erythrocyte and hemoglobin levels are also higher in children who have the type of congenital heart disease in which there is a mixing of venous and arterial blood. Some cells, such as muscle cells, adapt to a change in activity by increasing or decreasing their size.

Survival of the cell and maintenance of its function are dependent on conditions in its immediate fluid environment. It is from this environment that the cell obtains a continued supply of nutrients and into which it discharges its wastes and unstable materials. For all cells, this immediate environment is a pool of water in which a variety of substances such as sodium chloride and glucose are dissolved. For unicellular organisms, such as the amoeba, the fluid environment is a pond or puddle of water. For man and other large multicellular organisms, blood, lymph, and interstial fluid form the immediate environment of the cells. These fluids are known as the internal environment, in distinction to the external environment, or the world outside the skin and mucous membranes, since cavities lined with mucous membranes are in reality outside the body proper. The fluids composing the internal environment not only serve individual cells as such, but are the medium by which all body cells are united to and affected by the activities of all other cells within the entire organism.

What term is used to indicate the mechanisms for maintaining the constancy of the internal environment?

Because of the importance of the internal environment to the activities of cells, many adaptions are involved in maintaining its constancy, within well defined limits. These mechanisms were named homeostasis by Cannon.[7]

Although the complexity of the internal environment of cells has only recently been explored, the idea that it had an influence on human behavior is a very ancient one and is found in many civilizations. Regardless of the civilization into which a man is born, his level of intelligence or education, or

[7] Walter B. Cannon, *The Wisdom of the Body,* W. W. Norton & Company, Inc., New York, 1932, p. 24.

the period of history in which he lives, man has always tried to explain his own nature, his environment and his place in the latter. It is natural that the relationship to his fellow man, and the nature of evil and illness in particular should have occupied him then as it does now. For example, the Navaho Indians believe that health will be granted them when they "live in accord with the mountain soil, the pollen and the plants."[8]

Hippocrates, and later Galen, taught that man was composed of four humours. Man was healthy when these humours were in correct balance; disease was the result of unbalance. This doctrine is based on the concept that the universe is composed of four elements: fire, water, earth, and air. Man, as part of the universe, was seen as composed of the four humours that corresponded to the four elements of the earth: blood (fire), phlegm (earth), yellow bile (air), and black bile (water). This theory was expanded by later physicians. They believed that when one humour dominated the others, it determined the physical and emotional characteristics of a man. Terms derived from this concept are still used to describe the behavioral characteristics of people. Thus, a jolly, optimistic person, inclined to be fat, is said to be sanguine; one who is slow-moving, and is not easily aroused, is described as phlegmatic; one who is easily angered or quick-tempered is choleric; and one who is depressed, peevish, or solitary is melancholic.

According to Bettman,[9] this theory of body fluids was not challenged until 1858, when *Cellular Pathology* was published by Virchow. As a result of this work the cell was recognized as the important entity in health and disease. In 1878 Claude Bernard introduced the concept that cells live in the fluid that bathes them. This fluid—blood, lymph, and tissue fluid—he called the *Milieu intérieur*. He believed that all vital activities have but one objective, the maintenance of the stability of the *milieu intérieur*.

Cannon further elaborated and extended the scope of the work of Bernard. Like Bernard, he considered the stability of the internal environmet its most important feature. He emphasized that although the blood and other fluids were constantly absorbing materials from the external environment and from the cells, the composition of these fluids was maintained constant within limits. In describing his concept of how the constancy of the internal environment was maintained, he states: "The coordinated physiological processes which maintain most steady states in the organism are so complex and so peculiar to living things—involving as they may, the brain and nerves, the heart, lungs, kidneys and spleen, all working cooperatively—that I have suggested a special designation for these states, homeostasis."[10] He elaborated further that the term does not imply stagnation but rather variation within limits. Conditions are maintained constant within limits as long as the individual is capable of making appropriate adaptations to change.

---

[8] Rene Dubos, *Mirage of Health,* Harper and Brothers, New York, 1959, p. 4.
[9] Otto L. Bettman, *A Pictorial History of Medicine*, Charles C Thomas, Springfield, Illinois, 1956, p. 72.
[10] Cannon, *Op. cit.*, p. 24.

What are some of the factors in the maintenance of homeostasis?

The maintenance of homeostasis depends on a variety of elements. Substances required by cells must be available in adequate quantity. Material supplies include water, oxygen, and a variety of nutrients, including sources of calories, tissue-building materials, electrolytes, and regulators not synthesized or present in the body. The intake, storage, and elimination of excesses of supply are regulated so that the level of each substance is maintained within well defined limits. Conditions that must be maintained within limits include osmotic pressure, blood pressure, level of glucose in the blood, cation-anion balance and concentration, hydrogen ion concentration, and body temperature. Conditions in the external environment must be such that man can adapt. For example, man's capacity to adapt to extremes of temperature, high altitude, starvation, and physical trauma is limited.

Because of their size and complexity, multicellular organisms require specialized structures to supply cells with needed materials, to remove the waste products of metabolism, and to maintain the consistency of the internal environment. The healthy organism is capable of responding to disturbances in such a manner that damage is prevented or repaired. The kinds of structures that fulfill this function include the following:

1. Structures that absorb required substances from the external environment and, when necessary, modify them so that they can enter the internal environment. For example, oxygen is absorbed into the blood unchanged. The air from which oxygen is taken, however, requires conditioning. Nutrients usually require reduction to simpler forms before they can be absorbed and provision for elimination of indigestible substances is also necessary. Materials enter or leave the external environment through semipermeable membranes that separate the internal from the external environment. These semipermeable membranes act to protect the internal environment from too rapid change or from the entrance of potentially harmful or nonusable particles.

2. Structures that transport materials from points of entry to cells and from cells to points of elimination or exit such as the heart and blood vessels.

3. Structures that store or eliminate excesses of intake and by-products of metabolism. For example, glucose is stored as glycogen in the liver and muscles; much of the excess is stored as fat. Excess sodium is normally excreted in the urine.

4. Structures that make possible movement in the external environment. They enable the individual to seek food and water, to alter the environment to suit his needs, to overcome or avoid danger, and to find a mate.

5. Structures that reproduce themselves—to replace wornout cells, to repair injury or to produce a new organism.
6. Structures that protect the organism from injury.
7. Finally those structures that regulate and integrate the activities of all individual cells and aggregates of cells so that the organism functions as a whole.

The regulation and integration of bodily processes require that the organism has (1) receptors that function in such a way that the organism recognizes disturbances in its internal or external environment, and (2) structures that communicate information about these disturbances to a center or centers which receive it, evaluate it, and initiate messages which are communicated to the appropriate effector cells. The effector cells are muscle or gland cells. Upon stimulation, they act to correct the disturbance. In following chapters the mechanisms for the maintenance of, and disturbances in, various homeostatic conditions will be discussed in some detail.

How are homeostatic mechanisms regulated?

According to Cannon, the regulation of homeostatic mechanisms is primarily controlled by the sympathoadrenal system. Danger or its symbols, whether in the external or internal environment, result in activation of the sympathetic nervous system and the adrenal medulla. Changes occur that prepare the organism for flight or fight. Cannon also states that the sympathoadrenal system is responsible for regulating the processes whereby the resulting disturbances are repaired. According to his view, the parasympathetic nervous system is largely concerned with the regulation of activities relating to nutrition.[11]

According to present-day knowledge, the autonomic nervous system under the control of the hypothalamus does have an essential role in the maintenance of homeostasis. Despite some exceptions, the sympathetic and parasympathetic divisions of the autonomic nervous system appear to have opposing functions. Excessive activity of one or the other may produce symptoms of dysfunction. One avenue by which the emotional state of the individual affects physiological activity is through the autonomic nervous system.

In addition to nervous control of homeostatic mechanisms, hormones also play an important role. Their production is directly or indirectly subject to control by the hypothalamus. In some instances the action of a hormone enhances the action of the nervous system. For example, epinephrine and norepiniphrine support the action of the sympathetic nervous system. Although the function of the adrenal steroids has not been completely elucidated, their presence is essential to the reaction of the body to changes in

11 Cannon, *Op. cit.*, pp. 263-85.

either the internal or external environment and to the response of the body to injury. They play a role in the regulation of a variety of homeostatic activities. In the absence of the adrenal steroids, the individual reacts ineffectively to even moderate changes in activity, environmental temperature, illness, and physiological, psychological, or other stresses. The adrenal steroids have been demonstrated to play a role in the regulation of water, mineral, and glucose metabolism.

Other hormones such as insulin, thyroxin, parathormone, and antidiuretic hormone also function in homeostasis. Insulin is necessary for the utilization of glucose and possibly the storage of fat. Thyroxin regulates the rate of cellular metabolism and parathormone the level of calcium in the blood. The antidiuretic hormone participates in homeostatic regulation of water by increasing the rate at which water is reabsorbed by the renal tubules. No mention has been made of the role of the anterior pituitary in governing its so-called target glands or of its function in growth. The purpose has not been to review in detail all the structures that function in the control of homeostasis, but rather to indicate the complex nature of its regulation. The suggestion is made that the reader review the functions of the autonomic nervous system and the various hormones and their relationship to each other in a textbook of physiology.

What are some of the body's defenses against injury and how do they function in protection?

For the organism to continue to maintain and restore homeostasis, it requires both defenses against injury and mechanisms whereby damage can be repaired. In health, physiological adjustments involving either an increase or decrease in some bodily activity prevent excessive change. Change in one direction is counteracted by the initiation of a mechanism acting in the opposite direction. Thus, too great change is prevented. Other defense mechanisms protect the organism from the loss of its substance and from the entrance of harmful, or potentially harmful, agents. The intact skin and mucous membrane serve to do both. The skin protects underlying tissues from loss of water and from the effects of radiant rays as well as from other agents in the external environment. It also offers protection against the entrance of harmful chemical and living agents into the organism. Because the skin is in direct contact with the external environment, it plays an important role in the regulation of body temperature.

Body walls of the skull and thorax protect vital organs such as the brain, heart, and lungs, from injury. Secretions by glands serve to wash ducts and mucous surfaces and to dilute and remove irritants of all types. Some, such as the gastric juice, are bactericidal. Many reflexes, such as dodging, blinking, vomiting, sneezing, and coughing, prevent contact with injurious agents or remove them after they have gained entrance into a body structure. Certain cells, including those of the reticuloendothelial system, destroy harmful elements by digestion or by altering their chemical structure so that their toxicity is reduced.

Protection is also afforded by the fact that cells, as well as organs, function within limits. They often have a greater capacity for function than they are called upon to use in the ordinary course of events. For example, the relationship of anabolism to catabolism in the cell can be adjusted so that one equals the other, despite the excessive or deficient intake of food. Some organs have more tissue than is required to meet functional requirements. The fact that a healthy person has more kidney tissue than he requires to maintain kidney function is well known. The same is true of the heart, lung, and liver.

Even after cell or tissue injury, the body responds to limit the damage and to restore the organism to health. For example, an excess of water intake is normally followed by diuresis, and the volume of water in the body is quickly returned to normal. Injured tissues quickly respond by undergoing changes tending to limit the degree of injury and to prevent its spread. Under appropriate circumstances, cells can replace injured cells by undergoing hyperplasia. Some cells are also able to increase in size and strength when they are stimulated by increased demands.

The organism's capacity to meet its physiological needs results from the fact that the cells, tissues, organs, and systems, as well as the entire organism, can respond to disturbances in the environment in such a manner that injury is prevented, or damage is corrected.

What are Cannon's four features of homeostasis?

To summarize and to clarify the concepts of homeostasis, the four features of homeostasis as they are outlined by Cannon will be stated and then applied to one condition of homeostasis, the maintenance of blood pressure. The characteristic features of homeostasis are:[12] (1) to maintain constancy in an open system continually subjected to disturbance some mechanism to prevent change is required; (2) to maintain a steady state requires that any tendency to change is automatically met by increased effectiveness of mechanisms to resist change; (3) regulation of any homeostatic condition may require one or more mechanisms acting at the same time or successively; and (4) homeostasis does not happen by chance, but is the result of organized self-government. These postulates are illustrated by citing the instance of Mr. Brave. He was awakened at night by pain in the upper abdomen and a feeling of nausea. Shortly after awakening, he vomited what he and his wife described as a bowlful of bright red blood. Both were frightened. Mrs. Brave immediately called the family doctor, who suggested that Mr. Brave be taken to the hospital immediately. When he was admitted to the hospital his blood pressure was 120/76. This was his usual blood pressure and is well within the normal range. Let us suppose that he had lost 450 ml of blood.

[12] Cannon, *Op. cit.*, pp. 299–300.

*How can the fact that the blood pressure is within normal limits
after a person has lost a large volume of blood be explained in
terms of Cannon's postulates?*

The maintenance of blood pressure is dependent on agencies acting to
elevate it, balanced against those acting to lower it. Arterial blood pressure
depends on the relationship of the blood volume to the size of the chamber
(blood vessels) that holds it, and the force with which the blood is driven into
the arteries. The viscosity of the blood is also a factor in that a viscid fluid
offers more resistance to being moved than does a thin or watery one. All
these factors can be altered so that blood pressure is raised or lowered or
maintained. In terms of the first postulate, the loss of blood tends to disturb
the relationship between the volume of blood and the size of the chamber in
which it is contained. Since Mr. Brave is able to maintain his blood pressure
within normal limits, there must be some mechanism operating to counteract
the effect of blood loss.

The second postulate suggests further that as blood continues to be lost and
the tendency for the blood pressure to fall is increased, the mechanisms
elevating blood pressure must become increasingly active. For example, the
heart beats more rapidly and the arterioles increase the resistance to the flow
of blood by constriction. The heart responds to the increase in resistance by
contracting with increased force. For the time being, blood pressure is maintained. A point of considerable importance is that some persons may maintain
their blood pressure for a time despite large losses of blood, only to have it
fall suddenly to a dangerously low level. This emphasizes the necessity for
acting on the knowledge that, although individuals differ in their capacity to
adapt, there are limits to this capacity. No single measure of the status of a
patient should be considered to be infallible or apart from other evidence.

The third postulate states that there must be a number of agencies acting to
regulate any homeostatic condition. They may act together or successively.
The regulation of the blood pressure is quite complicated. Review of physiology reveals that both the heart and blood vessels are regulated by the
autonomic nervous system and by hormones as well as by other chemicals,
such as angiotensin, the activity of which depends on a substance secreted by
the kidney. Blood volume is also regulated by a number of mechanisms. All
of these will be discussed in detail later in connection with shock and hypertension. A number of factors play a role in preventing the fall of Mr. Brave's
blood pressure.

Postulate four states that the changes following disturbances in homeostasis
do not happen by accident, but that disturbances in physiological processes
call forth specific responses. This implies that there are receptors stimulated
by change, and when these receptors are stimulated, a set of reactions is
initiated to correct the disturbance. To illustrate by analogy, in any city in
which the services are organized to meet the needs of the community, a call to

the fire department brings forth firemen and fire-fighting equipment. Unless the fire is a big one or is in a critical area, the amount of equipment delivered to the fire is likely to be limited to one truck and the equipment provided by one outfit. It may or may not bring the police. In the instance of Mr. Brave, the stimulus initiating changes in his behavior was the loss of blood and what the loss of blood meant to him. Receptors sensitive to the level of the blood volume initiated impulses which resulted in the activation of mechanisms to maintain or to prevent the fall in his blood pressure. Thus Mr. Brave was protected against the harmful effects of blood loss.

At this point, it should be clear that Mr. Brave was able to maintain automatically his blood pressure because of multiple agencies acting to overcome the blood pressure-lowering effects of blood loss. In addition to those cited above, other mechanisms served either to reduce blood loss or to protect him from its effects. Contraction of blood vessels at the site of bleeding, combined with the tendency of the blood to clot, served to protect Mr. Brave from further blood loss. Even the fact that he felt faint was protective. Because of this feeling he lay down, decreased his activity, and eliminated the need to move blood against gravity. His anxiety was protective because it spurred him to do something about his situation. In general, then, homeostasis was maintained because Mr. Brave was able to regulate supplies and processes in such a way that excesses were eliminated and deficits corrected.

With this review of homeostasis, it should be evident that its maintenance depends on the capacity of the individual to adapt, that is, to respond to changes in his environment, in such a fashion that injury is prevented or damage is repaired. The environment is defined to include all internal and external factors affecting existence, growth, and welfare. For man it includes not only the fluid environment of his cells, but his external environment as well—physical, emotional, intellectual, and social. Some of the aspects of environment may be temporary and some permanent; whatever they are they affect the entire organism.

As has been indicated, in health the needs of the cells are met more or less automatically by the integrated and coordinated activity of all the cells, including those in specialized facilities. In illness the capacity of the individual to cope with disturbances in his environment in such a manner that his needs are satisfied is reduced. In patients with medical-surgical diagnoses, the incapacity frequently lies in an inability to meet one or more physiological needs. Many of the activities of the nurse in the care of medical-surgical patients are directed toward: (1) gathering information about the nature of the internal environment of the patient; (2) modifying the external environment of the patient so the adaptations the patient is required to make are within his capacity to make; (3) supporting the efforts of the patient to adapt or to respond; and (4) providing him with the materials required to maintain the constancy of his internal environment.

*What are some of the factors contributing to
biological adaptation?*

The preceding discussion considered in some detail the manner in which each individual adapts to the fluctuations in his environment. Not only are changes in function possible, but over a period of time alterations in structure may occur. The capacity to modify structures so that the organism is better suited to a particular environment is one of the truly remarkable features of living organisms. How this comes about is not completely understood. Observations have made it clear, however, that biological adaptation is one of the most necessary characteristics of life. Some traits confer on certain individuals an advantage over other individuals; that is, they favor their adaptation and survival in a particular environment and make them more likely to reproduce their kind than individuals who do not possess such traits.

There are numerous examples of successful structural and functional adaptations in nature. Birds adapted to living in the desert conserve water by excreting solid urine. Certain sea birds have developed salt-excreting glands that enable them to drink sea water. Despite having kidneys that are less efficient in removing salt from their internal environment than man's, they are able to maintain the concentration of salt in their extracellular fluid at about the same level. Man, having no comparable structure, is unable to use sea water. When he drinks sea water, he dehydrates himself by using body water to eliminate the excess salt into his urine. The dehydration is further increased by the diarrhea that results from the high concentration of magnesium in the sea water.[13]

Another example of an environmental condition favoring the survival of organisms with certain traits is observed in England. In rural areas a certain species of moth is commonly found to be of light coloration. In industrial areas, the dark variety predominates. There the trunks and branches of the trees are blackened with soot and the light-colored moths are conspicuous on the blackened trunks and branches. They are therefore more easily identified by birds than the dark-colored ones, and hence are eaten by the birds as they appear and do not have much opportunity to multiply while the dark species escape notice and survive.

Occasionally an abnormality serves as an asset in a particular environment. Sickle cell anemia is one such condition. For some reason it confers, or is associated with, some characteristic that increases resistance to malaria. In malarious areas of Africa sickle cell anemia is advantageous to the individual because it increases his chances of survival. In nonmalarious areas, such as the United States, it decreases rather than increases chances for survival.

At times the capacity of certain organisms to adapt has been a disadvantage to man. For example, the fact that mosquitos have developed resistance

[13] Knut Schmidt-Nielson, "Salt Glands," *Scientific American,* CC, January, 1959, pp. 109-19.

to DDT and other insecticides enables them to survive and makes the eradication of malaria difficult. A similar case is *Staphylococcus aureus,* of which strains resistant to penicillin have come to predominate. For a brief time, infections caused by this organism were brought under rapid control, but the capacity of the *Staphylococcus* to adapt has enabled it to survive. Not all species, however, have been successful in adapting to change. The mammoth dinosaurs are extinct because they were unable to adapt to changes from a tropical to a temperate climate or, what appears to be more likely, to a reduction in the amount of food available.

In general, man has the capacity to adapt to a wider range of conditions than do other organisms. There are a number of explanations for the superiority of man in adapting to different conditions. He is able to modify his external environment to his own needs, as well as to foresee his future needs and to make plans that enable him to meet them. Though many species are restricted geographically to a limited area, man can roam the earth or live out his life span in the place where he was born. In either situation he alters his environment to suit his needs. His capacity to adapt the environment to his needs increased greatly when he began to use shelter, clothing, and fire, and to cultivate plants and to domesticate animals as sources of food and of power. In modern times the adaptations of the environment have been further increased by the achievement of a high degree of refinement and efficiency in industrial and agricultural methods and tools.

What are some of the ways by which man adapts to the environment?

In addition to adapting his environment to his needs, man adapts in all aspects of his life. These adaptations may be temporary or permanent. Examples of a temporary biological adaptation that is protective include the capacity to tan the skin. Tanning on exposure to the sunlight offers some protection to the deeper layers of the skin. Persons whose skin does not tan run the risk of sunburn on each exposure to the sun. The fact that the races that developed in the tropics have dark skins while those in northern countries have fair skins is believed to represent a more permanent type of adaptation of the skin to environmental conditions.

Many other examples can be cited of ways in which man has adapted to climate, to geographical location, to physical activity, and to disease. Body build appears to be influenced by climate and by the type of activities in which the individual customarily engages. The short, stocky frame of the Eskimo and the layer of fat under his skin serve to prevent heat loss. The heavy muscles of the manual laborer or the professional wrestler illustrate an adaptation to activities requiring muscular activity. Enlargement of the myocardium in essential hypertension is another illustration of biological adaptation to increased work. One of the factors enabling man to live at high altitudes is that he adapts by increasing the number of erythrocytes and the quantity of hemoglobin in his blood.

Man adapts to some pathogenic microorganisms by developing an immunity to them. For some microorganisms, such as the virus causing smallpox, he has been able to develop a vaccine which causes his body to produce antibodies which protect him from the disease. Others, either because they have diminished in virulence or because man has developed some resistance to them, do not cause as much damage—incidence or severity, or both, of the diseases caused by them have lessened.

A universal adaptation, that is, one that is common to all groups of people, is to the type of food available in an area. Whatever plant or animal is most abundant is utilized as the principal food in the diet. In some areas of the world one or possibly two of the following plants are utilized as the basic or central nutrients in the diet: potatoes, rice, and wheat. In others the principal food is corn, a fruit, or meat. The manner in which food is prepared reflects its abundance or scarcity and the means that are available to prepare it. For example, meat may be added to vegetables or sauces for flavor or to make a little go a long way. Since man takes his food habits with him, wherever he goes, he may continue to select and to prepare foods in a certain way despite changes in his environment or in the availability of specific foods. In fact, changes in food habits are made only with difficulty. A common observation is that persons migrating from one area of the world to another adopt a new language, but continue to cling to old food habits.

Under what circumstances may adaptive responses be elements in the etiology of disease?

Although the capacity to adapt structure and function is essential to the survival of the individual or species, it can also be the cause of disease or injury. Among the first to make the relationship between adaptive responses and the etiology of disease was Claude Bernard. He proposed that disease could result when a response was faulty in degree or magnitude or when in correcting one defect other responses were initiated which resulted in injury. As an illustration, direct injury to cells causes an inflammation. When the degree of this response is excessive, swelling may be such as to impede the flow of blood and tissue nutrition may be so greatly impaired that cells die from a lack of nutrients and oxygen. When a sufficient number of parenchymal cells are killed, scar tissue proliferates. As a consequence of the inflammatory process and scar tissue formation, more harm may be done to the involved organ than the initial injury caused.

As another example, hypoxia acts as a stimulus to the formation of erythrocytes. Possibly, in some instances, the disease polycythemia vera is initiated by hypoxia. The capacity to increase the number of circulating erythrocytes at high altitudes or in certain congenital defects of the heart is homeostatic. In the absence of an appropriate stimulus and when the number of cells formed is excessive and continued, the condition is maladaptive.

Another concept of the relationship of adaption to disease causation was introduced by Selye, who proposed that the organism undergoes certain stereotyped general and local adaptive reactions to injury irrespective of its cause. To the extent to which these responses are appropriate in kind and degree, they assist the sick person in coping with the injury and its effects. Although Selye classified the phases of the adaptive response to illness under different names, they have come to be called the stage of injury or the alarm reaction, the "catabolic" phase and the "anabolic" phase. (See Chapter 3 for a discussion of the response of the body to injury.) Selye further suggested that certain diseases are "diseases of adaptation." According to Selye, these diseases are not the result of some external agent such as a microbe, but they result from the inability of the body to cope with injury by appropriate adaptive responses.[14] These diseases may involve the body tissues or the structures regulating the metabolic responses to injury. Thus in addition to the body tissues, the nervous system, the anterior hypophysis, or the adrenal cortex may be involved. Disturbances in adaptation may be manifested during any stage of its metabolic response to injury. Thus disturbances in adaptation occur during the stage of the "alarm reaction." Evidence of shock is not at all uncommon among individuals who have experienced injury of various types —psychological as well as physical. In certain acute fulminating infections, such as an infection caused by the meningococci, the "alarm reaction" may be profound. On examination the adrenal cortex is found to be destroyed with hemorrhage into the cortices of both glands.

Disorders of adaptation may also occur during the other stages of the "adaptive" syndrome. Thus there are disorders of adaptation during the "catabolic phase" of the general adaptation syndrome. Lesions similar to, but not identical with, those induced by the injection of large doses of aldosterone into animals are observed in a great variety of human diseases. These include disseminated lupus erythematosus, diffuse collagen diseases, dermatomyositis, psoriasis, acute and chronic nephritis, ulcerative colitis, as well as in a number of allergic states such as asthma and allergic rhinitis, and certain psychiatric states.

Similarly, disorders may result from failure of adaptation during the anabolic response to injury. Many patients, particularly those with wasting diseases, go through the early stages of illness satisfactorily only to falter in the anabolic (restoration-of-body-tissue) stage. The malnourished and seriously burned or injured patient may have a prolonged anabolic phase. Ill health in chronic illnesses, such as rheumatic fever or arthritis, may also be prolonged by failure to adapt during the anabolic phase of illness.

From the work of Selye and other investigators, there are now known to be

[14] Hans Selye, "The Stress of Life," McGraw-Hill Book Company, Inc., New York, 1956, p. 128.

changes occurring in the body that represent the body's reaction to injury. Inasmuch as they are appropriate in kind and degree, they facilitate survival and recovery. When they are excessive, inappropriate, or inadequate they can be sources of disease.

What are some of the factors influencing the capacity of the individual to adapt?

A number of factors influence the capacity of any individual to adapt. One of these is his genetic constitution. Recent studies indicate that the biochemical activities of cells are genetically controlled. This means that the genes determine the potential and the limits for the growth and development of both structure and functions in the individual. Through the influence of genes on the biochemical activities of cells, they affect the capacity of the organism to adapt to changes imposed on it from within or from without. The effects of genes range from the activity of enzyme systems in cells to body build and the pigmentation of the skin. Genes also play a role in the transmission of abnormalities. Some of these abnormalities are incompatible with life. Some are evident at birth; some appear early in life; and others do not make their appearance until late in life. An abnormality may be seriously handicapping or produce little or no disability. An example of a disorder in which a defective gene has been identified is the sickle cell trait. In other diseases, such as diabetes mellitus and essential hypertension, heredity appears to be a factor, but the exact nature of transmission is less certain.

The adaptive capacity or potential for adaptation is determined by heredity. In some individuals the capacity for adaptation is so limited that survival is impossible. Whether or not the individual who has sufficient adaptive capacity to survive achieves his potential depends on a variety of factors. A very important one is the extent to which his physiological as well as psychological needs have been met in the past, most particularly in his early life. Basic to the survival and development of each individual is an adequate supply of required materials. As stated in Chapter 1, an inadequate intake of high-quality proteins in infancy and early childhood predisposes to liver disease. A child who is seriously deprived of love is susceptible to failure to develop emotionally. How well an individual achieves his adaptive potential also depends on how he has learned to satisfy his needs and to react to stress as well as some of his experiences throughout his lifetime. Experiences along the way may predispose the individual to health or to disease later in his life. For example, repeated streptococcal infections may predispose a person to rheumatic fever and the rheumatic fever to a reduction in the capacity of the heart to adapt. As a result of the effects of repeated illness, as well as of the attitudes of his parents and others during periods of illness or health, he may come to prefer illness to health. His schooling may well be interrupted and his incentive to learn impaired. Because of a series of interrelated factors an individual whose hereditary potential was more than adequate, fails to develop his intellectual and possibly his physical potential.

Age is another factor influencing the adaptive capacity of an individual. The latter is generally greatest in youth and young middle life and least at the extremes of life. In infants and young children the capacity to adapt is limited by the fact that not all organs and systems are fully mature. At birth the kidneys, nervous system, and immunological systems are not fully developed. For example, the kidney of the young infant is not able to concentrate urine as efficiently as during youth and adult life. As a consequence of the immaturity of his nervous system and lack of experience he is unable to evaluate his external environment and to modify it in terms of his needs.

In the beginning the child's safety and welfare depends to a large extent on others. One of his more serious deficiencies is the immaturity of his immunological system. The very young child is more susceptible to and more seriously affected by infectious agents than older children and adults. His immunological system has to develop before it recognizes harmful agents and reacts to them by forming antibodies. As a result of the immaturity, the safety and welfare of the infant, and to a lesser extent the child, depends upon others.

In the later years of life adaptive capacity declines. All the factors in this process are not fully understood. One seems to be a lessening of the reserve capacity of vital organs. There is also a decrease in response to agents of disease such as bacteria. Infections, such as pneumonia, may be accompanied by few of the changes ordinarily associated with this disease. Fever may be absent or the temperature only slightly elevated.

What are the characteristic features of adaptation?

Whatever the power of the individual to adapt, adaptation is characterized by a number of features. As stated previously, one is that adaptation involves the entire organism. To clarify this concept it was related to Mr. Brave, who was awakened by a feeling of nausea and vomited a large amount of bright red blood. After he vomited, he saw the blood and was frightened. He called his wife who called his physician who asked him to go to the hospital— which is a social response to medical knowledge and equipment. Mr. Brave's fear or anxiety was so great that he did not delay putting himself under the care of his physician. Neither was it so great that he was immobilized. His body was also reacting. His sympathoadrenal medullary system constricted his peripheral blood vessels. He looked pale, felt cold, dizzy, and faint. He lay on the bed until the ambulance arrived. His heart and respiratory rates increased. Although the picture is not complete, enough has been presented to emphasize the point that Mr. Brave reacted as a whole individual.

A second feature of adaptation is related to time. Given time, an organism is able to adapt to a greater degree of stress than it can when it is called upon to adapt suddenly. In the instance of Mr. Brave, had he lost small amounts of blood over a period of time he would have been able to tolerate a lower hemoglobin level than when he lost blood rapidly. With a slow loss of blood he would probably have tolerated a hemoglobin of 4 gm (25 per cent) or less, without exhibiting manifestations of marked circulatory distress when he was resting. In contrast, with a rapid loss of blood, a hemoglobin of 50 per cent is accompanied by manifestations indicative of a serious impairment in the blood supply to vital tissues. There are a number of explanations for the differences in behavior of an individual following the slow and rapid loss of blood. Small losses of blood have little or no effect on blood volume. When the loss at one time is somewhat larger, but within the capacity of the blood vessels to constrict and thereby maintain a satisfactory relationship between the size of the chamber holding the blood and the blood volume, blood pressure is maintained. The loss of blood is accompanied by an increase in the concentration of the blood in relationship to the interstitial fluid. Since the concentration of the blood is greater than the concentration of the interstitial fluid, fluid moves from the interstitial space into the blood. As fluid moves from the interstitial space into the blood, interstitial fluid becomes more concentrated than the intracellular fluid. To restore the normal osmotic relationship between the interstitial and intracellular fluid, intracellular fluid then moves from the cell to the interstitial fluid. These shifts in body fluids provide fluid to restore or maintain blood volume. Although the fluid maintains the blood volume, it dilutes the constituents in the blood, and the quantity of hemoglobin per unit of blood falls. Other evidence of dilution of the blood includes a decrease in the hematocrit and in the erythrocyte count. One of the most important effects of dilution of the blood is a reduction in its oxygen-carrying power. With a sufficient decrease in the oxygen-carrying power of the blood, signs and symptoms of circulatory distress appear. They include palpitation, rapid heart rate, shortness of breath, and possibly dizziness. Depending on the extent to which the hemoglobin level is diminished, these manifestations may appear with activity and disappear with rest or be present much of the time.

In addition to the responses tending to restore and maintain blood volume, a decrease in the oxygen tension of the blood directly or indirectly stimulates the production of erythrocytes by the bone marrow. If the reaction of the bone marrow is insufficient to maintain the level of erythrocytes and hemoglobin, body cells adapt by decreasing their rate of cellular anabolism.

A third feature of adaptation is that the more flexible the organism is in its capacity to adapt, the greater is its capacity to survive. If, for example, the only mechanism available to adapt to the loss of blood was by constriction of blood vessels, man would be much more vulnerable and much less able to survive injuries involving blood loss than he is. Flexibility is as significant in psychological and social adaptation as it is in physiological responses. An illustration of the cultural adaptation to available materials and climate is observed in the building of houses. Among the materials utilized in the building of houses are snow, wood, cement, cinders, sand, clay, aluminum, steel, glass, and skins of animals. Houses vary in size from one room to a hundred or more. Depending on climate and availability of fuel, they may be airy or almost airtight. Their shapes are varied. In fact, any adequate description of the varieties in manner in which man has adapted materials to his need for shelter would be impossible to list in this volume.

A fourth feature of adaptation is that the organism generally uses the mechanism that is most economical of energy. The fact that adaptation also requires energy should not be overlooked. Adaptation is usually integrative in character. Whatever adaptation is made, it is usually the best that the organism can do at a given time. In illness there is always some decrease in the capacity of a person to adapt. The sick person is not at his best, and allowance should be made for his inability to cope with his environment and the resultant frustration of his needs.

A fifth feature is that the adaptive response may be either adequate to the situation or deficient; it may be excessive or inappropriate. To illustrate, following a meal, the blood sugar rises. In the healthy individual, as the blood sugar rises insulin is secreted and glucose is removed from the blood by the liver and converted to glycogen. Some glucose may be temporarily stored in the muscles and areolar connective tissues. Approximately two hours after a meal, the level of sugar in the blood drops to, or slightly below, the fasting level. As the level of glucose in the blood drops, mechanisms responsible for its fall are counteracted and the level of glucose in the blood rises to the normal range for the fasting blood glucose. (One of Cannon's characteristics of homeostatic mechanism.) An elevation in the level of glucose which is sustained above the upper limits of normal is usually due to a relative or absolute lack of insulin. Factors other than the secretion of too little insulin by the islet cells in the pancreas enter into the production of hyperglycemia, that is, an abnormal elevation in blood glucose. They will be discussed later. When too much insulin is secreted or injected, the blood glucose falls excessively and the person suffers from symptoms of hypoglycemia.

To sum up, adaptation enables all living organisms to respond to changes in their environment in such a manner that injury is prevented or damage is repaired. Although all living organisms possess the power of adaptation, not only species, but individuals of the same species vary in their capacity to adapt.

If the concept is accepted that in health the individual is in a dynamic state of equilibrium with the forces in his internal and external environment that tend to disturb it, what is disease?

Throughout his existence man has tried to explain disease. In the early phase of scientific medicine, physicians examined the elements that composed the body and tried to explain disease in terms of how these elements were disturbed. Later, as science progressed, the cell theory of disease was proposed. Today disease is beginning to be described and explained in molecular terms. Undoubtedly, as time passes this theory too will prove to be inadequate and new theories will have to be proposed and tested. In later chapters, references will be made to both the cellular and molecular theories of disease.

In contrast to health, disease is a state in which the individual is no longer in a state of equilibrium with the forces in his external and internal environment. Francis[15] expresses the above concept of disease in the following statement: "Disease is a reaction to stress which extends beyond the bounds of individual reserve and adaptability." Engel[16] defines disease as "failures or disturbances in growth, development, and adjustments of the organism as a whole or of any of its systems." Engel (*Ibid.,* p. 477) also emphasizes the importance of defining disease as a natural phenomenon.

To clarify differences between a state of health and of disease, the essential features of each are summarized below.

What is Health?

1. In health, structure, function and reserve are adequate.

2. Disturbances in the environment (internal and external) are within the capacity of the organism to respond to or to adapt to successfully. The organism is able to cope successfully with changes in its internal or external environment.

3. Responses to disturbances in environment are adequate and appropriate. They protect from injury.

4. As a result of a dynamic state of equilibrium, constancy of the internal environment is maintained within limits.

5. Adaptation is successful in preventing damage or in repairing it and in maintaining adequate functioning.

6. Survival, growth, reproduction and productivity are facilitated.

What is Disease?

1. In disease, structure, function or reserve are inadequate. (May be one or all).

2. Disturbances in the environment (internal and external) are outside the capacity of the organism to respond to or adapt to successfully, at the time of death, all adaptive powers are lost.

3. Responses to disturbances in the environment are inadequate, excessive, or inappropriate. They may be sources of injury.

4. Results in failure to maintain constancy within limits, that is, function is outside limits.

5. Disequilibrium in one area may lead to disturbances in function in other areas.

6. Adaptation is unsuccessful in some respects, that is, there is failure of adaptation at some level, including survival.

---

[15] Francis, *Loc. cit.,* p. 994.
[16] George L. Engel, "A Unified Concept of Health and Disease," *Perspectives in Biology and Medicine,* III, Summer, 1960, p. 459.

Though illness is characterized by a reduction of the adaptive capacity of the sick person, except at the time of death failure of adaptation is, of course, not complete. In the succeeding chapters, the manner in which adaptation breaks down in illness and how the nurse uses knowledge of the characteristic features of adaptation as well as of the nature of adaptive failure to protect and support the efforts of the patient will be considered. Kreuter's definition of nursing care is repeated here to emphasize this aspect of the practice of nursing. She states, "Nursing care is acting and interacting with the patient through physical and personal contact for his welfare and intervening in his behalf between him and those stresses in the physical environment and in the social climate that impinge upon him."[17] As the patient is restored to health, that is, as his capacity to adapt is restored, he is encouraged and helped to resume responsibility for meeting his own needs.

What are some of the factors placing strain on the adaptive capacities of the organism?

In the preceding section some of the factors influencing the capacity of the organism to respond to disturbances in its environment in ways that prevent disequilibrium have been considered. However, success depends not only on the capacity of the individual to react appropriately, but on the nature of the agent eliciting the response and on the interaction of both elements. Moreover, neither health nor disease results from a single factor. Rather both health and disease are the consequence of the interaction of many factors within the organism and its environment—physical, biological, psychological, and social.

Agents or conditions placing strain on the adaptive capacity of the individual have been adapted from Engel.[18] They are of four general types: (1) agents causing injury by their physical and chemical properties; (2) physical and chemical agents required for cellular process which result in injury when they are supplied in insufficient quantities;[19] (3) living agents including microorganisms and parasites; and (4) psychological stress.

The disease-producing power of a pathogenic agent depends on the following: (1) its nature and characteristics; (2) its ability to maintain life and potency; (3) its ability to gain entrance and to establish itself in the host; (4) its source and reservoirs; and (5) vehicles and conditions for its dissemination. These factors are of importance in diseases caused by physical or chemical agents as well as those caused by living organisms. Knowledge of these factors contributes to the prevention, control, and treatment of disease, as well as to the identification of a disease-producing agent and its removal from the environment or the reduction of its effects. The application of the

---

[17] Frances Kreuter, "What Is Good Nursing Care?" *Nursing Outlook*, V, May, 1957, p. 302.

[18] *Op. cit.*, p. 477.

[19] Some required substances can also cause injury when they are ingested in excessive quantities.

above to physical and chemical agents is made in Chapter III and to living agents in Chapter IV. In addition to the above certain other factors influence whether or not pathogenic agents are able to cause injury. Highly virulent microorganisms may overwhelm the host before he has an opportunity to mobilize his defenses. A chemical agent may be so concentrated that many cells are injured and death is inevitable. A physical injury may be so violent that all vital processes are immediately and completely depressed. For example, a head-on collision in an automobile may result in the sudden death of all its occupants. A single exposure of a susceptible individual to influenza is usually sufficient to cause disease.

Explain the concept "necessary and sufficient" as it applies to the etiology of disease.

Unlike the examples cited above, some agents do not cause disease on a single exposure and sometimes do not result in disease after repeated exposures. Not only do some etiological agents require repeated exposures over a period of time, but the development of a particular disease may depend on the presence of one or more other factors. These observations have led to the concept of "the necessary and sufficient cause."[20] According to this concept, some diseases do not develop in the absence of a specific agent. This specific agent is therefore necessary or must be present if a specific disease is to develop. The agent itself may or may not be pathogenic enough, that is, be powerful enough, to induce disease. For example, the disease tuberculosis does not develop in the absence of the *Mycobacterium tuberculosis.* Therefore, the *Mycobacterium* is a necessary etiological factor in tuberculosis. As a rule, tuberculosis does not develop on a single exposure to the disease, but requires multiple exposures. Moreover, other conditions such as undernutrition and youth are frequently required to provide sufficient conditions for the development of tuberculosis. In epidemiological terms, tuberculosis requires both a necessary and a sufficient cause for disease to occur.

In many of the chronic degenerative diseases the "necessary" condition for their development is not known, if such a factor exists. They appear to be the result of multiple factors, some of which have their origin in the internal environment and others in the external environment. Before disease develops the sum total effect of pathogenic agents must be sufficient to damage the cellular machinery and cause disease. Because the chronic degenerative diseases require months or years to develop, assessment of the degree to which possible pathogenic agents are responsible is difficult.

For example, the continued inhalation of tobacco smoke is associated with a number of harmful effects and shortens the life span in human beings. Among the important diseases having a higher incidence among persons who smoke cigarettes than among nonsmokers are coronary artery disease; cancer of the lung, mouth, lip, larynx, pharynx, and esophagus; and pulmonary

[20] Edward S. Rogers, "Man, Ecology, and the Control of Disease," *Public Health Reports,* LXXVII, 1962, p. 755.

diseases including pneumonia and influenza.[21] Agreement has not been reached about how tobacco smoke produces its harmful effects. Since not all persons who smoke develop the above disorders and some who do not smoke do, tobacco smoke is not a necessary condition in their development. It can be assumed, however, that in persons who do develop one of the above disorders, cigarette smoking combined with other factors is "sufficient" to cause disease.

Not all of the factors contributing to the development of chronic disease are necessarily of a physical or chemical nature nor are they of extrinsic origin. Apparently, the genetic constitution of an individual predisposes him to some diseases and protects him from others. Psychological and social stresses can also impose strain on the capacity of the individual to cope with physical and chemical agents. Therefore, when multiple factors appear to be involved in the causation of disease, the extent to which each factor—physical, chemical, genetic, microbiological, psychological, and social—is responsible in a given individual varies. When these and other factors combine so that the total effect is sufficient to interfere with cellular processes, disease results. In the person whose genetic constitution predisposes him to a given disease, less in the way of other factors is required than in individuals who are not so predisposed. Conversely, an individual who is not predisposed to a given disease can develop it, if one or more other etiological factors are sufficiently intense.

As indicated above, psychological stress places strain on the adaptive capacity of the individual and therefore is believed to predispose to disease. Engel[22] states that psychological stress includes all factors making demands on the organism and which require work or activity of the nervous system before any other system is activated. According to Engel,[23] for a situation or process to cause psychological stress, it must be capable of being "perceived, experienced, and represented in the mind of the subject." Psychological stress results from the meaning that a situation has for a person, rather than from the direct injury of cells. The person undergoing psychological stress does not have to be able to describe the entire situation responsible for his discomfort. Neither do all elements in the situation have to be on a conscious level; it must, however, be capable of being manifested to the individual and/ or observer in psychological terms. Causes of psychological stress are many and varied. Engel groups psychological stresses into three general categories. They are: (1) the loss of something of value to the person; (2) pain and fear of pain; and (3) the frustration of drives. During the course of a somatic illness one or more, if not all, of the above contribute to the psychological stress experienced by the individual.

Among the things a person is likely to value sufficiently to experience psychological stress when they are lost or their loss is anticipated are: per-

[21] E. Cuyler Hammond, "The Effects of Smoking," *Scientific American*, CCVII, July, 1962, p. 43.

[22] *Op. cit.*, p. 480.

[23] *Ibid.*, p. 481.

sons, values, job, a part of the body, a bodily function, body image, social status or role, goals, and hopes. A common reaction to the loss of something of value is grief or depression. The man whose wife dies or deserts him experiences grief. Likewise, Mr. Cocky, who takes great pride in his muscular strength, experiences severe grief after he develops a serious paralyzing disease. He not only has lost something he values, his muscular strength, but he will lose his job, and his role in the family as the breadwinner will be altered. In fact he will probably experience some losses in all aspects of his life.

A second cause of psychological stress is pain and fear of pain. A human being tries to avoid pain and injury and he reacts to threats to himself in much the same manner whether the danger exists in the external world or only in his imagination. One writer has said that man is the only living being that can frighten himself with his own thoughts. Whether a danger is real or imaginary the individual mobilizes his defenses to prepare himself to make appropriate adjustments. In the practice of nursing, psychological stress can be minimized by appropriately preparing the patient for what to expect and by learning what he expects in the situation.

The third general cause of psychological stress is the frustration of drives. In the process of growing up the individual learns to master his drives so that he is able to fulfil his needs in the world of reality. In the development of mastery, both external and internal controls are applied. Sometimes a conflict arises from the manner in which the drive is controlled or from the way in which the individual regards a particular drive. Unless the conflict is resolved, the resulting psychological stress may be a precipitating factor in disease. The effects of psychological stress in illness are discussed in detail in Chapter 6.

Rogers[24] summarizes in schematic form factors that act as immediate and specific causes of disease and injury. These can be seen in Figure 2-2.

How may disease be studied?

One way in which disease may be studied is to focus attention on the disease. When this is done it is described in terms of: (1) the causative factors—such as direct, remote, necessary and sufficient, permissive, conditioning, inciting, predisposing, precipitating, and perpetuating; (2) the mechanisms whereby the disease-producing agent produces its effect—such as hereditary, biochemical, physiological, psychological, social; (3) the nature of its onset—sudden or gradual; (4) the characteristic signs and symptoms; (5) the predicted outcome or prognosis; (6) the preventive measures; and (7) the therapeutic measures. Although individuals who are sick are unique, diseases are not. They occur in classes or groups having common characteristics. Many persons may have the same disease. The cause and manifestations of a disease as well as the methods by which it is effectively prevented and treated are similar in individuals who have the disease. For example, smallpox is caused by a

[24] Edward S. Rogers, *Human Ecology and Health*, The Macmillan Company, New York, 1960, p. 166.

1. Conditions may vary in the Agent
   (of illness or injury):

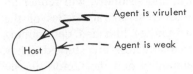

Agent is virulent

Host

Agent is weak

Some possible sources of variation:

Genetic constitution, nutrition, favorable growth conditions, dosage or intensity of impact

2. Conditions may vary in the Host:

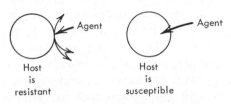

Agent

Host
is
resistant

Agent

Host
is
susceptible

Some possible sources of variation:

Genetic constitution, nutrition, balance of internal stresses and adaptations, age and sex, physical vigor or fatigue, specific immunity, knowledge and attitudes, personality

3. Conditions may vary in the Environment
   that brings the agent and the host
   together:

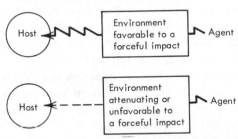

Host

Environment favorable to a forceful impact

Agent

Host

Environment attenuating or unfavorable to a forceful impact

Agent

Some possible types of variation:

Physical conditions—
   such as temperature, humidity, heat, light, shelter, traumatic hazards
Biological conditions—
   such as sanitation, parasites, disease vectors, nutrient value of foods available, crowding
Nonmaterial conditions—
   such as social and cultural patterns and values, emotional forces of many kinds

FIGURE 2—2. Schematic presentation of factors influencing the immediate and specific causation of illness or injury. (This model applies but approximately to some situations. The absence of something necessary to health, such as a nutrient from the diet, might serve as an agent. Also, in some chronic or mental illnesses, the role of the agent or precipitating event may be very obscure and actually of little individual consequence by contrast with the importance of an accumulation of events over time.) (Adapted with permission of The Macmillan Company from *Human Ecology and Health*, Fig. 23, p. 166, by Edward S. Rogers. Copyright © Edward S. Rogers, 1960.)

specific virus. Although manifestations vary in degree of severity, they are similar in all individuals who contract smallpox. Smallpox is effectively prevented by one attack of the disease or by vaccination. Treatment of the person who has smallpox is nonspecific inasmuch as no curative measures are available to shorten or modify the severity of the illness.

Another approach to the study of disease is to use the methods of epidemiology. Epidemiology may be defined very simply as medical detection. The same general methods are used in the identification of the person or persons responsible for a crime. A more comprehensive definition of epidemiology formulated by Frost[25] is: "It is the science which considers the occurrence, distribution, and types of diseases of mankind, in distinct epochs

[25] "Papers of W. H. Frost," K. F. Maxey, ed., *The Commonwealth Fund*, New York, 1941, p. 494.

of time, at varying points on the earth's surface, and secondly, will render an account of the relations of these diseases to inherent characteristics of the individual, and to the external conditions surrounding him and determining his manner of life." In epidemiology two general factors are studied. They are the effect of a disease on a group or community and the factors in the community contributing to its development. The term "epidemiology" had its origin in and relates to its use in identifying the community factors in epidemic diseases, that is, it was first used in the study of diseases caused by microorganisms. As the science of epidemiology developed, workers in the field have come to appreciate that the same techniques and questions are useful in the study of noninfectious diseases, such as mental illness and atherosclerosis. In the epidemiological approach to disease not only the sick, but the well, are studied. Answers are sought to questions such as: Who is sick? Who is well? What are the characteristics of those who are sick? Of the well? What are the etiological agents? What are the characteristics of each causative agent? What are the factors in the environment bringing the susceptible host and the etiological agent or agents together? The answers to these questions serve as the basis for other questions. Which of the factors that have been identified as contributing to the development of the disease can be controlled? How can this control be most effectively applied?

A third approach to the study of disease is to focus attention not on the disease per se but upon the person who is ill. In this approach some of the questions include: How has this disease come about? What effect does it have on the cells, tissues, and organs? Why did this particular person develop this particular illness at this time? What purpose, if any, does this illness serve the person? What purposes do the changes, physiological and psychological, serve in the adjustment of the individual to the causative factors in the illness?

To illustrate, a group of people become ill. Using the first approach, the disease is described as having a sudden onset; the cause is *Staphylococcus aureus*, which releases an enterotoxin; the enterotoxin induces acute gastroenteritis; the signs and symptoms associated with the gastroenteritis include severe nausea, vomiting, diarrhea, and prostration. In most persons who are affected, the symptoms last only a few hours. Of the 100 who developed symptoms, 98 recovered promptly. The other two died. Using the second or epidemiological approach, the persons who became ill were of all age groups above the age of 2 years. About two hours previous to the onset of symptoms they had all eaten ham at a community supper. Those who ate roast beef did not become ill. No one else in the community suffered the same symptoms. Further investigation revealed that the day was very hot and that the ham was sliced and was not refrigerated after it was cooked. The woman who sliced the ham had an infected finger. Both of the persons who died were elderly men.

In the third approach to the study of disease, attention is centered on each sick individual. The responses of each person are subject to investigation and evaluation. For example, both Marie Skinny and her date John Robust ate ham. Marie was only mildly sick, while John was severely ill. Marie convalesced slowly, while John recovered promptly. Elderly Mr. Claro died, while equally elderly Mrs. Claro suffered only a few minor symptoms. Questions arising include, why should John who was sicker than Marie recover more promptly than Marie? Why did Mr. Claro die and his wife recover? Some answers to these and other questions are easy to obtain. Others require extensive knowledge of the individual, his capacity for response, and what has happened to him throughout his lifetime. Because of insufficient knowledge, some questions cannot be answered at this time. The fact that John was sicker than Marie may or may not be completely explained by the fact that she ate sparingly of the ham while John ate not only his serving, but the remaining portion of Marie's. Certainly it does not explain why her recovery was prolonged. That Mr. Claro died may be explained in part by the fact that he had a diseased heart, but other factors may well have been of importance.

All these approaches to the study of disease and its effects are important. Knowledge of the manifestations of a particular disease is necessary to the recognition of illness and to the introduction of measures to limit its effects. The epidemiological approach aims at the identification of those elements within or without the individual that are subject to control and the institution of measures to protect the population from harmful agents. As a result of study of incidents such as the community supper cited above, laws governing the handling of food have been enacted. Educational programs have been instituted to inform people of the procedures that are necessary for their protection. The fact that food poisoning continues to occur when conditions combine not only to introduce the *Staphylococcus aureus*, but favor its multiplication, introduces the human factor. This brings the discussion to a summary of the third factor in the study of disease, that is, the individual. In the United States information is widely disseminated about the conditions favoring food poisoning. Why, then, should food be handled in such a manner that food poisoning occurs? The answers here are to be found in individual human beings. Each human being is an important factor in when, how, and why he becomes ill.

The incident of the community supper also serves to emphasize another concept that has been receiving increased emphasis in the literature. That is, any situation, including illness and recovery from illness, depends on the interaction of multiple factors. When the factors placing strain on the individual are within his adaptive capacity, he remains well. When they exceed his adaptive capacity, illness results. The nature of his illness, the degree of his illness, and the speed with which he recovers can also involve multiple factors.

What are some of the factors in the manifestation of disease?

In the following pages some generalizations will be made about the way in which a disease may be manifested as a basis for later discussions of the effects of specific disease conditions. A point that should be made before describing some of the manifestations of disease is that what is categorized as disease differs from one time in history to another, from one culture or group to another, and even from one person to another. For example, in the Andean Altiplano, goiter due to a lack of iodine was so common that an enlarged neck was regarded by the residents of the area as a normal condition. Among some groups in the United States, obesity among women and girls is believed to be indicative of health. Among others, an individual is not really ill unless he is incapacitated.

What terms are employed to describe different types of manifestations of disease?

Some of the effects associated with illness can only be experienced by the individual. Other effects can be observed by individuals, nurses, and physicians either directly or by the examination of a body structure or fluid with a special instrument. Those changes or effects that can only be experienced by the person are called symptoms. They may be communicated as complaints to others, but they cannot be observed by them, though the effects on the sufferer may be evident. Moreover, to be viewed as a symptom, a change must be perceived to be outside the range of what the person believes to be normal. It cannot be explained away by something the person did or as something to be expected. For example, one bright spring morning, Miss Winter donned a pair of low-heeled shoes and went for a long walk. The following morning, she had pain in the calves of her legs when she walked. Though the pain was severe, she did not think of it as a symptom of disease. Instead she asked herself, "How could I have been so stupid, as not to remember that I've been wearing shoes with high heels all winter?" Another example is that of Mrs. Ball, aged 83. Sometimes on a fine clear day, she has aches and pains in her muscles and joints. Though she complains bitterly about her discomfort, she does not consider her pain to indicate the presence of disease. Rather she says, "It is going to storm, you just wait and see. My aching joints are just a sign that I'm growing old and that the weather is about to change." In both these examples, pain and discomfort were not evaluated as symptoms of disease, but were interpreted as a normal event. Had Miss Winter experienced the same type and degree of pain in the absence of a satisfactory explanation, she would probably have perceived it as a symptom of disease.

Since a symptom is experienced only by the sufferer, the observer should be careful to describe it as exactly as possible. Often the words used by the patient are significant. In eliciting information from the patient, questions requiring answers include when, where, to what degree, and under what circumstances. Sometimes answers to these questions are evident. Sometimes they may have to be asked directly. The patient in pain whose fists are clenched and who has beads of perspiration on his brow may not need to be asked whether he is in pain. His general appearance indicates that he is. The patient may or may not communicate the symptom directly in words, as he may use gestures or bodily movements or some other method of indicating his discomfort. Furthermore, symptoms such as pain may be accompanied by physiological changes such as an increase in pulse or respiratory rate. Moreover the behavior of the patient may or may not be in keeping with the reported severity of the symptom. For example, Mr. Xeres states that he is having severe headache, yet he does not appear to be uncomfortable. His headache seems to be precipitated by a visit from his wife or boss. This type of information is of value to the physician who must make a medical diagnosis and institute a plan of therapy.

Other changes taking place in disease may or may not be experienced by the patient, but can be observed by others. These are called signs. Signs, such as edema or swelling, which are experienced by the patient, are also symptoms. Signs include a wide variety of changes, biochemical, functional, and structural. Among the biochemical changes may be included alterations in the levels of electrolytes, such as sodium or potassium, and nonelectrolytes, such as glucose and urea, in the blood and other body fluids. Structural changes range from death of body cells to alterations in the number or character and organization of cells in a tissue or organ. When cells die, enzymes concentrated in the cells may be released into the blood or other body fluids. For example, the level of lactodehydrogenase (LDH) in the blood rises after a myocardial infarction.[26] An elevation of the level of LDH in the blood does not by itself prove that an individual has had a myocardial infarction. When, however, LDH rises in combination with other signs and symptoms indicating myocardial infarction, it is considered to be significant. Some types of lesions are common to a variety of diseases. Others are characteristic of one specific illness. The latter is designated by the term pathognomonic. For example, Koplik spots are small white spots occurring on the buccal mucosa in the early stage of measles. Since they occur only in measles, they are said to be pathognomonic of measles.

Although a particular constellation of symptoms and signs is characteristic of certain diseases, many of them are common to a wide variety of disorders. By themselves they indicate that the individual is ill, but not how or why he is. Among the symptoms and signs occurring in many diseases are pain, including headache; fever or hypothermia, low body temperature; changes in the rate, rhythm, and character of the pulse and respiration; anorexia, nausea, vomiting, and diarrhea; general malaise, that is, a feeling of unfitness; weakness; changes in the level of erythrocytes and leukocytes in the blood; and changes in the quantity and concentration of the urine.

In summary, how the person who is ill behaves when he is ill and the effects that are produced by injury or disease are the result of the interaction of many complex factors which include: (1) the personality structure of the person and his pattern of reacting to stress or emergency situations, (2) the conditions defined by society as disease and the approved manner of behaving when

---

[26] Death of an area of heart muscle due to a failure in blood supply.

ill, (3) the nature of the agent placing strain on the adaptive capacity of the individual, and (4) the capacity of the individual to respond in ways that are constructive. These points are elaborated upon in later chapters.

What are the objectives of the health professions?

Three important objectives of the health professions are: (1) the maintenance and promotion of positive health or of a high level of wellness, (2) the prevention of disease, and (3) the care and hopefully the cure of the sick. When cure is not possible, the aim or goal in the care of the person is to maintain and support his strength and hope so that he remains a whole and, in so far as possible, a contributing member of society.

Each objective will be examined in terms of some of the problems, past and present, that contribute to and interfere with its achievement. From an examination of the past and present-day health problems, perhaps a foundation can

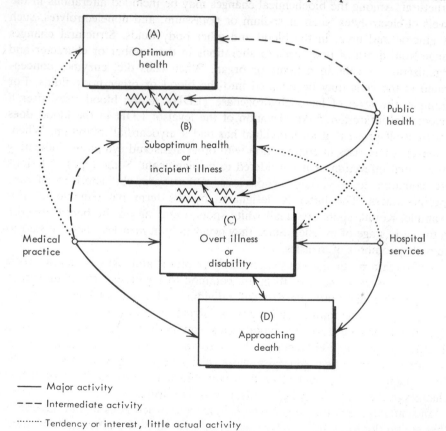

——— Major activity

— — — Intermediate activity

·········· Tendency or interest, little actual activity

FIGURE 2—3. Health status scale showing focus of major forms of health service. (Adapted with permission of The Macmillan Company, from *Human Ecology and Health*, Fig. 24, p. 176, by Edward S. Rogers. Copyright © Edward S. Rogers, 1960.)

be laid for thinking of birth, growth, and maturation, health, disease, and death as phases of life. Dunn[27] emphasizes the relationship of health and disease by saying ". . . it is essential to shift from considering sickness and wellness as a dichotomy toward thinking of disease and health as a graduated scale." What Dunn calls high-level wellness is at one end of the scale, while death is at the other. The problems that are presently known as disease, as well as those existing in the past, are related to conditions in the society of the time. Most of the health problems of today have always existed. As a matter of fact, writers such as Gordon[28] indicate that the broad categories of disease have not changed to any extent over the years. What has changed is the degree to which a given disease is a significant cause of morbidity and mortality. These changes have come about largely because of alterations in the relationship of man to his environment. Some present-day health problems result not so much from failure, but from accomplishment. For example, as infections and other conditions that were responsible for a high infant mortality rate have been brought under control, the ailments that are common in older adults have increased in incidence. Many, if not all, health problems have an ancient history. For example, evidence of coronary artery disease has been found in the mummies of ancient Egypt, but it was not recognized as a problem by the ancient Egyptians. What is indentified as a problem depends on its incidence in relation to other problems.

What is meant by the promotion of positive health or a high-level wellness?

Though the promotion of health is accepted as a desirable objective, very little is known about how to measure health or even how to achieve or to maintain it. In much of the literature little or no distinction is made between the promotion of health and the primary prevention of disease. Although knowledge and techniques are available that enable the physician to identify and categorize various diseases, there are little information and few techniques to aid him to distinguish among, and to classify, different degrees of health. If the goal, to promote a "high level of wellness," is to be accomplished, at least some health workers will need to shift their emphasis from death and disease to health and its fulfillment.[29]

How is health promoted?

For want of more definitive knowledge, conditions contributing to healthful living will be considered as facilitating the accomplishment of the objective

[27] Halbert L. Dunn, "High-Level Wellness for Man and Society," *American Journal of Public Health*, XLIX, June, 1959, p. 787.
[28] John E. Gordon, "Changing Accents in Community Disease," *American Journal of Public Health*, LIII, February, 1963, p. 141.
[29] Iago Galdston, *The Meaning of Social Medicine*, Harvard University Press, Cambridge, Massachusetts, 1954, p. 30.

"to promote health" and the measures more directly related to the prevention of specific diseases as facilitating the accomplishment of the objective "to prevent disease or disability from disease." The discerning reader will note that there is some overlapping between the two.

The Commission on Chronic Illness[30] lists the following as among the most important components of healthful living:

Nutrition—adequate, safe, and well-distributed food supplies as well as appropriate levels of personal nutrition.

Mental hygiene—beginning at an early age, it is important that the individual develop an equanimity in the face of the natural and inevitable frustrations of living; appreciation of the values of family life; acceptance of oneself and one's limitations.

Adequate housing—including proper safeguards against accidents for persons of all ages, and particular safeguards for children and for the aged handicapped.

Moderate and well-balanced personal habits—restraints in the use of alcohol and tobacco, sufficient rest and an appropriate amount of exercise, careful attention to personal hygiene.

A useful and productive role in society.

General education and education specifically for health.

A safe and healthful working environment.

Recreation, including access to recreational opportunities and facilities on the one hand, and proper balancing of recreational activities against satisfying work on the other.

A sense of personal security, related to such things as access to health services; legalized provisions for minimum wages and some sort of job security; provision for income maintenance during illness or following retirement.

To this list may be added another concept—that is, a system of values that will serve as a guide to action. Beginning at an early age, the individual should be helped to develop a sense of purpose in his life, that is, who and why he is, and where he is going. His goals should be based on a wholesome appreciation of the rights and dignity of his fellowman.

The promotion of health is both an individual and a social responsibility. Whenever a large group of people live in a limited area, regulations are necessary to protect the general welfare. The individual has a responsibility to cooperate in protecting not only his own rights, but those of others.

One of the best-known and -organized efforts in the field of health promotion is the well-baby clinic. The baby is examined regularly and the mother is given guidance in his care. Data are available by which the growth and development of the child can be measured. This information is useful in reassuring the mother that her baby is developing normally; in turn it may contribute to the mother's being more relaxed in the care of her baby. It may also be the basis for unnecessary anxiety, unless both the mother and the health worker know and accept the fact that there is much variation in the rate at which babies grow and develop. When the development of the baby is

[30] *Chronic Illness in the United States.* Vol. I. *Prevention of Chronic Illness,* Commonwealth Fund, Harvard University Press, Cambridge, Massachusetts, 1957, p. 9.

in some respect abnormal the mother can be aided in modifying his care, so that his health is promoted. For example, the baby may be gaining weight too rapidly. In addition to recognizing that obesity is undesirable, the mother may require support to modify his food intake. Attendance at the well-baby clinic also provides an opportunity to immunize the baby against certain diseases such as smallpox and diphtheria. Thus, through services provided to the baby and his mother, the healthy development of the baby is promoted.

Knowledge of the factors assisting in the promotion of health will undoubtedly increase in the future. Contributions from the fields of biochemistry, biophysics, psychology, sociology, and anthropology can be expected to provide a basis for a greater understanding of what health is and how it is measured and promoted than is now available. Among the questions being explored by social scientists are how to impart information about health so that it is effective, how to change attitudes, and how to improve communication between and among various groups.

As with other members of society, the nurse has a personal responsibility to promote her own health. As society expects the contributions of an individual to be commensurate with his education and opportunities, the nurse has more responsibility than the ordinary citizen to promote her own health. She also has a responsibility as a citizen to promote community projects such as improved housing and slum clearance that contribute to the general health and welfare of the entire community. As a professional nurse she also works with individuals and groups to help them raise their standards of health.

What is meant by the prevention of disease and how is it accomplished?

The second objective of the health professions is the prevention of disease. In the prevention of disease actions are taken to forestall the development of disease or injury. In already established diseases, procedures are instituted to prevent disability or to delay its progress.

In order to appreciate the tremendous contributions of preventive medicine, it is essential to be aware of some of the conditions in the world before the middle of the nineteenth century and some of the changes that have taken place in the Western world since that time. It is also imperative to understand that the conditions basic to health do not prevail throughout the world. In the larger part of the world the major health problems continue to be malnutrition, lack of sanitation, and inadequate medical care. In contrast, in the countries of the world where the supply of food is abundant, the sanitary facilities are adequate to the needs of the population, and a high standard of medical care is available, the problems are those with which Americans are familiar. These will be reviewed later in another context. Lest anyone conclude that the dangers to health in the external environment of man have been brought under final control, they should read *Time Magazine,* "Environment Versus

Man", (September 26, 1960, pp. 66-8). In this article the questions, "What is in the air? What is in the water? What is in the food?" are raised. Almost the entire January, 1964, issue of the *American Journal of Public Health,* including a supplement, is devoted to "Man—His Environment and Health."

How can the effects of the promotion of health and the prevention of disease be measured?

There are a number of ways in which the effects of the promotion of health and the prevention of disease can be measured. One of these is in terms of the infant and maternal mortality rates. Another is the average length of life or the life expectancy rate. In the last century the average life span has been remarkably prolonged. The extent to which it has been lengthened is made clear by examining some of the life expectancy rates of former eras. According to Dublin,[31] the average age to which each of the following lived was: (1) prehistoric man, 18 years; (2) the Romans, about 22 years; (3) American 1789, 35.5 years (Massachusetts or New Hampshire); (4) American 1900–1902, 49.2 years; and (5) American 1957, 69.3 years. Massachusetts and New Hampshire are identified because they were the only states that kept records at that time.[32]

What changes have contributed to this increase in longevity in the last century?

The gains in life expectancy are due to the development of modern industry and agriculture and to advances in knowledge of medicine and related sciences. In the early years of industrialization in England, living conditions were indescribably bad. One source of information is the novels of Charles Dickens. He not only wrote about the horrible social evils of the time, but he lent powerful support to the social reformers. Edwin Chadwick's "Report on the Sanitary Conditions of the Laboring Population of Great Britain"[33] focused attention on the dreadful living conditions in the cities of England. This report, which was published in 1842, gave rise to the modern public health movement in England, and it resulted in the first organized health department. Shattuck[34] made a similar contribution in the United States. With the development of sanitary and housing codes to protect the life and welfare of the people, laws were passed to protect the quality of food, the supply of water, and the work and home environment. Later as workers organized to promote and protect their rights, hours of work were shortened. Conditions under which women and children could work were defined. The

---

[31] Louis I. Dublin, *The Facts of Life from Birth to Death,* The Macmillan Company, New York, 1951, p. 389.

[32] *Statistical Bulletin,* Metropolitan Life Insurance Company, March, 1959.

[33] B. W. Richardson, *The Health Nations: A Review of the Work of Edwin Chadwick,* 2 vols., Longmans, Roberts and Green, London, 1887.

[34] Lemuel Shattuck, *Report on the Sanitary Commission of Massachusetts, 1850,* Boston, Dutton and Wentworth, Cambridge, Massachusetts, 1948.

right of the worker to a living wage was established. Machines not only enabled the worker to increase the production of goods, but by sharing in the rewards of increased production he was able to improve his standard of living and his health status. Members of groups such as fraternal organizations joined together to provide for insurance for their families in the event of death. Later, commercial insurance companies were formed for this purpose, and the types of insurance were expanded to cover other kinds of human disaster.

The relationship of health to economic status, education, and general standard of living has been demonstrated by the studies of Dublin[35] and others. For example, nonwhite Americans have a shorter life span than white Americans. College graduates live longer than non-college graduates. Clergymen, teachers, and lawyers live longer than the average. Walker[36] quotes a study being conducted by the National Office of Vital Statistics in which the death rate ratio is correlated with income. Those with the lowest income have the lowest life expectancy; those with the highest income have the longest life expectancy.

One further example will be cited. Each year in its annual report, the Department of Health of the City of Detroit summarizes the vital statistics for the city in a map. The divisions of the map correspond to the census areas of the city. In order to orient the reader to the map, the "Central City," which includes the downtown area, Figure 2-4, is the section bounded on three sides by the Grand Boulevard and on the fourth by the Detroit River. According to a study made by the Detroit Area Planning Committee of the United Community Services of Metropolitan Detroit,[37] approximately 260,000, or 15 per cent, of the population of the city of Detroit live in the area bounded by the Grand Boulevard. The extent to which overcrowding exists in this area is emphasized by a number of conditions. Much of the land space, which is 11 per cent of the total area of Detroit, is used for commercial and industrial purposes. Even more telling is the fact that the "Central City" contains only 4 per cent of the dwelling places of the community and 22 per cent of them are vacant. Much of the housing in the area is in various stages of deterioration and a not inconsiderable portion is unfit for human habitation.[38] Though the population in the area decreased in the period between 1950–1960, most of the decrease was in the adult population.

As is to be expected, the population of the "Central City" not only lives under inadequate and overcrowded conditions, but many individuals have marginal or inadequate incomes. It is estimated that in 1960, 41 per cent of the families receiving Aid to Dependent Children and 44 per cent of those persons receiving Old Age Assistance lived in this area.[39] Like other large

35 *Ibid.*, p. 100.
36 Gerald Walker, *This Week Magazine*, June 12, 1960.
37 *Social Services in Detroit's Central City*, September, 1960.
38 *Ibid.*, p. 6.
39 *Ibid.*, p. 8.

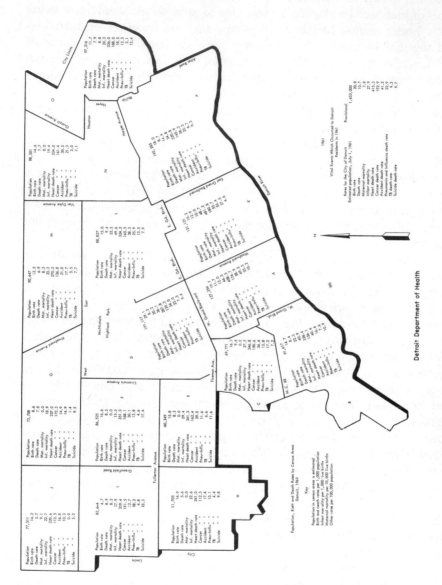

FIGURE 2-4. Vital events which occurred to Detroit residents in 1961. (Adapted. Courtesy the Department of Health of Detroit.)

cities, Detroit is working on slum clearance and on improving the standard of housing for all its citizens. In general, though, both in housing and in income, those living in the Boulevard area are poor in comparison to those living in the remainder of the city. Many of the problems of the area are compounded because few of the underprivileged have had an opportunity to acquire educations adequate to secure employment in a modern industrialized society.

What effect do the above factors have on the health of the population living in this area?

Granted that factors other than housing, education, and income have a bearing on the health status in the community, examination of the map reveals that on most counts the health of the people living inside the Boulevard suffers in comparison to the health of persons living in other areas of the city. Although the high rate of crime occurring in the "Central City" is not included on the map, it is a reflection of the mental health of the community. Both the maternal and infant mortality rates exceed the average for the city as a whole. The differences between the infant mortality rates in the "Central City" and outlying areas are particularly striking. The area with the highest infant mortality rate has a rate almost four times that of the lowest. As stated earlier, maternal and infant mortality rates are generally accepted as an index of the standard of health in the community. Differences in maternal mortality rates are not as great, since the highest rates occurred in areas adjacent to, but not in, the "Central City"; the lowest rates are observed outside it, however.

The over-all death rate is higher in the "Central City" than in any other part of the city. With the exception of cancer and suicide, the mortality rate for all diseases listed on the map is also higher. The differences in the mortality rates from tuberculosis are particularly striking. In census tract J, no persons were known to die from tuberculosis in the year 1961. In census tract K, 27.5 persons died per 100,000 population.

What do recent studies demonstrate relative to the relationship between socioeconomic status and health?

Although most studies performed in the past do show an inverse relationship between socioeconomic status and mortality, authorities are not all agreed about why this relationship exists. Nor do authorities agree as to whether the inverse relationship is limited to infectious diseases or is also true in chronic diseases. In order to examine the nature and extent of the relationship of socioeconomic status and mortality Stockwell[40] reviewed the 1949–1951 death records for the residents of Hartford, Connecticut, and Providence, Rhode Island, using two different approaches. By both methods, he confirmed that there was indeed a marked inverse relationship between socio-

[40] Edward G. Stockwell, "A Critical Examination of the Relationship Between Socioeconomic Status and Mortality," *American Journal of Public Health,* LIII, pp. 956-64.

economic status and mortality. He also found that the exact nature and extent of the relationship between the two factors vary between cities and with the methods used to study the relationship. In the light of the above, the conclusions about the relationship of the health of the population of the "Central City" of Detroit to the socioeconomic and educational status are probably valid. Neither the exact relationship nor all the factors involved have been established.

Another factor contributing to the improvement of life expectancy in the United States is the increase in food supply. Along with the industrial and social accomplishments of the nineteenth century, the capacity to produce food has been developed on a scale that was hitherto unknown. Modern methods of transportation and food preservation have made it possible for food to be distributed throughout the country and to be available in variety throughout the year. Thus, disorders that are caused by or predisposed to by a deficiency in the quantity or quality of food have decreased in incidence. Unfortunately an abundance of food favors overeating, which predisposes to obesity. Obesity appears to be one of the factors in the increase in incidence of the degenerative diseases such as atherosclerosis and diabetes.

Increased knowledge in medicine and in the basic sciences has paralleled improvements in conditions and standards of living. Some of the developments that have contributed much to the practice of medicine have had their origin in other fields of study. Many of the tools used in the identification of structures too small to be perceived by the naked eye and in making of precise measurements were developed by scientists in the basic sciences. Scientific discoveries in industry have also made contributions to preventive medicine. The many discoveries contributing to understanding the nature of disease and its control range from the grinding of lenses to be used to magnify heavenly bodies or objects too small to be viewed by the naked eye to the synthesis of chemicals such as salvarsan and sulfonamide. The principles of asepsis had their origin in the studies made by Pasteur, a chemist, to determine in the course of studies the cause of the souring of wine.

In what stages has knowledge of the prevention of disease developed? What was accomplished in each stage?

Review of the history of the development of knowledge of the prevention of disease reveals that progress was made in three stages. In the first stage the environment was rendered safe and the individual was protected from harmful influences in the environment. In this period applications of knowledge of bacteriology and immunology were made. Sanitation of food and water supplies and immunization against smallpox, diphtheria, and other diseases were important contributions of the first stage to the health of the public.

In the second stage some diseases were brought under control by the introduction of new drugs and vaccines. Drugs have made a significant contribution to the control of such diseases as tuberculosis, syphilis, and pneumonia. Hope that diseases such as tuberculosis and syphilis would be eradicated by the so-called wonder drugs has been replaced by the sobering knowledge that even today good control of any infectious disease depends on the constant application of all the available knowledge. Drugs have not proved to be the complete answer to the control of disease. Moreover, the value of an agent in the control or cure of an infectious disease is sometimes difficult to evaluate. To illustrate, the death rate from diphtheria, pneumonia, and tuberculosis had all dropped before modern methods of prevention and treatment were known. As infectious diseases have come under control, noninfectious diseases have increased in incidence. Whereas infectious diseases were the first as the cause of death in 1900, heart disease has now taken that place.

What is the challenge of the third and present era of prevention?

The challenge of the third and present era of prevention is, therefore, the prevention of noninfectious diseases. These are the diseases that have their highest incidence in maturity and the later years of life. In the present state of knowledge not too much is known about the primary prevention of some of the important noninfectious diseases. The approach to many of these diseases is to prevent or delay their progress; but even this is a significant contribution, for it not only lessens suffering and ill health, but it enables people who have these diseases to be productive for a greater part of their life span than they would otherwise be. It sometimes creates problems, too. For example, a man has a heart attack or is crippled by poliomyelitis. Following recovery and rehabilitation he frequently has a problem in securing work by which he can support himself.

In a discussion of current knowledge of prevention, Francis[41] classifies the area of true prevention as follows: (1) protection from exposure to harmful physical and chemical agents, (2) correction of dietary deficiencies and excesses, and (3) prevention of infectious diseases by specific measures and sanitary social procedures. He states that the first area applies primarily to occupational health. Certainly much has been done to create and enforce standards contributing to health and safety in factories and in other places of employment. Machinery is constructed with the safety of the worker in mind, and he is provided with clothing that is designed to protect him from the hazards of his particular job. In addition, educational programs are conducted to teach employees how to work safely and what to do in the event a fellow worker is injured. Campaigns are conducted to increase their interest and pride in their safety record. Workmen's compensation laws and various types of insurance protect the health of employees by establishing and enforcing safety standards. Insurance also provides a means of support for employees

[41] *Op. cit.*, p. 994.

and their families in the event of injury incurred while they are at work. Equally important to those who are permanently disabled is provision for their continued support.

What events have led to a beginning concern about the dangers to health resulting from the pollution of the air?

Recently, attention has been extended to evaluating dangers to the general public growing out of the pollution of the air by gaseous wastes. Impetus has been given to the study of this problem by the London and Donora air disasters. According to Breslow and Goldsmith,[42] public health authorities have been slow to recognize the potential dangers of air pollution. Because of public pressure they are, however, being forced to give their attention to it. According to Thomas,[43] urban air pollution stems from two different sources. One, the London type, is primarily coal smoke, which contains appreciable amounts of sulfur dioxide combined with a more or less dense fog. The other, the Los Angeles type, is primarily automobile exhaust gases. It contains none of the components of the London smog. The irritating and damaging compounds result from the action of sunshine on the substances contained in exhaust gas. Many cities have to cope to some degree with both types of air pollution. The prevention of air pollution is currently under study. According to Thomas,[44] prospects are good for understanding, and eventually controlling it.

A different but no less dangerous source of air pollution originates with explosions of atom and hydrogen bombs and from the use of radioactive materials in hospitals and in industry. The effects of ionizing radiation and some of the factors in its control will be discussed in a later chapter. One cannot, however, ignore the possible long-term effects of repeated exposure of large segments of the population to ionizing radiation. The pollution of the air, whether by coal smoke, automobile exhaust gases, or radioactive materials, illustrates how the external environment created by man threatens his health.

The second aspect of primary or true prevention, the correction of dietary deficiency or excess, will be considered in the chapter devoted to facilitating meeting the nutritional needs of people.

What is the third aspect of true prevention?

The third aspect of true prevention is the prevention of infectious disease by specific measures and by sanitary social procedures. Francis[45] emphasizes

---

[42] Lester Breslow and John Goldsmith, "Health Effects of Air Pollution," *American Journal of Public Health,* XLVIII, July, 1958, pp. 913-17.
[43] Moyer D. Thomas, "New Understanding from Current Atmospheric Pollution Research," *American Journal of Public Health,* XLIX, December, 1959, p. 1664.
[44] *Ibid.,* p. 1668.
[45] *Op. cit.,* p. 492.

that, contrary to common opinion, infectious diseases have not been eliminated. He cites the example of the resurgence of the problem with the *Staphylococcus*. Examples of diseases that recur from time to time, especially when control measures are neglected, include diphtheria and typhoid fever. Some time ago a radio news report included the announcement of the death of a young boy who had not been immunized for diphtheria. Two or three years ago diphtheria reached near epidemic proportions in a section of a large city where many children who had not been immunized lived. A number of these children died.

Not even smallpox, the first disease for which specific immunization or vaccination was known, has been eliminated. According to *World Health*,[46] the World Health Organization was notified of 242,000 cases in 1958 and 72,000 cases in 1959. The decrease in the number of cases from 1958 to 1959 is largely the result of a decrease in incidence in India and East Pakistan. Lest anyone think that smallpox in India or Africa has little to do with Mr. or Mrs. American, let him be reminded that by jet plane India and Pakistan are but a few hours away from any part of the United States.

Attempts are being made by the World Health Organization with support from UNICEF to eradicate malaria.[47] Leavell and Clark[48] state that it is still the leading cause of death in the world. There are some 250 million cases and between 2 and 3 million deaths from malaria each year. Efforts to eradicate malaria by eliminating the mosquito that carries the malarial parasite have been complicated by the fact that mosquitos develop resistance to insecticides and particularly to DDT. The problem is further aggravated by the recent finding that monkeys serve as reservoirs for the parasite. Only time will tell whether malaria can be eradicated. Probably, like other infectious diseases, it will be brought under control, but not eradicated.

A few diseases can be prevented by the use of specific drugs and antibiotics. Quinine and Atabrine hydrochloride[49] have been useful in the control of malaria in visitors to malaria areas. The use of silver nitrate and more recently penicillin in the prevention of infection of the eyes of the newborn infant by the gonococcus has done much to reduce the incidence of blindness. From recent studies, isoniazid (isonicotinic acid hydrazide) appears to be as useful in the prevention of tuberculosis as in its treatment.

Numerous studies indicate that the addition of fluorides, 1 part to a million parts of water, reduces dental caries by as much as 60 per cent. Despite the benefits of the procedure and the absence of harmful effects when used in the amounts stated, an organized opposition has succeeded in preventing the

---

[46] "Smallpox in the World," *World Health,* XIII, May-June, 1960, p. 37.
[47] *Everyman's United Nations, Op. cit.,* p. 388.
[48] Hugh Rodman Leavell, and E. Gurney Clark, *Preventive Medicine for the Doctor in His Community,* 2nd ed., Blakeston Division of McGraw-Hill Book Co., Inc., New York, 1958, p. 111.
[49] Trade name for quinacrine hydrochloride.

fluoridation of water in many regions of the country. According to *Public Health Reports* for June, 1960,[50] ". . . of the estimated 118 million people in the United States provided water from community supplies, 43 million drink water containing at least 0.7 parts per million of fluoride." Seven million drink water naturally containing 0.7 part per million or more of fluoride.

Certain diseases can be prevented by appropriate sanitary and social procedures. The importance of these procedures to health probably cannot be overestimated. One of the reasons that the Hebrews were able to escape safely from Egypt is believed to be due to their strict adherence to the sanitary laws of Moses. One of the first persons of early modern times to demonstrate conclusively the value of sanitation to the prevention of disease was John Snow, a London physician. Over 100 years ago he identified the source of a great cholera epidemic as the water obtained from the Broadstreet pump. Because of the methods he used to study the distribution of cases in the community, he is often referred to as the father of epidemiology. As a result of the application of the findings of Snow, London never again experienced an epidemic of cholera.

In the parts of the world where sanitary procedures are adequate the incidence of typhoid and other diarrheal diseases is minimal. In other regions, or when there is a break in sanitation, the incidence continues to be high. For example, in 1950 the writer was told by a health officer in a large city in South America that there were at least 50,000 typhoid carriers in that city. There were numerous victims of the disease in hospitals that were visited. Despite continued application of sanitary procedures, typhoid fever sometimes occurs in the United States. Woodward[51] reports an outbreak of typhoid fever extending from Minnesota to California. The source, though never proved, was probably from fresh vegetables such as lettuce or celery. Other vehicles serving to spread the *Salmonella typhosa* include contaminated water and milk. Even more recent and more disastrous was the epidemic of typhoid fever in a ski resort town in the Swiss Alps. This epidemic resulted from the failure to enforce the sanitary procedures required to protect water and food supplies from the *Salmonella typhosa.*

Evidence derived from epidemiological studies supports the hypothesis that infectious hepatitis is spread by water. Measures effective in destroying bacteria in water may not be adequate to rid it from the virus of infectious hepatitis.[52] The problems involved in the control of infectious hepatitis remain to be solved.

---

[50] "Status of Fluoridation in Community Water Supplies," *Public Health Reports,* LXXV, June, 1960, p. 560.

[51] Frank L. Woodward, "Implications of the Midwest Typhoid Fever Outbreak of 1956," *American Journal of Public Health,* XLVII, February, 1957, pp. 173-78.

[52] Robert Ward, *et. al.,* "Infectious Hepatitis—Studies of Its Natural History and Prevention," *New England Journal of Medicine,* CCLVIII, February 1958, pp. 407-16. David C. Poskanzer and William C. Beadenkoff, "Waterborne Infectious Hepatitis Epidemic from a Chlorinated Municipal Supply," *Public Health Reports.* LXXVI, Septemper, 1961, pp. 745-51.

Many city, state, and even federal laws have been enacted for the purpose of protecting the general public from agents causing injury and disease. Examples include laws or regulations to control traffic, housing and building construction, water supplies, food handling, the preparation and serving of food in restaurants, and sewage disposal. Pure food and drug laws protect the quality of food and drugs.[53]

One of the best-known laws regulating drugs is the Harrison Narcotic Act of 1914, which regulates the importation, manufacture, sale, dispensing or prescribing, and use of cocaine and opium and all their derivatives. The new synthetic preparations known to cause addiction are also included. Although the Harrison Act was intended to be regulatory, it is administered as if it were criminal or prohibitory in nature. In a discussion of the need for the reassessment of the problem of drug addiction, Murtagh[54] makes a plea for changes that will make it possible to treat the drug addict as a medical rather than legal problem. Although the intent of the Harrison Act is to protect society, it also has created problems in relation to drug addiction.[55] To protect the public health from unscrupulous drug manufacturers, the Federal Food, Drug and Cosmetic Acts were passed first in 1906, and revised in 1938 and 1962. The protection of the public from drugs such as Thalidomide is an excellent example of primary prevention.

To summarize, primary prevention depends on understanding and controlling the factors contributing to the development of disease. It also depends on the availability of procedures to remove noxious agents from the environment, to prevent their entry into the organism, or to neutralize their effects after they enter. Whether or not the appropriate techniques are available depends on both the status of knowledge and the resources available to procure the necessary supplies, equipment, and persons possessing the skills required to utilize current knowledge and techniques. For example, one of the deciding factors in whether a community can have sanitary water supply and a safe method of disposing of its wastes is whether or not it has or is willing to spend the money to build and to equip suitable facilities. Moreover, money is required to provide the necessary staff to operate the facilities after they are built, and persons with a variety of knowledges and skills are required to operate and maintain them so that they accomplish their purpose. Furthermore, the population must accept the need for these facilities and know how to use them. Use of a particular preventive measure depends in part on the knowledge of the group or individual that the measure is available and effective. The group must also accept a particular procedure as being necessary and desirable. Whether a facility or change in behavior will be adopted by a group of people

[53] See Louis S. Goodman and Alfred Gilman, *The Pharmacological Basis of Therapeutics,* 2nd ed., The Macmillan Company, New York, 1956, p. 17.
[54] John N. Murtagh, "Dilemma for Drug Addicts," *America,* CVIII, May 25, 1963, pp. 740-42.
[55] For a fuller discussion of the Harrison Narcotic Act, see Goodman and Gilman, *Op. cit.,* p. 1775.

depends on the degree to which its performance takes into account local customs, habits, and beliefs. For example, Towle[56] reported a study of the administration of vaccines by injection to a group of people living in India. He states that in the early part of the study most of the candidates for immunization were men. After making this observation, the investigators placed a screen in such a position that the women could be hidden from the view of men. Following this adjustment the number of women seeking immunization did not differ materially from the number of men.

How does the concept of prevention apply after a disease process is evidenced?

In those diseases in which knowledge is insufficient to prevent their development, emphasis is on the prevention of disability, or the delay of the progress of already established disease. Although disability may follow any illness, it is more frequently associated with chronic disease, that is, diseases that continue for a long period of time. Although the term "chronic disease" is well understood by the health workers, some persons prefer to use the phrase "long-term illness." Their objection to chronic illness is that it suggests hopelessness, rather than emphasizing the possibility of improving the situation of the individual. Chronic illness differs from acute illness in the intensity and length of course. Although the chronically ill person may have periods in which he is acutely ill (severe degree of illness and short, or limited, course), the degree of illness tends to be less marked and the course more prolonged than in an acute illness. Acute illness can terminate in full recovery or death, or develop into a chronic illness. In our present state of knowledge, prevention of disability due to the progress of chronic disease is frequently the most that can be accomplished. However, in many patients, limiting the damaging effects of a chronic disease and instituting a program which enables the person to utilize his strengths may make the difference between an active and useful life and one of complete invalidism.

The prevention of disability in the person who has a potentially disabling illness or injury involves knowledge of the factors in the development of the disability and what can be done to prevent or minimize it. Prevention of disability also depends on the ability to identify and help the person utilize his psychological, intellectual, physical, economic, and spiritual resources. It requires a knowledge of the facilities available in the community to assist him and knowledge of how to use them. With the imaginative and intelligent use of even limited resources, much can often be done to prevent unnecessary disability and to restore the disabled person to greater usefulness.

A number of factors have contributed to the marked increase in longevity of Americans during the last century. Industrialization, increased production

[56] Richard L. Towle, "New Horizon in Mass Inoculation," *Public Health Reports,* LXXV, June, 1960, pp. 471-76.

and distribution of food, increased knowledge in the fields of bacteriology, immunology, physics, chemistry, and physiology have contributed to increased understanding of ways to prevent and treat disease. Application of knowledge has been effective in bringing a limited number of infectious diseases under control. Their control, however, depends on the continued application of knowledge. Relaxation of or breaks in technique can be expected to lead to an increase in incidence. With reduction in the incidence and the severity of infectious diseases as well as improved standards of nutrition, there has been a marked decrease in the infant mortality rate. Improvement in the survival rate of infants is one of the important factors in the increase of life expectancy. With the lengthening of life, new problems have been created including an increase in the incidence of noninfectious diseases. Their control at this time is based largely on trying to identify and minimize the factors that contribute to their development and to their early identification, so that disability can be prevented and their progress delayed.

What problems contribute to and interfere with the achievement of the third objective of the health professions?

The third objective of the health professions is to care for the sick. Sooner or later in the life of every individual sickness becomes a reality. Depending on the nature of the causative agent or agents and the capacity of the individual to respond, he may be mildly or seriously ill. He may recover promptly or experience a lingering illness. He may die suddenly or slowly. He may recover spontaneously without, or even in spite of, treatment or he may die despite excellent and intensive therapy.

In the American culture there is a tendency to equate recovery from illness with success and chronicity or death with failure. This attitude toward illness undoubtedly contributes to emphasis on the leading causes of death as major health problems and to less stress on the causes and effects of morbidity, that is sickness. Little attention is paid by many individuals to health per se, as it is more or less taken for granted. As indicated earlier, the health professions are preoccupied with disease and death rather than with health and fulfillment.

Why should nurses be familiar with the major causes of death and morbidity?

Nurses should be familiar with the major causes of death and of morbidity because much of their professional life will be spent with sick people. Mortality statistics are the easiest health statistics to obtain, they are the most complete, and they provide certain types of useful data. Knowledge of the important causes of death can be used as a basis for making decisions about where money and effort should be concentrated in studying and treating disease. By use of comparisons between present-day causes of death and those of

50 or more years ago, trends in the incidence of disease during different periods of history can be identified and deductions can be made from them. Conclusions based on comparisons are valid, however, only when sufficiently exact data are available.

FIGURE   2 – 5

Leading Causes of Death by Rank—United States, 1900 and 1959[1]

		1900				1959		
Rank	Cause of Death	Deaths per 100,000 Population	Per Cent of all Deaths		Rank	Cause of Death	Deaths per 100,000 Population	Per Cent of all Deaths
	All causes	1,719.1	100.0			All causes	941.7	100.0
1	Influenza and pneumonia	202.2	11.8		1	Diseases of the heart	366.3	38.9
2	Tuberculosis (all forms)	194.4	11.3		2	Malignant neoplasms (cancer)	157.1	15.6
3	Gastritis, etc.	142.7	8.3		3	Vascular lesions affecting CNS	108.3	11.5
4	Diseases of the heart	137.4	8.0		4	All accidents	50.7	5.4
5	Vascular lesions affecting CNS	106.9	6.2		5	Certain diseases of early infancy	38.5	4.1
6	Chronic nephritis	81.0	4.7		6	Influenza and pneumonia	32.5	3.1
7	All accidents	72.3	4.2		7	General arteriosclerosis	19.7	2.1
8	Malignant neoplasms (cancer)	64.0	3.7		8	Diabetes mellitus	16.0	1.7
9	Certain diseases of early infancy	62.6	3.6		9	Congenital malformations	12.3	1.3
10	Diphtheria	40.3	2.3		10	Cirrhosis of the liver	11.0	1.2

[1] Rates for 1900 apply to the death registration states only. (*Progress in Health Services.* Health Information Foundation, New York. Source: United States National Office of Vital Statistics.)

Figure 2 - 5 illustrates how the incidence of disease causing mortality in the United States changed between 1900 and 1959.

Examination shows that influenza and pneumonia, which ranked first as a cause of death in 1900, had moved down to sixth place in 1959. Tuberculosis, which was in second place in 1900, was not among the first ten in 1959. There is considerable optimism at this time that with the application of present knowledge, the incidence of tuberculosis can be reduced to a point where it will not be a significant cause of mortality. By 1959 diseases of the heart and malignant neoplasms had taken first and second places, respectively. Accidents had moved from seventh to fourth place. Diabetes mellitus and cirrhosis of the liver had made their appearance among the ten most frequent causes of mortality. This table demonstrates clearly the changing nature of disease and correlates with the changes in living conditions that have occurred since the early part of the century.

Certain diseases brought under control in this period are not included in Figure 2-5. Among these are those that can be classified as diseases characterized by diarrhea and enteritis. Two diseases falling under this classification are infantile diarrhea and typhoid fever. In 1900 one of the hazards of life of the newborn infant was a disorder known as summer complaint or infantile diarrhea. Even today diarrhea during the first weeks and months of life of an infant is a serious disorder. With modern refrigeration and sanitation, the incidence is much decreased. Greater knowledge of water and electrolyte balance makes possible the saving of the lives of many of the babies who are afflicted.

The history of the control of typhoid fever can be traced through changes in its importance as a cause of death. In 1905 typhoid fever caused more deaths than any other infectious disease. Moreover, the death rate was higher than it needed to be, as the rate was much higher in the United States than in Europe. Although typhoid fever decreased steadily as a cause of death after 1900, not until 1919 was there a sharp drop in its incidence. Methods for the control of some diseases such as diphtheria have resulted in a reduction in the morbidity as well as the mortality from these causes. For others, such as measles, morbidity rates continue to be high, but mortality rates are lower than they were earlier in the century. Even this may be changed, as a practical method for inducing active immunity to measles has been announced.

Most Americans are aware that heart disease and cancer are the leading causes of death in the United States. What they may not know is that this is also true in the other countries of the world that have similar standards of living and medical care. *World Health*[57] compares the leading causes of death in 14 countries of the modern world. These are the countries in which there is sufficient food to meet the nutritional needs of the people. The sanitary and social procedures are such that people are protected from contamination of water and food with human excreta. Finally, medical care is available to meet the health needs of the population. In all 14 countries, heart disease is the leading cause of death. Malignant neoplasms are second, and vascular lesions third. In most countries accidents are high on the list, usually in either the fourth or fifth place. Pneumonia continues to be a problem in all countries, as it stands fourth or fifth as cause of death. When tuberculosis occupies a place in the first ten causes of death, it is toward the bottom of the list. In much of the rest of the world, that is, countries other than these 14, infectious diseases—malaria, tuberculosis, enteric diseases, and a host of others—continue to head the list.

[57] *World Health*, **XIII**, January-February, 1960, pp. 2-3. The Statistics were reproduced from the *Epidemiological and Vital Statistics Report of the World Health Organization 1959*, No. 12.

Another way to express the change in the health status is by comparing the expectation of life at birth. This information is summarized below.

Expectation of Life at Birth[58]

1900	47.3
1925	59.0
1950	68.2
1956	69.6
1960	

In the years between 1900 and 1956, more than 22 years were added to the life expectancy of man, more years than the total life expectancy of ancient man. In 1961, life expectancy at birth had increased to an average of 70 years, or approximately 23 years since 1900. By 1970, almost one half of the persons who reach 65 years of age will live to their eightieth birthday. In 1900, there were 3.1 million persons who were 65 years or older (about 4 percent of the population). In 1963, there were 17.5 million (9 per cent of the population), and the number is growing at a rate of about 1,000 persons a day.[59]

On the basis of a review of a limited number of mortality statistics, the assumptions referred to before are valid; namely, that in countries where the standards of living and levels of medical care are similar to those of the United States, the leading causes of death are also similar. As techniques are successfully applied in the control of infectious disease, life is lengthened. As longevity increases, mortality from noninfectious diseases also increases. Although authorities do not agree on what the possible length of the life span is, figures in the neighborhood of 100 years are usually cited. At no time in the recorded history of mankind have so many people lived to an age that approaches this goal and from this point of view the increase in the number of elderly in the population represents a victory. However, with the increase in longevity, other problems present themselves. How can the onset of the non-infectious diseases be prevented or delayed? How can disability be prevented? How can "life" be added to the added years? Questions are asked the elderly, such as how can they continue to be creative and productive members of society for as long as they live? These are questions that are of concern to nurses as well as to other members of the health professions. Despite the tendency to emphasize the negative aspects of aging, there are many aged people who live out their life span never experiencing any unusual problems. According to Haldeman,[60] at the time of the 1960 census less than 4 per cent of the persons over 65 years of age were living in nursing homes. One half of married persons were living with a spouse. The latter figure does not, of course, indicate the nature of the problems faced by persons who were living outside of nursing homes.

[58] *Ibid.*, p. 25.
[59] Jack C. Haldeman, "Nursing Homes, Related Facilities, and Programs," *Health Education and Welfare Indicators*, July, 1963, p. XIII.
[60] *Ibid.*, p. XIII.

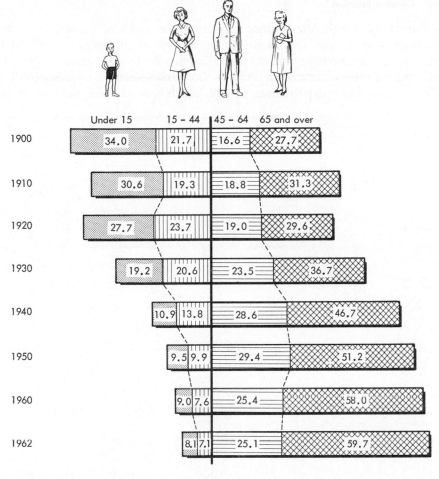

FIGURE 2—6. Age of death—a changing pattern. Percentage distribution—Michigan, 1900—1962. Since the beginning of the century an amazing and progressive change in the age at death pattern has occurred between the younger (under 45 years) and older (45 years and older) age groups.

	Under 45 Years	45 Years & Older
1900	56%	44%
1962	15%	85%

The trend has been a gradual decrease in each of the age groups under 45 years and a gradual increase in the combined age groups 45 years and older. In 1900 approximately one third of all deaths occurred under 15 years of age; the proportion has decreased to approximately one twelfth at the present time. In contrast, only slightly over one fourth of all deaths occurred in the 65, and over, age group in 1900; the proportion in 1962 has more than doubled.

During the last 32 years progress has been indicated by the fact that in 1962 the 65, and over, age group alone accounted for almost the same proportion of deaths as the combined age groups 45—64 and 65, and over, in 1930; approximately 60 per cent in each instance.

The above changes reflect (1) the decrease in deaths due to communicable diseases and other diseases of childhood, and (2) an increase in those due to chronic diseases in the older age groups. (Adapted. Courtesy of Statistical Methods Section, Michigan Department of Health.)

Morbidity statistics are another measure of the health of a community, but accurate statistics are difficult to obtain. Studies of the incidence of illness have to be very carefully planned if the findings are to have value. Sources of information about morbidity include hospitals, doctors' offices, medical clinics, state health departments, school health services, and sickness insur-

under 1 year		1-4		5-14	
Immaturity	907 20.8%	Accidents	182 29.9%	Accidents	290 39.8%
Congenital malformations	728 16.7%	Pneumonia & influenza	84 13.8%	Malignant neoplasms	133 19.2%
Postnatal asphyxia & atelectasis	705 16.1%	Congenital malformations	81 13.3%	Congenital malformations	46 10.4%
Birth injuries	510 11.7%	Malignant neoplasms	67 11.0%	Pneumonia & influenza	30 4.3%
Pneumonia & influenza	479 11.0%	Gastroenteritis & colitis	19 3.1%	Diseases of heart	15 2.2%
		Non-meningococcal meningitis	19 3.1%		
Total deaths 4,367 (100%)		Total deaths 609 (100%)		Total deaths 691 (100%)	
15-24		**25-34**		**35-44**	
Accidents	513 52.8%	Accidents	340 28.7%	Diseases of heart	748 26.5%
Malignant neoplasms	80 8.2%	Malignant neoplasms	176 14.9%	Malignant neoplasms	581 20.6%
Suicide	70 7.2%	Diseases of heart	142 12.0%	Accidents	369 13.1%
Homicide	43 4.4%	Suicide	105 8.9%	Vascular lesions of C.N.S.	152 5.4%
Diseases of heart	30 3.1%	Homicide	58 4.9%	Suicide	149 5.3%
Total deaths 971 (100%)		Total deaths 1,183 (100%)		Total deaths 2,826 (100%)	
45-54		**55-64**		**65 and over**	
Diseases of heart	2,390 37.8%	Diseases of heart	4,743 42.0%	Diseases of heart	19,152 45.8%
Malignant neoplasms	1,555 24.6%	Malignant neoplasms	2,746 24.3%	Malignant neoplasms	6,392 15.3%
Vascular lesions of C.N.S.	399 6.3%	Vascular lesions of C.N.S.	867 7.7%	Vascular lesions of C.N.S.	6,303 15.1%
Accidents	390 6.2%	Accidents	406 3.6%	Arteriosclerosis	1,385 3.3%
Cirrhosis of liver	225 3.6%	Diabetes	351 3.1%	Diabetes	1,330 3.2%
Total deaths 6,321 (100%)		Total deaths 11,287 (100%)		Total deaths 41,794 (100%)	

ance plans. Each of these represent limited rather than inclusive samples of the population. A number of national and local household surveys have contributed some useful information about the incidence of illness. According to *Progress in Health Services*,[61] the methods used in these surveys have changed so much in the course of time that accurate comparisons cannot be made between the information obtained from one survey and that from another. On the basis, however, of comparisons of data obtained in the various studies, the pattern of acute disabling illness remains about the same. The incidence, today as in the past, of acute disabling illness is highest in the young and decreases with age. In contrast, the incidence of chronic illness is lowest among the young and rises with age. According to the Baltimore Health Survey, 1952–1955, with the exception of the age group 15 through 24, the days of disability per person surveyed increased progressively with age. After the age of 65, they increased greatly. In both acute and chronic illness, females are found to have more days of disability than males. Respiratory infections are the most common cause of acute disabling illness, with infections of the gastrointestinal system being second. See Figure 2-8 for the incidence of acute disabling illnesses.[62]

Many disorders are accompanied by more or less extended periods of disability. Some diseases, such as arthritis, are not frequent causes of death, but are responsible for much human misery and loss of productivity. Problems under study include not only the factors in the causes of these diseases, but how to prevent their disabling effects. The chronic conditions that were most often reported by the National Health Survey for 1959 as causes of limitation of activity are summarized in *Trends*.[63] According to this publication, heart disease is the leading cause of disability. It is closely followed by arthritis and rheumatism. Orthopedic and back conditions, high blood pressure without heart involvement, mental and nervous disorders, and impair-

[61] Health Information Foundation, VIII, December, 1959, p. 10.
[62] U.S. National Health Survey, "Acute Conditions: Incidence and Associated Disability, United States, July 1957–June 1958, Series B-6, Washington, D.C., 1958," *Progress in Health Services*, Health Information Foundation, VIII, December, 1959.
[63] *Trends*, 1960 ed., U.S. Printing Office, Washington, 1960, p. 37.

FIGURE 2–7 (left). Leading causes of death by age groups—Michigan, 1962. Though data were secured for the state of Michigan, there is no reason to suppose that they differ materially from the rest of the United States.
Diseases of the heart lead as a cause of death among all age groups 35 years and over and constitute an increasingly larger percentage of the total deaths in each successively older age group. In 1962 they also appear among the first five leading causes of death in each group 5 years and over.
Accidents lead as a cause of death in all age groups under 35 years with the exception of infants under 1 year, and appear among the five leading causes in all age groups except under 1 year and the 65 and over groups.
Malignant neoplasms first appear in the age group 1 to 4 years as the fourth ranking cause of death. It is the second leading cause in the 5 to 14 year age group and maintains this position in all successive age groups. (Adapted. Courtesy of Statistical Methods Section, Michigan Department of Health.)

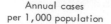

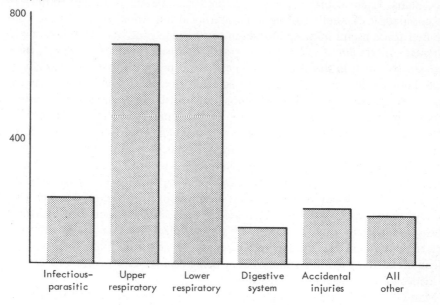

FIGURE 2—8. Incidence of acute disabling conditions by conditioned group. United States, July, 1957—June, 1958. (Adapted. *Progress in Health Services*, Health Information Foundation, New York.)

ment in vision follow in that order. The leading cause of complete disability is paralysis.

Other disorders[64] which are somewhat less common causes of limitation of activity include asthma and hay fever, paralysis of extremities and/or trunk, hernia, emphysema and bronchitis, impairment in hearing, diabetes mellitus, ulcer of the stomach and duodenum, malignant neoplasms, benign neoplasms, and tuberculosis. Some conditions, such as obesity and alcoholism, not only cause disability, but they predispose to disabling diseases. In a very real sense, they place the patient in a double jeopardy.

In our present state of knowledge little is known about the primary prevention of most of the diseases listed above. However, the situation is far from hopeless. With early diagnosis and adequate therapy much can be done to prevent their progression to disabling disease. Nursing has a number of contributions to make in the care of the chronically ill. Like the members of other health professions, the nurse is a case finder; as such, she can do much to encourage people to seek medical attention. People often bring symptoms to the attention of a nurse, because they hesitate to trouble a physician, or because they are worried and they feel safer telling a nurse. In her contacts with people, the nurse has an opportunity to observe conditions or symptoms

[64] *Trends, Ibid.*

that require medical attention. As a health teacher, the nurse has many opportunities to contribute to the health education of the patient and his family. By providing them with knowledge of what to expect, of what they can do and why, she makes a valuable contribution to the chronically ill. She provides nursing care that is planned to prevent unnecessary disability. Not by any means the least of her contributions is to convey to the patient a spirit of hope. Despite the unlikelihood of cure, much can and will be done to improve the lot of the patient.

What are the objectives of therapy in illness?

Therapy in illness is directed toward three objectives. They are: (1) to cure the sick person, (2) to modify the course of the disease so that its progress is slowed and disability is limited, and (3) to modify the effects of disease so that the person is maintained in as active and comfortable a state as is possible for as long as he lives. This includes assisting him to a peaceful death.

The accomplishment of the first objective depends on two factors—the availability of a method of treatment and the capacity of the sick person to respond appropriately. The tendency toward recovery may be so great that the patient gets well despite meddlesome or harmful treatment. An aspect of an appropriate response to treatment relates to the desire of the patient to accept treatment and to work toward recovery. The life of a seriously ill or frail patient may be saved by specific and energetic therapy combined with a strong desire to recover.

One approach to the cure of disease is to attempt to eradicate the disease-producing agent. Elimination of the etiological agent may be accomplished by administering a chemical or physical agent capable of reaching and destroying it or the diseased tissue without affecting healthy tissue. Examples include the use of antibiotic and chemotherapeutic agents to eradicate microorganisms causing disease and the use of X-ray or the radioactive isotopes in the treatment of malignant neoplasms. Surgery is also effective in eradicating disease by correcting structural defects or by removing diseased tissues.

Cure may also be effected by supplying a substance normally produced in the body in response to disease. An example of specific antisera is diphtheria antitoxin, which is successful in the treatment of diphtheria. In patients who respond to substances that are not usually harmful, relief may be effected by limiting the contact of the patient with the harmful agent or by counteracting his abnormal response. The person with hay fever can prevent or lessen the severity of an attack by eliminating substances to which he has a sensitivity from his environment. He may also lessen the severity of his reaction by taking an antihistamine or epinephrine.

When a disease is the result of the lack of a substance required in the body economy, cure may be effected by increasing the supply of the substance that is deficient. For example, scurvy is cured by adding ascorbic acid to the diet. Sometimes the physiological disturbance occurring as a result of disease is so severe that the body is unable to restore balance or overcome the disease without aid. In these instances, needed materials are supplied to support body responses or defenses. For example, the temperature of the body may rise to a level which, if continued, will produce cellular damage. Cold sponges or antipyretic drugs may be administered to reduce the temperature until such time as effective body controls are re-established.

That complete cure of disease is not always possible is well known. In some conditions such as acute poliomyelitis recovery from the acute infection may be complete, but there may be some degree of residual disability. In others, such as cerebrovascular accident, the patient may recover with or without disability, but the primary disease, atherosclerosis, remains. In these patients complete restoration to health may be impossible but the effects of the disease may be modified so that the person is restored, as fully as possible in his particular situation, to health. The accomplishment of this objective is one of the exciting challenges of today. Its achievement depends on the prevention of unnecessary disability, psychological as well as physical, the evaluation of the latter as well as of the patient's strengths and assets, and a program of education and work whereby the patient learns to use all his resources constructively. To accomplish this both the nurse and the patient must be aware of, accept, and work toward realistic or reasonable goals.

The prevention of unnecessary disability depends on the intelligent nursing of the patient during the acute phase of his illness. Months of therapy may be required to correct the effects, not of disease or injury, but of inadequate care. During the period of rehabilitation of the patient, nursing contributes to the progress of the patient in many ways. The patient is helped by an attitude of realistic optimism. He can be encouraged to try, even when his efforts are faltering. The nurse may find it difficult to decide when the patient should try to act for himself and when she should do things for, or help, the patient. In her sympathy for the patient she may forget that struggle is essential to growth or she may become impatient when the patient is discouraged or depressed. The chicken that escapes from the egg shell does so because it struggles. The chicken that does not struggle dies. The patient is helped in his struggle by the nurse's giving recognition to the fact that he is trying and that he is having difficulty. Recognizing his successes and helping him to accept his failures also contribute to his emotional support. For some patients a source of irritation may act as a stimulus. For example, elderly Mrs. Elm was irascible and depressed following a stroke, or cerebrovascular accident. Her nurse noted that she was a perfectionist who was greatly irritated by a crooked window shade or picture. Each day the nurse, unobtrusively but purposefully, pulled a window shade out of line. This seemingly minor event strengthened Mrs. Elm's feeling that nothing would be done correctly if she was not there, and she began to make an effort to recover. The nurse was successful in helping

Mrs. Elm because she was able to motivate her toward recovery. She concentrated on identifying what Mrs. Elm needed, and not on her failure to conform to her own expectations of how a patient should respond. Some judgment is required on the part of the nurse to assess the ability of the patient to perform so that he is not pushed beyond his capacity. Both thought and experience are required to learn when to wait and when to encourage the patient to continue his efforts. Physical and emotional readiness are both important factors in rehabilitation.

The family of the patient is also important to his rehabilitation. They can be a help or a hindrance depending on their relationship with the patient and on their understanding and acceptance of the program planned for the patient. The nurse can sometimes help them to accept what can be and is being done for the patient. They, too, need support to watch a patient struggle. They are more likely to be cooperative when they understand the plan of care for the patient and the what, how, and why of their contribution.

As a result of increased interest in rehabilitation, patients who have disorders associated with serious degrees of limitation of function are living more active lives than ever before in history. Some of them are self-supporting, drive cars, go to ball games and dances, take vacation trips, marry, rear families, and carry on lives that are as active as those of persons not physically handicapped.

For all persons the time comes when recovery and rehabilitation are no longer possible, for one of the realities of life is death. To some it comes quickly. To others it comes slowly in the form of a lingering illness. Some have a short life span, others a long one. In the American culture, extreme measures to prevent or to delay death for as long as possible are not at all unusual. Talk of death is avoided and elaborate efforts may be made to protect the sick from knowledge that death is a possibility. That these efforts sometimes, if not frequently, fail is indicated by the following letter written by Mrs. Carol Willis who was dying from cancer.[65]

Boston, Mass.

Dear Editors: The epidemic of articles by cancer victims in the last few years leads even the most unscientifically minded observer to conclude there must be some correlation between people dying of cancer and the urge to appear in print.

Without exception the cancer patient is portrayed as a martyr, deeply suffering, but led at last through his troubles to realize the big things in life. All his trivialities are swept away, he appreciates the wonders of nature as never before, a change has come over his character so he is now a reformed person, he has turned again to God and he keeps his temper.

I think that it is time we let down our hair and told the truth. We have the urge to rush into print all right, but we who are dying of cancer are not martyrs or saints or holy folk. Frankly, if the truth were told we embarrass our friends, and we often bore them.

[65] Carol Willis, "Letter," *Ladies Home Journal,* LXXXVII, January, 1960, p. 4. Reprinted by special permission of the *Ladies' Home Journal,* copyright 1960. Curtis Publishing Company.

Our first emotion is that of anger. We go through a "few nights of apprehension and hot weeping" but once over those we are surprised, shocked and angry, that this fate should be meted out to us—Us, of all people—seems hardly fair. We look around at our friends and neighbors and wonder why we have been singled out for this lingering, painful death. "Why me, O Lord, why me?" We forget that for every one of us who suffers others go free; we should be glad they are spared, not angry at our own destiny, deserved or undeserved. After all, why *not* us O Lord? We are no martyrs—heavens no.

Cancer is not a pleasant way to die. It is too endlessly prolonged, too excruciatingly painful. Yet through that last, the pain, we learn we can take more than we even thought possible. We may rail in spite of ourselves when pain mounts; but if it subsides enough to be bearable we feel happy and relieved, like a woman whose girdle felt so comfortable when she took it off. I am not recommending supreme pain as a method of increasing pleasure or making us grateful for small comforts, but it does make us more able to bear the later heights of pain we have to go through.

We embarrass our friends, for Emily Post has provided no rules for conversation with the dying. We know our friends guard their tongues, and they force us to watch our words even more. Mentioning that we won't be here next year, or even perhaps next month, is not in good taste. We have to talk about "when the children are grown" or "when this house gets too big for just the two of us," because the sensibility of our friends to death will not allow them to face what we face each minute; the fact of our dying.

We are quite likely to bore our friends with our preoccupation with illness. We are so wrapped up in ourselves we talk too much. For that reason, I never bring up my illness; but if I am seriously asked about it I am only too glad to talk. It is a great relief to unburden oneself occasionally, to have the fact that one is bearing pain appreciated. One of the kindest acts a friend can do for a dying man is to listen to him.

What do we answer to the casual, "How are you?" For a person who is dying to reply automatically "Fine" is ridiculous. I solved it by saying cheerfully, with a rising inflection, "Pretty good." Now that there is no longer any truthful affirmative answer I reply, as lightheartedly as I know how, "Coming along," and that takes care of that. We have to be particularly careful not to be a specter at the feast, lest we spoil others' pleasure.

I don't suppose I should admit this, but we are not saints. The canker of our death which always eats at us makes us impatient, intolerant of other people's troubles. In great pain it is hard for us to show sympathy with a bad cold, a hurt finger or a headache. Surprisingly enough, we usually come through well here, but don't be disgusted with us if we can't produce too much emotion over your problem. Yours will go, ours won't.

I'm afraid that I have to admit that I'm often testy, irritated over my children's complaints over trivialities, even sometimes upset by my husband's kindnesses when they are ill-timed. He is, naturally enough, concerned over his dying wife; it is far harder on him than on me. He has to go on living; all I have to do is to die, and die as well as I can.

Yet I, too, have cared for me for a long time, and I find it extremely hard to face the end of my personality, the complete extinguishing of everything I planned. Thus we are both inwardly upset, and sometimes show it outwardly. So is it any wonder that life, instead of being the beautiful idyl painted by cancerous writers, sometimes stoops to the petty details of existence?

I've gone through it all; the early times of Hope, the Facing the Truth, the

Grin-and-Bear-It stage, the Just Bearing It, and now the End-Is-Just-Around-the-Corner or Final Stage. I'm still angry about it all, for I think no one has ever loved living more or had more fun doing it than I, and I want it to go on and on. But if it can't, then I must be truthful and say there are a few advantages in living only half a lifetime. Besides the end of good, death also means the end of tribulations—no more holding in the stomach, no more P.T.A., no more putting up the hair in pincurls, no more cub scouts, no more growing old.

Sincerely,
Carol Willis

Mrs. Willis died two weeks after writing this letter. Her husband found it among her effects after her death.

Fielding,[66] in an essay on the uses of fear, expresses Mrs. Willis' feelings very beautifully.

When death comes slowly, fear may come fast: it can spread a conspiracy in a home: bright-eyed, stiff-smiling, and truly fearful. A silence is engendered which isolates the dying person far more surely than his malady. Two languages begin to be spoken: one in the sickroom and the other in the remainder of the house; the bedroom door may become an iron lattice filtering off the light and truth of the household from him who is in most need of them. But if the fear is described and accepted, the conspiracy shrinks to its proper dimensions; it is confined to the bed, to one man and the not-terrible whisperings of his demise. As Jacques de la Rivière said:
"Peace lies only in the irremediable."

Although Mrs. Willis' letter is a personal statement of her own needs and feelings, other dying persons can be assumed to experience similar feelings. Fielding's remarks about death also support this view. Because persons who visited Mrs. Willis were concerned with their own feelings, they were unable to perceive her need for someone to listen to her. Failure to accept death as a part of life or as a natural event cut off meaningful communication between Mrs. Willis and her visitors. By denying death, they placed on Mrs. Willis the burden of modifying her behavior, so that she did not make them uncomfortable.

What are some of the implications to nursing of Mrs. Willis' letter?

Conception, birth, health, disease, and death are all aspects of life. Of all, death engenders the greatest fear in most people. Even for persons who have great faith in an after life, death as the great unknown is often feared. It is feared not only by the person who is dying, but by the living. All cultures from the most primitive to the most complex have rituals that center around the dying and the dead. In the care of the dying, the needs, feelings, attitudes, and beliefs of the living as well as those of the dying should be considered.

[66] Gabriel Fielding, "The Uses of Fear," *Harper's Magazine*, CCXXIV, February, 1962, p. 94.

From both the moral and legal point of view nothing may be done for the purpose of hastening the death of a person. There is, however, no requirement that extraordinary measures be utilized in prolonging the life of a patient when only pain and suffering lie ahead. Rynearson[67] states that basic or indispensable care of the dying patient includes food, fluids, good nursing care, appropriate measures to relieve physical and mental suffering, and opportunity to prepare for death. Rynearson also summarizes criteria that should be met in the care of the dying. They are:

1. He should die with dignity, respect, and humanity.
2. He should die with minimal pain.
3. He should have the opportunity to recall the love and benefits of a lifetime of sharing; he and his family and friends should visit together, if the patient so wishes.
4. He should be able to clarify relationships, to express wishes—to share sentiments.
5. The patient and relatives should plan intelligently for changes which death imposes upon the living.
6. The patient should die in familiar surroundings if possible, if not, the quietus should take place in surroundings made as nearly homelike as possible.
7. Finally, but importantly, there should be concern for the feelings of the living.[68]

The burden of caring for the terminally ill patient is shared by the patient's family, his physician, nurses, social workers, and clergyman—minister, priest, or rabbi. When available, specialists in psychology, sociology, and anthropology can be helpful to those caring for the dying. Healthy people often hesitate about having a clergyman visit a seriously ill person for the first time. They fear that the patient will be frightened and give up hope of living. Some hospitals solve this problem by employing or arranging to have a clergyman visit all newly admitted patients, unless the patient specifically asks not to be visited by a chaplain. Visits are then continued as a regular service to the patient. Catholic patients usually expect to be visited regularly. Though non-Catholics find it hard to believe, most Catholics are comforted by having the last rites.

Much of the care that the patient receives is given by nurses. Some of the things that a nurse can do to ease the suffering of the patient who is dying are listed by Sister Mary Hubert in "Spiritual Care for Every Patient."[69] Although Sister Mary Hubert is writing about the spiritual care of every patient, her suggestions are most pertinent to the dying—whether death is imminent or a long time coming. Her first suggestion is kindness, thoughtfulness, gentleness, and a "personalized warm concern." Second, she suggests "frequent

---

[67] Edward H. Rynearson, "You Are Standing at the Bedside of a Patient Dying of Untreatable Cancer," *Ca: Bulletin of Cancer Progress,* IX, May-June, 1959, pp. 85-87.
[68] *Ibid.,* pp. 85-97.
[69] Sister Mary Hubert, "Spiritual Care for Every Patient," *The Journal of Nursing Education,* II, May-June, 1963, pp. 9-11, 29-31.

contacts"; staying away from the patient is easier when one is afraid or the patient is irritable and demanding, but only through contact with the patient can the nurse express her real concern for him or be kind or thoughtful. Third the nurse should understand her own attitude toward "the truths of human existence; life, suffering, old-age, and death." According to Sister Mary Hubert, suffering is one of the most frequently encountered facts of life and is the least understood. Her fourth suggestion, the encouragement of wholesome reading, may or may not be applicable. Certainly, encouragement of the patient to continue his interests and activities as long as he is able is to be recommended. Finally, by prayer—the nurse may pray with the patient, help the patient to pray, offer to say a prayer for the patient—the nurse may be able to convey to the patient her concern for him and his welfare.

What are some of the physiological and hygienic needs of the dying person?

The hygienic and physiological needs of the dying are also of great importance and they should not be neglected. In debilitated patients, improvement of nutrition may by itself bring about a marked change in the outlook of the patient and in his ability to be active. The same is true when anemia is corrected. Exercise is usually encouraged. It prevents the loss of strength that accompanies inactivity and improves the appetite as well as the morale of the patient. Florence Nightingale in *Notes on Nursing*[70] expresses the wish that as much attention were paid to the effect of the body on the mind as the reverse. Later she stated that one of the common causes of death in chronic illness is starvation.[71] This is no less true today than it was in Miss Nightingale's day.

Attention should be given to the maintenance of other functions such as fluid intake, respiration, and elimination. As the patient fails, more and more of the daily activities of living, such as bathing and mouth care and protection of his skin against breakdown will have to be assumed by others. Attention to details that give the patient comfort benefits not only the patient, but the members of his family.

An aspect of dying that has received little attention in nursing literature and is implied in Mrs. Willis' letter is that death does not always occur quickly. The final day or days of dying may follow weeks or months of gradually declining health. During this period, the patient not infrequently requires more and more physical care and emotional support. Because little or nothing can be done to effect cure, what could be done to relieve the anxiety of the patient and his family and provide physical comfort for the patient is neglected. The problem is intensified when doctors and nurses feel helpless or are angry with the patient for dying or with his demanding behavior.

[70] Florence Nightingale, *Notes on Nursing,* Harrison, 59, Pall Mall, London, 1860, p. 34.
[71] *Ibid.,* p. 37.

What aspect of the American culture helps to explain the nurse's feelings toward a dying patient?

In the American culture, the care of patients with fatal diseases or who are dying is made more difficult by the emphasis on cure as the primary objective of the health professions. In defining their role, patient, nurse, and physician all emphasize cure as an important criterion of success. When a patient recovers, nurses as well as doctors take credit for the patient's success. Moreover, patients, nurses, and doctors frequently expect not only that patients should get well, but that they should recover quickly and pleasantly. When they do not recover or they die, the nurse and/or doctor feels that he must have failed in some respect.

In addition to being an agent in the cure of the sick person, nurses also expect to comfort the sick and to relieve their suffering. When they are unable to do this, they may feel that as nurses they are inadequate and feelings of anxiety are aroused. With anxiety the defenses of the person against anxiety are invoked. The psychological defenses of sick and healthy are basically alike. Nurse and patient may both be using similar or different defenses against feelings of fear. Since the burden for adapting her behavior to the needs of the patient is on the nurse, she must have some insight into her own feelings about death and dying. When she has come to terms with her own feelings, she should be better able to concentrate on what the patient is feeling, even when he projects his negative feelings to her. She can allow the patient to talk about his feelings, be they of anger, remorse, guilt, or regrets. If, as Fielding says, the fear can be described and accepted, it can then be kept within bounds. Besides fear of death, it is not uncommon for healthy people to have mixed feelings toward the sick and disabled. Part of this feeling may be hostility. Nurses are taught to believe that they have kindly feelings toward their patients. One way the nurse may defend herself against her unacceptable feelings is by denial. She may grow angry with the patient and withdraw entirely or treat him in an impersonal or cold manner (the cool, starched look), or she may be excessively disturbed about the predicament of the patient. When this happens the nurse's own feelings of despair and hopelessness may cause her to withdraw from the situation by refusing to care for patients in the terminal phase of illness or her feelings may prevent her from being able to establish a supporting relationship with the patient because she frightens the patient. When the nurse feels too strongly, her feelings prevent her from being able to be sufficiently objective to form a relationship with the patient that will support him emotionally. Objectivity as used here is defined as follows: Objectivity enables the nurse to identify the patient's needs and to modify her own behavior, so that she can communicate with the patient in a meaningful way. The nurse may also feel guilty because she is healthy and can expect to go on living. Her negative feelings about the patient who is dying can interfere with her ability to communicate with the patient in a meaningful way.

As the condition of the patient deteriorates, he can be expected to become more and more dependent on those who are responsible for his care. How the nurse (or others) reacts depends on her ability to tolerate dependency in others. Chodoff[72] states that healthy persons often have ambivalent feelings with elements of hostility when they have contact with the helpless and disabled. In the patient who is in the terminal phase of a long-term illness such as cancer, there is no need for concern about the effects of long-term dependency on the nurse-patient relationship. The nurse must exercise judgment and sensitivity to the needs and feelings of the patient, so that he has done for him what comforts him and he is allowed and encouraged to do the things that he can and wishes to do.

Other problems to the nurse in the care of patients who die or are dying include the possibility that the nurse fears that the patient would not have died if she had acted quickly enough or in a different manner. When a patient dies unexpectedly or dies when the nurse is giving or assisting with his care, the nurse may feel that she was in some manner responsible. When a nurse is disturbed by any of the above questions, she will do well to discuss the problem with someone who can help her explore the various facets of the problem.

Although there is a tendency on the part of the healthy to avoid even thinking about death, it is not always unwelcome to the person who is dying. Poets have put into words what experienced doctors and nurses know, that is, death is not always unwelcome or feared.

Walter Savage Landor's poem "On Death"

> *Death stands above me, whispering low*
> *I know not what into my ear;*
> *Of His strange language all I know*
> *Is, there is not a word of fear.*

Alexander Pope in the first stanza of "The Dying Christian to His Soul" expresses a variety of feelings.

> *Vital Spark of heavenly flame!*
> *Quit, O quit this mortal frame!*
> *Trembling, hoping, lingering, flying,*
> *O the pain, the bliss of dying.*
> *Cease fond Nature, cease thy strife,*
> *And let me languish into life!*

John Donne, 1573–1631, in one of his sonnets says,

> *Death be not proud, though some have called thee*
> *Mighty and dreadfull, for, thou art not so;*

---

[72] Paul Chodoff, "A Psychiatric Approach to the Dying Patient," *Ca.* X, 1960. pp. 29-32.

For, those whom thou think'st thou dost overthrow,
Die not, poor death, nor yet canst thou kill me.
From rest and sleep, which but thy pictures be,
Much pleasure, then from thee, much more must flow,
And soonest our best men with thee doe go,
Rest of their bones, and soules delivery.
Thou art slave to Fate, Chance, kings and desperate men,
And dost with poyson, warre, and sicknesse dwell,
And poppy or charms can make us sleep as well,
And better then thy stroke; why swell'st thou then?
  One short sleepe past, wee wake eternally
  And death shall be no more; death thou shalt die.

Another aspect of the care of the dying that engenders negative feelings relates to the extent to which life should be prolonged or death prevented. Though nurses are not responsible for making the decision that a given treatment should be instituted, withheld, or continued, they are affected by these decisions. For example, the nurse may be troubled when therapeutic measures are instituted which, though they have as their objective the prolongation of the life of the patient, appear to increase his suffering. The physician is responsible for informing the family of the condition of the patient and suggesting to them courses of action. Much of the care of the dying patient is given by nurses. They cannot help but be affected by the decisions made relative to the patient.

What are some of the needs of the family of a dying patient?

As indicated above, not only the patient and the nurse are affected, but the family and his friends are affected. The family of the patient experiences feelings similar to those of the patient, and at the same time the patient requires their comfort, strength, and support. Even when family relationships have been good and family members have a basis for meeting the needs of the patient, they require comfort and emotional support. When the family relationships have not been good, the strain placed on the family by the illness may cause further difficulties. Particularly as the condition of the patient deteriorates, feelings of guilt and remorse may be awakened in family members. As a result they try frantically to compensate for past failures—real or imagined—in their relationship. Through their efforts to assist the patient, they try to reassure themselves of their devotion to the patient and of their own worth as human beings. The family needs support and a feeling that they are not alone. The nurse can help the members of the family fulfill their role by her acceptance of their behavior as having meaning, even when it seems to be unreasonable. The nurse cannot expect always to be able to change the behavior of the relatives of patients. She can show that she respects their feelings by listening to them and by treating them in a courteous, kind and thoughtful manner.

Summary

In the recent past there has been and is a tendency either to neglect the care of those who are in the terminal phase of an illness or to use extraordinary measures to prolong life. There is the beginning trend toward emphasizing that much can be done to increase usefulness and comfort during the period in which the health of the individual declines. In some instances the patient is fully informed of the nature of his condition and what may be expected from the treatment. Attention continues to be on what can be done and on conveying to the patient that something can and will be done to help him. The emphasis here is not on cure, though this possibility is recognized, but on comfort and support of the sick person. The criterion for evaluating success is not, so much, how many are cured, but how long an individual is maintained in a reasonably comfortable and useful state. In order to better meet the needs of patients who die slowly, studies should be done to determine what their needs are and how they can be met with emphasis on the nurse's role in this respect.

What are some other ways of evaluating health problems?

There are other ways of looking at the health problems that affect the practice of nursing. One is to examine some of the problems that arise out of illness and disability. These include some of the measurable costs of illness and disability to the community and to the individaul. Hospitals, health departments, clinics, and all the services for the prevention and treatment of illness are costly and, according to most predictions, will become more so. The individual wage earner who is ill often suffers complete or partial loss of income. He may have to go into debt to pay for his care or to care for the needs of his family. When the homemaker is ill and especially when there are children, a substitute mother may have to be employed. This may place a considerable financial burden on the family.

There are other losses that may be more difficult to measure than the direct costs of the illness. These include the loss of productivity of a worker and sometimes of those who depend on his service or the product that he produces for their work. Who can place a monetary value on the loss of the homemaker from the home or the teacher from the classroom? Few substitute mothers or teachers can pick up where their predecessor left off and carry on fully. The adverse effects from the death or disability of a parent on growing children include the gamut from insufficient food and clothing to effects resulting from emotional deprivation and premature cessation of schooling. These things do not always happen, but they can and do occur. For example, Mrs. Alphonse, the 35-year-old mother of ten children, has severe, crippling rheumatoid arthritis. The children range in age from a few months to 12 years. During the last year and a half, Mrs. Alphonse has been in the hospital most of the time. The children have been cared for by grandparents filling in for a series of housekeepers, most of whom leave after a few weeks. Though the children have not been neglected physically, who can predict the effects of the absence of the mother from the home and exposure to a continuing state of anxiety about the mother and the costs of her care?

In addition to the problems created for children by death or disability of a parent, other members of the family are also affected. Women are now living an average of about 8 years longer than their husbands. Among the problems that widows have to, or are likely to have to, face are: adjusting to single living; coping with real or feared inadequacy of income to meet their needs and those of dependent children; and remaining in or changing their living arrangements. Older widows with little or no family, few friends, and no interests outside their families may have little incentive to continue living. Their purpose and meaning of life may be gone. The older, friendless widow is often lonely. Unless she has or can find a way to support herself emotionally and financially, she may have to depend on her children or the community for both types of support.

Nurses cannot, of course, solve the economic and social problems arising out of illness, but they can sometimes be helpful to patients by being aware that they exist. They may also assist the patient by helping him to explore his resources and those in the community. With her special knowledge of the problems created by sickness, the nurse should be able to give constructive leadership to the community in its efforts to solve some of the problems arising as a result of illness.

What are some of the services provided by the community to cope with health problems? What are some of the trends in health care?

One of the most significant factors in the achievement of all objectives of health care is the quality and quantity of medical services available and utilized by the population. No single type of service will meet the needs of all persons or even the same person at different periods in his life.

Previous to the twentieth century, with the exception of the indigent, most persons who were ill were cared for in the home. With the tremendous increase in knowledge as well as the development of highly complicated tools and techniques, the sick were moved from the home to the office of the physician and to the hospital for care. Other factors contributed to this shift from the home to out-of-the-home care. Most families live in houses that are large enough to accommodate them when they are well, but do not provide sufficient space to isolate the sick from the well. In some families, the presence of a sick person may place considerable strain on all family members. When single persons live alone or all persons of a family work, no one is available to care for a sick person.

Although the modern hospital does have facilities for the care of sick people that could not possibly be made available to them at home, not all persons require a high degree of specialized care. To meet the needs of persons who require different types of care, a number of changes have been taking place both within and without the hospital. Within the hospital, patients may be assigned to different areas depending on the type and degree of illness. For example, patients undergoing a surgical procedure may be transferred from the operating room to a recovery room or to an intensive-care unit. With the concentration of patients having particular needs in a localized area, specialized equipment can be readily available and nursing personnel can develop a high degree of competence in the care of patients. This plan has some possible disadvantages. Unless provisions are made for continuing care, the patient may be transferred from one area of the hospital to another much as if he were going from one foreign country to another. What appears to the patient to be an abrupt change in expectations for him may increase his anxiety and his sense of depersonalization. With adequate planning and follow-through the patient does not have to experience these feelings. Certainly a real effort should be made to interpret a move from an intensive-care unit to a convalescent-care unit as a major step in progress from sickness to health. Provision should also be made for the personnel in the intensive-care unit to follow the progress of the patient.

Another possible danger in assigning patients to units on the basis of degree of illness is that patients who appear to be less acutely ill or convalescent will be neglected. Care may be concentrated on making provisions for meeting physical needs, the administration of medicines and treatments, and the performance of diagnostic tests. The transition from the care being given in the intensive-care unit to being responsible for meeting his own needs may be so abrupt that the patient becomes frightened. A patient who is undergoing diagnostic procedures is also likely to be more or less anxious about their effects and outcome. The period during which diagnosis is occurring may be highly stressful to the patient. Perhaps the most important statement to be made at this point is that the priority of needs differs with different degrees of illness, but that all sick people have needs. These needs should be identified and plans made to satisfy them.

With the trend toward the hospitalization of sick people and the modern advances in medicine, the cost of medical care has risen. To cope with the problem of cost, a number of voluntary health insurance plans have been developed. In general, these plans are one of three types: insurance to protect against an acute disabling illness, insurance to pay the cost of a major or catastrophic illness, and insurance to prevent the loss of income during illness. One form of income insurance is, of course, sick leave. An employed individual is allowed a set number of days each year when he may be absent from work without the loss of his wages or salary. In some situations, sick leave is cumulative. With the increase in the incidence of long-term illness, the latter types of insurance are of great importance.

Another trend stimulated by the cost of medical and hospital care is movement toward caring for less acutely ill patients in their homes. "Home care," as it is called, is a boon to the person who requires one or more professional services but does not require all the facilities of a hospital for the acutely ill. Home care plans have proliferated in the last few years, so that in many communities chronically ill persons can receive the care they require at home. To illustrate, Mrs. Albert, aged 35, has a chronic neurological disorder, multiple sclerosis. She has four young children ranging in age from 1 to 14 years. Though she required hospitalization at the onset of her illness, she is able to spend most of her time at home. In addition to medical supervision, she is visited daily by a visiting nurse who supervises her activity and exercise. A physical therapist visits her once a week, to supervise the nurse who is caring for her and to evaluate the effect of her program of activity. The nurse has taught Mr. Albert to administer a preparation of the adrenocorticotrophic hormone by intramuscular injection. The nurse has consulted the agency dietitian about how to help Mrs. Albert plan a low-fat diet. An occupational therapist is available but has not been consulted, because Mrs. Albert is kept busy supervising the children and the household. Since the Visiting Nurse Service also provides household aides, one is assigned to assist Mrs. Albert. Because the number of services and amount of care required by Mrs. Albert are great even home care is expensive. One of the values of home care which cannot be measured in terms of money is that Mrs. Albert fulfills within the limits of her ability her role as wife and mother. For many persons, home care may not play as vital a role, but it does make it possible for the person to live a more nearly normal life.

There is also a trend toward caring for patients in the terminal stages of illness at home and toward keeping the patient active as long as is practical. To do this the family must be emotionally and physically able to care for the patient at home. The willingness of the family to have the patient at home is perhaps the most important factor in determining whether the patient can be cared for at home. Mrs. Lottie Gamely is a good example of how a seriously disabled person may be cared for at home. Despite being bedridden and unable to turn in bed without help, she remained at home until the week before her death. During her last months she maintained her role as mother to her children—one aged eight, the other ten. Before they left for school in the morning she checked them in the same manner as do healthy mothers. She saw to it that they performed their household chores and did their homework. She comforted them and she disciplined them. Household help was, of course, required. Medical and nursing care was available and provided.

Besides remaining useful for a longer period of time, the patient's needs are often easier to meet with home care. Food prepared at home and in the manner to which the patient is accustomed is more palatable than hospital food. Visiting by friends and relatives is easier. The schedule and timing of the activities of the day are likely to be familiar. Medical and nursing supervision is necessary to the success of the care of the patient at home. This is required not only for the patient's safety but so that the strain on the family is not excessive. There is always the possibility that the patient will be neglected. There is also the possibility of the patient's becoming a sickroom tyrant. Neither is desired nor desirable.

Hospital personnel including physicians tend to minimize the problems faced by the chronically ill patient after he is discharged from the hospital. The result is that not all patients who require assistance at home are referred to the Visiting Nurse Service or other community agencies for guidance. The amount and type of assistance needed vary. Not all patients require as much help as Mrs. Albert or Mrs. Gamely; some require more.

Summary

In summary, the role of the nurse in the prevention of illness and conditions leading to illness and in its therapy includes:

1. Knowledge required for the recognition of conditions or situations that are favorable or unfavorable to health.
2. Skill in instituting preventive measures and in supporting community efforts to institute these measures.
3. Knowledge required to identify the symptoms and signs indicating illness. This knowledge is essential in the nurse's role as a case-finder.
4. Knowledge required to make judgments as to the urgency of the need of the patient for attention—Does he require the immediate attention of a physician? Should he be subject to careful observation? Can his needs be met at this particular time by the practice of nursing?
5. Knowledge required to make judgments as to the appropriate course of action, that is, to whom should the patient and his problem be referred?
6. Confidence to press for action when the condition of the patient appears to require it.
7. Knowledge and competence in the practice of nursing that is required to:
   a. Identify the nature of the patient's problem (i.e., problem that can be solved or alleviated by nursing).
   b. Modify his external environment so that the adaptations that the patient is called upon to make are within his adaptive capacity.
   c. Support the efforts of the patient to adapt and to respond.
   d. Provide him with the materials or supplies that he requires to meet his needs.
   e. Coordinate and integrate the activities of all those who have a function in care of the patient in order to facilitate movement toward the desired goals.

REFERENCES

Books

Abdellah, Faye G., Irene L. Beland, Almeda Martin, and Ruth V. Matheney, *Patient-Centered Approaches to Nursing,* The Macmillan Company, New York, 1960.
Bell, Walter, *The Plague in London,* Williams Clowez & Sons, London, 1924.
Cannon, Walter B., *The Wisdom of the Body,* W. W. Norton Co., Inc., New York, 1939.
Defoe, Daniel, *The Plague in London,* George Bell & Sons, London, 1889.
Duffy, John, *Epidemics in Colonial America,* Louisiana State University, Baton Rouge, 1953.
Eissler, K. R., *The Psychiatrist and the Dying Patient,* International University Press, New York, 1955.
Haggard, Howard W., *Devils, Drugs, and Doctors,* Harper & Brothers, New York, 1929.
Homburger, Freddy, *The Medical Care of the Aged and Chronically Ill,* Little, Brown & Company, Boston, 1955.
Leavell, Hugh Rodman, and E. Gurney Clarke, *Preventive Medicine for the Doctor in His Community,* 2nd ed., Blakiston Division of McGraw-Hill Book Co., New York, 1958.
Mumford, Lewis, *Technics and Civilization,* Harcourt, Brace and Co., New York, 1934.
———, *The Culture of Cities,* Harcourt, Brace and Co., New York, 1938.
———, *The City in History,* Harcourt, Brace and World, New York, 1961.
New York Academy of Medicine, *The Epidemiology of Health,* Health Education Council, New York, 1953.
Perkins, William Harvey, *Cause and Prevention of Disease,* Lea and Febiger, Philadelphia, 1938.
Sigerist, Henry E., *Civilization and Disease,* Cornell University Press, Ithaca, 1945.
Wohl, Michael G., *Long-Term Illness: Management of the Chronically Ill Patient,* W. B. Saunders Co., Philadelphia, 1959.

Articles

Abdellah, Faye G., and E. Josephine Strachan, "Progressive Patient Care," *American Journal of Nursing,* LIX, May, 1959, pp. 649-55.
Austin, Catherine L., "The Basic Six Needs of the Aging," *Nursing Outlook,* VII, March, 1959, pp. 138-41.
Bauer, Theodore, "Public Health and Chronic Disease," *Public Health Reports,* LXXIII, November, 1958, pp. 975-77.
Bierring, Walter L., "Preventive Medicine—Its Changing Concept, 1859–1959," *Journal of the American Medical Association,* CLXXI, December, 1959, pp. 2190-94.
Boek, Walter, and Jean Boek, "Health, Social Status, and the Life Cycle," *Journal of Chronic Diseases,* XIV, August, 1961, pp. 272-82.
Brown, Frances Gold, "Who Said Care of Long-Term Patients Is Routine?" *American Journal of Nursing,* LXII, May, 1962, pp. 58-61.
Burney, L. E., "Health Problems of the Aging: A Challenge to Preventive Medicine," *Journal of the American Medical Association,* CLXV, October 3, 1957, pp. 440-43.
Callahan, Enid Bailey, "Extending Hospital Services into the Home," *American Journal of Nursing,* LXI, June, 1961, pp. 59-61.
Chapman, Albert L., "The Chronic Diseases Affect Our Economy—A Look at the Future," *American Journal of Public Health,* LI, April, 1961, pp. 542-46.
Cherkasky, Martin, "The Montifiore Hospital Home Care Program," *American Journal of Public Health,* XXXIX, February, 1949, pp. 163-66.
Cherkasky, Martin, "Patient Services in Chronic Disease," *Public Health Reports,* LXXIII, November, 1958, pp. 978-81.
Chodoff, Paul, "Understanding and Management of the Chronically Ill Patient," *American Practitioner and Digest of Treatment,* XIII, March, 1962, pp. 165-70.
Committee on Indigent Care, "Organized 'Home Care Programs' in the United States," *Journal of the American Medical Association,* CLXIV, May 18, 1957, pp. 298-305.

Deaver, George G., Mary M. Jerome, and Winifred E. Taylor, "Rehabilitation," *American Journal of Nursing*, LIX, September, 1959, pp. 1278-81.

"Diseases of Ancient Man," *British Medical Journal*, I, March 24, 1962, pp. 852-53.

Flemming, Arthur S., "Fluoridation—A Statement," *Public Health Reports*, LXXIV, June, 1959, pp. 511-12.

Ford, Hamilton, "How to Approach a Geriatric Patient," *Geriatrics*, XVII, February, 1962, p. 110.

Ford, Loretta, "The Five Elements of Progressive Patient Care," *Nursing Outlook*, VIII, August, 1960, pp. 436-39.

Francis, Thomas, "Research in Preventive Medicine," *Journal of the American Medical Association*, CLXXII, March 5, 1960, pp. 993-99.

Frenster, John H., "Interaction of Load, Capacity, and Resistance in Body Processes," *Perspective in Biology and Medicine*, IV, Winter, 1961, pp. 152-58.

Frenster, John H., "Load Tolerance as a Quantitative Estimate of Health," *Annals of Internal Medicine*, LVII, November, 1962, pp. 788-94.

Glaser, Barney G., and Anselm L. Strauss, "The Social Loss of Dying Patients," *American Journal of Nursing*, LXIV, June, 1964, pp. 119-121.

Harpuder, Karl, "Basic Medical Principles in the Treatment of the Chronically Ill Patient," *Journal of Chronic Disease*, IV, August, 1956, pp. 170-76.

Horner, Ada L., and Muriel Jennings, "Before Patients Go Home," *American Journal of Nursing*, LXI, June, 1961, pp. 62-63.

Kaplan, J., "Day Center and Day Care Center," *Geriatrics*, XII, April, 1957, pp. 247-51.

Kariel, Patricia, "The Dynamics of Behavior in Relation to Health," *Nursing Outlook*, X, June, 1962, pp. 402-5.

Knutson, John W., "Fluoridation—Where Are We Today?" *American Journal of Nursing*, LX, February, 1960, pp. 196-98.

Lane, Harriett C., "Rehabilitation Nurse," *Nursing Outlook*, VI, March, 1958, pp. 157-59.

Lederer, Henry D., "How the Sick View Their World," *Patients, Physicians and Illness*, E. G. Jaco (ed.), The Free Press, Glencoe, Illinois, 1958, pp. 247-56.

Leeds, Morton, "The Role of the Professional in Working with the Senile," *Geriatrics*, XVII, February, 1962, p. 116-22.

Lissitz, Samuel, "Motivating Geriatric Hospital Patients," *Geriatrics*, XVII, May, 1962, p. 301.

MacLeod, Kenneth I. E., "Well Oldster Health Conference," *Nursing Outlook*, VI, April, 1958, pp. 206-8.

Morgan, Elizabeth, "A Push Anyone?" *American Journal of Nursing*, LVIII, June, 1958, pp. 831-33.

Nichols, Claude, and Morton Bogdonoff, "Programming the Care of the Chronically Ill," *New England Journal of Medicine*, CCLXVI, April 26, 1962, pp. 867-70.

"Report on Fluoridation in the United States," *Public Health Reports*, LXXIV, June, 1959, pp. 513-16.

Richards, Dickinson, "Homeostasis: Its Dislocations and Perturbations," *Perspectives in Biology and Medicine*, III, Winter, 1960, pp. 238-51.

Rogatz, Peter, and Guido Crocetti, "Home Care Programs—Their Impact on the Hospital's Role in Medical Care," *American Journal of Public Health*, XLVIII, September, 1958, pp. 1125-33.

Sargent, Emilie G., "Evolution of a Home Care Program," *American Journal of Nursing*, LXI, July, 1961, pp. 88-91.

Schwartz, D. "Nursing Needs of Chronically Ill Ambulatory Patients," *Nursing Research*, IX, No. 4, Fall, 1960, pp. 185-88.

Seegal, David, and Arthur Werther, "Progress in Control of Chronic Disease," *Public Health Reports*, LXXIII, November, 1958, pp. 971-74.

Sellers, A. H., "The Lengthening Life Span," *Canadian Journal of Public Health*, LI, May, 1960, pp. 171-85.

Selye, Hans, "The Physiopathoolgy of Stress," *Postgraduate Medicine*, XXV, June, 1959, pp. 660-67.

Shock, Nathan, "The Physiology of Aging," *Scientific American*, CCVI, January, 1962, pp. 100-10.

Smith, Genevieve Waples, "A Stroke Is Not the End of the World," *American Journal of Nursing,* LVII, March, 1957, pp. 303-5.

"Statements on Proposed Alternatives to Fluoridation of Water Supplies," *Public Health Reports,* LXXIV, June, 1959, pp. 517-20.

Statistical Bulletin, Metropolitan Life Insurance Company, XLI, January, 1960, p. 11.

Tillich, Paul, "The Meaning of Health," *Perspectives in Biology and Medicine,* V, Autumn, 1961, pp. 92-100.

Udell, Louis, "Philadelphia Plan for Home Care of Chronically Ill Persons," *Journal of the American Medical Association,* CLII, July 11, 1953, pp. 990-93.

Weisman, Avery D., and Thomas P. Hackett, "Predilection to Death," *Psychosomatic Medicine,* XXIII, May-June, 1961, p. 232-56.

Willard, Harold, and Frank Seixas, "Preventive Rehabilitation," *Psychosomatic Medicine,* XXI, May-June, 1959, pp. 235-46.

Wolf, Stewart, "A New View of Disease," *Journal of American Medical Association,* LXXXIV, April 13, 1963, pp. 129-30.

Wolf, Stewart, "Disease as a Way of Life," *Perspectives in Biology and Medicine,* IV, Spring, 1961, pp. 288-305.

Wolff, Harold G., "A Concept of Disease in Man," *Psychosomatic Medicine,* XXIV, January-February, 1962, pp. 25-30.

Woolever, Gloria M., "An Intensive Care Unit," *Nursing Outlook,* VI, December, 1958, pp. 690-91.

3 : The Effects of Injurious Agents on Cells

> The environment of the industrialized society is not only beclouded by products from the combustion of fuel, but it is also increasingly burdened by vast numbers of new chemicals of ambiguous potential used in medicine, agriculture, food processing, the cosmetic industry, and in vermin control. In addition, other products such as detergents, bleaches, and cleansing fluids—some highly toxic—are an essential part of the contemporary human environment.[1]

In the preceding chapter the various etiological agents were classified as those causing direct injury to cells and those inducing their effect indirectly through the mental apparatus. This chapter will be concerned with the effects of certain physical and chemical agents on cellular function and the implication of this information to the practice of nursing. Physical and chemical agents can have their origin in either the external or internal environment of the individual. Many of the harmful agents in the external and possibly in the internal environment are of man's own making. Moreover they are being created in increasing variety and potency. As a society we have been preoccupied with the hazards of exposure to ionizing radiation and have paid little attention to the possibility that other agents may be even more dangerous. Although some are, many of the noxious agents in the environment are not new. They are an augmentation of pre-existing natural hazards. For example, ever since lightning ignited a tinder-dry prairie or forest, man has been exposed to smoke. When man learned to use fire for his own purposes, he increased the intensity of his exposure to smoke. In man's early history he inhaled smoke from a campfire or a poorly constructed fireplace. Inventions such as the furnace and steam and diesel engines have increased the quantity of smoke spewed into the atmosphere. Though many cities have accomplished miracles in controlling the contamination of the air with smoke, much remains to be done. Whatever the quantity of smoke in the air, many persons expose their respiratory tissues more or less continuously during their waking hours to cigarette smoke. The harmful effects of this practice are well documented.

Knowledge of the nature and effects of physical and chemical agents on

---

[1] Wilson G. Smillie and Edwin D. Kilbourne, *Preventive Medicine and Public Health,* 3rd ed., The Macmillan Company, New York, 1963, p. 275.

cells is of increasing importance in the development of sound programs for the prevention of exposure to noxious agents as well as to the treatment of disease caused by them. General measures used in the control of potentially harmful physical and chemical agents do not differ very much in principle from those used in the control of microorganisms. Though the examples used to illustrate the points made in this chapter will be nonliving chemical and physical agents, living agents cause disease by their chemical and physical effects. Toxins formed by bacteria are poisonous chemicals. Control measures are based on information about sources of noxious agents, their vehicles for transmission, the forms in which they are harmful, and portals of entry as well as how they reach susceptible cells. Any information about the host making him or certain of his cells susceptible to a particular agent is also important. Most agents used in the therapy of disease are potentially injurious. Undesired effects may be induced by overdosage, or by failure of the mechanisms for inactivation or elimination. Some noxious agents do not cause any injury to the cell that is immediately apparent. Evidence that the individual was exposed to a particular agent may not appear for weeks or months or even years. Injury or death can also be the result of hypersensitivity or of unusual reaction to agents used in therapy. Sound and reasonable methods of control of chemical and physical threats to health and life depend on understanding their nature and sources of exposure. Moreover, the nurse requires this knowledge to protect not only patients, but herself.

Survival of the patient who has suffered cellular injury often depends on the protection of damaged tissues until healing has taken place. Although the physician plans the therapeutic regime, the nurse is frequently responsible for its effectiveness. She makes many of the observations that are used to evaluate the response of the patient to disease and treatment. She helps to interpret both preventive and therapeutic measures to the patient and his family.

Some of the objectives of nursing derived from knowledge of the nature and effects of agents directly injuring cells are:

1. To prevent injury to cells (or further injury).
2. To provide conditions essential to the recovery of the injured person.
3. To gather the information required to evaluate the progress of the patient.
4. To participate in community educational programs.

Although this chapter is devoted to a discussion of the effects of injurious agents on the structure, function, and response of cells to injury, the fact that the total organism reacts or responds to the injury should not be forgotten. Whatever the nature or level of the response, it is directed toward overcoming the harmful agent, limiting and repairing the damage, and restoring the cell, tissue, and individual to health. When the total response of the individual is adequate and appropriate to the injury, it is beneficial. The nature and extent of the response will depend on the nature and extent of the injury as well as the manner in which the individual perceives it and what his expectations are. Unless the injury is so great that death is sudden, the manifestations that are observed in the patient are often the result of complicated physiological and psychological changes set into motion by the effects of direct damage to cells. Thus, injury to one part of the organism may induce a whole chain of reactions and involve parts far from the site of the original insult including the entire individual. When these reactions are appropriate in quality and quantity to the injury, they promote recovery. They are, however, sometimes sources of injury.

What are some of the ways in which physical and chemical agents injure cells?

A wide variety of chemical, physical, and living agents are capable, under appropriate circumstances, of causing direct injury to cells. Some substances, such as cyanide, are highly potent, causing harm when present in minute quantities, while others, such as silica, require excessive amounts and/or prolonged exposure to be harmful. Deleterious effects are associated with either a deficit or excess of some substances requisite to health; for example, vitamin D can cause disease by either a deficit or an excess. Conditions within the individual may act to protect him from or increase his vulnerability to certain chemicals. For example, the drug Thalidomide was supposed to be a mild and relatively safe sedative. It was safe when administered to adults, unless the adult happened to be a prospective mother who was in the early stages of pregnancy. Even then the drug appeared to be safe for the mother, but an unusual number of infants born of mothers who had taken Thalidomide during the first six weeks of pregnancy were born with a deformity called phocomelia (seal limb). Although the reason for the susceptibility of the embryo to Thalidomide is not known, the drug arrests and deranges the development of the embryo exposed to it. It is generally thought that drugs which produce fetal deformities exert their action at the time the affected part is undergoing differentiation. Some infants are only slightly deformed, while others were born with multiple anomalies, including serious deformities of all four extremities and of the viscera.[2] The nature and extent of deformity depends on the time of differentiation in the embryo in relation to the ingestion of the drug and its action. The differences between the effects of Thalidomide on the adult and embryo serve to emphasize that the susceptibility of the individual can be a factor in the effect of a chemical agent. In this instance, immaturity was the critical factor. In other instances, it could be something else.

The results of the action of Thalidomide also illustrate another principle in biology; that is, a cell can perform only as its biological properties allow.

[2] Helen B. Taussig. "The Thalidomide Syndrome," *Scientific American*, CCVII, August, 1962, pp. 29-35.

Despite the effect of Thalidomide on growth and development, insofar as is known it has no power to alter structure after a given critical period in life. Chemical or physical agents can alter cell function, so that it is increased, inhibited, or fails. They can also alter cell structure, but they cannot make a cell perform a new function. For example, a muscle cell can be made to over- or undercontract or to fail to contract, but it cannot be made to secrete. Continued and unrelieved exposure of cells to agents increasing the activity of cells can be expected to result eventually in a failure of response. Simply stated, overstimulation leads to paralysis.

Knowledge of the manner in which the various physical, chemical, and living agents injure cells is incomplete. However, injury may be brought about: (1) by depriving the cell of something that it requires for its activities; (2) by crippling the cellular machinery, or, more specifically, by interfering with the action of the enzymes enabling the cell to utilize materials; and (3) by altering the nature of the proteins within the cells. The outcome depends on the degree of injury to the cell and its capacity to adapt. The outcome will be influenced by the nature of the injuring agent, its concentration, and the length of time that cells are exposed to it. When the injury to the cell is not too great, the process may be reversible and recovery complete. With greater injury, the process may be irreversible and death of the cell may follow.

How does the cell respond to an inadequate supply of materials or stimulation?

One of the important causes of injury to cells is depriving them of something they require for optimum function. There are two ways in which cells may be deprived. One is to reduce the supply of one or more essential nutrients below the quantity required to maintain function. The other is to deprive the cell of the stimulation it requires to function. The cell, like larger functioning units in the body, is capable of adapting to alterations in the conditions to which it is exposed. It is capable of adapting to a decrease in the supply of nutrients, or to a decrease in the functional demands made on it by decreasing its substance. As with other homeostatic mechanisms there are limits to which adaptation is possible. When the degree of deprivation is too great, the cell dies. The scientific term for the loss of substance, and with it a decrease in the size and strength of a cell or tissue, is "atrophy." Hopps[3] also includes a decrease in the number of cells in a tissue in his definition of atrophy. Atrophy of an organ leads to a decrease not only in its size, but in its functional capacity. For example, as a muscle atrophies it loses strength or becomes weak. In some instances atrophy can be prevented or reversed, if conditions leading to it are corrected soon enough. For instance, muscle

[3] Howard C. Hopps, *Principles of Pathology*, 2nd ed., Appleton-Century-Crofts, Inc. New York, 1964, pp. 171-72.

atrophy which accompanies insufficient exercise can be reversed and the muscle can be restored to its former strength by exercise.

What are the causes of atrophy?

Atrophy has many causes, some of which are physiological in origin. Others are the result of a pathological process. Atrophy is physiological or involutional when some tissue or organ diminishes in size as a result of the normal aging process. For the structure to maintain its youthful structure would be abnormal. For example, the thymus and lymphoid tissue normally atrophy at puberty. At the time of menopause, sexual organs, including the breasts of women, diminish in size. In old age all organs undergo some decrease in size. As a result elderly persons are not quite as tall as they were in their youth and they do not weigh as much. Shock[4] quotes a study made in Canada which illustrates the decline in weight from middle to old age. Men who weighed 167 lb at ages 35 to 40 years showed a decline in average weight to 155 lb at 65 years or older. They weighed 12 lb less at 65 than they did at 35 or 40 years of age. In a study made on a group of men in the United States, men who averaged 168 lb at ages of 65 to 69 years weighed, on the average, 148 lb at the ages of 90 to 94 years; that is, they lost approximately 20 lb during this period. Not only does the total body weight decrease, but individual organs decrease in weight after middle age. Shock[5] indicates that the average weight of the brain at autopsy drops from 1,375 gm (3.03lb) to 1,232 gm (2.72 lb) between the ages of 30 and 90. Mrs. Sabin illustrates these changes very well. At 95 years of age she weighs only 145 lb. Her highest weight was 215 lb. She has lost about 2 in. in height. Her skin is loose and wrinkled, her hair thin and sparse. With her loss of tissue she has lost strength. She is no longer as energetic as she was in her youth. She spends her days in her rocking chair.

What is a basis for classifying pathological atrophy?

Pathological atrophy is often classified according to its etiology or cause. Thus it is called: (1) disuse, (2) vascular or ischemic, (3) pressure, (4) neurogenic, (5) endocrine, or (6) generalized atrophy.

Disuse atrophy is one of the forms commonly seen by the nurse. In some instances, disuse atrophy can be prevented or limited by the practice of nursing. In disuse atrophy there is a wasting of tissue, especially that of the muscle and bone. Apparently the development and maintenance of the size, strength, and composition of muscle and bone are influenced by the amount of strain placed on them. This is supported by the principle that, in nature, parts develop in proportion to the stresses and strains placed on them. In a tree the

[4] Nathan W. Shock, "The Physiology of Aging," *Scientific American,* CCVI. January, 1962, p. 108.
[5] *Ibid.,* p. 108.

trunk is larger and stronger than the branches. The branches proximal to the trunk are larger in diameter than those distal to it. Patients are sometimes needlessly allowed to lose weight and strength for the want of exercise. Inactivity and immobilization lead to muscle and bone atrophy. The results of the demineralization of the bone are known as osteoporosis and can be seen on X ray. Sometimes the decalcification of the bone may proceed at such a rapid rate that calculi are formed in the urine. The weakness experienced by the patient who has been on bed rest is due in part to generalized atrophy. A striking example of disuse atrophy can be observed by comparing the size of a limb that has been recently encased in a cast with that of its mate which was free. To minimize disuse atrophy, unless there is some contraindication, bed patients should be encouraged to exercise. All patients should have arms and legs put through the normal range of motion each day. This can be done as they are bathed. The nurse should exercise reasonable judgment. Motion should not be forced beyond the normal range nor should it cause pain. Patients who are able should be taught to do exercises such as wiggling their toes, moving the legs up and down in bed, and doing muscle-setting exercises. When the patient's condition permits, activities such as boosting or raising himself up in bed, reaching, and turning help to maintain muscle strength. For patients who are paralyzed or who are unable to get out of bed, strain on muscles and bones may be increased by the use of the standing board. The circoelectric bed now makes this procedure easy to perform.

Two very closely related causes of atrophy are a deficient blood supply (ischemia) and pressure. The principal effect of pressure is to reduce the blood supply. There are many examples of pathology in which atrophy results from the reduction in the blood supply by pressure. For example, atrophy of the brain is associated with hydrocephalus, a condition in which cerebrospinal fluid accumulates within the ventricles in the brain. As the fluid accumulates, the brain tissue is stretched, and this creates pressure on the blood vessels and with it a lessening of the supply of blood to the brain. Another example is the atrophy of glandular structures such as the kidney or liver following obstruction of a ureter or the common bile duct. As a result of the blocking of the duct, urine accumulates in the ureter or bile in the bile ducts. The back pressure of fluid in a duct decreases the blood supply of the organ drained by the duct by distending the collecting ducts. The distended ducts press on blood vessels and reduce the blood supply to the affected organ. If ischemia of the organ is allowed to continue, changes in the parenchymal cells may occur and become irreversible. With a decrease in the number of parenchymal cells, there is a decrease in the functional capacity of the organ.

Loss of normal stimulation of tissues may be accompanied by atrophy. When a muscle loses its motor nerve supply, it wastes or atrophies. For example, in anterior poliomyelitis, destruction of the motor horn cells in the spinal cord deprives muscles of normal stimulation and the muscles become flaccid. The patient is said to have a flaccid paralysis. Muscles permanently deprived of their motor nerve supply eventually degenerate. Injuries to the sensory nerves may have a similar effect. Secretion by some of the endocrine glands is under the control of the anterior pituitary gland. Atrophy resulting in a loss of function of some of the endocrine glands may result from the failure of the anterior pituitary to produce its trophic hormones. Because of the negative feedback relationship of the anterior pituitary with its target glands, atrophy of a target gland can also be produced by the administration of large doses of its hormone.[6] To illustrate, atrophy of the adrenal cortex has been observed when large dosages of cortisone or hydrocortisone have been administered over a period of time.[7] When thyroxin is administered in the absence of a thyroid deficiency, the thyroid gland adapts by decreasing its secretion of thyroxin.

To generalize and summarize, in a broad sense, atrophy occurs when the stimulation or nutrition falls below that required to maintain the optimum number, size, and strength of the cells. The factors initiating atrophy may be physiological or pathological. As an adaptive mechanism atrophy permits cells to survive unfavorable conditions. The nurse through the practice of nursing can help to prevent atrophy by encouraging and assisting the patient to exercise, by preventing and relieving pressure, and by assisting the patient in maintaining his food intake.

How do cells adapt to an increase in nutrition and activity?

Just as cells have the capacity to adapt to lessened nutrition or strain by decreasing in size or number, they have the capacity to respond to an increase in nutrition and activity by an increase in size and/or in number of cells. The term "hypertrophy" is used to indicate an enlargement in the volume of parenchymal tissue. Hyperplasia denotes an increase in the number of cells. Whether cells undergo hypertrophy or hyperplasia depends in part on whether or not they are able to regenerate or reproduce themselves. Highly specialized cells, such as nerve, skeletal, and cardiac muscle, and, to a lesser extent, smooth muscle, do not proliferate and they thereby respond to stimulus for increased function by hypertrophy.

Both hypertrophy and hyperplasia are adaptive and they are beneficial when they enable the cell (organ) to meet increased demands for function. Furthermore, both are organized processes. Hopps[8] suggests that hypertrophy

---

[6] The relationship of the anterior pituitary to its target glands is essentially that of a system of negative feedbacks. The anterior pituitary produces a number of trophic (stimulating) hormones, each of which stimulates a specific endocrine gland. The gland so stimulated increases the secretion of its hormone. As the level of the hormone from the target gland rises, the secretion of the trophic hormone is depressed. The glands known to be under the control of the anterior pituitary are the adrenal cortex, the thyroid, and the gonads. The trophic hormones are ACTH (adrenocorticotrophic), TSH (thyrotrophic), and GSH (gonadotrophic). Some of the hormones secreted by the anterior pituitary, notably ACTH, have effects other than stimulation of target glands.

[7] Hopps, Op. cit., p. 174.

[8] Ibid., p. 175.

may be possible because the capacity of the cell for anabolism is greater than it generally uses. With a higher rate of anabolism there is an increase in the storage of materials in the cell and the cell becomes larger. In terms of function, hypertrophy increases the capacity of the cell to do work.

What is hyperplasia?

Hyperplasia, which involves the multiplication of cells, is a somewhat more complex process than hypertrophy. In hyperplasia two cells are derived from one cell. Hyperplasia is physiological. It occurs only in response to a need, the process is organized, and it is terminated when the need is met. Daughter cells are similar to those from which they derive, which means that they are differentiated. Hyperplasia is possible because cells have a built-in capacity to grow and to multiply.

The capacity of cells to undergo hypertrophy or hyperplasia varies greatly among different organs. Hopps[9] states that during pregnancy the muscle of the uterus may enlarge 100 times. The skeletal muscles and the myocardium increase their size by undergoing hypertrophy. The kidney and liver increase their size by undergoing both hypertrophy and hyperplasia.

What are some examples of hypertrophy? What purpose does hypertrophy serve in each of these?

There are many examples of hypertrophy. The bulging muscles of the wrestler or the weight lifter are examples of hypertrophy of skeletal muscles in response to increased work. The same adaptation may be observed in the person who has lost the function of his lower extremities and uses his arm and shoulder muscles as legs. Hypertrophy also enables the myocardium to move the blood against an increase in resistance such as is produced by stenosis of a heart valve or of the aorta or by arteriolar constriction in essential hypertension. These disorders are examples of adaptations to a pathological process enabling the organism to survive. Unfortunately, the capacity of the individual to nourish the increase in muscle tissue may not keep pace with the increase in size. Eventually the muscle becomes ischemic and fails.

Smooth muscle also undergoes hypertrophy when its work is increased. For example, as a result of hyperplasia of the prostate gland, the urethra is obstructed and resistance to the flow of urine is increased. The smooth muscle of the urinary bladder wall responds by increasing the size of the muscle fibers. For a time this results in a sufficient increase in force to move the urine through the narrowed urethra. In time, the bladder wall may reach several times its normal thickness. The capacity to undergo hypertrophy is adaptive. In this instance, the stimulus to hypertrophy is pathological. Hypertrophy of the pyloric muscle, with a narrowing or stenosis of the outlet of the stomach, occurs in infants of two to three weeks of age. The condition is usually of

[9] *Ibid.*, p. 177.

congenital origin. The infant manifests projectile vomiting, rapid loss of weight, and constipation or obstipation.

Hypertrophy can be expected to develop in any muscle in which the muscle is called upon to increase its work over that which it normally does. Hypertrophy is adaptive inasmuch as it enables the organ to perform a greater amount of work, but it is maladaptive when it narrows the lumen of a tube.

Hyperplasia and hypertrophy may occur together. Following the removal of one kidney, the other one enlarges. The enlargement is due to a combination of an increase in the size of the tubules and an increase in the number of cells lining them. The capacity of the bone marrow, the lymphoid tissue, and the reticuloendothelial tissue to undergo hyperplasia enables the organism to cope with infection, restore blood cells after blood loss or abnormal destruction of blood cells, and adapt to living at high altitudes.

The extent to which any organ or tissue can respond to a stimulus for an increase in function is limited. One of the factors in this limitation is the capacity of the body to increase the blood supply in proportion to the increase in the amount of tissue. To illustrate, hypertrophy of the myocardium is limited by the capacity of the coronary arteries to provide a supply of blood adequate to its needs. The increase in blood demands an increased supply of nutrients. Moreover, as the heart muscle enlarges, it may cause pressure against the small vessels and thereby decrease circulation. The consequence is an ischemic heart muscle, and, eventually, failure. In summary, hypertrophy and hyperplasia are adaptive responses to an increase in stimulation which may be either pathological or physiological. As a consequence of these responses an organ or part can increase the amount of work it performs. Without this adaptive capacity, life would be greatly shortened by many diseases and would not be possible in some environments.

What mechanism available to epithelial cells enables them to adapt to adverse environmental conditions?

Besides being able to adapt to environmental conditions by increasing the size and/or number of cells, some types of cells are also able to adapt by a process known as metaplasia. In metaplasia one type of tissue is changed to another type. Metaplasia involves two factors. First, the tissue must contain incompletely differentiated cells that have the potential for maturing into different types of cells. Second, the environment of the cells must be unfavorable to the type of cell normally found in the tissue. For example, the different types of epithelial tissues have their origin in a common cell, the basal cell. When conditions are unfavorable to a given type of epithelial tissue, it is transformed to another type that is better suited to the particular environmental conditions. The type of epithelial tissue that usually replaces other types is squamous cell epithelium. Conditions predisposing to epithelial cell metaplasia include chronic irritation by physical and chemical agents, certain vitamin deficiencies, and direct exposure of a mucous membrane to the external environment. For example, the mucous membrane in the trachea undergoes a transformation to squamous cell epithelium following a tracheostomy. The capacity to undergo metaplasia enables the cell or tissue to survive unfavorable conditions.

In addition to hyperplasia and metaplasia, what other alterations in growth sometimes occur?

Whereas hyperplasia enables the individual to adapt to a loss of cells by increasing the number and metaplasia enables cells to survive unfavorable conditions, cells may for a variety of reasons fail to develop or they may lose their capacity to proliferate. The failure of an organ or tissue to develop in the embryo is known as agenesis. Literally translated, "agenesis" means "without beginning." Occasionally an individual is born with only one of a pair of organs such as the kidney. This individual may very well live a normal life span. However, when neither kidney develops, life after birth is shortened to a few days or weeks. Agenesis of any organ is, of course, a possibility. When the organ is one that is essential to life, death occurs at or before birth.

The functional or reserve capacity of a tissue or organ may be inadequate either because of failure to develop sufficient tissue or because the tissue is destroyed by an injurious agent. This condition is known as aplasia (the adjective is aplastic), which means "without formation." A lesser degree of aplasia, in that some tissue is present, is hypoplasia. In hypoplasia, the amount of tissue is insufficient to meet the functional requirements of the body. For example, as a consequence of failure to develop or as a result of exposure to toxic agents, the bone marrow may be aplastic or hypoplastic. A child may be born with aplastic or hypoplastic bone marrow. He may develop a disease or be exposed to an environmental condition causing partial or complete destruction of the bone marrow. There are many agents capable of injuring bone marrow. Among them are X rays and radioactive materials and bone marrow poisons such as benzene. Evidence of an aplastic or hypoplastic bone marrow can be obtained from low blood cell counts and from biopsy of the bone marrow. As a consequence of hypoplasia, the individual not only is unable to adapt to conditions which require an increase in the number of blood cells, but may not be able to manufacture enough cells to meet his ordinary needs. The person whose bone marrow is aplastic can do neither. The capacity of the organism to adapt throughout life may be reduced by failure to develop an organ or structure, or by loss of the functional capacity of tissues.

Summary

The normal cell has the capacity to adapt to increased or decreased supply of materials or stimulation, by increasing its size and strength (hypertrophy) or by decreasing its size and strength (atrophy). The integrity of the structure is further protected by the capacity of some cells to proliferate (multiply) and to undergo hyperplasia. Certain cells have an additional power to protect themselves. They are able to differentiate into a type of cell better suited to the environmental conditions to which it is exposed. Failure of cells to proliferate whether owing to a low growth potential or to a deficiency or absence of tissue robs the individual of an important means of defending himself against cell injury.

What are some of the consequences of failure of the intracellular machinery?

Though alterations in supply or conditions to which the cell is exposed may be responsible for changes in cell structure and function, the machinery by which the cell utilizes nutrients may fail. The supply of materials required by the cell may be quite adequate, but the cell is unable to utilize them in a normal manner. This failure may result from: (1) the lack of an enzyme which catalyzes an essential step in the use of a nutrient (the lack of the enzyme may result from a defective gene), (2) the toxic effect of a chemical or bacterial poison on an enzyme or enzyme system, or (3) the effect of physical agents such as heat, cold, or radioactive materials on cellular machinery. When a cell is unable to utilize nutrients in a normal manner, the outcome depends on a number of factors. These include the nature and intensity of the injuring agent, the period of time over which the cell is exposed to the injuring agent, and the condition of the cell itself at the time of the injury. Depending on the interaction of these factors, the injured cell may recover fully, be crippled, or die.

Since these conditions are associated with a deterioration in the activities within the cell, and hence with its ability to function, they are called degenerations. In the various forms of degeneration, different substances accumulate within the cells. In some types of degeneration the name is descriptive of the substance that accumulates within the cell. In others, it is descriptive of the appearance of the cell. Thus, in fatty degeneration, fat accumulates within the cell. In cloudy swelling, changes take place that, as the name suggests, cause it to appear cloudy instead of clear.

Healthy cells may also be damaged by being overloaded with metabolites such as glucose or fat; the resulting condition is known as an infiltration. In degeneration and infiltration the cell is damaged. The specific effect depends on the tissue that is injured. Hopps[10] states that the sequence of events that follow cellular injury is as follows: first, the chemical activity within the cell is altered; next, cellular function is impaired; finally, the structure of the cell is altered. In sudden and overwhelming injuries there may be less structural change than in those that are of long standing. Knowledge of this fact is

[10] *Ibid.*, p. 82.

utilized when tissue is prepared for microscopic examination. It is quickly frozen or treated in such a way that structural changes are minimized. When the structure of the tissue and cells is preserved, the comparison made between it and so-called normal cells is meaningful. When a degenerative process is terminated during the phase in which cellular activity or cellular function is altered, it may be reversed and the cell restored to normal. This presupposes, of course, that the changes do not overwhelm the cellular enzymes, especially those in sensitive tissues, beyond the point of recovery. Once structural changes occur, the cell goes on to necrosis. When there are blood vessels, blood cells, and connective tissues in the area of the necrotic cells, they respond with inflammation.

What are some of the factors influencing the signs and symptoms developing after cells are injured?

The signs and symptoms accompanying cellular injury depend on the degree of injury to cells as well as the extent of injury. They are modified by the nature of the injuring agent. The signs and symptoms are, however, those that result from (1) the inflammatory response (see Chapter 5), (2) the effect of the injury on the tissues or organ, (3) disturbances that are secondary to those induced either by the inflammatory response or by the disturbances in function of the injured organ, and (4) the total body response to the injury.

Students who are interested in a more complete discussion of the various degenerations and infiltrations should consult a textbook on pathology.

What terms are used to indicate death of cells due to injury? Distinguish among them!

In those conditions in which cellular injury is sufficiently great or prolonged, death of the cell occurs. Throughout the course of life, body cells die and are replaced. For example, epithelial cells of the skin and mucous membranes, as well as blood cells, mature, live out their life span, and die. However, when a group of cells die not as a result of aging, but from some injury, the condition is known as necrosis. "Necrosis" is a general term denoting death of cells. Terms such as "gangrene" and "infarction" also imply death of cells, but have more specific meanings. Gangrene is ordinarily used to indicate the death of a large section of an organ or an entire organ or part. This term is frequently applied to a necrotic section of the bowel, to the appendix or gall bladder, or to an extremity such as a hand or leg.

Gangrene may be classified as wet or dry. Wet gangrene develops in those conditions in which there is fluid in the tissue. It is often associated with disorders in which there is an obstruction of the venous return from a tissue or organ. The explanation is as follows. Because venous pressure is relatively low in comparison to arterial pressure, veins are more easily obstructed than are arteries. With obstruction of the flow of blood through the vein, blood is prevented from leaving the part. For a time, the arteries supplying the part continue to deliver blood. The combination of obstruction of venous return and continued arterial blood flow results in an elevation of the filtration pressure of the blood in the capillaries. Fluid accumulates in the interstitial space, which further obstructs the venous return and interferes with lymphatic drainage. A vicious circle is initiated. As the venous pressure rises, filtration pressure also rises. This further adds to imbalance between the quantity of fluid leaving the vascular system and returning to it and leads to swelling. Eventually, tissue fluid pressure may equal the filtration pressure, and the blood flow to the area ceases. Venous stasis plus the diminishing arterial circulation to the tissues favors bacterial growth. With the growth of bacteria, tissues are liquefied and putrefaction occurs. As the products of bacterial growth and the necrotic tissue are absorbed, the patient becomes toxic. Inflammation with its signs and symptoms develops in the area adjacent to the necrotic tissue. Tissues in a confined space are particularly susceptible to wet gangrene such as in the patient who has an extremity encased in a cast or a circular bandage. He should be regularly and frequently observed for signs and symptoms indicating obstruction to the venous return, that is, for swelling, coldness, cyanosis or pallor, numbness and tingling, and failure to be able to move exposed fingers or toes. Because the wall of the cast is rigid, even moderate swelling may obstruct the venous return, and unless the condition is corrected, necrosis of tissue will result. This is also a danger to the patient with an abdominal hernia. A loop of intestine may be tightly caught in a hernial ring. This leads to obstruction of the venous return, and, unless treated immediately, to gangrene of the section of trapped bowel.

In dry gangrene, death of tissue results from obstruction of the arterial circulation. As a consequence, the tissue becomes dehydrated and shriveled. It is blackened and mummified in appearance. The area of dead tissue is usually clearly demarcated from the living tissue by a red zone of granulation tissue.

The term "infarct" is used to indicate a localized area of necrosis that results when the blood supply to an area falls below the ability of cells to tolerate it. Infarction may therefore result from the obstruction of an artery at a point where both the main blood supply and the collateral circulation are blocked. It may also occur when tissue requirements are raised above the capacity of diseased vessels to deliver blood. Although an infarction may occur in any tissue, those that require a large supply of blood and/or have a poor collateral circulation are particularly vulnerable. Organs in which infarctions are commonly found are the brain, heart, and kidney.

The consequences of an infarction depend on its location and extent. A large infarct in a vital organ such as the heart, lung, or brain may be responsible for sudden death. When the area that is infarcted is small enough for the function of the organ to be maintained, it may be healed by fibrous tissue substitution, that is, by the formation of scar tissue. Residual effects will depend on its size and location. The reserve capacity of the organ will, however, be reduced in proportion to the amount of loss of parenchymal tissue.

One point that cannot be overemphasized is that when the supply of blood to a tissue falls below a certain critical level in relation to the tissue's requirements for nutrients, death of cells occurs. The failure of blood supply is not always sufficient to cause death of cells. When the arteries supplying the area are only partly obstructed and/or the collateral circulation is sufficient to maintain life, the quantity of blood delivered to the tissue may be sufficient to meet its needs under some, but not all, circumstances. Tissues in which less blood is supplied than is required for full nutrition are said to be ischemic. In ischemia, there is a localized area of anoxia as a result of a deficiency in the arterial blood supply. Under some circumstances, sufficient blood is delivered to maintain life at rest or under limited activity, but not enough for the cells to adapt to all demands made upon them. Ischemia can be the result of any disorder that reduces the quantity or quality of blood being delivered to a tissue. Hypotension and anemia cause generalized ischemia of tissues. Occlusion of blood vessels, either external or internal, is more likely to cause localized ischemia. Tissues having double blood supply, or an adequate collateral circulation, may be ischemic rather than infarcted on occlusion of an artery supplying the area. In ischemia, tissue nutrition is adequate to sustain life, but insufficient to enable the tissue to adapt to all demands that may be made on it. The effects of ischemia depend on the degree to which the arterial blood supply is adequate to maintain tissue nutrition. Tissues may receive only enough blood to sustain life of the cells at rest, or the quantity of blood may be sufficient to sustain ordinary activities. Evidence of ischemia occurs only when unusual demands are placed on the tissue. For example the quantity of blood to the heart muscle may be so greatly reduced that any increase in activity induces pain. It may, on the other hand, be adequate unless the individual runs, lifts heavy weights, or becomes angry.

What are some of the causes of failure of arteries to deliver blood to tissues?

Since arteries deliver blood to tissues, any interference with the capacity of arteries to carry blood reduces the supply of blood delivered to the tissue. A reduction in blood supplied to tissues may result from abnormal constriction of an artery or arteries or from occlusion by disease. For example, in Raynaud's disease, arteries supplying the hands and/or the feet respond to cold or to other stimuli by constricting so greatly that no blood can pass through them to the tissue. As a consequence, the involved areas are blanched and painful. Since the attack is brief, tissue necrosis seldom occurs. Small areas of ulceration of the skin sometimes do develop. The frequency of attacks can be reduced by preventing exposure to inciting agents, such as cold.

A frequent cause of occlusive disease of arteries is atherosclerosis. Ischemia results as the capacity of the artery to deliver blood falls below the needs of the tissues. Diseased arteries cannot respond to an increase in the needs of cells for nutrients by dilating and thereby augmenting the flow of blood. The degree of ischemia is raised by any condition that increases cellular activity. Examples include exercise or elevation in the temperature of the part.

What are the causes of ischemia?

Ischemia results from any condition that prevents the organism from supplying tissues with nutrients and oxygen in required amounts. It usually involves some interference with the delivery of blood to tissues or in the capacity to increase blood supply in proportion to an increase in tissue requirements. Though the term is commonly used to indicate localized areas of tissue anoxia, hypotension is accompanied by generalized ischemia. Ischemia is therefore one of the serious consequences of shock.

Localized ischemia can be of extrinsic or intrinsic origin. Any condition that exerts pressure on blood vessels is capable of limiting their capacity to deliver blood. Common causes include prolonged sitting, the resting of a part of the body, particularly over bony prominences, against a firm surface, and casts and bandages that are too tight. Swelling of tissues, as the result of either edema or inflammation, reduces the capacity of vessels to carry blood. The effects of swelling develop more rapidly in solid tissue or those surrounded by a nonexpansible wall such as a cast or the skull. As explained earlier, any increase in tension in tissues lessens the capacity of veins to carry blood and therefore interferes with the removal of fluids from the area. Unless corrected, this leads to a decrease or even an interruption of arterial blood supply to the tissue. Neoplasms may also cause ischemia by pressing on either arteries or veins. Changes in the function or structure of blood vessels are frequent causes of ischemia. Veins and/or arteries may be implicated.

What are the effects of ischemia on tissue? What are some of the conditions modifying its effects?

Although marked and prolonged ischemia can be anticipated to lead to the death of cells, cells differ greatly in their capacity to tolerate undernutrition. The type of cell and the suddenness with which ischemia develops also influence the outcome. Cells maintaining a high metabolic rate, such as those in the brain and kidney, tolerate ischemia poorly. Cells adapt to slowly developing ischemia by reducing their metabolic rate and cellular substance; that is, they atrophy. This adaptation is successful *only* as long as the tissue nutrition is maintained at a level high enough to sustain the life of the cells and the cells are not stimulated to function beyond this point. Tissues rendered ischemic by one cause have a smaller tolerance for other ischemia-inducing conditions than do normal tissues. For example, Mr. Brown, who has occlusive vascular disease involving the arteries in his legs, is more susceptible to the effects of pressure on his heels than is his roommate, who has healthy arteries. When death of cells does occur, continuity of structure may be maintained by the formation of scar tissue. With the loss of parenchymatous cells, the reserve capacity of the organ is reduced and with it the capacity to adapt to changes in the environment.

Although ischemia is a factor in many illnesses, its effects on the skin and on muscle will be discussed at this time. Ischemia of the skin may result from a single or multiple causes. Whatever the etiology, it acts to cause a localized tissue anoxia. As stated earlier, external pressure on the skin, occlusive arterial disease, and failure of venous return are common causes. Generalized undernutrition, particularly of protein and ascorbic acid, increases the susceptibility to ischemia. For reasons not completely understood, tissues deprived of their sensory nerve supply have increased susceptibility to ischemia. Since the sensory nerve supply to the tissue is part of the warning system, its loss diminishes the capacity of the individual to detect and evaluate threats of injury to the tissue. For example, Mr. Book is paraplegic due to transection (severing) of the spinal cord. He is unable to feel anything below the level of his waist. He is unable to feel crumbs or wrinkles in his bed, the pressure of the bed covering or a brace, or the heat of a hot-water bottle. He is therefore unable to detect or to evaluate threats to the tissues below his waist. A loss in the sensory nerve supply to the skin may possibly interfere with reflex regulation of the diameter of arteries in relation to the needs of the tissue for blood. Another cause of ischemia is edema of the skin, which creates external pressure on blood vessels. Edema also renders the tissue more susceptible to ischemia from other causes.

Knowledge of factors contributing to ischemia of the skin is useful in the identification of patients who are susceptible to breakdown of peripheral tissues. There is evidence that some decubiti have their origin in deep tissues and that the breakdown of the skin occurs relatively late. To be effective, protective measures should be instituted before local evidence of tissue ischemia develops. The responsibility of the nurse in the prevention of ischemia and necrosis of skin includes the following activities: (1) provisions to limit or relieve pressure on susceptible tissue; (2) observation for signs and symptoms of impaired circulation and prompt introduction of measures for their relief; (3) attention to the patient's intake of food, with particular attention to protein and ascorbic acid intake; and (4) special attention (a) to undernourished and elderly patients, (b) to persons who are deprived of their sensory nerve supply, (c) to patients with extremities encased in casts or bandages, (d) to patients with edema of the sacrum, buttocks, or extremities, and (e) to unconscious patients. Measures to prevent excessive swelling, as well as observation for signs and symptoms indicating that circulation is impaired, have been previously emphasized.

As a basis for observing the patient, the signs and symptoms associated with ischemia of the skin vary with the cause and the suddenness with which it develops. Acute obstruction of the arterial circulation shuts off the blood supply to the tissue. When the venous return is adequate, the tissue becomes pale and cold, and pain is experienced in the area. Tissue breakdown follows unless the condition is rapidly corrected. When the venous return is obstructed, blood is delivered to the tissue, but is not removed. As has been previously stated, in arterial obstruction the problem is one of supply. In venous obstruction, it is one of pickup and return. In venous obstruction or insufficiency, the blood remains in the tissue longer than is normal. The hemoglobin loses its oxygen, the quantity of reduced hemoglobin in the area is increased, and the tissue takes on a bluish tinge, or is cyanotic. The increase in filtration pressure that accompanies venous obstruction increases the amount of fluid in the interstitial space and causes swelling. Pressure on sensory nerve fibers may cause numbness and tingling. Edema of the sacrum and buttocks should be regarded as evidence that the tissues in these areas are ischemic. In areas such as the buttocks, or over the heels and elbows, there may be a mild inflammatory response with reddening of the skin at the periphery of the area. For the patient who, by the nature of his illness or its treatment, is predisposed to ischemia of the skin and underlying tissues, a program of prevention of breakdown of tissues subjected to pressure should be instituted as early as possible.

What can the nurse do for the patient who presents signs and symptoms of tissue undernutrition?

Here, as in many areas, a few minutes devoted to prevention, when continued regularly, are worth days, weeks, or even months of cure. Once the skin breaks down, the first line of defense of the body is disrupted, and bacteria have a portal of entry. The situation may be further aggravated by the loss of tissue nutrients from the area.

The effects of pressure on the buttocks, sacrum, heels, elbows, and even the back of the head can be minimized by turning the patient regularly and by using devices that alter or distribute the weight of the body over a wide area. One device that, in the opinion of the writer, should be discarded is the doughnut. Though it relieves pressure on the tissue over the hole of the doughnut, pressure is concentrated on the tissues coming in contact with the doughnut. The purpose of pressure-relieving devices should be to remove all pressure or to distribute pressure evenly over a wide area. As an illustration, when a doughnut is placed under the heel, pressure on the center of the heel is relieved, but it is concentrated where the heel rests on the doughnut. The heels are much more effectively protected by placing a pad, a sheep pelt, or a thin pillow under the legs, just raising the heels from the bed. Care should be taken to prevent a ridge from pressing the tissue proximal to the heel. Provided the support extends far enough up the lower leg, preferably to the popliteal space, the broad surface on which the legs rest tends to distribute the weight of the legs and feet over a wide area and prevents the concentration of pressure at any one point. Unless the pressure-relieving device accomplishes this function, it is of little or no value. Furthermore, no one device should be depended upon to take the place of a regular program of moving and turning the patient. Pieces of sheepskin, or the newer synthetic substitute which is said to be less expensive, with the wool side toward the skin may be placed under the heels or for the patient to sit on. Sheepskin has a number of advantages. Since the body of the patient rests on the wool side, it not only acts as a cushion, but it contains oils that help to prevent excessive drying of the skin. The skin does not adhere to the wool as it does to cotton sheeting and this reduces the chances of injury to skin. Sheepskin is cooler than cotton over rubber or plastic sheeting. Since the requirements of cells for nutrients is increased with a rise in temperature, any device that prevents minimizing the rise in the temperature of the tissue contributes not only to the comfort of the patient, but to the protection of ischemic cells. Absorption of moisture by the wool helps to protect the skin from dampness. Sheepskin has a further advantage. It can be washed and reused and its initial cost is low.

Similar measures can be used to protect the buttocks and sacrum from the effects of pressure. In addition to those mentioned, an alternating pressure mattress is helpful. Turning frames render changing the position of the helpless patient relatively easy. However, whatever methods are used, their effectiveness depends on the nurse's identifying those patients who are most likely to tolerate pressure poorly or whose condition makes ischemia a real possibility. Since ischemia is only one factor in tissue breakdown, all conditions predisposing to it must also be identified and controlled. A program of care, planned to prevent the breakdown of the skin and underlying tissues, should include, in addition to procedures directed toward the prevention and relief of pressure, the following: (1) measures to keep the skin clean and dry, (2) bladder training and, if necessary to keep the patient dry, an external catheter such as a condom, (3) an optimum intake of food, and (4) prevention of tissue edema.

Ischemia of muscle is frequently the result of a partial or complete occlusion of an artery or arteries. The most marked manifestation in acute ischemia is pain. Although a lack of oxygen to the tissues may be responsible for the pain, just why pain occurs is not completely clear. There is, however, no doubt about the reality of pain. When occlusion is complete, the pain continues for a day or two and then subsides. When the ischemia is relative rather than absolute, the pain is initiated by any condition increasing the need of the muscle for oxygen or food. This can be physical exercise, such as walking or running, or it can be an emotional state, such as anger or fear. The pain is relieved by rest. The ease with which the pain is precipitated depends on a number of factors, one being the degree to which the circulation to the tissue is compromised. When the pain occurs in an extremity, it is sometimes referred to as claudication. When the myocardium is involved, the condition is known as angina pectoris. The basis for the pain is the same in both instances. Arteries supplying the muscle of the heart or the extremities are unable to adapt the supply of blood to the requirement of the tissues for nutrition.

When the ischemia of the muscle is complete, death of tissue or infarction occurs. The pain that follows the sudden obstruction of an artery supplying a muscle is variously described by patients as being boring, crushing, clamplike, or cramping. Unlike the pain induced by activity in the patient with a relative ischemia of a muscle, it is not relieved by rest. Necrosis of muscle and associated tissues ensues. The extent of the necrosis and the outcome will depend, of course, on the amount of tissue that is deprived of its blood supply and the adequacy of the collateral circulation. The symptoms and signs include those of inflammation—both general and local—and those arising from the effect the injury has on the affected organ. The general signs and symptoms, such as fever, leukocytosis, and increased sedimentation rate, usually start about the second day and continue for two or three days. Prolongation beyond this time usually indicates that complications are developing.

The responsibilities of the nurse in the care of patients with the occlusion of arteries supplying various organs will be considered later. However, these patients have a reduction in their capacity to adapt the supply of blood to the needs of the ischemic tissue. With impaired blood supply the tissue is susceptible to necrosis. Therefore, the tissue should be protected from conditions that increase its nutritional requirements. Any alteration in the activity in a tissue, whatever the cause, changes the need of the tissue for oxygen and nutrients. In general, inasmuch as is possible, ischemic tissues should be protected from conditions that place increased demands on them. When possible, measures to increase the flow of blood are instituted.

What are some of the effects of trauma on tissues?

In addition to ischemia, physical agents are one of the most common causes of cellular necrosis. They include a variety of agents—trauma, extremes of temperature, electricity, and radioactive rays. Although trauma is used to denote any type of agent that produces emotional or physical shock, it is used here to indicate a physical force. Trauma is capable of causing all degrees of tissue injury from relatively minor abrasions to crushing or disrupting of the continuity of tissues. Abrasions are lesions that result from the scraping of epithelial cells from the skin or mucous membrane by friction. They are produced by pulling or pushing the abraded area over a rough surface. The skinned knee of the child who falls on a sidewalk is an example. Abrasions of the skin can be caused by pulling a sheet from underneath a patient without lifting or turning him. The same effect can be produced by pulling (dragging) a patient over sheets when moving him. Obese or heavy comatose patients who are difficult to move and turn are most likely to suffer this treatment. Besides causing unnecessary discomfort, an abrasion robs the patient of one of his primary barriers to infection, that is, intact skin. In the care of the patient, attention should be given to the protection of the skin and mucous membranes from ill-advised friction, by rolling or lifting the patient as dictated by his condition and needs.

Injury to deeper layers of tissue is termed a "contusion" or "bruise." Contusions are caused by the application of force to tissue, thereby causing injury to the underlying structures. Contusion frequently results from striking a part of the body against a hard object such as a table or chair. In a contusion there may be extensive damage to soft tissues, including blood vessels, with subsequent bleeding into the tissues. The surface layer of skin or mucous membrane may or may not be ruptured. Particularly in debilitated patients, a bruised area may serve as the site favorable to the growth of pathogenic bacteria. Free blood in the tissues provides food for their growth, and swelling interferes with the body's ability to increase the number of leukocytes in the area. In all individuals, blood escaping into the soft tissue acts as a foreign body and induces an inflammatory response. Pain on pressure or movement of the tissue is usual.

In traumatic injuries involving the skull, the brain may be contused or bruised. Contusions of the brain occur even in the absence of skull fractures. The bleeding may create further injury by increasing intracranial pressure. Sometimes the volume of blood escaping from the blood vessels is insufficient to cause a significant increase in intracranial pressure, but the clot that forms attracts and holds water. Venous bleeding is likely to increase intracranial pressure more slowly than does arterial bleeding. Bleeding into the space between the dura and the skull also takes time to increase intracranial pressure. (See Chapter 13, Part B.) The dura is tough and resists separation from the skull. Days or weeks may elapse after the injury before signs of increased intracranial pressure are seen. An injury that is unique to the brain is that of the so-called "contrecoup," in which the bruise occurs at a site other than at the point at which the skull suffers trauma. A contrecoup injury is most likely to occur when the body has been in motion at the moment of injury and the head is brought to an abrupt stop by the injuring force. As an example, a contrecoup injury may occur when the head strikes the windshield in an automobile accident. The same type of injury may result from a fall. The course of events in the development of a contrecoup injury can be simulated by taking a full pail of water and walking rapidly—a sudden stop will cause the water to splash. Emergency-room nurses, as well as those caring for patients who have suffered head injuries, should be alert to the possibility that the brain has been bruised despite absence of obvious injury to the scalp or skull. Location of the site of injury depends on careful observation of the signs and symptoms presented by the patient. Changes in level of consciousness and of vital signs should be reported without delay. Because the brain is susceptible to edema after it is shaken (concussion) or bruised, the patient should be encouraged to lie quietly, and care should be taken to protect the head from jarring or sudden movements.

Lacerations, injuries in which there is a disruption of the surface-layer tissue, may also result from trauma. Lacerations not only disrupt natural defenses, but may be accompanied by contusions and bleeding. Attention should be paid to minimizing the contamination of the wound, and, if necessary, to controlling the bleeding. The wound may be contaminated with one or more microorganisms, including *Clostridium perfringens (B. welchii)* and *Clostridium tetani.*

Both *Clostridium tetani* and *Clostridium perfringens (B. welchii),* and other types of clostridia, are widespread in nature. Since they form spores, they are protected against unfavorable environmental conditions such as drying and change in temperature. They are anaerobic and grow on devitalized tissues. Once *Clostridium tetani* or *perfringens* is able to establish itself in a tissue and elaborate its toxin, it is able to maintain the conditions necessary to its growth. *Clostridium perfringens* and other gas-forming organisms cause extensive damage at the site at which they enter the tissue. Gas in the tissues is not always due to the clostridia, however, for certain other bacteria, notably gas-forming strains of *E. coli,* also may be responsible. In order to prevent conditions that favor the growth of these microorganisms, accidentally incurred wounds should be thoroughly cleansed and débrided of foreign bodies and necrotic tissue. In addition, many physicians believe that persons who have not been previously immunized against tetanus should receive tetanus antitoxin. There is, however, considerable debate at present over whether or not all people with accidentally incurred lacerations should receive tetanus antitoxin. Since tetanus antitoxin is contained in horse serum, individuals who are to receive it should be tested for sensitivity previous to its administration. Tetanus toxoid has been demonstrated to be effective in establishing an active immunity. Like other antigens, tetanus toxoid takes time to produce immunity. Since injuries in which tetanus is a possibility are common, immunization with tetanus toxoid is included in most immunization programs. Booster doses at regular intervals are necessary to keep up the level of immunity.

Unlike tetanus, there is at this time no effective way to protect individuals from gas gangrene by either active or passive immunization. Protection depends primarily on thorough cleansing and débridement of the wound. Sometimes despite thorough cleansing of the wound, gas gangrene develops. According to Hook,[11] the usual incubation period is from one to four days, though the range is from six hours to six weeks. The onset of gas gangrene is often heralded by a severe pain in the affected part. It also is accompanied by a sweetish, foul odor. Bubbles of gas may be seen in the drainage from the wound. Since gas gangrene progresses rapidly, the area around the wound should be inspected regularly. Though this is usually done by the physician, the nurse should be alert to symptoms and signs such as pain in the injured part and the characteristic odor, both of which indicate the possible development of gas gangrene. The physician should be notified promptly, as the life

[11] Edward W. Hook, "Other Clostridial Infections," *Principles of Internal Medicine,* 4th ed., eds. T. R. Harrison *et al.,* McGraw-Hill Book Co., New York, 1962, p. 996.

or limb of a patient may depend on the promptness with which treatment is instituted.

To summarize, trauma injures tissue by removing surface cells, by crushing tissues, including blood vessels, and by disrupting the continuity of tissue. The terms used to indicate the type of injury resulting from trauma are, respectively, "abrasion," "contusion," and "laceration." Trauma predisposes to further ill effects by disrupting the body's first line of defense against microorganisms: the intact skin and mucous membranes. By devitalizing tissues it renders them liable to infection by one or more types of clostridia. Prevention of infections by these organisms can usually be accomplished by passive and active immunization against *Clostridium tetani* and by thorough cleansing and débridement of the wound.

How do extremes in temperature injure tissues?

A second physical agent causing cellular (tissue) injury is a low temperature, or cold. According to Hopps,[12] healthy tissues can survive the gradual reduction of body temperature to 20° C. (68° F.). This, of course, refers to the temperature within cells and not the temperature of the external environment. Hypothermia has many interesting aspects, including the profound metabolic acidosis that occurs regularly and physiological hypotension. Esophageal temperatures below 78° F. are associated with an extremely poor prognosis. When tissue is actually frozen, further injury is caused by the formation of ice crystals. Exposure to moist cold over a long period of time damages capillary endothelium and increases its permeability. As fluid leaks into the tissues, the erythrocytes are concentrated in the capillaries with the result that they tend to pack in clumps and obstruct the flow of blood. When these changes occur in the feet, the condition is known as immersion or trenchfoot. Trenchfoot was a serious problem during World War II, as the men were exposed to cold, damp weather for extended periods of time. Although the men had waterproof boots, their feet were kept in a dampened condition by their tendency to perspire. Because the external environment was cold, their feet were both damp and cold, and the capillaries of the feet were injured, with the consequences described above. During the Korean conflict a new type of boot that was developed in Iceland was used to protect the feet.

Just as there are lower limits to temperatures which are tolerated by cells, there are also upper limits. Robbins[13] states that the range varies from 30° to 45° C. (88° to 115° F.). Hopps[14] states that temperatures over 108.5° F. are tolerated by tissues for only a short time. Though tissue damage may not be evident immediately, this does not necessarily mean that tissue has not been injured. Evidence may appear later. Just how heat damages the tissue is

---

[12] *Op. cit.,* p. 80.
[13] Stanley L. Robbins, *Textbook of Pathology with Clinical Applications,* W. B. Saunders Company, Philadelphia, 1957, p. 8.
[14] *Op. cit.,* p. 92.

not fully understood. A principle of chemistry applying to the effect of temperature on the tissue is that the speed of chemical reaction is directly proportional to the temperature. Chemical reactions proceed more rapidly at higher temperatures than they do at lower temperatures. This principle applies to reactions catalyzed by enzymes as well as to those in test tubes. With each degree of temperature elevation, the metabolic rate goes up approximately 7 per cent. Hypermetabolism may be accompanied by the accumulation of acid metabolites in the cells and by a relative anoxia and lack of nutrients to support metabolism. Another explanation is that since enzymes are protein in nature, they, like other proteins, are inactivated by excessive heat. Tissue proteins may also be coagulated. The fact that arteriosclerotic tissue tolerates increases in temperature poorly may be the result of the inability to supply nutrients and oxygen in amounts needed by the tissue. Because tissues can be and are injured by heat, the nurse should protect the patient from injury by being certain that applications of heat are within the tolerance of the tissues. Individuals who are fully conscious and whose sensory nerve and blood supply are adequate are less likely to be injured than persons who have a deficit in either nerve or blood supply. All patients should, however, be protected from the danger of burning. Patients whose arterial circulation is impaired should be protected from temperatures that are harmless to persons with a normal circulation. (See Chapter 9.)

Thermal burns are one of the important and common causes of injury to tissue. Few persons escape minor burns from time to time. Serious burns are one of the most difficult types of injury to treat successfully. Burning is the second most frequent cause of accidents occurring in the home and the fourth most frequent cause of injury.[15] Moyer[16] estimates that approximately 6,000 hospital beds are occupied the year around by persons who have been scalded or burned. Burns were responsible for approximately one third of the deaths at Hiroshima. Because of the high incidence of burning among children, burn centers are being established in the United States for the care of children who have been burned. According to some estimates at least one half of the burn injuries could be prevented by reasonable care. In the year 1963 72 persons living in one large city died as a result of burns. Thirty-nine of the deaths were due to careless smoking. Eighteen of the victims were children under six years of age. Thirteen of them had been playing with matches. Twelve persons were burned in fires resulting from drying clothing too close to a heater. This report does not include other causes of burning nor does it include the number of persons who, though burned, recover. Some of these individuals spend months in the hospital before they recover. Among other incidents in which carelessness or a lack of reasonable foresight resulted in

[15] *Vital Statistics,* Special Reports, Volume 44, No. 1, February 29, 1956.
[16] Henry N. Harkins, Carl A. Moyer, Jonathan E. Rhodes, and J. Garrott Allen, *Surgery, Principles and Practice,* 2nd ed., J. B. Lippincott Co., Philadelphia, 1961, p. 304.

serious burns are the following: A small child is scalded by pulling on the handle of a pan containing boiling water. A woman wearing a loose-sleeved negligee reaches over a lighted stove. A child or an adult steps into a tub of scalding water. An entire family dies in a fire having its origin in defective wiring. A 14-year-old boy is seriously burned in a fire started by the throwing of gasoline on smoldering rubbish.

How are thermal burns classified?

Over the course of history a variety of classifications have been employed to express the extent of tissue damage resulting from burns. The most recent classification is simply: (1) partial-thickness injury to the skin and (2) full-thickness injury to the skin. The older classification identifies burns by degrees of injury: first-degree burns—erythema; second-degree burns—death of the epidermis, with the appendages of the epidermis remaining viable in the dermis; third-degree burns—death not only of the epidermis, but of its appendages in the dermis; and fourth-degree burns—charring or carbonification of the skin.[17] First- and second-degree burns are partial-thickness burns. Third- and fourth-degree burns are full-thickness. The seriousness of a thermal burn depends not only on the depth of the burn, but on its extent.

Electricity causes cellular injury in a variety of ways. It may produce cellular necrosis by direct coagulation of proteins and by changes in the polarity of cells which result in an increase in their permeability. Furthermore, resistance to the passage of the electric current through a tissue results in the production of heat which has the same effect on the tissue as any other heat. The fact that the tissues are heated as the electric current passes through them is the basis for the use of diathermy. Depending on how the electric current is distributed through the tissue, diathermy may either heat a tissue or destroy it. In either instance a high-frequency alternating current is passed through the tissue from one electrode to another. See Figure 3-1. Death from

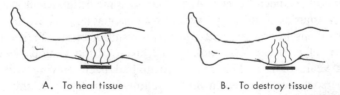

A. To heal tissue   B. To destroy tissue

FIGURE 3—1. Diffuse and concentrated distribution of electric current passing through tissue in diathermy. A. To heal tissue. B. To destroy tissue.

exposure to an electric current is usually due to its effects on the heart and brain tissue.[18] Exposure of the heart to 110-volt electric current alternating at 60 cycles per second can be expected to induce ventricular fibrillation, be-

[17] Moyer, in Harkins, *et al., Ibid.*, p. 285.
[18] Hopps, *Op. cit.*, p. 98.

cause one of the stimuli is bound to come at the end of the refractory period when the heart is most susceptible to fibrillation. In contrast, an electric current may be used to stop ventricular fibrillation or to initiate contraction in a heart that has stopped beating.

Radiation is another form of physical energy capable of injuring cells. Radiation may be classified as rays that can be seen, that is, light rays; those that can be felt, or heat rays; and those that cannot be detected by any of the five senses. All may also be classified as to their length. In the discussion which follows, the effects of ultraviolet rays and of ionizing radiation, neither of which can be seen, will be considered. According to some authorities, ultraviolet rays also induce ionization in exposed tissues.

Sunburn may be caused by the ultraviolet rays from the sun or from a lamp. These burns range from a mild erythema of the skin through second-degree burns. Fever and leukocytosis are not common unless the burns are severe. However, the cornea and conjunctiva of the eye are very sensitive to ultraviolet light and even shorter exposures may produce keratitis (inflammation of the cornea) and conjunctivitis. The eyes can be protected from ultraviolet light by the wearing of dark glasses. However, they do not protect the eyes from infrared rays. Persons who wear dark glasses should be instructed not to lie and look at the sun because of the danger of burning the retina. In the past, numbers of people have become partly blinded by staring at the sun during an eclipse. The pupil of the eye remains open because of the lack of light, and infrared rays concentrate on the retina, causing serious burns. Persons who tan can protect themselves from sunburn by gradually increasing exposure to the sun. Tolerance can be built up by starting with a limited exposure and extending the time by ten minutes or so each day. A number of factors modify the length of exposure to ultraviolet light which can be tolerated. Blondes and redheads are much more sensitive to ultraviolet rays than are brunettes. Some never tan. Young infants and children are susceptible to burning and are unable to protect themselves. Concentration of ultraviolet rays is increased by reflection. Therefore, exposure is greater during activities such as boating or swimming. Since ultraviolet rays pass through clouds, sunburn is possible on cloudy days. Though the shade from trees provides some protection against sunburn, protection is only partial. Exposed areas are therefore liable to sunburn even when a person is shaded by a tree.

Prolonged or extended overexposure of the skin to the rays of the sun intensifies the rate at which it ages. It also predisposes to carcinoma of the skin. The incidence of carcinoma of the skin is higher among those living in tropical climates than those living in temperate or arctic regions. It is also higher among farmers and sailors than among those who work indoors. Great-grandma's sunbonnet and long sleeves served a useful purpose; they protected her skin from the sun. Other factors such as the winds may increase the tendency to aging and carcinogenesis.

Why is knowledge of the effects of ionizing radiation
of importance to everyone?

Because of the extensive use of ionizing radiation, as well as its awesome potentialities, everyone should have some knowledge of its nature, uses, and dangers and of some of the methods man can use to protect himself from its effects. Since its discovery, the uses of ionizing radiation have greatly increased. It was first used primarily in medicine for diagnosis, treatment, and research. Now, industry is developing it as a source of power. Its capacity as an agent of destruction has been amply demonstrated and is well known. Depending on its use and the precautions taken in handling it, ionizing radiation can be either a boon to mankind or the source of his destruction. The latter possibility raises philosophical and ethical questions that are of serious import. Some of the problems arising out of the peaceful uses of atomic energy include the protection of those who work with it, as well as the protection of the general population from atomic wastes. Questions requiring answers include the following: What effects will raising the level of ionizing radiation in the atmosphere have on the length of life and health of the people now alive? What effects will it have on future generations? How can it be used and the population be protected?

Some answers or clues to answers to the above questions, as well as to others, are being obtained from experimental work with a variety of animals. Knowledge of both the effects of massive generalized doses of ionizing radiation as well as those of small, but repeated, doses on man are also being studied. The populations who were exposed at Hiroshima and Nagasaki and in the Marshall Islands have been and are being studied. Workers in laboratories where accidental spillage of radioactive materials has occurred have also been subjected to intensive and extensive study. Knowledge of the local effects of small, but repeated, exposure to ionizing radiation has been obtained from a variety of sources. One important source has been physicians who pioneered in the use of X-ray and radium. For example, *The AMA News* for August 10, 1959, carried an article about Dr. Emil Grubbe, aged 84, who had pioneered in the use of X-ray. The event that occasioned the article was that Dr. Grubbe had undergone his ninety-second operation for cancer. In this operation he had the first and fourth fingers of his right hand removed. Previously he had lost part of his left hand, nose, and jaw. Cancer had developed as a result of Dr. Grubbe's exposing himself to Crooke's tubes in 1895. Knowledge has also been obtained from the effects radiation has had on industrial workers. For example, girls were employed to paint the dials of watches with radium salts. In the process, they moistened the brushes that they used by placing them in their mouths. Radium and thorium contained in the paint were absorbed and stored in the bones of the girls. Eventually they developed cancer of the nasal sinuses and osteogenic sarcoma. Though from the point of view of the girls, their families, and society, the situation was a tragedy, it had one positive aspect. Useful information was gained about the long-term effects of low-level exposures to internal emitters of radiation.

Though this chapter is primarily devoted to agents that injure tissue cells and the manner in which cell function is altered, the use of ionizing radiation in therapy and diagnosis will also be included. Incorporation of this material in this chapter is justified because whatever the source or the reason for exposure to ionizing radiation, the effect on living tissue is the same. There is a transfer of energy, which, if the concentration is sufficient, will have a destructive effect on the growth and reproduction of cells.

Before discussing the effects of ionizing radiation, some of the terms used in the discussion will be defined.

Ionizing radiation "is an electromagnetic radiation (consisting of photons or particulate radiation including electrons, neutrons, protons) usually of high energy, but in any event capable of ionizing air, directly or indirectly."[19] Hardy[20] simplifies the definition. He says, "In simplest terms, ionizing radiation separates the target molecule into ions, or removes an ion from the molecule." Shields[21] defines ionizing radiation as follows: "Ionizing radiation may be defined as particles of electromagnetic waves moving so fast that they knock electrons from atoms or molecules of matter."

Alpha rays (alpha particles) "are particulate ionizing radiation consisting of helium nuclei traveling at high speed."[22]

Beta rays (beta particles) are particulate ionizing radiation consisting of electrons or positrons traveling at high speed."[23]

Gamma rays "are X rays originating in the nuclei of atoms."[23]

Roentgen rays "are X rays usually produced by bombarding a (metallic) target with high-speed electrons in a suitable device."[23]

X rays (sometimes X radiation) are electromagnetic ionizing radiation.[21]

Neutrons (or neutron rays) are neutral particles of electricity found in the nuclei of atoms.

Protons are positively charged particles of electricity.[25]

Isotopes are atoms of an element having an identical number of protons and orbital electrons, but differing in weight because the number of neutrons in their nuclei differs. All isotopes of the same substance have the same atomic number. They may be stable or unstable.[26]

[19] *Permissible Dose From External Sources of Ionizing Radiation,* Handbook 59, U.S. Department of Commerce, National Bureau of Standards, 1954, p. 2.

[20] James D. Hardy, *Pathophysiology in Surgery,* The Williams & Wilkins Co., Baltimore, 1958, p. 191.

[21] Shields, Warren, *The Pathology of Ionizing Radiation,* Charles C Thomas, Springfield, Illinois, 1961, p. 3.

[22] *Op. cit.,* p. 4.

[23] *Ibid.,* p. 3.

[24] *Ibid.,* p. 2.

[25] Armand Joseph Courchaine, *Chemistry Visualized and Applied,* 2nd ed., G. P. Putnam's Sons, New York, 1957, p. 14.

[26] *Ibid.,* p. 19.

Radioactive isotopes are those in which the nucleus undergoes spontaneous degeneration with the production of new elements and four types of rays— alpha, beta, and gamma rays and neutrons. Some radioactive elements such as radium occur in nature; others are produced artificially. In the process of degeneration, a radioactive isotope may form another radioactive isotope or it may decompose immediately to a stable atom.[27]

Half-life is the period of time it takes one half of the atoms of an element to disintegrate or to become stable. The half-life of different elements varies from a few seconds to several billion years.[28]

Rad is the unit of radiation dose. It is 100 ergs absorbed per gram of absorber. Therapeutic doses are measured in hundreds or thousands of rads. Diagnostic dosages are usually in millirads as it is desirable to minimize exposure.[29]

What are the sources of ionizing radiation?

Despite the tendency to think of ionizing radiation as something new, it has existed since the beginning of time. Sources of natural radiation include cosmic rays and the crust of the earth. Exposure is greater at high than at low altitudes and in regions containing uranium and thorium deposits. Although the extent to which the general population is exposed differs, everyone is and always has been exposed to radioactivity. To illustrate sources, the table of the gonadal dose of irradiation in the United Kingdom[30] follows:

Source	Annual Dose Rate (Millirads Per Year)
Natural background	85–106
Medical radiology (1957)	19
Miscellaneous source (TV, shoe X rays, etc.)	1
Occupational exposure (1959)	0.5
Fallout: Average value over five year period 1955–1959	2.4

From this table the reader can see that by far the greatest exposure to ionizing radiation is from natural sources. This does not mean, however, that radioactive rays may not do harm, because they may. Protection from the effects of ionizing radiation depends largely on controlling sources that are made and/ or used by man.

What is the effect of ionizing radiation on tissues?

All radioactive material, whether in the form of electromagnetic rays (gamma rays) or particles such as the alpha or beta particles or neutrons,

[27] *Ibid.*, p. 99.
[28] *Ibid.*, p. 100.
[29] Edith H. Quimby, *Safe Handling of Radioactive Isotopes in Medical Practice,* The Macmillan Company, New York, 1960, p. 10.
[30] *World Health*, XV, January-February, 1962, pp. 5-7.

has the same effect on tissues. Delario[31] states that all radiations directly or indirectly produce their tissue effect through ionization. Robbins[32] emphasizes that regardless of its source all ionizing radiation acts by a single mechanism that evokes an identical tissue change. Hopps[33] states that the tissue change resulting from exposure to ionizing radiation is degeneration. If the effect on the tissue is marked, cells undergo necrosis. Although the effect on cells is the same, the various rays and particles have differing powers to penetrate tissue or other materials. A curious fact is that the less they are able to penetrate, the more ion pairs they produce in the tissues through which they pass. Alpha particles which have the least penetrating power produce more ion pairs than do either beta particles or gamma rays. However, because gamma rays and neutrons have the greatest penetrating power, they are by far the most damaging type of radiation. Because alpha particles are filtered by air or a single sheet of paper, they are unlikely to have an opportunity to come in contact with much tissue. Likewise, the extent of damage caused by beta particles is limited by their poor power of penetration. They can and do cause superficial injuries when tissues are exposed to them. Furthermore, beta particles may cause serious injury when they are ingested or inhaled in large quantities as after an atomic explosion. Likewise they can affect tissues in the interior of the body when they are introduced by a cut or injection. Unlike alpha and beta particles, gamma rays and neutrons can traverse the entire body.

The various types of radiation, their sources, their tissue-penetrating power, and what protects against each of them as well as potential hazards are summarized in Figure 3-2.

How does degree of sensitivity influence the effect of ionizing radiation?

Although all living things are sensitive to the injuring effect of ionizing radiation, there is considerable variation in degree of sensitivity. For example, an earlier misconception about the effects of ionizing radiation was that it injured animals, particularly man, but has had little if any effect on plants. To test the validity of this belief, Woodwell[34] and others designed experiments in which they exposed plants to ionizing radiation. From these studies, they learned not only that plants are sensitive to ionizing radiation of an intensity sufficient to injure human beings, but that different plants have different degrees of sensitivity. For example, pine trees are more sensitive than oak trees and weeds are highly resistant. Moreover, when a forest is destroyed by ionizing radiation, it upsets the ecological system in the forest. As an illustra-

---

[31] A. J. Delario, *Roentgen, Radium, and Radioisotope Therapy,* Lea & Febiger, Philadelphia, 1953, p. 61.

[32] *Op. cit.,* p. 240.

[33] *Op. cit.,* p. 99.

[34] George M. Woodwell, "The Ecological Effects of Radiation," *Scientific American,* CCVIII, June, 1963, pp. 40-49.

F I G U R E   3 – 2

Type of Radiation	Sources of Particles or Rays	Mode of Exposure	Penetrating Power	Protection Against	Potential Hazards
Alpha particles	Helium nuclei traveling at high speed	Ingestion. Inhalation. Through breaks in the skin. Introduction into a body cavity or tissue in diagnosis or treatment	Minimal—completely absorbed or stopped by a few centimeters of air or a thin piece of paper	Very easily absorbed. Distance. Shielding. Rubber gloves. Filtration mask. Protective clothing	Because of limited penetrating power, alpha particles are essentially harmless unless inhaled or ingested
Beta particles	Electron particles of small mass carry a negative charge. Radioactive nuclei. Emitted by I_{131}, Gold$_{198}$, Ra$_{226}$	As above	Only a few millimeters of tissue at most. Two millimeters thickness of brass. One millimeter of lead	Easily absorbed. As above. Copper and aluminum filters	Local tissue injury at site of application including tissues to which beta particles are applied in the interior of the body. When ingested or inhaled in sufficient quantities causes injury as listed below
Gamma rays	1. Roentgen rays or X rays produced by bombarding a metallic target with high-speed electrons 2. X rays originating in the nuclei of atoms—e.g., Iodine$_{131}$, Gold$_{198}$, Radium$_{226}$	As above, plus exposure to rays in the environment Scatter X rays from diagnostic or therapeutic X rays	Great. Can traverse, that is, pass through, the entire body	Penetrates several inches of metal. Lead is commonly used for shielding. Concrete	1. Prompt effects A. Hematopoietic system B. Gastrointestal system C. Nervous system 2. Delayed effects A. Genetic aberrations B. Induction of malignant neoplasms C. Reduction in the life span D. Other effects such as: (1) Sterility (2) cataracts
Neutrons or neutron rays Uncharged particles	Cyclotron and from the so-called atomic pile. Atom bomb (nuclear fission and transmutation)	1. Explosion of atom bomb 2. Persons working with them 3. During therapy	Passes. In general very penetrating	Very penetrating—concrete slows down	See gamma rays

tion, white oak trees were more sensitive to irradiation than some of the insects living on them. Therefore, though not all trees were killed by radioactivity, those remaining died because they were stripped of their leaves by the proportionately larger numbers of insects. There were, obviously, many other similar imbalances. One implication of these studies relates to the disposal of atomic wastes. Life in any area exposed to sufficient radioactivity to injure man is liable to destruction.

Which tissues are most sensitive to ionizing radiation?

Although the effect of all forms of radiation is the same, tissues differ in their degree of sensitivity. No tissue, however, has absolute resistance. Knowledge of the order of sensitivity of tissues helps the nurse or physician to anticipate the effects that radiation will have on the different tissues and the signs and symptoms that will be manifested. Lymphoid tissue is most sensitive. Therefore, the most sensitive and earliest test of the effect of total body irradiation is the level of lymphocytes in the blood. The hematopoietic (blood-forming) cells of the bone marrow are next in degree of sensitivity. Leukopenia and thrombocytopenia are the first evidence of bone marrow depression. Anemia does not occur as early as changes in other cells, because the red cells have a longer life span than the leukocytes. Bone marrow studies provide evidence of the effect of ionizing radiation on bone marrow. The gastrointestinal epithelium and the germ cells are also highly sensitive. Nausea and vomiting follow injury to the gastrointestinal tract. When these are protracted, the patient may become severely dehydrated and undernourished.

What are some of the factors influencing the degree of sensitivity of tissues to ionizing radiation?

Not only do tissues vary in their sensitivity to ionizing radiation but the degree to which any tissue is sensitive can be altered to some extent. Any condition, such as hyperthyroidism or fever, elevating the metabolic rate increases tissue sensitivity. The reverse is also true. A decrease in metabolism is accompanied by a decrease in sensitivity. Sensitivity is also related to the degree of cellular differentiation and to the ability of the tissue to reproduce. The more highly differentiated a cell or tissue, the more resistant it is to the effects of radiation. The greater the capacity of the tissue to reproduce, the less its resistance is to the effects of radiation. This fact helps to explain the sensitivity of bone marrow and germ cells to irradiation. Cells undergoing reproduction are particularly sensitive when they are in the prophase of mitosis. Immature cells are more sensitive to irradiation than are mature cells.

The use of ionizing radiation in the treatment of malignant neoplasms depends on the differences in sensitivity between healthy and neoplastic tissues. The effects on neoplastic cells are similar to those on normal cells. The fact that cells in malignant neoplasms are less well differentiated and are less mature renders their cells more susceptible to ionizing radiation than healthy cells.[35] Just as healthy cells differ in their degree of sensitivity, so do those in neoplasms. Ionizing radiation is useful in the treatment of those neoplasms whose sensitivity is enough greater than that of the surrounding healthy tissue to make it possible to destroy the neoplasm without excessive damage to healthy tissue.

What factors must be taken into account in evaluating the possible effects of ionizing radiation?

Factors that must be taken into consideration when evaluating the possible total effects of radiation include the sensitivity of the tissues to irradiation, the function of these tissues, and the period of time over which the radiation is absorbed. The effects of a single large dose may be quite different from those that result from small repeated exposures over a period of time. The effects of irradiation also are modified by the size of the area exposed.

Why should the nurse have some knowledge of the effects of total body irradiation?

Because this is the era of the atomic bomb, as well as the limited use of total body irradiation in medicine, the nurse should have some knowledge of the effects of exposure of the entire body to ionizing radiation. Radiation of the entire body produces a number of effects that differ from those that accompany local exposure to radiation.[36] Moreover, in addition to injury from radioactivity, those who are in the area of an atomic bomb explosion may suffer from flash or thermal burns or be injured by falling debris. Though given less publicity and attention, the effects of blast and burns may be more serious and cause more injuries than those of ionizing radiation. They are also more difficult to protect against. The seriousness of injury from ionizing radiation depends on distance from the site of the explosion and the extent to which the persons are shielded. If a group of people are at the same point, those who are out in the open will suffer the greatest exposure. Next will be those who are shielded by natural objects or who are in buildings made of brick, concrete or metal. Those who suffer the least exposure will be those in tunnels, caves, and air raid shelters. Scientists believed that at Nagasaki and Hiroshima the explosion was an important factor in the injuries that were suffered. Those who were injured by ionizing radiation were found in a relatively small area. As a consequence, they believed that ionizing radiation released by the atom bomb would be harmful only to those in a limited area.

[35] Studies recently reported indicate that the cells in neoplasms proliferate less rapidly than normal cells. Instead of one of the daughter cells dying, both daughter cells proceed to multiply. In fact, it is well recognized that in general the proliferation of neoplastic cells is *less* rapid than that of normal cells.

[36] Total body irradiation has been employed to destroy leukemic cells or to depress the immunologic mechanisms. One of the serious problems in the care of these patients is the prevention of a fatal infection.

The Bikini test proved that they were wrong. Fishermen in a boat called the "Fortunate Dragon" 110 miles from the site of the explosion suffered from the effects of total body irradiation. Some died.

According to Shields,[37] irradiation of the entire body with massive doses, such as occurred in Hiroshima and Nagasaki, results in unconsciousness, and death occurs shortly after exposure. Unless the person who receives a dose of total body irradiation is so heavily irradiated that he dies from damage to the brain or he is burned or is struck by flying debris, he may not be immediately aware of the fact that he has been injured. Depending on the seriousness of the injury, symptoms may appear in a few minutes or be delayed for eight to ten days. The early symptoms may last for a brief period and then return sometime between the fifth and twentieth days. The effect is similar to that of skin reactions following local applications of irradiation.

Early symptoms are those of nausea, vomiting, and diarrhea. Increased capillary and cell permeability throughout the body leads to a progressive loss of fluid and electrolytes with the development of shock. Death occurs in a few days. Bleeding into the skin and mucous membranes occurs. It is evidenced by petechiae and ecchymoses of the skin as well as frank bleeding from the mouth and gastrointestinal tract. One of the factors in the bleeding is a depression in the level of circulating thrombocytes. The leukocytes also disappear from the blood, and this decreases the resistance of the person to infection. Because of their longer life span, erythrocytes do not disappear as rapidly as do the other blood cells. Ulcerations in the gastrointestinal tract provide portals of entry for bacteria. With the decrease in resistance, infection follows. Weakness and fever are a consequence of the infection and the malnutrition which result from the nausea and vomiting. In patients who survive, fever and weakness may persist for months. These patients have decreased resistance to all forms of stress including physical exertion and infection. Consequently during the period of recovery, patients should be protected from stress and from infection.

Other effects of radiation result from less intense exposures to ionizing radiation. They may follow the use of ionizing radiation therapy as well as its use in destruction. Some of the effects such as the induction of malignant neoplasms, the reduction in the life span, and genetic aberrations may take months, years, or generations to make their appearance. They may result from a single or multiple exposures.

Radiation due to total body irradiation can be summarized as:

1. Prompt effects (within a few days or weeks)
   A. None—exposure of entire body to less than 200 rad or superficial injury from exposure to alpha or beta particles
   B. Hematopoietic form (200 to 400 or 500 rads)
      (1) Lymphopenia

---

[37] *Op. cit.*, p. 16.

        (2) Leukopenia
        (3) Anemia
        (4) Loss of immune response
    C. Gastrointestinal form (400 or 500 to 1,000 rads)
        (1) Nausea, vomiting
        (2) Diarrhea
        (3) Ulceration and infection
    D. Central nervous system form (greater than 1,000 rads)
  2. Delayed effects (months or years)
    A. Genetic aberrations
    B. Induction of malignant neoplasms
    C. Reduction in life span
    D. Other effects
        (1) Sterility
        (2) Cataracts

Skin damage may result from exposure to any form of ionizing radiation. At the site of exposure, the first evidence of injury is erythema or redness occurring 24 to 48 hours after exposure. Later edema, vesiculation, and exfoliation (peeling) occur, leaving the skin denuded. Deep ulcers that heal poorly may form. Epilation, or loss of hair, and brittleness of the nails also occur.

In those who have received a lethal dose of irradiation, no treatment is known at this time which is effective in preventing death or in restoring the person to health. Those who have lesser exposures benefit from blood transfusions, antibiotics, protection from infection, maintenance of nutrition and of water and electrolyte balance, and emotional support. Because of widespread knowledge of the possible harmful effects of ionizing radiation, emotional support is essential. Lapp's[38] account of the 23 Japanese fishermen who were injured as the result of the Bikini explosion tells of the reactions of these men, their families, and the members of the community to the exposure of the fishermen to total body irradiation. It is well worth reading for it emphasizes the psychosocial effects of ignorance and misconceptions on the behavior of people as well as some of the very human effects of a catastrophe. The men were treated as if they were carriers of a contagious plague by their fellow townsmen.

Summary

Persons who are exposed to total body irradiation, as the result of either an explosion of an atom bomb or the accidental spillage of atomic materials, and those who are exposed to ionizing radiation over extended periods of time are liable to varying types of injury. Patients who are treated with ionizing

---

[38] Ralph E. Lapp, *The Voyage of The Lucky Dragon,* Harper and Brothers, New York, 1957 and 1958.

radiation may also be injured, but they are usually protected by screening of untreated areas and by the control of the size of the dose that is administered. Disorders that require extensive exposure of the body or exposure of sensitive tissues are likely to be accompained by evidence of tissue injury. The types of injury that may occur were summarized earlier, but will be repeated for the sake of emphasis. They include: (1) direct injury to the skin, (2) injury to the blood-forming organs, (3) the initiation of malignant neoplasms, (4) the production of cataracts, (5) decreased fertility, (6) harmful genetic mutations, and (7) decreased life span.

How is ionizing radiation utilized in medicine?

In the following section the use of ionizing radiation in the diagnosis and treatment of disease will be considered. In the hands of the well-trained physician who understands both the uses and dangers of ionizing radiation, it may be used to benefit the patient. In the hands of the untrained or the unscrupulous, there are few forces available to mankind that can cause more harm and human misery. The public is partly protected by laws regulating the use and availability of radioactive isotopes. They are not as well protected from the misuse of X radiation. The physician who has special training has credentials he can present, if necessary, to the patient. Should the patient have any doubt about the competence of a physician, he should ask to see the physician's credentials. The nurse as a citizen and as a health educator has a responsibility for educating the public about the uses and abuses of X radiation. She should have at least enough knowledge to appreciate its dangers and benefits. She should have some basis for protecting herself and for aiding others to protect themselves.

In selecting the source of radiation to be used in the treatment of a given patient, the physician considers many factors including the location of the tissue to be treated, the tolerance of adjacent tissues, and the rays or particles available for use. Therapy may be administered externally through the skin and tissues over the organ, or be applied directly to the organ, or be administered internally. Whatever method of application is used, the effect on exposed tissues is the same. When the dosage is small, it leads to moderate degeneration of cells. When it is large, cells undergo necrosis.

What are the local effects of external applications of ionizing radiation?

Ionizing radiation, whether applied as rays or particles, has a local as well as a general or systemic effect. Evidence of the local effect is presented by changes in the skin through which the radiation passes. Although modern methods of treatment lessen the number of patients having marked skin reactions, the application of radiation through the skin to neoplasms is always accompanied by some changes in the skin. The physician is responsible for preparing the patient and his family to expect reddening and possibly some desquamation of the skin. The fact that the nurse knows that this is expected and takes it as a matter of course is supporting to the patient. Any expression of surprise may lead to doubts as to whether the treatment is being properly applied or is producing the expected effect. Furthermore, the changes in the skin should be spoken of as a reaction, which of course it is, rather than as a burn. The term "burn" may suggest carelessness, which the term "reaction" does not. By her use of appropriate terminology the nurse helps to protect the patient from unnecessary psychological stress.

After a large dose of radiation, the skin develops an active erythema which disappears in a few days. A week or so later the erythema reappears. This time it develops gradually, but increases in intensity until it resembles a severe sunburn. Blistering and desquamation may take place. In severe reactions the area may be very painful and continue to be painful for about a month. Examination of the skin and underlying tissue reveals degeneration of cells in the epidermis. Small blood vessels, especially the arterioles, also undergo degeneration. Some of the vessels are thrombosed. Capillary permeability is increased, and the tissue is hyperemic.[39] In six or eight weeks the skin begins to regenerate. The appendages of the skin, such as the hair follicles and the sweat glands, do not regenerate. The resulting skin is thin and pigmented. The underlying tissue has a poor blood supply. When the injury is severe, skin atrophy, dryness, telangiectasis (dilated veins) and hyperkeratosis are common.

When the method used to administer radioactive rays or substances is such that damage to the skin is minimal, special care of the skin may not be required, If there is an obvious reaction, the skin requires special care. The tissue is susceptible to pressure, trauma, and infection. Gentleness is essential. Because the skin is fragile, washing should either be omitted or be limited to the use of clear water. Oily substances should not be placed on the skin unless specifically ordered by the physician. Oil prevents the evaporation of perspiration and predisposes to maceration of the skin by keeping it moist. The skin should be protected from the effects of pressure from bed coverings or clothing by the use of bed cradles and lightweight, loose clothing. With the exception of cornstarch, powders should not be applied to the skin exposed to irradiation during the period of therapy. Many commercially prepared powders contain zinc. The radioactive rays or particles ionize zinc or other ionizable substances. These ions produce further injury of the skin.

If the skin breaks down, it must be treated as an open wound, that is, aseptically. Patients who are being treated on an outpatient basis should be warned against exposure of the treated areas to the rays of the sun, as they increase the damage to the skin. The patient should also be instructed not to remove marks placed on the skin by the physician because they serve as guides to treatment. Nurses should assume responsibility for making certain

[39] Hopps, *Op. cit.*, p. 100.

that patients understand the instructions given by the physician. Repetition is necessary to learning for those who are under severe stress.

Why can the patient under treatment with ionizing radiation be expected to be under severe emotional and physical stress?

The patient who is under radiation therapy is likely to be under severe emotional and physical stress. The nature of his illness as well as the therapy itself contribute to this. His fears, whether they are realistic or based on misconceptions, are upsetting. He may express them in various ways. He may be overly cheerful or talkative, or withdrawn, or highly critical and demanding. Mrs. Huron reacted in the latter manner. She was admitted to a large city hospital from a smaller one in her own community, for deep X ray therapy following a radical mastectomy for adenocarcinoma of the breast. From the moment she was admitted she was excessively critical of the hospital, its facilities, and the nursing service. The nurse who was assigned to care for her found her criticism hard to bear because the nurse felt that everyone, including herself, was doing her best to be helpful As she bathed and cared for Mrs. Huron, she kept saying to herself, "There must be a reason, there must be a reason." In discussing the situation at a later time with her supervisor, the nurse pointed out that as she became more accepting of the behavior of the patient, Mrs. Huron became less demanding. In the instance of Mrs. Huron, the most difficult nursing problem arose not from the physical effects of the therapy, but out of her reaction to her total situation, including the meaning that the treatment had for her.

As with other patients who are under severe stress, patients may be helped by knowing that their feelings are appreciated by those who are responsible for their care. Other types of measures helpful in minimizing the effects of stress include: (1) accepting the behavior of the patient as the best he can do at the time, (2) preparing the patient for what to expect, (3) adapting the hospital routine to meet the needs and feelings of the patient, (4) giving care that adds to his physical comfort, (5) attending to his needs and wants promptly—all contribute toward reducing unnecessary stress.

What are some of the factors contributing to the development of irradiation sickness?

As was stated earlier, patients who are treated with ionizing radiation may have systemic as well as local reactions during treatment. Depression of the bone marrow is accompanied by leukopenia, anemia, and thrombocytopenia. One type of systemic reaction is sometimes referred to as irradiation sickness. A number of factors contribute to its development. They include the location and intensity of the treatment and the emotional state of the patient. Treatments over the abdominal organs are more likely to be accompanied by systemic reactions than are those over other parts of the body. The symptoms presented by the patient include anorexia, nausea, vomiting, and diarrhea. These symptoms are seldom of serious import, but they add to the discomfort of the patient. There are a number of theories about the cause of the symptoms in radiation sickness. One theory is based on the possibility that toxic substances are formed as a result of the injury to the cells or that metabolism in the cell is in some way deranged. Another theory is based on the belief that the symptoms are primarily the result of an emotional disturbance. Those who support the latter view point out that patients have many fears, some of which are aroused by the treatment itself and the meanings that it has. This theory is supported by the large number of agents used in the treatment of radiation sickness. Allen[40] lists 27 drugs and other agents that have been said to have benefited a large percentage of patients suffering from radiation sickness. He casts doubt on the specific value of any of them and suggests that their value lies in the "cheerful and enthusiastic attitude of the physician."

Whatever the cause of the symptoms, patients are usually very miserable. They have difficulty in eating and are often worried by this fact. They lose food and fluids through vomiting and diarrhea. When these symptoms are severe, they can lead to dehydration and electrolyte imbalance. Intravenous fluids may be necessary to restore hydration and electrolytes. The problem of maintaining the fluid and food intake of the patient during therapy is sometimes difficult to solve. For some patients the food intake may be increased by adjusting the times at which meals are served. The patient who is treated early in the morning may be able to eat in the late afternoon or early evening. Food likes and dislikes should be given special consideration. This is no time to try to reform the food habits of the patient. A bottle of "Coke" or ginger ale may not meet all his nutritional requirements but they do provide glucose and water. Adjustments made in the timing, or in the foods served, also help to convey to the patient the concern for his welfare. Whatever the initiating factor, vomiting and diarrhea, if severe or prolonged, can lead to disturbances in water and electrolyte balance that further aggravate symptoms. The objectives toward which the patient's care should be directed include: to minimize the undesirable effects of ionizing radiation and to provide the patient with support and comfort.

What nursing actions may be helpful to the patient who is nauseated and/or vomiting?

The nurse who recognizes and accepts that the patient is wretched may not be able to eliminate entirely his misery, but she can at least make it more bearable. Knowledge that the illness is self-limiting and that the symptoms will cease as soon as the treatment is completed may be helpful to some patients. Such simple actions as remaining with the patient when he vomits,

[40] J. Garrott Allen, "Radiation Injury from Local or Total Body Exposure," in *Surgery Principles and Practice,* Eds. Henry N. Harkins, *et al.,* J. B. Lippincott Company, Philadelphia, 1961, p. 309.

providing him with an opportunity to rinse his mouth after he has vomited, and the prompt emptying and thorough washing of the emesis basin contribute to his comfort. Sometimes suggestion can be used to help him. He can be told that if he lies quietly, when he feels nauseated, he will be less likely to vomit. He may be encouraged to swallow when he feels a wave of nausea. When suggestion is used, one should try to convey to the patient that this is a procedure that he may use to help himself. Success in the use of suggestion is based on confidence of the nurse that the action will be helpful. It also requires that the nurse spend time with the patient and that she convey to the patient her desire to be helpful. When the patient's and the nurse's efforts are unsuccessful, neither should be made to feel that he is to blame for the failure.

How does the method of application of ionizing radiation affect the nursing needs of a patient?

The nurse should also take into account the method by which radiation therapy is being applied. When therapy is given by X ray or cobalt-60 is used, the patient should be prepared to be placed in a room by himself. He should know that there is a small window in the room through which he can be seen at all times. There is also an intercommunication system which will enable him to talk to the person responsible for his treatment. In the care of patients in whom an applicator containing a radioactive element, such as radium or its salt radon, or cobalt-60, is placed directly in the organ, the nurse has additional responsibilities and objectives. They include: (1) to care for the patient in such a manner that the applicator stays in place, (2) to prevent the loss of the radioactive element, usually radium, (3) to notify the physician who is to remove the applicator at the proper time, and (4) to protect the personnel (and others) from the harmful effects of radiation.

The needs of the patient who has had an applicator containing radioactive material will be presented in the following example. Mrs. Erie was in the hospital for the diagnosis and treatment of a lesion on her cervix. When the diagnosis was established as carcinoma, her surgeon decided to treat it by placing a tube containing radium in the cervix. Radium, as well as most other radioactive isotopes, is a beta emitter. Due to its limited penetrating power, the tissue of the cervix can be heavily treated with a minimum effect on the surrounding tissue. Since radium is scarce and expensive, radon, a gas produced by radium, may be placed in tubes and implanted in the tissues. Since the half-life of radon is less than four days, it may be left in the tissue. In the instance of Mrs. Erie, however, radium was used. Mrs. Erie was taken to the operating room for the insertion of the radium. On her return she was to lie quietly and to avoid unnecessary movement in order to prevent the dislocation of the applicator, or, stated positively, to keep the applicator in the position in which it was placed. An indwelling catheter had also been inserted, so that she would not have to use the bedpan for urination.

Particularly when the cervix is subjected to intensive radiation, surrounding regions may also be affected. Irradiation of the rectum causes proctitis. This condition may be exquisitely painful. Mrs. Erie was fortunate in not developing this complication.

Mrs. Erie's physician had explained to her why she needed to lie still. Because she was a very conscientious person, she scarcely moved. As anyone who has tried knows, lying in one position is very tiring. Mrs. Erie's back ached and she was generally uncomfortable. To reduce the backache, the nurse slipped her hand under the small of Mrs. Erie's back. She helped her move her legs and encouraged her to move her arms. She answered Mrs. Erie's light promptly and visited her frequently. The nurse performed those tasks for Mrs. Erie that Mrs. Erie could not do for herself. One of the objectives that the nurse considered very important was to make what was for Mrs. Erie a trying time less difficult. To protect herself, the nurse maintained a distance of at least a yard between herself and the patient when she was not actually giving care.

In addition to providing care for the patient, the nurse has a responsibility to prevent the loss of radium. The specific procedures in the prevention of the loss of radium vary from institution to institution and with the part of the body into which it is placed. However, there should be a regular system for informing all who care for the patient that the patient is under treatment. There should also be a system for saving and checking dressings after they are removed and before they are discarded. If the applicator containing the radium escapes the cavity in which it was placed, it should not be replaced, but the physician should be notified immediately. If the radium is applied in an area where it may be dislodged by movement, the patient must remain quiet until it has been removed.

In addition to the use of X ray and radium, artificial radioactive isotopes may be used in the diagnosis and treatment of disease. Whether any special precautions are required in the care of patients receiving artificial radioactive isotopes depends on the size of the dosage that the patient receives, the length of the half-life of the isotope, and the route by which it is excreted.

One of the most frequently used radioactive isotopes is iodine[131] The value of iodine[131] in the diagnosis and treatment of diseases of the thyroid has been established. Iodine[131] may be administered in very small or tracer dosages to determine the degree of activity of the thyroid gland, or the presence of distant metastasis in malignant neoplasms of the thyroid. It may be administered in larger dosages in the treatment of malignant disease of the thyroid or to reduce the activity of the gland in hyperthyroidism. Its use is based on the fact that after iodine is absorbed from the gastrointestinal tract into the blood, thyroid tissue removes it from the blood and concentrates it. In hyperthyroidism more iodine is trapped by the thyroid than by the normal gland. In the absence of the thyroid or when it is hypoactive, iodine is excreted in the urine in increased amounts. Though iodine is largely a beta emitter, enough gamma rays are formed that the Geiger-Müller counter can be used to locate it. Because of the minute quantities of iodine[131] used in diagnosis, special protective measures for personnel and visitors are not required. When it is used in therapy, larger quantities of iodine[131] are used and protective measures are necessary. These are discussed later.

Other radioactive isotopes used in diagnosis and treatment are isotopes of phosphorus and gold. Radiophosphorus is used in the treatment of polycythemia vera and of certain solid tumors. Radioactive gold is injected into certain body cavities to reduce pleural effusion or ascites. In research, radioactive elements have been and are used to trace the course of biochemical activities of cells. Radioactive rubidium is being used to study the microcirculation of the heart muscle. Many other studies yielding valuable information have been and are in progress.

The most common form of ionizing radiation employed in medicine is X ray. Though X rays are utilized in therapy, they have their most frequent use in diagnosis. X rays, like light rays, sensitize photographic plate on contact. Since they penetrate body tissues in inverse proportion to the density of the tissues, dense tissues filter out a higher proportion of the X rays than do less dense ones. Therefore, when a body containing tissues of varying densities is placed between the source of X rays and a photographic plate, dense tissues appear as light areas on the plate and less dense tissues appear as darkened areas. In order to outline hollow organs such as the esophagus or stomach, contrast can be obtained by filling the organ with a radiopaque substance such as barium sulfate or an iodine-containing compound. Contrast can also be obtained by removing the fluid from a cavity and replacing it with oxygen or air. X rays of the brain or spinal cord are made by removing the cerebrospinal fluid and then replacing it with air or oxygen.

X rays may also be focused on a special screen after they pass through the body. This procedure is known as fluoroscopic examination. It is used to follow the progress of certain procedures such as cardiac catheterization and the reduction of fractures.

In the use of ionizing radiation in therapy, the physician has to consider the fact that exposure to ionizing radiation delays wound healing. When ionizing radiation is administered previous to a surgical procedure, time must be allowed for the tissue to recover. Following surgery, treatment must be delayed to allow time for healing to take place. For example, when X ray therapy is employed for a patient who has been treated surgically, treatment is delayed until wound healing is well under way.

Other problems may arise in the use of ionizing radiation, because organs in the area of treatment may be injured. Proctitis is possible when the cervix is treated with ionizing radiation. Pnuemonitis may accompany exposure of the lung to ionizing radiation. Bone necrosis is also a possibility in the therapy of cancer of the breast or uterus.

Two latent effects that are particular hazards to the person who handles and works with radioactive materials are radiation-induced cancer of the skin and leukemia. The instance of Dr. Grubbe has already been cited. He, along with others who pioneered in the use of X ray and radium, developed carcinoma of the skin of the hands. In some instances the neoplastic changes occurred fairly early. In others it was delayed for years. Leukemia is twice as frequent among physicians as it is in the general population. In Great Britain, where more stringent precautions are taken to prevent exposure of physicians, the incidence of leukemia among physicians does not differ greatly from its incidence in the general population. Employed by those who know and respect its dangers as well as its uses, it can be controlled and utilized to benefit mankind. In the hands of the ignorant or careless it may be a lethal weapon both for the user and for his victims. Protection from the hazards of radiation is important both for those who work with it and for patients. As stated previously, standards have been set for the protection of both workers and patients from the harmful effects of radioactivity. Some of these have been enacted into law.

The following principles, if acted upon by nurses and others, serve as guides to protection. Nurses are responsible for protecting patients and their relatives as well as themselves and their assistants. Ionizing radiation may injure tissue without producing immediate effects. When the degree of injury is small, the effects may not be evident for weeks, or even months or years. Its effects are cumulative. Some tissues are more sensitive than others. Because of the sensitivity of the gonads to radiation, special precautions should be taken to protect them in both patients and personnel. The effects on the gonads include the possibility of mutations of germ cells and of sterility.

Effective protective measures are based on shielding, distance, and time or length of exposure. The extent of each of these and the measures that are necessary depend on whether the source emits rays or particles. Since rays have the greatest power of penetration, lead-impregnated walls or materials are required for protection. Most radioactive isotopes are beta emitters. They have only limited power of penetration. To affect deeper tissues they must be taken into the body by ingestion or inhalation or be introduced by injection. Otherwise, their effect is primarily on the skin. Knowledge of what happens to the isotope in the body as well as its half-life is also important. For example, when radium salts or strontium 90 are ingested, it is stored in bone. Since both have a long half-life, they may initiate changes that result in cancer of the bone or in leukemia. Last, the quantity of radiation to which the individual is exposed can be determined. This is of particular importance in personnel employed in radiotherapy, including nurses who are responsible for patients who are receiving radioisotope therapy. Badges containing material sensitive to radioactivity are worn. They are examined at regular intervals. Should they indicate excessive exposure, procedures can be initiated to find the cause and to limit the exposure of the individual who has been exposed excessively.

Nurses who are responsible for the care of patients receiving ionizing radiation need to be concerned for their own protection only when patients are receiving treatment with radium or radioactive isotopes. As stated earlier, the principal source of harm from beta-emitting particles is from ingestion or inhalation of these materials. Protection is afforded by distance, shielding, the length of exposure, and checking. Provided the nurse is conscientious about carrying out appropriate protective measures, she does not have to worry about being harmed.

For nurses who do not work in X-ray departments or in radioisotope laboratories, the usual sources of contact with ionizing radiation are limited to (1) radioactive isotopes that are to be administered to or introduced into a patient, and (2) the patient who is being treated, and his excretions. In the handling of radioactive materials protection is afforded by shielding and distance. They are transported in lead containers with long handles, which enables the person to keep the container at a distance. If the material is to be ingested, the patient removes the glass from the lead container and drinks the "cocktail" previously prepared in the isotope laboratory. After the glass is emptied, it is rinsed by the patient and replaced in the container. Radium is also transported in a lead-covered case and kept at a distance by a long handle.

In the care of patients receiving internal therapy with radioisotopes, the nurse protects herself by limiting the time she spends with the patient and by the way in which she handles equipment. Bed linens or other materials that are subject to contamination are handled without shaking so that a minimum of dust is raised. Thorough hand washing and keeping the nails short and clean are important. The 23 Japanese fishermen referred to previously were found to have large amounts of radioactive materials under their fingernails. Measures such as wearing monitoring badges are for the protection of the individual against the cumulative effects of repeated exposure. They also serve to remind personnel of hidden danger. Since some of the isotopes such as I^{131} are excreted in the urine and feces, the nurse should check to determine whether urine or feces should be collected and saved for the duration of half-life of the isotope. Contamination of linen, the floor, or equipment should be checked by the radiation department. They should also supervise the cleaning of the floor should it be contaminated. The patient should either be confined to bed or be in a private room. In working with radioactive materials, the nurse should remember that an unsafe act may endanger not only herself, but many other persons. Finally, relatives and visitors of patients should be instructed so that they can visit safely and comfortably.

Fields[41] lists the essential rules for handling patients who are receiving radioactive isotopes. Quimby[42] also discusses the use of radioactive isotopes in medicine and the precautions that should be taken in hospitals. Many of

[41] Clinical Use of Radioisotopes, 2nd ed., Ed. by Theodore Fields and Lindon Seed, Year Book, Chicago, 1961, pp. 341-51 and 362-74.
[42] Edith H. Quimby, Safe Handling of Radioactive Isotopes in Medical Practice, The Macmillan Company, New York, 1960, pp. 11-35, and 56-97.

the points relative to protection have been previously made, but will be repeated for the sake of emphasis. Protection should take into account the length of the half-life of the isotope, the size of the dosage administered to the patient, and the route of excretion. To illustrate, the effective half-life of iodine[131] is six days. When it is administered as a tracer dose, the amount given is very small. It is excreted in the urine. No precautions need be observed in the care of the patients, but the urine should be saved in special bottles for checking. Because the drug is given by mouth, breakfast is limited to toast and coffee and other food is restricted for three hours, as this is the length of time required for the absorption of iodine. The study also requires that the patient should not have been receiving an iodine-containing drug within the past two weeks. Because the patient who is treated with iodine[131] receives a larger quantity of the isotope, precautions should be observed in his care. The precautions include the wearing of rubber gloves when giving direct care and the protection of the mattress and pillows with rubber covering. Linens used by the patient should be saved and checked. The urine of the patient should be saved and sent to the laboratory for checking. Should any be spilled, the radiological laboratory should be called to superintend the cleaning up.

The rules for the handling of patients receiving radioactive isotopes are usually made by the radiologist and/or the health physicist. They are applied by those who care for patients. The measures required are simple, but they will be ineffective unless they are strictly followed. Quimby[43] cites a well-known observation that persons are likely to be very careful when they first work in a new project and to become careless later. Certainly knowledge of how to protect oneself should make the nurse more comfortable in the care of patients and, in turn, improve the quality of the care of the patient. In caring for a patient who is undergoing radiation therapy, the nurse should work quickly without seeming hurried. An attempt should be made to reduce the patient's feeling of isolation by frequent short visits. Diversional therapy such as reading, radio, television, or handiwork may be helpful to those patients who feel well enough to enjoy them.

The bibliography contains references that contain more specific directions for the management of patients under treatment with radioactive isotopes.

What group of chemicals are radiomimetic?

A number of synthetic chemical compounds have biological effects similar to those of the radioactive substances. Because of the nature of their effects they are said to be "radiomimetic." Among the radiomimetic agents are the nitrogen mustards, a group of chemicals all containing the chlorethylamine group ($-NHCH_3 CH_2Cl$). The reactivity of the chlorine atom is essential to the effect of a nitrogen mustard. When the compound is dissolved in body fluids, the chlorine atom splits off, leaving a reactive intermediate that easily

[43] *Ibid.*, p. 35.

combines with many of the molecules within the cell. The result of this attachment of the straight-chain group (NHCH$_3$ CH$_2$ -) to the molecules within the cells is known as alkylation, and the chemicals having this effect are called alkylating agents. Alkylating agents have probably had their greatest benefit in the discovery of new knowledge about cellular processes. They have been used in the palliative treatment of cancer, but because they destroy normal cells in the bone marrow as well as malignant cells, their use is limited. The alkylating agents are unable to discriminate between healthy and malignant cells. At best they induce remissions, not cures. Alexander[44] suggests that knowledge gained from the study of radiomimetic agents ought to stimulate greater attention to the chemicals, old and new, that people encounter in their daily lives. These chemicals may be greater threats to health and life than atomic radiation.

What are some of the chemical agents of extrinsic origin that cause injury to cells? What are some of the toxic effects of chemical agents?

In addition to physical agents such as extremes of temperature and electricity, chemical agents may destroy tissues and cells. Chemical injury of tissue can be caused by a variety of substances. Their effects may be direct or indirect. For example, cyanide is a highly effective poison, because it blocks the action of the respiratory enzymes in the cell. As the result of this action, cells are unable to release the energy from nutrients that they require for their activities. Death from cyanide poisoning is certain and occurs in a matter of minutes. The only method of prevention is to avoid the inhalation or ingestion of chemicals containing cyanide.

Certain chemicals coagulate cellular proteins. Examples include phenol and formaldehyde.

Carbon monoxide is also a powerful poison, but it causes its effect indirectly. Despite the presence of carbon monoxide in air contaminated by gases containing products of combustion, it seldom reaches dangerous levels except in confined spaces such as houses, where defective heating devices are used, or tunnels for automobile traffic. The poisonous effect of carbon monoxide is due to the ease with which it combines with hemoglobin. Hemoglobin has 300 times the affinity for carbon monoxide than it has for oxygen. Consequently, when carbon monoxide is present in the blood, it readily combines with hemoglobin. The hemoglobin is, therefore, not available to carry oxygen, and cells are deprived of their oxygen supply. In the treatment of carbon monoxide poisoning, patients are placed in an environment containing a high concentration of oxygen. When the partial pressure of the oxygen in the alveoli is increased, the quantity of oxygen going into solution in the blood is also

[44] Peter Alexander, "Radiation-Imitating Chemicals," *Scientific American,* CCII, January, 1960, pp. 99-108.

increased. More important, however, is the effect of the law of mass action; that is, the speed or rate of chemical reaction is proportional to the concentration of each of the reacting substances.[45] According to the law of mass action, the quantity of oxyhemoglobin can be increased by increasing the amount of oxygen available to combine with the hemoglobin. When patients who have suffered carbon monoxide poisoning are treated with high concentrations of oxygen, a mask is the most satisfactory method of administration. When other methods are employed, particular attention should be paid to ensuring adequate concentrations of oxygen. When oxygen is administered by catheter, it should be replaced at least every six to eight hours or more frequently, if necessary, to maintain its patency. When it is administered in a tent, the canopy should be kept well tucked in, in order to maintain the concentration of oxygen in the inspired air at a high level. In addition every effort should be made to maintain the patency of the airway. (See Chapter 7.) To be of value the oxygen must be inhaled and have an opportunity to be absorbed.

How do fat solvents cause injury?

A group of toxic chemicals that are employed in industry and in the home are the solvents. Solvents are chemicals tending to have their effect in fatty tissues. Benzene, because of its affinity for bone marrow, causes death relatively quickly. Other fat solvents such as chloroform or carbon tetrachloride are concentrated in the liver, kidney, and brain, and produce tissue necrosis in the affected organs. Because fat solvents are volatile and are used in the dry-cleaning industry, special precautions are necessary to protect workers from injury. Protection of patrons from the danger of fat solvents was one of the problems that had to be solved before "do-it-yourself" dry-cleaning establishments could be made relatively safe. Precautions should also be taken by those who use these agents at home. Directions on containers should be followed explicitly. One way to limit the quantity inhaled is to work out of doors. Dry-cleaning fluids should be stored out of reach of children, and bottles of "spot removers" should be stored away from medicines and food. Had Mr. Curly and his wife followed this rule, he might have been spared a long hospitalization and permanent renal injury. One night he awakened with indigestion. He went to the medicine cupboard and drank what he thought was a popular remedy for indigestion. Instead it was a dry-cleaning agent. As a result of the toxic effect of the solution and delay in treatment, Mr. Curly experienced gastroenteritis, injury to the liver, and permanent and serious injury to the kidneys.

A third source of chemical poisons is bacterial toxins and enzymes. See Chapter 4.

A fourth group of toxic chemicals are the heavy metals such as mercury,

[45] Courchaine, *Op. cit.,* p. 246.

arsenic, and lead. Although mercury harms cells in other parts of the body, death is usually from its effect on the kidney. Small quantities of mercury in the form of organic compounds are used as diuretics, because they inhibit enzyme systems concerned with the reabsorption of chloride ions by the tubule cells in the kidney. Toxic dosages of mercury salts cause necrosis of the renal tubules and result in failure of kidney function.[46]

The effects of arsenic are widespread; it damages the brain, heart, bone marrow, and kidneys. One of the interesting points about arsenic is that in times past, it was the favorite agent in fact and fiction to eliminate one's enemies.[47] Arsenic is an ingredient in insecticides, rat poisons, and crabgrass killers. Children should be protected from the danger of accidental poisoning by proper handling and storage of supplies of arsenic-containing compounds and by the substitution of less toxic agents. Though mercury and arsenic in appropriate forms and dosages have therapeutic uses, lead does not. As with the other heavy metals, the effects of lead are widespread. Moreover, it may result in poisoning not only as a result of its use in industry, but from the contamination of the air, food, and drinking water. Young children who chew everything that they can get into their mouths are particularly likely to be exposed to lead poisoning. *Time Magazine* (82, August 19, 1963, 36) cites an outbreak of lead poisoning among children living in the slums of Chicago. Fourteen children aged one to five years have died. More than 40 others have been seriously ill. Most of these children have permanent brain damage. The source of the lead is materials in the environment of the child—nails, flakes of old paint, painted plaster, or any surface covered with a paint containing lead. The child chews the lead-containing material. A little lead appears to do no harm, but it is stored in the bones, where it accumulates. In the hot summer months when more vitamin D is available, the turnover of calcium and lead from the bones to the blood is more rapid than in colder months of the year, thus raising the level of lead in the blood. Other factors may also be involved. The effects on the nervous system, especially the brain, are marked. To prevent lead poisoning the use of paints containing lead should be avoided. Treatment with disodium calcium versenate, if instituted early, is effective in removing the lead and in preventing brain damage.

The treatment of arsenic, gold, mercury poisoning with Bal[48] is based on the observation that they all inhibit the same essential catalytic action. Nurses should be familiar with the location of the nearest poison center. If the container from which the poisonous material was taken is available, the name of the product and/or its constituents can be given to the center by telephone so that proper treatment can be initiated promptly.[49]

---

[46] Louis S. Goodman and Alfred Gilman, *The Pharmacological Basis of Therapeutics,* 2nd ed., The Macmillan Company, New York, 1955, p. 971.

[47] *Arsenic and Old Lace.*

[48] Trade name for dimercaprol, U.S.P.

[49] For a more complete discussion of the action of heavy metals see Goodman and Gilman, *The Pharmacological Basis of Therapeutics,* or some other pharmacology textbook.

A fifth type of poisonous chemical is methyl alcohol, commonly called wood alcohol. It is a highly toxic substance that produces its effect indirectly. It is converted first to formaldehyde and then to formic acid. Methyl alcohol is thought to be toxic by virtue of conversion to formaldehyde. Formic acid itself is nearly innocuous. Acidosis results from the inhibition of aerobic metabolism (in particular the enzyme lactic dehydrogenase) with accumulation of organic acids, especially lactic acid. In nonlethal doses, methyl alcohol causes blindness by injuring the retina. During prohibition, poisoning from methyl or wood alcohol was not uncommon. An article in a recent newspaper indicated that the number of illegal stills in operation has been increasing and with them there has been an increase in the number of persons poisoned by wood or methyl alcohol. Ethyl alcohol differs from methyl alcohol in one respect: it takes smaller amounts to induce inebriation. Although the effects of the long-term excessive use of ethyl alcohol are not within the scope of this chapter, alcoholism is an increasing problem in the United States. Despite its absence from mortality tables, many authorities consider alcoholism to be one of the major health problems. Alcoholism is not a new problem, nor is it one that is unique to industrialized societies.

A sixth type of noxious chemical is the insecticide and rodent and weed killers, all of which are man-made. Each year more of these chemicals are added to the list of substances available to kill insects, bees, and rodents. Because some of these chemicals are highly toxic and chemically stable, they are threats to both man and nature. They are prepared in the form of dusts, sprays, and aerosols. Currently about 350,000,000 lb of pesticides are used each year in the United States. Because of the large quantity used, there has been an increase in the level of certain toxic compounds in the environment. Pesticides have on occasion caused the widespread destruction of wild life. Acute insecticide poisoning is responsible for about 150 deaths a year. About half the deaths are among children. In the state of California alone as many as 1,100 instances of acute insecticide poisoning have occurred among agricultural workers in a single year.[50] Aerosol preparations carry with them an additional danger, as the containers can explode if damaged or heated. Because these chemicals are relatively new there has been little or no time to evaluate their long-term effects on human health. Depending on the form in which they are employed, these chemical agents may be inhaled, be ingested, or contaminate the skin. For example, in Hamlet, U.S.A., for three consecutive nights just preceding a Fourth of July celebration the entire town was dusted with DDT powder to kill the mosquitoes. Great billowing clouds of dust blanketed the area, thus exposing all the inhabitants to a potentially toxic chemical. Similar programs are carried out in large cities for the control of Dutch elm disease. There is growing concern about the extent to which residues in food constitute a health hazard.

In the area around Hamlet, U.S.A., many of the wells have been rendered

[50] "Science and the Citizen," *Scientific American*, CCIX, July, 1963, p. 64.

unfit for use by either human beings or animals by chemicals containing nitrogen. Over a period of years commercial fertilizers containing large quantities of nitrogen have been employed in enriching the soil. Because nitrogenous compounds are highly soluble, each rain carries them further into the subsoil. Eventually the nitrogenous chemicals reach the water supplying the wells. Although the high nitrogen content of drinking water does not appear to harm mature animals, it causes a serious illness in immature animals, including human infants.

In order to evaluate the possible hazards of chemical weed killers, pesticides, and insecticides, and to formulate principles governing their use, a number of experts have been studying the problem. Among them have been members of FOA and WHO meeting jointly to consider problems in relation to their use. In the United States, the President's Science Advisory Committee prepared a report calling for reforms in the use and control of chemical pesticides. Among the recommendations made by the committee are that: (1) the government transfer responsibility for all the health aspects of the pesticides to the Department of Health, Education and Welfare, (some are now controlled by the Department of Agriculture); (2) a data-gathering system be developed to monitor pesticide levels in the environment; and (3) the federal agencies cease area spraying with long-lived insecticides, except when required to control vectors of disease. The third recommendation has been put into effect. Moreover, this committee commended Rachel Carson for alerting the public to the hazards associated with the indiscriminate use of pesticides.[51]

Another possible chemical hazard about which there is little real information is the chemicals that are added to food to preserve it or to improve its palatability or appearance. These chemicals may be added at the time a food is processed or during the growing stage. As a simple example, coloring is used to create pink ice cream or green lime sherbet. Stilbestrol is administered to chickens or beef cattle to improve the quality of the meat and to lessen the cost of weight gain. Although none of these practices are believed to be hazardous to man, over the years they may be.

Drugs are chemicals which, when administered in appropriate amounts, are expected to be beneficial. For some, the margin between the effective therapeutic dose and the toxic dose may be wide. For others, the margin may be very small. At one time, it was believed that there was a threshold of exposure to certain physical and chemical agents below which no harmful effects occurred. Scientists, therefore, tried to establish safe levels of exposure. It is now known that some agents have delayed effects which may be manifested months or years after the initial exposure to the substance. As a consequence, the concept of safe level of exposure has been replaced by the "permissible dose." Basically, permissible dose means that the possibility that exposure to a particular agent will cause harm is slight. At times the condition of a person alters the quantity of the drug that he can tolerate. For example, acetylsali-

[51] *Ibid.*, p. 64.

cylic acid (aspirin) is a drug found in every medicine chest—and possibly in almost every purse. Few people are aware of the toxic potentialities of aspirin. Yet when a child finds a bottle of a hundred or so aspirin tablets, and eats them, the acetylsalicylic acid can cause fatal acidosis. Occasionally an individual is so sensitive to aspirin that one 5-gr tablet can cause serious effects or even death. A laxative taken to treat a digestive upset may cause the perforation of an inflamed appendix. The concept that certain drugs are safe and that within limits all drugs are safe is being replaced by the concept that safety is a relative matter. Furthermore, safety cannot always be judged by the immediate effects of a drug.

Some of the hazards associated with the exposure of the population of cities and industrial areas to pollution of the air was presented in Chapter 2. Water in these areas is also rendered unfit for human use and dangerous to fish by detergents and industrial wastes. In industry, a variety of chemicals are potential sources of danger against which workers require protection. They include arsenic, thallium, beryllium, aliphatic hydrocarbons, nickel, chromium, asbestos, and benzol. Although a number of sources of injury to cells have been cited, there are others and the number will undoubtedly be increased in the future. According to Lee,[52] a conservative estimate of the number of new potentially toxic chemicals added each year is at least 500. Since many chemicals are stable (they do not deteriorate into harmless compounds) and are highly toxic, increasing attention is being devoted to regulating their use and to devising ways of protecting the population from unnecessary exposure to them.

As emphasized in succeeding chapters, failure to maintain the concentration and distribution of components of body fluids within limits has an adverse effect on cellular function. Marked alterations are incompatible with life. Cellular function and structure depend on the regulation of physical and chemical conditions within the organism so that neither too much nor too little is present.

No discussion of noxious chemicals is complete without some mention of the effects of cigarette smoking. Over the last decade or so increasing attention has been devoted to the question of the relationship of cigarette smoking to the genesis of disease. Hammond[53] discusses a number of studies, including one of his own, that were made to discover answers to the above question. One of the reasons for interest in the problem was that the incidence of bronchogenic carcinoma, a disease that had once been relatively rare, was known to be rising rapidly. Hammond[54] discovered in his study that not only was the incidence of cancer of the lung higher among cigarette smokers, but the total death rate from all causes among this group was far higher than

[52] Douglas H. Lee, "Environmental Health and Human Ecology," Supplement to *American Journal of Public Health,* Part 2, LIV, January, 1964, p. 8.

[53] E. Cuyler Hammond, "The Effects of Smoking," *Scientific American,* CCVII, July, 1962, pp. 39-51.

[54] *Ibid.,* p .42.

among nonsmokers. He states that this finding is the most significant of all. Though the death rate is lowest among nonsmokers, those who stop smoking have a longer life expectancy than those who continue to smoke. There is also an adverse relationship between the number of cigarettes smoked and the life expectancy. The more cigarettes smoked, the shorter the life span. Since the results of Hammond's study will be discussed in chapters including content on cancer and coronary artery disease, this material will not be further considered here.

In January, 1964, the Surgeon General of the United States released a report based on a long series of major research projects establishing smoking as a significant health hazard.

What are some of the physical or chemical agents of intrinsic origin that may cause injury to cells?

In the preceding discussion, some of the physical and chemical agents found in the external environment that have a deleterious effect on the structure and functions of cells have been presented. Cellular injury also may be caused by physical or chemical agents of intrinsic origin. It may result from the abnormal distribution or concentration of one or more body constituents or from the failure of one or more steps in the utilization of substances within the cell. The latter is usually due to the lack of one or more enzymes or to some condition interfering with their action. As a consequence, substances which are necessary to the body economy or which are the product of a step in metabolism accumulate within or around the cells. Chemically inert substances may act as foreign bodies. In common with foreign bodies of extrinsic origin, chemically inert substances provoke an inflammatory response. In addition, those that are chemically active may also alter chemical and physical conditions within the cell and have an adverse effect on the activity of cellular enzymes. The effects of the accumulation of normal or abnormal products within or around cells can be summarized as follows: (1) As they accumulate they occupy space, thereby encroaching on normal cellular constituents. (2) They alter the physical and chemical conditions in and around the cell, thereby interfering with the activity of enzymes. Some of these conditions are reversible when detected early. If they are allowed to progress, they lead to death of parenchymal cells and all that their loss implies.

Although there are many possible disturbances in intermediary metabolism, among the most common are those involving fat, amyloid, and calcium. Disturbances in the metabolism of glucose are discussed elsewhere. Disturbances in the metabolism of fat or lipids are most frequently of one of two types. One or both types may be present in a tissue at one time. Although the mechanisms by which they affect tissue are different, they are both known as fatty infiltration. In the first type, adipose tissue cells undergo hyperplasia. They are found in organs or in parts of organs where they are not normally present. They infiltrate the tissue rather than the cells. In the other, fat particles enter (infiltrate) cells and displace cellular elements. In severe obesity, adipose tissue cells undergo hyperplasia and infiltrate tissues in which they are not normally found For example, some fat is ordinarily found around the base of the heart; however, in severe obesity adipose tissue cells infiltrate the muscle. They do not enter the muscle cells, but they lie between muscle fibers. They neither cause cellular degeneration, nor provoke an inflammatory response. Because of their number, they occupy space and interfere with function by their presence or mechanical effect.

Adipose tissue may also fill space left by the atrophy of the parenchyma of organs. Replacement of parenchymatous tissue by adipose tissue sometimes follows normal involution of organs, such as the thymus at puberty. It is also associated with pathology. Atrophy of muscle, especially when it results from a loss of the nerve supply to the muscle, may be accompanied by an increase in adipose tissue. When this happens the affected extremity may maintain its normal size, despite the loss of muscle tissue. Of course, with the loss of muscle, the function of the extremity is lost.

Persons who are obese and in whom loss of weight is desired are placed on a weight-reduction regime. Before a strenuous program is introduced, the patient should undergo a medical evaluation so that his general state of health, as well as the reasons for his overweight, can be determined. Central to any weight-reduction program is the development of a pattern of eating compatible with continued optimum weight. There are many ways in which the nurse may be helpful to the patient. One is to aid in the interpretation of the diet plan. Another is to encourage and support the patient so that he does not become discouraged. Physicians differ in their opinions about the most successful way to initiate, secure, and maintain weight reduction. Even the matter of "crash" diets is far from settled. In particular, Duncan has found that a total fast of from two days to two weeks may be desirable, but must be supervised.

In the other type of fatty infiltration, lipids enter the cells of the organ and displace normal elements of the cell. One organ in which this type of fatty infiltration occurs is the liver. Though fatty infiltration of the liver may develop rapidly, it usually develops slowly. In the United States, the most common cause of fatty infiltration of the liver is the malnutrition accompanying chronic alcoholism. In chronic alcoholism the principal source of calories is ethyl alcohol. The etiology of fatty liver is disputed. The current most popular theory is that alcohol affects the DPN$\rightleftharpoons$DPNH system so that DPNH[55] is greater than DPH; entrance of acetyl Co A into Krebs cycle is impaired, and the two carbon fragments are shunted toward fat synthesis. In parts of the world where the supply of high-quality proteins is deficient and malnutrition is made more severe by diarrhea, a disease called

[55] DPN is an abbreviation for diphosphopyridine nucleotide. The reduced form is abbreviated to DPNH.

kwashiorkor is common among young children. One of its striking features is fatty degeneration of the liver. One of the problems in the care of the patient who is alcoholic is to encourage him to eat foods such as meat, milk, eggs, and cheese. In regions where high-quality proteins are not available in sufficient quantity, the first problem is to supplement the available diet with protein and to do this inexpensively. The other is to teach mothers how and why the new food should be used.

Ingestion of poisons, such as phosphorus, is followed by the rapid development of fatty degeneration. Though the liver is perhaps the most common site of fatty degeneration, other organs such as the heart muscle may be affected. Fatty degeneration of the heart is a serious complication of diphtheria and of marked and longstanding anemia, particularly pernicious anemia. Phosphorus poisoning has become infrequent, since phosphorus is no longer used in matches. Diphtheria is easily prevented by immunization. Patients with pernicious anemia can be protected by adequate treatment of their anemia. In the latter two conditions, the nurse contributes through participating in public and individual education and by assisting with the required procedures.

Despite the importance of disorders characterized by fatty infiltration of vital organs, the disease with the highest incidence in which disordered metabolism of lipids is strongly implicated is atherosclerosis. The general effects of this disorder were discussed earlier in the chapter. They will be further considered in Chapter 9.

What are some effects of chronic infection?

Although the problems created by infections and infectious disease will be presented in another chapter, many longstanding infections are accompanied by a common type of degenerative change in cells. In longstanding infections such as empyema, tertiary syphilis, and tuberculosis, a starchlike substance known as amyloid is deposited in the cells of the body. The organs most likely to be affected are the kidneys, spleen, liver, and adrenal glands. Similar to fatty degeneration, amyloid degeneration usually develops slowly and does not cause acute cellular degeneration or stimulate an acute inflammatory response. It does result in atrophy of the cell, probably as a result of interference with cellular nutrition. Symptoms resulting from the failure of function depend on the extent of damage to the affected organs. Though a number of organs may be involved, death is usually from renal failure.

Like other body constituents, calcium and phosphorus are subject to disturbances in their metabolism. Normally they exist in the blood plasma in a concentration very close to saturation. About one half of the plasma calcium is in an ionized form and the other half is bound to protein and is therefore in a colloidal form. The latter serves as a reserve supply which can be added to or subtracted from as needed. Phosphorus also exists in the plasma in differing states. These include the phospholipids and ester lipids and inorganic phosphorus in the form of mono- and dibasic phosphate ions. There is a reciprocal relationship between the levels of calcium and phosphate ions in the blood. When the level of one is raised, that of the other is depressed. The product of their levels must be kept below a certain point or precipitation of calcium occurs.

Knowledge of the factors entering into the regulation of calcium and phosphorus is incomplete. Because of their reciprocal relationship, anything that affects the level of one also affects the level of the other. Their levels in the plasma, however, represent a balance between intake and output. Absorption of calcium from the gastrointestinal tract is increased by vitamin D_2, or calciferol. Calciferol also increases the excretion of phosphates in the urine. Although authorities are not in complete agreement as to the action of parathormone, it is believed to regulate the excretion of phosphates by the kidney and absorption of calcium from the gut and bone. When the level of phosphates in the plasma falls, the calcium level rises. The source of the calcium is either from absorption from the gastrointestinal tract or from the bone. Although discussion of the metabolism of calcium and phosphorus in the bone is not planned here, the bone serves as an important reserve supply of both.

Abnormal calcification may take place when tissue is diseased or in certain types of disturbances of calcium and phosphorus metabolism. There are many conditions in which calcification of diseased tissues occurs. The ultimate effect depends on the tissues affected and the effect that the calcification has on the functioning capacity of the involved or related organs. For example, calcification of fibrous tissue in an old tubercle or thrombus is an expected reaction of the body to a particular type of injury. It is also regarded as beneficial rather than harmful. Calcification of the medial layer of middle-sized arteries results in the so-called pipestem arteries. This type of calcification is relatively harmless. In contrast, calcification of the pericardium, which sometimes follows tuberculosis or pneumococcal pericarditis, causes great harm. The firm wall formed around the heart limits its ability to dilate and therefore to fill during diastole. This condition is known as constrictive pericarditis. Calcification of the heart valves following the healing of rheumatic fever contributes to their rigidity and deformity and to their failure to open or close properly.

Disturbances in the metabolism of calcium and phosphorus may result in the calcification of normal tissues. As was stated earlier, calcium and phosphorus are in the blood in a nearly saturated solution. Any condition increasing the level of one or the other, or that decreases their solubility, favors precipitation. For example, calcium is more soluble in an acid than in an alkaline solution. Consequently, calcification is more likely to occur in those tissues where alkaline conditions exist. According to Hopps[56] these are most likely to be in the stomach, lungs, and kidneys. In the stomach, following secretion the cells secreting hydrochloric acid are left with an excess of

[56] *Op. cit.,* p. 125.

hydroxyl ions and are therefore relatively alkaline. In the kidney tubule, cells are in an alkaline state after the excretion of acid phosphate. The effect on the patient depends on which organ is calcified. Other conditions favoring calcification of normal tissues are hyperparathyroidism, the excessive intake of calciferol, and primary disease of bone associated with excessive decalcification of the bones. In nursing, knowledge that excessive intake of vitamin D may result in pathology should serve as a basis for instructing parents and patients to limit the dosage of vitamin D to that prescribed by the physician. This is the instance where some is good, but more is definitely not better.

Another pathological condition resulting from the precipitation of calcium and phosphorus and sometimes other blood constituents is the formation of concretions or stones. The terms used to indicate their formation or presence are lithiasis and calculi. Stones are formed in hollow organs and their ducts, primarily in the biliary and urinary tracts. Though their composition varies, they are generally composed of calcium, phosphorus, and organic matter. The formation of stones depends on two factors: (1) a focus, usually of organic materials, and (2) a soluble substance in solution which precipitates on the organic particles such as bacteria, epithelial cells, or tissue debris. The substance that precipitates depends on the constituents of the fluid in the hollow organ or duct. For example, calculi formed in the gall bladder may be composed of cholesterol, calcium, or bilirubin or a mixture of two or more of these substances. Those formed in the urinary tract are most likely to be of calcium oxalate.

The effects of lithiasis depend on such factors as the size of the stones and the structure in which they are located. Small stones generally cause more trouble than large stones, because the small stone is more likely to move into a duct and cause obstruction and muscle spasm. The muscle spasm is accompanied by severe cramping pain, which is referred to as colic. The patient with a stone in the common bile duct accompanied by pain is said to have biliary colic. The patient with a stone in the ureter has renal colic. In both instances, the pain is thought to be due to the muscle spasm induced by obstruction and stretching of the tube. The pain, which is often accompanied by some degree of shock, is severe, often exquisitely so.

If the stone remains in the duct, it also causes obstruction. The consequences of the obstruction depend, in part, on its location. An obstruction in the cystic duct from the gall bladder may cause pressure on the blood supply of the duct and be followed by gangrene of the gall bladder and spillage of bile into the peritoneal cavity. Obstruction of the common bile duct or a ureter interferes with the drainage of the liver or the kidney, respectively. This leads to pressure and stasis and, if unrelieved, to infection and eventually to the atrophy or necrosis of the affected organ. Other effects will depend on the function of the organ.

At this time there is no known method of dissolving calculi that are already formed. Because fat in the stomach initiates a reflex initiating contraction of the gall bladder, patients who are subject to biliary colic are advised to restrict their intake of fat. The nurse can assist the patient by helping him to learn what foods to include or reject from his diet. For patients who have, or who are predisposed to, renal calculi, teaching them to maintain an adequate, or even a high fluid intake, may help to keep the urine diluted and thus prevent the formation of stones. When a patient is admitted in acute colic, measures should be taken to relieve his pain as rapidly as possible. This usually involves the injection of an analgesic such as morphine or Demerol hydrochloride[57] and an antispasmodic such as atropine sulfate, scopolamine hydrobromide[58] and/or papaverine hydrochloride. Prescription of the drug or drugs to be used is, of course, the prerogative of the physician. The nurse is responsible for making the needs of the patient known to him and for instituting prescribed therapy as soon as possible.

How do body fluids cause cell injury?

One further source of injury to cells is the patient's own secretions and body fluids. As stated earlier, blood escaping from blood vessels causes damage by occupying space, by irritation and by increasing the number of osmotically active particles in the area. There is usually an inflammatory response in tissues into which there has been bleeding. Interstitial fluid or lymph, when it accumulates in excessive quantities, interferes with tissue nutrition because it occupies space.

Digestive juices are also capable of causing cell injury when they escape from the gastrointestinal tract, or when the balance between the resistance of the mucous membrane lining the tract and the digesting action of the secretion is upset. Gastric, pancreatic, and intestinal juices contain protein-splitting enzymes. When they come in direct contact with cells, these enzymes break down the protein constituents of cells into polypeptides or amino acids and thereby disrupt the structure of cells. The digesting action of the various secretions is modified by the pH. In health, gastric juice is acid, and secretions in the intestine are alkaline. A prolonged or marked lowering of the pH of the gastric juice is a frequent finding in peptic ulcers, that is, in ulceration of the distal end of the stomach and the proximal portion of the duodenum. Although ulceration may occur anywhere along the alimentary canal, the stomach, the proximal portion of the duodenum, and the large intestine are the most common sites. Ulcerative disease of the large bowel is often disabling. Not all the factors responsible for ulceration along the alimentary canal are understood. In many instances multiple factors probably interact to disturb the balance between the digesting action of the juices in the stomach or intestines and the efficiency with which the mechanisms for the protection of the mucous lining act. The results of this failure are disruption of cell struc-

[57] Trade name for meperidine hydrochloride.
[58] Also known as hyoscine hydrobromide Bp.

ture and the formation of sores opening to the surface of the mucous lining of the alimentary canal. The size and depth of the ulcers vary with the location, acuteness of the condition, and other factors.

Specific therapy of ulceration along the gastrointestinal tract is directed toward providing conditions favorable to healing. To the extent to which the ulceration is related to the patient's way of life, healing and continued good health may also depend on the identification and control of predisposing factors. Thus Mrs. Johns, who has an active duodenal ulcer, is admitted to the hospital for treatment. She is thereby removed from her usual environment. In addition a therapeutic regime is instituted to accomplish two general objectives. One is to decrease the motor and secretory activity of the alimentary canal and the other is to decrease the digesting power of the gastric juice. As soon as Mrs. Johns is well enough, a program of instruction is begun that will help her learn to manage her life and disease so that the possibility of future ulcerations are decreased. The problems associated with the therapy of the patient with peptic ulcer are described more fully in Chapter 10.

Digestive juices also have a destructive action on cell proteins of structures outside the alimentary canal. Pancreatic enzymes, when activated by a reflux of bile into the duct of Wirsung, digest the pancreas. This serious condition may be induced by obstruction of the ampula of Vater by biliary calculi, or by scar tissue. Fistulae, especially those from the small intestine, usually heal with great difficulty. Sometimes they are of great size. Healing is facilitated by preventing digestive enzymes from coming in contact with body tissues. This is not easy.

An abnormal opening such as an ileostomy or colostomy allows the intestinal contents to escape onto the abdominal wall. Unless appropriate measures are instituted, breakdown of the skin is inevitable. The situation is more acute when the feces are fluid than when they are solid, as the watery state brings the enzymes in contact with the skin. The proper application of an ilestomy or colostomy bag reduces this possibility to a great extent. Other measures are discussed elsewhere.

Continued exposure of the skin to urine predisposes to its breakdown. The skin does not tolerate being wet over long periods of time as this predisposes the skin to maceration and lessens its resistance to destructive agents. In addition, with standing, urea contained in urine is decomposed by bacteria to ammonia, a highly irritating substance. When urine escapes onto the skin, prevention of cell destruction depends on the conscientious use of measures designed to prevent urine from coming in contact with the skin or to remove it by washing the exposed areas of the skin with soap and water and changing the bed linen promptly.

Summary

In this chapter some of the causes and effects of injury to cells have been presented. Emphasis has been on the nature of the pathological changes rather than on the agents causing the injury. Agents leading to cellular injury may have their origin in the external or the internal environment of cells or from within the cell itself. Injury to the cell may result from a deficiency of, or an excess of, or imbalance among substances required by the cell or substances useful to the organism in its activities. Cellular injury may be induced by agents interfering with machinery of the cell for utilizing nutrients, or by alteration of the nature of the proteins within the cell. Within limits, cells are capable of adapting to unfavorable conditions. They do this by undergoing atrophy or hypertrophy or hyperplasia or by altering the character of cells. Furthermore, the cells reverse the changes induced by injury provided the structure of the cell itself is not altered.

In relation to tissue injury, the nurse has a responsibility to prevent injury to cells and tissues by forestalling conditions leading to further injury. The responsibilities of the nurse encompass a variety of activities ranging from public education to the direct care of the sick. Public education includes activities such as how to protect children from accidental poisoning and what to do should poisoning occur or be suspected. Some of the activities in the care of the sick to prevent injury or to protect already injured tissues have been indicated. More will be included in later chapters.

REFERENCES

Books

Apperly, Frank L., *Patterns of Disease,* J. B. Lippincott Co., Philadelphia, 1951.
Best, C. H., and H. B. Taylor, *The Physiological Basis of Medical Practice,* 7th ed., The Williams & Wilkins Co., Baltimore, 1961.
Bland, William H., Franz K. Bauer, and Benedict Cassen, *The Practice of Nuclear Medicine,* Charles C Thomas, Springfield, Illinois, 1958.
Boyd, William, *A Textbook of Pathology,* 7th ed., Lea & Febriger, Philadelphia, 1961.
Harkins, Henry, *et al.,* eds., *Surgery: Principles and Practice,* 2nd ed., J. B. Lippincott Co., Philadelphia, 1961.
Harmer, Bertha, and Virginia Henderson, *Textbook of Principles and Practice of Nursing,* 5th ed. The Macmillan Company, New York, 1955.
Hopps, Howard C., *Principles of Pathology,* 2nd ed., Appleton-Century-Crofts, Inc., New York, 1964.
Kulowski, Jacob, *Crash Injuries,* Charles C Thomas, Springfield, Illinois, 1960.
Lapp, Ralph E., *The Voyage of the Lucky Dragon,* Harper & Brothers, New York, 1957.
McLaughlin, Harrison L., *Trauma,* W. B. Saunders Co., Philadelphia, 1959.
Quimby, Edith H., *Safe Handling of Radio Active Isotopes in Medical Practice,* The Macmillan Company, New York, 1960.
Smullen, Willard C. (ed.), *Basic Foundations of Isotope Techniques for Technicians,* Charles C Thomas, Springfield, Illinois, 1956.

Articles

Artz, Curtis, and Byron Green, "Essentials of Burn Therapy," *Surgical Clinics of North America,* XXXVIII, December, 1958, pp. 1461-74.
Baker, Thomas, "Open Technique in the Management of Burns," *American Journal of Nursing,* LIX, September, 1959, pp. 1262-65.
Bardsley, Christine, Helen Fowler, Edith Moody, Elizabeth Teigen, Elizabeth and Joan

Sommer, "Pressure Sores," *American Journal of Nursing,* LXIV, No. 5, May, 1964, pp. 82-84.

Bugher, John, "Radiation and Human Health," *American Journal of Public Health,* XLVII, June, 1957, p. 682.

Campbell, Rose M., "The Surgical Management of Pressure Sores," *Surgical Clinics of North America,* XXXIX, April, 1959, pp. 509-30.

Costa, P. J., and Mary Jane Dews, "Mushroom Poisoning," *American Journal of Nursing,* LVI, August, 1956, pp. 998-1000.

Davis, J., Jr., "We Cure Bed Sores with Sheepskin," *R.N.,* XXII, October, 1959, p. 59.

"Decubitus Ulcer," *Journal of the American Medical Association,* CLXV, November 9, 1957, p. 1780.

Eckelberry, Niel, "Electric Burns," *American Journal of Nursing,* LV, July, 1955, pp. 836-38.

Elser, Joan Riemer, "Acute Barbiturate Intoxication," *American Journal of Nursing,* LX, August, 1960, pp. 1096-99.

Garb, Solomon, "Survival in a Thermonuclear War: III. Important Aspects of Nuclear Radiation," *New York State Journal of Medicine,* LX, September 1, 1960, pp. 2731-34.

Hasterlik, Robert J., "Radiation Injuries: Their Nature and Diagnoses," *Medical Clinics of North America,* XLIV, January, 1960, pp. 193-202.

Hebb, D. O., "Motivating Effects of Exteroceptive Stimulation," *American Psychologist,* XIII, March, 1958, p. 109.

Heron, W., B. K. Doane, and T. H. Scott, "Visual Disturbances after Prolonged Perceptual Isolation," *Canadian Journal of Psychology,* X, 1956, p. 13.

Heron, Woodburn, "The Pathology of Boredom," *Scientific American,* CXCVI, January, 1957, pp. 52-56.

Hicks, Mary L., and Ina June Cannell, "Decubitus Ulcers," *American Journal of Nursing,* LVIII, July, 1958, pp. 1008-10.

McIntyre, Patricia Hope, "Total Body Irradiation," *American Journal of Nursing,* LXI, September, 1961, pp. 62-65.

Owen, Charles A., "The Diagnostic Use of Radioactive Isotopes," *Post-graduate Medicine,* XXIV, November, 1958, pp. 449-54.

Owen, Charles A., "The Diagnostic Use of Radioactive Isotopes," *Post-graduate Medicine,* XXIV, December, 1958, pp. 669-73.

Owen, Charles A., "The Diagnostic Use of Radioactive Isotopes," *Post-graduate Medicine,* XXV, February, 1959, pp. 196-201.

Powell, Clinton C., "Medical Aspects of the Control of Radiologic Health Problems," *American Journal of Public Health,* XLVII, February, 1957, p. 179.

Powell, Clinton C., "Radiation Hazards," *American Journal of Public Health,* XLIX, January, 1959, p. 1.

Puck, Theodore T., "Radiation and the Human Cell," *Scientific American,* CCII, April, 1960, pp. 142-52.

Putt, Arlene M., "Radiation Accidents," *Nursing Outlook,* IX, June, 1961, pp. 350-415.

Rhodes, Verna, and Anna Shannon, "Nursing Care of the Burn Patient," *American Journal of Nursing,* LIX, September, 1959, pp. 1265-68.

Snively, W. D., "The Body's Response to Burning," *G.P.* (General Practitioner), XX, September 19, 1959, pp. 132-44.

"Symposium of Surgical Therapeutics," *Surgical Clinics of North America,* XXXIX, February, 1959, p. 1.

Worman, Leonard W., Carol J. Yount, and Lois E. Jacobs, "The Care of Patients with Gunshot Wounds," *American Journal of Nursing,* LXIII, February, 1963, pp. 93-96.

4 : The Control of Infections

From the most ancient times peoples have taken measures to protect themselves against the introduction of diseases from without.
Among the most elaborate codes of this kind in the written history of
man are the regulations enunciated in the Hebrew scriptures, chiefly
in the Book of Leviticus.[1]

Man lives in a world populated with other forms of life, many of which
threaten his existence. Not all living forms are directly visible, though their
effects can be observed. Neither are all forms of invisible life, or microbes,
harmful. As a matter of fact, relatively few microorganisms are harmful or
disease-producing. Many are highly beneficial to man.

Disease producing microorganisms are called pathogens, and the diseases
they cause are called infectious diseases. The process involved in the development of an infectious disease is called an infection. Most authorities define
infection as a condition resulting from the entrance of microorganisms into
the tissues of the body causing injury and subsequently tissue reactions.
Dubos[2] disagrees with this definition; he prefers to use the term "infection" to
mean that microorganisms are present in the tissues, whether or not there is
evidence of detectable pathology.

*What are some of the general characteristics of
infectious diseases?*

Although infectious diseases have a number of similar characteristics, they
are also very different from one another. One characteristic common to all is
that they are caused by pathogenic microorganisms. The microorganism may
be a virus, bacterium, yeast, mold, protozoan or other parasite. The microbe
is capable of being transmitted from a reservoir, usually another human being,
but it may be an animal, to a susceptible host. The infectious disease may
occur with great frequency and be readily transmissible, such as the common
cold or measles, or it may occur infrequently and only under special conditions. It may be self-limiting, that is, run a relatively predictable course and be
self-terminating; or it may have no point at which it terminates naturally but
continue indefinitely. It may induce a more or less permanent immunity or be

---

[1] *World Health,* November-December, 1958, p. 7.
[2] René J. Dubos, "The Evolution and the Ecology of Microbial Diseases," *Bacterial and Mycotic Infections of Man,* 3rd ed., J. B. Lippincott Company, Philadelphia,
1958, pp. 14-27.

characterized by repeated attacks. The infectious process may be relatively mild or wreak great destruction. For some reason not understood, different microorganisms have a predilection for specific organs or tissues of the body. The period of time required by different microorganisms to establish themselves in the body and induce disease varies from hours to many months and possibly years.

Terms relating (more or less specifically) to infectious diseases are defined below:

Communicable disease is an illness caused by a specific infectious agent or its toxic products, which is transmitted directly or indirectly from an infected person or animal to a susceptible host.

Carrier is an apparently well person in whom pathogenic microorganisms live and multiply without apparent ill effect.

Contamination indicates the presence of pathogenic or disease-producing microorganisms on inanimate objects. The term "contamination" is often used to indicate the possibility rather than the known presence of microorganisms.

Endemic is a disease continuously present in a community.

Epidemic is a temporary and significant increase in the incidence of a disease at a given time.

Pandemic is a world-wide epidemic.

Sporadic means that disease occurs occasionally and its incidence is low.[3]

What are the nurse's responsibilities in the control of infectious diseases?

References are made to certain aspects of infectious disease in other chapters. In this chapter, information has been selected to further the understanding of the nurse of some of the important problems involved in the control of diseases caused by microorganisms. No attempt will be made to describe in detail all of the infectious diseases to which man is heir. A number of diseases that are problems in the United States will be selected to illustrate points being made, but not all information about each disease will necessarily be included. Emphasis is on the control of an infectious disease, rather than on the care of the patient who is sick with one or another of the infectious diseases. The nursing of the person who is ill with an infectious disease has two general aspects, the care of the person who is sick and the prevention of the spread of disease to the nurse and others. As in the control of infectious disease in the community, measures employed can be classified as:[4]

[3] For a more complete list of definitions see *Control of Communicable Diseases in Man,* 9th ed., An Official Report of the American Public Health Association, 1960, The American Public Health Association, 1790 Broadway, New York.

[4] Gaylord W. Anderson, Margaret G. Arnstein, and Mary R. Lester, *Communicable Disease Control,* 4th ed., The Macmillan Company, New York, 1962.

1. Preventing spread.
2. Increasing the resistance of the new host.
3. Minimizing the ill effects of cases that have not been prevented.

To fulfill her responsibilities in the control of infectious disease the nurse requires a body of knowledge that will enable her to perform as follows:

1. She must keep abreast with changes in knowledge of the factors in the control of infectious disease.
2. She must develop procedures and practices based on the knowledge required for the protection of patients, personnel (including self), and the community.
3. She must evaluate, or participate in the evaluation of, practices employed in the control of infectious disease.
4. She must accept changes in established procedures when change or changes are indicated.
5. She must carry out procedures that are for the protection of all concerned.
6. She should develop and/or participate in the hospital or agency educational program.
7. She should participate in the hospital or agency program to control infection:
   a. By identifying problems in the control of infection.
   b. As a participating member of the committee on infections.
      (1) She should report to the committee problems in the control of infections.
      (2) She should report to the nursing staff the deliberations of the committee.
      (3) She should make suggestions in the committee on the problems and possible solutions.
   c. By making suggestions to the nurse member of the committee on the problems and proposing suggestions as to how the problems might be solved.
8. She must recognize that in the present state of knowledge the control of some of the troublesome infections is complex and complicated.
   a. Nurses should be prepared and willing to cooperate in investigating the source of infections and in correcting conditions that appear to be responsible.
9. She must act as a case finder.
10. She should participate in community programs of prevention.
11. She should participate in the education of the public in supporting the rational use of antimicrobial agents.

The above is indeed an imposing list of responsibilities. To fulfill them, the nurse requires knowledge, experience, interest in learning, and a willingness to alter her practice when new discoveries indicate the need for change. In addition, the effective control of an infectious disease frequently depends not on the nurse alone, but on the cooperation of a large proportion of the community.

What concept must be implemented if change is to be brought about?

One of the essential elements in the effective control of infectious disease is application of the concept: A change in practice is difficult if not impossible to effect, unless the person who desires to bring it about understands what the beliefs and values are that support existing practices. Understanding of this concept is important in the United States because of the diverse character of the population. Furthermore, more and more nurses are traveling to distant lands to assist people to improve their health practices. Since not all persons have the same beliefs or system of values, one of the elements in the success of nurses working with peoples from different cultures is the ability to put into practice the above concept.

What are some of the general beliefs about the causes of disease?

One way to approach the problem of differences in belief about the nature of infectious disease is to trace the historical development of ideas about disease. In the world of today, there are groups of people who are in all stages of knowledge in respect to the cause and control of infectious disease. Knowledge of what a person or a people believe to be the cause and proper treatment of disease is important if one is to secure cooperation. Sometimes the measures employed by a group of people have a sound basis, though there may be little or no understanding of why a practice is successful. Their practices are based on observation and interpretation of apparent cause-effect relationships and not on scientific knowledge. For example, bubonic plague is still endemic in Kurdistan. When villagers observe that the rat population is increasing, they move out of their houses into huts located in the middle of a field some distance from the village. Villagers start watching the rats more closely in September, for the plague season starts then and continues until May.[5] The observation that rats have something to do with the spread of disease is valid, since plague is transmittd from sick rats to human beings by fleas. Moving from the village to a hut in the center of the field is successful in limiting the spread of the plague because it removes people from the source of the infection, the sick rat carrying the transmitter of plague, the flea. The move is made, however, not because the people understand the above relationships, but because the increase in the rat population is regarded as an omen of an impending epidemic of a deadly disease.

[5] Pierre Gascar, "Died of the Plague: Ramsara's Daughter, 14 Years," *World Health,* XI, May-June, 1958, p. 12.

Over the course of history of mankind, ideas about the cause of disease have included the following:

1. Disease is due to the malign influence of supernatural powers.
2. Disease is punishment for sin and the result of the wrath of an essentially righteous god.
3. Disease is part of the natural order and can be explained on a rational basis.
4. Disease is due to the epidemic constitution of the atmosphere, miasmic influences, and filth.
5. Disease is due to a germ.
6. Disease, in some instances at least, requires not only the necessary condition (a microbe), but a sufficient cause.

This list of theories could be further expanded.

None of the above has been entirely relegated to the past. The first, or demonic, theory, though probably the oldest theory of the causation of disease, has not been entirely eliminated. Usually this theory is expressed in one of three ways. Living persons (witches) have the power to cause disease in other living persons. This power may be exercised in different ways: the individual may cast a spell on someone whom he dislikes; or he may have some power such as an evil eye. The witches were persons who were believed to have an evil influence because of supernatural powers. Even today one may hear an expression of the belief that one person is able to harm others as a result of supernatural powers. Sam Thrill says, "You had better stay away from me, I always bring other people bad luck."

A second form of the demonic theory is that disease is caused by the spirits of disembodied dead. This idea is the basis for some of the burial rites practiced by primitive peoples. It is not unknown today, however.

A third expression of the demonic theory is that disease results from superhuman abilities of inanimate objects. Stones, trees, animals, and natural events are ascribed special qualities which enable them to act in a malevolent fashion.

When a demon is held to be responsible for disease, prevention and treatment are directed toward the demon rather than the person who is sick. The principal methods employed are exorcism, evasion, and sacrificial propitiation. The individual who is possessed of a devil is beaten or he is given a vile-tasting medicine. Trephining (making a hole in the skull) was originally performed to provide an avenue of escape for the demon who had taken over the body of the sick person. Evasion, or avoiding the demon, is achieved by rituals which are prescribed to prevent contact between the potential victim and the evil spirit. The people of Kurdistan, by moving from the village to the field, were practicing a form of evasion. Sacrifices are made to appease the god who is believed to cause the epidemic. The sacrifice is really a bribe. The man makes the sacrifice, not to atone for wrongdoing, but to prevent an evil spirit from harming him.

How does the second theory of disease causation differ from the first?

A second theory of disease causation is that disease is incurred by the wrath of an essentially righteous god as a punishment for sin. Winslow[6] states that this concept of disease causation reached its height among Semitic peoples and is best expressed in the Old Testament. This belief, however, was not limited to the Hebrews. The Hindus believed the epidemic of plague (1896–1897) was a punishment imposed on them by their god Silva.[7] "Sin-caused" disease was treated by making atonement sacrifices to the offended god. Earlier modes of treatment, i.e., magical practices to appease demons, were condemned in this era. The theory of disease as a punishment for sin introduced a new concept as it is based on a law of the universe in which the law is spiritual rather than material.[8]

The first known reference to the idea that events in the universe can be explained on a rational basis appeared in the sixth century B.C. in the writings of the Ionic Greeks. Again in the words of Winslow,[9] "The Hebrews gave us a universe of moral law; but the Greeks clearly visualized for the first time in human history a universe of natural law." Thus the Greeks introduced a new way of thinking about disease. They stressed observation as a tool for learning about disease and advocated looking at the patient, rather than assuming that his disease was something imposed on him from without by another being.

What is the basis for the theory that disease is due to the epidemic constitution of the atmosphere, miasmic influences, and filth?

In the period between Hippocrates and Pasteur, emphasis was on epidemic constitution of the atmosphere, miasmic influences, and filth. According to this theory, disease is propagated by the air, diseased persons, and goods transported from infected places. One or more of these agents was employed to explain epidemics occurring in various parts of the earth. For example, when plague was destroying a large part of the population of the world, the pandemic was explained on the basis that the immediate cause was a malign conjunction of planets over the Indian Ocean. They produced "corrupt vapors, raised up and disseminated through the air by blasts of heavy and turbid southerly winds."[10] References to atmospheric conditions as factors

[6] Charles Edward Armory Winslow, *The Conquest of Epidemic Disease,* Princeton University Press, Princeton, 1943, p. 36.
[7] *Ibid.,* p. 39.
[8] *Ibid.,* p. 35.
[9] *Ibid.,* p. 55.
[10] *Ibid.,* p .182.

in the cause of disease are not unknown at the present time. Natural disasters, inasmuch as they disrupt measures taken to protect water and food supplies, can be sources of epidemic disease. What the individuals do at the time, however, depends what they believe about the source of illness during disaster. If one believes that the cause of the illness is borne on a "turbid southerly wind," nothing much can be done to avoid disease. If, however, one believes that, when water and sewage pipes are broken, there is a possibility of drinking water being contaminated with pathogenic microorganisms contained in human feces, then measures such as boiling water or treating it with chlorine appear to be rational.

What is meant by the term "miasmic influences"?

By miasmic influences is meant that the air is poisoned or polluted by vapors rising from swamps, marshy grounds, and putrid or decaying matter. Because miasmic influences were held to be particularly dangerous at night, houses were often tightly sealed during the hours of darkness. Application of the theory of miasmic influences to the care of the sick resulted in sealing the sick person and his entire family into their house. As a result of sealing the house, disease-producing air was prevented from escaping into the atmosphere. This also prevented contact between the sick person and the members of his family, as well as between inanimate objects used in his care and members of the community. Because it usually increased the degree of contact among family members, sealing the house practically ensured that every family member would contract the disease. In the recent past persons who were ill with certain infectious diseases, as well as their human and animal contacts, were confined for the longest usual incubation period. Although current practices vary somewhat in different legal jurisdictions and with different diseases, restriction of the movement of persons is usually limited to those who are sick with the disease. The movement of contacts, that is, persons who are exposed and who are susceptible, may be limited during the longest usual incubation period. If, by the end of the incubation period, the contacts are well, restriction on their movements is lifted. Such practices as placarding the house have been discontinued.

Why was the theory that epidemic diseases were due to the epidemic constitution of the air, miasmic influences, and filth reasonable prior to the mid 19th century?

The theory that epidemic diseases were due to the constitution of the air, miasmic influences, and filth may appear to be strange. Considering, however, the state of knowledge and the conditions under which people lived during the Middle Ages, the theory was reasonable. It is difficult, if not impossible, for the modern-day middle-or upper-class American to imagine the conditions of filth under which people lived. People living in cities were crowded together.

Provisions for safe water and food supplies, as well as for the disposal of human wastes, were limited and exceedingly primitive. Because of the lack of modern sanitary facilities for human excreta, filth was everywhere.[11] Though it is now known that pathogenic microorganisms are discharged in the body excreta and are spread by flies or by contact with the excreta, this was not known in the early nineteenth century. In keeping with the ideas of the time, diseases such as typhoid and cholera were believed to be transmitted by emanations from the filth. Facilities for bathing and for maintaining general cleanliness were lacking. Furthermore, similar conditions still exist in some parts of the world. While traveling, the writer observed people using the same ditch as a source of water for drinking and cooking, for washing clothes, and for disposal of excreta. Overcrowding and limited provisions for personal and community hygiene are not unknown in certain large cities of the United States.

Not only did social conditions in the past provide a reasonable basis for the theory that infectious diseases were due to the state of the external environment, but a number of pandemics occurred. In Europe of the Middle Ages, epidemics of plague, syphilis, and cholera killed vast numbers of people. In the famous London plague of 1665, 68,596 Londoners died. Such a terrifying event called for drastic action. Consequently, it is not surprising that, besides sealing the family and person dying from plague into the house, dogs and cats were killed, as they were believed to be the source of the disease. Because of lack of knowledge of the source of plague or its mode of transmission, flea-infested rats were allowed to run free.

By the end of the eighteenth century, plague, which had been a major threat to the populations of Europe for 400 years, was no longer a serious problem. It had been recognized as being contagious and measures appropriate to its eradication were undertaken.

Although there were a number of serious pandemics during the Middle Ages and Renaissance, they have not been confined to these periods in history. References are made in the Old Testament to ancient pestilences sent by God to punish people for having sinned against Him. The last great pandemic occurred during World War I when influenza spread to all corners of the earth. More people died as a result of influenza than from battle injuries. In the United States, few people escaped, and because of the rapidity with which influenza spreads, entire families were ill at the same time.

Measures instituted to control the spread of disease during each pandemic depended on the state of knowledge and the prevailing theories of disease causation. Although some of the practices, based on the belief that the constitution of the air and filth caused disease, were irrational in the light of present-day knowledge, some were sound. The observation that disease and

---

[11] For an account of the sanitary conditions in England and other parts of the world, Winslow (*Op. cit.*, pp. 236-66, "The Great Sanitary Awakening") is highly recommended.

filth were associated led to the great sanitary movement, first in England and shortly thereafter in America. By the beginning of the nineteenth century the modern public health movement had been born. The fathers of this movement were lay people and social reformers, not physicians. Among the names referred to with some frequency in the literature are John Howard (18th century) and Edwin Chadwick (early 19th century). Neither was a physician. John Howard was a sheriff who discovered that the conditions in the jails for which he had responsibility were appalling. When one reads about the sanitary procedures that he instituted, they appear to be elementary. At the time they were put into effect, however, they were most progressive. Walls were to be whitewashed each year. The walls were to be washed and cells ventilated regularly. Hot and cold water was to be made available to the prisoners for bathing. Clean clothes were also to be lent to prisoners, if necessary.

Chadwick, who was a social reformer, studied living conditions in the slums of London. His studies led to administrative reform and to laws relating to conditions affecting the health of the poor. His report, *Condition of the Labouring Population of Great Britain,* was published in 1842. It served as the basis for the sanitary reform that spread over the civilized world.

Shortly after Chadwick's report was published, another event transpired which contributed to knowledge of the practical importance of cleanliness to health and recovery from disease. Florence Nightingale went to Turkey where war was in progress in the Crimean Peninsula. (1853–56). Aided by 37 assistants, she was able to reduce the death rate of soldiers hospitalized in Scutari from 42 to 2 per cent. Miss Nightingale had knowledge neither of germs nor of antibiotics. Previous to Miss Nightingale's appearance, cholera and dysentery ran rampant among the men who were hospitalized. She and her assistants used soap, water, clean linen, and humane care, with the result that she accomplished more than the entire British Medical Department in saving the lives of British soldiers. Though Miss Nightingale was the first to reduce the death rate among soldiers by reducing the incidence of infection, she was not the first to note the disastrous effects of infections among soldiers. An early Greek historian, Thucydides, wrote, "Appalling too was the rapidity with which men caught the infection; dying like sheep if they attended one another; and this was the principal cause of mortality."

Not too long after the close of the Crimean War, the American Civil War (1861–1865) was fought. As in the Crimean War, infectious diseases were responsible for a high rate of mortality. Dysentery, typhoid fever, and tetanus killed more men than the wounds of battle. Approximately 300,000 men died and two-thirds of them died, not from wounds, but from disease.

What events led to the germ theory of disease?

At the time Miss Nightingale was saving lives in Scutari by instituting hygienic and humane care, Pasteur was disproving the theory of spontaneous generation and developing the germ theory of disease. As is usually true when new ideas are proposed or discoveries are made, Pasteur was not solely responsible for either accomplishment, as the theory of spontaneous generation had been questioned earlier. What is important, however, is that, as a result of the work of Pasteur, the idea that living beings, no matter how small, had their origin, not from dead or decaying matter, but from other similar beings, was accepted. Translated into the germ theory of disease, a specific microorganism is a necessary condition in the development of each infectious disease. Anthrax does not devlop unless the anthrax bacillus is present. The natural culmination of the germ theory of disease was Koch's postulates. They are a set of criteria which can be utilized to prove that a specific microorganism does or does not cause a specific disease. In the period following the discoveries of Pasteur and Koch, the attention of scientists was on identifying the specific agents responsible for disease. The sanitary movement, which was introduced by the social reformers, now had a scientific basis.

The germ theory, along with related accomplishments, encouraged the hope that for each disease a specific causative agent could and would be identified. With knowledge of the cause, specific preventive and curative measures would follow; in some instances, this has happened. For example, although diphtheria has probably existed in epidemic form since the earliest times, it was not until 1826 that a French physician, Bretonneau de Tours, placed the clinical diagnosis of diphtheria on fairly firm ground. The diphtheria bacillus was seen and described by Klebs in 1883 and established as the cause by Löffler in 1884. Thus it is frequently referred to as the Klebs-Löffler bacillus. From his observations of patients and animals with the disease, Löffler postulated that the bacillus secreted a diffusable toxin which was responsible for many of the effects of the disease. After this theory was proved by other investigators, the toxin was used to stimulate animals (the horse) to produce antitoxins. The antitoxin was found to provide passive immunity against diphtheria and, when administered early in the course of the disease, to hasten recovery and to prevent serious complications.

Unfortunately, the relationship between cause, prevention, and cure does not fall so neatly into place with many infectious diseases. An effective preventive measure was available for smallpox before its cause was known, and although the disease can be prevented, there are no specific methods available for its treatment. Vaccines have been developed that are effective in the prevention of a number of other diseases, including poliomyelitis, tetanus, and whooping cough. There is no method available to cure either poliomyelitis or whooping cough. Both must run their course. Tetanus can be treated with antitoxin, provided treatment is instituted early enough. For many infectious diseases there are no specific methods that are effective in either prevention or cure.

Only a few of the accomplishments of the nineteenth century have been reviewed. As one reads about them, one cannot help but be impressed with their tremendous significance to health. The first half of the century laid the foundation for a sanitary revolution. In the second half, the reason for sanitation was discovered and the germ theory of the causation of infectious disease was formulated and demonstrated to be valid.

What discoveries have contributed to a reduction in the incidence of infectious disease?

In the nineteenth and twentieth centuries, a variety of discoveries has contributed to the reduction in the incidence of infectious disease. Included among the more important discoveries are the following:

1. Sanitary measures could effectively control the spread of enteric diseases.
2. Some diseases were caused by microorganisms, and techniques were developed, such as staining and culturing, for identifying them.
3. Immunity to some diseases can be induced:
   a. By injecting antibodies specific for the disease (temporary or passive immunity)
   b. By introducing antigenic substances (active acquired immunity)
   c. By having the disease (active acquired immunity)
4. Some diseases can be cured by antimicrobial agents. For example, penicillin cures syphilis.
5. Some diseases are transmitted by an insect vector, and in some instances the microbe also spends part of its life cycle in the insect.
6. Some pathogenic microorganisms inhabit carriers and can be disseminated to susceptible persons and cause disease.
7. Some airborne diseases are spread by droplets and others by droplet nuclei.

All of the above are of significance in any program of control of infectious disease. Each will be considered later in relation to the control of specific microorganisms.

How important are infectious diseases as causes of morbidity and mortality? Which are most important as causes of morbidity? Of mortality?

Despite the emphasis on the decreasing incidence of some infectious diseases, they continue to be important causes of both morbidity and mortality. The ubiquitous common cold and other acute respiratory infections are the most common causes of short-term disability in the United States. Acute gastrointestinal infections are second in frequency. Infectious diseases such as tuberculosis are also important causes of long-term morbidity. Since they rank fourth in the causes of death, infections continue to be significant factors in mortality. In more than 100,000 of the deaths reported each year, infections are stated to be the underlying cause.

Throughout the course of history, five infectious diseases—plague, smallpox, cholera, typhus, and yellow fever—have been the great killers. None has been entirely eradicated, as there are pockets of infection for each of the above in various parts of the world. As long as reservoirs of infection remain, there is always the possibility that one of the above can become epidemic.[12] Egypt has experienced four sizable epidemics of typhus. The latest one began in 1956. Although not included as one of the great killers in history, diphtheria was also responsible for the deaths of large numbers of persons. As with other infectious diseases, control of diphtheria depends on the continued application of appropriate measures, that is, the immunization of susceptible persons with toxoid.[13]

Though the five diseases listed above are no longer widespread, a number of others continue to be important causes of disability and death. Among them are malaria, tuberculosis, syphilis, yaws, schistosomiasis, and hepatitis. In many regions of the world, infections caused by the cocci, *Escherichia coli, Pseudomonas,* and *Klebsiella* are the cause of increasing concern.

What is the current scientific theory of the causation of infectious diseases?

Despite a large body of knowledge about microbial agents and how they reach their potential hosts, many questions remain to be answered. One of the most intriguing is: Why can virulent pathogenic agents be present in the tissues of man and not at the same time be accompanied by evidence of clinical disease. According to Dubos,[14] the most difficult question in medical microbiology is not, "How do microorganisms cause disease?" but rather, "Why do pathogens so often fail to cause disease after they become established in the tissues?" Though the answers to these questions are still incomplete, enough is known to be able to say with confidence that infectious diseases are similar to many other diseases; their development depends on the host, the etiological agent or agents, and the factors in the environment that bring the agent and host together. In certain instances, exposure of a susceptible person (nonimmune) to a microorganism known to cause a specific disease, such as measles or smallpox, almost always results in that disease. In many others, for example, tuberculosis, only a small percentage of those who are infected develop the disease (tuberculosis). The development of tuberculosis requires not only the presence of the *Mycobacterium tuberculosis,* but conditions within the host favoring its ability to establish itself and to cause

[12] WHO, What It Is, What It Does, How It Works," *World Health,* XV, July-August, 1962, pp. 4-9.
[13] Toxoid is a toxin altered by removing its toxophore, but retaining its haptophore group. It therefore has immunizing properties but is nontoxic to the recipient.
[14] René J. Dubos, "The Evolution and the Ecology of Microbial Disease," *Op. cit.,* p. 14.

disease. Dubos, in discussing the relationship of the condition of the host to the development of disease, states that during World Wars I and II, the incidence of tuberculosis rose in Europe. Following the close of each war, those who developed the disease frequently improved without the benefit of treatment. Apparently conditions occurring during the war affected the resistance of certain individuals to tuberculosis. In addition to variability in the resistance of the host, microorganisms may also vary in virulence. As an illustration, the diphtheria bacillus appears to vary in virulence from time to time.

For a variety of reasons, the incidence of specific infectious diseases varies from one part of the world to another. Because of similarities in sanitary procedures, standards of living and medical care, and climate, similar diseases are problems in the United States and western Europe. Diseases due to inadequate sanitation, such as typhoid fever, cholera, and dysentery, have been brought under control. Experience in the United States and in Zermat, a town in the Swiss Alps, indicates, however, that any real lapse in the application of methods of control can result in an outbreak of typhoid fever.

Among the infectious diseases having a high rate of morbidity in the United State are some of the acute infectious diseases of childhood—such as measles, mumps, and chickenpox; acute infections of the respiratory system—the common cold, influenza, pneumonia; and acute infections involving the gastrointestinal system. Other more serious infectious diseases include syphilis, tuberculosis, staphylococcal infections, and infections caused by the normal inhabitants of the alimentary canal. Rheumatic fever, though not due directly to infection, is the most important result of beta hemolytic streptococcic infection.

In other regions of the world, factors such as climate predispose to, or eliminate, the possibility of diseases such as malaria. Although there is a large number of infectious diseases, a few are of great significance because they affect a large number of people and have serious effects. In terms not only of the number of people involved, but also of its debilitating effects, malaria continues to be the number one health problem in the world. According to the "Little Dictionary of Infectious Diseases,"[15] 250 million people had malaria in 1955, and 140 million had it in 1962. In 1958, Ethiopia experienced an epidemic of malaria. Three million of the population of 18,000,000 had the disease and 100,000 persons died. Most of those who were sick were between the ages of 5 and 20 years, but some were younger. In some families, every member was ill.[16]

Not only is the mosquito a vector for the malarial parasite, but it requires the mosquito for part of its life cycle. In eradication projects,[17] attempts have

[15] World Health, XV, July-August, 1962, p. 5.
[16] "Malaria Epidemic Strikes Ethiopia," World Health, XIII, May-June, 1960. p. 39.
[17] The objective of eradication is to wipe out, or abolish, an infectious disease. In contrast, the objective of control is to prevent a disease from becoming a problem, that is, epidemic.

been made to eliminate the mosquito by spraying malarious areas with insecticides such as DDT (dichlordiphenyl-trichlorethane). Unfortunately, some mosquitoes have become resistant to DDT, thus greatly complicating the problem of eradication.

Among other diseases causing ill health and disability are leprosy, trachoma, yaws, and onchocerciasis, or river blindness. There are approximately ten million persons throughout the world who have leprosy. About 500 million persons have trachoma, which causes total blindness in about 1 per cent of its victims and economic blindness in about 4 per cent. Yaws is a widespread, disfiguring disease affecting large numbers of people in Asia. Onchocerciasis is due to a minute worm transmitted to man by a black fly. When these worms invade the eye, they cause blindness. Some 200 to 300 million people are believed to be infected.[18]

The purpose of presenting this brief survey of some of the more important infectious diseases in the world of today is not to provide the nurse with the information required to work in a program of control, but to emphasize that infectious diseases continue to be a real threat to the populations of the world. They are important as causes not only of mortality, but of serious degrees of morbidity. In areas where diseases such as malaria and bilharziasis are endemic progress in raising standards of living is impeded because of the large number of people who are affected with these serious and debilitating diseases.

In all infectious diseases, three factors are involved in control—a host, a parasite, and the conditions in the environment that bring the host and the parasite together.

For the purpose of this discussion, the host is a person or human being. Any living being of plant or animal origin can, however, act as a host. The mosquito is an intermediary host in the transmission of the malarial parasite. The parasite is a microorganism—virus, rickettsia, bacterium, or animal parasites such as a protozoan or worm, or fungus. Although parasites are generally regarded as enemies, they are as much a part of nature as man and they have the same type of homeostatic needs as higher organisms. Similar to higher organisms, they require oxygen and nutrients for metabolism and favorable conditions in their external environment.

What kinds of relationships may exist between microorganisms and their host?

Before a healthy baby enters the birth canal, he is free of microorganisms. Beginning with birth and continuing throughout his lifetime he acquires, and develops a relationship with, a variety of microorganisms. Depending on the host and microbe, their relationship varies all the way from one of mutual benefit to the production of serious disease in the host. The state in which a

[18] *Op. cit., World Health,* XV, pp. 5 and 8.

host and microbe live in a mutually beneficial relationship is known as symbiosis. For example, microorganisms living in the alimentary canal obtain their nutrients from its contents. They also synthesize vitamin K, a nutrient their human host cannot synthesize. The relationship is symbiotic because man and microbe both profit from the arrangement.

A second type of relationship between the host and his microorganisms is called commensalism. The microorganisms are dependent on the host, but they neither injure nor benefit it. The microorganisms of the normal flora in the gastrointestinal tract have been generally classified as commensals. Though these organisms are generally harmless, there is increasing evidence that under certain conditions they can cause infectious disease. According to McDermott,[19] the microorganisms forming the normal flora of the gastrointestinal tract are more important in the cause of infectious disease than is the *Staphylococcus*. Apparently the condition of the host is a factor in determining the type of relationship between it and the commensals.

A third type of relationship is known as parasitism. In this relationship, one organism derives significant benefit from the other. In the instances in which the commensals cause disease, they become parasitic. Of the organisms living in a parasitic relationship with the host, some are able to live independent of the host as well as with it. These are known as facultative parasites. Staphylococci and streptococci are examples of facultative parasites. Other microorganisms are dependent on the host for survival and for propagation. They are known as obligatory parasites. An example is the *Treponema pallidum*. It dies very quickly after leaving the body; it has never been cultivated, with certainty, outside the human body.

What are some of the causes and effects of disturbing the ecological equilibrium between man and microorganisms?

The relationship existing between man and his microbes is an excellent example of the concept that adaptation is basic to survival. As a result of adaptations, both man and microorganisms exist in a state of ecological equilibrium. Anything tending to disturb the equilibrium in favor of man (the host) leads to a reduction in the incidence of disease. Any disturbance in the state of equilibrium favoring the microorganism increases the incidence of disease. Survival of the microbe depends on its maintaining and reproducing itself without destroying its host. Microorganisms have been successful in doing this. For example, when a group of people are exposed to a microorganism for the first time, both the attack and morbidity and mortality rates are high. In another group, who have lived with the same microorganism for a long time, both the attack and the mortality rates tend to be low. The late Theobold Smith summarized this point in a much quoted statement, "When-

[19] Walsh McDermott, "Inapparent Infection: Relation of Latent and Dormant Infections to Microbial Persistence," *Public Health Reports*, LXXIV, June, 1959, p. 485.

ever you find a parasite that has affected a given host over a long period of time, you will find that the infection does not interfere with the survival of the host and is of low virulence." Dubos[20] cites a number of examples of populations that suffered great losses on their first exposure to smallpox. After smallpox was introduced into North America, whole villages of Indians were decimated. Historians believe that, had it not been for smallpox and other acute communicable diseases, the Indians would have been able to resist colonization more effectively than they did.

The results of the adaptation of man to his microbes, and vice versa, are also illustrated by the effects of tuberculosis among successive generations of Indians living on the Qu Appelle Valley Reservation.[21] In the first and second generations, many individuals experienced acute forms of the disease. By the third generation, though the disease was still epidemic, it showed a tendency to localize in the lung. Glandular involvement, a manifestation of high susceptibility, had fallen to 7 per cent. In the fourth generation, evidence of tuberculosis occurred in less than 1 per cent of the schoolchildren. Although an ecological equilibrium developed between two living organisms, it is not permanent. Thus the incidence could be disturbed at any time by a change in the susceptibility of the host or in the virulence of the microorganism.

Interest in the factors influencing the ecological equilibrium between host and his microorganisms has been stimulated by a number of observations. The incidence of diseases caused by microorganisms that were once believed to be relatively harmless has risen greatly. Microbes that were once susceptible to antimicrobial agents are now resistant to them. More attention is being paid to the observation that, in some individuals, the host is an important factor in whether or not an infection develops and in its outcome. Therefore a question that is being asked with increasing frequency is, "Why does the host develop or resist disease?" Perhaps one of the reasons that this question has been neglected is that it is a difficult one to answer. Another is that man prefers to look outside himself for answers to troublesome questions.

What are some of the possible reasons for the increase in the incidence of disease due to the commensals?

Man has for centuries been able to alter his external environment and adapt it to his needs. Now he is able to alter his internal environment as well. Through the use of antimicrobial agents, he has been able to change the nature of the normal flora of his gastrointestinal tract.

All living organisms live in ecological equilibrium with other living organisms. This concept is as true of microorganisms as of multicellular plants and animals. The members of an ecological system live in competition with each other. Competition is particularly keen for food. The growth and multiplication of one species may suppress the growth and multiplication of an-

[20] René Dubos, *Mirage of Health,* Harper and Brothers, New York, 1959, p. 77.
[21] *Ibid.,* p. 71.

other species. For example, despite the bad reputation of the fox as a chicken thief, he functions in nature to control the population of rodents. When, because of disease or overhunting, the fox population is decreased excessively, the population of rodents rises. When, in contrast, the population of foxes exceeds the supply of food, they become susceptible to disease and raid neighborhood chicken yards. Death from starvation may also help to reduce their number.

In the gastrointestinal tract many microorganisms live in a state of equilibrium not only with their host, but with each other. Apparently, when this equilibrium is not disturbed, the growth of some species tends to suppress that of others. Exactly how this is accomplished is only beginning to be understood. When the balance among the microorganisms is disturbed, some species may grow and multiply in excess and may therefore cause disease. For example, the tetracycline antibiotics, such as Aureomycin,[22] inhibit the growth and multiplication of the gram-negative bacteria forming part of the normal flora of the intestinal feces. Tetracycline-resistant organisms include yeasts, fecal streptococci, *Proteus,* and *Pseudomonas.* There are instances reported in the literature in which death was caused by *Candida albicans,* a yeast. As the bacterial count diminishes, the microorganisms that are resistant to the tetracyclines flourish and the total count of microbes may actually increase. Goodman and Gilman emphasize that the point of particular significance is that strains of microorganisms resistant to antimicrobial agents increase.[23]

Not only do microorganisms of different species apparently suppress the multiplication of other organisms, but different strains of the same organism may have the same effect. In addition, a slight change or difference in an individual of a species may alter its ability to survive in different types of environments. A previously cited example was that of the light and dark moths. The light-colored ones are adapted to survive in a rural environment, whereas those with dark coloration are better adapted to survive in industrial (sooty) cities.[24] The *Staphylococcus aureus* exhibits the same type of behavior. When penicillin was first introduced, infectious disease caused by the *Staphylococcus aureus* responded to it. After a time the observation was made that some infectious disease caused by the *Staphylococcus aureus* did not respond to antimicrobial therapy. Reasons suggested for this failure include the possibility that susceptible strains underwent mutations. The new strain or strains were then resistant. Another possibility is that reduction in the number of susceptible strains favored the growth and multiplication of resistant strains.

In a paper titled "Inapparent Infection," McDermott suggests two other possibilities for the increase in the incidence of certain infections.[25] During his

[22] Trade name for chlortetracycline.
[23] Louis S. Goodman and Alfred Gilman, *The Pharmacological Basis of Therapeutics,* 2d ed., The Macmillan Company, New York, 1956, p. 1381.
[24] H. B. D. Kettlewell, "Darwin's Missing Evidence," *Scientific American,* CC, March, 1959, pp. 48-53.
[25] McDermott, *Op. cit.,* pp. 485-89.

lifetime, man acquires and carries certain microorganisms. Some of these organisms may be in a dormant or in a latent state. McDermott distinguishes between dormant and latent infections as follows: In a dormant infection the microorganisms can be demonstrated to be present, but they are not causing disease. Carriers of *Salmonella typhi* and *paratyphi* and *Corynebacterium diphteriae* are classical examples. McDermott also suggests that the organisms comprising the respiratory and intestinal flora, the so-called commensals, may also be viewed as dormant infections. McDermott uses the term "latent infection" for situations in which organisms cannot be demonstrated to be present by methods now available, but in which overt disease later develops. A familiar example is that of herpes simplex (cold sores). The virus remains within the cells of the body. Cold sores appear only when conditions are right, that is, when the person has a fever, is overexposed to sunlight, or is menstruating.[26]

Tuberculosis sometimes recurs in persons who have been "cured" of the disease. Although the recurrence may be the result of an exogenous infection, it is believed that it is often the result of what may be called a self-infection. McDermott states that he is of the opinion that microorganisms are able to assume a state in which they are protected from the effects of microbial drugs.[27] In this state, with the methods now at hand, the presence of microorganisms in the tissue cannot be demonstrated. However, the protective state allows them to survive. When conditions again favor their resuming the vegetative state, they do so. Perhaps one of the reasons for the increasing incidence of tuberculosis among people over 50 years of age is that the microorganism was acquired earlier in their lives. At the time it entered the body it assumed a latent state. Later when the condition of the host was favorable, the *Mycobacterium tuberculosis* multiplied and caused active disease. Though tuberculosis has been used as an example, this capacity to assume a protective state is not limited to the *Mycobacterium tuberculosis*. All the reasons for microorganisms going into the dormant or latent state are not known. In some instances drug therapy may be a factor. The capacity to become latent is a mechanism by which microorganisms adapt to survive.

What information about a pathogenic microorganism is required to control its spread?

In order to answer the questions, "Who protects whom from whom?" and "How?" certain information about the pathogenic microorganism is required. Among the characteristics of a microorganism which should be considered are its capacity to survive outside a living organism, its infectivity and invasiveness, as well as its pathogenocity and virulence. It is also necessary to know what the reservoirs are and how the organism escapes from the infected individual and is transmitted to and enters the new host.

[26] *Ibid.,* p. 489.
[27] *Ibid.,* p. 490.

What are some of the factors that enable microorganisms to cause disease in a susceptible host?

One factor having significance in the capacity of pathogenic microorganisms to cause disease is their number. It is possible for a single organism to establish itself and cause disease, but an increase in the number of microorganisms is generally believed to increase the chances of disease. Some of the characteristics of microorganisms that may influence their ability to survive and to establish themselves include their: (1) morphology, (2) physiology, (3) nutritional and temperature requirements, (4) toxin production, (5) viability, and (6) resistance to destructive agents. Knowledge of such characteristics as morphology, physiology, and nutritional requirements are helpful means by which to identify microorganisms. Identification is essential to appropriate methods of treatment and control. Knowledge of temperature requirements, viability, and resistance to destructive agents is also necessary to the control of a microorganism. These points will be further clarified in the discussion of specific microorganisms.

The next link in the chain in the infectious process is the reservoir or source of a microbe. In a strict sense, a reservoir is a storage receptacle. In microbiology the term is used to indicate not only a storage site, but a place where microbes grow and propagate. Reservoirs of pathogenic microorganisms include the tissues of people, animals, and insects, as well as human wastes, and food and water contaminated by them.

Human reservoirs include apparently well persons who harbor pathogenic microorganisms, persons in the prodromal stage of illness, and those who are mildly, as well as those who are seriously, ill. The apparently well person whose mucous membranes or secretions are found to contain virulent microorganisms is called a carrier. The reasons that some individuals become carriers are not well understood. Diseases in which carriers serve as reservoirs include typhoid fever, diphtheria, and infections caused by the *Staphylococcus* and *Streptococcus*. After recovery of the individual from typhoid fever, the biliary tract can continue to act as a source of typhoid bacilli. Virulent diphtheria bacilli, staphylococci, or streptococci can be found on the mucosa of persons who have not experienced an apparent infection.

Persons who are ill with an infectious disease are reservoirs or sources of virulent microorganisms. The number of germs available for dissemination does not necessarily correspond with the stage or degree of illness. For example, the most infectious stage of measles is the prodromal stage, that is, before the rash appears and when the eyes and nose are weepy. The degree of illness apparently does not prevent the individual from being a source of microbes. Therefore a person who shows little evidence of illness or one who has symptoms only a short period of time can still be a source of infection. For example, not all persons who have poliomyelitis during an epidemic are diagnosed as having the disease. Fewer still become paralyzed. Yet persons who are not aware of having had poliomyelitis can be demonstrated to have antibodies in their blood. Terms such as "inapparent infection," "missed cases," and "abortive cases" are used to describe the situation in which an individual apparently reacted to a virulent microbe without experiencing the expected manifestations of the disease. The extent to which communicability is related to degree of illness is not known.

In addition to people, animals may serve as reservoirs of infection. Although animal reservoirs are not as important in the United States as they once were, some diseases such as Rocky Mountain spotted fever, tularemia, and psittacosis are transmitted to human beings by animals. In some parts of the world they are of considerable significance. Diseases such as plague and malaria are examples previously cited. Diseases of animals to which human beings are susceptible are known as zoonoses. The zoonoses are important not only because they are animal diseases that are transmissible to man, but because they add to the problem of disease control. As an example, a tick is the reservoir for the rickettsiae causing Rocky Mountain spotted fever. Besides man, a number of animals, some of which are wild, are susceptible to this disease. Obviously the eradication of all infected animals is difficult. Another disease difficult to eradicate is yellow fever because wild monkeys serve as reservoirs. Besides living reservoirs, inanimate substances may be sources of pathogenic microbes. As examples, food and water can be reservoirs for some microorganisms such as the *Staphylococcus, Streptococcus,* and typhoid bacillus.

In order for the infectious process to succeed, a microorganism must not only have a reservoir, but it must have a mode of escape from it. The avenues of escape from the reservoir include the respiratory, gastrointestinal, and urinary tracts, and open lesions of the skin. In some instances escape of the microorganism from the reservoir depends on some living organism other than the host. This organism is often an insect.

The most common natural avenue of escape for microorganisms is the respiratory tract. Droplets of secretions containing microorganisms located on the respiratory membranes are driven out with the expired air and by coughing, talking, and sneezing. Although large droplets quickly settle to the floor, the moisture surrounding small droplets may evaporate, leaving the nucleus containing bacteria or viruses suspended in the air. These droplet nuclei may be held aloft or wafted in air currents for considerable periods of time or for appreciable distances.[28]

Most of the pathogenic microorganisms discharged from the gastrointestinal tract are expelled with the feces. In addition to the normal flora of the intestinal tract, which can under certain circumstances cause disease, the feces may contain organisms causing typhoid and paratyphoid fever, cholera, and

[28] For a complete discussion of transmission of respiratory infections among human beings, see Richard L. Riley and Francis O'Grady, *Airborne Infection,* The Macmillan Company, New York, 1961.

amebic dysentery. Worms or their eggs may also be contained in the feces and, when ingested, cause ill health. The control of infectious diseases involving the gastrointestinal tract has been accomplished largely by providing sanitary facilities for the discharge of feces and by controlling water and food supplies. The same facilities also serve to prevent the dissemination of microorganisms contained in the urine. Open lesions serve as a route of escape either by direct contact with a sore or by contact with its discharge.

Once a microorganism has escaped from the host, it must have a vehicle for its transmission to a susceptible host. The simplest mode of transmission is direct contact. The microorganism is passed directly from one person to another either by droplets, by droplet nuclei, or by a body surface of the susceptible host coming in direct contact with infected tissue. For example, Mary Sue arises in the morning with the "sniffles," which she interprets as a cold. After she goes to school she sneezes, spraying droplets of nasal and pharyngeal secretions in all directions. Children in the room inhale the droplets as well as droplet nuclei, and within a few days many of the children have colds. The usual mode of transmission of syphilis is by the tissues of the susceptible host coming in contact with a lesion containing the *Treponema pallidum*.

Microorganisms may also be passed indirectly from one person to another by means of air currents, contaminated dust, hands, water, food, or objects. The indirect transmission of microorganisms will be illustrated in the discussion of staphylococcal infections. Some microorganisms such as the typhoid bacillus may be transmitted on the feet or bodies of insects such as the fly. To be transmitted indirectly, microorganisms must be able to survive for at least a time outside the body of the host. Organisms such as the *Treponema pallidum* and the gonococcus are fragile and survive for only brief periods outside the body. They are therefore unlikely to be transmitted by indirect contact. In contrast, the typhoid and tubercle bacilli are capable of living for extended periods of time outside the host. They can therefore be expected to be transmitted indirectly.

Besides requiring a portal of exit from the reservoir and a vehicle for transmission, microorganisms must be able to find a portal of entry into the new host. The same structures, that is, the respiratory tract, mouth, skin, and mucous membranes, that are sites for the escape of microorganisms are also portals for their entry into the host. However, before a microorganism can cause disease, it must get past the defenses which guard each of these structures. The reader is referred to Chapter 5. Even when the microorganism makes its way past these defenses, the specific resistance of the individual may be sufficient to overcome the microorganism so that disease does not occur.

The character of the microorganism also influences its disease-producing capacity. Terms used to describe attributes of microorganisms, which enable them to cause disease, include pathogenicity, virulence, and invasiveness. The term "pathogenicity" refers to the capacity of a microorganism to cause disease. The meningococcus is pathogenic for man, but under natural conditions is not pathogenic for animals.

Despite the tendency to use the term "virulence" as a synonym for pathogenicity, it adds the concept of degree of disease-producing capacity. For example, some strains of staphylococci have a greater power to produce disease, that is, greater virulence, than others. Certain viruses, such as those causing influenza, increase in disease-producing power or virulence when they pass rapidly from one susceptible person to another.

Invasiveness refers to the capacity of microorganisms to enter the tissues of the host, multiply, and spread to adjacent tissues or to distant parts of the body. Microorganisms vary greatly in their power to invade and disseminate themselves throughout the body. At one end of the scale are the toxin producers, such as the organisms of tetanus and botulism, and at the other end are the highly invasive organisms of plague and anthrax. Burdon states that most microorganisms that have any degree of invasiveness have some sort of capsule or protective covering.[29] The capsule appears to protect the microorganism against the defense mechanism of the host. An example of a microorganism whose invasiveness depends on its capsule is the pneumococcus.[30] Without its capsule, it is quickly destroyed by the phagocytes. Even viruses have a protein "capsule" surrounding the central core of DNA (desoxyribonucleic acid). The protein capsule attaches itself to the cell, but only the DNA enters. After the DNA multiplies within the cell, the cell must build protein to surround the DNA before the cell ruptures and releases the virus. Without the protein capsule, viruses cannot cause disease.[31]

Once microorganisms are established, how do they cause disease?

As indicated earlier, pathogenic microorganisms may be present in the tissues without causing manifestations of disease. For clinical evidence of the disease to appear the organism must not only establish itself in the host, but multiply in sufficient numbers to overcome host resistance and to induce certain tissue responses. Whether or not the microbe is successful in causing disease will depend on the relationship of its virulence, invasiveness, and numbers to the nonspecific and specific resistance of the host. Once the microorganism is successful in establishing itself, that is, once it becomes adapted to a susceptible host, it may then induce local and systemic effects, by one or more mechanisms. Some bacteria, such as the diphtheria bacillus, secrete water-soluble toxins that are distributed by the blood to all regions of the body. Exotoxins are responsible for the systemic manifestations of disease

[29] Kenneth L. Burdon, *Microbiology,* 5th ed., The Macmillan Company, New York, 1964, pp. 127-28.
[30] *Ibid.*
[31] Gunther S. Stent, "The Multiplication of Bacterial Viruses," *Scientific American Reader,* Simon and Schuster, New York, 1953, p. 354.

in botulism, tetanus, diphtheria, and gas gangrene. Exotoxins are highly specific, as each exotoxin acts as an antigen stimulating the body to produce a specific antitoxin (an antibody) that neutralizes a specific toxin. The exotoxin not only stimulates the antibody-producing mechanism of a victim of a disease, but it can be used to stimulate an animal, such as a sheep or a horse, to produce antitoxin. Serum obtained from an animal treated with toxin, therefore, contains the specific antibody or antitoxin, and it can be used to confer a passive immunity, that is, to neutralize toxin in the blood of an infected host. To protect a person who has a disease caused by an exotoxin-forming microbe, the antitoxin must be given early, for once a toxin has combined with cellular constituents, antitoxin is of little or no benefit. Persons with a disease, such as diphtheria or tetanus, must receive antitoxin at once if they are to benefit. Nurses acting as case finders may be responsible for getting patients under medical care. In the recent epidemic of diphtheria in one large city, a school nurse was credited with recognizing the possibility that the children who were sick had diphtheria. When her suspicions were verified, sick children were treated with antitoxin, and measures were undertaken to prevent the spread of diphtheria to others by immunizing schoolchildren and other contacts. A modified toxin can also be used to stimulate the production of antitoxin by the individual. The toxin may be modified by the addition of antitoxin or by a chemical such as formalin. Because the immunity produced as a result of disease or vaccination is relative rather than complete, Anderson and Arnstein suggest that the term resistance might be preferable.[32]

Though the general manifestations occurring in tetanus, diphtheria, and botulism differ, the specific exotoxins produced in each of these diseases cause injury to the nervous system. The exotoxin of diphtheria also injures the myocardium. Each of the exotoxins varies in degree of toxicity; however, exotoxins are among the most highly poisonous substances known.

The local effects of microorganisms producing exotoxins vary. The *Clostridium botulinum* does not cause injury by the growth of microorganisms in the alimentary canal or in the tissues, but by an exotoxin produced by the microorganism growing in bland vegetables canned at temperatures insufficient to kill *Clostridium botulinum* spores. There is no local growth of microorganisms to cause injury. Fortunately, the exotoxin is easily destroyed by boiling bland vegetables such as home-canned corn, beans, or peas for five minutes before they are eaten. Commercially canned vegetables are rarely sources of botulism because they are subjected to high temperatures during the process of canning. *Clostridium tetani* also causes little local effect. It does not grow on living tissue and is a strict anaerobe. Tetanus has been known to occur after small or insignificant wounds have healed. For the *Clostridium tetani* to grow, however, there must be some necrotic tissue. In diphtheria the local manifestation consists of superficial ulceration of mucous membrane, usually located in the nasopharynx, pharynx, or larynx. The ulcerated tissue is

[32] Anderson, Arnstein, and Lester, *Op. cit.,* p. 38.

covered by a membrane, which may extend through the glottis into the larynx and tracheobronchial tree, where it can cause death by suffocation.

In addition to exotoxins, bacteria also form substances known as endotoxins. Endotoxins differ from exotoxins in that they are not liberated in appreciable amounts during the life of the bacterial cell, but they are released as the cell degenerates. Endotoxins also differ from exotoxins in that they are not specific to a given microorganism. They appear to be a fairly homogeneous group of substances that probably cause injury by a similar chemical grouping.[33] Hardy states that endotoxins with similar properties can be obtained from a wide variety of unrelated species of microorganisms.[34] In experimental animals these endotoxins cause similar physiological effects. Among these changes are severe shock and fever. The implications to nursing of both of these conditions have been discussed elsewhere.

Many microorganisms have the power to invade healthy tissues. Not all the factors that enable microorganisms to invade tissues and to disseminate themselves throughout the body are known. Some of the substances formed by bacteria which facilitate their spread are not directly toxic. They play a role in the infectious process by protecting microorganisms from the defense mechanisms of the body or by enabling them to spread throughout the tissue. For example, many pathogenic staphylococci produce a substance called coagulase. Coagulase plus certain factors in the blood serum contributes to the formation of fibrin clots in small blood vessels supplying the infected area as well as to the formation of fibrin walls around areas of tissue infected by the *Staphylococcus*. The fibrin wall serves to protect the *Staphylococcus* from the defenses of the body and from antistaphylococcic drugs and therefore favors their persistence in the tissues.

Clostridium welchii produces collagenase and lecithinase. These substances dissolve collagen and lecithin and thereby facilitate the spread of microorganisms throughout the tissue.

Hemolysins and leukocidins dissolve erythrocytes and leukocytes, respectively. Streptokinase has the opposite effect of coagulase. It breaks down coagulated plasma and for this reason is thought to be an important factor in the spread of organisms such as hemolytic streptococci throughout the body. It has been used experimentally to digest blood clots formed in blood vessels in disease.

A group of enzymes, formed by certain bacteria and known as hyaluronidases, act as spreading factors because they have the power of increasing the permeability of tissues. Hyaluronidase is sometimes added to fluids administered subcutaneously to increase tissue permeability and, as a consequence, to increase the rate at which the fluid is absorbed.

The outcome of the struggle for survival between an individual host and an

[33] Burdon, *Op. cit.,* p. 247.
[34] James D. Hardy, *Pathophysiology in Surgery,* Williams and Wilkins Co., Baltimore, 1958, p. 132.

invading microbe depends on many factors. These include the state of the defense mechanisms of the host and his capacity to respond promptly and appropriately to microorganisms. The microorganism must be able to find a vehicle or mode of transmission, a portal of entry, and tissue that provides an environment suited to its needs, and be able to establish itself, grow, and multiply. Whether or not it induces general or local evidence of disease also depends on a number of factors. It must be able to produce an exotoxin which is not neutralized before it combines with susceptible tissues, or produce other substances that enable it to destroy tissue cells. These cells may be either parenchymal or blood cells, particularly leukocytes.

Though microorganisms forming exotoxins tend to remain at the site at which they enter the tissue, other microorganisms behave differently. Some multiply at the point at which they enter the host. They break down the local tissue defenses and spread to contiguous tissues before being disseminated by the blood and lymph. Others have little or no effect at the site of entry, but are carried to distant points by blood and lymph. The microorganism may be free in the blood or it may be a passenger in a macrophage, because the macrophage was successful in ingesting the microbe but unable to destroy it. Macrophages may disseminate the *Mycobacterium* tuberculi throughout the body because they are able to ingest, but not destroy, them. Whatever the specific mechanisms, microorganisms can be distributed to, and set up secondary infections far from, the point of origin. The routes by which microorganisms and their products may be disseminated throughout the body are summarized on page 195.

The manner in which the body is protected and defended against injury is referred to in other chapters. Because of the importance of defense mechanisms in the prevention of and recovery from infectious disease they are outlined below.

1. Defenses against the entrance or effects of potentially harmful agents in the external environment.
    a. Ability to respond to changes in the environment in such a manner that injury is prevented or to adapt the external environment to prevent injury
    b. Protective structures and functions
        (1) Mechanical factors
            (a) Intact skin and mucous membranes
            (b) Flow of secretions
            (c) Body structure (bony cages)
            (d) Peristalsis
        (2) Structural adaptations to changing conditions
            (a) Hypertrophy
            (b) Atrophy
            (c) Hyperplasia
            (d) Metaplasia

    (3) Reflexes, such as
        (a) Vomiting
        (b) Sneezing
        (c) Coughing
        (d) Blinking-tearing
        (e) Diarrhea (in some instances)
    (4) Ciliary action
    (5) Emergency functions of normal body structures
    (6) Reserve capacity of vital organs—margins of safety
    (7) Character of secretions
2. Defenses against spread.
  (First line of defense having been penetrated)
  a. Localizing factors—act to prevent distant spread
    (1) Hyaluronic acid
    (2) Phagocytes—principally macrophages
    (3) Lymph nodes
    (4) Local tissue reaction (inflammation)
    (5) Local action of antibodies
  b. General defenses (assumes that the second line of defense has been penetrated)
    (1) Phagocytoses
        (a) Macrophages
        (b) Microphages
    (2) Excretion by the kidney and liver—liver also detoxifies potentially harmful substances
    (3) Responses of hormonal and nervous system
        (a) The concept of stress—including metabolic changes that accompany disease and injury
    (4) Development of immunity—formation of antibodies
3. Tissue repair.
4. In all stages, the availability and intelligent use of preventive and therapeutic resources contributes to protection against and recovery from disease.

One characteristic of self-limiting diseases not previously discussed is that if the disease is to survive, the organism must pass from one susceptible person to another rapidly enough to keep the infection going. Infectious diseases that are self-limiting, such as measles or the common cold, tend to die out in nomadic tribes. In urban societies, epidemics of measles tend to occur every second or third year. In a measles year, most of the susceptibles develop measles. Then the incidence of measles drops to a low level until the proportion of susceptibles to nonsusceptibles rises and another measles epidemic occurs. Some microorganisms appear to gain in virulence when they pass rapidly from one person to another. At the beginning of an epidemic, such as of influenza, the disease is relatively mild but later it becomes more severe.

What are some of the factors influencing the susceptibility of the host to infection?

Reference has already been made to factors influencing the susceptibility of the host to infection. Each individual has a variety of physical and physiological defenses against agents in his external environment. He also has an internal defense system that enables him to limit the spread of microorganisms beyond the point or area of entry. When he is unable to prevent a disease-producing microbe from establishing itself and causing disease, his defense mechanisms may still be adequate to overcome eventually the microorganisms causing the disease. These defenses are summarized in outline above in the chapter. According to Dubos, how the individual reacts to infection depends on his immunological past, his constitution, and his environment.[35]

With a few exceptions, resistance to disease develops with age. As is stated in the discussion of the development of immunity, the body is not able to form antibodies until shortly before or after birth. Burrows[36] states that prophylactic immunization of infants is ineffective for at least two or three months. Babies are, however, temporarily protected by antibodies from their mothers. By the time children have reached puberty, they have developed an immunity to many diseases. Burrows emphasizes that, although youngsters become immunized to a number of diseases by the age of puberty, this immunity is a coincidence and is not due to a cause-and-effect relationship.[37] For some reason not understood, susceptibility to tuberculosis begins to be evident in the teens and wanes in the late twenties. A second peak begins about the age of 50 and continues through the last three decades of life. Age also is an element in susceptibility to staphylococcic infections as they are more common in the very young and in the old.

There are many other factors appearing to influence susceptibility to infection. For some of these, that they do is based more on observation than on a clear understanding of why they do. For example, sex influences susceptibility to infection. Males appear to be more susceptible to pneumonia and epidemic meningitis than are females, while females are more susceptible to scarlet fever and typhoid fever. Seasonal variation in the incidence of some infections is common knowledge. The common cold becomes more frequent in the late fall and early winter. One explanation is that in the late fall and early winter people move indoors and houses are closed, and the closeness of contact among the occupants is increased. The incidence of poliomyelitis is highest in summer and early fall. General physiological well-being also influences susceptibility to infection. Cortisone and its related analogues diminish resistance

---

[35] René Dubos, *Bacterial and Mycotic Infections of Man, Op. cit.*, p. 26.
[36] William Burrows, *Textbook of Microbiology*, 18th ed., W. B. Saunders, Philadelphia, 1963, p. 321.
[37] *Ibid.*, p. 322.

to the spread of microorganisms in the tissue by suppressing the inflammatory response.[38] The use of cortisone in the treatment of a variety of diseases is believed by some authorities to contribute to the increase in infections caused by microbes of the normal flora. Persons whose adrenal cortices hypersecrete the glucocorticoids also have an increased susceptibility to infection.

An association between nutritional status and the incidence of certain infections is well known. The lack of resistance particularly to skin infections of the poorly controlled diabetic patient is common knowledge. Ischemia predisposes to infection of tissues. The observation that the incidence of certain infections rises when the nutritional level of a group falls is well documented. During both World Wars I and II the incidence of tuberculosis in Europe rose. Following each war, the incidence fell. Although undernutrition was only one of the factors, the diseases that were common in the concentration camps in Europe during World War II were skin ailments, bronchopneumonia, staphylococcal infections, and pulmonary tuberculosis.[39] These conditions were due to the microorganisms that were common in the European community. The conditions under which the people lived combined to reduce their resistance and render them susceptible to the microbes with whom they lived. Following the war many of these people improved with little or no treatment. In other words, balance between man and his microorganisms was restored, so that they could live together in a state of peaceful coexistence.

What are some of the factors in the environment that bring the agent and the host together?

Besides a pathogenic microorganism and a susceptible host, conditions in the environment must be such as to bring the two together if an infectious disease is to develop. Many of these factors have been alluded to earlier. Bilharziasis has increased in incidence as a result of vast systems of irrigation constructed to improve living standards. Some authorities say that it is the most common and important parasitic disease in man as it affects the young and causes a high degree of disability. Conditions required for the propagation of the snail in which the *Schistosoma* (a flatworm) spends part of its life cycle are provided. The eggs of the organism are voided or defecated into the water by infected persons. They hatch, and the larvae enter a suitable freshwater snail. After a period of time, free-swimming larvae leave the snail. They pierce the skin of a person wading, working, or swimming in the water. From the site of entry, they are carried by the blood to the liver, where they mature. The essential point here is that customs and habits, i.e., discharging human excreta wherever convenient and the provision of suitable conditions for the propagation of a pathogenic microorganism, provide the conditions in the

[38] Ernest Jawetz, Joseph L. Melnich, Edward A. Adelberg, *Review of Medical Microbiology*, 4th ed., Lange Medical Publications, Los Angeles, 1960, p. 109.
[39] Dubos, *Bacterial and Mycotic Infections in Man, Op. cit.*, p. 23.

environment required to transmit the disease. The practices of working, wading, and swimming provide the final conditions necessary to spread the disease. Control of bilharziasis could be effected by the sanitary disposal of urine and feces.

A variety of conditions in the environment facilitate or prevent the transmission of a pathogenic microorganism to man. They include such factors as sanitary procedures, housing, and the adequacy of health facilities. For those diseases to which immunity can be developed, the proportion of susceptibles to nonsusceptibles is a significant factor in the control of spread.

As a summary, the six factors listed by Anderson, Arnstein and Lester[40] as being essential to the infectious disease process are reproduced below. They are:

Essential Factors in Susceptibility	*Summary of Components of Essential Factors*
1. A causative or etiological agent	Viruses
	Rickettsia
	Bacteria
	Spirochetes
	Protozoa
	Fungi
2. A reservoir or source of the causative agent	Human beings
	Animals, including insects
3. A mode of escape from the reservoir	Respiratory tract—sputum
	droplets
	droplet nuclei
	Alimentary canal—feces
	Genital tract—secretions
	Urinary tract—urine
	Skin lesions—drainage
	Blood
4. A mode of transmission from the reservoir to the potential new host	Vehicles—air
	dust
	food
	water
	blood
	fingers
	insects
5. A mode of entry into the new host	Respiratory tract; mouth; skin or mucous membrane
6. A susceptible host	

40 Anderson, Arnstein, and Lester, *Op. cit.*, p. 19.

The outline (pages 210-11) summarizes the operation and interrelationship of the factors which produce three of the infectious diseases which plague man.

Factors affecting the susceptibility of the host to any type of illness have been considered elsewhere. One critical characteristic is the degree to which the individual is or is not immune to the pathogenic microorganism. Immunity is seldom absolute. Whether or not disease results from exposure to a pathogenic microorganism depends on the interaction of the host and the microorganism.

These steps or links in the chain in the infectious disease process have been listed because, if any one is absent or missing, infection or infectious disease will not occur. One aspect in the practice of nursing is the prevention of the spread of infectious disease not only to others, but to the nurse. In the prevention of the spread of infection, one of the first questions that the nurse should ask and answer is, "Who should be protected from whom?" For example, Mr. Allen (burned) required protection from those in his environment. The same is true for Mrs. Jason (major surgery). In contrast, after Mr. Allen's wounds were observed to be infected by the *Staphylococcus aureus,* personnel and other patients required protection from infection. When applying the question of "Who should be protected from whom?" preparatory to making a nursing care plan for Miss Hercules (diagnosis of infectious hepatitis), the answer would appear to be that persons who are healthy require protection from her. To answer the question, "How?" other information is required.

What are the elements in the development of infectious diseases?

In the following outline elements entering into the development of an infectious disease are summarized.

1. Characteristics of *mechanisms of defense* of the host
   a. Anatomic and physiologic barriers to the entrance of microorganisms
   (1) Intact skin and mucous membranes
   (2) Structures and functions that protect the entrances to the respiratory and gastrointestinal tract
   (3) Character of secretions and body fluids
      (a) Low (acid pH inhibits bacterial growth)
      (b) Lysozyme produced by leukocytes found in tears, saliva, and other body fluids. It lyses bacteria and is bactericidal
      (c) Properidin system
      (d) Bactericidins
      (e) Agglutinins
      (f) Opsonins

   (4) Anatomic barriers within the tissues
    (a) Continuous matrix
    (b) Fibrin barrier
  b. Cells
   (1) Microphages (neutrophils—highly mobile, quickly respond-ing, somewhat vulnerable)
   (2) Macrophages
  c. Antibodies
   (1) Antitoxic—directly neutralize toxins
   (2) Antibacterial or antiviral are antibodies that combine with a specific substance at the surface of a virus or bacterium and produce a new surface about which leukocytes can spread and more easily ingest the microorganism
  d. Inflammatory response
  e. Outcome
   (1) No infection or disease
   (2) Develop infection
    (a) Carrier state
    (b) Inapparent infection
    (c) Aborted infection
   (3) Infection followed by apparent disease
    (1) mild (2) severe (3) fulminating
   (4) Recovery
    (a) Long-time increase in resistance or immunity
    (b) Short-time or limited increase in resistance
   (5) Death
 2. Characteristics of microorganisms
  a. Factors that limit spread
   (1) Failure to escape from reservoir
   (2) Failure to achieve vehicle or mode of transmission
   (3) Failure to find portal of entry
   (4) Low virulence or power of invasion or inadequate numbers
  b. Factors favoring disease-producing potential
   (1) Escapes from reservoir, gains a vehicle for transmission, finds a portal of entry
   (2) Number, virulence, and invasiveness is sufficient to overcome local body defenses. Reaches tissue in which the environment is favorable to its adaptation so that it can grow and multiply and maintain a satisfactory rate of multiplication
   (3) Characteristics of microorganisms or their products that en-hance pathogenicity
    (a) Polysaccharide capsule inhibits phagocytosis
    (b) Toxin production
     (b^1) Exotoxin
     (b^2) Endotoxin

     (c) Other substances
       (c^1) Coagulase
       (c^2) Streptokinase

c. Routes of spread
  (1) Intercellular spaces—direct extension to contiguous tissues
  (2) Lymphatics
     (a) Arrest at lymph node
     (b) Spreads from the lymph node through lymphatics to blood stream
  (3) Blood stream
  (4) Ingested by macrophages but not destroyed—carried to other parts of the body
  (5) Spillage or escape from a hollow organ
     (a) Direct extension
     (b) Perforation of the hollow organ

d. Outcome
  (1) Death of the microorganism
  (2) Establishment of infection without disease
     (a) Carrier
     (b) Inapparent infection
  (3) Infection with disease
  (4) Escape from reservoir and continuation of the cycle.

What is the course of infectious disease?

In a discussion of infectious diseases, some attention is usually given to the course of infectious disease, which is usually divided into three stages or periods. The first, or incubation, period is the time which elapses between the entrance of the microorganism into the body and the appearance of clinical signs and symptoms. In terms of the microorganism, the incubation period is the time it takes it to adapt to the host and achieve a rate of multiplication sufficient to cause evidence of disease. The length of the incubation period is different for each acute communicable disease, but is constant for a particular disease. As examples, the incubation period for measles is 10 to 14 days and not longer than 21 days. In meningococcus meningitis, it varies from 2 to 21 days. In those diseases in which not only a specific microorganism (a necessary condition) but other factors (sufficient cause) enter into their development, the length of the incubation period may be difficult to determine. For example, the virus of herpes simplex may be present in the tissues for an extended period of time without any indication of its presence. When the individual develops a cold or has a fever, a cold sore appears. The length of the incubation period for tuberculosis is also variable. It depends upon such factors as age, state of nutrition, and other factors.

The next stage is the period of illness. As with the incubation period, the length of the period of illness is predictable for a given disease, but varies from one type to another. A self-limiting disease may run its course in a few hours or extend for a few weeks at most. The old saying, If a cold is treated it lasts two weeks and if it is not treated it lasts 14 days, applies here. Most of the acute communicable diseases are of relatively short duration. Some diseases such as tuberculosis may continue to be active for months or years. As in noninfectious diseases, the degree and severity of illness vary from one individual to another. Some individuals have antibodies in their blood indicating that they must have reacted to a given microorganism, but they have no knowledge of ever having had the disease. Other individuals experience mild attacks, while in still others, the course of the disease is so rapid and so severe that the patient becomes ill and dies within a few hours. When the course of a disease is unusually rapid and the manifestations are unusually severe and uncontrollable, it is said to be fulminating.[41] For example, John Harvey felt fine yesterday. This morning he awakened with a shaking chill, feeling very ill. He had a fever which continued to rise. Despite every effort to reduce the severity of illness, he died less than 24 hours after the onset of his illness. He was diagnosed as having fulminating pneumococcal pneumonia, type III. At the onset of his illness he was not a weakened old man, but a healthy and robust young one. Despite the possibility of an infectious disease being fulminating, the tendency toward recovery in a given period of time is strong in most acute communicable diseases.

The onset of the acute communicable diseases is usually marked by a prodromal period. During the prodromal period the individual has early manifestations of the impending illness, but does not have the specific signs and symptoms of a specific disease. One of the problems in the control of diseases such as measles is that the manifestations indicating the onset of illness are similar to those of the common cold. Moreover, the individual is more infectious during the prodromal phase than he is later. This morning when Mary Sue went to school with "just a cold," she might well have been in the prodromal phase of measles or another acute communicable disease.

Following the onset of illness, the individual experiences a period in which the specific manifestations of the particular illness are evident and he is more or less sick. Depending on the nature of the disease and the person who is ill, he may go into the period of convalescence and complete recovery; he may develop complications; or he may die.

What are some of the characteristic manifestations in acute infectious disease?

During the period of illness most patients have fever. The fever may be constant, intermittent, or remittent. A fever is said to be constant when the amount of variation is less than 2°. It is remittent when it varies more than 2°,

---

[41] The term "fulminating" can be applied to any disease in which the manifestations are unusually severe and which progresses in a short time to death.

but does not drop to normal. It is intermittent when the temperature varies above and below normal levels. The type of fever, the degree of elevation, and the length of time it persists are reasonably characteristic for each disease. For example, in untreated pneumococcal pneumonia, the temperature of the patient rises rapidly following a shaking chill. It can be expected to remain elevated to from 38.8° C. (102° F.) to 40° C. (104° F.) for five to nine days. The fever then falls rapidly, that is, by crisis, to below normal. Unless the patient develops a complication, the temperature does not again rise above normal, and from that point on, the patient can be expected to recover rapidly. When the temperature does not fall within the expected period of time, or if it rises above normal after the crisis, a complication such as lung abscess or empyema is suspected. Accurate determination and recording of the temperature are important in assessing the progress of the patient toward recovery. Although some deviation from the expected pattern does not always indicate that the patient is developing complications, it may.

Along with fever, the patient can be expected to have an elevation in pulse and respiratory rates. Other signs and symptoms are more or less characteristic for each disease. The state of illness is terminated when the body has formed sufficient antibodies to enable its defense mechanisms to overcome the causative agent. For example, in diphtheria the antibodies that are formed neutralize the exotoxin. With the neutralization of the exotoxin, the phagocytes are then able to overcome the diphtheria bacilli.

In some infectious diseases, notably typhoid fever, the patient may appear to be making a normal recovery, only to have a recurrence of symptoms. Usually the course of the second illness is not as severe, nor does it last as long as the original attack. Recurrence of infection in patients treated by antimicrobial agents also happens. Apparently the antimicrobial drug suppresses but does not kill the microbe. The recurrence is due to the multiplication of the microorganism following the termination of drug therapy.

Not all infectious diseases are self-limiting. The period of illness in some diseases, such as tuberculosis, may depend as much or more on conditions within the person who is ill as it does on the virulence and invasiveness of the microorganism.

During convalescence, which follows the period of illness, the patient returns to health. Its length will depend on how long the patient has been ill as well as on how well his general condition was maintained during the illness. Some illnesses are more debilitating than others. For example, though the period of illness from influenza may not be unduly long, patients often complain of being weak and easily fatigued for considerable periods. In the past when patients who had typhoid fever were starved, convalescence was delayed until their nutritional status was improved. Attention to nutrition during the period of illness as well as in the period of convalescence is important.

The requirements of the patient who has an infectious disease should be evaluated in the same manner as for persons with other illnesses. Particular attention should be paid to the person who is isolated. Many, but not all, patients who are isolated feel rejected by nursing and medical personnel. Because drainage from an ulcer on her leg contained virulent staphylococci, Mrs. Lilac was placed on isolation precautions. Since no single rooms were available, the curtains were drawn about her bed. At 11 o'clock in the morning a nurse opened the curtains to speak to Mrs. Lilac. Her breakfast tray was still sitting on her bedside table and her bed was in complete disarray. When the nurse spoke to Mrs. Lilac, she burst into tears. As she sobbed, she spoke of her feelings of desolation at being deserted. "You would think that I had leprosy or something. What do I have that makes everyone afraid and avoid me? It must be awfully bad."

Not all patients who are isolated, however, feel neglected. Mrs. Solo, who was also screened from other patients in a large ward, thanked the nurse for making it possible for her to have privacy. The differences in the responses of the two patients related to differences in their perception of a similar situation.

The nurse, too, should examine how she feels about the particular illness. It is not uncommon for nurses to express fear of diseases such as tuberculosis or syphilis. Nurses should also know how they feel about people who have these diseases. Although one cannot always completely change one's feelings, they are easier to control when one knows what they are. Some fears arise from ignorance of the manner by which specific infectious diseases are spread and from not knowing what is necessary and what can be done to prevent their spread.

The role of the nurse in meeting the physiological needs of patients has been discussed in other chapters. During the period when the patient is acutely ill, attention should be directed toward conserving the energy of the patient, providing comfort, relieving symptoms associated with fever, and maintaining the fluid intake of the patient and, if possible, his intake of food. Rest should be provided and unnecessary stimulation avoided. Since fever activates the herpes virus, cold sores on the lips and face of the patient may cause him discomfort. Camphor ice or some type of bland or mildly stimulating ointment, prescribed by the physician, should be applied as necessary. Unless the patient breathes through his mouth, his mouth will remain clean and moist if his fluid intake is adequate; however, he should be given whatever assistance he requires to maintain his fluid intake. During illness and convalescence, the patient should be protected from unnecessary exposure to other infectious agents.

During convalescence, the needs of the patient will not be particularly different from those of the patient undergoing a surgical procedure or some other severe stress. Some patients, especially those having had typhoid fever or diphtheria, may continue to discharge virulent bacteria. Precautions designed to protect others may therefore have to be continued during the period of convalescence.

What kinds of activities or procedures are required for the control of acute infectious diseases?

Activities that are useful in the control of infectious disease are directed toward the accomplishment of three objectives. These objectives, as stated by Burrows, are: (1) to reduce or to eliminate the reservoir of infection; (2) to break the chain between the reservoir and the susceptible host; (3) to reduce the number of susceptible people in the community.[42] Anderson and his associates[43] add to the list of objectives: to minimize "the ill effects of cases that have not been prevented."

As stated earlier, the reservoirs of infection include human beings who are carriers or who are ill with the infectious disease, animals including insect carriers, and human wastes. Human beings are isolated or quarantined during the period of illness and for as long as they carry virulent microbes. In some infectious diseases, the number of human reservoirs may be reduced by treating the disease. One of the reasons, though not the only one, for treating patients who have tuberculosis in hospitals is to remove them from the community, where they may be a source of infection to others. Therapy of the patient who has tuberculosis has two aims. One is to eradicate the reservoir. The other is to help the patient learn a way of life that will enable him to live in healthful coexistence with the *Mycobacterium tuberculosis.* Even before the days of the antituberculosis drugs, the tuberculosis process was arrested in many patients by a program of rest—both mental and physical—a nutritious diet, and attention to individual factors in each patient. The atmosphere in the sanitarium is calm and unhurried. Because the individual patient is a key factor in his recovery, he is taught early the nature of his disease and what his part is in recovery and in maintaining health. He also learns how to protect others. The program of therapy serves to assist the patient not only to arrest the tuberculous process, but to learn a way of life that will enable him to keep his disease under control.

Surgical therapy has made a contribution to the eradication of the reservoir in tuberculosis. Some surgical procedures result in temporary or permanent collapse of the affected area in the lung. In either event the purpose is to assist the body in healing diseased tissue. When the disease process is localized in one organ or part of an organ, the diseased tissue may be removed surgically. For example, when tuberculosis involves one kidney and not the other, the diseased kidney is usually removed. In pulmonary tuberculosis, a part of or an entire lung may be removed. In some instances, portions of both lungs may be excised. Eradication of the reservoir by surgical removal of the infected tissue is not limited to tuberculosis, as persons who are typhoid carriers can sometimes be cured by cholecystectomy.

The most recent addition to measures available to eradicate the reservoir

---

[42] Burrows, *Op. cit.,* p. 349.
[43] *Op. cit.,* 4th ed., p. 47.

have been chemical antimicrobial drugs. The drugs listed by Goodman and Gilman that have been used in the treatment of tuberculosis include: (1) derivatives of sulfones, (2) streptomycin sulfate, U.S.P. and its relatives, (3) para-aminosalicylic acid (PAS), (4) derivatives of thiosemicarbazone, and (5) isoniazid.[44] When antituberculosis drugs were first introduced, the hope was entertained that man now would have a means of effectively and easily eradicating tuberculosis. Drugs used in the treatment of tuberculosis have fallen short of the original expectations. Goodman and Gilman list the reasons as follows: (1) Like other antimicrobials, the antituberculosis drugs are primarily bacteriostatic rather than bactericidal. Their effectiveness depends, therefore, on a combination of the action of the drug and the effectiveness of the defense mechanism of the patient. They may therefore suppress, rather than eradicate, the infection. (2) The *Mycobacterium tuberculosis* has a tendency to become resistant to the more effective antimicrobial drugs. (3) Many of these drugs are toxic to the patient in dosages that are most effective in eradicating the mycobacterium tuberculosis.[45] Since the introduction of the antituberculosis agents, the mortality rate from tuberculosis has fallen sharply. The morbidity rate has fallen, but not as significantly. Some authorities, such as Bloomquist, suggest that this may be due in part to the breakdown of tuberculous lesions in patients with arrested tuberculosis. Bloomquist is of the opinion that emphasis in the control of tuberculosis should be on treatment of patients with tuberculosis.[46]

Case finding is important, but is not an end in itself. It is done so that patients who have tuberculosis can be identified and brought under treatment. The initiation of prompt and effective treatment, not only with antimicrobial drugs, but with measures designed to improve the resistance of the host to tuberculosis, is imperative. "Cure" of persons with active tuberculosis must be accomplished so that the reservoir of tuberculosis in the community can be reduced before the *Mycobacterium* of tuberculosis becomes resistant to antimicrobial agents.

Antibacterials are also useful in the eradication of reservoirs in other infectious diseases. Among diseases treated with success are syphilis, gonorrhea, and bacillary infections, as well as infections due to the pneumococcus, meningococcus, and hemolytic *Streptococcus*.

Animals also act as reservoirs of disease. Animal reservoirs may be reduced or eradicated by killing diseased animals. For example, in the past, bovine tuberculosis was a problem in dairy cattle. After methods for the identification of tuberculous cattle were developed, programs were instituted to identify and to destroy diseased animals. Farmers, however, were resistant to the program of testing because diseased animals were destroyed. To farmers, the problem was a matter not of public health, but of economics. They

[44] Goodman and Gilman, *Op. cit.,* p. 1250.
[45] *Ibid.*
[46] Edward T. Bloomquist, "Chemotherapy, a Public Health Measure Against Tuberculosis," *Public Health Reports,* LXXV, November, 1960, p. 1069.

did not find it easy to accept as a fact that healthy-looking cows were diseased and must be sold for a price far below their value as producers of milk. The program has, however, been effective in eradicating bovine tuberculosis among cattle and therefore among human beings. When the reservoir of disease is in one or more species of wild animals, the problem of eradication becomes exceedingly difficult. Eradication of the *Anopheles* mosquito eliminates not only a reservoir of malaria infection but its mode of transmission as well.

Sewage serves as a reservoir for some types of microorganisms. One of the problems in urban living is the disposal and disinfection of human wastes. As populations concentrate in an area in larger and larger numbers, the problem of protecting people from their own excreta increases. Articles are beginning to appear in journals devoted to public health on the inadequacy of present facilities and the need for dealing with this problem. In one midwestern state, many of the wells are presumed to be contaminated because the water has a high nitrogen content from barnyard wastes. The high level of nitrogen in the water is of itself dangerous to babies and to immature animals. There is also the possibility that the water in these wells contains pathogenic microorganisms.

Though a considerable discussion has been, and will be, devoted to the value and methods of breaking the chain of events that lead from the reservoir to the susceptible host, community efforts are highly important. They include such activities as the filtration and chlorination of water supplies, the pasteurization of milk, the supervision and inspection of food and food handlers, and the destruction of insect vectors.

The third method in control of disease is to reduce the number of persons in the community who are susceptible to the disease. This may be done by administering antibodies (passive immunity) or by stimulating the person to form his own antibodies Sometimes antibodies are administered to persons sick with a disease in order to modify the course of the disease. Whether or not the person develops an active immunity depends on the time the anti-serum is administered in relation to the onset of the disease, as well as other factors. The immunization procedures that are most effective are those most nearly like the natural process. Immunizations for smallpox in which living, but attenuated, viruses are administered and for diphtheria, in which attenuated toxin is injected, are at the present time the most successful. Killed organisms are not usually as effective as live ones. The new poliomyelitis vaccines also are apparently effective in controlling poliomyelitis. These vaccines not only raise the level of resistance of the person to the poliomyelitis virus, but this resistance lasts for some time.

A problem that has to be solved before a vaccine can be administered to human beings is that it be both effective and safe. One of the recent issues in the field of public health has been over whether the live, but attenuated, poliomyelitis virus is as safe as the killed virus; there is some evidence that it is more effective. The most important test that a vaccine must pass is that it is safe. Although there is no such thing as absolute safety, the element of risk should be far below the risk involved in having the disease.

Influenza vaccine, which induces a temporary immunity, is useful in preventing the rapid spread of influenza throughout a community. Vaccines, such as those for typhoid fever, typhus fever, and yellow fever, are often advised for persons traveling into communities where these diseases are endemic.

Authorities in public health point out that the control of an infectious disease does not depend on the eradication of all the reservoirs of infection or the immunization of all who are susceptible. They do not underestimate the desirability of this goal, but they are aware of how difficult total eradication is to attain. The spread of an infectious disease can be quite effectively controlled provided a sufficient proportion of the population is immune to it. In a community of persons who are susceptible to a given infectious disease, when one person develops it, it spreads by geometrical progression; that is, one person infects two persons and two people infect four, and so on until all susceptible persons in the community develop the disease. Of course, this formulation is theoretical, not actual, as one person may be the source of infection for none or for many persons. If, in contrast, only half of the people in a community are susceptible, then of each two persons exposed only one develops it. Instead of spreading rapidly through the community, the infectious disease spreads slowly.

Anderson et al.[47] state that diphtheria can be controlled in a community, provided 50 per cent of the children are immune. For this percentage to be effective in the control of diphtheria, the children must be distributed among all age groups. An occasional case of diphtheria will develop, but the disease will not become epidemic. The community runs a risk of an epidemic when the number of susceptibles is allowed to rise.

What means are available to identify persons who are susceptible to a certain infectious disease?

Although tests are not available in all instances, the identification of persons who have reacted to specific microorganisms or their antigens is useful in the selection of persons for immunization procedures. For many diseases, such as measles and smallpox, no special test is necessary, since all persons are presumed to be susceptible unless they have had a known attack of the disease. The immune reaction, a slight swelling and reddening at the site of inoculation, in smallpox, indicates that the person who was vaccinated was already immune at the time.

The tests that are available for the identification of persons who have or have not reacted to specific antigens are of two types. In one, a specific toxin is injected into the skin to identify the presence or absence of neutralizing

---

[47] Op. cit., 4th ed., p. 81.

antibodies. In the other, antigenic material is injected intradermally to identify skin-sensitizing antibodies. For example, the Schick test is used to identify persons who have antibodies against diphtheria toxin. A minute quantity of toxin is injected into the skin. Persons lacking the neutralizing antitoxin develop, within 24 to 48 hours, a swollen, reddened lesion at the site of injection. These persons are said to have a positive Schick test and are susceptible to diphtheria. Those who do not react to the toxin have sufficient antibodies to neutralize the toxin. This does not necessarily indicate, however, that they have a high level of immunity to diphtheria, though they may.

In contrast, in tuberculosis, antigenic material is injected to demonstrate the presence or absence of a tuberculous infection, by determining whether or not there are skin-sensitizing antibodies in the skin. The test is based on the fact that the tissues of an individual who acquires a tuberculous infection react to the proteins of the tubercle bacillus in a characteristic way. The primary use of tuberculin testing is to determine the size of the reservoir of tuberculosis in the community. Two sources of material are available for tuberculin testing. One is an extract of the tubercle bacillus, which is called old tuberculin, or simply OT. The other is purified protein derivative, or PPD. It is prepared by growing tubercle bacilli on special synthetic media. Whether the material is injected into the skin (Mantoux), scratched into the skin (Von Pirquet), or applied as a patch test (Vollmer), an area of induration is interpreted as a positive reaction and a nonindurated area as a negative reaction. A positive reaction indicates that the person has at some time reacted to the tubercle bacilli; that is, he has experienced a tuberculous infection. As a consequence, his skin contains sensitizing antibodies which react with the injected antigenic material to produce a hypersensitivity reaction. Since a positive test does not indicate whether or not the person presently has active tuberculosis, those who have positive tuberculin tests should then have a chest X ray.

How is an infectious disease diagnosed?

The diagnosis of infectious disease is based on four types of findings, not all of which are present in every instance. The first and most definitive diagnostic finding is the identification of the causative organism. Somewhat less certain, but highly useful in diagnosis, are the manifestations of illness presented by the patient. Third is the identification of specific types of responses to microorganisms. One type of response, the formation of sensitizing antibodies, has been previously discussed in relation to tuberculosis. Another is changes that have taken place in the blood serum in response to a microorganism.

In a number of infectious diseases the identification of the causative organism is essential not only to proper treatment of the patient, but to the protection of noninfected individuals. For example, a diagnosis of tuberculosis carries with it the possibility that long-term treatment will be required and the possibility that others will be infected. Because the tubercle bacillus can usually be obtained from sputum or gastric washings, a diagnosis of tuberculosis is usually considered to be tentative until the bacillus has been identified. Positive verification may require that a body fluid—sputum, gastric washings, or urine—be injected into a guinea pig.

Among other infectious diseases in which a positive diagnosis can be made by the identification of microorganisms are typhoid fever, bacterial and amebic dysenteries, bacterial pneumonias, and staphylococcal and streptococcal infections. The nurse frequently is responsible for collecting body discharges to be examined for pathogenic microorganisms. She should handle the discharges and containers in such a way that the outside of the container is kept clean, and she should protect her hands from contact with potentially contaminated material. Finally, she should thoroughly wash her hands after the collection procedure has been completed.

Although many of the manifestations in infectious disease are similar from one disease to another, the pattern of signs and symptoms is fairly characteristic for each disease. Frequently there are one or two effects that are pathognomonic of a particular disease. For example, swelling at the angle of the jaw and pain on swallowing sour food, such as pickles, are characteristic findings in mumps. When the patient is at least moderately ill and there are other patients in the community with the same infectious disease, the problem of diagnosis may be relatively easy. When the manifestations presented by the patient are not very marked and there are but few other sick persons, then the problem of diagnosis may be difficult.

A third method used in the identification of the presence of specific infections is the serological test. In persons who are infected by the *Treponema pallidum,* certain immunochemical changes take place in the blood which can be determined by appropriate procedures. Since similar changes can be temporarily induced by a number of other disorders, such as infectious mononucleosis, malaria, and virus pneumonia, a patient can have a positive serological test and not have syphilis. For example, patients who have a diagnosis of lupus erythematosis frequently have a positive serological test despite the absence of syphilis.

Skin-sensitizing antibodies are also formed in response to certain other microorganisms. For example, the pathological changes that occur in blastomycosis are often similar to those of tuberculosis. A patient may be found on X ray to have pathology similar to that of tuberculosis and yet to have a negative Mantoux test and no tubercle bacilli in his sputum or gastric washings. Injection of antigenic material into his skin from the organism causing blastomycosis may reveal sensitization to it.

To this point, the factors that influence the nature of man's relationship to the microorganisms in his environment have been presented. Although man has been able to control a few microbes, he has not been able to eradicate them. In the past, applications of the germ theory have led to remarkable progress in controlling some diseases. In recent years, the germ theory is being extended to include the fact that man is as important as the germ.[48] Infection remains a problem to the health of the public and therefore to nursing. The infectious diseases that are problems differ in nature, but the questions to be asked are, however, similar.

Why is knowledge of the virus diseases of increasing importance?

Diseases attributed to viruses are becoming an increasing problem. Furthermore, the study of viruses is of interest not only to those in the field of health, but to biological scientists as well. Viruses are known to be responsible for at least 50 human diseases and are responsible for a high percentage of cases of acute morbidity. Diseases in which they are a necessary condition also result in permanent disability and death. The possibility that viruses are a factor in the development of cancer in human beings is now under investigation. They may therefore make a greater contribution to disability and death than is now appreciated. Virus diseases are not limited to human beings. There are viruses that infect many living organisms—bacteria, plants, animals, and man. From their studies of viruses, biologists and biochemists hope to gain insight into how cells proliferate, how viruses interact with the cells that they infect, how viruses reproduce, and what factors cause them to vary in character.

Study of viruses has lagged behind that of other microorganisms. At least three factors have contributed to this difficulty. One factor is that viruses are ultramicroscopic in size. Not until the development of the electron microscope were scientists able to establish that viruses existed as particles. Pictures have not yet been made of all viruses that have been identified by other means. According to Andrews,[49] there are no pictures of the virus or viruses causing the common cold.

A second factor adding to difficulty in the study of viruses is that they propagate only within living cells. The study of viruses was greatly advanced by the discovery by John F. Enders, Thomas H. Weller, and Frederick C. Robbins that the virus of poliomyelitis could be grown in animal as well as in human tissue culture. Techniques have been developed so that many viruses can now be grown in fertilized eggs and in cultures of embryonic cells. The difficulties encountered in the development of a suitable media for the growth of viruses is described by Andrews.[50] The fact that it took almost 14 years of work before a suitable medium was developed indicates that the process was not easy.

[48] René J. Dubos (ed.), "The Evolution and the Ecology of Microbial Diseases," *Bacterial and Mycotic Infections in Man, Op. cit.,* pp. 14-15.
[49] Christopher H. Andrews, "The Viruses of the Common Cold," *Scientific American,* CCIII, December, 1960, p. 90.
[50] *Ibid.,* pp. 88-102.

A third difficulty in the study of viruses arises out of the fact that human viruses rarely grow readily in animals. In order to grow and multiply, they have to adapt to the animal host. Burnet, in discussing this problem, states that although scientists working in different laboratories start with the same virus, they may not be working with exactly the same one at a later time. As a result, their findings may be at variance.[51] The capacity of viruses to alter their character in nature also has great practical significance. For example, epidemics of influenza vary greatly in the extent of the epidemic and in the severity of the disease. One explanation is that the influenza virus changes in virulence from time to time. Another possibility is that the number of persons who are susceptible to influenza may also vary from one epidemic or pandemic to another.

Much of the information about the relationship of the virus to the host has been obtained from the study of bacteriophages, that is, viruses that attack bacteria. Burnet[52] also reviews some of the results of studies of the way in which the influenza virus infects the cells of a mouse or ferret. Studies made on the composition of viruses indicate that they are composed of a protein which forms a shell around a central core of nucleic acid. According to Andrews, the nucleic acid in the larger viruses is usually desoxyribonucleic acid (DNA). In the smaller ones it is usually ribonucleic acid (RNA).[53] In some viruses, the protein shell has been demonstrated to contain RNA. The protein shell and the central core have different functions.

What are the functions of the protein shell and how are they accomplished?

According to Stent,[54] the protein shell has two functions: it protects the DNA and is responsible for the pathogenicity of the virus. For example, a bacteriophage approaches a bacterium; it attaches itself to the bacterial cell. Enzymes in the wall of the virus break down certain molecules in the protein wall and in the bacterium and allow the DNA to flow into the cell. Inside the cell the DNA multiplies itself until there are 200 particles. Then protein shells are constructed around each particle and the infected cell ruptures. Should the cell rupture before the DNA is encapsulated by its protein shell, the DNA is soon destroyed by the body defenses. Moreover, DNA by itself is not able to enter a host cell; it therefore cannot cause disease.

What are some of the implications of the physical and chemical characteristics of viruses to nursing?

Some of the physical and chemical characteristics of viruses have practical implications in the practice of nursing. Most viruses are destroyed by heating

[51] F. M. Burnet, "The Virus," *Scientific American Reader,* Simon and Schuster, New York, 1953, p. 338.
[52] *Ibid.,* p. 337.
[53] Andrews, *Op. cit.,* pp. 90-91.
[54] Gunther S. Stent, "The Reproduction of Viruses," *The Physics and Chemistry of Life,* Simon and Schuster, New York, 1955, pp. 134-42.

to 60° C. (140° F.) for 30 minutes. An important exception is the virus that causes serum hepatitis. It is able to withstand heating to 60° C. for four hours. It is also highly infectious. As little as 0.01 ml of plasma can carry enough virus to cause disease or to contaminate a batch of pooled plasma. Persons without a history of hepatitis may be carriers of the virus. The virus of infectious hepatitis, while less resistant to heat, may also be transmitted in blood plasma. For this reason authorities generally recommend that needles, syringes, and pipettes and other articles that are contaminated by blood be sterilized by autoclave for 15 minutes.

The virus of infectious hepatitis also withstands residual chlorine of 1 part to 1 million. The resistance of the virus of infectious hepatitis is of significance, as the virus leaves the body in the feces and is ingested from food and water. In large cities, however, the water supply can usually be counted upon to be safe. The swimming pool in the back yard can be a source of infection unless care is taken to keep it clean and to disinfect the water. Poorly constructed and overcrowded camp sites are also hazardous. Some epidemics of hepatitis have had their origin in oysters obtained from contaminated water and eaten raw.

How are viruses classified? What are some of the characteristic responses to viral invasion?

Viruses may be classified according to certain characteristics. On the basis of four characteristics—size, nucleic acid composition, resistance to ether, and excretion in the feces—viruses are classified as herpes viruses, arboviruses, myxoviruses, adenoviruses, enteroviruses, and pox viruses. To these six groups, Andrews[55] states that possibly the common cold viruses should be added as a seventh group. Briefly, an example of a pox virus is smallpox. The herpes viruses include not only those found in herpes simplex and herpes zoster (shingles), but those found in chickenpox as well. The term "arborvirus" is a shorthand term for viruses carried by arthropod insects. A commonly cited example is yellow fever. The myxoviruses cause a variety of diseases in which the patient has symptoms similar to the common cold. The virus causing influenza is a myxovirus. The term "adenovirus" obviously gets its name from the fact that these viruses affect glands. The viruses of this group induce symptoms of an acute respiratory infection, including acute sore throat. The enteroviruses, as the name suggests, inhabit the intestine, and, according to Andrews,[56] there are 57 varieties. The three strains responsible for poliomyelitis are the best known and most destructive of the enteroviruses.

When viruses are classified according to the symptoms that they induce, they can be placed in two large groups: that is, those that induce generalized effects and those in which the primary effects of the virus are localized. Generalized diseases include smallpox, measles, chickenpox, and yellow fever.

[55] Andrews, *Op. cit.*, p. 91.
[56] *Ibid.*, p. 92.

Many types of tissue serve as the primary site for infection in virus disease. The nervous system, the respiratory tract, the skin and mucous membranes, the eye, the liver, the salivary glands, and the lymph glands are all known sites of infection.[57]

Cellular responses induced by viruses are of two types and can occur alone or in combination. Tissue invaded by a virus may undergo hyperplasia. A familiar example is the common wart. This ability to induce hyperplasia in tissues suggests the possibility that viruses may play a role in initiating some types of neoplasms. Hyperplasia may be followed by necrosis of cells. The lesions formed in smallpox are characterized by hyperplasia followed by necrosis. Necrosis can occur alone. The lesions in the anterior horn cells in poliomyelitis are characterized by necrosis.

Viruses are capable of causing all degrees of infection. In an epidemic of diseases such as poliomyelitis, antibodies can be demonstrated in the blood of those who have not been ill, as well as of those who have been. Depending on the epidemic, only some who are ill are paralyzed. The fact that the person is ill may be obvious, but the character of his illness may not be. Some virus infections are accompanied by different manifestations in different persons. For example, during an epidemic of common colds, some persons may have symptoms that are more or less typical of a cold while others have symptoms of gastroenteritis.

Many viruses are capable of inducing immunity. For some virus diseases, vaccines have been prepared that are successful in establishing immunity. The best known and most successful is the vaccine for smallpox. The diseases in which the virus has to travel through the blood stream to cause disease are the ones in which antibodies are most successful in preventing a second attack. For those in which the virus directly infects cells, as in influenza, it is more difficult to establish a lasting immunity. Diseases in which a variety of viruses appear to be involved, such as the common cold, may never be entirely preventable by immunization. Possibly this is not undesirable. Scientists have discovered that for a time after one virus infection, an animal is not susceptible to infection by another. Why this happens is not known.

What are some of the nursing responsibilities in the care of a patient having a virus infection?

In the care of the patient with a virus infection, the nurse has two general responsibilities. One of these is to meet the needs of the patient for nursing. The other is to prevent the spread of the disease to herself and others. The same principles apply to the spread of virus infections as to others caused by microorganisms. The fact that viruses are relatively resistant to conditions in the external environment should be taken into account when planning an

[57] For a detailed classification see Ernst Jawetz, Joseph L. Melnick, and Edward A. Adelberg, *Review of Medical Microbiology,* 5th ed., Lange Medical Publications, Los Angeles, 1962, pp. 238-40.

effective method for preventing their spread. The only viruses that consistently leave the body in feces are enteroviruses, but the adenoviruses may. Others are spread in respiratory secretions. Andrews states[58] that his experiments demonstrate that the common cold is spread by droplets rather than droplet nuclei. If this is true, a properly worn mask on the person who has a cold should be reasonably effective in preventing the transmission of it to his contacts.

In the last ten years or so, more than 300 viruses that cause human and animal disease have been identified. The circumstances that made this possible are the electron microscope and the development of methods to culture viruses in tissue culture. Great as the advances in knowledge have been, much is left to be learned. In addition to knowledge of viruses as causative agents in disease, through their study scientists hope to learn more about the fundamental processes of cell growth and multiplication. Perhaps the latter is even more important than the former.

What unique considerations should influence the nurse in planning care for a patient with an infectious disease?

To illustrate the factors that the nurse should consider when planning the care of a patient with an infectious disease, the preceding content will be applied to the care of patients with syphilis, tuberculosis, and staphylococcal disease and has been summarized in figure 4-1. The discussion of these diseases will be, for the most part, limited to the facts that the nurse should consider in the control of syphilis and staphylococcal diseases. The first to be discussed is syphilis. The necessary condition, that is, the direct cause of syphilis, is a delicate and fragile spirochete known as the *Treponema pallidum*. Although there are instances in the literature in which scientists have claimed to have grown the *Treponema pallidum* in pure culture, others have not been able to duplicate these experiments. Therefore, there is doubt as to whether or not it has actually been grown on artificial media.[59] Because of the inability to grow the *Treponema pallidum* in the laboratory, its physiological characteristics are unknown. As was stated earlier, the *Treponema pallidum* is a fragile organism. It is rapidly killed by drying and by a temperature of 42° C. (107.6° F.). This is one of the factors believed to account for the value of fever therapy in the treatment of syphilis. It is also susceptible to cold, to soap and water, and to weak disinfectants.

To summarize the characteristics of the *Treponema pallidum,* then, it is a fragile organism and is not adapted to conditions differing from those existing within the living human being. When a nurse cares for a patient who has syphilis, and she asks the question, Who is to be protected from whom? the answer is that the nurse *may* require protection. More information is required,

[58] Andrews, *Op. cit.,* p. 102.
[59] Jawetz, *et al., Op. cit.,* 4th ed., p. 194.

FIGURE 4−1

Summary of the Interrelationship of Factors Which Produce Three Infectious Diseases in Man

Interrelated Factors	Pathogenic Agent		
	Staphylococcus (Numerous Strains)	Treponema Pallidum	Mycobacterium Tuberculosis
Distribution	World-wide (ubiquitous)	Widespread, throughout the world	World-wide; incidence varies in countries and segment of population
Nature-characteristics			
a. Ability to survive outside living organism	More resistant to drying than most non-spore formers	Fragile—exists outside host only moments. Susceptible to penicillin. Adequate treatment usually terminates communicability within 24 hours	Capable of long-term survival outside host; resistant to disinfection; acid-fast. Susceptible to sunlight
b. Infectivity-invasiveness			
c. Pathogenicity-virulence	Often resistant to antibiotics		
d. Reservoirs—human and animal	Human beings, carriers as well as the obviously infected, possibly animals, contaminated objects and articles	Man—organism contained in exudate from obvious or hidden lesions of primary and secondary syphilis—chancre, moist condylomata, blood, semen, vaginal secretions during the infectious stages	Primarily man, but in some areas diseased cattle
e. Vehicles and conditions of transmission	Airborne droplets, or droplet nuclei; contact with contaminated articles	Direct contact by kissing, sexual intercourse, fondling of children, during primary and secondary stages of syphilis	Contact with persons with active disease; via droplets and droplet nuclei, or via exudate or secretions from infected organs; milk from diseased cattle. Usually requires extended and intimate exposure.

FIGURE 4–1. Continued.

Summary of the Interrelationship of Factors Which Produce Three Infectious Diseases in Man

Interrelated Factors	Pathogenic Agent		
	Staphylococcus (Numerous Strains)	Treponema Pallidum	Mycobacterium Tuberculosis
Human Host			
a. Age, sex, race b. Heredity, personality c. Habits, customs d. Defenses—general and specific	Fair degree of immunity or resistance; susceptibility general, especially in newborn, elderly, and debilitated	Susceptibility is universal as there is no natural immunity	Some family contacts avoid infection for a long period of time. Susceptibility highest in children under three years of age. Higher among the undernourished
e. Portal of entry	Skin, wounds, respiratory tract	Mucous membrane, breaks in skin	Respiratory and gastrointestinal tracts; lung lesions probably most important
f. Portal of exit	Open lesions	Chancre, mucous patches, moist condylomata	Respiratory tract

Environmental Factors Which Bring Agent and Host Together:
A. Physical environment—lack of sanitary procedures, cleanliness, or asepsis
B. Socioeconomic factors—insufficient income, crowded housing, inadequate health facilities, lack of information and/or motivation.
C. Biological—animals and insect vectors.

Chain of events necessary in the process of infection:
A. Pathogenic agent.
B. Satisfactory reservoir.
C. Susceptible host.
D. Portal of exit—entry.
E. Means of transmission.

To Prevent Transmission of Infection, Answer These Questions About Each Agent:
A. Who is to be protected from whom?
B. How can protection be established?
C. How can protection be maintained?

however, before the nurse can answer the question positively. If protection is required, then the next question to be asked is, From whom or what is protection required? Since the organism is delicate and survives for only a brief period of time outside the host, objects that come in contact with the patient do not remain contaminated for long. This is especially true if the objects are dry. Since the *Treponema pallidum* is sensitive to heat and to weak chemical disinfectants, elaborate measures are not required to disinfect objects or materials with which the individual comes in contact.

In syphilis, the reservoir or source of the *Treponema pallidum* is the person who has syphilis in an infectious stage. The location of the reservoir depends on the stage of the disease. The reservoir, the mode by which the spirochete escapes from the reservoir, the mode of transmission, and the portal of entry will be discussed at the same time. The portal of entry is usually the skin or mucous membrane or through the placenta from the mother to the fetus. Transmission is by direct contact. It is usually by sexual intercourse or kissing. The length of the incubation period, that is, the time between the entrance of the spirochete into the body and the appearance of clinical evidence of disease, varies from two to ten weeks; different authorities cite different figures. In any event, some time after the individual is exposed, a sore or ulcer, called a chancre, develops at the site where the organism entered the body. Because of the nature of its transmission, the chancre is likely to be located on the genitalia or the lip. Though the lesion is often described as a painless ulceration surrounded by a hard, raised edge, it may be painful and varied in appearance. The chancre is highly infectious, as it teems with spirochetes. The spirochetes can be identified under the microscope by dark-field examination. Though spirochetes may be found in the blood during this stage, the primary source of infection is the chancre. Since the *Treponema pallida* are transmitted by direct contact and by the blood, protective measures should have as their purposes the prevention of contact with the chancre and prohibition of the patient serving as a blood donor. At present most patients with primary syphilis are not treated in the hospital, but receive treatment in the office of a physician or in an outpatient clinic. The essential point in prevention is that care should be taken to avoid direct contact with the chancre or with blood of the patient.

Should a patient having a chancre on the lip or tongue require mouth care, gloves are indicated. Gloves should also be worn when performing procedures such as catheterization or vaginal douches. The purpose of wearing gloves is to prevent contact between the hands of the nurse and the lesion. By avoiding contact, a link in the chain from the causative organism to the susceptible host is broken. Reason also suggests not handling with the bare hands anything that has recently been in contact with the lesion such as a wet dressing or a douche nozzle. However, elaborate precautions are undoubtedly unnecessary. Since the *Treponema pallidum* requires about the same conditions for its survival as do human cells, it dies soon after it leaves the host.

Fortunately, the length of the period of communicability can now be shortened by treatment of the patient with penicillin. According to Goodman and Gilman, the spirochetes disappear from both the primary (chancre) and secondary surface lesions (described below), in 6 to 60 hours; the average is 12.[60] Therefore, when patients are adequately treated, they are no longer infectious after two or three days.

Whether or not treatment is given, the chancre heals. Some weeks later, in untreated patients, the secondary stage follows. In some patients this stage is so mild that it passes unnoticed, while in others the symptoms may be severe. Symptoms characteristic of the second stage include a generalized rash on the skin and mucous membranes, fever, sore throat, and malaise. According to Heyman, the rash may be widespread, even involving the palms of the hands and the soles of the feet.[61] The rashes on the mucous membranes of the mouth, anus, and genitalia are more significant than in other areas because these rashes tend to break down and form small superficial erosions called mucous patches. They, like the chancre, are teeming with spirochetes. The lesions on the anus and genitalia may hypertrophy and form moist condylomata.

Because the lesions on the mucous membranes are open and are full of spirochetes, the patient is highly infectious. The fragility of the microbe, however, limits the mode of transmission to direct contact. Although authorities such as Anderson, Arnstein, and Lester[62] concede that transmission by fomites—food or toilet seats—is theoretically possible, it is highly unlikely. Babies born of syphilitic mothers may develop congenital syphilis, though they may not if the mother has had syphilis for several years or is adequately treated prior to, or during, the early stages of pregnancy. Babies born of syphilitic mothers do not have the first stage of syphilis. They may be stillborn or, if born alive, be in the secondary stage, or they may present no evidence of having syphilis. The lesions of the baby with secondary syphilis are also full of spirochetes.

Whatever the age of the patient, the nurse is the person who requires protection. This protection requires that contact with the lesion or lesions containing spirochetes be prevented as long as the patient is infectious. Rubber gloves should be worn to prevent the nurse from having direct contact with infectious lesions until the patient is rendered noninfectious by treatment. In the general care of adult patients, there may be few occasions when gloves are required. They should, however, be worn when handling a newborn baby who has secondary lesions. In the absence of effective treatment,[63] congenital infections are not usually communicable for more than one or two years. Patients who acquire syphilis after birth remain communicable for a

[60] Goodman and Gilman, Op. cit., p. 1242.
[61] Albert Heyman, "Syphilis," Principles of Internal Medicine, 4th ed., Ed. T. R. Harrison, et. al., McGraw-Hill Book Co., Inc., New York, 1962, p. 1071.
[62] Anderson, Arnstein, and Lester, Op. cit., 4th ed., p 463.
[63] Anderson, Arnstein, and Lester, Op. cit., 4th ed., p. 462.

period of from two to five years. Heyman[64] states that the disease is most communicable during the first four years after infection. Mothers may transmit the infection to the fetus for as long as ten years after they are infected. The ability to transmit the *Treponema pallidum* to others, of course, depends on continuing infection. Patients remain infectious only if they are not adequately treated.

Following the secondary stage of syphilis, the disease becomes latent. During this period there are no clinical signs and symptoms indicating that the person has the disease. The only way the majority of cases can be recognized is by serological testing.

Serological tests are based on the presence of an antibodylike substance, sometimes called reagin, in the serum of a patient who has been infected by the *Treponema pallidum*. Among the serological tests used in the past and the present are the Wassermann, Kline, Hinton, Kohlmer, Kahn, Mazzini, and VDRL (Venereal Disease Research Laboratory). Some, such as the Hinton, Kahn, Kline, Mazzini, and VDRL, are flocculation tests. These tests are based on the knowledge that when normal blood serum is treated with lipid antigen, the particles remain dispersed. In serum containing reagin, aggregates or clumps of material are formed, particularly when it is shaken or centrifuged. Tests such as the Wassermann and the Kohlmer are complement fixation tests. As in the flocculation tests, a positive reaction depends on the presence of reagin in the blood serum.

Some of the individuals who have syphilis will never have more sign of it than a positive serological test. However, in others the *Treponema* invades some body structure, usually the cardiovascular system or nervous system. The period in which clinical symptoms are absent is called the latent stage of syphilis. As much as 20 to 30 years later the patient develops symptoms of the disease. The latent period in syphilis is not always long. Recently a patient was admitted to a local hospital with acute tertiary, or third, stage of syphilis. The course of the disease had been telescoped from the first to the third stage in just a few weeks. The physician who cared for this patient had not seen a similar patient in 20 years. Usually when syphilis is introduced into a new population, it runs a rapid course. Winslow[65] indicates that toward the end of the fifteenth century syphilis swept over Europe as an epidemic of great deadliness. An endarteritis is the characteristic lesion of late syphilis and, according to Hopps,[66] the spirochetes probably lodge in the vasa vasorum. This results in an endarteritis which causes an ischemia of the wall of the blood vessel. The effects on the tissues and the clinical symptoms will depend on the location of the lesion. The results of late syphilis are often serious because they are incapacitating.

In the past the late lesions of syphilis were not thought to contain the

[64] Heyman, *Op. cit.*, p. 1072.
[65] Winslow, *Op. cit., The Conquest of Epidemic Disease*, p. 124.
[66] Howard C. Hopps, *Principles of Pathology*, 2nd ed., Appleton-Century-Crofts, Inc., New York, 1964, p. 270.

spirochete. Because patients with late syphilis improve following treatment with penicillin, this is regarded as evidence that spirochetes are in the tissues in a form that cannot be recognized by measures now available.[67] During the late stage of syphilis, the reservoir for the spirochete is the organ or tissue that is infected. The danger of infecting others by ordinary means is considered to be nonexistent. Because of the possibility of the blood containing the *Treponema pallidum,* patients in any stage of syphilis are not permitted to be blood donors.

To summarize, when a nurse cares for a patient who has a diagnosis of syphilis, she should first learn whether or not the patient is in an infectious stage of the disease. If he is not, no special precautions are necessary. If he is, she should then ask herself, Who is to be protected from Whom? From what and for how long is protection necessary? The answers to these questions would then serve as a basis for her actions. Nurses are frequently unnecessarily worried about the possibility of a patient's being infectious. When the nurse is in doubt, she should discuss her fears with the head nurse or with the patient's physician.

She should not delay seeking appropriate advice. If there is a real possibility that she has been infected, the sooner she is treated the better. Moreover, the problem should be resolved so the nurse can be spared needless worry.

Miss Slender illustrates the above situation. When handling wooden side rails from the bed of a patient in the tertiary stage of syphilis, she scratched a finger on a jagged edge of the side rail. From her knowledge of syphilis, her intellect told her she was not in any danger. Yet she was frightened. After worrying for a day or so, Miss Slender told her head nurse what had happened. Because Miss Slender was anxious, the head nurse told Miss Slender what she already knew, that she was not in danger. However, since she was concerned, the head nurse suggested that Miss Slender consult her physician. When Miss Slender saw her physician, he, too, told her that she was in no danger, but he administered penicillin as a prophylactic measure.

One point that requires emphasis when discussing nursing of the patient who has acquired syphilis is the nurse's own feelings about the disease and its mode of transmission. The nurse should be particularly careful to avoid making moral judgment and to avoid allowing her own values to interfere with care of the patient. The aim in treatment should be to enlist the cooperation of the patient so that he will continue treatment and be helped to prevent the late effects of the disease. Moreover, the protection of others depends on early and adequate treatment of the disease.

In answering the question, Who protects whom? the answer includes more than the protection of the nurse from the infection. It includes the protection of the patient from the destructive effects of the disease and the prevention of the infection of others.

[67] McDermott, *Op. cit.,* pp. 485-89.

One problem that should be of concern is that the incidence of infectious syphilis, especially among teen-agers, is rising in the United States.

In the November, 1960, *Public Health Reports* a brief report is made about Seminars conducted on venereal disease during 1960 by the United States Public Health Service.[68] Among the conclusions that have pertinence to nursing practice were the following:

1. The knowledge and skills are available to reduce the incidence of syphilis to the point where this disease can be kept under control by nominal expenditures of money, time, and effort.
2. Action must be taken promptly.
3. The basic action is to find the newly infected person before he has a chance to infect four others and to bring him under treatment.
4. Case finding requires the use of all community resources, including the patient. Another paper in the same issue of *Public Health Reports* describes a program for training nurses to interview patients, so that they can participate effectively in case finding and in case holding.[69]
5. The suggestion was also made that informational and educational efforts should also be strengthened.

Summary

Briefly, the causative agent in syphilis is the *Treponema pallidum*. It is a delicate organism that is well adapted to the internal environment of the human being. It is susceptible to, that is, easily destroyed by, conditions that vary in any degree from these conditions. The reservoir is the person who is infected. The period of greatest communicability is the first four or five years after the infection is acquired, though occasionally it may be as long as ten years. Transmission is by direct contact with tissues, including blood containing the spirochete. Prevention depends on sterilizing the reservoir or protecting others from contact with it. To eradicate the reservoir of infection, persons who are in the communicable phases of the disease must be identified and brought under treatment before they have had an opportunity to infect others. This is in their own interest as well as for the welfare of others. They must also be treated until they are cured. This requires follow-up and education. Nurses participate in all these activities.

What infection has come into prominence in recent years as a significant cause of morbidity and mortality?

In 1957 Letourneau stated that staphylococcic infections were the most important problem facing hospitals.[70] Although not everyone would agree that this problem supersedes all others, the large number of papers appearing

---

[68] *Public Health Reports,* LXXV, November, 1960, pp. 989-10.
[69] *Ibid.,* pp. 1000-6.
[70] Charles Letourneau, "Nosomial Infections," *Hospital Management,* LXXXIII, February, 1957, p. 41.

in the literature indicate that staphylococcic infections have been, and continue to be, regarded as a serious problem. As stated earlier, certain other common organisms are responsible for a rising incidence of infection. Reimann[71] states that though death rates from pneumonia and hemolytic streptococci have been reduced, these gains have been more than offset by infections caused by staphylococci, aerogenes, *Proteus,* and *Pseudomonas.* From recent papers in scientific journals, monilia might well be added to this list. The problem of staphylococcic disease is not a limited one, but is world-wide. Reports of investigations of various aspects of the problem are published in many languages and come from many countries of the world. In the hospital the problem is not confined to one area, but is hospital-wide. In a survey made by Godfrey and Smith[72] staphylococcic infection was found to be epidemic on medical and surgical wards. Seventeen per cent of the surgical patients had staphylococcic infections. Of these, 2.6 per cent of the surgical patients had severe staphylococcic disease. The number of patients having staphyloccic infections was less on the medical wards than on the surgical wards, but the percentage having severe disease was greater. Twelve per cent had staphylococcic disease and 7.3 per cent had serious infection. Staphylococcic disease is also a cause of death. In the study cited above, 10 to 29 patients with staphylococcic disease died, and in three of the patients the disease was probably the cause of death. Numerous studies have been reported on the problem of staphylococcic infection in nurseries of newborn infants.

The extent of the problem has been, and is, difficult to determine. Not all infections are reported and not all infections that are acquired in the hospital are manifested while the patient is in the hospital. The classic example is that of the newborn baby who acquires the infection during his sojourn in the hospital nursery. At the time he is discharged from the hospital, he appears to be healthy. A few days to a week or so later he develops impetigo or some other skin manifestation of staphlyococcic disease. About 14 days later his mother develops a breast abscess. This, of course, is not inevitable as not all mothers who breast-feed babies with staphylococcic disease develop breast abscesses. Those who do not breast-feed their babies are not likely to develop abscesses. Since the breast abscess in the mother develops after the disease appears in the baby, authorities believe that the mother is infected by the baby. Furthermore, the spread of the disease is not limited to the mother, for other members of the family develop impetigo, furuncles, and other manifestations of staphylococcic disease. In this way the community is seeded with resistant staphylococci.

[71] Hobart A. Reimann, "Variation of Staphylococcus Microccocus Pyogenes," *American Medical Association Archives of Internal Medicine,* CVI, September, 1960, pp. 341-44.
[72] Mary E. Godfrey and Jan Maclean Smith, "Hospital Hazards of Staphylococcic Sepsis," *Journal of American Medical Association,* CLXVI, March 8, 1958, pp. 1197-1220.

Why are staphylococcic infections regarded as serious?

The problem of infection in hospitals is not new. Hospital-acquired infection has been a problem for centuries. Not until the introduction of antisepsis and asepsis in the late nineteenth century were infections brought under some degree of control. The present concern about infections is due to the observation that the incidence of infection in hospitals is higher than it was previous to the introduction of antimicrobial drugs. According to Reimann,[73] between the years of 1935 and 1947 the death rate from infections at the Boston City Hospital fell steadily. Since 1947 it has increased steadily. In 1957 there were four times as many patients with staphylococci in their blood stream as there were in 1935 and twice as many as in 1947. Reimann continues by saying that, prior to 1937, infections from gram-negative bacilli were rare and they have increased at even a more rapid rate than have those caused by staphylococci.

Unlike some microorganisms having a predilection for certain tissues or organs, resistant staphylococci are able to establish themselves and cause disease in many tissues. Less serious manifestations, such as pimples, impetigo, and furuncles, involve the skin. Small breaks in the skin such as those caused by a cut may be followed by a localized area of infection. Wound infections following a surgical procedure may be limited to a stitch abscess or may be disseminated throughout the entire wound. Other serious forms of staphylococcic disease include pneumonia and septicemia. A few years ago the writer observed a young woman who developed a staphylococcic septicemia following an illegal abortion. Abscesses were distributed throughout her body, including her brain.

The increase in the incidence of staphylococcic disease is attributable to a number of factors. Because the rise has been marked since the introduction of antimicrobial drugs, the role of these agents in the development of strains of staphylococci that are resistant to them is stressed. Associated with the use of antimicrobial drugs was a relaxation of antiseptic and aseptic techniques, as a result of the belief that antimicrobial agents could be used to prevent infection and that, if infection should occur, antimicrobial agents could be used to promptly cure it. Furthermore, there seemed to be evidence to support this belief. For example, when penicillin was being tested for safety and effectiveness in the treatment of infections in human beings, a young man who had undergone surgery developed a blood stream infection (septicemia) caused by the *Staphylococcus aureus*. Despite the severity of his illness, the physician who was in charge of the experimental use of penicillin told the surgeon that he could cure the patient. The surgeon then asked, "What do you expect, a miracle?" There was in fact a miracle, for the young man did recover fully. News of the recovery of this man, as well as of others, was reported in

[73] Hobart Reimann, "Infectious Disease," *American Medical Association Archives of Internal Medicine,* CVI, November, 1960, pp. 679-705.

scientific and lay journals. Newspapers and magazines carried dramatic stories detailing the recovery of persons who had been ill and had recovered because they were treated with a "wonder drug." Penicillin proved to be effective in the treatment of pneumococcus pneumonia, hemolytic *Streptococcus* infections, meningitis, and, when properly used, gonorrhea and syphilis.

About 1954 hospitals and physicians became aware that patients were developing infections that did not respond to the usual methods of treatment. Since then thousands of papers from all over the world have been written outlining the nature and extent of the problem. Since the findings that are presented by one investigator are at variance with those of others, answers to the problem await the future. There is, however, little doubt about the fact that pathogenic staphylococci remain an important factor in the cause of both morbidity and mortality in the United States and in the world. What happened? Perhaps the survival of resistant strains is another illustration of the concept that adaptation is basic to survival, that is, adapt or die. The staphylococci "chose" to adapt and therefore to survive. Staphylococci were favored in adapting by the fact that they are a hardy species. Moreover, some antimicrobial agents are bacteriostatic in action rather than bactericidal. Thus the antimicrobial agent inhibits the growth and multiplication of the organism, but it does not kill it. The weakened microorganism is rendered more susceptible to destruction by the host's defense mechanisms.

Evidence that antimicrobial agents have played a role in the selection of resistant strains comes from a number of sources. A number of investigators state that resistant strains of staphylococci are more prevalent among patients and personnel in hospitals where antibiotics are used freely than in hospitals where they are not. In mental hospitals, where antimicrobial agents are rarely used, the prevalence of resistant strains is similar to that found in the general population. Mudd presents evidence which convincingly supports the hypothesis that the rise of resistant staphylococci is in direct proportion to the use of antimicrobial drugs.[74] The indiscriminate use of antimicrobial drugs had its origin in the fact that, in the beginning, the limitations on their effectiveness were not known or understood.

Widespread publicity in the newspapers and magazines encouraged people to believe that the drugs were both safe and effective. That some people continue to believe in the efficacy and safety of antimicrobial agents is illustrated by the case of Mrs. Heron, who recently commented to a friend as follows: "I told my friend that she should go to her doctor and tell him that she must have some penicillin for that cough. After all, she [the person with the cough] knows more about what she needs than the doctor does." Patients often express doubt and disappointment when the doctor hesitates or refuses to prescribe an antimicrobial drug. In our culture, patients tend to demand

[74] Stuart Mudd, "The Staphylococcus Problem," *Scientific American,* CC, January, 1959, p. 43.

that all that is available at any time be used. In addition, emphasis in advertising on "the quick and easy" leads the public to expect that if there are not ways of treating illness that bring prompt and effective relief, there ought to be. It is imperative to help the patient and his family understand that his treatment is appropriate and that recovery takes time and the combined effort of the patient, nurse, physician, and all others concerned with the care of the patient to effect relief. Sometimes the desire of the patient to have something done can be met in part by quality nursing. Through effective use of her supportive or expressive role, the nurse may be able to reduce tension in the group—that is, between the patient and the physician. If she is successful, she may be able to help the patient work and wait for recovery. (See Chapter 6.)

Another factor believed to have contributed to the problem of staphylococcic disease is that there has been some slackness in aseptic practices. Though these will be discussed in more detail later, most authorities emphasize that they should never be relaxed, no matter what antimicrobial agent is available. Staphylococci are ubiquitous. The control of their spread is complicated by the fact that they are disseminated not only by patients with staphylococcic disease, but by healthy carriers. Whether or not disease develops depends not only on the causative agent, but on a susceptible host and the interaction between the two. Little is known at this time about the latter aspects of the problem.

In our present state of knowledge, however, control of staphylococcic disease is concentrated on limiting the spread of virulent staphylococci. The nurse should understand that the available procedures are not always completely successful in preventing disease. Because many of the practices in hospitals have been developed empirically, they may need to be studied to determine whether or not more effective methods are required. This does not mean, however, that more complicated methods are needed.

In a recent study performed by a group of students, less than 20 per cent of persons washed their hands after caring for a patient. They progressed directly from one patient to another without washing their hands. Whatever methods are decided upon should be clear and easily followed by everyone. One unsafe act may endanger not only patients, but nurses and other hospital personnel. In the past there has been a tendency to blame the spread of infectious diseases on the nurse. Present knowledge indicates that many factors contribute to the spread of staphylococci. Whenever an increase in the incidence of staphylococcic disease occurs, an effort should be made to discover its source or sources, not for the primary purpose of finding a scapegoat, but to identify and correct the cause. Although the eradication of infection from the hospital is desirable, as with other infectious diseases control is a more practical goal. A rate of about 1 per cent is generally considered to be what is possible to achieve.[75]

[75] Jean A. LaLiberte, "Staphylococcal Disease—A Challenge to the Hospital," *American Journal of Public Health*, XLIX, September, 1959, pp. 1181-83.

In limiting the spread of resistant staphylococci, the first question that arises is, "Who protects whom and from what should they be protected?" Without knowledge of the links in the chain in the infectious process from the causative agent to the susceptible host, an adequate answer cannot be given.

What are the characteristics of the causative organism?

Although the *Staphylococcus* is a strain of *Micrococcus,* it is generally referred to by the former term. According to Burdon, two species are recognized, the *Staphylococcus epidermidis* and the *Staphylococcus aureus.*[76] The *Staphylococcus epidermidis* forms white colonies when grown on agar and the *Staphylococcus aureus* usually forms orange or golden-yellow colonies. *Staphylococcus aureus* is also known as *Staphylococcus pyogenes.* Large numbers of staphylococci are found on the skin at all times, the most common species being the *Staphylococcus epidermidis.* Since it has a low virulence even when injected, its presence is not viewed with concern. Because the *Staphylococcus aureus* is usually found in the nose, and is more abundant on the hands and face than on other parts of the body, Burdon suggests that its principal habitat may be the nose.[77] Furthermore, most strains of *Staphylococcus aureus* are potentially pathogenic. Healthy persons whose anterior nares are colonized by virulent *Staphylococcus aureus* are carriers.

What are some of the characteristics of Staphylococcus aureus that facilitate their survival?

Staphylococci get their name from the fact that they form grapelike clusters in stained smears. They are gram-positive and stain easily. They are easily cultivated on simple culture media. They grow well at room as well as body temperature. They are aerobic, but will grow under anaerobic conditions. These cultural characteristics help to explain why certain strains of *Staphylococcus aureus* are frequently implicated in food poisoning. Foods containing mixtures of egg and milk, such as cream pies, provide a good culture medium for the *Staphylococcus aureus.* If food is contaminated and allowed to stand at room temperature, the *Staphylococcus* multiplies and in five to seven hours produces enough enterotoxin to cause gastroenteritis. To prevent poisoning from food contaminated by the *Staphylococcus aureus,* bakeries and restaurants are required to refrigerate all cream pies and other cream-filled desserts. Housewives should do likewise in the home. Since time is required for the *Staphylococcus* to elaborate the enterotoxin, there is no danger from foods that are eaten as soon as they are prepared.

After the ingestion of the enterotoxin, the incubation period is short. It varies from 45 minutes to six hours. The more virulent the enterotoxin, the

[76] Burdon, *Op. cit.,* p. 471.
[77] *Ibid.,* pp. 470-71.

sooner symptoms appear. Acute prostration and even death may occur in debilitated patients. The main feature in therapy is to restore the fluid and electrolyte balance of the patient. As indicated above, prevention is based on prompt and adequate refrigeration of susceptible foods. Since the enterotoxin is heat-stable, heating the food after enterotoxin is formed is of no avail. The only procedures of value are to prevent the contamination of food and to refrigerate it if it is not eaten as soon as it is prepared. The sanitary handling of food lessens the chances of introducing microorganisms and refrigeration minimizes bacterial growth. In addition to their ability to grow and multiply in simple culture media, staphylococci are able to survive for extended periods of time outside the host. Their great resistance to drying is emphasized by Colbeck.[78] His assistants were able to make cultures of staphylococci from sealed test tubes containing dried cultures which had not been subcultured in five years. The staphylococci were pathogenic. Eighteen hours after opening the tubes, Colbeck developed boils on two fingers; organisms recovered from the boils were the same phage type as those in the test tubes. Since the phage type was rare in Vancouver, the assumption was made that the source of the staphylococci was the old dried culture.

To determine whether virulence of staphylococci is altered by exposure to drying, Colbeck[79] smeared pus obtained from a subcutaneous abscess of a rabbit on a glass slide. The slide was kept at room temperature and 50 per cent humidity for varying periods up to 11 days. There was a marked tendency for microorganisms to die off between the seventh and the eleventh days. Colbeck concluded, however, that the virulence of the staphylococci that survive was unchanged. Whether or not disease developed in animals that were injected with cultures made from material on the slides depended on the number of organisms present.

In addition to being resistant to drying, staphylococci are also able to withstand temperatures up to 50° C. for one-half hour or more.[80] To kill them, chemical germicides such as phenol or mercury chloride in solutions of 1 to 2 per cent require about 15 minutes. They are, however, highly susceptible to gentian violet and other aniline dyes.

The capacity of *Staphylococcus aureus* to survive outside the host, combined with its ability to develop resistant strains, makes it a formidable foe. Procedures designed to prevent the spread of staphylococci from one person to another must take these facts into account. The implications of the above will be discussed further in relation to modes of transmission.

As has been stated earlier, not all virulent staphylococci are alike in all characteristics. In fact, one of the problems with them has been that there are a multitude of types. They can, however, be classified into four main groups according to the types of bacterial viruses (phages) that attack them. Like other living organisms, bacteria have diseases. Some attempts have been made

[78] John C. Colbeck, "The Hospital Environment—Its place in the Hospital Staphylococcus Infections Problem," *American Journal of Public Health,* L, April, 1960, p. 472.
[79] *Ibid.,* p. 471.
[80] Burdon, *Op. cit.,* p. 260-77.

to utilize this knowledge in the treatment of bacterial disease, but they have been limited. Just about the time the antimicrobial drugs were first introduced, interest in the possibility that phages might be useful in the control of bacterial infections was beginning to develop. Though this possibility remains to be exploited, phages are now useful in the identification (typing) of staphylococci. According to LaLiberte,[81] about 60 per cent of virulent staphylococci can be typed by this method. The test is performed by inoculating agar phages with a culture of the organism. The phages, which have been assigned a number, are then dropped on the plate and the plates are incubated. Since the phage destroys susceptible bacteria, clear zones indicate the bacteria that are attacked by specific phages and the phage type is assigned from this information. Some strains are attacked by more than one phage. Phage typing is useful not only in identifying the strain of staphylococci causing disease in a patient, but in tracking the source and routes of infection.[82] In other words, phage typing is an epidemiological and research tool. Phage typing is not usually performed until other studies have been made.

There are four main groups of phages and many different types. The groups are numbered with Roman numerals from I through IV. Staphylococci susceptible to group III phages were the first to develop resistance to antibiotics. In the last few years those susceptible to group I phages have appeared more commonly than those susceptible to group III. According to Mudd,[83] phage 80 and a close relative 81, and frequently referred to by the shorthand 80/81, have been implicated in staphylococcic disease in many parts of the world.

Not only is the *Staphylococcus* extraordinarily resistant to adverse environmental conditions, but it possesses the capacity to produce a wide variety of substances that assist it in establishing disease. These include a variety of hemolysins, leukocidin, and hyaluronidase. Most strains of staphylococci now causing infection also produce a penicillin-destroying enzyme known as penicillinase. They almost all produce substances called coagulases. One of the first tests done to identify the character of staphylococci obtained from a patient or carrier is to determine whether or not it is coagulase-positive; most pathogenic staphylococci are coagulase-positive. Mudd[84] states that under certain circumstances staphylococci may have extracellular capsules. Previous reference was made to the fact that some strains elaborate an enterotoxin that is responsible for one type of food poisoning.

What are the characteristics of a lesion caused by a virulent strain of Staphylococcus? *What kinds of infections are caused by pathogenic staphylococci?*

Invasion of a tissue by a virulent strain of *Staphylococcus* is followed by the formation of an abundant purulent exudate or pus, which is character-

[81] LaLiberte, *Op. cit.,* p. 1182.
[82] J. E. Blair and M. Carr, "Bacteriophage Typing of Staphylococci," *Journal of Infectious Diseases,* XCIII, July-August, 1953, p. 1.
[83] Mudd, *Op. cit.,* p. 42.
[84] *Ibid.,* p. 45.

istic of a lesion occurring in staphylococcic disease. Langmuir[35] classifies staphylococcic disease as follows: (1) impetigo and pyoderma of infants, (2) mastitis in postpartum patients, (3) wound infection in surgical patients, and (4) infections in debilitated patients that are superimposed on other conditions. This classification does not include skin manifestations of the disease that may occur in adults or older children, such as furuncles, carbuncles, infected decubiti, and paronychia.[86] Other infections include pyelonephritis, endocarditis, parotitis, and pneumonia. Pneumonia that accompanies a terminal illness is usually due to a staphylococcal infection. Infection of bone, either directly as in a compound fracture or as a metastatic infection from a locus such as a furuncle, is known as osteomyelitis. It is often a serious and persistent infection that has a tendency to recur during the lifetime of the individual. Manifestations of staphylococcic disease are not limited to those cited above. Staphylococci have a remarkable ability to establish themselves in a wide variety of tissues.

Briefly, impetigo is a superficial skin infection that may be caused by either hemolytic staphylococci or group A hemolytic streptococci.[87] It occurs most commonly in infants and children and creates a problem when it infects nurseries of newborn infants. The newborn infant has not had an opportunity to develop immunity to infection and is highly susceptible.

Wound infections in surgical patients may be minor or they may be serious. A small stitch abscess may heal promptly following the evacuation of pus. As in other infections caused by staphylococci, the infection may be localized to the wound or it may spread from the wound to surrounding tissue, causing cellulitis, and it may spread to distant points. As it spreads through the lymphatics, it may produce a lymphadenitis. Eventually it may enter the blood, where it multiplies and is carried to distant sites where metastatic abscesses may be formed.

As indicated above, staphylococcal infections may be primarily a localized disease or a systemic infection. Localized disease can be converted into a systemic infection by disruption of the local lesion or failure of the body's defense mechanisms to prevent spread. In systemic disease, pathogenic microorganisms and/or their products are disseminated throughout the body. A variety of serious disorders are therefore possible. They include pyemia, septicemia, hemorrhagic nephritis, and staphylococcic pneumonia that terminates fatally.

[85] Alexander D. Langmuir, "Ecologic and Epidemiologic Aspects of Staphylococcic Infections in Hospitals," *Journal of the American Medical Association,* CLXVI, March 8, 1958, pp. 1202-3.

[86] A paronychia, or runaround, is an infection of the nail bed. It usually results from an infection of a hangnail.

[87] Ivan L. Bennett, Jr., "Localized Infections and Abscesses," in T. R. Harrison, *et al.,* ed., *Principles of Internal Medicine,* 3rd ed., McGraw-Hill Book Co., Inc., New York, 1958, p. 961.

What are some of the factors facilitating the spread of
virulent staphylococci?

A virulent *Staphylococcus* is highly communicable. It passes readily from the carrier, or the person with staphylococcic disease, to his contacts. Persons who share the environment with an individual who has a staphylococcic infection are likely to become carriers of the same strain of organism. They may become nasal carriers or develop lesions characteristic of disease.

The second link in the chain of factors leading to an infectious process is a reservoir or source of the causative agent. Unlike the *Treponema pallidum,* which is fragile and dies soon after it escapes from the human host, the *Staphylococcus* is not only able to survive after its discharge from the host, but it appears to maintain its virulence. Although the human host is the primary source of coagulase-positive staphylococci, the nature of the organism enables it to survive in the air and on articles in the environment of the infected person. The host may be either a healthy person who carries coagulase-positive staphylococci in the mucosa of his anterior nares or a person who is ill with staphylococcic disease. In the person who is sick with staphylococcal disease, coagulase-positive staphylococci are found both in the anterior nares and in the lesion associated with the disease.

Three general groups of people in the hospital act as reservoirs for staphylococci. The first group includes patients who are admitted for the treatment of a septic condition or who are carriers of pathogenic staphylococci. The second group includes those patients who are negative at the time they are admitted, but who acquire a staphylococcic infection after their admission to the hospital. The person may become a carrier or develop staphylococcic disease. The third group is comprised of the various members of the hospital personnel. They, too, may act as carriers or develop overt disease.

As might be expected, the incidence of carriers among hospital personnel is higher than it is in the general population. The carrier rate in the community as reported by Blair[88] has been reported to range from 30 to 50 per cent. Figures cited by different authorities as to the percentage of hospital personnel who harbor staphylococci in their anterior nares vary somewhat. Wise[89] reports that about 80 per cent of hospital personnel were found to carry some strain of staphylococci in their anterior nares. Of these, 50 per cent were coagulase-positive. About 12 per cent of the people working in the hospitals carry the organisms responsible for the majority of hospital-acquired infections. Burnett and associates[90] made nasal cultures on 640 members of hospital personnel. Forty-one per cent were found to harbor coagulase-positive

[88] John E. Blair, "The Staphylococci," *Bacterial and Mycotic Infections of Man,* 3rd ed., ed. René J. Dubos, J. B. Lippincott Co., Philadelphia, 1958, p. 327.

[89] Robert I. Wise, "Principles of Management of Staphylococcic Infections," *Journal of the American Medical Association,* CLXVI, March 8, 1958, 1178-82.

[90] W. Emory Burnett, *et al.,* "Program in Prevention-Eradication of Staphylococcic Infections," *Journal of the American Medical Association,* CLXVI, March 8, 1958, pp. 1183-84.

staphylococci. Only 4 per cent were of the phage type 42 B/52/81. This type was responsible for 69 per cent of hospital infections.

A study reported by Dowling and his co-workers[91] illustrates how resistant microorganisms are disseminated. On admission to the hospital, 41 per cent of patients were found to carry resistant staphylococci. A group of patients were cared for by personnel of whom 92 per cent carried resistant staphylococci. By the time the patients were discharged 90 per cent of them had acquired resistant staphylococci. After these patients returned to their homes, 50 per cent of their household contacts acquired resistant staphylococci. After seven weeks at home, 59 per cent of patients continued to carry resistant organisms.

The results of a number of studies on carriers indicate that some persons do not easily become carriers. In some persons who do, the carrier state is persistent, while in others it is intermittent. The reasons for these differences are not well understood. In general, the highest rate of carriers is found among those persons in the hospital who are in closest contact with patients. The lowest rate is found among those who are farthest from the patient. As a consequence, the rate is highest among nurses and physicians and lowest among office personnel.

Not only may the carrier state be a problem to the nurse, but she, too, sometimes develops staphylococcic infections. In a study by Davies[92] on the incidence of staphylococcic infections among nurses at the London Hospital, he found that 16.4 per cent of the admissions of nurses to the infirmary were for staphylococcic infections. In the six years prior to the year in which the study was made, the percentage was 18.2 per cent. The study showed that the average length of time lost by each nurse was 8.5 days. Davies states that all the infections were of the soft tissues, and were of the type that probably involved transmission by direct contact. The lesions were found on the face, neck, axilla, and upper limb. Almost 98 per cent of the organisms were resistant to penicillin. Davies questions the use of the scrubbing brush, since many of the lesions were on the hands. Vigorous scrubbing may disrupt the skin and thereby provide a portal of entry for microbes.

Numerous studies indicate that the environment of the patient with staphylococcic disease is heavily laden with staphylococci. Colbeck[93] states that bacteriological examination often reveals that objects such as blankets, bath basins, toilet seats, and other fomites in the hospital are heavily laden with microorganisms. Walters et al,[94] in a study of the water in bedsides carafes, found that the water was often heavily contaminated with a variety of micro-

[91] Harry F. Dowling, Mark H. Lepper and George G. Jackson, "Clinical Significance of Antibiotic-Resistant Bacteria," *Journal of the American Medical Association,* CLVII, January 22, 1955, p. 327.

[92] D. M. Davies, "Staphylococcal Infections in Nurses," *Lancet,* I, March 19, 1960, pp. 644-45.

[93] Colbeck, *Op. cit.,* p. 469.

[94] Carl W. Walters, *et al.,* "Bacteriology of the Bedside Carafe," *New England Journal of Medicine,* CCLIX, December 18, 1958, pp. 1198-1202.

organisms. Colbeck's[95] study of the air in the room of the patient indicated that when the air was not in motion, it was not an important source of microorganisms.

By this time the answer to the question of who is to be protected from whom begins to emerge. The broad answer is, "That depends." It depends on whether the patient or the nurse carries the microorganism. It also depends on whether the patient has been in the hospital for some time or is newly admitted.

The third link in the chain of the infectious process is that the microorganism must have a portal by which it escapes from the reservoir. The *Staphylococcus* may, of course, be discharged into the external environment from the nose during talking, sneezing, and coughing. Septic wounds open to the outside, along with purulent discharges, serve as means by which microorganisms may be discharged into the external environment.

The next step in the infectious process is that of the mode or vehicle of transmission. Because of the resistance of the staphylococci to destruction, they may be transmitted by either direct or indirect contact. Authorities do not agree as to the importance of each of the various mechanisms of transmission. There appears to be some evidence that the size of the dose of microorganisms plays a role in their ability to produce disease. Instances are, however, reported in which infection resulted from a very small dose. Because more than one vehicle may be involved in the transmission of staphylococci from a reservoir, the usual possibilities will be discussed. No attempt will be made to establish one as being of greater importance than others.

The air may become directly or indirectly contaminated and serve as a vehicle of transmission. Coughing, sneezing, and talking have been demonstrated to be accompanied by the discharge into the air of droplets of moisture of varying sizes. Because large droplets settle rapidly, doubt is now cast on the importance of droplet infection as a vehicle of transmission. Droplet nuclei are, however, believed to be important because tiny dried particles or nuclei are suspended in the air. Because they are buoyant, they remain in the air currents and are carried by the air wherever the air goes. Riley[96] cites three studies in support of the theory that droplet nuclei and dust serve to transmit infection. Air may also be contaminated by dust particles which can carry pathogenic staphylococci. Colbeck[97] states that the number of colonies of staphylococci cultured from the air can be doubled by moving a blanket rapidly from the top to the foot of the bed once a minute for five minutes. Blankets and sheets may be contaminated by drainage from a wound. The air is then contaminated by dust shaken from the bedding during procedures such as changing or straightening the patient's bed.

Not all investigators agree about the extent to which clothing and bed

[95] Colbeck, *Op. cit.,* p. 470.
[96] Richard L. Riley, "Airborne Infection," *American Journal of Nursing,* LX, September, 1960, p. 1247.
[97] Colbeck, *Op. cit.,* p. 470.

linens of patients with staphylococcic disease act as vehicles of transmission. There is, however, general agreement that they are heavily contaminated. Burnett, *et al*[98] state that among hospital personnel, student nurses seem to be most vulnerable. Since their infections were found to be on exposed areas, this suggests transmission by contact. From this brief review of the mechanisms of transmission of the *Staphylococcus,* the fact that they are multiple and complex should be evident.

The fifth link in the chain of the infectious process is that to cause disease the microorganism must have a point at which it enters the susceptible host. The intact skin serves as a barrier to the entrance of microorganisms. Blair[99] states that the healthy skin tends to rid itself of organisms that settle on it. Although the manner in which the disease process takes place in the skin is poorly understood, Blair presumes that there must be some decrease in local resistance, combined with some trauma, to render the tissue susceptible to the infection. The person who has a break in his skin has, of course, a demonstrable point at which microorganisms may enter. Along with the break there is often some condition that renders the tissue vulnerable to infection.

The last, although by no means the least, important link in the chain is the susceptible host. Though there is some knowledge of the factors contributing to resistance and susceptibility, there is much that is not known. As has been indicated earlier, age is a factor in staphylococcic disease; those at the extremes of age are considered to be most vulnerable. Healthy adults usually have considerable resistance to staphylococcal infections. Persons with debilitating diseases are, however, very susceptible. Influenza predisposes to staphylococcic pneumonia. One possible explanation is that the cells in the mucosa lining the tracheobronchial tree that are invaded by the influenza virus may be disrupted, thus providing a portal of entry for *Staphylococcus.* Since not all persons having influenza develop pneumonia, there must be other contributing factors. Total body irradiation reduces resistance to staphylococcic disease. Therapy with cortisone or its analogues may have a similar effect. At this time not too much is known about the development of immunity to the *Staphylococcus.* In the present state of knowledge, though the resistance of the host is believed to be a significant factor in the development of, and recovery from, staphylococcal infection, specific information is limited.

The knowledge necessary to answer the questions, Who is protected from whom? From What? How? is briefly summarized below. The causative organism, the *Staphylococcus,* is everywhere. It is resistant to drying and to other destructive agents. It grows on simple media at room temperature as well as at body temperature. There are many strains, some of which are known to be pathogenic. So-called nonpathogenic strains are normal inhabitants of the skin. Virulent strains of staphylococci have a tendency to develop resistance to antimicrobial drugs. Many of them produce a penicillin-destroying enzyme called penicillinase. Most, if not all, disease-producing staphylococci produce

[98] Burnett, *Op. cit.,* pp. 1183-84.
[99] Blair, *Op. cit.,* p. 321.

a substance called coagulase. Coagulase is capable of clotting blood serum. In staphylococcic disease, it clots the blood in the small veins in the affected area. Coagulase also deposits fibrin on the staphylococci in the area. This interferes with their ingestion and destruction by phagocytes.[100] Various strains form other toxins and enzymes. Among them is leukocidin, which destroys leukocytes, a variety of hemolysins which lyse erythrocytes, and enterotoxin, which is responsible for one form of food poisoning. The lesion of staphylococcic disease is characterized by the formation of an abundant purulent exudate. Though skin lesions are a common manifestation in staphylococcic disease, abscesses may be widespread throughout the body. Staphylococcic disease varies in severity from a minor and localized lesion, such as a stitch abscess, to a virulent and deadly disease, such as pneumonia. The problem of the control of the *Staphylococcus* is aggravated by its high degree of communicability and by the fact that it tends to colonize the anterior nares of healthy persons, with the result that they become carriers.

In studies of an epidemic of staphylococcic disease, phage may be used to trace its course. The typing is based on the fact that about 60 per cent of the strains of staphylococci are attacked by one or more bacterial phages or viruses. Staphylococci are classified in one of four groups depending on which phages destroy them.

The reservoir, or source, of staphylococci is a human being who has staphylococcic disease in which the lesion is in contact with the external environment. The patient may also carry the same strain of staphylococci in his anterior nares. The healthy carrier is also a source of resistant staphylococci. Because of the ability of the *Staphylococcus* to exist outside the host, fomites may harbor virulent organisms.

The methods of transmission of the *Staphylococcus* are varied and complex. Anything coming in contact with a patient or carrier may be a vehicle for its transmission. Air contaminated with droplets of moisture, droplet nuclei, or dust may serve as one vehicle of transmission. The hands of carriers of antimicrobial-resistant staphylococci, as well as fomites—dust, food, bed linens, instruments, walls, mattresses and pillows, furniture, and clothing of patients with draining lesions—may all serve as vehicles for the transmission of staphylococci.

The problem of how the microorganism enters the susceptible host is not clear in all cases. Breaks in the integrity of the skin, particularly if accompanied by some trauma to the surrounding tissue, serve as possible sites for the *Staphylococcus* to enter the tissue.

A susceptible host is another factor in the development of staphylococcal infection and disease. Not all carriers behave in the same way. In some the carrier state is persistent, in others it is intermittent. Others do not become carriers or are carriers for only brief periods of time. The reasons for differences in the carrier state are not known.

Certain conditions or states appear to predispose to the development of

[100] Jawetz, *Op. cit.,* 5th ed.. p. 134.

staphylococcic disease. These include the extremes of age, surgical procedures, debilitating disease, total body radiation, and therapy with adrenal cortical hormones. At this time, factors in the development of immunity to staphylococcic disease, and even whether such immunity is possible, are not known.

Much remains to be learned about the factors contributing to the spread and development of staphylococcic disease. The findings in some studies conflict with those of other studies. Perhaps this should be expected when a problem is as complex as this one. Because of limitations of knowledge, perfect control does not seem to be possible at present. The over-all infection rate should not, according to some authorities, be over 1 per cent. Methods that are used in the control of staphylococci should take into account the hypothesis that the number of microbes may be a factor in pathogenesis. They should also take into consideration the human element. Procedures that are decided upon should be as simple as is possible to accomplish the purpose. Highly elaborate procedures may be theoretically effective, but fail because they are difficult and time-consuming. Second, when procedures are decided upon, an educational program as to the why and how is also necessary. Procedures should also be subjected to investigation of their practicality and effectiveness.

Although the operating room and the newborn infants' nursery are often referred to as the most important areas in the control of hospital-acquired staphylococcic infection, all areas are of importance. One of the most commonly used measures in the control of airborne infection is the wearing of masks. Masks are worn to accomplish two different purposes. One is to prevent the contamination of the external environment by microorganisms from the respiratory tract of the person wearing the mask. In terms of the links in the chain of the infectious process, the mask stands between the point at which a microorganism leaves the reservoir and the point at which it finds a vehicle for its transmission. This is the basis for wearing a mask in the operating room or in the newborn infants' nursery. A mask may also be used to guard a portal of entry. In this instance, a nurse or doctor wears a mask to protect himself from microorganisms discharged by the patient. According to Riley,[101] masks are more effective in preventing the escape of microorganisms from the reservoir into the external environment than they are in preventing the inhalation of droplet nuclei. The reason that masks are more effective in preventing the escape of microorganisms than they are in preventing their entrance is that they catch the droplets of moisture in the expired air. Droplet nuclei, which form as the moisture evaporates, are smaller in size and are therefore more difficult to trap. Although it is accepted that the construction of a mask and the way it is worn determine its effectiveness, instances are all too frequent in which masks are improperly worn. Riley[102] states: "Further-

[101] Riley, *Op. cit.*, p. 1248.
[102] Richard L. Riley, "Protective Measures," *Nursing Outlook,* VII, January, 1959, p. 39.

more, proper use of the mask depends on individual initiative and a high level of understanding, cooperation, and discipline."

Blair[103] describes in detail the construction of a face mask and outlines the procedure for wearing it. In general the mask should be constructed of a number of layers of material of dense porosity. It should be made of absorbent material so that it takes up moisture as it passes through. It should be clean when applied and discarded when removed. It should be replaced before it becomes wet. Most authorities suggest that a mask should not be worn longer than an hour or an hour and a half. It should cover both the nose and the mouth. It should be tied firmly in place. Some surgeons, such as Adams,[104] advocate the wearing of double-thickness masks. Howe[105] recommends that two masks be worn and that they be changed at one-and-one-half-hour intervals in long operations.

Although masks have been the most widely used device to control airborne infection, other measures are available. The concentration of microorganisms in the air can be reduced by ventilation. One of the measures advocated by Florence Nightingale in the care of the sick was ventilation. It is still frequently neglected. Outdoor air may be laden with soot and dust, but it usually carries few microorganisms. Particularly in the operating room, air-conditioning systems may be used to remove the respired air and add clean air. Hart[106] recommends that ultraviolet light be used to sterilize the air in the operating room. One point that is too often neglected in the control of airborne infection is keeping doors closed. Air currents carry droplet nuclei wherever they go. The control of airborne infection is difficult. The methods that are most readily available are using masks, providing ventilation, and controlling the circulation of air. Since the concentration of microorganisms in the air can be increased by moving blankets and other bed linens rapidly in the air, the shaking of coverings should be avoided. These latter procedures are under the control of the nurse.

The hands may act as vehicles in the transmission of virulent staphylococci. The source of their contamination may be discharges from the nasal mucosa of carriers or discharges from open lesions. Contamination of the hands may therefore result from direct contact with a lesion or its discharges or from contact with dressings covering septic wounds, bed coverings, or the clothing of the patient. Measures should be carried out to prevent the hands from being contaminated or to remove any microorganisms present on them.

To protect the person who is changing the dressings over draining wounds, rubber gloves should be worn. The dressings should also be discarded in such

---

[103] Esta McNett Blair, "Oh for a Mask," *Nursing Outlook*, VII, January, 1959, pp. 40-42.

[104] Ralph Adams, "Prevention of Infection," *American Journal of Nursing*, LVIII, March, 1958, p. 345.

[105] Chester W. Howe, "Prevention and Control of Post Operative Wound Infection owing to Staphylococcus Aureus," *New England Journal of Medicine*, CCLV, October 25, 1956, pp. 787-94.

[106] Deryl Hart, "Bacteriocidal Ultraviolet Radiation in O.R.," *Journal of the American Medical Association*, CLXXII, March 5, 1960, pp. 1019-27.

a manner that no one handles them after they are removed. For example, they may be placed on several thicknesses of newspaper and wrapped so that the outside of the package is kept clean. Whatever technique is utilized, it should be based on the certainty that discharges from infected lesions are teeming with virulent microorganisms.

Since it is impossible to prevent contamination of the hands in all instances, hand washing is essential to the removal of microorganisms. To be effective, it must be performed properly. Benson[107] describes in detail the hand-washing technique used at the Clinical Center, National Institutes of Health, Bethesda, Maryland. It will not be repeated here. The procedure described by Benson is for use on medical and surgical wards and not as part of the preparation for surgical operations. Hand washing, properly performed, is an essential step in interrupting the chain of events in the infectious process.

Because of the nurse's close contact with the patient and the resistance of staphylococci to destruction, the clothing of the nurse may become contaminated. For this reason, the nurse wears a gown during the time she cares for the patient. In some hospitals anyone who changes or assists in the changing of dressings on septic wounds also wears a mask, gown, and gloves. To limit the danger of the spread of virulent organisms from one patient to another, individual dressing trays or sets are recommended for each patient.

In a report of a survey of current aseptic practices in hospitals Thomas,[108] concludes that until further work is done, the following practices should be observed by nurses caring for patients with staphylococcic disease:

(1) Wearing a mask constructed as described in the article.
(2) Wearing it tied as securely as possible over the nose and mouth.
(3) Wearing it until such time as the care of the patient is completed, that is, through the removal of the contaminated linen from the room and the finishing of all work in the room of the patient.
(4) Discarding the mask immediately on leaving the room.
(5) Removing the gown that has been worn as part of the protective clothing.
(6) Washing the hands thoroughly, so that the nose that has been supposedly protected by the mask will not subsequently become infected by the hands.

One large area in the control of staphylococcic disease comes under the heading of housekeeping. Studies performed by a large number of investigators indicate that blankets, mattresses, bed linens and other articles in a patient's environment become laden with resistant staphylococci. Sheets and pillowcases are usually sterile after they are laundered; soiled linen may, however, release virulent organisms in linen chutes and may be sources of infection for laundry workers. Each hospital should have a method for handling contaminated linen so that the worker is protected. Bed linens on the beds of patients with heavy discharges should be changed frequently enough to prevent heavy contamination with microorganisms. The time-worn custom

---

107 Margaret E. Benson, "Handwashing—an Important Part of Medical Asepsis," *American Journal of Nursing,* LVII, September, 1957, pp. 1136-39.
108 Margaret W. Thomas, "Nursing Procedures in Management of Staphylococcal Infections," *American Journal of Public Health,* L, April, 1960, p. 499.

of storing blankets in a common cupboard should, if it has not already been, be eliminated. Blankets should be washed and sterilized after the discharge of a patient. Because wool blankets withstand washing poorly, some hospitals are replacing them with blankets made of washable fabrics. In some hospitals, blankets are oiled to encourage particles to adhere to the fibers.

In some hospitals, mattresses and pillows are encased in plastic coverings. Because staphylococci are resistant to drying, plastic coverings should be sterilized between patients. Ordinary washing is not likely to be effective. In some hospitals, mattresses and pillows are sterilized between patients. Adams[109] emphasizes that a light cleansing with a brush dipped in lysol solution has little or no effect on organisms buried in the mattress (or in a plastic cover either). Lend[110] is reported in *Time Magazine* to have found old pillows carrying not only enormous numbers of bacteria, but a wide variety of gross contaminants such as food and false teeth.

General cleaning techniques should include wet mopping, or mopping with a mop treated with a substance that causes dust to adhere to it. The same general procedure should be observed in dusting. In the past the use of vacuum cleaners has been frowned upon, because they stir up dust. Recently, there have been some references to types in which this factor is controlled.

The control of the spread of staphylococcic infections is neither quick nor easy. The procedures that are available are not glamorous; no newspaper is likely to headline them as producing a miracle. They are based on the application of principles of hygiene and antiseptic and aseptic techniques. Everything that comes in contact with a patient with staphylococcic disease, be it an oxygen tent or a mask or a bed sheet, should be treated as being contaminated. Measures employed in the control of staphylococcal infections should be based on the knowledge that the offending microorganism is ubiquitous and that it is resistant to drying.

Summary

Staphylococcic infection and disease are a very old problem. The discovery of the sulfonamides and then of penicillin and other antibiotics encouraged the hope that man could be victorious in his struggle with microorganisms. The appearance of strains of staphylococci that are resistant to antimicrobials has led to a resurgence of the problem. As a result, the importance of considering all of the steps in the infectious process when planning the control of a microorganism is being re-emphasized. Nurses are not responsible for staphylococcic infections becoming a problem. They are not solely responsible for their control. They do have a responsibility to participate on the infections committee, to cooperate in control measures, and to study ways to improve methods of control. They also have a responsibility to participate in educa-

---

[109] Ralph Adams, "Prevention of Infections in Hospitals," *American Journal of Nursing*, LVIII, March, 1958, p. 345.
[110] *Time Magazine*, November 14, 1960, p. 56.

tional programs in the institution so that more effective control measures can be instituted and effected. Specific methods useful in the destruction of micro-organisms have not been discussed. References have been included in the References for those who are interested. The infections that are most prevalent at this time in the United States are different from those of the past. There are many questions and few definitive answers. For this reason the nurse must expect, and be prepared to take, responsibility for continued learning. In protecting herself and others she should ask the questions, Who is protected from whom? Why? From what? How? Even when answers to these questions appear to be adequate, they should be continuously explored in an effort to obtain more adequate ones.

In addition to her role in the care of patients in hospitals, the nurse has a responsibility to educate persons in the hospital and out in the community in the use of hygienic measures to prevent the spread of infectious diseases. The following quotation, taken from "An Official Report of the American Public Health Association," *Control of Communicable Diseases in Man,* 9th ed., 1960, p. 12, appears to cover the personal practices required to limit the spread of communicable disease.

Education in personal cleanliness—This phase includes the various means available to impress upon all members of the community, young and old, and especially when communicable disease is prevalent or during epidemics, by spoken and printed word, and by illustration and suggestion, the necessity of:

a. Keeping the hands clean by sufficiently frequent soap and water baths.
b. Washing hands in soap and water immediately after voiding bowels or bladder and always before eating.
c. Keeping hands and unclean articles, or articles that have been used for toilet purposes by others, away from the mouth, nose, eyes, ears, genitalia, and wounds.
d. Avoiding the use of common or unclean eating, drinking, or toilet articles of any kind, such as cutlery and crockery, drinking cups, towels, handkerchiefs, combs, hairbrushes, and pipes.
e. Avoiding exposure of persons to spray from the nose and mouth, as in coughing, sneezing, laughing or talking.
f. Washing hands thoroughly after handling the patient or his belongings and wearing a protective overall apron while in the sickroom.

Other measures in the control of infectious diseases, such as immunization and the maintenance of a sanitary environment, are, of course, of continuing significance. At the present time, infectious diseases remain controlled only as long as effective measures are enforced.

REFERENCES

Books

Anderson, G. W., M. G. Arnstein, and Mary R. Lester, *Communicable Disease Control,* 4th ed., The Macmillan Company, New York, 1962.

Cady, Louise Lincoln, *Nursing in Tuberculosis,* 2nd ed., W. B. Saunders Co., Philadelphia, 1961.

Clifton, C. E., *Introduction to the Bacteria,* McGraw-Hill Book Co., New York, 1958.

Control of Communicable Diseases in Man, 9th ed., American Public Health Association, New York, 1960.

Control of Infections in Hospitals, American Hospital Association, Chicago, Hospital Monograph Series No. 12, 1962.

De Kruif, Paul, *Microbe Hunters,* Harcourt, Brace & Co., New York, 1926.

Diagnostic Standards and Classification of Tuberculosis, National Tuberculosis Association, New York, 1961.

Duffy, John, *Epidemics in Colonial America,* Louisiana State University, Baton Rouge, 1953.

Faddis, M. O., and J. M. Hayman, *Care of the Medical Patient,* McGraw-Hill Book Co., New York, 1952, pp. 38-45.

Hopps,, Howard C., *Principles of Pathology,* 2nd ed., Appleton-Century-Crofts, Inc., New York, 1964.

New York State Department of Health and the American Public Health Association, *Guide for the Prevention and Control of Infections in Hospitals,* Albany.

Riley, Richard L., and Francis O'Grady, *Airborne Infections,* The Macmillan Company, New York, 1961.

Rivers, Thomas M., and Frank L. Horsfall, Jr., *Viral and Rickettsial Infections of Man,* 3rd ed., J. B. Lippincott Co., Philadelphia, 1959.

Rogers, Edward S., *Human Ecology and Health,* The Macmillan Company, New York, 1960.

U.S. Department of Health, Education and Welfare, *Hepatitis,* Public Health Service Publication No. 446, Health Information Series, No. 82, U.S. Government Printing Office, Washington, D.C., 1959.

Winslow, C. E. A., *The Conquest of Epidemic Disease,* Princeton University Press, Princeton, 1943.

Articles

Adams, Ralph, "Prevention of Infections in Hospitals," *American Journal of Nursing,* LVIII, March, 1958, pp. 344-48.

Andrewes, Christopher H., "The Viruses of the Common Cold," *Scientific American,* CCIII, December, 1960, pp. 88-105.

Bearn, A. G., and James German, "Chromosomes and Disease," *Scientific American,* CCV, November, 1961, pp. 66-76.

Beck, Ann, "Issues in the Anti-vaccination Movement in England," *Medical History,* IV, October, 1960, pp. 310-21.

Beerman, Herman, *et al.,* "Syphilis," *Archives of Internal Medicine,* CVII, January, 1961, pp. 121-40.

Benson, Margaret, "Handwashing—An Important Part of Medical Asepsis," *American Journal of Nursing,* LVII, September, 1957, pp. 1136-38.

Benzer, Seymour, "The Fine Structure of the Gene," *Scientific American,* CCVI, January, 1962, pp. 70-84.

Berntsen, C. A., and W. McDermott, "Increased Transmissibility of Staphylococcus to Patients Receiving An Antimicrobial Drug," *New England Journal of Medicine,* CCLXII, March 31, 1960, pp. 637-42.

Blair, John E., and E. T. Bynoe, "Variation in Three Staphylococcal Typing Phages," *Public Health Reports,* LXXIII, May, 1958, pp. 465-66.

Blair, John E., and Miriam Carr, "Staphylococci in Hospital Acquired Infections," *Journal of the American Medical Association,* CLXVI, March 8, 1958, pp. 1192-96.

Bliss, Eugene L., "Reaction of the Adrenal Cortex to Emotional Stress," *Psychosomatic Medicine,* XVIII, January-February, 1956, pp. 56-74.

Burnet, F. M. "Theories of Immunity," *Perspectives in Biology and Medicine,* III, Summer, 1960, pp. 447-58.

Burnet, Sir MacFarlane, "The Mechanism of Immunity," *Scientific American,* CCIV, January, 1961, pp. 58-61.

Burnett, W. Emory, H. Taylor Caswell, Kenneth M. Schreck, Elsie R. Carrington, Normal Learner, Howard H. Steel, R. Robert Tyson, and William C. Wright, "Program for Prevention and Eradication of Staphylococcic Infections," *Journal of the American Medical Association,* CLXVI, March 8, 1958, pp. 1183-84.

Carrington, Elsie R., and Alice M. Sroat, "Epidemic Puerperal Breast Abscess," *American Journal of Nursing,* LVIII, December, 1958, pp. 1683-86.

Caswell, H. Taylor, "Staphylococcal Infections Among Hospital Personnel," *American Journal of Nursing,* LVIII, June, 1958, pp. 822-24.

Davies, D. M., "Staphylococcal Infections in Nurses," *Lancet,* I, March 19, 1960, pp. 644-45.

DiSandro, Edith H., "Eastern Viral Encephalitis," *American Journal of Nursing,* LX, April, 1960, pp. 507-8.

Dougherty, William J., "Epidemiology," *American Journal of Nursing,* LX, April, 1960, pp. 508-10.

Dubos, René J., "Infections into Disease," *Perspectives in Biology and Medicine,* I, Spring, 1958, pp. 425-35.

Edwards, J. H., "The Genetic Basis of Common Disease," *American Journal of Medicine,* XXXIV, May, 1963, pp. 627-38.

Evans, Alfred S., "Sneezes, Wheezes and Other Diseases," *GP,* XXIII, February, 1961, pp. 82-89.

Godfrey, Morey E., and Ian Maclean Smith, "Hospital Hazards of Staphylococcic Sepsis," *Journal of the American Medical Association,* CLXVI, March 8, 1958, pp. 1197-1201.

Harder, Helen I., and Margaret Panuska, "A Program to Control Staphylococcal Infections," *American Journal of Nursing,* LVIII, March, 1958, pp. 349-51.

Horne, R. W., "The Structure of Viruses," *Scientific American,* CCVIII, January, 1963, pp. 48-56.

Jacob, Francois, and Elie Wollman, "Viruses and Genes," *Scientific American,* CCIV, June, 1961, pp. 92-107.

Jones, Gordon W., "The Year Virginia Mourned," *Bulletin of the History of Medicine,* XXXV, May-June, 1961, pp. 257-65.

Kaitz, Alan L., and Elizabeth J. Williams, "Bacteriuria and Urinary Tract Infections in Hospitalized Patients," *New England Journal of Medicine,* CCLXII, March 3, 1960, pp. 425-30.

Kloetzel, Kurt, "Clinical Patterns in Severe Tetanus," *Journal of the American Medical Association,* CLXXXV, August 17, 1963, pp. 559-67.

Knox, R., "New Penicillins," *Guys' Hospital Reports,* CX, February, 1961, pp. 134-47.

Langmuir, Alexander D., "Ecologic and Epidemiologic Aspects of Staphylococcic Infections in Hospitals," *Journal of the American Medical Association,* CLXVI, March 8, 1958, pp. 1202-3.

Lentz, John William, *et al.,* "Venereal Disease Control in the Twentieth Century," *Nursing Outlook,* X, November, 1962, pp. 722-26.

Lester, Mary R., "Staphylococcal Infections," *American Journal of Nursing,* LIX, December, 1959, pp. 1805-28.

McDermott, Walsh, "Inapparent Infection," *Public Health Reports,* LXXIV, June, 1959, pp. 485-99.

Meyers, Mary E., "A Hospital Asepsis Committee," *American Journal of Nursing,* LIX, October, 1959, pp. 1432-33.

Minchew, B. Harvey, and Leighton E. Cluff, "Studies of the Epidemiology of Staphylococcal Infection in Hospitalized Patients," *Journal of Chronic Diseases,* XIII, April, 1961, pp. 354-73.

Mudd, S., "Practicability of Enhancing Specific Resistance to Staphylococcic Infection," *Journal of the American Medical Association,* CLXXIII, July 23, 1964, pp. 1360-61.

Nahmias, Andre, and Theodore C. Eichhoff, "Staphylococcal Infections in Hospitals; Recent Developments in Epidemiologic and Laboratory Investigations," *New England Journal of Medicine,* CCLXV, July 13, 1961, pp. 74-81 and, July 20, 1961, pp. 120-28.

Nelp, W. B., "Multiple Candida Abscesses Resulting from Insulin Injections," *New England Journal of Medicine,* CCLXVIII, March 21, 1963, pp. 664-65.

New York State Department of Health and the American Public Health Association, *Guide for the Prevention and Control of Infections in Hospitals,* Health Education Service, Albany, 1957.

Paul, John R., "Polio Virus Vaccines," *American Journal of Nursing,* LX, January, 1960, pp. 60-62.

Rakich, Jennie H., Margaret W. Thomas, and Mary Lester, "Nurses Are Asking About Staphylococcal Infections," *American Journal of Nursing,* LX, December, 1960, pp. 1766-69.

Riley, Richard L., "Airborne Infections," *American Journal of Nursing,* LX, September, 1960, pp. 1246-48.

Rose, Anthony H., "New Penicillins," *Scientific American,* CCIX, March, 1961, p. 66.

Spencer, Steven M., "The Hospitals Fight Their Toughest War," *Saturday Evening Post,* May 17, 1958, pp. 23-24, 107-11.

Thompson, La Verne, "Viruses—Old and New," *American Journal of Nursing,* LIX, March, 1959, pp. 349-51.

Waksman, Selman, "Antibiotics—20 Years Later," *Bulletin of the New York Academy of Medicine,* XXXVII, March, 1961, pp. 202-12.

Waksman, Selman A., "Role of Antibiotics in Nature," *Perspectives in Biology and Medicine,* IV, Spring, 1961, pp. 271-87.

Ward, Robert, and Saul Krugman, "Viral Hepatitis," *Disease-A-Month,* June, 1961, 524, (entire issue).

Wise, Robert I., "Principles of Management of Staphylococcic Infections," *Journal of the American Medical Association,* CLXVI, March 8, 1958, pp. 1178-82.

Wroblewski, Felix, "Enzymes in Medical Diagnosis," *Scientific American,* CCV, August, 1961, pp. 99-107.

5 : The Response of the Body to Injury

> As the essence of things must always remain unknown, we can learn only relations, and phenomena are merely the result of relations.
>
> Claude Bernard

Man has a remarkable capacity to respond to changes in his internal and external environment in such a manner that function is maintained within physiological (and psychological) limits. As long as disturbances do not threaten or exceed the adaptive capacity of the individual, energy is available for growth, for reproduction, and to alter conditions in his external environment. When, however, conditions in the environment are such that the survival of the organism is threatened, energy is utilized to escape from, or to overcome, the enemy or injuring agent and to make necessary repairs. Many of the manifestations commonly observed in the sick patient are the result of his response to injury. Many, though not all, authorities believe these responses are homeostatic. When they are effective, they prevent or limit injury to cells, repair damage induced by the injuring agent, and restore the organism to health. Similar to other homeostatic mechanisms, responses to injury may be excessive or deficient in degree or they may be inappropriate to the stimulus.

The stimulus that initiates one or more of the responses to injury may be actual damage to cell structure or a symbol or symbols that imply danger to the individual. To illustrate, fire, by raising the environmental temperature above that tolerated by the tissue, injures the tissue by burning it. Cells in the burned area are affected by the products released by injured or killed cells and respond in ways that are protective. The pain associated with even a small burn acts as a stimulus for responses involving the entire organism. When more than a limited area of tissue is burned, the individual can be expected to respond on all levels of organization, from the biochemical level to the highest integrative centers in the brain. Some of these same reactions can be elicited by a situation in which fire is perceived as being a source of danger to the individual. Seeing a flame where none should be elicits behavior similar to that in which actual burning has occurred. Even a fire siren may be a cause for alarm in an individual who has recently experienced a severe burn.

Many of the responses occurring during illness are to injury or danger, rather than to the specific agent. They are, therefore, nonspecific, rather than specific. Though there are modifying factors, the magnitude of reaction is usually in proportion to the extent of the danger or injury. There are, of course, patterns of response that can be attributed to particular etiological agents. Certain aspects of a nonspecific response may be modified by the nature of the causative agent. For example, during the prodromal stage of the acute infectious diseases of childhood, the child is ill, but the nature of his illness may be unclear for several days. Unless he develops a rash or some other feature of a specific disease, his illness will be attributed to a cold or a virus. The final outcome in any illness depends on two general factors: the nature and extent of the injury and the appropriateness of the response of the individual. These points will be further expanded in this chapter.

Some understanding of the physiological mechanisms by which the organism responds to injury is essential to nursing directed toward meeting the needs of patients. During the early stages of an acute illness or following a serious injury, the energy and resources of the patient are concentrated on survival. During this period, suitable objectives in the nursing of acutely ill patients include:

1. To prevent further injury.
2. To ascertain the degree and extent of injury as a basis for modifying the nursing care of the patient.
3. To support the patient and modify his environment and nursing care so that he can use his energy to recover (survive).
4. To observe the reactions of the patient so that his care can be altered as his needs change and, inasmuch as is possible, complications can be prevented.
5. To provide the patient with materials and services required during the various phases of illness.

Later, as the patient recovers, emphasis shifts from protecting the patient to increasing his activity so that he assumes more and more responsibility for his own needs.

Despite the emphasis to this point on the response of the organism after it is injured, it is also protected against injury. Many protective mechanisms are discussed in other chapters. Body structure and functions protect vital structures and prevent noxious agents from entering the body proper. Function is maintained within limits by a variety of regulatory mechanisms. The tissues are capable of responding to threats of injury, so that injury is prevented or damage is repaired. Through the use of his intellect, man evaluates and modifies his environment so that he protects himself against many potential dangers. Through the enactment and enforcement of laws, he regulates his own behavior and that of his fellows so that all are protected from disease and injury. Some of the factors that influence what and how he does this are discussed in Chapter 2.

*What are some of the ways the body is protected
against injury?*

Body structure is protective. Boney cages shelter vital organs such as the brain, heart, and lungs. The eye is recessed in the skull and is further guarded by the nose and the outward jutting of the brow. Injury great enough to disrupt the continuity of bones is almost always accompanied by some injury to underlying or surrounding structures.

Barriers against the entrance of foreign matter into the body include sensory receptors that are stimulated by conditions in the external environment; the intact skin and mucous membranes; mechanisms for conditioning air as it passes through the respiratory tract and for the removal of particles that do reach the alveoli; and mechanisms for the rejection of irritating substances from the gastrointestinal tract. The hydrogen ion concentration of secretions in the stomach, mouth, and vagina offers some protection against microorganisms. Since secretions by glands in these organs is stimulated by irritation, there is an increased volume of fluid to dilute and wash away noxious agents.

Reflexes such as coughing, sneezing, vomiting, dodging, and blinking initiate activities enabling the individual to remove or avoid harmful agents. Often protection involves a number of mechanisms. For example, a particle of dust gains access to the cornea of the eye where it stimulates sensitive nerve endings in the cornea. Exquisitely severe pain demands relief, and the person suffering it is prompted to initiate measures for the removal of the foreign body. Simultaneously the lacrimal glands are stimulated to secrete tears. They dilute the foreign material (when this is possible) and wash it away by flooding. Blinking of the eyelids distributes the tears over the eyeballs and tends to prevent the entrance of new particles. A person in whom the cornea and sclera are insensitive to pain or who cannot secrete tears lacks a primary defense mechanism. To prevent irreparable injury to the affected eye, this person must institute a regular schedule of procedures that substitute for the ones that have been lost. Since he does not suffer pain when a foreign body enters his eye, he must develop the habit of inspecting the sclera for redness several times a day. He should also consciously blink his eyes at regular intervals. He may have to bathe his eyes with saline solution. He should try to identify sources of injury and then utilize appropriate measures to protect himself against them. For example, on windy days or when there is the possibility of exposure to dust, he should wear goggle-type glasses.

The fact that all body structures have the capacity to respond to changes in the environment in ways that are protective and that they function between limits also aids in the prevention of injury. Since this is a concept that is emphasized throughout, it will not be further expanded here.

Despite protective structures and the capacity to respond to the environment so that injury is prevented, injury to cells does occur. When cells are injured, survival depends on the capacity of the organism to react in such a manner that the injury to cells is limited and any damage is repaired. As with other homeostatic mechanisms, there are limits to the capacity of any individual to respond to injury. The damage to the total organism or to a vital structure may be so great that death occurs within a matter of minutes. At the other end of the scale, because human beings are learning, remembering, and feeling organisms, they sometimes respond to symbols of danger when no real threat exists. Responses to imaginary dangers may be as incapacitating as responses to physical injury.

In injury or illness of a serious nature, not only the cells in and around the site of injury, but those throughout the entire organism participate in the response. Many of the manifestations observed in illness arise from the local and general reactions of the organism to cell damage. They are initiated by a noxious agent that is sufficiently potent to cause direct injury to cells or to alert the mental apparatus to the possibility of serious danger.

What is the ultimate goal of the homeostatic responses to injury?

As stated earlier, the ultimate goal of the homeostatic responses of the individual to injury or to dangers perceived as sources of injury is survival. The attainment of this goal involves escaping from, or overcoming, noxious agents and repairing disturbances or damage that results. At the time the individual is threatened with, or suffers, severe injury or illness, a whole series of integrated reactions are initiated involving the neuromuscular, neuroendocrine, circulatory, respiratory, and reticuloendothelial systems. Structures and functions that are not immediately useful to survival are suppressed. The significance of the above to nursing will be indicated as the various responses are discussed.

Although a causative agent may alter in some ways the character of a particular response, the essential features of responses to injury are the same for all agents. In other words, the organism has stereotyped ways of behaving when injured or threatened with injury. They are for the most part nonspecific. There are, however, some mechanisms such as antibody formation that are specific. Although a given antibody is specific for a particular microorganism or its toxin, the process by which it is formed is automatic, and the body can respond to a variety of foreign substances by forming antibodies. Like other homeostatic mechanisms, responses to injury or danger are self-limiting; that is, they are terminated when the disturbance initiating them has been corrected. They, too, may fail as the response may be excessive, deficient, or inappropriate to the kind or amount of injury. When any of the above occurs, the response itself may be a source of injury.

What are some of the factors influencing the magnitude of an individual's response to injury?

In general, the magnitude of a response to injury varies with the extent of the injury. Some agents inflict more damage and provoke a greater reaction than others, and injuries to certain body structures are accompanied by a greater response than are others. The characteristics of the person who is ill also influence his response. Persons who are at the extremes of age usually respond less vigorously than do children and young adults. The response of persons in middle life is not as vigorous as that of young adults, but it is greater than that of the elderly. There are, of course, exceptions. Mrs. Malone, aged 96, is one. She recently experienced and recovered from pneumonia. At the height of her illness, she had a fever of 102° F. It is not uncommon for persons of advanced age to have little or no elevation in temperature in disorders commonly causing fever in younger persons. Males usually respond more vigorously than females, but the fact that vigorous young men respond actively does not mean that they have a higher recovery rate from serious illness than women do. In fact, there is some evidence that the reverse is true.[1] As might be expected, the well-nourished react more actively than the poorly nourished, and vigorous, healthy persons more than debilitated or sickly ones. In general, the vigor of homeostatic responses to illness or injury is greater in those with a good adaptive capacity and less in those whose adaptive capacity is deficient.

How does the ability of man to alter his position in space create problems during illness?

One of the primary and earliest responses to threat of, or actual injury is the alteration of position in space. There are, obviously, many other types of stimuli that result in movement. At the very minimum, this response depends on a receptor connected by nerve cells and fibers to an effector. Receptors contain cells that are sensitive to changes in the internal or external environment. The retina of the eye contains receptor cells that are sensitive to light. Effector cells are capable of some overt activity. They are of two general types, muscle and gland cells. Between the receptor and effector cells are efferent (sensory) nerve fibers that convey messages from the receptor cells to centers, groups of cells, in the spinal cord and brain where "decisions" are made. (See Chapter 13, Part B.) From the centers, messages are sent by way of efferent pathways to a few or to many effector cells. Alteration of position in space requires not only intact neuromuscular units, but an adequate skeletal system. Joints must be functional so that areas of the body can be moved, and the bones must be sufficiently rigid to be moved by the muscles.

Response to danger or to injury by alteration of position in space may be manifested in one or more of three ways. One is to flee or run away. A second is to remain and fight the enemy. A third is to become immobile or freeze, by contracting opposing sets of muscles. Each type of reaction is appropriate in different situations. On awakening, Mr. Allen notes that his apartment is on

[1] Robert Elman, *Surgical Care,* Appleton-Century-Crofts, Inc., New York, 1951, pp. 27-29.

fire and that the blaze is sufficiently large that fighting it is out of the question; to try is to court disaster. Immobility is even more inappropriate. To flee as quickly as possible is the only reasonable course of action. Under other circumstances, such as in the presence of a lion or a poisonous reptile, immobility is the only response likely to be successful.

Frequently the manner in which the individual reacts is entirely automatic. Sometimes a person is able to control the impulse to act and to make a conscious decision as to the most appropriate course of action. An illustration of more or less automatic behavior occurred when Mr. Allen, who had taken his son John with him as he left his burning apartment, found that John had returned to the apartment to get his clothing. Although Mr. Allen had to go through flames, he returned to the apartment. Despite suffering painful burns, he was able to rescue his son and to protect him from the fire. He had no recollection of his actions or of what had happened to him. Had his reaction not been more or less automatic, he probably would not have been able to save his son.

An illustration of a situation in which a young woman was able to increase her chances of survival was recently reported in the newspaper. This young woman was trapped in a walk-in freezer. Despite feelings of panic, she remembered having heard someone say freezing could be delayed by continued movement. In order to maintain her self-control and to keep herself moving, she concentrated on counting the cans of food stored in the refrigerator. Fortunately, her mother missed her before she suffered serious injury. She survived because she was able to act intelligently and therefore to modify her behavior and to utilize her resources constructively. One factor that was very helpful to her was the certainty that her mother would miss her soon enough so that she would be rescued in time.

Despite the value of "flight, fight, and freeze" to the past survival of the human species, the number of situations in which it now serves a useful purpose is quite limited. In fact, fight and flight are both modes of behavior that are disapproved of in the American culture. Persons who fight in public are censured or jailed for disturbing the peace. Those who openly flee are called cowards. This leaves only one mode of behavior, that is, immobility brought about by the contraction of opposing sets of muscles in circumstances eliciting a fight-or-flight response. Some persons actually are in a state of more or less constant muscular contraction. They behave as if they are in a constant state of danger. Persons who have a large number of muscles contracted are likely to appear tense or strained. In some persons, contraction may be limited to a group of muscles such as those of the back or neck. Sustained muscular contraction, even in the absence of motion, requires the expenditure of energy, and it results in fatigue and muscular pain. In some instances, it may predispose to disease.

In illness, sustained muscular contraction is a not uncommon source of suffering. Headache is one of the most common complaints of people who are ill. One of the factors in its development may be spasm of the head and neck muscles. Backache is another frequent discomfort. It results from sustained contraction of back muscles. Many other aches and pains of illness result from the effects of muscle tension. In a number of diseases, and following injury, a characteristic feature is increased muscular tension or even muscular spasm. For example, the person whose thyroid hypersecretes is in a continuous state of increased muscular tension. A small sudden noise initiates a startle reflex out of proportion to the stimulus. Disorders in which muscle spasm is a factor in pain include: acute poliomyelitis, fractures, rheumatoid arthritis, peritonitis, biliary or renal colic, and menstrual cramps.

What measures are employed in the prevention and treatment of increased muscular tension?

Measures used in prevention and treatment of muscular tension vary. They are usually directed toward one or more of the following objectives: (1) to lessen the degree of muscular spasm; (2) to relieve the pain; and (3) to remove the cause. Measures that relieve muscle spasm are likely to relieve the pain associated with it. For example, the application of moist or dry heat over an area of a painful muscle is a well-known practice in folk medicine. In acute poliomyelitis, muscle spasm and pain may be relieved by the application of moist heat. In rheumatoid arthritis, use of salicylates with or without the application of heat will often afford relief. Diathermy is also employed to relieve pain by the application of heat. (See Chapter 3 for explanation.) Under some circumstances, muscle spasm can be relieved by the application of traction, that is, by the application of a force opposing muscle contraction. After a period of time the muscle becomes fatigued and relaxes. As an example, traction is frequently employed in the treatment of fractures (broken bones) in which the ends of the bones are displaced. Traction may be applied to lessen muscle spasm by fatiguing the muscle. As the muscle relaxes, the two ends of the bone return to their normal position with the two parts of the bone in normal alignment and the ends of the bone just touching each other. Should the traction be removed, the muscles again contract and displace the fracture. When traction is utilized in the treatment of a fracture, everyone, including the patient and members of his family, should understand why it must be continuously applied. They should also know what conditions must be met for it to be effective. Under no circumstances should it be removed or lessened without a prescription of the physician. Traction may also be prescribed in the treatment of muscle spasm associated with pressure on nerve roots. For example, it is used to relax the muscles of the back in low-back pain or to relax the muscles of the neck when pain is due to pressure on nerves supplying the spastic muscles. When a patient is placed in traction, the nurse should know why the traction is applied and whether it may or may not be released.[2]

[2] See the References for descriptions of the types and methods of applying traction.

When pain results from the spasm of muscles in ducts or tubular structures such as a ureter or the common bile duct, an analgesic or muscle-relaxing drug may be required to relieve the pain. Thus morphine or one of its substitutes with or without a smooth-muscle relaxant such as papaverine is usually administered to relieve the pain.

Because muscle tension frequently accompanies illness and its treatment, the nurse should develop the habit of looking for evidence indicating its presence as well as for conditions that predispose to its development. She should also develop skill in the performance of nursing measures that prevent and/or relieve muscle tension. Most of these are not difficult to perform and require little complicated equipment. They do require a conviction on the part of the nurse that they are important to the welfare of the patient. One of the most important aspects is attention to the position and body alignment of the patient, not only when he is in bed, but when he is up and about and sitting in a chair. Weak and flaccid muscles should be supported and protected from overstretching. When supports are required, they should support, rather than be held in place by, the patient. They should extend along the length of the part and they should be adjusted so that strain is not placed on another structure. For example, when a sling is applied to support an arm, it should extend the entire length of the forearm. It is not enough to support the arm at the wrist.

One of the most frequent causes of discomfort in the patient confined to bed is back pain. It can often be prevented by use of a firm mattress or by the simple procedure of placing a board under the mattress. Frequent changes in position also aid in the prevention of prolonged strain on back and other muscles. When a patient is required to lie on his back more or less continuously, a support under the lumbar curve of the back may prevent stretching of back muscles. A properly placed footboard and a cradle to prevent bed covering from weighing on weakened extremities are other measures that may be utilized to protect muscles from spasm or overstretching.

No matter how comfortable a position is at the start, it becomes less so as time elapses. There should therefore be a regular schedule for changing the position of weak and helpless patients. At the time their position is changed, the arms and legs should be put through the normal range of motion. Exercise not only promotes muscular relaxation by relieving strain on muscles used by the patient to maintain his position, but it acts as a stimulus to relaxation. A well-given back rub will further contribute to muscular relaxation. Any attention to the comfort of the patient should facilitate relaxation. It is difficult to relax when one has to look at a bright light, listen to a leaking faucet, or be too cold or too warm, and not be able to correct the situation. The nurse should be alert to possible sources of irritation and take appropriate steps to prevent or eliminate them from the environment of the patient. Since the psychological and social climate of the patient has an effect on his physiological status, these too may be the source of muscular tension. At this point, Florence Nightingale's injunction is appropriate.[3]

"Apprehension, uncertainty, waiting, expectation, fear of surprise, do a patient more harm than any exertion. Remember, he is face to face with his enemy all the time, internally wrestling with him, having long imaginary conversations with him. You are thinking of something else. 'Rid him of his adversary quickly,' is a first rule with the sick." There are many sources of muscular tension in the course of an illness, and no effort will be made to enumerate them all. The nurse should develop the habit of looking for evidence of it. When a patient looks relaxed and comfortable, he probably is. When he appears to be tense or in poor position, he is likely to be uncomfortable. The nurse should also be alert to conditions in the environment of the patient—physical, psychological, or social—that are likely to induce tension. She should then act to correct them.

The following illustrations represent two relatively common nursing problems whose solutions are not very complicated. The first is the case of Mr. Allen, who was introduced earlier. For the first two or three days after he was burned he paid little attention to his surroundings and showed no concern for anyone but himself. About the third day, he began to ask about his son John, whom he had removed from his apartment at the time of the fire. Despite everyone's effort to reassure him that John was not badly injured and would soon be discharged from the hospital, he was obviously worried. Arrangements were, therefore, made for John to visit him. When he saw that John's burns were really of a minor nature, he was much relieved. This one visit did what verbal reassurance could not do; it convinced Mr. Allen that John was alive and would completely recover from his injury.

About a week or ten days after Mr. Allen was burned, skin grafts were applied to his upper arms and neck, and he was instructed to lie still for three days as any movement might disrupt the contact between the skin graft and the underlying tissue. Since Mr. Allen understood and accepted the importance of remaining immobile to the success of skin grafting, he concentrated on lying quietly. Although he maintained the desired position, he experienced considerable muscular tension. Since the nurse knew that Mr. Allen would be expected to lie in the same position for three days, she checked his mattress to be sure that it was firm and provided adequate support for him. To encourage Mr. Allen to relax, his back was rubbed at two-hour intervals by inserting a hand between the mattress and the lumbar region of his back, and he was assisted in performing leg exercises. He was encouraged to wiggle his toes and to flex and extend his foot at the ankle. The nurse made a real effort to anticipate his needs and to visit him frequently. Since he was in a large ward, she encouraged ambulatory patients to stop briefly to see if he needed anything. As is frequently true when the arms are immobilized, one of his greatest sources of discomfort was an itching nose. When the nurse observed

[3] Florence Nightingale, *Notes on Nursing*, New Edition, Harrison, London, 1860.

him wiggling his nose, she offered to scratch it for him. During the period immediately following skin grafting, the objective given precedence in Mr. Allen's nursing care was to minimize the sources of physiological and psychological stress so that he could use his energy for recovery. His environment and nursing care were planned to meet this objective. Even so, he experienced more or less discomfort. Despite the inability of the nurse to eliminate all of Mr. Allen's discomforts, she was able to minimize them and to make the experience more tolerable.

The second patient is Mrs. Carney, who had a radical amputation of the left breast. Her left arm was to be elevated in order to prevent swelling of the hand and arm. To prevent swelling, the positioning of the arm must be based on the fact that water runs downhill. Therefore, distal parts should be higher than proximal parts. In terms of the particular structures the hand should be higher than the elbow and the elbow higher than the shoulder. Unnecessary muscle tension can and should be prevented by arranging and balancing supporting apparatus, including pillows, so that it supports Mrs. Carney's arm. Briefly stated, supports should support.

The capacity to alter his position in space has been one of the significant factors in the survival of man. It has enabled him to overcome danger, to find or produce food, to find a mate, and to alter his environment so that it is better suited to his needs. In illness, the neuromuscular system reacts to the implied as well as to the real injury. Inasmuch as this response is appropriate, it contributes to survival. Even when muscle tension is appropriate, it adds to the fatigue and pain of illness. When the response is inappropriate or excessive, it increases the suffering of the patient, and it may be a factor in the development of undesired complications or sequelae.

Summary

The nurse can help to lessen the severity of the neuromuscular response and its attendant discomforts by:

1. Removing noxious stimuli from the external environment that the patient, if able, would eliminate or remove himself. Some examples include: bright lights, loud or sudden noises, overheated or underheated surroundings, inadequate ventilation, dripping faucets, blaring radio or television sets, overtalkative people, untidy surroundings.
2. Giving attention to the position of the patient, changing his position regularly.
3. Providing for a comfortable bed.
4. Relieving muscle tension by putting extremities through the normal range of motion and rubbing the back.
5. Performing therapeutic procedures to relieve muscular spasm such as warm, moist packs, administering prescribed pain-relieving medications, and supervising traction.

6. Identifying the implications that the illness has to the patient and the use of appropriate resources to relieve him. Preparing the patient for what to expect and what is expected of him.
7. Modifying care of the patient in relation to the severity, extent, and phase of his illness. This implies accepting him and his behavior.

The seriously ill patient who is fighting for his life should not be required to make decisions or to be responsible for meeting his own needs. The patient is allowed and encouraged to be sick. He should be bathed, moved, turned, and assisted out of bed as his condition demands. He should be held responsible neither for deciding when he requires care nor for carrying it out. When the nurse gives care she should, of course, exercise judgment about its timing. When caring for a very ill patient, his welfare may demand that certain aspects of care be omitted or be given at a particular time. With some sick patients the nurse may have to say firmly and kindly, "I have come to give you a bath. You look miserable and the bath will help you to feel better," or "It is time for you to be turned to your other side or to get up." As the patient recovers, responsibility is shifted to him as he is able to assume it.

Disease, surgical therapy, and other forms of injury elicit both systemic and local responses. A knowledge of the nature and effects of the response to injury is basic to adapting the supportive treatment to the needs of the patient. Unless the nature of the various responses of the body is understood, the care provided for the patient may interfere with, rather than promote, his recovery.

The various types of systemic and local responses or reactions to injury are outlined below.

1. Systemic responses.
    1.1 Neuroendocrine responses
        1.11 Sympathoadrenal
        1.12 Pituitary—adrenal axis (anterior pituitary—adrenal cortex)
        1.13 Posterior pituitary
        1.14 Other glands secreting hormones
            1.141 Thyroid
            1.142 Gonads
            1.143 Islands of Langerhans
    1.2 Antibody formation
    1.3 Fever
    1.4 Leukocytosis
2. Local tissue responses at site of injury.
    2.1 Inflammation
    2.2 Phagocytosis
    2.3 Proliferation of cells
        2.31 Hyperplasia
        2.32 Wound healing

As has been repeatedly emphasized, man reacts as a whole to his environment. Any threat to his survival can be expected, therefore, to initiate changes in the activity of his neuroendocrine system that alert him to danger. It also alters his visceral and metabolic processes in such a manner that energy is made available for fight or flight and materials are supplied to repair injured tissues.

What is the role of the sympathoadrenal medullary system in response to injury?

The following generalization provides a framework for predicting the types of changes that occur as a result of the response of the sympathoadrenal medullary system to injury. Functions that are of little or no immediate value to survival are suppressed, and those facilitating escape from, or overcoming, the enemy and providing materials for repair of damaged tissues are augmented. Although understanding of the responses of the total organism to injury has been greatly extended since Cannon first published his flight-fight theory, much of the recent work is an extension rather than a replacement of this theory. According to Cannon, the automatic responses of an individual who is facing or who has undergone injury prepared him for flight or fight. These responses are under the control of the sympathoadrenal system. Stated briefly, when survival of the organism is threatened, the sympathoadrenal system takes over, and the function of the parasympathetic division of the autonomic nervous system is inhibited.[4] Since both the parasympathetic and sympathetic divisions of the autonomic nervous system are represented in the hypothalamus, they are believed to be regulated by it. Inasmuch as the hypothalamus is interconnected with other centers including higher centers in the nervous system, the autonomic nervous system is integrated into the total nervous system. Consequently the autonomic nervous system can be activated by events in the external as well as in the internal environment.

In general, the sympathoadrenal and parasympathetic nervous systems have opposing effects on automatic or visceral functioning. The sympathoadrenal system supports those functions that are essential to meeting emergency situations and depresses those that are not immediately useful. Thus it increases the rate and output of the heart, elevates the blood pressure, and suppresses the action of the alimentary canal and lessens the contraction of the urinary bladder. Stimulation of the sympathetic nervous system also causes sweating. The innervation of sweat glands is somewhat peculiar. Though anatomically they are part of the sympathetic nervous system, they are cholinergic; that is, the chemical mediator for the postganglionic fibers supplying sweat glands is acetylcholine. Depending on their orientation, some authorities classify the nerve supply to the sweat glands as parasympathetic, while others consider them to be under the control of the sympathetic nervous system.

---

[4] Because of the role of the autonomic nervous system in the regulation of all visceral functions, it will be referred to many times.

Some of the effects of activation of the two divisions of the autonomic nervous system are summarized below:

Selected Actions Resulting from Activation of the Sympathetic and Parasympathetic Divisions of the Autonomic Nervous System

Site of Effector Cells	Activation of Sympathetic Division (Thoracolumbar) Tends to	Activation of Parasympathetic Division (Craniosacral) Tends to
Heart	Increase rate and output	Decrease rate and output
Coronary arteries	Dilate	
Blood vessels in nose, salivary glands, and pharynx	Constrict	Dilate
Cutaneous vessels	Constrict	
Bronchi	Dilate	Constrict
Gastrointestinal motility and secretion	Decrease (decreased peristalsis and muscle tone) Constrict sphincters	Increase Relax sphincters
Glycogenolysis by liver	Increase	
Glands	Decrease secretion	Increase secretion
Sweat glands	Increase (some authorities classify this as a parasympathetic function)	
Pupil of eye	Dilate	Constrict
Ciliary muscles	Lessen tone. Eyes accommodated to see at a distance	Contract ciliary muscles. Eyes accommodated to see near objects
Mental activity	Increase	

One effect of increased sympathoadrenal activity deserving emphasis is that the seriously ill or injured patient is frequently unusually alert. Furthermore, this effect may be overlooked in planning and effecting nursing care. Whereas a high degree of alertness is protective in a hostile environment, it may be an unnecessary source of stress to the patient who is under professional care. In fact, the climate surrounding the patient ought to be such that the patient can trust others to be responsible for his care. Conversations in the vicinity of the patient should take into account the possibility that the patient may be overly alert. Nothing should be said that is likely to increase the anxiety of the patient. A useful rule is not to talk in the presence of the patient without including him in the conversation. (See Chapter 6.) Furthermore, noise, jarring, and other forms of unnecessary stimulation should be avoided, as the patient is likely to be unusually sensitive to them.

In addition to usually having opposing effects, there are other differences in the manner in which the sympathetic and parasympathetic systems respond to stimulation. The sympathoadrenal system tends to act as a unit, whereas stimulation of one part of the parasympathetic nervous system does not involve all of the organs innervated by the parasympathetic division. Anatomical differences help to account for differences in the way the parasympathetic and sympathetic nervous systems respond.

The parasympathetic nervous system consists of the third, seventh, ninth, and tenth cranial nerves and branches of the second, third, and fourth sacral nerves. There are no interconnections among the fibers forming these nerves. In the parasympathetic system, the ganglia lie in, or very close to, the organ that they stimulate with the result that preganglionic fibers are long and postganglionic fibers are very short. There are very few connections among ganglia. (See Figure 5-1.)

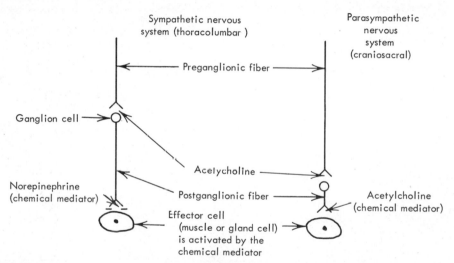

FIGURE 5—1. Peripheral structure of the sympathetic and parasympathetic divisions of the autonomic nervous system.

The preganglionic fibers of the sympathoadrenal system originate from cells in the thoracolumbar portions of the spinal cord. The preganglionic fibers synapse in ganglia (groups of cells) lying peripheral to the spinal cord. Depending on their location, these ganglia are known as vertebral, collateral, or terminal. The location of the various ganglia can be seen in the accompanying diagram.

In the diagram the reader will also note that preganglionic fibers of the sympathoadrenal system branch widely and provide pathways for the communication of messages to the variously located ganglia. Preganglionic fibers branch in the vertebral ganglia. Some of the branches synapse with ganglionic cells, while others pass through the ganglia to higher or lower vertebral ganglia or to collateral ganglia; that is, preganglionic fibers branch and

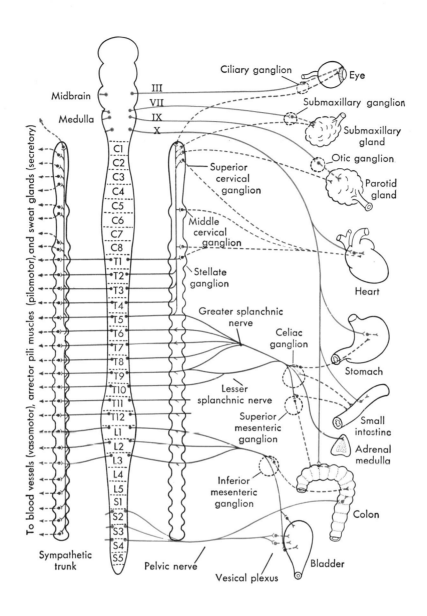

Ciliary ganglion — Eye

Midbrain

III
VII
IX
X

Medulla

Submaxillary ganglion

Submaxillary gland

Otic ganglion

Parotid gland

To blood vessels (vasomotor), arrector pili muscles (pilomotor), and sweat glands (secretory)

C1
C2
C3
C4
C5
C6
C7
C8
T1
T2
T3
T4
T5
T6
T7
T8
T9
T10
T11
T12
L1
L2
L3
L4
L5
S1
S2
S3
S4
S5

Superior cervical ganglion

Middle cervical ganglion

Stellate ganglion

Greater splanchnic nerve

Celiac ganglion

Lesser splanchnic nerve

Superior mesenteric ganglion

Inferior mesenteric ganglion

Heart

Stomach

Small intestine

Adrenal medulla

Colon

Sympathetic trunk

Pelvic nerve

Vesical plexus

Bladder

synapse with cells in more than one ganglion. Preganglionic fibers are generally relatively short and postganglionic fibers are long. One exception is the fibers supplying the adrenal medulla. The adrenal medulla is similar to peripheral sympathetic ganglia as it is supplied with preganglionic fibers.

Another relationship exists between the sympathetic nervous system and the adrenal medulla. The chemical mediator between the sympathetic postganglionic fiber and the effector cell—muscle or gland—is norepinephrine. Norepinephrine, as well as epinephrine, is secreted by the adrenal medulla. Both these chemicals augment and prolong the action of the sympathetic nervous system.

The activity of the sympathoadrenal system can be expected to be increased in any patient who suffers an injury or illness threatening his survival. Major surgery, severe burns, overwhelming infection, frightening sounds or sights, myocardial infarction, pain, and many other conditions stimulate the activity of the sympathetic nervous system. Most, if not all, persons have experienced symptoms resulting from stimulation of the sympathetic nervous system. Mr. Brave (bleeding peptic ulcer), Mr. Allen (burned), Mrs. Carney (amputation of breast)—all had symptoms and signs indicating stimulation of the sympathetic nervous system. Both Mr. Brave and Mrs. Carney perspired profusely. All these patients had an increase in pulse rate. Mr. Brave complained that his heart pounded (palpitation). All breathed at a rapid rate. Though both Mr. Brave and Mrs. Carney lost blood, neither had an appreciable drop in blood pressure. Despite a loss of considerable volume of fluid into the burned area, and possibly in other tissue, Mr. Allen's blood pressure was maintained within normal limits. All three patients had some depression in gastrointestinal activity. In Mrs. Carney, diminished gastrointestinal activity was of short duration. Mr. Allen, in common with other patients who are seriously burned, was predisposed to acute gastric dilitation. Consequently oral fluids were withheld for two days. When oral fluids were first prescribed, he was given 30 ml per hour for four hours. Since he did not complain of feelings of fullness, or of nausea, he was rapidly promoted to a full fluid and food intake.

Some degree of hyperglycemia may result from increased sympathoadrenal activity. On the third day after Mr. Allen was burned, his fasting blood sugar was 180 mg per 100 ml of blood. Since he was not known to have diabetes mellitus and his blood glucose returned to physiological limits after a few days, the elevation probably indicated an increase in the release of glucose from glycogen by the liver. Other factors, including increased secretion of glucocorticoids by the adrenal cortex, may have contributed to the increase in the level of the blood glucose.

Mr. Brave had some evidence of so-called paralytic ileus. His abdomen was distended and silent (absence of peristalsis). To prevent overdistention of his stomach, his physician prescribed nasogastric suction until peristaltic activity was re-established. On admission to the hospital, Mr. Brave was cold to the touch and he was pale; he appeared to be alert and anxious. These manifestations can all be ascribed to increased sympathoadrenal activity. Probably most patients have some increase in activity of the sympathoadrenal system at some stage of their illness. Even when illness is relatively minor, uncertainty about its cause or outcome may be a sufficiently potent stimulus to bring this about. When diagnostic or therapeutic procedures are perceived as indicating the possibility of a serious disease, or inducing pain, the likelihood of sympathoadrenal stimulation is further increased.

When a patient exhibits signs and symptoms indicative of increased sympathoadrenal activity, the nurse should seek answers to the following questions. Do the manifestations presented by the patient indicate that his illness is becoming more severe or that he is developing a complication? Are they the result of some physical or emotional stress associated with his illness or his personal life? Is there something in the environment of the patient that probably explains their presence? Has the patient undergone, what is for him, an unusual degree of activity? Are the symptoms and signs transitory or do they persist? As an illustration, suppose that Mr. Brave has an increase in his pulse and respiratory rate. Since he has a history of hemorrhage, he may be bleeding. Depending on other circumstances the nurse will investigate for additional evidence that he is bleeding or will modify his care in some way. Perhaps a visitor has stayed too long or Mr. Brave is anxious because his wife, whom he expected at 2, has not arrived by 5 o'clock. If Mr. Brave is out of bed for the first time after several days of bed rest, the nurse will assist him to bed. She may then allow him to rest for a short period of time and then recheck his pulse and respiration. If indicated, she will take his blood pressure. Whatever the stimulus is, Mr. Brave is responding to it by increasing his circulatory and respiratory rates. Appropriate action on the part of the nurse depends on taking into consideration the possible causes and acting in light of the one or ones that appear most reasonable.

What types of nursing activities contribute to reducing the intensity of the sympathoadrenal response to injury?

Care planned to reduce the activity of the sympathoadrenal system should be based on two factors. One is that, within limits, physical activity tends to lessen the degree of activity of the sympathoadrenal system, and the other is that implied or imagined threats can act as stimuli initiating or augmenting its action.

Much of the nursing care given to relieve muscle tension will also tend to minimize sympathoadrenal activity. Care that increases the comfort of the patient promotes muscle relaxation. Within limits, physical activity has a similar effect. One of the values of early ambulation is that it decreases the intensity of the sympathoadrenal response. Patients whose condition allows them to get out of bed and to walk soon after injury or major surgical procedures usually have less pain and an earlier return of gastrointestinal activity than do those who are confined to bed for longer periods of time.

Not only does the sympathoadrenal system participate in the response of the individual to present and actual dangers to his survival, but it is activated by fear or anxiety initiated by implied or imagined threats to his well-being. When the nurse is successful in developing a trusting relationship with the patient, she can lessen the opportunities for him to imagine or magnify dangers in the situation. (See Chapter 6.)

What effect does removal or inactivation of the sympathetic nervous system have on the requirements of the patient for nursing?

Sympathectomy by surgical or chemical means is employed in the therapy of diseases of blood vessels in which vascular spasm is believed to be a factor. It is most commonly used in the treatment of essential hypertension, severe Raynaud's disease, and occlusive arterial disease involving the extremities. In surgical sympathectomy, a few to many pre- or postganglionic fibers of vertebral sympathetic ganglia are interrupted and a section of the fiber is removed. The number and location of the fibers to be excised depends on the disorder under treatment. Preganglionic fibers to collateral or terminal sympathetic ganglia may also be interrupted. In splanchnicectomy the preganglionic fibers to the celiac ganglia, the superior and inferior mesenteric plexuses, may be severed and removed. Instead of surgical interruption and excision of sympathetic fibers, a similar effect may be obtained by chemical means. There are a number of drugs that inactivate the autonomic nervous system by blocking the transmission of impulses through autonomic ganglia (ganglionic blocking agents). The most frequent use of these drugs is in the treatment of essential hypertension. These drugs act by reducing the number of impulses reaching blood vessels and thereby reducing vascular tone and blood pressure. One undesirable effect of extensive surgical and chemical sympathectomy is that they limit the capacity to adapt the diameter of the blood vessels to changes in position. Blood pressure falls when the affected person assumes the upright position after having been in the recumbent position. The patient should therefore be instructed to assume the upright position slowly. When postural hypotension is severe, excessive pooling of blood in the legs may be prevented by wrapping them from instep to groin with elastic bandages.

When the dosage of ganglionic blocking agent is large, transmission through parasympathetic ganglia may also be blocked and be responsible for a number of annoying effects. Some of these effects are due to a lessening of peristalsis, which predisposes to fecal impaction, as well as to considerable abdominal discomfort and distention. A minor, though, in some patients, a troublesome, effect of the action of ganglionic blocking agents is dilatation of the pupil of the eye. Inability to constrict the pupil renders reading difficult, if not impossible, as the print tends to blur when the affected person tries to read. Although the sympathetic nervous system is not essential to life, inactivation of it results in some lessening in the capacity of the individual to adapt to changes in his environment.

Summary

One of the factors in the survival of man has been his capacity to respond to threats of, or actual, injury by attacking or removing himself from danger. Many of the processes involved in these responses are under the control of the sympathoadrenal system. Since the sympathoadrenal system can be activated by any change in the external or internal environment that is perceived to be a threat to survival, most serious illnesses are accompanied by increased sympathoadrenal activity. Trauma, including surgical therapy, is, of course, a stimulus to increased sympathoadrenal activity. The effect on the patient is a decrease in those activities not immediately essential to survival and an increase in those that are. Thus the individual is more alert, his pupils are dilated, and he has increased muscle tension as well as an increase in heart and respiratory rate, increased sweating, and a rise in blood sugar. Activities not immediately essential to his survival are depressed. Thus the alimentary canal is less active or may be temporarily paralyzed. Many of the discomforts and problems accompanying illness are due to alterations in the activity of the autonomic nervous system. They should therefore be anticipated and dealt with by appropriate measures.

What are the metabolic responses to injury? What factors appear to be responsible for them?

In addition to muscular and visceral responses in illness that are largely regulated by the nervous system, there are also metabolic reactions to tissue injury. Though not all of the factors regulating the metabolic response have been identified, several are known to play a definite or a permissive role. Even in these responses, the nervous system may participate in their initiation and regulation. Whereas muscular and visceral responses enable the organism to fight or flee his enemy, the metabolic responses provide materials to repair the damage suffered by the tissues. Authorities disagree as to whether these changes are adaptive or maladaptive. Though knowledge is increasing about the regulation of the metabolic changes occurring during illness, it is still incomplete.

What is the role of the thyroid hormone in the metabolic response to injury?

Although thyroid hormone is essential to health, there is little evidence that it plays a special role in response to illness or injury. According to Hardy,[5] the

5 James D. Hardy, *Pathophysiology in Surgery,* The Williams & Wilkins Company, Baltimore, 1958, p. 14.

hypothesis that the activity of the thyroid gland is increased following injury is reasonable. However, experimental evidence to support this hypothesis is lacking. Some of the metabolic changes occurring following injury could be explained by an increase in thyroxin.

What is the effect of injury on the secretion of the gonads?

Following a serious injury the activity of the gonads may be depressed. Some, but not all, women miss one or more menstrual periods following surgery.

What is the role of the neurohypophysis (posterior pituitary) in the response to injury?

The posterior hypophysis appears to play a role in reactions to injury. Unlike the anterior hypophysis, it has neural connections with the hypothalamus. Consequently stimuli activating the autonomic nervous system may result in increased secretion and release of the antidiuretic hormone. Most patients undergoing major surgery or experiencing major trauma or serious burns do have some degree of water retention in the immediate postoperative or postinjury period. Urine that is eliminated tends to be concentrated. Depending on the severity of the injury and other factors, the patient undergoes a period of spontaneous diuresis approximately 6 to 24 hours after injury or surgery. Retention of water by the kidney can be explained by an increase in the secretion and release of the antidiuretic hormone. This response enables the body to protect its blood volume despite the loss of blood and other fluids. Since the advent of intravenous infusions, it also predisposes to pulmonary edema and to overloading the circulation unless care is taken to balance intake with output. (See Chapter 8.)

What is the role of the adrenal cortical hormones in the metabolic response to injury?

Despite knowledge that the adrenal cortical hormones are required for survival, definite knowledge of their mechanisms of action is lacking. It has been known for some years that patients with adrenal cortical insufficiency are unable to cope successfully with even mild stress.Though the adrenal gland has been known to be essential to life for more than 100 years, it was not until the 1920's that scientists agreed that the cortex rather than the medulla was the essential structure. It is also known that when these persons are adequately treated with adrenal cortical hormones they react to injury as well as and in the same manner as persons who secrete theirs naturally. Following injury, many persons can be shown to have an increase in secretion of adrenal cortical hormones. Because of this observation, some authorities suggest that the action of adrenal cortical hormones is permissive; that is, they are required for certain reactions to occur, but do not themselves cause the reaction. Other authorities suggest that this observation may result from the more efficient use of the adrenal cortical hormones. Evidence favoring the causative in distinction to the supporting role of the adrenal cortical hormones is that some of the metabolic changes occurring following injury can be induced by the administration of large dosages of the adrenal cortical hormones. Whatever future studies reveal, there is no doubt that the adrenal cortical hormones are essential to the maintenance of homeostasis and to survival following injury. The actions of the adrenal cortical hormones are described in detail in Chapter 13, Part A.

Despite a lack of definitive knowledge of the mechanisms by which the adrenal cortical hormones act in regulating the response to stress, some hypotheses have been suggested. One of the most widely known has been proposed by Hans Selye. He suggests that the anterior pituitary-adrenal cortical hormones play a primary role in the response to injury. He has written voluminously for both scientists and the lay public.[6]

Explain Selye's theory of how the body responds to injury.

Selye's theory of how the body responds to injury is highly elaborate. Essentially, however, he proposes that the responses of the tissues during injury are the result of the reaction of sensitive tissues to an increase in secretions of the adrenal-pituitary axis. Much of the data on which this theory is based have been obtained by subjecting rats to varying types of physical, chemical, and psychological injury. From these studies, he postulated that no matter what agent was used to cause injury, certain nonspecific stereotyped reactions occur in the stressed organism. Like Cannon,[7] he believes that homeostatic responses may cause disturbances in the internal environment. Selye also postulates that certain diseases may result from prolonged overactivity of homeostatic mechanisms. These he calls the diseases of adaptation. He includes among the diseases of adaptation the collagen fiber diseases and degenerative vascular diseases[8]

According to Selye, increased endocrine secretion particularly from the adrenal pituitary axis is responsible for the response of the organism to injury. This response may be general or local or both. In either instance, it is nonspecific, since it may be elicited by any agent causing injury. The general response which Selye calls the "adaptation syndrome" takes place in three stages. They are: (1) the alarm reaction, (2) the stage of resistance, and (3) the stage of exhaustion. The alarm reaction consists of two phases: (a) shock and (b) countershock. During the stage of shock and countershock the organ-

---

[6] Since the secretion of the adrenal cortical hormone, particularly the adrenal corticoids, is regulated by adrenocorticotrophin (ACTH), the two glands cannot really be separated. Other factors also influence the secretion of aldosterone.

[7] Walter B. Cannon, *The Wisdom of the Body*, W. W. Norton Co., Inc., New York, 1939.

[8] Hans Selye, "General Adaptation Syndrome and the Diseases of Adaptation," *J. Clinical Endocrinology*, VI, 1946, pp. 117-230.

ism undergoes metabolic and other changes that result from the effects of the injury and the response of the body to it. During countershock, the organism is restored to its preinjury condition. In the stage of resistance the organism is adapted to the injuring agent. It can tolerate greater exposure to the injuring agent than can the nonadapted organism. Eventually if the stress is continued, the animal loses its adaptation and goes into the stage of exhaustion. The stage of exhaustion is comparable to the shock of the earlier period.

Whether or not the animal goes through all phases of the adaptation syndrome depends on its capacity to react, as well as on the intensity and continuance of the injuring agent. Any injury may be so severe that the vital processes of an individual are depressed to such an extent that death occurs immediately. Or he may die because his adaptive capacity is inadequate to cope with the injury. In contrast the individual may add to the damage by overreacting. Finally, when an injury is limited to a single insult and is within the adaptive capacity of the individual, recovery may be complete.

Selye believes that adrenal cortical hormones not only affect the general responses of the organism, but also modify the local response of tissue to injury. Further, the type of change in the tissues depends on whether the mineralocorticoids (aldosterone) or the glucocorticoids (cortisone) predominate. According to Selye, the mineralocorticoids are prophlogistic; that is, they stimulate the connective tissue to proliferate and enhance its inflammatory potential. In contrast, the glucocorticoids are anti-inflammatory or anti-phlogistic. They inhibit proliferation of connective tissue and suppress the inflammatory process with the result that there is a reduction in the quantity of scar tissue formed in repair. Thus they may be prescribed in the treatment of rheumatic fever, rheumatoid arthritis, and other disorders in which an excessive or prolonged inflammatory response may lead to crippling scarring. Selye is of the opinion that the growth hormone from the anterior pituitary sensitizes the tissue to the mineralocorticoids. Other investigators do not agree that the changes in metabolism following tissue injury are due solely to the action of the adrenal cortical hormones.

Although the mechanisms of action of the adrenal cortical hormones in response to injury are not known, these hormones are essential to the general response. Furthermore, cortisol and its analogues are known to modify and are used therapeutically to modify the local reaction of certain tissues to injury.

What is the source of information about the nature of the metabolic response to injury?

Many of the extensive studies of metabolic responses of human beings to injury have been made on young men undergoing a surgical procedure, but some studies have been made on individuals who have suffered fractures or burns. There is no reason to suppose that patients who are seriously ill with nonsurgical diseases do not also have metabolic reaction. Response to injury is believed to be universal, and many, though not all, authorities believe it to be homeostatic.

Knowledge of the systemic response to injury, disease, or surgical therapy is essential to determining the requirements of patients who have suffered injury or acute disease. Unless the reactions of the patient are understood, treatment may interfere with rather than support the responses that promote recovery. These responses appear to have three objectives. They are: (1) to maintain the stability of the organism during stress, (2) to repair damaged tissues, and (3) to restore the body to normal composition and activity. The care of the patient should therefore be planned to assist him in achieving these objectives.

What changes in metabolism occur during the period of convalescence following surgery or other trauma?

Though there is overlapping between the various phases, Moore[9] describes convalescence as taking place in four phases. During the first phase there is rapid catabolism of lean tissue and fat. For about 6 to 24 hours after major surgery or a severe injury, water and sodium chloride are retained in the body. Until the patient is eliminating water and salt at a normal rate, overloading is possible. The danger of overloading is greatest among patients with heart disease or who are elderly. In the period immediately following major surgery or injury, careful attention should be paid to the rate at which solutions are introduced intravenously, to the type of solution, and to the relation of intake to output. Nitrogen, potassium, and phosphates are lost in the urine. Clinically the patient is characterized by all the reactions to an acute injury. Hemorrhage, pain, and fear augment the reaction. The patient has tachycardia and a slight fever which persists for two or three days. Unless he is storing water, he loses weight as the result of tissue catabolism.

The changes in nitrogen metabolism that are a part of the stress response have been extensively studied. As a result of this response, lean tissues undergo catabolism and large amounts of nitrogen and potassium are lost in the urine. The catabolic response cannot be reversed and may be intensified by forced feeding. It can also be induced by the administration of corticotrophin,[10] or the adrenal corticoids. It occurs in any adrenalectomized animal who is maintained on the adrenal cortical hormones.[11]

In nondiabetic persons who have a healthy liver, marked changes in glucose metabolism are not usually evident during stress, whereas the person who is diabetic usually has an elevation in blood glucose unless measures are taken to prevent it. The adrenal cortical hormones and insulin are physiological

[9] Francis D. Moore, *Metabolic Care of the Surgical Patient,* W. B. Saunders Company, Philadelphia, 1959, p. 27.
[10] Also known as adrenocorticotropin.
[11] James D. Hardy, *Pathophysiology in Surgery,* The Williams & Wilkins Company, Baltimore, 1958, pp. 15-16.

antagonists. During stress the tolerance of the diabetic person for glucose is lessened. For a period following surgery, the diabetic patient requires more insulin than he does at other times. Following injury, considerable amounts of fats may be utilized as fuel. In patients who have diabetes mellitus, regular checking of the urine for glucose and acetone is therefore important.

Phase II, which Moore[12] calls the turning point, begins about the fourth day and continues for two or three days. Catabolism of tissue substance decreases, and preparations are made for anabolism. Clinically the patient appears improved. His appetite and spontaneous activity increase. He begins to be a bit less self-centered and more interested in the affairs of others. He shows some concern for his wife or for his roommate or for the man down the hall.

In phase III, or anabolic phase, which begins seven to ten days after an extensive injury, the person who has been injured restores his lean tissue. This phase involves the reconstruction of the lean tissues lost during the catabolic phase of illness. During this period, the person requires a generous dietary intake, and if he does not receive it, convalescence will be retarded as he will fail to gain the necessary weight, strength, and vigor. Wound healing continues normally, despite postoperative starvation.[13] Progress through phase III, depends, however, on an adequate intake of calories and protein. Unless adequate calories and protein are available during this period, the recovery of the patient may be seriously delayed. A patient may require between 2,000 and 3,000 calories per day. Progress means not only that wound healing occurs normally, but that the patient gains weight and strength. Attention must be paid to the food intake of patients following surgical treatment, severe trauma, burns, and severe infections. The glass of milk in the refrigerator for a between-meal or evening snack is important and contributes to recovery provided it is consumed by the patient. Further, since many surgical patients are discharged some time between the seventh and tenth days, attention should be given to preparing them so that they understand the importance of eating sufficient amounts and variety of food. Eating may not be a serious problem for those whose appetite is good, but in the elderly or chronically ill, a real effort may be required to assure adequate food intake. In the patient who has been seriously burned, losses of protein during phase I may have been very great. Infection of the burned areas may have aggravated that loss. For example, despite the fact that Mr. Allen ate quite well, his food intake was augmented by tube feeding to the point where his gastrointestinal tract was unable to tolerate food. Despite heroic efforts to maintain his caloric and protein intake, he lost 20 lb during the first few weeks of his illness.

During phase IV, which may last for weeks or months, there is a return to full body weight and function. Fat deposits are restored, and the patient

---

[12] *Op. cit.,* p. 42.
[13] Francis Wilson, D. Moore, and Jepson, in G. A. Smart, ed., *Metabolic Disturbances in Clinical Medicine,* Little, Brown & Co., Boston, 1958, p. 80.

returns to work. During this phase the appetite of the patient may be very good. When he reaches his desired weight he may have to consciously limit his food intake in order to prevent an excessive gain in weight.

What are some of the factors appearing to modify the intensity of metabolic response?

The intensity of a metabolic reaction varies with a number of conditions. For example, the catabolic response is greatest in well-nourished young males. A less intense response occurs in females, the elderly, and the poorly nourished of either sex. The degree and type of trauma also influence the reaction. Minor trauma induces a less intense response than major trauma. Following minor trauma phase I is shorter. Phase II is scarcely noticeable, and the other two phases are passed through quickly. Burns and bone injury elicit a more vigorous response than can be predicted on the basis of the degree of injury. Extensive injury to soft tissues also adds to the severity of the reaction. There is evidence that a marked and prolonged metabolic response to injury predisposes to the development of decubiti. Among the seriously injured, tissue breakdown may occur in a matter of hours. Care that can ordinarily be counted on to prevent the development of decubiti may be ineffective. Under these circumstances they result not so much from neglect as from the vigor of the metabolic response of the patient. Because seriously injured patients are predisposed to decubiti, protective measures should be instituted immediately. Since tissue breakdown can be far advanced before external evidence such as reddening of the skin occurs, preventive care should not be delayed. Protection of the tissue from prolonged pressure and other preventive measures should be instituted as early as possible and carried out faithfully.

The metabolic response to injury can be intensified by apprehension and pain, and by other factors such as chilling, fever, and infection. The nurse has a responsibility to provide an emotional and physical environment that reduces undesirable stimuli to a minimum. Preoperative preparation of the patient for what to expect after operation, prompt attention to the relief of pain, gentleness in handling the patient, a quiet, nonstimulating environment, realistic expectations for and acceptance of the behavior of the patient—all should reduce the strain on the patient. The patient should be protected from well-meaning friends and relatives, who stay too long or talk too much, who are too boisterous or come in too large numbers. The writer has seen newly operated and seriously ill patients exhausted by too many visitors or by those who remained too long. Conversely, a relative or friend whose presence comforts or quiets the patient should have an opportunity to visit the patient or be encouraged to remain. When the necessity arises to lessen the number of visitors or the length of time that they stay, the interpretation should be in terms of the needs of the patient. The feelings of the visitor should also be respected. The nurse may need to take initiative and use her ingenuity in accomplishing the reduction in the number of visitors. When necessary, something can be arranged to do to or for the patient that requires the visitors to leave. The nurse may also suggest to the visitors that cards and letters are greatly enjoyed. However, the regulation of visiting should be based on the needs and condition of the patient.

Occasionally the problem of no visitors to a patient arises. The patient may be far from home or have no surviving relatives or friends. Visits from the doctors and nurses are then especially welcome. If a Grey Lady or Cherry Lady or other volunteer service worker is available, she may be utilized to meet needs of the patient that are ordinarily met by the family. In addition to visiting the patient she may write letters for him, read to him, shop for minor necessities, and the like. Of course, what the volunteer does should be adapted to the requirements of the patient. A friendly and sympathetic person who sits quietly by his bed may make a significant contribution to a seriously ill patient.

To summarize, as a result of severe injury, major surgery, or serious illness, the person undergoes a variety of responses that are integrated by the neuro-endocrine system. Among the changes are a series of metabolic responses by which the organism provides the materials for repair and restores itself to normal. These changes have been studied more extensively in patients who have been treated surgically than in patients with acute or chronic disease. The metabolic changes are characterized by a series of catabolic and anabolic changes that proceed through well-defined phases. In the earlier phases of the reaction elements associated with an intense reaction are youth, male sex, and good nutrition. Elements associated with a less intense reaction are advanced age, female sex, and undernutrition. Extensive surgery, burns, and fractures are accompanied by more intense and prolonged reactions than is minor injury or surgery. Apprehension, pain, and other circumstances associated with operative procedures intensify the response to injury. Through the intelligent practice of nursing, the emotional and physical climate of the patient can be controlled so that harmful stimuli are minimized. The nurse should give attention to those observations indicating the state of the water and electrolyte balance. As soon as the patient is able to eat, his food intake should be noted and attention given to those patients who eat poorly. Patients who suffered wasting diseases before surgical treatment require special attention to improve their nutritional status. Intelligent application of the knowledge of the changes taking place after injury can shorten the convalescence of the patient.

Just what initiates or ends the metabolic responses is not known at the present time. The metabolic changes following surgery or injury are assumed to be the result of homeostatic mechanisms which function to maintain the circulating fluid volume so that tissues may be supplied with nutrients and oxygen. The catabolic changes liberate both water and materials from which energy may be obtained to maintain body processes. The changes occurring in the later phases of the response to injury restore the body to preinjury condition.

What is meant by the term immunity and what are some of the factors in its development?

Whereas many of the responses to injury are nonspecific, most individuals also have, or are able to develop, resistance to specific microorganisms. The term "immunity" signifies a characteristic of the host which confers resistance to a specific agent. Immunity varies in degree from complete insusceptibility to almost complete susceptibility. For example, human beings do not develop the disease known as chicken cholera, but they are highly susceptible to measles. After experiencing an attack of measles, they become relatively immune. Few persons have measles more than once. Moreover, a relative degree of immunity can be induced in human beings and other animals by exposure to modified forms of microorganisms or their products. A temporary or passive immunity to measles may be conferred by the injection of gamma globulin made from the pooled serum of persons having had measles. A vaccine containing measles virus has been prepared which is said to stimulate an active immunity to measles.

What are the types of immunity?

Immunity has been classified as natural and acquired. Natural immunity is defined as the resistance to disease with which one is born. Little is actually known about the mechanisms involved in natural immunity. It is of three types: species, racial, and individual. Man's immunity to chicken cholera and relative immunity to avian (bird) tuberculosis are a species immunity. Man is also susceptible to diseases to which animals are immune. For example, man is susceptible to the *Treponema pallidum* (syphilis) and to gonococci (gonorrhea) but animals are not.

Within one species, genetic differences determine the degree to which individuals of a given race or strain are resistant to certain diseases. This has been demonstrated among mice in which strains have been developed that are highly susceptible to viral and resistant to bacterial infections.

As with any biological phenomenon, individuals within any genetic or racial group exhibit great differences in degree of resistance to infection. There are always a few individuals who, despite repeated exposure to virulent microorganisms, fail to contract the disease. In the same group there will also be a few persons who will fail to develop an immunity after having a disease to which most persons become immune. Among factors known to influence susceptibility or resistance to infectious diseases are nutritional status, hormonal balance, and exposure to ionizing radiation.

What are the types of acquired immunity and how do they differ?

In contrast to natural immunity, acquired immunity is usually attained after birth. It is of two types, passive and active. In the passive type of acquired immunity, resistance to disease is gained by administering antibodies against a particular bacterial or viral agent that has been formed in another individual. For example, passive immunity to diphtheria or pneumococcus pneumonia of certain types can be conferred by the injection of horse serum containing the appropriate antibodies. Similarly passive immunity to measles can be attained by injection of gamma globulin obtained from individuals who have had measles. Because the antibody molecules are continuously breaking down and are not being replaced, passive immunity is temporary. It is greatest immediately following the administration of antibodies and lasts for only a few weeks at the longest. Passive immunity is most beneficial in the prevention and modification of those bacterial diseases such as diphtheria in which the major effects are caused by an exotoxin. The antibody (antitoxin) combines with the toxin and inactivates it. Passive immunity is also of value in preventing or modifying the course of certain virus diseases such as red (rubeola) and German (rubella) measles. Gamma globulin may be administered to prevent measles in susceptible infants or children who are sick with some other disease. Prevention of German measles is most important in women who are in the first trimester of pregnancy as the incidence of deformities is believed to be higher among infants born of mothers who have measles during the first three months of pregnancy.

A naturally occurring type of acquired passive immunity results from the transfer of antibodies from the mother to the child in utero. This immunity may be reinforced by antibodies contained in the mother's milk, particularly in the colostrum. Immunity is effective for only about four to six months.

The second type of acquired immunity is active immunity, which develops as a result of the individual's reaction to microorganisms and their products. Active immunity may be induced by the presence of a clinical or subclinical infection, by the administration of living or dead microorganisms or their products, or by the injection of antigenically active materials obtained from them. For example, active immunity to poliomyelitis may be attained by having the disease whether or not paralysis occurs. In the absence of paralysis, poliomyelitis is said to be subclinical. It is effective in inducing immunity, however. Immunity may also be induced by the administration of either living or dead poliomyelitis virus. Active immunity to diphtheria or tetanus may be achieved by the injection of attenuated toxin or by the administration of antigenically active material (toxoid).

What is known about the "anatomy and physiology" of immunity?

Despite the demonstration by Jenner in 1798 that active immunity to smallpox could be induced by introducing lymph containing the cowpox virus into the skin, the anatomy and physiology of immunity are still not completely understood. One element contributing to the failure to elucidate the mechanisms by which immunity is developed has been the lack of suitable tools for the task. Essentially the development of immunity depends on the capacity of the tissues or certain tissues of the body (1) to recognize certain substances as foreign or antigenic and (2) to form substances (antibodies) capable of neutralizing or otherwise destroying them. In current language, the tissues or the cells comprising them are able to distinguish between "self" and "nonself." Self in this instance refers to the individual's own tissue proteins, while nonself refers to other large molecules and the tissue proteins of other individuals of the same or different species.

A number of terms employed to describe or indicate aspects of normal and abnormal immunological responses are defined below:

Antigen is a substance which, when introduced into the body, stimulates the formation of antibodies.

Allergen is a substance that gives rise to hypersensitivity or allergy.

Hapten is an incomplete antigen. Requires another substance to become antigenic. Can react with an antibody, but does not by itself stimulate antibody formation.

Antibody is a substance formed in the body as a result of contact with an antigen.

Immunity implies a protected state.

Allergy is an altered reaction of tissues to repeated contacts with antigenic agents. The tissues behave differently on exposure to a material than they did on earlier exposures.

Hypersensitivity is used interchangeably with allergy.

Normergy is a normal tissue response to a given substance.

Hypoergy is a deficient tissue response to a given substance.

Hypergy is an exaggerated tissue response. In allergy the tissues hyperact.

Atopy is an allergic disease of the wheal and erythema type and in which there is usually a family history of allergic disease.

Reagin is a skin-sensitizing antibody occurring in the skin of some persons who are allergic. Reaction characterized by a wheal and flare respond about 20 minutes after the intradermal injection of antigen.

Histamine is a powerful vasodilator. Experimentally it has been demonstrated to produce asthmalike symptoms. Powerful stimulator of secretion of hydrochloric acid.

Serotonin is a powerful smooth-muscle constrictor and vasoconstrictor. Serotonin is formed in the argentaffin cells of the gastrointestinal tract and is transported by the blood platelets. It is found in the brain and other tissues.

What theories have been developed to explain the mechanism by which immunity is developed?

In the development of immunity, an antibody is formed in response to an antigen. Antibody is a globular protein which has been identified by its physical behavior as beta and gamma globulins. They react specifically with the antigen which stimulated their production. Antibodies are classified according to their location as circulating, or humoral, and cellular.

An antigen may be any one of a variety of substances, a part of a virus, bacterium, or foreign tissue cell, or a fragment of a foreign tissue cell, or a large molecule such as polysaccharide. Lipids and nucleic acids are capable of becoming antigens after they combine with protein. With the exception of the erythrocytes and tissues sequestered from the blood stream, such as parts of the brain and the lens of the eye, antigens stimulating the formation of antibodies are usually derived from another species or individual.

Although man has been known to be capable of becoming immune to a number of infectious diseases for a long time, the details of the mechanism of immunity is only beginning to be understood. A great variety of large molecules, many of them protein in nature, though they may be polysaccharides or some substance that is active only after they are attached to proteins, are antigenic. Antigenic substances stimulate the body to synthesize antibodies; antibodies act in some manner to protect the body from the antigen. Two principal theories are advanced to explain the formation of antibodies. One, the instructive theory, suggests that the antigen directs or determines the form of the antibody. The other, the selective theory, states that antibody-forming cells "know how" to form antibodies, that this knowledge is genetically derived, and, further, that the synthesis of antibodies does not differ from the formation of other body proteins. The antigen acts merely to stimulate the appropriate cells to form antibody.

Occasionally an individual is born who has congenital agammaglobulinemia, a disorder in which there is a failure in the synthesis of gamma globulin. It is probably due to a defect in the formation of plasma cells. Agammaglobulinemia falls into three categories:

1. Primary congenital—sex-linked, recessive—male children.
2. Primary acquired—no clear-cut hereditary basis and may appear in either sex at any time in life.
3. Secondary—to neoplastic disease, e.g., Hodgkin's, other malignant lymphomas, multiple myeloma, and chronic lymphatic leukemia.

Syndrome of primary agammaglobulinemia includes:

a. Recurrent pyogenic infections.
b. Gastrointestinal symptoms (diarrhea, large, bulky foul-smelling stools, and flat oral glucose tolerance curves).
c. Reticuloendothelial disorders.
d. Arthritis and arthralgia.

The ability of tissues to react to antigenic agents by synthesizing antibodies and to distinguish between self and nonself has many applications in the field

of medicine. On the positive side, the capacity of tissues to react to foreign
substances by forming antibodies enables the individual to become immune to
(protected against) a variety of infectious agents. On the negative side, it increases the hazards of blood transfusion, limits the extent to which tissues of
one individual can be successfully transplanted to another, and is responsible
for a number of diseases. As examples, because the body is able to form antibodies against the virus causing smallpox, immunity to smallpox can be developed. Before blood can be safely transfused into an individual, the blood from
the donor and the recipient must be matched to eliminate the possibility of the
recipient's serum containing antibodies against the antigen in the donor's
erythrocytes. Unless the donor is an identical twin or the recipient has
agammaglobulinemia, the chances of tissue transplanted from one individual
to another "taking" are negligible. The tissues of one individual act as antigens in another; that is, the tissues of the recipient recognize the tissue as
"foreign" and form antibodies against it.

What is the course of events by which the body reacts to the transplantation of foreign tissue?

Following the transplantation of tissue, there is a more or less typical and
predictable sequence of events. For a few days the transplanted tissue remains
viable and its blood supply appears to be developing. Then the donor tissue
dies. Examination of the rejected tissue reveals thrombosis of its blood supply. Even when thrombosis is prevented by administration of an anticoagulant
to the recipient, the graft eventually dies. There is a considerable body of
evidence to support the hypothesis that the rejection of homografts is the
result of an immunological response. There is something about, or in, the
cells, tissues, and body fluids that recognizes that the donor tissues are genetically different from themselves. The cell that is probably responsible for
immunological activity is the lymphocyte. The recipient responds as it does
when it is exposed to other foreign proteins; it forms antibodies against them.
Evidence supporting the hypothesis that failure of homotransplantation has
an immunological basis includes: (1) the period of time elapsing between the
grafting of tissue and its rejection by the recipient is within the limits required
for antibody formation; (2) a second tissue graft from the same donor is
rejected more quickly than the first; (3) the larger the homograft, the more
quickly it is rejected; (4) measures suppressing antibody formation, such as
total body irradiation, prolong the length of life of the graft; and (5) antibodies reacting against the donor cells appear in the blood plasma of the
host.[14]

To achieve success in the transplantation of homografts, some method
must be found to suppress for as long as necessary the individual's immunological defense mechanisms. Interest in this problem is far from new. Neither

[14] James D. Hardy, *Pathophysiology in Surgery,* Williams & Wilkins Company, Baltimore, 1958, pp. 118-19.

is it limited to research scientists. Nurses ought to have some understanding of why answers are difficult to obtain. At some later time, knowledge of the immunological defense system may be sufficiently great that the mechanism can be more easily suppressed or stimulated than is possible at the present time. Parenthetically, the immunological defense system can now be suppressed by total body irradiation, but when this is done the individual becomes susceptible to the microorganisms in his environment.

Under what circumstances does the immunological defense mechanism become an etiological factor in disease?

Like other homeostatic mechanisms, the immunological defense system can be a source of disease. One abnormality, agammaglobulinemia, in which the individual is unable to form antibodies against foreign materials, has been previously mentioned. A far more frequent malady is allergy, a disorder in which tissues respond by forming antibodies against agents that are not usually antigenic.

The word "allergy" was introduced in 1907 by von Pirquet to describe the altered reaction of tissues after repeated contact with microorganisms and antigenic agents such as foreign serums, tuberculin, and vaccine virus. Subsequently, the term "allergy" has come to include a large group of conditions in which the tissues or organs of a person respond on repeated contacts with a foreign material in a way that is different from the manner in which other members of the same species react. Allergy differs from beneficial immunological reactions in that it does harm to body tissues. Crowle[15] refers to allergy as an immunological mistake. It is immunity gone wrong. Examples of allergic conditions include hayfever, vasomotor rhinitis, allergic asthma, urticaria, drug reactions, infantile eczema, contact dermatitis, and experimental anaphylaxis. In some people disorders such as migraine headaches and gastrointestinal disturbances can be shown to be due to hypersensitivity to a drug or food.

A large number of disorders are classified as being of allergic origin. There are, however, some significant differences among the different types of allergic disorders. Not all the facts about their mechanisms have been clarified. Allergic disorders are classified as immediate or delayed, depending on the length of time elapsing between exposure of a person who is sensitized to a substance and his reaction to it. The immediate reaction is also called the anaphylactic type; the delayed reaction is called the tuberculin type. Allergic disorders usually result from a response to an extrinsic antigen. In one group, the autoimmune diseases, the immunological defense mechanism reacts against its own tissues, as it does to foreign antigens. For some reason an individual forms antibodies against his own tissues.

[15] Alfred J. Crowle, "Delayed Hypersensitivity," *Scientific American,* April, 1960, p. 129.

*What are some of the common antigens? What are some of the
factors influencing the antigenicity of various substances?*

Antigens vary in their capacity to induce antibody formation from those
that are seldom antigenic to those that almost always are. Horse serum induces hypersensitivity in a high percentage of instances on the first exposure
to it. Poison ivy will eventually induce hypersensitivity, if exposure continues
to be repeated. As indicated earlier, large molecules are more likely to be
antigenic than small molecules. Chemically, antigens are usually proteins or
polysaccharides, though they may be lipids or nucleic acids. According to one
hypothesis, polysaccharides do not become antigenic until they attach themselves to a protein molecule. Lipids and nucleic acids must be attached to a
protein molecule to be allergenic. A vast variety of substances are therefore
potentially antigenic. Some of the more common ones are the plant pollens,
animal danders, sea foods, berries, eggs, chocolate, and wheat. Foreign
serums, tuberculin, and vaccine viruses as well as drugs such as penicillin,
streptomycin sulfate, heavy metals, sulfonamides, iodides, and barbiturates
are also common offenders. Antigens may be introduced in the body by
injection, inhalation, ingestion, or contact with the skin.

*What are some of the factors influencing the tendency to
become allergic?*

Just as antigenic agents vary in potency, individuals vary in their capacity
to become allergic or hypersensitive. Many of the common forms of allergy
depend on a hereditary factor. What is inherited is not the allergic manifestation, but the tendency to become allergic. For example, a parent has asthma;
his child develops urticaria. Physical, chemical, and emotional factors also
play a role in the development of allergy. They may be significant not only in
inducing hypersensitivity, but in prolonging a particular allergic response.
Some persons appear to be hypersensitive to certain substances on their first
contact with them. Others evidence great resistance to even common allergens. For example, some babies are unable to tolerate wheat or eggs from
their first exposure to them. One theory advanced to explain this observation
is that antigenic material is transferred from the mother to the fetus in utero.

Until recently most antigens were believed to be foreign substances that
were introduced into, or entered, the individual from his outside environment.
Some individuals, for reasons that are poorly understood, appear to lose their
ability to identify their own tissues as being of themselves, for they react to
certain of their own tissues as they would to foreign antigens. Diseases in
which the body may possibly form antibodies against its own tissues are called
autoimmune diseases. Though this theory offers an attractive explanation for
the changes, occurring in certain diseases such as glomerulonephritis, rheumatic fever, multiple sclerosis, lupus erythematosis, periarteritis nodosa, and

rheumatoid arthritis, it is largely unproved. One disorder usually cited as being due to a hyperimmune response is Hashimoto's disease of the thyroid. A number of observations have been made that lend support to the theory that tissues can become antigenic and thus stimulate the formation of antibodies against themselves. In diseases such as glomerulonephritis and rheumatic fever, the onset is frequently preceded by a streptococcal infection occurring approximately two to three weeks earlier. How the infection or the products of bacterial growth induce changes in tissue cells is now known. It has recently been shown that *Streptococcus* and the myocardium possess a common antigen—a body response to the streptococcal infection is also a response against myocardial tissue. Antibodies are formed in response to this antigen; they combine with the antigen and injure tissue cells. The damaged cells release histamine and possibly serotonin, both of which cause secondary changes which are possibly more damaging than the initial injury.[16] Further destruction of healthy tissues may result from the contraction of scar tissue formed to replace dead tissue. One of the puzzling things about these diseases is that once they are initiated, there is no sure way known to stop their progress.

There is also experimental evidence to support the theory that disease can result from the individual's becoming hypersensitive to his own tissues. Merrill[17] describes an experiment in which changes similar to those of acute glomerulonephritis are induced in the kidney of a rat. Kidney tissue is removed from a rat; then it is finely ground and injected into a duck. After the duck has produced antibodies in its blood plasma, some of the blood of the duck is removed and the plasma is injected into the rat from which the kidney tissue was taken. The kidney of the rat reacts to the antibodies by undergoing changes similar to those of glomerulonephritis.

Although animal experiments have value as they provide evidence that a condition can be induced, there is no certainty that what happens in one species will occur in another. Experiments of the above type are, of course, impossible in human beings. Merrill has, however, obtained evidence to support the theory that glomerulonephritis results from an allergic response. For some years he has been working on the problem of transplanting a healthy kidney into persons with renal failure. Though he has been successful in transplanting a kidney from one identical twin to the other, in two instances in which glomerulonephritis had been responsible for the renal failure in the recipient, the transplanted kidney also developed the disease. Since skin grafting was successful in both these individuals, Merrill concludes that the recipients formed antibodies that reacted with the kidney tissue of the donor.[18]

[16] "Histamine and Serotonin Release: A Possible Common Basis for Allergic Reactions," *The Relation of Histamine and Serotonin to the Allergic State,* Schering Corporation, Bloomfield, New Jersey, January, 1961, pp. 3-4.
[17] John P. Merrill, "The Transplantation of the Kidney," *Scientific American,* CCT, October, 1959, p. 62.
[18] *Ibid.,* p. 48.

In the more usual conception of allergy, the tissues most likely to become hypersensitive are those in contact with the external environment, that is, the skin and the respiratory and gastrointestinal tracts. When there is a high concentration of antibodies in the circulating blood, circulatory collapse may follow re-exposure to the antigen. The tissues in which allergic responses are manifested are sometimes referred to as shock tissues. It is not known whether they have a greater tendency to become sensitized or whether they become sensitized because they have greater exposure to allergens.

What are some of the known differences between the immediate and delayed types of hypersensitivity reactions?

Hypersensitivity reactions are of two types, immediate and delayed. Under some circumstances an individual may have both types of reaction. In the immediate type of reaction, antibodies called circulating, or humoral, antibodies are found in the blood stream and a reaction occurs on contact with an allergen. The delayed reaction takes several hours or days to develop. In the delayed type of reaction, antibodies are not found circulating in the blood stream, but they are found in the cells of the lymphatic system.

The immediate type of hypersensitivity reaction may be manifested as a localized lesion or a systemic response. Factors influencing the nature of the clinical manifestations may depend on the site and rate of the reaction. Jawetz, et al.,[19] state that the mechanism for the systemic reaction (anaphylactic shock) may be postulated to occur something as follows: (1) soluble antigen antibody complexes attach themselves to certain cells, (2) cells are injured by these complexes, and as a result they release histamine, serotonin, and possibly other chemicals, and (3) these chemicals act on sensitive cells in shock organs (these differ in various species). Many of the clinical manifestations may be due to the effects of the chemicals released as a result of cell injury.

What are the causes and effects of systemic shock?

In man, the clinical manifestations of systemic shock (anaphylactic shock) result from the effects of cell injury and of the chemicals released by the injured cells. These effects include increased capillary permeability, generalized contraction of smooth muscle, generalized itching, and decreased coagulability of blood. Vagal tone is increased with the result that the glands supplied by the vagus are stimulated. Obvious effects include profuse tearing and sneezing. There is also an increase in the secretion of mucus along the tracheobronchial tree. As will be seen later, this mucus adds to the problem of maintaining an adequate airway.

The results of increased capillary permeability are possibly even more seri-

[19] Ernest Jawetz, Joseph L. Melnick, and Edward A. Adelberg, *Review of Medical Microbiology,* 5th ed., Lange Medical Publications, Los Altos, California, 1962.

ous. The localized lesion of allergy is the wheal, or hive; it is due to increased capillary permeability. There is a localized area of swelling which is reddened and hot, and this is accompanied by itching. Hives may, and frequently do, accompany a generalized response. As capillary permeability increases, fluid is lost from the blood into the interstitial spaces and causes edema, which may be noted as swelling of the face, eyelids, and lips. Edema of the larynx also occurs, and when it is severe it is an immediate threat to life, as it impairs ventilation and may completely obstruct the airway. A second effect of increased capillary permeability is a decrease in blood volume. With a decrease in blood volume the blood pressure falls thereby predisposing to hypoxia of tissues as a result of diminished circulation. Because the capillaries are dilated, the skin is flushed or red. From the above, it should be obvious that increased capillary permeability threatens the life of the individual by predisposing to laryngeal edema and loss of blood volume. Since the manifestations develop rapidly, the patient should be observed for flushing of the skin and any puffiness of the face, mouth, or eyelids. Any patient in whom these signs appear should be treated immediately.

A third systemic effect is a generalized contraction of smooth muscle. In man, contraction of the musculature of the bronchi causes labored breathing characteristic of asthma. Increased contractions of the gastrointestinal musculature causes vomiting and diarrhea.

Generalized itching is important, not because it threatens the life of the individual, but because it serves as a warning that a general systemic reaction is developing. When a patient has received a potentially antigenic drug such as penicillin, itching should be regarded as indicating the patient is developing a systemic response. The fact of itching should be immediately reported to the patient's physician.

In addition to the manifestations described above, there is a decrease in the coagulability of the blood which is due to the release of heparin by the blood platelets. The level of the platelets in the blood diminishes.

Among the hypersensitivity reactions of the immediate type are many of the disorders commonly associated with allergy. Included in this group are conditions such as anaphylaxis, serum sickness, Arthus' reaction, hay fever, asthma, urticaria, angioedema, and certain gastrointestinal allergies.

Of these, the one that is most immediately threatening to life is anaphylaxis.[20] According to Cooke and Sherman the manifestations in an anaphylactic reaction are the same in any given species no matter what antigen is used. The symptoms do, however, vary from species to species. Most of the manifestations can be explained on the basis of smooth-muscle spasm and increased capillary permeability, which have been previously described. In man the usual effects are urticaria (hives), asthma, and failure of the peripheral circulation. In severe attacks, death may occur in half an hour or less. In the past, the

[20] Robert A. Cooke, and William B. Sherman, "Allergy," *Pathologic Physiology*, ed. William A. Sodeman, W. B. Saunders Co., Philadelphia, 1961, pp. 270-74.

most frequent cause was heterologous serum, that is, serum obtained from an animal of another species. Today with the widespread use of drugs such as penicillin and streptomycin sulfate the possibility of anaphylaxis has been greatly increased. Before any drug is administered to a patient, he should be asked whether he has any history of allergy in himself or his family, and whether he has ever, to his knowledge, been treated with the drug to be used. Because of the common practice of treating infections in cows with penicillin, milk may contain penicillin. Persons who drink milk may be sensitized to penicillin without ever having been treated with it therapeutically. For reasons not well understood, drugs applied to the skin are more likely to induce sensitivity reactions than those ingested or injected. When there is reason to suspect that an individual may be allergic, he should be tested for skin-sensitizing antibodies. When a patient inquires about the nature of a drug that he is receiving, the nurse should at least ascertain the reason for his question. In some hospitals, only the physician tells the patient what drugs have been prescribed. The practice of withholding information from a patient about the drugs he is receiving is being questioned in some quarters. Some physicians now request the pharmacist to indicate on the label of the container the generic or trade name of drugs prescribed for and taken by the patient. Should the patient state that he is allergic to a given drug, it should be withheld until the physician has been notified. Even drugs such as aspirin, can, in the occasional individual, be highly antigenic. When agents such as heterologous serum are administered, the patient should be skin-tested before the serum is administered, and a syringe containing epinephrine should be prepared so that it will be immediately available should symptoms develop. In all patient areas, emergency equipment including epinephrine, a tourniquet, an airway, oxygen, and intravenous equipment should be immediately available.[21] Despite the infrequency of anaphylactic reactions, they can cause death unless they are treated immediately. Patients who are treated as outpatients should remain at least one-half hour after the injection of any agent.

The danger to the individual who receives an antigen to which he has been sensitized can be illustrated by Mrs. Johns, who had a serious reaction to penicillin. Fortunately for Mrs. Johns, she had not left her physician's office when she experienced systemic or anaphylactic shock. The reaction might have been prevented had either the physician who prescribed the penicillin or the nurse who administered it questioned her about her previous experience with penicillin. Failure to do so very nearly cost Mrs. Johns her life. Almost immediately following an injection of penicillin, she developed hives and had great difficulty in breathing; in a matter of a few minutes her blood pressure dropped sharply and she became unconscious. The physician injected epinephrine and applied artificial respiration. As soon as an ambulance could be obtained, she was taken to a hospital. When her condition improved, the doctor learned that she had had penicillin on two previous occasions. After

    [21] Richard A. Kern, "Anaphylactic Drug Reactions," *Journal of the American Medical Association*, CLXXIX, January 6, 1962, pp. 19-22.

the second injection she had had swelling, reddening, and itching at the site where it was injected. She had not remembered to tell her doctor of this. Unlike horse serum, skin tests to determine sensitivity to penicillin are unreliable.[22] The only protection of the patient lies in regular questioning of each patient before therapy with penicillin is initiated.

Although there is a tendency to view an inflammatory response at the site where a drug is injected, either subcutaneously or intramuscularly, as being of bacterial origin, it may be the result of an allergic response. Such an allergic response is known as an Arthus phenomenon. At one time this reaction was thought to be limited to rabbits, but it occasionally occurs in human beings. It is therefore possible that the inflammatory response that Mrs. Johns had experienced following an earlier injection was due to an antigen-antibody reaction rather than to a bacterial infection. Any swelling and redness at the site of injection of a drug should be recorded and reported to the physician.

A second type of systemic reaction to foreign substances is serum sickness. It differs from anaphylaxis in that the reaction develops in a nonsensitized person about 6 to 12 days after he receives an antigenic material such as a foreign serum. Though the patient may be, and often is, acutely ill, serum sickness is not as likely to threaten the life of the individual as is an anaphylactic reaction. Edema of the glottis may occur, but this is unusual. When serum sickness develops, some of the antigenic material remains after antibodies against it have been formed in sufficient amounts to cause a significant antigen-antibody reaction. In patients who have had the same type of serum, such as horse serum, on some previous occasion the reaction is likely to occur earlier than it does in the nonsensitized person. The characteristic manifestations of serum sickness are urticaria, itching, fever, swollen and painful joints, and lymphadenopathy. Since the advent of chemotherapeutic and antibiotic agents, serum is infrequently used in the treatment of disease. However, when it is employed, serum sickness occurs in as high as 90 per cent of those who receive serum. The manifestations of serum sickness are not, however, unique responses to serum. Similar signs and symptoms are manifested in persons with allergic responses to various antigens, including a wide variety of drugs, among which are chemotherapeutic and antibiotic agents. Although the consequences of allergic responses to drugs and serum can be observed and described, the course of events in the blood and tissues that are responsible for the reaction is not known. In a discussion of serum sickness, Thomas[23] states that after injection, a foreign serum can be detected in the blood. Six to twelve days later a precipitating antibody appears. Following the appearance of the antibody, the antigen begins to disappear from the blood. Authorities generally accept a relationship between the appearance of antibodies and the manifestations of serum disease.

Serum sickness is a benign and self-limiting disease lasting from approxi-

[22] Goodman and Gilman, Op. cit. p. 1348.
[23] Lewis Thomas, "Serum Sickness," in Cecil-Loeb A Textbook of Medicine, ed. Paul B. Beeson and Walsh McDermott, 11th ed., W. B. Saunders, Philadelphia, 1963, p. 463.

mately one to three weeks. When the nervous system is involved, causing weakness, the course is likely to be prolonged, but the patient can be expected to recover completely.

The treatment of serum sickness is symptomatic. The urticaria usually responds to small doses of epinephrine. It can also be controlled by antihistamines and ephedrine sulfate or hydrochloride. With the control of urticaria, itching is also relieved. Calamine lotion is sometimes prescribed to be applied locally to the urticarial lesions. Pain in the joints responds promptly to aspirin or other salicylates. When the patient is acutely ill, adrenal steroids are usually prescribed by the physician; the patient can be expected to respond quickly. Since there is the possibility that the patient may suddenly develop laryngeal edema and require a tracheostomy for the maintenance of his airway, a tracheostomy set should be at hand during the acute stage of illness. When the cause of the illness is serum, employed to prevent either diphtheria or tetanus, the patient should be encouraged to be immunized with the appropriate toxoid to prevent a repetition of his illness.

There is a group of common human allergies, including nonseasonal vasomotor rhinitis, hay fever, infantile eczema, urticaria, and angioedema, as well as some migraine headaches and gastrointestinal disorders, having a number of features in common. They all appear to be based on a common predisposing hereditary factor. The characteristic lesion in the allergic tissues is the wheal or hive. In many instances, symptoms and signs appear promptly on exposure to the allergen. Injection of the offending allergen into the skin is followed by the immediate type of response.

There are some instances, however, in which individuals who are predisposed by heredity to become allergic do not develop signs and symptoms following exposure to an allergen for 12 to 24 hours. For example, Silas Cornflower has a positive family history for allergy, as his mother had urticaria when she ate strawberries or sea food. Injection of minute quantities of antigenic material from either strawberries or sea food results in a raised swollen area at the site of injection (wheal). Mr. Cornflower has asthma when he is exposed to dog dander, but his symptoms do not develop immediately on exposure. They are delayed for 12 to 24 hours after he is in close proximity to a dog. Skin tests do not show the immediate type of reaction. The mechanism in the delayed type of immunological responses must be different from that in the immediate type. How it differs is not known.

In hay fever (seasonal vasomotor rhinitis) and nonseasonal rhinitis the mucous membranes lining the nose, related structures, and conjunctiva are affected. The manifestations include tearing and redness of the eyes, burning of both the eyes and nasal mucosa, sneezing, watery discharge from the nose, and obstruction to the passage of air by congestion of the nasal mucosa. The severity of symptoms varies from mild to so severe that the patient cannot get sufficient rest. Seasonal and nonseasonal vasomotor rhinitis differ principally in the antigens to which the person is sensitive. They include pollens—ragweed is a common offender, and is responsible for seasonal vasomotor rhinitis —house dust, animal danders, drugs, foods, and the products of infection. With the exception of ragweed, all the other materials cause nonseasonal vasomotor rhinitis. Besides causing varying amounts of discomfort, vasomotor rhinitis predisposes to allergic asthma. In allergic asthma, the basic lesion is the same as in other allergic responses of the immediate type, but the lesions occur in the bronchial tubes. Three factors are commonly considered to be responsible for allergic asthma. They include: (1) the inhalation of allergens, causing seasonal or nonseasonal asthma, (2) infection of the respiratory tract causing intermittent or chronic symptoms, and (3) a combination of the first two. The same antigens causing allergic rhinitis may also be responsible for allergic asthma. Because of the variety of factors involved in allergic asthma, it may be seasonal, nonseasonal, or chronic.

Because the bronchi are involved in allergic asthma there are three responses contributing to the development of symptoms: (1) increased capillary permeability in the mucosa lining the bronchi, (2) spasm or contraction of bronchial musculature, and (3) increased secretion of mucus. All these changes contribute to the interference with breathing—the major manifestation in asthma. At the onset of an attack, the patient is likely to feel that he is about to suffocate and his behavior may suggest that he is in a state of panic or acute anxiety. For example, Mrs. Pine, who had been hospitalized for the treatment of asthma, developed an acute attack. She turned on her light. Before the nurse had time to reach her room, she called out for the nurse to hurry. Mrs. Pine appeared to be frightened and she did not want to be left alone. The feelings of suffocation accompanying an attack of asthma probably always engender feelings of fear and anxiety and may prolong the attack, once it is under way. Whatever the cause, cell injury results in the release of histamine and serotonin. Any serious threat to oxygen supply and to the removal of carbon dioxide can be expected to have a similar effect.

Emotional factors may also trigger attacks of asthma. As an illustration, one morning Mrs. Pine thought that she had been given a drug to which she was allergic and she developed a full-blown attack of asthma. What had actually occurred was that a laboratory assistant had drawn blood. The attack had been triggered by a thought rather than a material substance. It was no less severe, however. She required the same treatment as any patient experiencing an acute attack of asthma. During the attack Mrs. Pine sat with her feet hanging over the edge of the bed. She was supporting herself with her hands and arms in a winglike position. This position enabled her to make maximum use of her accessory muscles of respiration. Because bronchi dilate with inspiration and are smaller with expiration, air is trapped in the lungs causing them to be distended and the chest to be in a continuous state of expansion. Therefore, the efforts of the patient are directed toward forcing air out of the lung during expiration. Expiration appears more labored than inspiration. Her (Mrs. Pine's) respirations were accompanied by a wheeze that was audible to her and to those who were nearby. Coughing was stimulated by an increase in the secretion of mucus. Therapy for an acute asthmatic attack is directed toward depressing the allergic response and dilating the bronchi, decreasing the anxiety of the patient, and correcting the conditions predisposing to asthma. When at all possible someone should stay with the patient who is in an acute attack of asthma. When only one person is available, the most reasonable course of action is to prepare and administer the prescribed drug or drugs. Some of the same drugs that are effective in treatment of anaphylactic shock are also useful in relieving an acute attack of asthma. These drugs include epinephrine, ephedrine sulfate or hydrochloride, aminophyllin U.S.P., B. P., isoproterenerol hydrochloride and Tedral.[24] In a very acute attack, epinephrine is usually administered.

Skin reactions characteristic of the immediate type of allergy include infantile eczema, erythematous rashes, exfoliative dermatitis, and hives. The rashes accompanying measles and scarlet fever are examples of erythematous rashes. Some drugs such as phenobarbital also may be responsible for rashes that are similar in appearance to those associated with infectious diseases. Treatment with drugs such as arsphenamine, gold, penicillin, iodine, and quinine may be accompanied by exfoliative dermatitis, a generalized and serious form of dermatitis in which all or nearly all of the surface of the skin is covered with blebs or blisters, filled with serous fluid.[25] The patient presents many of the same problems as the one who has been seriously burned. Protein-containing fluid is lost into the blisters and drains from the lesions after the surface tissue is disrupted. After the blisters break, the underlying area is vulnerable to infection. Because of the injury to the skin, its function in the regulation of body temperature is disturbed. All in all, the patient with exfoliative dermatitis has an extremely poor prognosis.

Urticaria or hives of the skin is most frequently associated with allergy to foods. Drugs may also be responsible.

Wheal and erythema reactions occurring along the gastrointestinal tract, combined with the contraction of smooth muscle, cause symptoms such as nausea, vomiting, and diarrhea. Gastrointestinal allergies are likely to be due to ingestants such as sea food, wheat, or eggs.

The hemopoietic system may become hypersensitive to drugs. Either a delayed or immediate type of hypersensitivity reaction may be involved. Bone marrow depression results in thrombocytopenia, (diminished number of thrombocytes in the blood) and agranulocytopenia (diminished number of granular leukocytes in the blood). With a decrease in the number of thrombocytes in the blood, the individual is predisposed to hemorrhage. Lowering of the number of leukocytes predisposes to infection.

From the preceding discussion, it should be obvious that there are a num-

[24] Trade name for compound containing: Theophylline 0.13 gm; ephedrine hydrochloride 24 mg; phenobarbital 8 mg.
[25] A number of terms are used to describe blisters. Blebs, vesicles, and bullae all imply blisters. Bullae are large blisters.

ber of systemic and local allergic responses of the immediate type. The nature of the manifestations depends on whether or not the response is systemic or localized to an organ or part. The organs in which the manifestations are most prominent are those in direct contact with the external environment: the skin, the airway, and the gastrointestinal tract. The bone marrow may, however, be a primary site of reaction as well. In anaphylactic shock, the blood vessels throughout the body are affected. Two factors that seem to influence the nature of the response are the rate and site of exposure to an allergen (antigen). Most of the manifestations are due to increased capillary permeability and to contraction of smooth muscle. Vascular collapse and obstruction of the airway as a result of edema of the larynx are the two most serious threats to the life of an individual. No person should be treated with a foreign serum or other type of antigenic agent without first determining whether or not he has been treated with it at some earlier time. Patients receiving horse serum should be tested previous to its administration, by the injection of horse serum intradermally (into the skin). A reddening or flare indicates that the patient has been sensitized to horse serum.

How does the delayed type of hypersensitivity response differ from the immediate type?

One of the most easily identifiable differences is that in the immediate type antibodies are found in the blood, while in the delayed type they are probably located in cells. A difference that can be directly observed is the time elapsing between the injection of antigenic material and the appearance of a wheal. Unlike the immediate type of response, the lesion of the delayed type of hypersensitivity reaction takes several hours to appear. It is similar inasmuch as the area is red, hot, and swollen. The swelling is firmer and lasts longer than it does in the immediate type of reaction. When the reaction is severe, tissue cells may be killed and cellular necrosis may be evident. The initial damage may result from the combination of the antigen and the antibody. Further injury may be caused by substances released by the necrotic cells. With cellular injury, tissues also respond by inflammation. This response will be discussed later in the chapter. The classical example of the delayed type of hypersensitivity is the response of the tissues to tuberculin. Anyone whose tissues have been sensitized to the *Mycobacterium* of tuberculosis and has had a Mantoux or similar test has experienced the delayed type of allergic skin reaction. When this reaction is marked, there is some degree of tissue necrosis.

Whereas examples of the immediate type of allergic response include anaphylaxis, Arthus' reactions, serum sickness, hay fever, urticaria, angioedema, asthma, and certain gastrointestinal allergies, the allergies of the delayed type include contact dermatitis, poison ivy, drug allergies, and allergies of infections such as tuberculosis. According to Crowle,[26] the cavities

[26] Crowle, *Op. cit.,* p. 133.

forming in the lungs in tuberculosis appear to be the result of a delayed hypersensitivity reaction. Changes occurring in the tissues in a variety of other infections such as syphilis are believed to be due to hypersensitivity reactions. Symptoms in conditions such as athlete's foot may be the result of delayed hypersensitivity to the organism causing the disorder. Following the administration of heterologous serum and certain drugs, including penicillin, changes take place in blood vessels that are characteristic of a delayed type of allergic response. The pathological changes in the blood vessels resemble those of periarteritis nodosa.

One of the most common examples of delayed hypersensitivity is contact dermatitis. Because of the frequency with which it occurs and its increasing incidence, contact dermatitis will be discussed in some detail. As a result of repeated contacts with a wide variety of antigenic agents, including detergents, the skin becomes sensitized to an antigen. Pillsbury[27] states that though the changes occurring in the skin in dermatitis are relatively constant and follow a basic pattern, the agents that initiate or prolong dermatitis are numerous. The signs of dermatitis, in the order in which they appear, are as follows: (1) erythema and swelling, (2) oozing and/or vesiculation, (3) crusting and scaling, (4) thickening and evidence of repeated excoriation (the results of scratching), and (5) hyperpigmentation, scratch papule formation, and lichenification.[28] The first three groups of signs occur during the acute phase, the latter two during the chronic phase of the disorder. According to Pillsbury and Shelley,[29] acute contact dermatitis may be due to primary irritation by a toxic substance or it may result from a hypersensitivity reaction. The eventual outcome depends on the early identification and elimination of the cause. When contact dermatitis is allowed to persist, secondary changes follow and tend to prolong it.

What kinds of information can be gained by injecting antigenic material into the skin?

As was previously stated, various body tissues may be sensitized to specific antigens. Since antibodies are frequently found in the skin, and it is conveniently located, the skin may be used to identify those individuals who are or are not sensitive to a specific antigen. Examples include the identification of persons who have been sensitized to horse serum before the administration of tetanus or other types of antitoxin. Skin tests are used to check the effectiveness of immunization procedures. The Schick test is useful in determining whether or not the individual is immune to diphtheria. In tuberculosis, epidemiologists use skin tests to trace its distribution in the community. Skin tests are sometimes useful in establishing a diagnosis. For example, the ap-

[27] Donald M. Pillsbury and Walter B. Shelley, "Diseases Affecting the Skin," *Principles of Internal Medicine*, 4th ed., T. R. Harrison *et al.*, McGraw-Hill Book Co., New York, 1962, p. 1926.
[28] Lichenification is the process whereby the skin becomes leathery and hardened.
[29] *Op. cit.,* p. 1926.

pearance of the lung is similar in tuberculosis and histoplasmosis. When antigenic material obtained from the two organisms is injected into the skin, a response at the site of one and not the other is helpful to the physician in making the differential diagnosis.

Skin tests may be performed by injecting a dilute solution of the desired antigen into the skin or by placing a small quantity of the solution on the skin and abrading or scratching it with a hypodermic needle. The scratch test is believed to be safer than intradermal injection because the rate of absorption of the antigen is slower. In the intradermal test, 0.1 to 0.2 ml of a given dilution of the antigen is injected into the skin. In patients known to be or suspected of being hypersensitive, the dilution should be appropriately large. The patient or a member of the family should be asked if he has had the particular type of injection previously and, if he has, how he reacted to it. Skin reactions, similar to other allergic responses, may be immediate or delayed. The immediate reaction occurs within a few minutes after the antigenic material is injected and lasts only a short time; the area should therefore be subject to continuous observation. With a positive reaction, the skin becomes red or flushed. Careful observation of the site where antigenic material is injected is important, if an immediate response is to be detected. When the patient is to receive an antigenic agent such as tetanus antitoxin (horse serum), detection of a positive response may prevent the patient from developing a serious response or even be lifesaving. A person who is found to be sensitized to horse serum and who requires tetanus antitoxin can be temporarily immunized by small but increasing doses of antigenic material. The first dose may be no larger than the initial test dose. The safety of the patient depends on identifying the fact that he is sensitive and on rigid adherence to the schedule for increasing the dosage and for its timing.

The skin reaction in the delayed type of hypersensitivity takes several hours to appear. It may or may not have been preceded by the immediate type of reaction. The skin at the site of the injection is red, hot, and swollen. The swelling is firm. The lesion lasts longer than it does in the immediate reaction.

In some skin tests, such as the Schick test, reddening of the skin indicates that the individual has not developed antibodies against the antigen. Antibodies protect the skin from the antigen rather than sensitizing it.

Upon what principles is the therapy of patients with allergic diseases based?

Because allergic resonses, however they are manifested, are the result of an immunological mechanism, preventive and therapeutic measures are based on similar principles and are directed toward the achievement of three objectives. The site of the response and the requirements of the individual patient influence the selection of specific preventive and therapeutic measures. These factors also influence the decision as to which objective takes priority at a given moment in time. The primary objectives are: (1) to prevent or limit the exposure of the patient to antigens to which he may be, or is known to be, hypersensitive; (2) to relieve or mitigate the effects produced by a hypersensitivity reaction; and (3) to increase the resistance of the patient to a specific antigen.

The accomplishment of the first objective, that is, to prevent or limit the exposure of the patient to antigens to which he is known to be, or may be, hypersensitive, depends on knowledge of what the common allergens are, what their sources are, how they are transported in the environment, and how they gain entrance into the organism. Actually, this is the very knowledge that forms the background for the prevention of the spread of infectious agents causing disease. Since not all persons are allergic to the common allergens, knowledge of the particular antigens to which the patient is hypersensitive is also useful. Some of the substances to which people are frequently hypersensitive have been previously mentioned. Hypersensitivity to horse serum is so common, and so easily developed, that all persons are presumed to be sensitive to it unless they are shown not to be by skin testing. The use of skin testing in the identification of substances to which individuals are hypersensitive has also been discussed. Although skin testing is of value, it also has limitations. A reddened area indicates that the patient has antibodies for that antigen in his skin but it does not necessarily mean that he will have an allergic response when he is exposed to it. Why this is true is not known. Neither does the absence of a reddened area necessarily mean that the person is not hypersensitive to a particular antigen. Some persons have a high degree of hypersensitivity to an antigen, despite the absence of a positive skin reaction.

Because skin tests do not necessarily give complete information about the antigens to which an individual is hypersensitive, other methods have to be used in their identification. Perhaps the most important of these is the observation of a cause-effect relationship between contact with an antigen and the development of an allergic reaction on the part of the patient. Patients are often aware of these relationships. For example, Mrs. Cornflower knows that each time she eats strawberries, she develops hives. In some instances an individual such as Mrs. Cornflower knows that if she eats one strawberry she becomes deathly sick. Her cousin Frank is able to eat a small serving of strawberries three or four times during the summer, but he has hives if he eats them more frequently. Nurses can help in identifying antigens when they observe and report events that are coincident. For example, Mrs. Batelman was hospitalized for treatment of an acute attack of allergic asthma. Following her recovery, her physician decided to remove some nasal polyps obstructing her breathing. Nasal polyps are a common sequela in allergic rhinitis. As part of her preparation for polypectomy, Mrs. Batelman was given ephedrine sulfate. Shortly thereafter, she began to wheeze and to show signs of a developing asthmatic attack. Despite the impending attack of asthma, the surgeon removed the polyps and the ephedrine was continued. Each time Mrs. Batelman received ephedrine, wheezing and difficulty in breathing were intensified. The nurse observed the apparent cause-effect relationship between the ephedrine and the difficulty in breathing exhibited by Mrs. Batelman. She brought her observation to the attention of the physician, who discontinued the drug. Mrs. Batelman's breathing improved and other evidence of asthma also cleared rapidly. Despite the usefulness of ephedrine sulfate in relieving asthmatic attacks in most individuals, in the instance of Mrs. Batelman it acted to trigger its onset.

Cause-effect relationships are frequently more difficult to establish than in the illustration cited above. In order to collect data, the patient may be instructed to keep a diary or a record of his activities, including what he eats, and to describe any abnormal responses .For example, Mrs. Bobbin learned from keeping a diary that she was allergic to an insecticide used to kill mosquitoes. She developed asthmatic symptoms each evening after an insecticide containing pyrethrum was sprayed just outside the porch where she sat in the evening.

When a food is suspected to be allergenic, a diary may be employed or the patient may be placed on an elimination diet. The elimination diet may be approached in different ways. The patient may be instructed to eliminate one food at a time and observe his response or to eliminate all commonly allergenic foods and then add them to his dietary, one at a time. Before adding a new food, he should note any response to the one just previously included in his dietary. Occasionally all foods except those which are rarely antigenic may be removed from the dietary and then the above procedure followed. The success of any type of elimination diet in discovering foods antigenic to the patient depends on the patient and/or the person who prepares his food understanding why the diet is prescribed and what is entailed in its preparation. It must be understood that it is the specific food, and not its method of preparation, that is important. The food must be eliminated in all forms. The following example has its origin in the days before electricity was supplied to every farmhouse. Mrs. Farwell brought her three-year-old son, Bobby, to University Clinic for the treatment of atopic eczema. In an attempt to identify the offending allergen, the physician prescribed a diet from which all forms of wheat were to be eliminated. Mrs. Farwell was duly instructed and appeared to be interested and cooperative. A week later she returned with Bobby. He was no better. The physician checked with Mrs. Farwell to determine whether she had carried out the instructions. He asked her if Bobby had had any bread. She replied, "No, none at all. I toasted every bit of it." Mrs. Farwell did not have a toaster and she did not usually toast bread unless a member of the family was ill. She believed that toast was more easily digested than untoasted bread and was therefore more suitable than bread for a sick person. The making of toast was a cultural response to illness.

Patients sometimes eliminate foods from their dietary because they are, or believe that they are, allergic to them. Although the avoidance of one or two specific foods is not likely to cause malnutrition, the exclusion of many foods may, and this possibility increases in proportion to the number of foods eliminated. Occasionally an individual appears for medical attention who has eliminated almost all types of food from his dietary. It is quite important that persons for whom elimination diets are prescribed understand that the diet is temporary.

In addition to assisting in various ways with the identification of antigenic agents, the nurse is often responsible for the preparation of an environment which is as nearly free of antigenic agents as is possible. She may also be helpful to the patient in planning his home environment. Leavell and Clark[30] suggest that extremes be avoided in adapting the home to the needs of the allergic person. The same general points apply whether the patient is in the hospital or at home. Frequently, stripping the bedroom of the person who is allergic of unnecessary dust-catching furniture and draperies is all that is required. Overstuffed furniture, draperies, pillows, mattresses with ordinary covering, and rugs serve as reservoirs for the accumulation of dust, and they should be removed or covered with an impervious material. Mattresses can now be purchased with plasticized coverings which prevent them from accumulating dust. They do not require further covering. The rest of the house may be furnished as desired. For older children and adults, airborne allergens are of considerable importance. House dust and pollens are common antigens. When furniture is purchased for the home, ease of cleaning should be kept in mind. In both the hospital and in the home the mattress should be covered with plastic material or the covering should be plasticized. Leavell and Clark[31] suggest that the patient use a dacron[32] pillow. Sponge rubber may be used, but in time it tends to take on dust, and some persons are allergic to rubber. Allergic patients often take their own pillows with them to the hospital. Despite the possibility of the patient's losing his pillow, this should be permitted and a concerted effort should, of course, be made to prevent its loss.

The air may be a source of dust and pollens. Leavell and Clark[33] emphasize that hot-air systems without adequate filters circulate considerable dust. For persons who are allergic to dust, filters should be installed in systems circulating air. They require regular cleansing or replacement. Many persons who are sensitive to pollens can reduce exposure enough to keep themselves fairly comfortable by sleeping in an air-conditioned room. When this is not possible, a window fan combined with a paper or glass-wool filter will give some relief by reducing the pollen count and cooling the room. Keeping the windows closed will also reduce the pollen count in the house. For patients

[30] Hugh Rodman Leavell and E. Gurney Clark, *Preventive Medicine for the Doctor in His Community*, McGraw-Hill Book Company, New York, 1958, p. 280.
[31] *Ibid.*, p. 280.
[32] Synthetic fiber.
[33] *Ibid.*, p. 280.

who have severe hay fever or asthma, and who are able to afford it, a trip to an area in which the pollen count is low may be indicated. Before the advent of air conditioning, certain areas of the United States were havens for hay fever sufferers. Persons who are sensitive to fungi are advised to avoid damp climates. Damp basements can be dried by the use of electrically operated dehumidifiers. Anyone who has worked in the emergency room of a large city hospital cannot escape being impressed by the number of patients who come in for treatment of asthma on a warm, moist summer evening. In fact, physicians and nurses can sometimes be heard to say, "This is an asthma night." Many persons who are allergic learn to identify substances and circumstances that activate their symptoms and can plan to avoid them.

Animal danders are another common cause of hypersensitivity. Hypersensitive persons should be advised against acquiring a dog or cat if they do not already have one. When there is a pet in the home its effect can be tested by removing it for a month or so. If the condition of the patient is improved, then, of course, the patient and his family should be advised to dispose of the pet. Should there be no difference in the patient's condition, there is no reason to do so.

In the control of contact dermatitis, the same general principles hold. The first step is to identify the offending antigen or antigens and then to make a plan whereby contact with it or them can be avoided. Because of the variety of contactants, this is not always as easy to do as to narrate. The importance of prompt action cannot be overestimated. Secondary changes including infection may cause more problems than the original dermatitis. Sometimes, as in the instance of a housewife who is allergic to detergents, protection merely involves wearing rubber gloves when using detergents or substituting soap for them. To avoid dermatitis, she may have to wear gloves every time she uses a detergent.

At other times the problem is more complicated. For example, streptomycin sulfate has been found to induce hypersensitivity in a high proportion of those who work with it either in its preparation in factories or in hospitals. This problem has been minimized since streptomycin sulfate is now supplied in disposable syringes. According to Goodman and Gilman[34] sensitivity reactions to streptomycin sulfate are more common among physicians and nurses than they are among patients who receive the drug. Goodman and Gilman[35] also state that skin reactions to penicillin are most common after topical applications. Contact dermatitis can occur in persons who handle penicillin, but this does not occur as commonly as it does with streptomycin sulfate. The amount of either of these drugs required to cause a reaction in sensitive persons may be infinitesimal. In one hospital where nurses had become sensitized to streptomycin sulfate, it was necessary to assign them to units where patients did not receive streptomycin.

[34] *Op. cit.*, p. 1370.
[35] *Ibid.*, p. 1348.

On occasion, a nurse may develop a sensitivity to other drugs. In the experience of the writer one nurse was so highly sensitive to morphine that she developed a dermatitis each time she prepared even a single dose of it. In order to continue in the practice of nursing she had to arrange to be relieved of any responsibility for administering morphine, or being near where the drug was prepared. In nurses who develop contact dermatitis, the problem of control is often difficult. Any measures that can be taken to prevent its development are well worth taking. When the possibility of exposure to a sentitizing agent exists, thorough washing with soap and water will serve to remove the agent and thereby reduce the intensity of the contact. For example, after exposure to poison ivy a shower should be taken as soon as possible. Although both soap and water should be generously applied this should be accompanied by minimum rubbing of the skin as the antigen of poison ivy does not induce sensitivity unless it is rubbed into the skin.

To summarize: The first step in the accomplishment of the objective, to limit or prevent the exposure of the patient to substances to which he is hypersensitive, is to identify the offending agent or agents. In some instances this can be accomplished by skin tests. In others, the antigenic agents cannot be identified by skin tests, but may be by establishing a cause and effect relationship. This requires a form of medical detective work. The patient and others, including the nurse, try to identify the conditions associated with the onset of symptoms. The relationship of various elements to the patient's allergic manifestations can be tested by eliminating possible antigens one at a time from his environment and observing the results. In instances in which there is doubt, a suspected antigen may be further tested by its reintroduction into the environment of the patient. Once the causative agent is identified, the next step is to plan how contact with the agent can be reduced or eliminated. Points to be considered include the nature of the antigen, its source or reservoir, vehicles by which it is transmitted, and portals of entry. The degree of sensitivity of the person is also a factor. In the person who is highly sensitive to an antigen, all exposure may have to be prevented. In the person who is less sensitive, restrictions on exposure may be less stringent.

When an allergic patient experiences an acute response to an allergen, his symptoms may be such that he is incapacitated or his survival threatened. At this time the second objective, to relieve or mitigate the allergic response, takes priority. The urgency of the situation depends on the type and acuteness of the reactions of the patient. Prompt and energetic treatment may be necessary to save the life of a patient in anaphylactic shock or in status asthmaticus. Protection from further exposure to foreign serum or an antigenic drug and palliation of his symptoms may meet the major requirements of a patient with serum or drug sickness. The patient with hay fever (allergic rhinitis) may be miserable, but his life is not usually in danger.

Drugs have an important role in the prevention and relief of allergic responses of various types. One of the most generally useful drugs in the therapy of allergic disorders is epinephrine. It is believed to act directly on effector cells, stimulating some and inhibiting others. Since the action of epinephrine is similar to that of the sympathetic nervous system, it is said to be sympathomimetic. It antagonizes the effects of the parasympathetic nervous system (cholinergic), other cholinergic chemicals, and histamine. In disorders such as anaphylaxis and acute asthma it may be lifesaving. Epinephrine should always be in readiness in situations where an anaphylactic response is a possibility. Because of its powerful bronchial dilatory action, it is often effective in the relief of asthmatic attacks that are resistant to other drugs. It affords symptomatic relief in urticaria, serum sickness, hay fever, angioneurotic edema, and other similar allergic disorders. It may be administered by subcutaneous, intramuscular, or intravenous injection or by inhalation. The usual range of dosage for subcutaneous injection for adults is from 0.2 to 0.5 ml of a 1:1000 aqueous solution. Despite the fact that epinephrine is dispensed in ampoules containing 1 ml, a nurse should not give more than 0.5 ml without special instructions from the physician. Smaller dosages are indicated when the patient is receiving the drug for the first time. Patients with hyperthyroidism and hypertension are especially susceptible to the effects of epinephrine, and it is contraindicated in these conditions. In any patient, an overdosage of epinephrine predisposes the patient to ventricular fibrillation.

When epinephrine is administered by inhalation, the exact dosage is difficult to control. To deliver epinephrine to the bronchi requires that the solution be converted to a fine mist. It also requires that the solution be at least 1 part epinephrine to 100 parts of water. Goodman and Gilman[36] make the following recommendations. An atomizer or nebulizer should be made entirely of glass or plastic. When the patient uses a hand-operated atomizer he may need considerable practice to coordinate squeezing of the bulb with inspiration. Proper coordination is necessary to deliver and distribute the drug through the tracheobronchial tree. Oxygen may be used in a nebulizer to convert the solution to a fine mist and distribute it to the desired area. Whether an atomizer, a mask, or a nebulizer is used, the drug is inhaled through the mouth. Goodman and Gilman[37] emphasize that the patient should be cautioned against overusage, as it causes dryness of the throat and irritation of the tracheobronchial tree. Should irritation of the airway occur, the patient may have to discontinue inhalations for several days. The nurse should note the frequency with which patients inhale epinephrine, and if it seems excessive, she should caution the patient or bring her observation to the attention of the physician. Because swallowing epinephrine causes epigastric pain, the patient should be taught to wash his mouth after each administration. Sometimes the mucus that is expectorated is pink, but changes in the color of the drug are responsible and this does not necessarily indicate bleeding.

[36] *Ibid.*, p. 498.
[37] *Ibid.*, p. 498.

Ephedrine sulfate may be used to relax the smooth muscle of the bronchi in asthma. It has an advantage over epinephrine because it can be administered orally. Theophylline U.S.P. is also prescribed because it relaxes the smooth muscle in the tracheobronchial tree.

The antihistaminics are a group of drugs providing relief in a number of allergic disorders. Among those in which antihistaminics are most beneficial are hay fever, serum sickness, urticaria, drug reactions, and angioneurotic edema. According to Goodman and Gilman,[38] the antihistaminics have been disappointing in the treatment of asthma. The antihistaminic drugs have two general effects believed to be important in the treatment of allergy. They are supposed to counteract the effect of histamine by displacing histamine from receptor sites in the cell. This effect is called the blocking action of the antihistaminic drugs. Some authorities question the validity of this concept of their action. The chemical structure of some antihistamines bears little superficial resemblance to histamine. Therapeutic dosages of these drugs cause some depression of the central nervous system; they have a sedative effect in some persons and in others they cause restlessness, insomnia, and nervousness.

Cortisone and ACTH have proved to be useful, not only in the relief of symptoms in acute attacks of asthma, hay fever, allergic dermatitis, and drug reactions, but also in the treatment of chronic states. In some patients the relief lasts only as long as the drug is administered; in others relief may continue for months or longer.

Itching is frequently referred to as a troublesome symptom of allergic dermatoses. While itching does not threaten the life of the patient and does not always incapacitate him, it can cause him a good bit of discomfort. It may also reduce his efficiency or be incapacitating. Since the introduction of antihistaminic drugs, itching is often easier to control than it was in the past. In the care of the patient, the nurse may add to the comfort of the patient by the prevention of overheating of the room, as sweating increases itching. A cool environmental temperature reduces itching, while a warm one increases it. When wet dressings are ordered, at least 20 layers of gauze or an equal thickness of turkish toweling should be used. Dressings should be applied loosely and kept well soaked. One of the frequently used solutions is aluminum subacetate, or Burrows' solution, a mild astringent. To prevent increasing the concentration of the solution, water should be used to remoisten dried dressings.[39] When the patient is able to moisten his own dressings, he may be given some of the solution or water and a syringe so that he can keep his dressings moist. Though a nonporous material may be placed under the dressing to protect the bed, it should not be wrapped around the dressing, as interference with evaporation decreases heat loss and predisposes to elevating the temperature of the involved area. Before selecting material to protect the

---

[38] *Ibid.*, p. 663.
[39] When a solution is used repeatedly to moisten the same dressings, the concentration of the solution increases. Water evaporates but the solute does not and its concentration, therefore, rises.

bed, the nurse should ascertain whether or not the patient is allergic to the material to be used.

Since most of the injury to the skin in allergic conditions is caused by scratching, every effort should be made to prevent and relieve the itching. The fingernails should be cut short. Sometimes the patient gets some relief by scratching the bed. Few symptoms are more unpleasant than itching. A patient with a severe dermatitis is likely to be irritable, because he is uncomfortable and has difficulty in obtaining rest and sleep. Whenever lotions or salves are applied to the skin in dermatitis, the nurse should observe the skin for signs of increasing irritation, that is, redness, swelling, or vesiculation, as some patients develop a sensitivity to the chemicals used in therapy.

Since contact dermatitis is likely to be a recurring problem, the patient should be taught to identify and to avoid agents in his environment to which he is sensitive. He should also be encouraged to institute palliative measures as soon as he notes the characteristic lesions on his skin. Scratching is to be avoided, as it excoriates the skin and predisposes to more itching as well as to infection. For many persons, contact dermatitis is a long-term problem. As in many other chronic disorders, control depends on the willingness and ability of the patient to carry out the preventive and therapeutic program.

What are the elements in the accomplishment of the third objective—to increase resistance to an antigen?

To accomplish the third objective, that is, to increase the resistance of the patient to a specific antigen, the patient may be given small but increasing doses of an antigen over a period of time. The procedure for raising the resistance of the patient to a specific antigen is known as desensitization. In addition to the desensitization of a patient to foreign proteins, as previously discussed, some patients with hay fever benefit from being treated with offending pollens. Therapy is usually started two or three months before the expected onset of symptoms. According to Sherman,[40] the injected antigen stimulates the formation of what is known as the blocking antibody. The blocking antibody is distinct from the pre-existing sensitizing antibody. Increased tolerance for the antigen appears to be due to the blocking antibody.

Since emotional factors may predispose to, precipitate, perpetuate, or contribute to the development of complications, their significance in each patient may require evaluation. When emotional factors are of importance, the patient may require assistance in learning to identify situations aggravating his disorder and either avoid them or modify his reaction to them. For example, Mrs. Cornwall usually develops an asthmatic attack when she smells, or imagines she smells, cigar smoke. Since the physician believes that emotional factors are probably involved in precipitating and prolonging Mrs. Cornwall's asthmatic attacks, he explores this possibility with her.

[40] William B. Sherman, "Hay Fever," in Cecil-Loeb, *A Textbook of Medicine, Op. cit.,* p. 437.

The discussion thus far has dealt with the immunological tissue responses of the body, factors that incite them, and methods of predicting and controlling them. The capacity of the organism to produce antibodies is one of its mechanisms of defense against foreign invaders. It arises out of the capacity of the cells of the body to distinguish self from nonself. Although the self-recognition system is not fully developed at birth, it develops shortly thereafter. As with other mechanisms of defense, immunological responses are useful when they are initiated in response to truly harmful agents and in the amounts required by the situation. They are harmful when they are initiated in response to harmless substances or when the response is deficient or excessive. Abnormal immunological responses are of two types, immediate and delayed. In the immediate type of hypersensitivity, antibodies circulate in the blood stream. Many of the diseases of allergy are of this type. In the delayed type of hypersensitivity, antibodies are believed to reside in the cells of the reticulo-endothelial system, including lymphoid cells. Conditions such as contact dermatitis, poison ivy, and tissue reaction to the tubercle bacillus are of the delayed type. Recent experiments provide evidence to support the theory that many chronic diseases may result from delayed hypersensitivity. This group of diseases is also referred to as autoimmune diseases. Among the autoimmune diseases are rheumatic fever and glomerulonephritis. Perhaps information gained from studies of how to suppress the immunological response to foreign tissue will contribute to a better understanding of diseases in which hypersensitivity is important. With new knowledge successful methods of prevention and control may be developed. This is a whole new and exciting field in medicine.

In the care of patients with the diseases of allergy, nurses have an opportunity to assist in the identification of agents that act as antigens, they care for patients during acute phases of illness, and they help to prepare the patient to live with his disorder.

To this point the body defenses that have been under discussion have been those that involve the body as a whole. In addition to these responses, cells at the site of injury also react to injury in a characteristic and more or less stereotyped fashion. Similar to the more widespread responses, the local reactions to injury serve to limit the area of injury, to prepare the area for repair, and finally to replace the damaged tissue. The reaction which serves to limit the area of injury and to prepare it for repair is known as inflammation. When the quantity of tissue that is damaged is small and the growth potential of cells in the area is adequate, healing is primarily by regeneration of the normal tissue. When the quantity of tissue that is lost is large or the cells are unable to multiply, repair depends on the formation of fibrous connective or scar tissue. The healing of Mr. Allen's burns offers a good example. All of his burned areas reacted by becoming inflamed. In the areas in which the damage to skin was limited to the first and second degrees or, according to the newer classifications, to a partial thickness, epithelial cells remaining in the skin of the injured area underwent hyperplasia. Healing was, therefore, by replacement of the normal tissues. In the parts burned to the third degree, classified as a full-thickness burn, tissue damage was so great that epithelial tissue was either absent or inadequate to restore the continuity of the skin by hyperplasia of epithelial tissue. Healing was, therefore, by the formation of scar tissue.

The local reaction of the tissues that serves to limit the area of injury and prepare it for repair is inflammation. Because inflammation is one of the most common responses of the body to injury, a knowledge of the mechanisms involved in inflammation provides a basis for understanding the changes that occur in a wide variety of diseases. Essentially the response of the tissue injured by an antigen-antibody reaction is one of inflammation. Even in those conditions in which inflammation is not considered to be an aspect of the disease, it may play a role. For example, in some patients who have cancer, the body responds to the neoplastic cells (new growth cells) much as it does to a foreign body, with the result that surrounding tissues are inflamed.

What has been the historical development of knowledge of inflammation?

Basic knowledge of the acute inflammatory process can be presented by tracing the history or the evolution of the understanding of inflammation. Almost 20 centuries elapsed between the time the cardinal signs of inflammation were first described and the fundamental nature of the response was understood. This is not to imply that knowledge of the process is yet complete, for it is not. Similar to knowledge in other areas, progress has been uneven and sometimes delayed by false steps and interpretations. Hopps[41] states that in the first century A.D., Celsus described the four cardinal signs of inflammation as rubor (redness), calor (heat), dolor (pain), and tumor (swelling). About a century later Galen added a fifth cardinal sign—loss of function. It was not until almost the end of the eighteenth century that John Hunter first established inflammation as a mechanism of defense. Cohnheim, a student of Virchow's, recognized the part that blood vessels play in inflammation. He also described the margination and emigration of leukocytes. The part played by the leukocytes in phagocytosis was established by the Russian zoologist Metchnikoff when his study of inflammation was published in 1901. Though knowledge of the biochemical changes in the inflammatory process was, and still is, incomplete, with the discoveries of Metchnikoff understanding of the fundamental nature of the process was established.

What is inflammation?

Inflammation may be defined as an active and aggressive response of tissue to injury. It involves the blood vessels, the fluid and cellular compo-

[41] Howard C. Hopps, *Principles of Pathology*, 2nd ed., Appleton-Century-Crofts, Inc., New York, 1964, p. 130.

nents of the blood, and the surrounding connective tissue. It is a useful response, because it serves to destroy or neutralize the injurious agent and to prepare the tissue for repair. As will be seen when the process is described in more detail, inflammation may be accompanied by harmful effects, by virtue of its location, or by an ineffective, excessive, or inappropriate response.

Despite a tendency to think of inflammation as a response initiated primarily by bacterial infections, it can be induced by any agent causing injury to tissue cells, including mechanical and other forms of physical injury, as well as by chemical and other living agents and allergic reactions. The injuring agent may have its origin outside the body (extrinsic) or within the body (intrinsic). An example of a condition in which there is an inflammatory response to an intrinsic substance is atherosclerosis. Cholesterol and other lipids accumulate in the intima of blood vessels and stimulate an inflammatory response in one or more arteries.

What part do blood vessels play in inflammation?

One way to learn about inflammation is to place the web of a foot of a frog or a rabbit's ear chamber under a microscope and then observe the changes occurring in the blood vessels before and after the tissue is injured. Cells can be injured by placing a drop of a chemical irritant, such as croton oil or a concentrated acid, on the tissue to be examined. If the observer watches carefully, the vessels may be seen to constrict momentarily. Constriction is extremely transitory and is of no consequence as far as accomplishing the purposes of inflammation. Following constriction, arterioles, then venules, and finally capillaries dilate, and more blood vessels come into view. The blood can be seen to be coursing rapidly through the vessels and the tissue becomes bright red. The active increase in the flow of blood through the tissue is known as hyperemia.

Associated with the greater blood flow is an increase in the filtration pressure of the blood and in the permeability of the capillaries with the result that a large volume of fluid, known as the inflammatory exudate, is moved into the interstitial space. In minor injuries, the increase in capillary permeability may be small so that little extra fluid escapes into the injured area. Neither is there an increase in the rate at which larger molecules in the blood plasma diffuse from the blood into the injured area. In more severe injuries, large molecules, most particularly proteins, escape into the inflammatory exudate in increased quantities. The effects of this loss of protein are not serious when the inflamed area is small. However, when the area is large, or when the loss continues over an extended period of time, the consequences may be serious. As an illustration, the patient who is burned may lose enormous quantities of proteins as well as of water and electrolytes into the burned area. Moreover, the absorption of chemicals released at the site of the burned or injured tissue may increase the permeability of capillaries throughout the body causing a generalized edema. Loss of fluid leads to a decrease in blood volume and concentration of the blood of the patient.

The extent to which fluid escapes into the tissue of the patient who has been burned can be illustrated by Mr. Allen. Examination of the intake and output record reveals that during the first 48 hours after he was burned, the ratio of his fluid intake to output was 13,000 ml to 2,000 ml. Even when another 2,000 ml is added to his output to account for fluid lost by other avenues, he still lost at least 10 l of fluid into the burned area. In addition to water, he lost protein and electrolytes. According to Artz and Reiss,[42] the average human blister fluid contains 4 gm of protein per 100 ml of fluid. Because serum albumin is smaller in molecular size than the other blood proteins, a higher proportion of albumin is lost into the inflammatory exudate than of either globulin or fibrinogen.

The increase in filtration pressure plus the greater permeability of the capillaries upsets the balance between the quantity of fluid leaving the capillary and the quantity returning, in favor of the fluid escaping from the capillaries. The disequilibrium is further aggravated by the loss of protein from the blood plasma to the interstitial fluid. As protein is added to interstitial fluid, it increases its colloid osmotic pressure. When the quantity lost from the blood is large, the level of protein in the blood falls and with it the colloid osmotic pressure of the blood. The three factors contributing in varying degrees to the production of the inflammatory exudate may therefore be summarized as: (1) the elevation of the filtration pressure of the blood, (2) the increased permeability of the capillaries, and (3) the increase in the colloid osmotic pressure of the tissue fluid in the area. The result is inflammatory edema.

Why do the blood vessels dilate during the inflammatory process?

As is often true, it is easier to describe what happens than to explain why it happens. However, the current explanation is that on injury, cells release a chemical or chemicals acting either directly or reflexly to dilate the blood vessels and to increase their permeability. Sir Thomas Lewis first described such a substance which, because of its similarity to histamine, he called the H-substance. Hopps[43] states that present evidence indicates that the substance is probably a mixture of histamine and serotonin. Menkin[44] has isolated a substance from the inflammatory exudate which he calls leukotaxin. It increases capillary permeability and, in addition, attracts leukocytes.

During the early phase of the inflammatory reaction, the blood moves rapidly through the tissues. Later, depending on the severity of the injury,

[42] Curtis P. Artz and Eric Reiss, *The Treatment of Burns,* W. B. Saunders Co., Philadelphia, 1957, p. 31.
[43] *Op. cit.,* p. 132.
[44] Valy Menkin, *Biochemical Mechanisms in Inflammation,* Charles C Thomas, Springfield, Illinois, 1956, p. 11.

blood flow slows. The factors contributing to slowing include: (1) the increased concentration of the blood in the capillaries that results from the loss of fluid into the inflamed area, (2) the increase in tissue fluid pressure which counteracts the increase in filtration pressure of the blood, and (3) possibly increased resistance to the flow of blood by the blood cells that adhere to the vascular endothelium.

With the slowing of the flow of blood, cells, especially the leukocytes, settle out of the main stream and line the vascular endothelium. This is known as the pavementing of leukocytes. Normally, the blood cells are carried in the center of the stream with the leukocytes in the center and the smaller cells or erythrocytes surrounding them. The erythrocytes are separated from the vascular epithelium by a layer of plasma. In the inflammatory process, red cells tend to adhere together in clumps (blood sludge) that are larger than the leukocytes. They replace the leukocytes in the center of the stream. The leukocytes migrate peripherally, adhere to and enter the capillary wall, and pass through it by the process known as emigration. Although leukocytes are usually attracted to the inflamed area, they are occasionally repelled. The factors responsible for the direction of the movement of leukocytes are known as chemotaxis. Attraction of the leukocytes with movement in the direction of the irritant is called positive chemotaxis. When leukocytes are repelled by the irritant so that they move away from it, this is known as negative chemotaxis.

Retardation of the blood flow may be so great that the blood moves forward only when the heart is contracting. This is one cause of a throbbing sensation. As long as some blood flow to the tissues is maintained, the process may be reversed and the tissues restored with little or no permanent harm. Blood flow, however, may be stopped by the formation of blood clots (thrombosis) in small vessels and by the pressure of inflammatory edema. Swelling due to inflammatory edema is a particular hazard in tissues that have little space for distention, such as the brain or an extremity encased in a bandage or plaster cast. As the inflammatory edema increases, pressure on the small blood vessels increases, thereby decreasing their capacity to carry blood. The problem is aggravated by the fact that the venous return is restricted first, so that although blood continues to enter the tissue, it adds to the swelling. Unless the condition is corrected, tissue pressure eventually exceeds the arterial pressure and the blood flow to the tissue ceases. When an extremity is involved, swelling, pain, numbness and tingling, bluish discoloration of the skin, coldness, and inability to move the part are warning signs. When the brain is affected, signs of increasing intracranial pressure develop. (These are discussed in Chapter 13, Part B.) Proper elevation of the extremity encased in a cast will often support the venous return enough to prevent excessive swelling.

To illustrate, Mrs. Willow suffered a fractured tibia in a traffic accident. The fracture was reduced and the leg was encased in a cast. She was placed in a bed in which the mattress was slightly depressed at the foot of the bed. A nurse found her crying with pain and begging for a "shot." Instead of administering an analgesic medication, the nurse examined Mrs. Willow's toes and found them to be cold, blue, and swollen. She could move her toes only with difficulty. The nurse then elevated Mrs. Willow's leg so that gravity aided the venous return.[45] She also told Mrs. Willow that she expected that her pain would be relieved shortly by the elevation of her foot and leg, but if it was not, she would call her physician and obtain a prescription for a pain-relieving medication. Should elevation fail to relieve the pain, the physician would also be appraised of this fact. Should the cast be too tight, the cast might have to be cut to relieve the pressure. In about half an hour the nurse returned to see Mrs. Willow. She was comfortable and about to begin eating her breakfast. Her toes had improved in color and she could wiggle them.

What factors determine the character of the fluid exudate?

The character of the fluid exudate depends on the severity of the injury. In less severe injuries there may be very little exudate and what there is may differ very little in composition from normal interstitial fluid. The more severe the injury is, the greater is the capillary permeability and the larger are the particles escaping into the interstitial fluid. The greater the degree of injury to the blood vessels, the more components of the blood are found in the inflammatory exudate. In mild injuries the fluid exudate is serous in nature; that is, it is similar in appearance and composition to the blood serum. In more severe injuries the exudate contains large amounts of fibrin, and in the most serious ones it contains large numbers of red blood cells. The latter is the so-called hemorrhagic inflammation. The presence of large numbers of erythrocytes in the inflammatory exudate is responsible for so-called "black" smallpox or meningitis. The fibrinogen escaping into the exudate is converted to fibrin and forms a sort of meshwork structure in the inflamed area. It also obstructs small lymph vessels and capillaries. Authorities disagree about the function of the fibrin. Some, such as Menkin,[46] believe that it prevents dissemination of organisms by providing a mechanical barrier to their spread. Hopps[47] states that the fibrin probably acts to delay the spread of microorganisms by providing a sort of maze through which bacteria must pass before they can escape into the surrounding tissue. This also increases the likelihood of the bacteria coming in contact with phagocytic cells. The fibrin network may contribute to the difficulty of removing all microorganisms from tissues, even when the microorganisms are sensitive to antibiotics. The network acts to protect microorganisms by limiting their exposure to therapeutic agents. Until the inflamed area is well walled off, it should be protected from trauma.

[45] The nurse applied a law of thermodynamics in which it is stated that energy runs downhill.
[46] *Op. cit.,* p. 111.
[47] *Op. cit.,* p. 139.

What is the role of the cellular elements in the inflammatory exudate?

Although cells playing an active role in the acute inflammatory process have phagocytic action, they are classified in different ways. Cells carried in the blood, such as the polymorphonuclear leukocytes, are called wandering cells. Those found in tissues, such as Küpffer cells in the venous sinuses of the liver, are referred to as fixed cells. Cells may also be classified according to their size as microphages and macrophages. The microphages, which are the most abundant type of phagocyte, are free in the blood. Microphages are of two types, the polymorphonuclear leukocytes, or granular leukocytes, and the lymphocytes. The granular leukocytes include the neutrophils, the eosinophils, and the basophils. Of these the neutrophils are most important in acute inflammation, the eosinophils are increased in allergy, and the function of the basophils is not known.

Neutrophils, similar to other granular leukocytes, have their origin in the bone marrow. Although neutrophils are short-lived cells, living only three or four days, the healthy bone marrow is capable of replacing them in large numbers. Some drugs, such as aminopyrine, sulfanilamide, and nitrogen mustards, depress the bone marrow, so that following their administration the production of granulocytes may be diminished or even absent. As discussed in the preceding chapter, radioactive materials, including X rays, have a similar effect. The capacity of the bone marrow to tolerate chemical and physical agents depressing its activity places a limitation on their use in treatment. Injury to the bone marrow by aminopyrine and sulfonilamide occurs when it is hypersensitive to a particular agent. Not all persons, therefore, experience depression of the bone marrow after ingestion of these agents. In contrast, nitrogen mustard and ionizing radiation have similar, though not identical, effects on cells. The nitrogen mustards contain two or more alkyl groups which react with some of the constituents of cells. Radioactive materials injure the cells by ionizing substances within them. Though cells vary in sensitivity, all cells are injured when they receive a large enough dose of either type of agent.

When the number of neutrophils is markedly deficient, the condition is known as agranulocytosis. A better terminology would be granulocytopenia. Granulocytopenia is a serious disorder because the capacity of the person to protect himself against microorganisms is impaired. Evidence of a loss of the capacity of tissues to protect themselves is seen as ulcerations in the mouth, pharynx, gastrointestinal tract, and vagina. When infection develops in the patient with agranulocytosis, his prognosis is very poor. Special precautions should be taken to protect persons with agranulocytosis from infection.

What is the role of the neutrophil in inflammation?

The neutrophil plays an important role in the inflammation, both when it is alive and after it dies. It is actively phagocytic when alive. After it dies it releases proteolytic enzymes which digest not only other dead cells and bacteria, but itself. Thus neutrophils aid not only in overcoming the injurious agent, but also in ridding the area of debris. The latter process is an essential step in the preparation of the tissue for healing. Wood[48] postulates that dead neutrophils release a substance which is pyrogenic (fever-producing) when absorbed into the blood stream in sufficient amounts. If this hypothesis is correct, the neutrophil contributes not only to the local reaction, but to the total response of the individual.

What is the role of the lymphocyte in inflammation?

The lymphocyte is the second most abundant leukocyte. It is smaller than the granulocyte and has a large nucleus with relatively little cytoplasm. It does not appear to be phagocytic to particulate matter.

Monocytes, though phagocytic, are less so than either granulocytes or macrophages. According to Hopps,[49] their important functions are to develop into macrophages and to produce antibodies.

The plasma cell is not ordinarily found in the circulating blood. It is most commonly found at the site of chronic infections. (It probably also produces antibodies.)

How do macrophages differ in structure and function from microphages?

Macrophages, which may either be fixed or wandering, are large phagocytic cells having a number of important functions. They act as scavengers. They phagocytize foreign bodies, cellular debris, and the more resistant organisms, such as the *Mycobacterium tuberculosis* and fungi. They are called upon to remove such substances as silica, talc, mineral oil, and sutures. They are essential to the reaction in tuberculosis as they form the epithelioid cells. They fuse to form giant cells, which are also found in the tubercle (the specific lesion of tuberculosis). They are necessary to the formation of fibrous connective tissue, as they mature into fibroblasts.

Fixed macrophages are large branching cells that comprise an important group of phagocytic cells found in the reticuloendothelial system. These cells are distributed throughout the body, particularly in areas where blood flow is slow, such as in venous sinuses in the liver (Küpffer cells), the spleen, and the bone marrow. They also are found in the lymph sinuses in lymph nodes. A third type of macrophage, the histocyte, is found in solid tissues. Apperly[50] compares the fixed microphages to the rural police, as they are scattered through the body at strategic points. They are highly phagocytic. They digest bacteria, foreign substances, worn-out red blood cells, and other cells, as well as remove certain dyes. They are also believed to form antibodies.

[48] W. Barry Wood, "Fever," *Scientific American,* June, 1957, p. 68.
[49] *Op cit.,* p. 188.
[50] Frank L. Apperly, *Patterns of Disease,* J. B. Lippincott Co., Philadelphia, 1951, p. 59.

Summarizing the role of leukocytes in inflammation, leukocytes are essential to the inflammatory response. They function by phagocytosis (digestion) of foreign bodies, bacteria, and the products of inflammation. Some of them form antibodies. Macrophages not only have a high phagocytic power, and form antibodies, but they contribute to the repair of the damage by maturing into fibroblasts and forming collagen. Without the power of phagocytosis the organism is at the mercy of any foreign invader. Not only do leukocytes increase in number in the injured area, but the number in the circulating blood is usually increased in all but minor injuries. The leukocyte count may reach 30,000 cells per cubic millimeter of blood or rise even higher in severe systemic reactions to infection or tissue injury. In acute inflammation, the rise is usually in the neutrophils, particularly in the less mature forms. As neutrophils mature the nucleus undergoes segmentation; therefore, the percentage of segmented cells drops when the number of neutrophils rises rapidly. In a few infections such as acute infectious mononucleosis and whooping cough, the lymphocyte count rises.

The number of leukocytes may also fall (leukopenia) in a number of infections. Infections in which this is true include typhoid fever, brucellosis, and malaria. As was stated earlier, the count may be depressed in overwhelming infections or in any condition having a toxic effect on the bone marrow.

Why does Leukocytosis occur?

The reasons for leukocytosis are not known. It occurs not only in acute bacterial infections, such as pneumonia, but in conditions in which there is death of tissue, such as myocardial infarction and advanced malignant neoplasia. With leukocytosis there is often an associated increase in the sedimentation rate. The degree of increase in leukocyte count or sedimentation rate provides clues to the severity, but not to the specific nature, of the illness. Whether or not the level of the leukocytosis is in keeping with the apparent severity of illness is also significant. The obviously sick patient with a falling leukocyte count has a poor prognosis, for it indicates that the response of the patient is inadequate to the degree of illness.

In the preceding pages, the nature of the changes taking place in the blood vessels and in the blood cells occurring in inflammation have been considered. These changes have two purposes: (1) to destroy or localize the injuring agent, and (2) to prepare the tissue for repair.

How is the irritant localized and destroyed?

The dilitation and increased permeability of the blood vessels bring fluid to the area which contains antibodies and other substances to neutralize the toxins or to destroy the irritant. This fluid also dilutes the toxins and helps to restore homeostatic conditions by reducing the hydrogen ion concentration. It contains nutrients required for the release of energy and for the repair of cells.

The leukocytes in the exudate phagocytose and destroy the irritant and the cellular debris.

What is the sequence of events that follows acute injury of the tissue?

The early changes which have been discussed proceed somewhat as follows: The tissue is injured by an inflammant—heat, cold, radiant rays, chemicals, trauma, microorganisms, or some combination of these. Almost immediately the blood vessels in the area dilate and capillary permeability increases. The extent to which these changes take place depends on the severity of the injury. Blood flow increases and there is an outpouring of fluid and leukocytes. The polymorphonuclear leukocytes move toward the irritant and surround it. When the inflammatory response is initiated by bacteria able to reproduce themselves, the bacteria may at first overcome the leukocytes. Leukocytes, however, are poured into the area and eventually they turn the tide in favor of the body. In the process, however, tissue cells, bacteria, and leukocytes are killed. Fibrinogen which escapes from the blood is converted to fibrin. It forms a meshwork in the area. Antibodies are formed in increasing quantities and support the action of the phagocytes by neutralizing bacterial toxins. The wall of leukocytes surrounding the irritant deepens. The leukocytes are supported by a net formed of fibrin. The inner zone of leukocytes is composed of polymorphonuclear cells with lymphocytes, monocytes, and macrophages at the periphery. The area is bathed by a fluid rich in antibodies and nutrients. Obstruction of small blood and lymph vessels helps to block the spread of microorganisms. If the response is successful, the few bacterial cells escaping from the area are phagocytosed in the blood and lymph. The central mass in the inflamed tissue is composed of dead cells and living and dead leukocytes and bacteria. These are digested. The entire zone of inflammation is called an abscess. The abscess may rupture spontaneously or be opened. Drainage of the abscess to the outside facilitates healing by aiding in the removal of materials that would otherwise have to be digested and absorbed before healing can begin. Rupture of the abscess into a serous cavity, such as occurs in perforation of the appendix, leads to the dissemination of the contents of the abscess as well as those of the intestine into the peritoneal cavity, thus predisposing to localized or generalized peritonitis. Perforation with the development of peritonitis is one of the most serious complications in acute appendicitis. When leakage from the appendix is minimal, the body may be able to wall off the area with the formation of an appendiceal abscess.

Rupture of an abscess into the pleural space results in a condition called empyema, a disorder that is often resistant to treatment. Although the term "empyema," when used by itself, usually refers to an accumulation of pus in the pleural cavity, it actually means a collection of pus in any natural body cavity. Therefore an accumulation of pus in the gall bladder is also empyema.

Understanding the nature of the walling-off process of inflammation is of importance in the practice of nursing. Premature or improper opening of an abscess may interfere with the mechanisms of the body for limiting spread of microorganisms and lead to their widespread dissemination. Manipulation of boils and pimples should be avoided until they have a well-defined area of pus in the center. Then they should be opened under surgical conditions. Care should be taken not to squeeze a pimple or a boil forcefully and the extruded pus should be prevented from coming in contact with the surrounding skin. Pus contains living bacteria and proteolytic enzymes that are able to digest both dead and living tissue. The combination of protein-digesting enzymes and viable bacteria predisposes to infection of the tissues with which they come in contact. Anyone changing dressings, covering draining wounds should protect himself by using instruments to handle the dressings or by wearing gloves.

In addition to draining at the surface, an abscess may terminate in other ways. When an abscess is small or the injury to the tissue structure is minimal, the products of inflammation may be digested and absorbed into the circulation. This process is known as resolution. Following pneumonia, healing takes place by resolution. Enzymes released by the degenerating leukocytes digest and liquefy the material in the alveoli. Much of the exudate is removed by coughing. Following recovery from uncomplicated *pneumococcal* pneumonia there is no evidence of past disease. The lung is restored to its original condition and there is no evidence of scar tissue having been formed.

Still another way an abscess may terminate is for it to drain to the surface of the body through a sinus or tract. A sinus differs from a fistula in that a sinus is a tract draining an abscess, while a fistula is a tract between two hollow organs or between a hollow organ and the outside. An example of a sinus is a tract from a mediastinal abscess to a bronchus. An example of a fistula is a tract or passageway between the rectum and the vagina, or from the colon through the abdominal wall to the outside.

Ulcers and erosions may also result from an inflammatory process. They are alike inasmuch as the surface layer of tissue, skin, or mucous membrane is lost. They differ in that an ulcer extends through the covering membrane, while an erosion involves only the covering membrane. Examples of ulcers include peptic ulcers and varicose ulcers. A common site of an erosion is the cervix uteri. In the formation of ulcers and erosions, the body mechanism for maintaining the integrity of tissue breaks down and the tissue destruction follows. In most people the tissue lining the stomach and duodenum is protected from the digesting action of gastric secretions. Any condition that upsets the balance between tissue resistance and protection from the digesting action of the gastric secretions so that digestion is favored predisposes to peptic ulcer formation. Varicose ulcers are essentially the result of inadequate tissue nutrition.

*What are some of the factors affecting the possible outcome
of an inflammatory response?*

The outcome of an inflammatory response depends on many factors including the agent responsible for injury to the tissues, the effectiveness of the
individual's mechanisms of defense, and the specific tissues that are involved,
as well as the nature and extent of the injury to the tissues. Factors influencing
the capacity of an individual to respond to injury include his age and general
state of health and of nutrition. When microorganisms are responsible, the
body may or may not be able to localize them. Some bacteria are difficult to
localize because they manufacture an enzyme, hyaluronidase, that destroys
hyaluronic acid. Hyaluronic acid is a mucopolysaccharide that forms a gelati-
nous substance between cells and in the tissue spaces. It is also a component
of the capsules of certain types of streptococci, pneumococci, and certain other
microorganisms as well as of synovial fluid, vitreous humor in the eye, and the
umbilical cord (Wharton's jelly). In the joints, hyaluronic acid acts as a
lubricant, and in the tissues it acts as a jellylike cement substance and a means
of holding water in the interstitial spaces.[51] Because hyaluronidase destroys
the tissue hyaluronic acid and therefore allows greater spreading of materials
in the tissue spaces, hyaluronidase is called the spreading factor. Production
of hyaluronidase by such organisms as the *Staphylococcus* and *Streptococcus*
enables them to break down the continuity of the tissue as well as the fibrin
clots formed in the area of infection. When microorganisms are successful in
disrupting barriers to their spread, they are then able to penetrate the surrounding tissue and cause cellulitis. With a breakdown of the local barriers to
their spread, organisms may also enter the lymph and blood channels. Fibrin
clots in the small venous and lymph channels may delay the entrance of
bacteria into the general circulation. Lymph nodes in lymph channels also act
as traps to remove the phagocytosed bacteria. When bacteria enter and are
circulated in the blood, the condition is known as bacteremia. When bacteria
not only are transported by the blood, but multiply, the condition is called
septicemia. In some diseases, such as typhoid fever, bacteremia occurs in a
phase of the illness. In others, such a pneumonia, the appearance of bacteremia is an unfavorable prognostic sign. Septicemia is always a serious and
often fatal disorder. In either bacteremia or septicemia, microorganisms may
be distributed through the body and set up sites of infection distant from the
original infection.

How may inflammation be classified?

Any condition that modifies the nature of the inflammatory response or is
useful in identifying something about it can be used as a basis for classification. Inflammation may be classified according to: (1) the causative or

[51] Harold A. Harper, *Review of Physiological Chemistry*, 8th ed., Lange Medical
Publications, Los Altos, California, 1961, p. 371.

etiological agent, (2) the characteristic type of exudate, (3) the location or site in which it occurs, and (4) the length of time the process has been in existence. Any classification of inflammation according to cause includes an endless variety of physical, chemical, and living agents. Some have their origin in the external environment and some in the internal environment of the individual. Only a few of the possible causative agents will be discussed. Essentially they all act to injure tissue cells. The surrounding tissue then responds in the manner that has been previously discussed. How the various types of agents injure cells was presented in the preceding chapter. Physical agents that are common initiators of the inflammatory process are heat, cold, radiant rays including ultraviolet and infrared rays, radioactive rays, and trauma. Chemical agents also act as irritants. They may be either extrinsic or intrinsic in origin or result from a combination of the two. Examples of extrinsic chemical irritants include strong acids and bases, insect bites, allergens, and the toxins manufactured by microorganisms.

Chemical irritants of intrinsic origin are substances that are produced in the body. They may be normal substances, such as pancreatic juice that escapes from the gastrointestinal tract and comes in contract with tissues not protected from the digesting actions of its enzymes. Large areas of necrosis of the abdominal wall may occur in those who have the misfortune to have a fistulous tract from the small intestine to the surface of the body.

Perhaps the most common example of a body fluid that is "out of place" is blood. The body responds to blood that escapes into tissue from a break in a blood vessel as it does to a foreign body. Frequently soreness is the first sign of bleeding into a tissue. Soreness at the site of an intramuscular injection may result from the rupture of a small blood vessel during the insertion of a needle. Bruises caused by bumping furniture or other hard objects often pass unnoticed for a day or so and then come to attention because the area is painful.

Inflammation also develops in the tissue surrounding dead or necrotic tissue. In the degeneration of the dead tissue products are formed that act as irritants. When the death of tissue is due to the loss of its blood supply, the necrotic area may also serve as a site for the development of infection. The tissue, robbed of its blood supply, is no longer able to supply phagocytes to control microorganisms in the area. They are therefore able to establish themselves and grow and multiply in the tissue. For example, following infarction due to the obstruction of a branch of the pulmonary artery by an embolus, Mr. Ash developed pneumonia. The original focus for the infection was in the infarcted tissue.

Products of metabolism may also act as irritants. They may be abnormal either in quantity or in kind or in the manner in which the body handles them. In gout, because of a defect in the metabolism of purines, uric acid crystals accumulate in the tissues about joints. The resulting inflammatory process is exceedingly painful. Since, according to folklore, gout is the result of high living, which it is not, persons who develop gout are often subjected to cruel jokes and ridicule. Hopps[52] states that relatively little study has been devoted to diseases in which the chemical irritants are derived from the body itself.

What are the characteristics of each type of exudate?

The inflammatory process may be classified according to the nature of the exudate. The exudate may be purulent, serous, serosanguineous, fibrinous, hemorrhagic, or catarrhal.

Purulent exudate

A purulent exudate is commonly known as pus. Although a number of other agents stimulate the production of a purulent exudate, it is most commonly associated with the so-called pyogenic bacteria. In these infections the exudate is rich in leukocytes. The purulent exudate or pus contains a large number of leukocytes, together with tissue debris and the products of digestion by proteolytic enzymes released by dead and dying leukocytes. The thick creamy pus found in the spinal fluid of the patient with meningococcic meningitis is an example of a purulent exudate associated with a pyogenic infection. Another more common example is the pus associated with staphylococcal infections of the hair follicle or a wound. The material occurring in the center of a pimple or boil (furuncle) is a purulent exudate.

Serous exudate

A serous exudate is a watery, low-protein fluid derived either from the blood or from the cells lining serous cavities and joint spaces. Perhaps the most common example of a serous exudate is the fluid found in the blisters or vesicles associated with second-degree burns. Mr. Allen had some blistering of his skin as a consequence of burns. The blisters contained a serous exudate. Another example of a serous exudate is the fluid which accumulates in the pleural cavity as a result of some types of pleurisy. This type of pleurisy is known as pleurisy with effusion. It is frequently caused by tuberculosis or by a malignant neoplasm in the lung.

Infections involving the peritoneum or the pericardium may likewise result in the production of a serous exudate. Pericarditis with effusion is likely to cause serious impairment in cardiac function. Relatively small amounts of fluid prevent the heart from dilating fully during diastole and interfere with the filling of the heart. This results in congestion of blood in the systemic venous circulation and reduces the quantity of blood available to circulate to the tissues.

Fibrinous exudate

In the more severe acute inflammatory processes, damage to capillaries may increase permeability to the extent that large molecules such as fibrinogen escape in the exudate. A fibrinous exudate is characteristic of certain

[52] *Op. cit.,* p. 142.

types of infections, such as pneumococcal pneumonia. The alveoli are filled with a fibrinous exudate containing large numbers of leukocytes. When the inflammatory process extends to the pleura, it causes the so-called fibrinous pleurisy. The fibrin on the surface of the pleura is sticky. Pain during breathing results from the pleural surfaces rubbing together. Though fibrinous pleurisy is an early finding in pneumonia, it also occurs in the absence of pneumonia.

Hemorrhagic inflammations

In very severe inflammatory reactions, damage to the blood vessels may be so great that erythrocytes escape into the exudate. This may be observed as minute hemorrhages into the skin that are known as petechiae, which appear as small reddened areas in the skin. One disorder in which they are commonly found is subacute bacterial endocarditis. In fulminating infections the damage to blood vessels may be so great that bleeding into the subcutaneous tissues takes place. This gives the skin a dusky hue. The color of the skin is responsible for the black smallpox or meningitis of fact and legend.

Catarrhal inflammation

Catarrhal inflammation occurs only in those tissues in which there are mucous glands—that is, in mucous membranes. The term is really a misnomer, but it continues to be used because of force of habit. The exudate from mucous membranes contains large amounts of mucinous material. It is one of the most frequent types of exudate because it is associated with inflammations of the respiratory tract. The clear mucinous exudate accompanying a common cold is an example. Mucous secretion may be increased by the exposure of the respiratory tract to chemical irritants such as those contained in smoke or smog.

In addition to classifying inflammation according to the type of exudate, what other classifications are used?

Inflammatory processes may also be classified according to the tissue or organ in which they are located. Students can recognize that the inflammatory process is involved when the suffix "itis" is added to the combining form indicating a tissue or organ. Inflammation of the trachea and bronchi, whatever the causative agent, is known as tracheobronchitis. The term "myositis" indicates that a muscle is inflamed. Myocarditis is used to indicate that the heart muscle is inflamed. Nephritis indicates that the site of inflammation is the kidney. None of these terms indicate the cause of the inflammatory process. The only information provided is that a particular organ is the site of an inflammatory process.

The inflammatory process may also be classified as to the length of time it has been in existence. This classification gives some clue as to the degree of activity of the process. Thus the term "acute," "subacute," and "chronic" are used. Acute inflammations are those of recent origin and in which the process is active. The common cold is an example of a condition in which there is an acute inflammatory process. A recently incurred burn is another. An example of a condition that may go from the acute to the chronic stage is acute hemorrhagic nephritis. The kidney may recover fully following the acute phase of the disease or it may fail to do so and go into the subacute phase and finally into chronic nephritis.

Not all inflammatory processes are highly active at the beginning. Some inflammants are only mildly irritating and cause damage to cells by prolonged exposure to them. Such an irritant is silica. When it is inhaled into the lung, it sets up a simple inflammatory process in which the macrophage plays an important role. Since silica is indigestible, it cannot be destroyed by the macrophage. Marcrophages, however, can wall it off by forming fibroblasts which mature into fibrous connective tissue. One particle of silica will not require a very large scar, but many particles do. Therefore, to prevent serious scarring of the lung, workers who are exposed to silica dust in the course of employment require measures which reduce the chances of inhaling dust.

How are the signs and symptoms caused in inflammation?

The signs and symptoms in inflammation depend in part on the degree of response of the host, the nature of the inflammant, and the site of the injury. Mild irritants, including psychogenic stimuli triggered by a symbol of injury, may produce only a transient inflammation lasting only a few minutes or hours, while severe injury may last for days, weeks, or even months. The response may be limited to a small area or may involve the entire organism.

The cardinal signs of inflammation are increased heat, redness, swelling, pain, and loss of function. The rise in the temperature of a part is due mainly to an increase in blood supply, though there may also be some increase in the metabolic rate. With the increase in blood flow in the area, the temperature approaches that of the interior of the body. The increase in blood in the area is also responsible for the redness. Although the increased quantity of blood in the area contributes to the swelling, swelling or inflammatory edema is mainly due to the accumulation of the exudate in the tissue. Swelling causes pain because of pressure on sensory nerve endings. Some authorities believe that toxic metabolites also are a factor in pain.

Loss of function is partly due to pain, as motion increases pain. Muscle spasm in the injured area also serves to splint or limit motion of the part. For example, following spillage of the contents of the gastrointestinal tract into the peritoneal cavity, the muscles of the abdominal wall contract and act as a physiological splint. Even cuts involving skin over or near a joint induce some muscle spasm and a disinclination to move the joint because of the pain.

As a space-occupying mass, an area of inflammation may impinge on the circulation to an organ or obstruct a hollow organ or duct. For example, a localized area of inflammation of a structure within the cranial cavity may raise the intracranial pressure enough to deprive the entire brain of an adequate supply of blood. It may also cause pressure on the area of the brain where it is situated. An abscess in the mediastinum may interfere with swallowing by obstructing the esophagus from without. An abscess in the neck may obstruct the trachea by local pressure on it. In none of these examples does the inflammatory process directly involve the affected structures, but it causes its effects as a space-occupying mass.

In the description of inflammation thus far, emphasis has been on the local responses of tissues to injury. When only a relatively small number of cells are damaged, most, if not all, of the physiological response is in the region of injury. When, however, the products of inflammation are absorbed into the blood stream in sufficient quantities, the whole organism becomes involved. Although the nature of the etiological agent influences the severity and timing of the general physiological manifestations, they are not unique to a single class. Therefore the manifestations of illness resulting from the escape of the products of inflammation into the general circulation can be observed in Mr. Allen (burns), Mr. Hoffer (myocardial infarct), and Mrs. Carney (radical mastectomy—major surgery) as well as Miss Mallow, who has pneumococcal pneumonia.

What are the generalized symptoms and signs that accompany inflammation?

One important group of symptoms includes fever and the symptoms and signs that commonly accompany fever. The degree and character of fever vary with the causative agent. Following a major surgical prodecure or an acute myocardial infarction, the temperature rises a degree or two and remains elevated for two or three days. It should then return to normal and remain within the normal range. If it does not, or the temperature rises higher than expected, this usually indicates that a complication is developing. Since the pattern of fever varies with each acute infectious disease, no attempt will be made to describe them here. The pulse and respiratory rate are usually, though not invariably, accelerated in proportion to the increase in temperature. Weakness and general malaise—a general feeling of unfitness—are common. Anorexia, or loss of appetite, is frequent; headache, backache, and generalized aching are not uncommon. Nausea may occur, with or without vomiting or diarrhea. Leukocytosis and an increase in the erythrocyte sedimentation rate occur in a wide variety of acute conditions—with and without infection. Some infections, such as pneumococcal pneumonia, may be preceded by a chill in adults or by a convulsion in infants and young children. In other conditions, such as advanced tuberculosis, subacute bacterial endocarditis, and malaria, chills and fever may alternate with sweating (diaphoresis).

If the inflammatory process (1) continues for more than a few days, (2) is severe, (3) is associated with fever, or (4) is associated with the loss of considerable quantities of tissue substance or nutrients, weight loss may be marked. During fever, the metabolic rate is increased about 7 per cent for each degree of fever. With continued fever, the patient needs a substantial intake of calories to prevent weight loss. In long-continued inflammatory processes, particularly when associated with infection, the production of erythrocytes by the bone marrow may be depressed; normocytic anemia is a common finding in chronic infections.

Summary

Inflammation is one of a living organism's most important mechanisms of defense against injury. Inflammation is a defensive response to an injurious agent. It involves blood vessels; blood cells, particularly the leukocytes; tissue cells; and cells of the reticuloendothelial system. It serves to neutralize, destroy, and limit the spread of inflammants, and to prepare the tissues for repair.

The signs and symptoms accompanying the inflammatory process result from the response of the injured tissue and the person to injury as well as from the nature and severity of the injury. Inasmuch as the inflammatory process is a space-occupying mass, it may interfere with the function of organs. The signs and symptoms will depend on the extent to which function is disrupted. When sufficient products of the inflammatory process are absorbed, signs and symptoms indicating that the whole person is sick follow.

The specific therapy of any patient who has suffered cell injury and an accompanying inflammatory response will, of course, depend on such factors as the nature of the etiological agent, and the extent of the injury and its location, as well as on the adaptive capacity of the individual. In general, therapy will be directed toward: (1) assisting the patient to overcome or eliminate the causative agent, (2) supporting the inflammatory response, and (3) providing substances required for the repair of the injured tissues. Attention is also given to the prevention of further injury so that the individual may be restored to health.

In planning the therapy of the patient a number of principles serve as guides in the selection of specific measures. The first principle, when appropriately used, is that rest favors healing. How rest of an organ or part is achieved depends on its location and function. Both these factors—location and function of the affected part—are important in determining the degree of rest that it is possible to achieve. To illustrate, Mr. Carlos fractured his leg. Maintaining his leg at rest was relatively easy. It was placed in a cast or in traction with the two ends of the bone held in apposition. Mr. Carlos remained in bed until sufficient healing occurred. Even after he was out of bed he did not bear weight on his leg until healing was well under way or the leg was immobilized by a cast or brace. By way of contrast, despite the desirability of rest to the liver in the treatment of hepatitis, only relative rest can be secured. Mr. Devon, who had a diagnosis of infectious hepatitis, was placed on a high-carbohydrate, high-protein, and low-fat diet. He was maintained at bed rest for several weeks in order to provide rest for the liver.[53] Mr. Hoffer, who suffered a myocardial infarction, was also treated by bed rest for four weeks in order to reduce strain on the heart; then his physical activity was gradually increased.[54] Immediately following myocardial infarction, Mr. Hoffer was fed, bathed, and, inasfar as possible, protected from psychological and social stresses. Though bed rest is used less extensively than in the past, it is still believed to be an important form of treatment in infectious disease, in acute glomerulonephritis, and in acute rheumatic fever.

Bed rest is not without its hazards. As emphasized earlier, rest or lack of use of the body is accompanied by a loss of body substance and strength. Visceral and circulatory functions are depressed with the result that gastrointestinal function is disturbed and clotting of blood in vessels is favored. Respiratory excursions are lessened and this predisposes to atelectasis and pneumonia. Despite these and other disadvantages, the indications for rest may be sufficiently great for the physician to prescribe it. When bed rest is prescribed, the nurse has the responsibility to select appropriate nursing measures so that physical and psychological rest are achieved.

A second principle is: survival depends on an adequate circulation of blood to and from the tissue. The effectiveness of the inflammatory response as well as the life of the cells depends on (1) a continued supply of nutrients, leukocytes, antibodies, and other substances required by the tissue and (2) the removal of products of tissue metabolism as well as those of the inflammatory process. Heat in the form of dry or moist heat may be used to dilate the blood vessels. Since each tissue has a thermal death point, care should be taken to prevent burns. Moist heat is more dangerous than dry heat because it prevents evaporation. A temperature of from 40.5° to 46° C. (105° to 115° F.) is very hot.[55] Exposure of the tissue to 85°C. for as little as ten seconds is sufficient to cause burning. With each degree that the temperature of tissue is raised, the metabolic rate goes up about 7 per cent. Patients with arterial diseases such as arteriosclerosis are sensitive to heat because they have a limited capacity to increase the delivery of nutrients to their tissues by dilating their arteries. Their ability to judge the temperature may also be defective. Should moist heat be applied to a patient with a diagnosis of arteriosclerosis, the temperature of the solution should be prescribed by the physician and the temperature of the solution should be checked with a thermometer. The dressings should be removed if the patient complains of pain and the physician should be

---

[53] Authorities disagree about the necessity for bed rest in the treatment of hepatitis.
[54] The time selected is to illustrate a point and is not intended to reflect any particular practice in treating patients following myocardial infarction.
[55] *A.M.A. Handbook of Physical Medicine and Rehabilitation,* Blakiston Co., Philadelphia, 1950, p. 174.

notified. These patients should also be taught to check the temperature of bath water with a thermometer before stepping into the bathtub.

Heat is sometimes applied to extremities of patients in the form of a light cradle. Tissues can be protected by using a cradle in which the heat is controlled thermostatically. The temperature should be maintained between 30° and 34° C. (between 86° and 95° F.) as this is the temperature at which maximum vasodilation can be expected.[56] When a cradle with a thermostatic control is not available, the patient can be afforded some measure of protection by using light bulbs of 25 watts or less. Despite great care some patients have pain due to muscle ischemia at environmental temperatures that are very little above ordinary room temperature. When this is true, the heat should be discontinued and the physician notified.

Maintenance of the venous return is also important to the nutrition of tissues. In inflammation, distention of tissues by the inflammatory exudate causes pressure on veins, thereby interfering with the venous return. Elevation of an extremity is an important measure in promoting venous return. (Water runs downhill.) An elastic stocking or bandage is also useful in supporting the venous circulation. Should signs and symptoms that accompany impaired circulation occur in an extremity encased in a cast or bandage, measures to relieve the situation must be instituted promptly, if tissue injury is to be prevented. When elevation of the part is not successful in reducing the swelling, then the bandage or cast must be removed. Though this is the responsibility of the physician, the nurse has the obligation to bring the situation to the attention of the physician with sufficient promptness and clarity that the patient is protected.

Care directed toward the maintenance of the circulation of inflamed tissue is important. Observation of the signs and symptoms indicating the status of the circulation in the tissue is imperative if indications that the circulation is failing are to be detected early and appropriate measures instituted in time.

A third principle in therapy is to provide the patient with specific assistance in overcoming the causative agent. This principle applies primarily to those conditions in which the causative agent propagates itself, or is a foreign body. At this time the main group of causative agents falling into the first category are microorganisms. Perhaps at a future time delayed hypersensitivity reactions will also be classified in this group. There are two general, but specific, ways of attacking microorganisms or their products. One is to give the patient specific antibodies formed by an animal or another human being. The other is to administer a chemical that acts to weaken or to kill the microorganism. The use of specific therapy in the treatment of infectious disease will be further expanded in the chapter on infections.

The fourth principle is to modify the tissue response in inflammation so

[56] R. W. Wilkins, "Peripheral Vascular Diseases Due to Organic Arterial Obstruction," Cecil-Loeb, A Textbook of Medicine, 11th ed. Paul B. Beeson and Walsh McDermott, W. B. Saunders Co., Philadelphia, 1963, p. 782.

that tissue injury is prevented. As in other body responses, the inflammatory reaction may be deficient or it may be excessive. In the first case, recovery may be threatened because the body is unable to overcome the irritant and prepare the tissue for repair. In the latter, the tissue is damaged by the excessive reaction. Agranulocytosis has been previously cited as an example of a condition in which the body response to injury may be inadequate. In individual patients in whom the inflammatory response is excessive, tissue damage may result. The control and effects of excessive swelling have been discussed. Necrotic areas are often repaired by fibrosis. Scar tissue may cause deformity of the affected tissue or organ. In disorders such as iritis, arthritis, and rheumatic fever, residual injury can sometimes be lessened by modifying the severity of the inflammatory response of the tissues. By limiting the exudative phase of the inflammatory response, tissue swelling is lessened. This contributes to the maintenance of the circulation to the tissues and therefore helps to prevent tissue necrosis. In the absence of tissue necrosis, fibrosis does not occur. To illustrate, in the treatment of iritis (inflammation of the iris of the eye) cortisone, hydrocortisone, or one of their synthetic analogues may be placed in the eye to reduce the severity of the inflammatory reaction and, as a consequence, the amount of scarring. Although authorities do not agree as to how the corticoids act, they reduce in some way the exudative response in inflammation. As a result, there is less tissue damage and a reduction in the amount of scar tissue formed in healing. Corticoids and salicylates are used in the treatment of arthritis and rheumatic fever for essentially the same reason.

The fifth principle is that healing cannot proceed until the inflammatory debris, foreign bodies, blood clots, necrotic tissue, and the like are removed. In simple inflammations, the products of inflammation may be digested and absorbed into the blood stream. The blood vessels and tissue may be repaired leaving little or no evidence of the past inflammation. In pneumonia, the exudate in the lung may be coughed up and the tissue repaired without leaving any sign of the past infection. In boils, wound infections, empyema, and other similar infections, as well as those in which foreign bodies are present in the tissue, recovery may be hastened by the evacuation of pus, tissue debris, or foreign bodies. The removal of necrotic tissue and foreign bodies is called débridement; sometimes, as with a boil, this may need to be done only once. In other disorders, such as a serious wound infection, repeated opening of the wound may be required to facilitate drainage. Such wounds may be irrigated with isotonic saline or some other solution to remove debris and pus. When irrigation is done, enough force should be used to remove the purulent material. Care should be taken to prevent contamination of other areas of the skin of the patient and of the nurse.

The final principle in the treatment of the patient with an inflammatory response is that procedures should be instituted which help to support the patient in his reaction to his condition. The support should be both emotional and physiological, as one augments the other. No one is at his best when he is ill and he should not be expected to be. Moore and his associates[57] found that apprehension and fear before a surgical procedure were associated with a mild catabolic response. Attention to the needs of the patient and prompt relief of unnecessary pain should help to minimize suffering. Attention should be given to supplying the nutritional needs of each patient. There is evidence to indicate that in undernourished patients phagocytic ability is less than in those who are well nourished. Nutrients are necessary to the formation of antibodies and to the replacement of nutrients lost in the inflammatory exudate. Tissue substance lost as a result of the catabolic response to tissue injury must also be replaced by the food intake of the patient.

Water intake should be sufficient to replace that which is lost. Insensible perspiration may be increased by one l or more in fever. Drenching diaphoresis may be responsible for the loss of one l or more of water. A urine output of less than one l usually indicates that the fluid intake of the patient is inadequate. This presupposes a normally functioning kidney.

Rest and reassurance may also be important ingredients in the care of the patient. The doctor usually orders the degree of activity which is allowed the patient, but the nurse is the one who tries to modify his environment so that he is able to rest. Reassurance is discussed in a chapter devoted to meeting the emotional needs of the patients.

Provided that the body is successful in removing, destroying, or neutralizing the injurious agent, the tissue goes on to repair the damage that has been done. Essentially the nature of repair is the same whether the continuity of the tissue is disrupted by a spontaneous process or by a carefully planned incision.

The question of whether repair is the final stage of inflammation or is a separate response to injury is really of little importance. What is significant is that repair is a response to injury in which the body attempts to restore the injured tissue to normal. How this is accomplished depends on the severity and type of the injury as well as on the tissues that have been injured. There are three general ways in which repair may take place. Hopps[58] calls these healing by recuperation, by regeneration, and by replacement with scar tissue.

In the discussion of possible outcome of inflammation, the point was made that when injury to the tissue is minimal, the products of inflammation are absorbed and the tissues are returned to their former condition. Hopps[59] defines the restoration of tissue to its former state as recuperation.

When the injury is more severe and cells are destroyed, repair may be accomplished by regeneration, a process in which cells are replaced by similar cells. Actually, regeneration of tissues such as the skin is a constant process. As the surface cells of the skin are shed, they are replaced by underlying cells, which are in turn replaced by cells at the base of the skin, each of which

[57] Wilson, Moore, and Jepson, *Op. cit.,* p. 76.
[58] *Op. cit.,* p. 217.
[59] *Ibid.*

undergoes mitosis and divides into two. The process is carefully controlled, so that only as many cells are produced as are needed to replace those that are desquamated. Mr. Allen healed his tissues, which were burned to the second degree, by the regeneration of epithelial cells.

Regeneration of cells and tissues depends on two fundamental properties. One is the capacity of cells to proliferate or multiply. The other is the capacity of the organism to organize new cells into a functional pattern. Scientists have long been intrigued by the fact that animals, such as the salamander, are able to regenerate limbs following amputation. Recent findings indicate that one of the factors in the regeneration of an organ is the ability of cells forming different types of tissue to regenerate at the same rate. In man different types of tissue cells reproduce at different rates. The problem is complicated by the fact that fibrous connective tissue regenerates more rapidly and under less favorable circumstances than do other types of tissues. Therefore, even in tissues having the capacity to regenerate, healing may take place by scarring, rather than by regeneration.

Not only is man incapable of regenerating limbs, but the capacity of his tissues to regenerate varies. As has been stated previously, highly specialized cells such as those in nerve and muscle tissues are incapable of regeneration. Injuries are repaired by replacement with microglia (a connective tissue in the nervous system) and fibrous connective tissue. By way of contrast, tissues having their origin in the mesenchymal tissues (those that form the supporting structures for the parenchymal or functioning cells) have a great capacity for regeneration. Surface and glandular epithelium, bone, and lymphoid tissue are also able to regenerate adequately.

The capacity to produce an adequate number of differentiated cells is only one aspect of regeneration. Another is the capacity to organize these cells into functioning units with the necessary blood, lymph, and nerve supply. A good example of an organ in which the capacity to regenerate fails, not because cells do not proliferate, but because the body is unable to properly organize them into functioning units, is the liver. The liver is susceptible to injury by a wide variety of agents: microorganisms; chemical poisons, such as chloroform or carbon tetrachloride; and undernutrition, as the liver is particularly susceptible to a lack of protein and of vitamin B in the diet. The liver fails to recover following injury not because liver cells do not have an adequate capacity to regenerate, but because the body is unable to organize the cells around ducts. Despite the capacity to replace damaged liver cells, the resulting tissue is likely to be of little use. In a way, the liver is repaired much as a jerry-built house is constructed—a cell here and one there without thought as to where it should be placed to accomplish its function.

The third way in which repair is achieved is by the substitution of fibrous connective tissue for the injured tissue. When fibrous connective tissue is used in repair, it serves as a patch that preserves or restores the continuity of the tissue. It does nothing more. Therefore, when an injury to a vital organ is repaired by the substitution of fibrous connective tissue, the result is a decrease in the functional reserve in that organ. For example, a myocardial infarct heals by the formation of scar tissue. The extent to which the cardiac reserve is diminished will depend on the size of the scar. Following an attack of glomerulonephritis, scar tissue is formed to heal the kidney. The scarring may do more damage than the original disease process because as the scar tissue matures, it contracts and obstructs the flow of blood to the kidney. Functioning tissue dies as a consequence of loss of blood supply. In patients who die from the effects of glomerulonephritis, the kidney is frequently found to be a contracted mass consisting mostly of scar tissue.

Under what circumstances is repair by substitution of fibrous connective tissue likely?

The circumstances under which repair by the substitution of fibrous connective tissue occurs are: (1) when conditions in the internal environment are unfavorable to mitosis, (2) when the quantity of tissue destroyed is too large for it to be replaced by regeneration of the cells in the area, (3) when highly specialized tissues have been destroyed, (4) when the rate at which parenchymal cells multiply is slow, and (5) when tissues are subjected to repeated injury.

As has been implied, healing by the formation of fibrous tissue serves a number of purposes. It restores the continuity of tissue after too great destruction of tissue. It walls off foreign bodies and disease processes such as tuberculosis. It reinforces weakened structures such as aneurysms of the aorta and other large arteries.[60] Fibrous connective tissue also plays an important role in the healing of thrombosis, infarctions, osteomyelitis, and nephritis as well as of many other conditions. When thrombi form in veins, fibrous tissue serves to hold the clot at the site of formation and to repair the damage. Following an infarction, scar tissue maintains tissue continuity.

Similar to other homeostatic mechanisms, tissue repair by the formation of scar tissue is beneficial when the process is initiated by an appropriate stimulus and is sufficient to correct the damage caused by injury. Likewise it may also be the source of harm. The principal harmful effects of scar tissue are: (1) the unnecessary replacement of parenchymatous tissue; (2) interference with the function or drainage of an organ; or (3) the cutting off of the blood or nerve supply to an organ; and (4) the formation of an excessive quantity of scar tissue.

Certain of the characteristics of scar tissue account for some of its potentially harmful effects. It is composed largely of collagen. When collagen is subjected to slight or moderate stress,[61] it tends to shorten or contract. When it is subjected to much stress, it tends to lengthen. Contraction of the scar does no harm when it is in the abdominal wall and the quantity of scar

[60] An aneurysm is a bulge or outpouching in the wall of an artery. It usually results when the wall is weakened by a disease such as arteriosclerosis or syphilis. As it distends, the wall of the artery thins and is further weakened. Fibrous connective tissue strengthens the wall.

[61] Hopps, *Op. cit.,* p. 301.

tissue is not excessive. However, when scar tissue is formed in or around an organ, it can be expected to interfere with the function of the organ as it matures, as sometimes happens in the healing of third-degree burns or in arthritis. In these patients, attention to maintaining the extremities in the appropriate position so that deformities due to contractures can be prevented may be a lasting service to the patient.

Scar tissue located in areas where it is subjected to repeated strain may lengthen or extend. Sites which are subjected to considerable pressure include the wall of the heart and the arteries. Especially when an infarct in the wall of the heart is large or when the heart is subjected to repeated infarction and the quantity of scar tissue is large, the collagen fibers in the scar may be stretched by the pressure created as the heart contracts. Since they are not elastic, once they are lengthened they do not return to their former state. This results in a bulge or aneurysm. This bulge reduces the mechanical efficiency of the affected ventricle. Instead of only one area of relatively low pressure, that is, the artery, there are two, the artery and the distensible area in the wall of the heart. As the heart contracts, blood enters both the artery and the aneurysm. This increases the work of an already weakened heart. For reasons that will be discussed later, this may also decrease the ability of the heart to maintain its own blood supply.

What are the factors that favor tissue repair?

Many of the general factors favoring tissue repair have already been indicated. They may be summarized as: (1) a limited amount of injury and a high regenerative capacity of tissues; (2) an abundant supply of blood to the tissue as well as an adequate supply of protein and ascorbic acid; and finally (3) good health and youth. Regarding the latter point, the most important practical difference between healing in the young and in the old is that the young tend to heal more rapidly than the old. Most of the other factors have been discussed previously. The need for a good blood supply is obvious. Protein is necessary to supply the amino acids required for the formation of new tissue. Some authorities are inclined to interpret the metabolic response following injury as an adaptation by which the organism provides the tissues with the materials needed for healing. Others regard this response as maladaptive. Since the metabolic response is greater in the young and healthy than in the old and feeble, perhaps this is one reason that they recover more quickly than do the old and feeble. Ascorbic acid, or vitamin C, is necessary for the formation of collagen—an essential element in fibrous tissue.

The presence of diseases such as uncontrolled diabetes mellitus or atherosclerosis delays repair. Though there is some disagreement among authorities about the effect of anemia on wound healing, it probably is not an important factor.

Local conditions in the injured tissue also have an effect on the healing of the injured tissue. The exact nature of the stimulus to cellular proliferation is not known, but it is believed to be due to a local factor or factors. As was emphasized in the discussion of inflammation, healing is delayed or prevented until the wound has been cleared of infection and any dead space has been obliterated. In the past, healing has been delayed by the introduction of foreign substances at the time the wound was made or treated. At various times throughout history, antiseptics and germicides have been placed in wounds to destroy microorganisms. It is now known that any agent potent enough to kill bacteria also kills body cells. Furthermore, before healing can proceed normally, all foreign material must be removed. Because it acts as a foreign body when introduced into a wound, talcum is no longer used to powder gloves. A form of treated cornstarch has been substituted for it. Though it is much less likely to produce a foreign-body reaction, cornstarch can and does. Therefore, it should be used as sparingly as possible in powdering the gloves. The outer surface of the gloves should be washed before the operation is started.[62]

The mechanism of injury also has a bearing on healing. A clean, incised wound free from infection is the most favorable to healing. Crushing wounds, fractures, especially those with much soft-tissue damage, and infection of wounds delay healing. They also are attended by the possibility of excessive scar tissue formation.

So that the reader may have some understanding of what is happening in a patient who is healing an area of injured tissue, the healing of a clean, incised wound will be briefly described. The process of healing all injuries is essentially the same. The principal differences between the healing of a clean, incised wound and an infected one, or one in which the tissue is subjected to longstanding injury, are in the quantity of scar tissue required to heal the defect and, as a result, healing is delayed. In a clean, incised wound only a small scar is required, which may form quickly; in other wounds, scarring may be extensive and delayed.

Preparatory to, and during, healing a number of things must be accomplished. The damaged cells and tissue debris must be removed. Bleeding must be stopped. The gap between the two severed edges of tissue must be bridged. As the surgeon makes the incision he works carefully. Though a small clot of blood or fluid exudate is necessary to fill the defect between the two sides of the wound, a large clot delays healing. Therefore, the surgeon carefully ligates (ties) the ends of each blood vessel as it is cut. Small vessels seal themselves by the formation of blood clots, which on retraction of the vessel form an effective plug in its end. The surgeon also facilitates healing by the careful approximation of like tissues to like tissues. As he completes his part in the healing of the wound, nature takes over.

Authorities usually describe healing as occurring in three phases. There is considerable overlapping among the various phases. They may all be going on at the same time in different parts of the wound. The first phase, which lasts

[62] Henry N. Harkins, "Wound Healing," *Surgery: Principles and Practice*, 2nd ed., Henry N. Harkins, *et al.*, J. B. Lippincott Co., Philadelphia, 1961, pp. 15, 16, and 220.

from three to five days, is variously called the initial, the lag, the catabolic, and the inflammatory phase. These terms all have some virtue in that each describes some change or condition that is present in the tissues. The term "lag" has been used, because the strength of the wound diminishes during this time. The term is, however, misleading because it implies that no changes are occurring in the tissue. This is not true, for exudation is increased and leukocytes accumulate in the area. Blood vessels dilate and the area becomes hyperemic. The fluid exudate and/or blood fills the space between the two edges of the wound and not only causes the edges of the wound to stick together, but provides a meshlike framework for fibroblasts and budding capillaries. Materials essential to tissue repair accumulate. Fibroblasts appear and there is an increase in collagen. Without collagen, wound healing does not take place. Harkins[63] emphasizes that collagen does not form unless the proper materials and conditions are present. Capillary buds also begin to appear. Their formation coincides with the general catabolic response of the body as a whole. During this phase the patient looks and acts ill. Moore[64] calls this the stage of injury or the adrenergic corticoid phase.

After four or five days the leukocytes begin to disappear from the wound. About this time the fibroblasts can be observed to be actively proliferating. During this phase collagen is formed and the newly formed tissue is highly vascular. Because of its appearance, the new tissue is called granulation tissue. As the collagen fibers mature, they tend to shorten or contract. Early in the process of wound healing, epithelial cells migrate and later proliferate to cover the wound surface. With large wounds the epithelial covering may be very thin and delicate. Care should be taken when the wound is dressed to protect these newly forming cells, lest they be destroyed. In time, the scar, which was a bright pink, pales or fades, because the blood vessels are squeezed out. The result is a mature scar, or a cicatrix.

When a wound is infected, suppuration occurs and healing is delayed. At one time infection was so common that surgeons thought it was necessary to healing. The type of pus that was believed to favor healing was called laudable pus. When pus is present, the wound is said to heal by second intention. Healing is delayed and more granulation tissue is required to fill the defect than in the absence of infection. Occasionally, either because of the nature of the wound or because of its disruption, secondary closure is necessary. This is known as healing by third intention.

Currently, knowledge of the factors involved in wound healing is incomplete. Questions as to what initiates the process and what terminates it have not been answered. In experiments with rats, Selye has been able to prevent scar tissue formation by the administration of cortisone, and to augment its formation by administration of desoxycortisone. Exactly how cortisone, hydrocortisone, and related analogues act is not known. In rats, the different

[63] Ibid., p. 9.
[64] Francis D. Moore, Metabolic Care of the Surgical Patient, W. B. Saunders Co., Philadelphia, 1959, p. 28.

adrenal cortical hormones depress or enhance the inflammatory response that follows tissue injury.

Earlier in the chapter the changes occurring in the tissue in response to injury were described. In the table that follows, changes that take place in the body as a whole and in the wound are summarized and correlated with the signs and symptoms which can be expected in the patient and his needs during each phase. The length of each phase varies with the extent of injury to the tissue as well as with the capacity of the individual to respond. The summary is based on the changes occurring in a patient who has a clean, incised wound such as is made in the performance of abdominal surgery. Changes are less marked in conditions in which the extent of injury to tissue is less and is more marked in those in which there is greater injury to the tissue.

During the twentieth century techniques have been perfected and the knowledge of the changes that take place in the body as a whole, as well as in the wounded tissue, has increased. With expansion in the fields of physiology and biochemistry, clues are being uncovered that can be expected to lead to a knowledge of the factors that initiate the healing process, regulate its course, and terminate it. Interest is also centered on the biochemical changes that take place in the body as a whole following injury and during illness. The preceding discussion re-emphasizes that the body acts as a unit. Biologically it gives priority to the injured tissue. As the understanding of these changes becomes more complete, care of the patient following injury can perhaps be planned to support body responses rather than to interfere with them. In other patients, such as those with glomerulonephritis or rheumatic fever, this knowledge may make it possible to limit the inflammatory response, including subsequent scarring, so that tissue structure and function may be preserved.

In this chapter, mechanisms by which the organism responds to injury have been presented. Inasmuch as these responses are appropriate and adequate, the survival of the organism is facilitated.

Though the role of the nurse has been indicated throughout the chapter, objectives of her care may be summarized as follows: (1) To control, or to teach the patient to control, agents causing injury of the tissue. This includes many activities: the prevention of fires and automobile accidents, the protection of an allergic person from the antigen or antigens to which he is susceptible, the maintenance of asepsis in the operating room and cleanliness in the areas where patients reside, and the prevention of sunburn. (2) To provide the necessary conditions for the tissue response to be adequate to the needs of the situation. This too involves a variety of activities ranging from those that have to do with supporting the arterial or venous circulation to providing the necessary nutritional elements. Although points were illustrated in many instances by relating the content to events occurring in patients treated by surgical therapy, all persons who are ill undergo similar responses. They may be less obvious and are sometimes of a lesser degree. All illness, however, of whatever degree is compounded of injury and the response of the individual to the injury.

FIGURE 5–3. Summary of Some of the Responses to Injury

Phase I	Neuro-endocrine	Psychological	Circulatory	Metabolism	Water and Electrolytes	Blood
A. Onset		Anxiety, fear Guilt, shame Frustration *Denial *Aggression: ill-tempered, irascible *Passivity: pitiable, complains, obsequious *Elation: neurotic level of function *Indecisiveness, vacilation ↓				
B. Injury 2-4 days patient looks and feels sick	Sympatho-adrenal Medullary Response (1-12 hours) ↑Norepinephrine ↑Epinephrine	Surrender, abdication of responsibility Listless, sleeps, "regressive integration" *Egocentricity *Constriction of interests or lack of interest *Emotional dependency, with ambivalence toward those on whom dependent *Hypochondriasis	Tachycardia ↑Cardiac output ↑Systolic blood pressure Vasoconstriction ↑Diastolic blood pressure Splenic contraction to maintain blood volume ↑Blood volume	↑Hepatic glycogenolysis, hyperglycemia	↑Water loss from: Lungs Skin ↑sweating	↑Platelets and fibrinogen ↓Prothrombin time Results in acceleration of blood clotting ↑Sedimentation rate (varies with blood content) of fibrinogen
Catabolism exceeds anabolism	Adenohypophysis (anterior pituitary) ↓ ACTH ↓ Adrenal cortical response ↑Glucocorticoids ↑Cortisol (peak 6 hours)			↓Adrenal cholesterol and ascorbic acid ↑Gluconeogenesis ↓Cellular glucose utilization ↑Protein catabolism ↓Protein synthesis		Leukocytosis Eosinophils disappear Hyperglycemia

318

Respiration	Alimentary Canal	Other	Wound	Needs of the Patient
↑ Rate and depth Bronchial dilation ↑ Oxygen consumption As a result of anesthesia, drugs, unconsciousness, immobility, and other effects of illness, increased secretion into and interference with mechanisms for clearing the tracheobronchial tree predispose to obstruction of the airway	Peristalsis decreased or absent for 12-48 hours No appetite	Skin: ↑ sweating (cholinergic) Immobilization and splinting of wound with pain Resistance to movement; tries to find a comfortable position Hypothermia first 12 hours or so, then fever should not be over 100° F. for 24-48 hours, and then return to normal	Lag or inflammatory Phase Strength of wound is low Exudation of fluid into the wound —contains leukocytes and antibodies. Exudate also contains protein, mucopolysachrides, and ascorbic acid from which collagen fibers are formed During this time tissue debris and foreign materials are removed. This phase may be prolonged by the accumulation of blood, pus, or any other material in the wound that must be removed before wound healing can take place	The specific regime for each patient is prescribed by his physician. Oral food and fluids are withheld until peristalsis is restored. Encourage deep breathing, coughing, and turning, exercises of the extremities, and ambulation. Patient requires assistance and support. Protect from unnecessary stimulation, provide for periods of rest and quiet, use analgesics and other measures to prevent unnecessary pain. The nurse should assume responsibility for the care of the dependent patient. Observe vital signs, urinary output in relation to intake, and if intake is exceeding output to an unexplained degree, report observation to the physician. Note time, onset, degree of elevation of fever. Should it be over 37.7° C. (100° F.) or continue at or above this level longer than usual 24-48 hours, this indicates that an infection may be developing; for example, incipient infection is often characterized by a marked rise in body temperature to 38.3° C. (101° F.) or higher All abdominal and chest wounds should be supported when the patient coughs. Excessive and ineffective coughing should be avoided as it may lead to the disruption of an abdominal wound

FIGURE 5-3. Summary of Some of the Responses to Injury—Continued

Phase I	Neuro-endocrine	Psychological	Circulatory	Metabolism	Water and Electrolytes	Blood
				Negative-nitrogen balance Nitrogen excretion in urine increased. May lose 7-15 gm per day in ordinary soft-tissue injury ↑Fat mobilization (from fat depots) ↑17-hydroxy-corticosteroid excretion ↑17-ketosteroid excretion in urine ↑11-oxysteroid excretion		
	↑Adrenal androgens (slight) Mineralo-corticoids ↑Aldosterone					
	Neurohypophysis ↓ ↑ADH			Rapid weight loss	Sodium retention Potassium excretion Water retention resulting in oliguria for approximately 12 hours after injury Diuresis may begin in 1-2 days Diruesis of water and salt	

Phase II	Neuro-endocrine	Psychological	Circulatory	Metabolism	Water and Electrolytes	Blood
Turning point 3-7 days Patient begins to look and feel better	Adrenal medullary signs past Adrenal cortical secretion returns to normal	Ambition with weakness "I feel better today." Interested in surroundings, grooming and visitors	Normotension Normal cardiac output	↓17-hydroxy-corticosteroid excretion ↓Nitrogen excretion Wound begins to acquire tensile strength (stitches out)	Potassium excretion Body water still slightly high	Eosinophils Normal leukocytes

Respiration	Alimentary Canal	Other	Wound	Needs of the Patient
		↓Gonad, secretion, amenorrhea, ↓ libido		

Respiration	Alimentary Canal	Other	Wound	Needs of the Patient
Normal	Bowel sounds return Appetite improves	Temperature returns to normal	Chemical and morphological changes occur in the wound leading to the formation of scar tissue and the healing of wound.	During this period the patient may feel better than he actually is. He should be protected from overactivity and overstimulation. Food intake should be encouraged. High-quality proteins and food containing ascorbic acid are of particular importance. The patient should be encouraged to be up and walking.

FIGURE 5 – 3. Summary of Some of the Responses to Injury—Continued

Phase III	Neuro-endocrine	Psychological	Circulatory	Metabolism	Water and Electrolytes	Blood
Muscular strength 2-5 weeks	Normal	Reintegration of personality Relinquishes: *dependence *egocentricity *provincial reactions *rebellion against dependency *wants to go home *ambulation no longer painful *ambition with increasing strength	Normal	Positive nitrogen balance Weight gain Anabolism exceeds catabolism Resynthesis of muscle tissue	Normal	Normal

Phase IV	Neuro-endocrine	Psychological	Circulatory	Metabolism	Water and Electrolytes	Blood
Fat gain several months	Normal	Normal strength Returns to work	Normal	Postive nitrogen balance carbon and energy balance	Normal	Normal

Respiration	Alimentary Canal	Other	Wound	Needs of the Patient
Normal	Absorption capacity returns	Needs adequate diet and exercise May attempt premature overwork	Wound broader, raised red scar, tensile integrity established and function of soft tissues resumed	Patient should not return to work involving heavy muscular exercise until this phase has been completed. Normal strength returns

Respiration	Alimentary Canal	Other	Wound	Needs of the Patient
Normal	Normal	Looks underweight, at beginning Clothes fit loosely May tend to overeat Normal sexual function returns	During this time the wound loses its convex and reddened appearance. It becomes a concave, thin white line	The patient is able to return to his ordinary occupation. The patient's food intake should exceed his energy output until desired weight is regained. When this has been accomplished, food intake should be balanced with energy output so that obesity is avoided

[1] Henry D. Lederer, "How the Sick View Their World," *Patients, Physicians and Illness*, ed. E. G. Jaco, Free Press, Glencoe, Illinois, 1958, pp. 247-56.

[2] Francis D. Moore, *Metabolic Care of the Surgical Patient*, W. B. Saunders Company, Philadelphia and London, 1959, pp. 25-48.

[3] Ruy Perez-Tamayo, *Mechanisms of Disease*, W. B. Saunders Company, Philadelphia, 1961, pp. 452-57.

REFERENCES

Books

Apperly, Frank L., *Patterns of Disease,* J. B. Lippincott Co., Philadelphia, 1951.
Boyd, William, *A Textbook of Pathology,* 7th ed., Lea & Febiger, Philadelphia, 1961.
Cannon, Walter B., *The Wisdom of the Body,* W. W. Norton Co., Inc., New York, 1939, pp. 244-62, 263-85.
Harkins, Henry, *et al., Surgery: Principles and Practice,* 2nd ed., J. B. Lippincott Co., Philadelphia, 1961.
Hollander, Joseph, *et al., Arthritis,* Lea & Febiger, Philadelphia, 1950.
Hopps, Howard C., *Principles of Pathology,* 2nd ed., Appleton-Century-Crofts, Inc., New York, 1964.
Larson, Carroll, and Marjorie Gould (revisors), *Calderwood's Orthopedic Nursing,* 4th ed., C. V. Mosby Co., St. Louis, 1957.
Lawrence, H. Sherwood, *Cellular and Humoral Aspects of the Hypersensitive States,* Hoeber-Harper, New York, 1959.
Menkin, Valy, *Biochemical Mechanisms in Inflammation,* 2nd ed., Charles C Thomas, Springfield, Illinois, 1956.
Netter, F. H., *The Ciba Collection of Medical Illustrations.* Vol. I. *Nervous System,* Ciba Pharmaceutical Co., Summit, New Jersey, 1953.
Perez-Tamayo, Ruy, *Mechanisms of Disease,* W. B. Saunders Co., Philadelphia, 1961.
Shaffer, Joseph H., *Mechanisms of Hypersensitivity,* Little, Brown, and Co., Boston, 1959.
Swartz, Harry, *Allergy: What It Is and What to Do About It,* Rutgers University Press, New Brunswick, 1949.
Wolstenholme, P. E. W., and Maeve O'Connor, eds., *Symposium on Cellular Aspects of Immunity,* Little, Brown & Co., Boston, 1960.

Articles

Barckley, Virginia, Agnes Bettinger, Lucille A. Guenther, and Rosalie M. Ross, "Arthritis and a Narrow Perspective Do Not Mix," *Nursing Outlook,* VI, November, 1958, pp. 638-39.
Brown, Charles, "New Blocking Agents," *American Journal of Nursing,* LVII, July, 1957, p. 877.
Bovard, Everett, "A Concept of Hypothalamic Functioning," *Perspectives in Biology and Medicine,* V, Autumn, 1961, pp. 52-60.
Cave, Edwin French, "Back Pain Caused by Conditions Other Than Intervertebral Disk Injury," *Medical Clinics of North America,* XLII, No. 6, November, 1958, pp. 1589-1601.
Cole, Milton B., and Arthur A. Reynolds, "The Management of the Patient with Bronchial Asthma," *Southern Medical Journal,* LIV, January, 1961, pp. 17-24.
Crowle, Alford J., "Delayed Hypersensitivity," *Scientific American,* CCII, April, 1960, pp. 129-38.
Edwards, Leon C., and J. Englebert Dunphy, "Wound Healing. I. Injury and Normal Repair," *New England Journal of Medicine,* CCLIX, July 31, 1958, pp. 224-33.
Edwards, Leon C., and J. Englebert Dunphy, "Wound Healing. II. Injury and Abnormal Repair," *New England Journal of Medicine,* CCLIX, August 7, 1958, pp. 275-85.
James, Harriet D., "Use and Abuse of Corticotrophin and the Corticosteroids in the Treatment of Asthma," *Medical Clinics of North America,* XLIV, March, 1960, pp. 531-38.
Lancet, I, "Penicillin Hypersensitivity," March 26, 1960, p. 688.
Landrum, Faye L., "Nursing in an Allergist's Office," *American Journal of Nursing,* LVIII, May, 1958, pp. 677-78.
Marrazzi, A. S., "Messengers of the Nervous System," *Scientific American,* CXCVI, February, 1957, pp. 87-94.
McLean, James A., "Hay Fever," *American Journal of Nursing,* LXI, July, 1961, pp. 85-87.

Mueller, Harry Louis, "Serious Allergic Reactions to Insect Stings," *American Journal of Nursing,* LX, August, 1960, pp. 1110-12.

O'Brien, George F., "Collagen Diseases," *Medical Clinics of North America,* XXXIX, January, 1955, pp. 125-39.

Patterson, Roy, "Allergic Emergencies," *Journal of the American Medical Association,* CLXXII, January 23, 1960, pp. 303-5.

Smyth, Charley J., *et al.,* "Rheumatism and Arthritis," *Annals of Internal Medicine,* LIII, No. 7, December 30, 1960, pp. 1-368.

Stuart, George J., "Psychosomatic Allergy," *Southern Medical Journal,* LIV, February, 1961, pp. 169-71.

"Symposium on Rheumatic Diseases," *Medical Clinics of North America,* XXXIX, March, 1955.

Unger, Leon, "The History of Allergy," *Journal of the International College of Surgeons,* XXXIV, October, 1960, pp. 536-46.

Wells, Roe E., "Physiologic Concepts in the Treatment of Bronchial Asthma," *Medical Clinics of North America,* XLIV, September, 1960, pp. 1279-95.

6 : The Psychosocial Aspects of Illness

Canst thou not . . . raze out the written troubles of the brain,
And with some sweet oblivious antidote
Cleanse the stuff'd bosom of that perilous stuff
Which weighs upon the heart?

Shakespeare, *Macbeth*, Act V, Scene 3

In the preceding chapters, the concept was developed that human beings have physiological and psychosocial needs which must be met if the individual is to survive, grow, reproduce, and be productive. Each person has a physical structure which not only enables him to react to changes in his physical, interpersonal, and social environment, but also determines the limits to his capacity for adaptation. The capacity for adaptation to changes in the environment varies from individual to individual and in the same individual from time to time. In this chapter, the content has been selected to provide the nurse with knowledge of some of the factors to be considered if the psychosocial needs of patients with medical-surgical disorders are to be met. It is not within the scope of this book to discuss the causes and effects of serious disturbances in the interpersonal or social behavior of the individual. In most individuals, however, illness which requires medical attention causes some disturbance in the individual's interpersonal and social functioning. These disturbances arise out of the meaning that the illness has for the person, emotionally as well as intellectually. How he behaves will also depend on his family and cultural background. Likewise, how others treat him when he is ill will depend on the meanings they attach to his illness and his behavior.

In order to provide a common understanding, the terms "psychology," "social," and "culture" are defined.

Psychology is defined as a science that is primarily interested in the study of the individual as a thinking, remembering, imagining, feeling, and reacting person. It is concerned with those aspects of behavior that have their origin in the mental apparatus. This behavior may be either expressive or coping. Expressive behavior reflects some state of the individual. It is usually unconscious and nonmotivated. An illustration is that of a child skipping home from school on an early spring day. The child's behavior indicates joy and peace with himself and the world. He has not made a conscious decision to skip, nor does he expect to gain anything by it. Coping behavior, on the other hand, is purposeful, motivated, and usually learned. It is directed toward modifying the environment in some way. The same child is hungry when he arrives home from school. He goes to the refrigerator, selects a bottle of milk, and decides on making a peanut butter sandwich. There is some cold roast beef, but he has learned from past experience that he is not to take cold meat without his mother's permission. The child's behavior is directed toward relieving his hunger. Satisfaction requires that he select from a number of choices. The psychological needs of the patient are those that arise out of what he thinks, remembers, imagines, and feels about his illness. His reactions will be expressed through his behavior—expressive and coping.

Social is an adjective used to describe relationships of one person to another, either singly or in groups. Sciences such as sociology and cultural anthropology are those that deal with social actions and the behavior of human beings. Together with psychology, they are classified as the behavioral sciences. Sociology is broader than cultural anthropology in that it includes the study of social class, social organization, human ecology, social pathology, urban or rural sociology, the family, community, and race relations. Cultural anthropology is the science of the culture of man.

Culture, as defined by Biesanz,[1] is "the learned portion of human behavior and the man-made part of the environment." Mead[2] defines culture as a "body of learned behavior which a group of people, who share the same tradition, transmit entire to their children, and in part, to adult immigrants who become members of the society." Biesanz emphasizes that culture is peculiar to man while society is not. This is illustrated by the fact that animals such as the wolf and bison organize themselves into herds or packs (animal societies). These societies are characterized by a division of labor and a system for protecting the group from intruders.[3] In other words, the term *society* is used to indicate the structural relationships among a group of men or animals. Culture is an abstraction, meaning a way of life. Though all cultures have common characteristics, they are also variable. One of the important sources of differences among cultures is the geographical environment.

In recent years, interest has increased in extending knowledge of the psychological and cultural factors that influence the acceptance, use, and rejection of medical care. Many of the questions that have been and are being investigated are familiar to nurses. For example, why do some people seek medical attention at appropriate intervals while others do not? Even among those who appear to accept advice and to follow instructions, cooperation may appear to be more complete than it actually is. This point is illustrated by Mrs. Puffy, who had been visiting the outpatient clinic every three weeks for the past six

---

[1] John Biesanz and Mavis Biesanz, *Modern Society,* Prentice-Hall, Inc., Englewood Cliffs, New Jersey, 1954, p. 27.

[2] Margaret Mead (ed.), *Cultural Patterns and Technical Change,* United Nations Educational, Scientific and Cultural Organizations, Paris, 1953, pp. 9-10.

[3] Biesanz, *Op. cit.,* p. 29.

months. Her visits had been for the purpose of regulating her dosage of Cytomel.[4] Each time, she asked to have her prescription renewed. Because she was not responding to treatment, her physician planned to institute a series of examinations to determine the nature of her medical problem. When the physician left the examining room to make arrangements for the tests, the nurse asked her if anything had interfered with her taking her medication. The patient then explained that she had not taken the Cytomel for three months, as what she really needed was something to treat the "cold in her chest." The medication that she was receiving had not benefited it. The behavior among those who do not seek medical attention, or who ignore or reject advice, also varies. Some seek attention so late in the course of illness that little can be done to restore health or to reverse the disease process. Others seek attention and then openly or quietly refuse to follow recommendations or to permit themselves to be treated.

Answers to questions such as the following may provide clues as to how to extend the use of available community services. For example, why did Mr. and Mrs. Early respond to an extensive educational program by having their children immunized for poliomyelitis and diphtheria, while Mr. and Mrs. Grail did not? Why does Mrs. Far consider herself to be ill when she has a cold while Mrs. Hops continues about her ordinary activities and appears to resent any comments about her cold? What determines the patient's pattern of behavior when he is ill?

Because illness involving hospitalization is usually regarded as a crisis situation by the patient and his family, the patient can be expected to experience fear and anxiety. Furthermore, psychologists say that the person who is ill can be expected to behave as he does in the other crisis situations in his life. If this is true, then each patient should be expected to behave in an individual manner. If this concept is accepted, why do those who care for Mrs Jolly consider her behavior as cooperative, courageous, and sensible, and describe her as a fine woman who is to be admired because she takes adversity without a murmur? Why, on the other hand, is Mrs. Irate's seemingly irrational behavior equated with stubbornness, ignorance, or stupidity? Why is she looked upon as childish, demanding, and lacking in self-control and self-discipline? Why does Mr. Robbin resist every suggestion or effort to help him and make what seems to be excessive or impossible demands on the staff? Why does Mr. Quiet accept the care offered to him without question and make no extra demands on the nursing staff? Why is he described as a good patient? Why do many nurses like to care for Mrs. Jolly and Mr. Quiet and avoid, when possible, the care of Mrs. Irate or Mr. Robbin? Why was Mrs. Carol satisfied with hospital care while Mrs. Severly felt that the care she received was unfeeling and inadequate?

---

[4] Cytomel (sodium liothyronine, U.S.P.) is the active isomer of triiodothyronine, prepared for oral administration in 5 and 25 μg tablets. It is used in the treatment of patients with hypothyroid states, and is believed to facilitate entry of iodine into the cell. Its toxicity and side effects are generally those of hyperthyroidism. See a textbook of pharmacology for further details.

Other questions arise out of the observation that there appears to be a relationship between the way a person perceives his illness and his chances for recovery. For example, why should Mr. Energetic strive to recover from a severe stroke, while Mr. Dolmis, who appears to have had a small stroke, makes little effort to recover?

A complete answer to any one of these questions is, of course, impossible without much more information about each individual and his life situation. However, these illustrations suggest three general questions, Why do people behave the way that they do? What purpose does their behavior serve? How can this knowledge be used in the practice of nursing?

A general answer to these questions is that people behave as they do in order to meet an obvious (overt) or hidden (covert) need. Failure to satisfy a need results in behavior that is directed toward its satisfaction. Much of the behavior that results in the satisfaction of needs is learned. This is true even in the satisfaction of physiological needs such as the need for food. What a person eats and enjoys, and how he prepares it, depend on his family and cultural background. Whether he prefers steak broiled, pounded and fried, in sukiyaki, or in spaghetti sauce depends on past learning. How he behaves when he is in a situation when food is not available in the form or the amount that he prefers or wishes also depends on past learnings.

Knowledge of the family and cultural pattern is helpful in the identification of the patient's needs that can be met by nursing and in the selection of the manner in which care is provided. Obviously, a nurse cannot be expected to know or anticipate all the variations in the expectations of patients that arise out of their family and cultural pattern. She should have enough understanding of her own culture and of herself that she knows what her values, goals, and expectations are. An analogy may be drawn for the learning of languages. The learning of one language is said to facilitate the learning of another. Perhaps the same can be said of culture. With knowledge of the characteristic features of several cultural patterns, the nurse should be prepared to consider the possibility that a patient's behavior has its origin in his culture. Instead of the patient's behavior being abnormal or peculiar, the nurse may find that he is acting according to the dictates of his culture and that from his standpoint his behavior is natural and reasonable.

According to Biesanz,[5] all cultures have the following similarities: (1) language—a system for communication is essential to the continuation of a culture; (2) a system for utilizing the natural resources so that food, clothing, and shelter are provided; this necessitates a technologic and an economic system; (3) a social structure based on at least age and sex and usually on many other differences; (4) a means of ensuring desirable behavior and of perpetuating the society; (5) an explanation of the nature of the universe and man's place in it; this may be mythological or scientific; (6) a religion—this involves rituals for dealing with the supernatural and with problems such as death; (7) a way of communicating thoughts, ideas, emotions, and esthetic

[5] Biesanz, *Op. cit.*, pp. 30-31.

experiences; this may be through unwritten folklore or through written literature, music, and art; (8) play and recreational activities. Cultures vary in the
way in which they achieve each of the above.

Which of the characteristic elements of culture have the most
significance for the practice of nursing?

The elements of a culture that have significance in the practices of nursing
are: (1) religion, (2) patterns of family organization and child care, (3) care
during the following: birth, sickness, and death, (4) values as they relate to
age and sex, (5) language, (6) food habits, (7) orientation to time, (8)
patterns of sleep and personal hygiene, (9) patterns of modesty, and (10)
means of communicating satisfaction and dissatisfaction. Circumstances that
influence cultural and subcultural differences in the United States include:
(1) place of residence—such as city or country, north or south, and segregated or integrated, (2) socioeconomic status, (3) place of birth (America or
foreign country), and (4) level of education including professional education.
As the level of education of all people rises, differences among people tend to
become less marked. In other words, education becomes the great leveler.

These elements serve as the basis for the way in which a given culture plans
for and meets the problems that arise out of illness. They also affect the way
in which an individual within a culture regards illness and what he does to
prevent illness or to treat it. In other words, each person brings to every
situation (1) a set of values, (2) a set of expectations, (3) a code of behavior—a set of rules or standards that guide his conduct, (4) customs or
ceremonies he observes, and (5) manner and vocabulary by which he communicates with other people—nonverbal as well as verbal. An important
aspect of communication in nursing is the manner in which satisfaction and
dissatisfaction are expressed. Without this information the nurse may have
difficulty in determining whether or not the patient's needs are being met.

To illustrate and clarify the preceding statements, a folkway that is characteristic of middle- and upper-income groups in Western society is described
below. The situation is one in which Mr. and Mrs. Host invite Mr. and Mrs.
Guest for supper on Sunday. The language and the manner in which the
invitation is extended provide information about the party, such as degree of
formality, purpose, and who is likely to be invited. Depending on these and
other factors, each person will bring to the party a unique set of expectations
about how the guests and host and hostess should behave and be treated, and
what constitutes hospitality. They also have a set of rules or standards to
guide their conduct, customs or ceremonies they observe, and even a terminology for communicating with each other. Mr. Host expects that Mr. and
Mrs. Guest will or will not arrive at the time they are invited. Mr. Host, who
places high value on time, may feel that Mr. and Mrs. Guest ought to arrive
on time, but it is very likely he may not expect that they will. Mr. Host

alters his own behavior in respect to his expectations as to the time the guests can be expected to arrive. When the expectations of both the host and the guest are the same, few problems arise. When they differ, the guest may arrive and find his host in his shirt sleeves and the hostess in the bathtub, or find that the roast is dried out. If the purpose of the party is to celebrate a special occasion, the best china may be used and a formal menu planned. On the other hand, if the party is planned on the spur of the moment, and the invited guests are old friends, the everyday china and a simple menu, with everyone helping in the preparations, may be the order of the day.

The hosts and guests also have ways of expressing their satisfaction or dissatisfaction with the party and with each other. They may be sincere or they may cover their true feelings. When they say, "Good night," they may express pleasure despite the fact that the evening was dull.

Though this illustration could be expanded further, enough detail has been presented to make the point that each individual has a set of expectations, a code that guides his behavior, customs he observes, and a terminology for expressing his meanings. A party is more likely to be a mutually satisfying experience when the host and guests have a similar set of expectations or the host is aware of and takes into consideration the fact that the guests' expectations differ somewhat from his own. Moreover, when a host invites a comparative stranger to his home he attempts to learn something about his habits and customs, and to apprise him of what to expect so that he can plan in terms of his needs. If he values the guest's friendship or esteem, he does not show disrespect for him by ignoring a practice that has value or meaning to the guest. For example, he does not serve meat to a Catholic on Friday or pork chops to an Orthodox Jew. At the same time, the guest does not expect a host to serve a cocktail before dinner when the host disapproves of alcoholic beverages. In the care of the sick, the host-guest relationship differs inasmuch as the sick person is under stress. He is therefore likely to be less able to adapt to varying situations. When the nurse is also under stress, there are two people in the situation whose capacity to adapt is impaired.

Knowledge of the elements of culture should be helpful to the nurse in anticipating the individual patient's needs and in personalizing his care. In the chapter devoted to meeting the nutritional needs of the patient, attention will be devoted to the cultural aspects of food. Because of the limitations of the scope of this book, American patterns of child care and of childbirth will not be included.

An essential consideration in the care of each patient is his religion. A simple definition of religion is that it is man's idea of God and of his relationship to Him. It also includes the ways in which man shows his respect and love for God. Respect for the individual requires that his right to practice his particular religion be respected. The nurse, physician, social worker, and teacher must accept the person's right to his own religious beliefs, just as others must respect the nurse's right to her own religious beliefs. Many patients who are ill turn to their religion for comfort and solace. The nurse can be helpful to the patient by making it easy for him to see his pastor or a clergyman of his faith and by learning what is important to him, so that she can anticipate his religious needs. She can also be of assistance by showing her respect for his dignity and, with care marked by compassion, sympathy, and charity, contribute to meeting his spiritual needs. Charity means that the nurse is not only touched by the patient's suffering, but that she acts to relieve it. She contributes to the patient's spiritual welfare by supporting his faith and hope that his suffering is not in vain. She does what she can to ease his suffering and to keep his hope alive. She does not abandon or desert him. References are given at the end of chapter to which the nurse may refer for more specific information about the major faiths.

Although all the possible patterns of family organization cannot be described in detail, knowledge of who is the head of the family, who takes the responsibility in time of crisis such as illness, how the members of the family regard each other, and similar information may be helpful. In the United States, we have three kinds of family life, generally; patriarchal, matriarchal, and equalitarian. The latter is a product of the twentieth century and is not generally seen in other cultures. In the patriarchal family the husband makes the decisions. In the matriarchal family the wife or mother is the head of the family and therefore makes the decisions. In the equalitarian family, decisions are made jointly. To illustrate, the submissive wife is behaving appropriately in the patriarchal family when she accepts her husband's decisions. When she is ill or requires medical attention, she should not be expected to behave in the same way as the woman who has been the head of a family or who has supported herself for the same length of time. She should not be expected to acquiesce to a plan of therapy or change without having an opportunity to ask her husband.

A certain amount of disruption of the family is to be expected when a member is ill. The degree of disturbance will depend in part on the role of the person who is ill in the family. According to Parsons and Fox,[6] illness of the mother in a family is more disturbing to the rest of the family than is sickness of either the father or one of the children. They believe that this is true because the mother provides the primary emotional support for the other members.

Until recently, the trend toward hospitalization of the sick has increased. This has been particularly true for those who are seriously ill or for whom the illness is prolonged. Reasons given for caring for patients in hospitals include the fact that specialized services and equipment are available and that the patients can be given care that would be impossible for them to have at home. Sometimes this is true. Sociologists also suggest other reasons for caring for

[6] Talcott Parsons and Renée Fox, "Illness, Therapy and the Modern Urban American Family," *Patients, Physicians, and Illness*, ed. E. Gartley Jaco, The Free Press, Glencoe, Illinois, 1958, p. 239.

the sick in specialized institutions. One of these is that it serves to protect the family from the disrupting effects of having a sick person in their midst. In a small two- or three-bedroom house the continued presence of a seriously ill person may place great physical and emotional strain on the family. A trend is developing, however, toward returning the sick to their homes earlier than has been the general practice in the immediate past. The success of this plan depends, among other things, on the patient, the nature of his illness, the family strengths, the attitudes of the members of the family toward each other and toward the illness, and their acceptance of the patient and the plan to care for him at home. It also depends on the provision of the kinds of services to the patient and his family that make it possible for him to be cared for, or to care for himself, at home. These services include medical and nursing care, physical therapy, housekeeping, and occupational therapy. Ambulance service may be provided to return the patient to the hospital for a needed service such as an X ray or for hospitalization. In some instances, home care is easier for the patient and family to accept, when they are assured that the patient will be readmitted to the hospital promptly should this be necessary.

Not all cultures care for their sick in the hospital. In fact they may look upon the hospital as a cold and formal place that can in no way substitute for the presence of a loving family. For example, Saunders cites the instance of the young girl whose family would not permit her to be hospitalized for the treatment of tuberculosis, because they believed that the sick should have the care and support of the family. The fact that the girl was capable of infecting the family was of no importance to them. Neither did they believe that she might be given better care in the hospital than at home.[7] In other cultures, support is provided by one or more of the members of the family going to the hospital with the patient and staying until he is well. They may cook his meals and provide for his personal care. Probably one of the greatest values of this practice derives from the fact that the patient shifts his concern for his welfare to his family. They are there. They will be responsible. They will take care of him.

Practices in the care of the dying and the dead vary in different cultures all the way from placing the dying outside the village limits or deserting them to taking extraordinary measures to preserve life. Though the desertion of the sick and infirm seems cruel, in primitive societies this may be necessary to the survival of the living. There are also those who question the kindness of taking extreme measures to continue life in the seriously disabled or diseased person.[8] In the American culture there is a tendency to protect the young from knowledge of death and from the dying. Many who die die in hospitals, where they are separated from family members by equipment, procedures, and personnel. Most students of nursing have had little, if any, experience

[7] Lyle Saunders, *Cultural Differences and Medical Care*, Russell Sage Foundation, New York, 1954, pp. 16-17.
[8] "Way of Dying," *Atlantic Monthly*, January, 1957, pp. 53-55.

with death. Many adults are fearful in the presence of the dying person. Mrs. Carol Willis was well aware of this when she said, "We embarrass our friends." She also said that one of the needs of the dying person is for someone to listen. As long as the nurse is primarily concerned with her own fears about death and dying, she cannot be a sympathetic listener.

The attitude of those caring for the sick aged may be adversely influenced by the fact that, in the American culture, youth is the idealized state. In some cultures youth is considered to be a handicap and age is respected because it brings with it experience and wisdom. In these cultures the aged are given status rather than being relegated to the background.

Another factor that is significant to the status and role of an individual in his group is his sex. In some cultures the male has a higher status than the female, though the reverse is true in some cultures. In most cultures the relationships between the sexes are defined, as are the occupations and activities that are fitting for, or expected of, one and not the other. Appropriate behavior is also defined in terms of sex. For example, in the Anglo-American culture women may cry without losing status. Men may not. In a society such as ours, what is acceptable behavior is subject to change. Not too many years ago nice women did not smoke or wear trousers in public. Now they do both. To satisfy the patient's needs requires some knowledge of how he regards his role and what he considers is and is not proper for him to do.

Language is, of course, necessary to communication. Even when two people speak the same language, difficulties in communication may arise out of the fact that though they use the same words they may not have the same meanings. Inflection, tone, and nonverbal behavior may also contribute to giving a variety of meanings to words. When people who are trying to communicate speak different languages, some other means of communication must be used. In case there is a person who speaks the patient's language, he should be used as an interpreter. Suitable provisions must also be made to communicate with the patient who is unable to speak because of a defect in his nervous system or organs of speech. Sign language or writing may be used. Although nonverbal communication is always important, it becomes increasingly significant when caring for patients who are unable to make their needs known or to understand the language spoken by their attendants. Kind, gentle care given with a true concern for the welfare of the patient will do much to overcome the barriers created by the lack of a common language.

How does a person's orientation to time influence his expectations and behavior during illness?

Some problems in the care of patients arise out of differences in orientation to time and the value placed on it. Orientation to time may be to the past, present, or future. This is illustrated in the literature of various peoples. For example, in our literature the ant spends the summer busily storing supplies for the coming winter months, while the improvident grasshopper dashes around enjoying himself. It is quite shocking to Americans to learn that there are cultures in which the ant is viewed as the foolish one, and the grasshopper wise. From the latter point of view, the present is what one has. Why expend effort for a time that may never be. A third orientation to time was held by some Chinese in bygone days. They believed that the future is behind one and therefore cannot be seen. They are said to have built pleasure gardens along the side of the streams where they sat facing downstream contemplating the past.

That not all Americans have the same view of time is borne out in a study by Koos.[9] In this study he found that respondents from class I (upper) looked toward the future; those from class II (middle) were primarily occupied with the present; while those in class III (lower) had little hope in either the present or the future. In general, middle-class Americans look at the present as better than the past, and the future is expected to be better than either. In another study, Saunders found that Spanish-speaking Americans who live in the southwestern part of the United States lived in the present or immediate past rather than in the past or the future. He states that this creates a problem in their medical care. How can they know whether they want a clinic appointment next week when they do not know how they will be feeling at that time? According to their perception of time, this is a logical conclusion. When they are talked into making clinic appointments, they may or may not keep them. If on the day of the appointment they feel well, they see no reason to keep it.[10]

Because of the trend in the American culture to consider the future important, Americans provide for old age and for illness and death by buying some type of insurance. People who fail, or are unable, to do this are generally considered to be improvident. As a result of the depression which began in 1929, the fact that industrial workers were not always able to protect themselves against unemployment was recognized. In 1935 the Social Security Act was passed. It had three provisions based on the principle that society has an obligation to provide for the security of its people. The first provision was for unemployment compensation to be handled by the states. The second was establishment of an annuity which was to be paid at age 65 or on retirement of its members. The third provided for special categories of needy persons including the aged, the blind, the crippled and disabled, and dependent children. In this way the government has assumed responsibility for helping people provide for the future.

The other dimension of time is the value placed on it. Time is sometimes equated with success by Americans. It is generally believed to have value in achieving success, as it can be used with profit or it can be wasted. Sayings in

[9] Earl L. Koos, *The Health of Regionville,* Columbia University Press, New York, 1954, pp. 21-24.
[10] Saunders, *Op. cit.,* pp. 117-22.

the American language such as "Time waits for no man" or "Time is money" indicate this. When one is employed by another, he sells his time rather than his productivity. He punches a time clock when he arrives at and when he leaves his place of employment. An employee is usually paid for the number of hours rather than units of work. There is a tendency to judge efficiency in terms of the individual's ability to appear to be busy at any given moment. Even nurses are judged by this standard. The nurse is employed for 40 hours per week. The nurse who is busy is commended. The one who is not occupied or appears to be using her time in a frivolous manner, such as visiting or talking to patients, is frowned upon.

Because of the emphasis placed on the value of time in the American culture, it is not surprising that the sick person places great value on having his medications and treatments at the time they are scheduled and that he judges the quality of his care in terms of how closely the schedule is kept. He also wants to know when his care is to be given and to be apprised of changes as well as the reason for change. From the point of view of the nursing staff, these points may not seem to be important. Because of the emphasis placed on the value of time in the American culture, failure to utilize this knowledge in the care of the patient may be a source of unnecessary psychological stress to the patient and, because the patient is unhappy, it may subsequently be a source of psychological stress to the nurse. For example, Mrs. Benrus who was hospitalized for an extended period of time was allowed to spend her weekends at home provided she arrange to have a nurse administer Acthar[11] by intramuscular injection at eight in the morning and eight in the evening. When the nurse was even a few minutes late, Mrs. Benrus became very agitated, thus placing a strain on the nurse. In this instance the nurse recognized the importance of time to Mrs. Benrus and made an effort to arrive a few minutes early.

Some knowledge of the sleep patterns of the person may be useful when providing care. For example, the person may be accustomed to having a room of his own, or to sharing his bed with another. If the first person is in a large ward, he may have difficulty in sleeping, while the second may be lonely when he is by himself. This does not mean that the nurse may be able to alter the situation, but she can be understanding of the patient's difficulties. Perhaps more attention should also be given to the patient's habits of personal hygiene than is often done. Not all people come from areas where a daily bath or shower is possible. Some even live where taking a bath entails a good bit of effort and planning. Old people, especially old men, may suffer itching of the skin when they bathe more than once or twice a week. Conversely, there are

[11] Acthar (adrenocorticotrophic hormone) is a trade name for an extract of anterior pituitary glands, prepared for parenteral use in doses of 10, 20, 25, 40, and 80 U.S.P. units. It acts by stimulating the adrenal cortex to secrete all of its glucocorticoids and mineralocorticoids at an increased rate. The average adult dose is 40 to 50 U.S.P. units daily. See a pharmacology textbook for further information about the action and toxicity of adrenocorticosteroids.

those who bathe at least once daily and are upset when they cannot. This point can be illustrated by two brothers, Allen and Bert, who were seriously ill. Allen was much upset because his nurse insisted on giving him a bath every morning. Bert was upset for an entire day because he did not have a bath. In neither instance did the patient's physical welfare depend on whether or not he had a bath. Other aspects of personal hygiene that are sometimes neglected and at other times forced upon reluctant or protesting patients include the opportunity to brush their teeth, to have their hair combed, to wash their hands after using the bedpan, and to have back care. The point here is to try to learn something about the personal habits and expectations of the patient. When something in the nature of the illness of the person necessitates a change, then, of course, the cooperation of the patient should be enlisted. The nurse should assess those aspects of hygienic care which are essential to the welfare and peace of mind of the patient and modify the care of the patient accordingly.

There are innumerable ways in which persons can express their satisfactions and dissatisfactions. Though either may be expressed directly, they may also be expressed indirectly. For example, a patient may smile and say that everything is fine and be sincere, or he may feel quite differently. Sometimes the nurse may detect something in the patient's tone of voice, expression, or position that tells her that everything is not fine. He may not wish to hurt her feelings, or he may want her approval, or he may feel that she is not really interested, or he may even feel that it is not safe for him to express his dissatisfaction directly. He may also express his dissatisfaction indirectly by being demanding or hypercritical. Sometimes only after the nurse has made considerable effort to develop a trusting relationship will the patient express his true feelings.

Place of residence is another factor that influences the cultural and subcultural differences in people. In the United States there is less difference between city and country people than there once was. However, differences do continue to exist particularly in those instances where a group is segregated or isolated, either by choice or by custom, from the remainder of the population. For example, some religious groups, such as the Mennonites and Amish, settle in communities in order to protect and maintain a way of life that is essential to the practice of their religion.Though the situation is changing slowly, Negroes living in rural areas in the South are isolated from the white population. One preliminary study of the behavior of hospitalized Negro patients being cared for by white nurses has been reported by McCabe.[12] While she is careful to state that her conclusions are tentative, effective care of these patients appears to depend on the nurse's being aware of the patient's expectations of the nurse's behavior, as well as her own expectations. McCabe also indicates that to evaluate success in meeting the needs of Negro patients from

[12] Gracia S. McCabe, "Cultural Influences on Patient Behavior," *American Journal of Nursing*, LX, August, 1960, pp. 1101-4.

southern rural areas, the nurse must know how they express satisfaction or dissatisfaction with their care. She emphasizes the importance of not stereotyping patients.

Despite the general conviction of Americans to the contrary, socioeconomic status does influence the expectations, aspirations, and way of life of Americans. Recent statistics indicate that it even influences life expectancy in that the lower the income, the shorter the life expectancy. It seems safe to conclude that anything in the life of the individual that is different from that of other individuals contributes to differences in expectations, codes regulating behavior, modes of expressing and satisfying needs, and the language used. If the point that individuals differ appears to be overstressed, it is because not only patient satisfaction, but that of the nurse, depends, in part, on the identification and satisfaction of individual expectations of patients.

How does a person's system of values affect his expectations during illness?

One of the important aspects of culture is its system of values. Ruesch states that many of the values held in America have their origin in the fact that until very recently America was a pioneer country. Moreover, the early settlers were Puritans who placed a high value on plain living, industry, self-control, will power, cleanliness, consistency, honesty, and the assumption of responsibility. In settling the country, survival often depended on such characteristics as strength, initiative, and hard work. There was little time for pleasure. Entertainment was organized around important events in life such as a wedding, a death, or a house building.[13]

According to Ruesch, the American value system is based on the four premises "equality, sociality, success, and change." The ideal that all men are equal has its origin in the Judeo-Christian belief that all men are equal in the sight of God. This represents a change in culture. In the ancient world the attitude toward man was very different. In the words of Edith Hamilton,[14] "In Egypt, in Crete, in Mesopotamia, wherever we can read bits of the story, we find the same conditions: A despot enthroned, whose whims and passions are the determining factor in the state; a wretched subjugated populace; a great priestly organization to which is handed over the domain of the intellect." The founders of our nation made their views clear in *The Declaration of Independence* when they said, "We hold these truths to be self evident; that all men are created equal; that they are endowed by their Creator with certain inalienable Rights, that among them are life, liberty and the pursuit of happiness." Lincoln re-emphasized the belief in equality of men in the opening sentence of *The Gettysburg Address*. One of the important issues in the world

[13] Jurgen Ruesch and Gregory Bateson, *Communication,* W. W. Norton & Co., Inc., New York, 1951, pp. 94-134.
[14] Edith Hamilton, *The Greek Way,* W. W. Norton & Co., Inc., New York, 1930, p. 19.

today stems from whose rights come first, the individual's or the state's, and from whom these rights are derived.

In application of the premise of equality to the practice of nursing, nurses are taught to give the same quality of care to all patients whatever their background, social condition, or disease. Because all patients are individuals, as are nurses, and each one is different from all others, perhaps the nurse can come closer to reaching the ideal of equality of care if she can accept the patient as a human being, recognize his dignity, identify behavior that provides clues to his needs, consider the meaning of his behavior, and plan his care to meet his needs. To do this, the nurse requires some knowledge of her own system of values.

The second premise on which Ruesch[15] says the American value system is based is that of sociality. By this is meant that the American tends to be guided in his actions by the opinion of his peers. He forms social groups in which he works to accomplish the goals of the group. He is responsive to the pressure of the group and is very much aware of his status in it. When called upon to make a decision, he tends to think in terms of "What will the neighbors think?" As might be expected, health care and the way the individual behaves when he is sick is influenced by dependence on his neighbors' approval or disapproval of his actions. Koos's study cites the example of a woman who called a physician to see her child with the chickenpox, not because she felt it was necessary, but because she did not want her friends to think that she was neglecting him.[16] Children and adults are dosed with vitamins and patent medicines, not because there is objective evidence that they are required, but because everyone is taking the preparation.

The tendency of Americans to form social groups is also evident in the health and welfare field. Organizations in the health field extend from those that are dedicated to research and investigation of the causes of, and education of the public about, the nature of a single disease, to those in which a group of people associate themselves together in order to provide emotional support as they work toward the accomplishment of a single goal such as the loss of weight.

Moreover, the value of group action is held to be so great that Americans voluntarily tax themselves for the financial support of numerous organizations. They do this by contributing to the individual organization or to the Community Chest. Individuals who devote time and effort to these organizations are accorded special status in the community. They may be both approved and envied by their peers. Certain values influence defining of the goals of these groups. For instance, the strong help the weak as long as the weakness is the result of age or some circumstance that is not within what society considers to be the control of the individual. Americans also place a high value on independence. Children are trained early to be independent. Dependence is ac-

---

[15] *Loc. cit.*
[16] *Op. cit.*, p. 71.

cepted as a part of illness, but the patient is expected to work toward independence. If the individual is to be given continued assistance, he is expected to make an effort to alter his situation for the better.

The need to be a part of a group and for status is also seen in the behavior of hospitalized patients. Patients who are hospitalized for long periods form social groups on both an informal and formal basis. In some hospitals where patients are hospitalized for the treatment of tuberculosis or mental illness, committees are formed which serve many purposes. They provide a channel through which the patients' grievances are brought to the attention of the administration. They may act as a quasi-official governing body, or to prepare and distribute a ward or hospital paper. They may also be utilized to help patients work out their problems and to prepare them for life outside the hospital.

Nurses need to be aware that patients' need for status in the group and acceptance by members of the group may be violated by practices the patient does not understand or for which he is not prepared. To illustrate, Mr. Long had been hospitalized for weeks for a condition which had been treated by the removal of one lobe of one lung. Throughout the period he received excellent nursing care and had recovered to the point where he was ready for discharge in a few days. The decision was made to assign an aide rather than a nursing student to provide his nursing care. Later in the morning when the head nurse visited him, she was surpised at the violence with which Mr. Long objected to being cared for by an aide. She listened quietly—she hoped. Mr. Long finally concluded his statement by saying that he expected that Miss Student was caring for a patient who needed her more than he did. Miss Head Nurse agreed and said that Miss Student would also visit him later in the day. This patient's feelings of rejection might have been prevented by an explanation previous to the time the change was made.

Sometimes the patient achieves status by having an unusual condition or by having an unusual variation of an illness. On the other hand, the fact that he is different or does not conform to the usual pattern may cause him to be anxious. After he recovers, he may boast to the neighbors that he had an illness that his doctor had never seen before. But during the illness, the fact that he did not conform to the norm may have caused him concern or may have been the cause for shame.

The American places a high value on a healthy body, youth, and physical attractiveness. He tends to look down on those who are physically weak, deformed, or unsightly. At times a patient may be unable to accept a necessary treatment, because of the effect that the treatment will have, or that he believes it will have, on his appearance, his capacity to function, or his acceptance by the group to whom he belongs. The need to conform to the expectations of the group is also illustrated by the concern of parents that their children meet norms which are considered to indicate that the children are developing normally. This sometimes results in unnecessary anxiety on the part of parents and pressure on children. That children also are sensitive to pressure from their peer group to conform is illustrated by the instance of six-year-old Joey, a dark brunet, who played with light, blond children. That he was aware of this difference was made clear when he said to his mother, "Mommy when you were getting a boy, why didn't you get a light one?"

The recognition of the value that Americans place on the approval of their peers as well as of their tendency to work in groups and conform to group pressures has significance in the practice of nursing. It is an important factor to consider when the condition of the patient demands a change in his pattern of living. It also relates to that aspect of the role of the nurse in which she functions to relieve tension among the members of the therapeutic team. In this role she contributes to the care of the patient by helping each member of the team feel good toward each other. It is also well to remember that in the American culture, for many people, to be liked is more important than to like. As a consequence, failure of the patient's physician or nurse to express approval may be interpreted by the patient as disapproval or as an indication he is not progressing satisfactorily. Despite the fact that the patient is recovering as expected, he may need to be reassured by the physician that he is recovering satisfactorily. The nurse may be helpful to the patient by listening to the patient's doubts and pointing to evidence of progress. When the patient expresses more than usual concern, this should be reported to the physician as well as recorded.

The third premise on which the American value system is based is that of success. Success is a yardstick by which the value of an individual is measured. This means that there is generally a high value placed on achievement. There is little respect for those who rest on their oars or who are not considered to be productive. There is a tendency to believe that failure results from a lack of effort and that mastery of any problem or difficulty is possible if sufficient effort and/or money is expended. Thus the chronically ill person, or the one who has lost his job, loses status because he has not expended sufficient effort to stay well or be restored to health, or to keep or to get a new job. This point of view may help to explain the fact that many health workers in America, including nurses, prefer to care for the acutely ill who get well quickly and to avoid the care of the chronically ill, that is, those who fail to recover fully or quickly. While the individual is expected to try hard to achieve, his effort must not show. People whose efforts to succeed are obvious are frowned upon. The student who studies diligently and obviously is labeled a grind or some equally derogatory term. Another aspect is that, in the achievement of success, the end tends to justify the means. That is to say, an act is not bad in itself. It becomes bad only when the person is caught. As a consequence, mastery and virtuosity are not valued as highly as they are in some societies.

There is also a tendency to measure success in the various aspects of life. A baby is not just a baby who is thriving, but he is the biggest, the smallest, the fattest, the cutest, the cryingest, or the most voracious eater of any baby on the block. Mr. Lip was not just sick with pneumonia, but he was the sickest, had the highest temperature, and made the quickest recovery of any patient in the hospital. One of the measures used to indicate success in life is the tendency to emphasize the length of life rather than the quality or richness of it.

The fourth premise is that, for the American, life is not static, but is in a process of change. The result is that the American is geared for action and ready for change. He values adaptability and moves from one job to another to get experience, better pay, or higher status. He hopes by change to improve his chances of ascending the ladder of success. Popular magazines frequently carry articles about the mobility of American society, its causes and effects. Associated with change is anxiety, for anxiety is necessary to prepare the individual for change.

The patient's attitude toward change is reflected in his expectations as to what constitutes adequate and appropriate medical care. He is willing to spend money to finance research into the causes and prevention of illness, but he finds it difficult to understand why answers may be slow in coming. He looks anxiously for signs indicating that he is improving, and when he does not find them or he learns that he cannot expect to recover quickly, he tends to be downcast. He also has great faith in the value of machines and drugs in his treatment. He is likely to feel somehow cheated if they are not necessary or used.

As a basis for a discussion of the role of the sick person in the American culture, some values that relate to Ruesch's four premises which motivate Americans, that is, equality, sociality, success, and change, have been discussed and illustrated. There are other values that are important to many individual Americans. Since the values held to be important by the individual influence his behavior, personalizing of patient care depends on having some knowledge of what they are. The nurse should remember, however, that not all Americans value the same things. Studies that have been reported indicate that even in fairly homogeneous communities, the values held differ from one socioeconomic group to another. For example, Hollingshead and Redlich[17] report that the type of psychotherapy which patients expect differs with each socioeconomic group. Patients from the upper socioeconomic groups expect and profit from insight therapy. They expect to learn about why they act as they do and to learn to modify their behavior. Those in the lower classes expect an authoritarian attitude on the part of the psychiatrist. They want the psychiatrist to tell them what to do. Hollingshead and Redlich qualify this by stating that there are individuals in the upper classes who cannot profit from insight therapy, while there are those from the lower classes who can. The authors of this study further state that psychiatrists, both because they come

---

[17] August B. Hollingshead and Frederick C. Redlich, *Social Class and Mental Illness,* J. B. Wiley & Sons, Inc., New York, 1958, p. 345.

from the middle and upper classes and because they are trained to use insight therapy, seemed to find it difficult to work with patients from the lower classes.

Studies of the attitudes of nurses toward patients such as the one reported by MacGregor[18] also indicate that nurses view patients in light of their own values. MacGregor concluded that the students' image of the upper-class patient tended to be that of a "spoiled, demanding, condescending person who may regard the nurse as a servant." The students' view of the middle- and lower-class patient was that of "a person who is more appreciative, respectful, and less demanding." These examples are cited not in criticism of either psychiatrists or nurses, but to emphasize the point that each individual tends to evaluate the behavior of others in light of his own values and standards. This happens even when both individuals are from a similar, though not identical, culture. Of necessity this discussion has been brief, but perhaps enough detail has been presented so that the nurse can appreciate that each person tends to perceive his situation in light of his past learnings and experiences. It is easier to accept others who have similar values and standards of behavior than it is to accept those who differ. This is as true for nurses and physicians as for patients. Individualization of the patient's care demands that the nurse try to see the situation through the eyes of the patient and communicate that she is trying. She should also realize that she can never do this completely.

Why is some knowledge of culturally established rules governing the behavior of the sick and those who care for them essential in the practice of nursing?

In addition to having values that are important in other aspects of the life of the individual, each culture or subculture establishes rules about what it regards as sickness and the behavior and responsibilities of those who are ill as well as of those who care for them. This can be illustrated by the studies made by Zborowski[19] of the responses of Jewish, Italian, and Old Americans to pain which led him to conclude that knowledge of culture is essential to the effective care of these patients. He found that the Jewish and Italian patients were more overtly emotional in expressing pain than were the Old Americans. Jewish and Italian patients differed in their response to treatment, however. When appropriate measures were instituted, the Italians were relieved of their pain and happy with the result. Jewish patients, on the other hand, were concerned about the possible implications of their pain to their future health and were reluctant to take pain-relieving medications. They were fearful that drugs might produce ill effects which would be manifested at some future

---

[18] Francis Cooke MacGregor, *Social Science in Nursing,* Russell Sage Foundation, New York, 1960, p. 101.

[19] Mark Zborowski, "Cultural Components in Response to Pain," *Journal of Social Issues,* VIII, 1952, pp. 16-30.

time. To relieve Jewish patients' pain it was necessary to relieve their concern about what was causing the pain and to reassure them about possible delayed effects of the pain-relieving medication, or about their illnesses. Though the observed behavior appeared to be similar for Italian and Jewish patients, the meaning was different. To be effective, the treatment had to take the meaning of the pain into account.

Zborowski[20] also found that the patient of Old American stock was similar to the Jewish patient inasmuch as he tended to be concerned about the implications of the pain to his future recovery. He differed from the Jewish and Italian patient in that he was undemonstrative in his reaction to pain. He also gave the impression of trying to report on pain; that is, he appeared to be trying to be an objective observer. When he was in severe pain, he tended to withdraw from society. He might cry, but when he did he preferred to cry alone. He was observed to have a different pattern of behavior when he was with his family and friends than when he was with members of the professional staff. In the presence of his family and friends he tended to minimize his pain and to avoid complaining. On the ward he tried to cooperate with the staff and to behave as he thought he was expected to. He considered himself a part of the team—doctor, nurse, and patient—in which every member had a part to play and each member was expected to do his share.

Not only does each man's beliefs, customs, and value systems affect the way he behaves when he is ill, but they also affect how he thinks he should be treated and how those who are responsible for his care feel about him and what they do for him. As in other areas involving human beings, multiple factors are often involved and seemingly simple behavior may have complex meanings which are interrelated with other factors. Furthermore, the interpreter interprets in his own frame of reference. The patient who moans and groans when he has pain may be suffering from pain that is well-nigh unbearable, or he may feel that this is the way to bring his pain to the attention of those who care for him or that his family expects him to behave in this way. He may be concerned about the pain itself or the implications for his future. The nurse who cares for the patient may have been brought up to believe that pain should be borne silently, or that it is appropriate to express it, or that once it is treated one should be satisfied. The manner in which the nurse treats the patient, and the extent to which she is able to be helpful to him, will depend in some measure on her understanding of the meaning that the situation has to the patient. Respect for the rights and dignity of man and the right of each person to participate in plans that concern his welfare are values that are sometimes lost in the conflict over other values.

An attempt has been made to establish the importance of knowledge of the beliefs, customs, and values of the providers of care as well as of those who receive it. It is not possible to discuss all aspects of the American culture, let alone the characteristics of its subcultures. One point that has not been intro-

[20] *Ibid.,* pp. 16-20.

duced is that professional education creates certain barriers between those who serve and those who are served. As a result of a professional education and experiences, the individual acquires a different set of values, attitudes, vocabulary, and ways of behaving in regard to illness. As part of his education the professional person should learn to transcend the barriers. One way to do this is through the use of language. For example, a public health nurse talked about dressings in explaining to a group of workmen about provisions in their company-sponsored insurance plan for home care. The union supervisor reminded her that the men did not understand what dressings were but that they would understand if she called them bandages. This example illustrates how lack of a common vocabulary is a barrier to understanding.

What are some of the culturally determined expectations common to nurses belonging to the middle class American culture?

Nurses, as well as patients, are people who have needs that require satisfaction. They, like other people, learn to satisfy their needs in ways that are socially acceptable to the family, group, and culture into which they were born. When they enter a school of nursing they bring with them the values, ideals, goals, and ways of behaving they have learned. Depending on their past experiences, they bring to nursing a set of expectations for what patients ought to be like and how they ought to behave. When the student is from the Anglo-American culture, she is likely to expect that patients will respond to treatment by getting well quickly and that patients will express satisfaction with and be grateful for their care. The nursing student also brings to nursing a set of expectations based on values she has learned. This includes what she believes a good nurse is, does, and ought to be able to accomplish. Through the course of her nursing program, the goals of the student and expectations for herself and for patients are modified or changed to conform more closely to those of her mentors. As in other areas of nursing, all nurses should be able to improve their ability to identify and meet the psychosocial needs of patients through study, evaluation, and practice.

By this point the fact that illness and health have social and cultural definitions as well as biological and physiological ones should be clear. As a result of family, group, and cultural patterns the individual learns what to regard as health or sickness. He learns what he should do about sickness—what kinds of measures can be expected to be effective in warding it off or in curing it. He learns what his responsibilities are when he is ill and what he should expect from others including his family and the members of his culture who have special knowledge and skill in matters of health and disease. Those who are given status by a society by virtue of having special knowledge and skill in treating illness also have expectations, values, and ways of behaving that they accept as being appropriate. The more nearly those of the patient and the nurse or other professional persons agree, the more satisfactory services are likely to be and the more likely both individuals are to achieve satisfaction. Conversely, the greater the disparity between the client and the giver of service, the greater the possibility that the service will not be provided in a way that is satisfactory to the recipient. Moreover, this disparity can be a source of psychological stress to the patient.

As has been emphasized, the meaning that an illness has for an individual and what he does to prevent or to treat it are conditioned by the beliefs, customs, and values which he acquires from his family and the society in which he lives. These factors determine what man as a thinking, remembering, imagining being regards as illness and what he should do about it. Illness is, however, a personal as well as a cultural experience. When a person is ill, he responds in a variety of ways: intellectually, emotionally, physically, and physiologically. The degree of his response depends on a variety of factors some of which include the causative agent, the way in which the person perceives the threat to his well-being, and his biological, intellectual, and emotional resources. Some of his responses will be voluntary, others involuntary. Some of them will be highly individual. Whatever they are, they will be of value to the degree to which they are constructive and integrative and result in action which enables him to protect himself against, or to eliminate, danger. They are pathological to the degree that they are disorganized, inappropriate, exaggerated, and ineffectual.

In the discussion of the psychological aspects of illness, the following points will be considered:

1. The levels of psychological reactions in illness.
2. A review of a concept of emotional homeostasis.
3. A definition of psychological stress.
4. Some of the causes of psychological stress in illness.
5. How people react during the various phases of illness.
6. What some of the aspects of emotion are and how they relate to psychological stress.
7. Ways in which the nurse may seek to relieve psychological stress in illness.

What are some of the intellectual responses to illness?

In illness, each individual reacts as he does in other crises in his life. His reactions are often complex. Psychological responses involve the individual's intellect and his emotions. Through the use of his intelligence, man is able to foresee the consequences of his actions and to plan to avert injury or to correct the damage that has been done. Inasmuch as he is able to acquire knowledge and to grasp and identify the significant factors in his situation, and to use his capacity to reason and think, to modify his behavior, or to adapt the environment to his needs, his intelligence is useful to him. However, like other factors that concern human beings, how well any person uses his intelligence depends on numerous factors, including his educational background and his emotional state. Hence, a highly intelligent and well-educated person, even a physician or a nurse, may act irrationally as well as rationally in a crisis situation such as illness. Intelligence is useful to an individual inasmuch as he uses it objectively, to identify the nature of the threat and to plan to protect himself from it or to eliminate it. It fails him inasmuch as the knowledge on which he bases his decisions is inadequate or inaccurate, or not applicable, or his emotional state is such that he is unable to use his knowledge. This is not to imply that education and intelligence are not of value to the person when he is ill, because they are. Moreover, the point that intelligence is not synonymous with either education or years of schooling is worth making. Some persons who are intelligent, but who have had little opportunity to go to school, are well educated. Because of the tendency to equate schooling with education and with intelligence, quite intelligent but unschooled persons may be treated as if they were unintelligent. They may then respond as if they were truly stupid. When the patient's level of education is similar to that of his attendants, communication is facilitated. They are more likely to have similar vocabularies and values than when their backgrounds differ widely. When there are differences in background, the degree of success with which attendants meet the needs of the patient is related to the extent to which they take into account these differences.

Any illness that is serious enough to cause a person to seek medical attention is likely to provoke a variety of emotions: fear, anxiety, anger, helplessness, hopelessness, or even relief and pleasure. Sometimes feelings are contradictory; the person may be anxious about the cause of his illness or its symptoms, but be relieved because his illness justified some of his actions. Illness can be used to explain a failure or to escape an unpleasant duty. For example, illness may be used to explain failure in an examination or a patient's irritation with his nurse. Or it may be used to justify the refusal of an invitation to a party that the person feels he should attend. The fact may be that he dislikes the hostess or the type of party. Illness, however, provides a socially acceptable excuse for not attending.

What is meant by the concept of emotional homeostasis?

Although the concept of homeostasis was introduced by Cannon to explain the constancy of internal physiological environment of cells in the body, psychologists have adapted the concept to encompass the emotional state. As with physiological homeostasis, emotional homeostasis depends on having certain needs fulfilled. Whereas the supplies required to satisfy physiological needs are materials such as oxygen or water, those required to meet psychological needs are nonmaterial. They are the conditions, situations, actions, or effects of actions which the individual perceives, experiences, and represents in his mind as having meaning. Depending on the situation and its meanings the person feels safe and protected, esteemed by others and himself, and loved. Conversely, he may feel threatened, unsafe, unesteemed, endangered, and unloved. The satisfaction of psychological needs depends on the organism having structures that function in such a manner that he is able to perceive and evaluate threats to his welfare. Psychological homeostasis implies, as does physiological homeostasis, the presence of processes or mechanisms that are regulated to maintain or to restore emotional, or psychological, stability in a changing environment.

Agents that endanger psychological homeostasis may have their origin in either the internal or external environment of the individual. They are similar to agents that threaten physiological homeostasis in that they may result from an excess or deficit of supply. They differ from agents that threaten physiological homeostasis in that the individual responds not only to the agent itself, but to what it symbolizes. Consequently, fear and anxiety can be engendered by harmless things. The individual feels and behaves in the presence of the symbol as he would if he were in the presence of the thing it represents to him. As a consequence of this phenomenon, much of what man fears is learned.

To illustrate, Mrs. Simon is afraid of cats. Despite her knowledge that cats are for the most part harmless, when she sees a cat she feels and acts terrified. She has all the signs and symptoms that are commonly associated with terror. She has no memory of what the situation was that was responsible for her fear, but to her the cat—any cat—is a symbol of danger which is just as real as was the original one.

As in physiological homeostasis, individuals differ in their capacity to adapt. Many factors contribute to this difference. Some of these may be inborn, others learned, while others may result from disease. For example, the capacity of the brain-injured child or adult to adapt to frustration is less than that of a healthy person. This must be recognized and the environment adapted, so that expectations are kept within the person's ability to function. Though the capacity to tolerate psychological stress differs from one individual to another, all people have a limit. As stated earlier, there are many factors in illness that contribute to psychological stress.

How is psychological stress defined?

As a basis for the discussion of the causes of psychological stress, Engel's definition of stress is quoted.

"Psychological stress refers to all processes, whether originating in the external environment or within the person, which impose a demand or requirement upon the organism, the resolution or handling of which necessitates work or activity of the mental apparatus before any other system is involved or activated."[21]

[21] George L. Engel, "A Unified Concept of Health and Disease," *Perspectives in Biology and Medicine,* III, Summer, 1960, p. 480.

Any condition or situation which requires adaptation may place strain on the adaptive capacity of the individual. This may be true because the capacity of the individual is limited or because the condition to which he is required to adapt is extreme. This applies to psychological as well as physiological agents. Psychological stresses place strain on the adaptive capacity of the organism by acting on the brain and mental apparatus.[22] Although other agents that place strain on the adaptive capacity of the organism may produce psychological stress, this action is secondary. Their primary effect is on biochemical processes, cells, organs, or system. Psychological stress may also, and often does, involve structures other than the mental apparatus, but its primary effect is on the mental apparatus. Whatever the cause of the disturbance, agents that act as stimuli result in the initiation of mechanisms of response that serve to reduce or relieve the discomfort. In general these mechanisms enable the individual to attack or to withdraw from the danger or to play dead (possum). References have been placed at the end of the chapter for those students who wish to review the psychological mechanisms utilized by people to defend emotional homeostasis.

Although Engel's classification of the causes of psychological stress was included in Chapter 1, it is repeated here. They are: (1) the loss of something that is of value to the person, (2) injury or threat of injury to the body, and (3) the frustration of drives. These, obviously, are interrelated. In illness all these elements contribute in some degree to cause psychological stress in patients.

During illness the individual may lose or be threatened with the loss of something that has value to him. He is almost certain to suffer painful procedures or to fear that he will. The fear is often made worse by the fact that he does not know what to expect and therefore fears the worst. In the process of growing up the individual learns to master his drives so that his needs can be met in keeping with reality. Sometimes the manner in which he regards his drives is a source of conflict. During illness these conflicts may be intensified. Whatever the specific source of psychological stress in illness, it leads to unpleasant feelings such as anxiety, anger, helplessness, hopelessness, guilt, shame, and disgust. To counteract these feelings and to restore emotional homeostasis, psychological defense mechanisms that have been relatively effective in the past will be initiated. When defense mechanisms such as rationalization, projection, sublimation, displacement, or denial are ineffective or unavailable to restore emotional homeostasis, physiological and/or behavioral changes follow.

What will actually be disturbing to any patient during illness and how he will react are highly individual matters. There are, however, some causes of psychological stress that occur frequently enough that they should be considered when each patient's needs are assessed. The first of these is the patient's concept of himself. This self-concept includes all the ideas, conscious and

[22] *Ibid.*, p. 480.

unconscious feelings, beliefs, and attitudes that the person has about himself and his possessions. In his concept of himself he answers the questions, "Where am I?" "What am I?" and "Who am I?" Among the many things that the person may or may not value about himself are his body image or picture of himself; his feeling of being intact or whole; his role and status in his family, community, and job; his adequacy and acceptability as a marriage partner; his success and sense of fulfillment; and his hope that tomorrow will be better than today. He may value his family, home, state, and country. Other values that may be threatened during illness include the way in which he regards financial, physical, or emotional dependence and independence; how he feels about relinquishing control over events that relate to his welfare, as well as the way in which he ordinarily relates to other people.

Because they threaten the self-concept of the individual in some way, certain types of disease are more likely to cause psychological stress than are others. These include those that cause disfigurement, especially of the face, or the loss of a part that is easily identified, such as an extremity. Diseases or treatments that threaten the organs of reproduction are also sources of anxiety. Some diseases such as venereal diseases are regarded as bringing disgrace on the person and his family. In some groups tuberculosis and cancer are also perceived as a cause for shame. Mental illness and mental retardation fall in the same category. Other diseases such as heart disease or cancer are associated in the minds of many people with death. In addition cancer is generally equated with an extended and painful illness.

How may the differences in the definition of the role of the sick person be a source of psychological stress?

Another source of psychological stress to the patient and his attendants is the difference in their respective concepts of what is appropriate for the role and behavior of each other in illness. An example cited earlier was that of the differences in behavior of persons in pain. The role of the sick person in the American culture has been studied and defined by sociologists. One such definition is by Parsons,[22] who defines illness as a "socially institutionalized role-type" characterized in the American culture by some incapacity to carry on the normally expected role and tasks. He summarizes the American culture view of illness as follows:

1. The person is exempted from his role obligations.
2. He is not held responsible for being ill.
3. This state is held to be legitimate, if
4. He accepts the need for help and cooperates with those who help him.

The meaning of each of these will be clarified later in the chapter in relation to patients.

[22] Talcott Parsons, "Definitions of Health and Illness in the Light of American Values and Social Structure," *Patients, Physicians, and Illness*, ed. E. Gartley Jaco, The Free Press, Glencoe, Illinois, 1958, p. 176.

Conflict, with psychological stress as a consequence, not uncommonly arises between the patient and his attendants over differences in their interpretation of their respective roles. The conflict may be further aggravated by the tendency in the American culture to evaluate the expression of emotion in terms of good (desirable) or bad (undesirable). Thus anger, or the expressions of anger, are bad, and people who express anger are treated as bad people. This view neglects the fact that emotions are the substance of life. They give it color and meaning. Emotions are useful when they are directed toward the accomplishment of socially acceptable goals. Their usefulness is impaired when they are inappropriate to the situation, or excessive or deficient in degree. Anger, when properly controlled and directed toward the accomplishment of goals, may serve as a spur to the correction of an injustice. When it is uncontrolled, or excessive in amount, it may lead to the destruction of an individual or a nation.

Another source of anxiety to patients is the expense of illness. Direct costs are of greatest concern to those whose incomes are limited and who do not have hospital and sickness insurance. This is especially true if in the past they have always been able to meet their financial obligations. Added to the cost of hospitalization and medical care is loss of salary, and extra expenses such as the money needed for the care of children during the mother's absence or while she works to add to the family income. Even relatively short illnesses may make serious inroads on a limited income. This is particularly evident in the case of the elderly who are without hospital insurance and are living on restricted incomes. Other costs of illness include the demands which are made on family members to visit and comfort the sick person or to provide care for him when he is ill at home. When an illness is short-term, this may be minimal. In long-term illness the financial burden placed on the family may be very great. The nurse is not responsible for the cost of illness, but she should be aware that it may be a problem to the patient. She can alert the patient's physician to the fact that the patient is worried. Depending on the nature of the situation, the problem may be referred to a social worker. In communities where home care plans are available, some patients may be cared for at home. This may be both less expensive and more satisfactory to the patient. Patients are not always aware of services that are available in the community. The nurse may serve the patient by bringing them to the attention of the patient and/or his family. Even when nothing can be done to alleviate the patient's situation, knowledge that someone knows about and appreciates his problem may be comforting.

Another cost to the patient and his family is the pain and suffering and the fear of pain and suffering that is a real part of every illness. Here nursing can do much through using appropriate measures to relieve or prevent unnecessary pain and to explain to the patient what he can expect and what he can do to help himself. Studies which have been made indicate that patients who know that they will receive a pain-relieving medication when they have pain require less medication than those who do not.

Further sources of anxiety include the diagnostic and therapeutic procedures that are performed by as many strangers as there are procedures. There is always the possibility that the patient knows or believes that a procedure may be harmful as well as helpful. The patient's anxiety may be increased by the manner in which procedures are performed. No list of the situations in which the performance of a procedure may add to a patient's anxiety can ever be complete. However, awareness of some of the common ways in which anxiety is prevented or provoked should be helpful. Moreover, the nurse who is aware that patients are likely to suffer some degree of anxiety should be alert to clues that indicate that his anxiety is being increased by a procedure or is out of proportion to the situation. To illustrate, Mrs. Tall was to have a urea clearance test on Tuesday. On Monday the physician told her about the test and that she would be moved to the treatment room for the duration of the test. Later in the morning, the nurse found Mrs. Tall weeping. As the nurse attempted to comfort Mrs. Tall, she learned that the patients called the treatment room the death room. The belief had its origin in the fact that the artificial kidney was in this room. The patients had observed that some of the patients who went into the room died, hence the name "death room." The nurse reported Mrs. Tall's feelings to her physician, who replied, "That is the reason that she looked so forlorn when I told her about the test." He arranged to perform the procedure in Mrs. Tall's room, and of course, told her that the plans were changed to that extent. In this instance it was possible to change the aspect of the procedure that was most threatening to Mrs. Tall. This may not always be true. When it is not, the nurse can still be helpful by conveying to the patient that she recognizes his feelings and is sympathetic with them.

There are many other ways in which the performance of the various aspects of the patient's care can be a source of psychological stress and thus produce unnecessary anxiety. They include: (1) failure to prepare the patient for what to expect including when it can be expected, (2) lack of skill and awkwardness in the handling of equipment and the patient, (3) unnecessary roughness or hurrying of the patient, (4) failure to give necessary physical support, (5) lack of needed supplies, (6) uncertainty about how to proceed, (7) changes in the performance of the procedure that the patient does not understand, (8) failure to observe the patient's modesty pattern by adequate screening or by covering the parts of the body that the person ordinarily covers when in the presence of others, (9) entering his room without knocking, (10) and making careless or thoughtless remarks in the presence of the patient which suggest dangers that may or may not exist.

Although the point has been made previously that illness involves relinquishing, to a greater or lesser degree, the ability of the person to control events in relation to himself, it bears re-emphasis. The patient is told when he is to go to bed, when to get out of bed, when and what he shall eat, and when he will bathe. He may be asked to perform procedures that he does not feel able to do. For example, Mrs. Mel had a hysterectomy following several days of severe hemorrhage. The day after the surgery was performed Miss Nurse entered the room and said, "Now it is time for you to get up." Mrs. Mel responded by asking, "How can I get up? I have all these tubes and I feel too weak." She had three tubes, one into her stomach, one into her urinary bladder, and another connected into a needle in a vein in her left arm. "Doctor's orders," said Miss Nurse. "All patients get up the day after surgery. Just turn on your side and swing your feet over the edge of the bed and raise up as you do so." Mrs. Mel got up, because she felt that she was helpless to alter the situation. She also felt that Miss Nurse was harsh and unfeeling. Mrs. Mel's feeling that she was called upon to perform activities for which she was unprepared and without adequate physical and emotional support is all too common. Some expression on the part of the nurse that indicated that she appreciated how Mrs. Mel felt and that she could and would help her might have reduced Mrs. Mel's fear. The nurse might also have assisted Mrs. Mel in turning and in assuming a sitting position, after first explaining to her why it was necessary for her to be out of bed so soon after surgery.

The nurse should also be aware of the fact that some people find the need to depend on others very difficult, or even impossible, to tolerate. Thus when they find themselves in a position where they are dependent on others, they become increasingly anxious. If their anxiety is very severe, they may be unable to tolerate any degree of dependency and may either ignore symptoms of illness or refuse necessary treatment. They may deny the presence of the illness. Some of these patients can tolerate dependency if they are allowed some control over what happens to them. This requires close cooperation among those who work with the patient. For example, the patient for whom complete bed rest and no visitors except his wife and no telephone calls are prescribed, may find his situation more bearable if he is allowed to have a limited number of telephone calls or if he can select one other person who is permitted to visit him. When what is acceptable to the patient is different from what the doctor has prescribed, the change in the patient's regime must, of course, be planned with the physician.

A word of caution; the nurse should be sure that the patient's problem has been really identified. For example, Mr. Eighty-year-old, who had had a cerebrovascular accident, was a great problem to the nursing staff because he refused to stay in bed. The doctor ordered that restraints be used to keep him in bed. Miss Freshman, who was assigned to care for him, noticed that Mr. Eighty got out of bed when he needed to urinate. Thereafter he stayed in bed, because plans were made in terms of his need—to have a urinal at regular intervals. No restraints were necessary.

To summarize some of the causes of psychological stress in illness, six patients will be presented.

First there is Mr. Tompkins, admitted to Ward X. By this very act he was separated from his responsibilities as an executive and father. It also established the fact that he was incapable of carrying on his normal role and activities. Correct sickroom behavior on the part of Mr. Tompkins and his visitors included the avoidance of talking about his business or the trouble that Junior was having in school. In fact, visitors were expected "to cheer him up." Anyone who violated this code was immediately labeled as harmful to his welfare. His employer assured him that he was not being held accountable, by providing him with sick leave and medical and hospital insurance and by assuring him that his job would be waiting for him when he recovered. His co-workers took up a collection for flowers and as individuals sent him cards.

Last, he was accepted as a sick person capable of being helped, if he recognized that he was ill and placed himself in the hands of professional people and followed their orders and suggestions. He was considered cooperative or uncooperative to the degree to which he did not, or did, question his care, follow orders, and the like. If he was "cooperative," he won for himself the title of "good patient" and the approval of the personnel concerned with his care. To the degree that he questioned his treatment and did not follow orders and suggestions, he was labeled "uncooperative." Depending on his behavior, he was titled demanding, unreasonable, stubborn, impossible, or neurotic. Under these circumstances he was held responsible for his condition and care was withheld or given in such a way as to remind Mr. Tompkins of his responsibility as a patient. That this tactic seldom succeeds in doing anything except to make the patient feel misunderstood is rarely recognized. The patient often continues to exhibit the offending behavior or may even increase the intensity of his efforts to be recognized as an individual. The staff, failing to recognize the defensive nature of the patient's behavior, continues to remind him of his responsibility as a patient by withholding care or by giving it reluctantly.

The diagnosis—peptic ulcer—afforded Mr. Tompkins a certain amount of status in the community. It was assumed to indicate that he was hard-working and successful. Therefore, he was allowed the privilege of being hospitalized without loss of status. He could refuse to do certain things commonly expected of persons in his employment or social group. He could refer to his ulcer with modest pride. In fact, among some groups it is one badge of success.

Next there is Mr. Hearty, who was hospitalized following an acute myocardial infarction. His illness constituted a serious threat to his self-concept. He had always taken great pride in the fact that he was strong and healthy. He boasted to his friends about never having lost a day at work. He had always perceived being sick as a sign of weakness. The onset of the myocardial infarction was accompanied by a severe pain under the sternum. He felt frightened, angry, and helpless. He tried to tell himself that the pain would go away. When it became very severe, he called his doctor. After his admission to the hospital Mr. Hearty made many demands on the nursing staff for attention. When he turned on his light, he expected it to be answered immediately. Through his behavior, he indicated that he wanted what he wanted when he wanted it. By his behavior he supported his feeling that he had some control over his situation. Though he vented his hostile feelings on the nursing staff and his wife, he did not feel safe in attacking his physician. He covered his hostile feelings toward the doctor by telling stories and making light of his situation. As Mr. Hearty began to improve and the physician was able to reassure him that his heart was healing, he began to press for changes in his medical regime and in the management of the nursing unit. In fact, he did this from the beginning, for he refused to use a commode and insisted on going to the bathroom. Part of his reaction to injury, then, was to try to reconstruct the world in which he found himself.

It was evident that Mr. Hearty's behavior did not conform to that expected in the American cultural pattern. This could lead to a feeling on the part of his family and nurses that Mr. Hearty dislikes them as people. With these feelings, they could find it difficult to meet his needs. Conversely, if they are able to accept Mr. Hearty as a sick man whose behavior is in keeping with his manner of coping with other crises in his life, they may then be able to identify his needs and provide a therapeutic environment for him. Even when the nurse recognizes that the patient's behavior has a cause and serves a purpose, acceptance of the patient who violates the "rules" may not be easy. Knowledge of the possible sources of conflict should facilitate their identification and serve as the basis for making appropriate adjustments in the patient's environment.

In the room next to Mr. Hearty was Mr. Quiet. He, too, was in the hospital for the treatment of a myocardial infarction. At the onset of the pain under his sternum, he, too, felt frightened and helpless. In contrast to Mr. Hearty, however, he was described as a good patient because he conformed to the cultural definition of the sick person. After consulting his physician, he went to the hospital, where he cooperated in care; that is, he followed the doctor's orders exactly. He lay quietly, permitting himself to be fed and bathed. He seldom asked for anything, and when he did, he was both patient and polite. Instead of reacting by attack, he responded to his fears and feelings of helplessness by withdrawal and by regression. He was able to be dependent on others for his care. Though his nursing care provided very well for his physical needs, his psychological needs were in danger of being overlooked. He was worried, not so much about whether he would die, but about whether he would be able to return to his work as a riveter in an automobile plant and what would happen to his wife and five children if he were not able to work. He had always been able to provide for his family. He had hoped to be able to send his sons to college. Because Mr. Quiet was undemanding there was also danger that he would be left alone for long periods. One of the elements in establishing a therapeutic environment for Mr. Quiet is to provide for regular visits and a climate in which he feels comfortable in expressing the thoughts that trouble him.

Each of the next two patients had an above-the-knee amputation of a leg.

Though the surgical procedure was similar for both patients, their psychological reactions were quite different. The first patient is Mrs. Oeski, an elderly Polish woman. She appeared to have little concern about the loss of her leg, per se. She was, however, very worried because she was afraid that she would no longer be able to go up and down stairs. This was serious, for though her home had a "company" kitchen and dining room on the first floor, they were seldom used. The kitchen that was used in everyday living was in the basement. Her concept of herself as a homemaker appeared to be more threatened than that of her physical self. She worked hard to learn how to use her prosthesis so that she would be able to walk up and down stairs. Her family were also interested in what they could do to make it possible for her to go up and down stairs. Because of Mrs. Oeski's personal resources and goals and the support given to her by her family, she was able to be rehabilitated to the point where she could continue her homemaking role. The fact that she had a strong goal was very helpful.

Down the corridor from Mrs. Oeski was Mr. Young. His amputation followed an accident in which a basket of ingots had fallen on his right leg and crushed it. For days afterward he lay with his face to the wall refusing to eat, to be bathed, or to perform any activity that was considered necessary to his welfare. Though he guarded against anyone seeing him weeping, the nurses were sure that he did cry. He lacked interest in his children and in events that had been of interest to him previously. His general appearance was that of a dejected or depressed person. It was assumed that he was mourning the loss of his leg.

If nurses are to provide a therapeutic environment for Mr. Young, they must recognize the fact that grief very frequently follows the loss of a part or function that the person values, and accept that the patient may need to mourn for a lost part in order to facilitate his recovery. They must also recognize that his behavior violates two of the tenets of the sick role in the American culture pattern. He does not cooperate with those responsible for his care, nor does he make an effort to recover. His behavior is also inappropriate for a man; he cries. If Mr. Young's nurses are able to accept his behavior as having meaning and serving a purpose, then they may be able to provide an environment in which he is able to express his grief and examine his feelings. With this help, he may be able to move forward toward making plans for his recovery and rehabilitation.

Mary Belle Smith represents another psychological problem in illness. She had rheumatic fever at ages three and seven which was followed by mitral stenosis. As a consequence, she spent little time in school and was generally protected by her family. At age 23 she had a mitral commissurotomy, which, according to the surgeon, was a success. Mary Belle, however, continued to be an invalid and resisted all efforts at rehabilitation. Her self-concept remained unaltered and she was unable to cope with life except as an invalid. It was the only method she had of relating to others. Mary Belle's reaction, though not the one desired, is not unique. Kaplan,[23] in a study of patients having cardiac surgery, found that some did not recover, despite the correction of their physical disability. In some instances the patient continued to be a cardiac invalid; in others he developed other disabilities. According to Kaplan, the patient who uses heart disease as a means of adapting psychologically to the problems in his life is less likely to be benefited by surgery than is one who does not. This reaction is not unique to patients with heart disease. Studies of patients with other diseases such as arthritis and duodenal ulcer affirm the above.

Sometimes patients reject themselves or appear to do so by making self-derogatory remarks. They may be asking the person to whom they address their remarks to disagree. For example, Mrs. Busy says to her neighbor, "I'm lazy and never accomplish anything"; she expects Mrs. Neighbor to say, "You are the best and hardest-working woman in the neighborhood," rather than to agree with her. Mrs. Busy may very well want to be reassured that her efforts are appreciated and that they add up to something. Sometimes the person wants to be assured that what happened did not happen or that it is interpreted in a charitable fashion. For example, Mrs. Terrly had a hysterectomy. As she passed through the stage of excitement in her recovery from a general anesthetic, she cried, screamed, and thrashed about in bed. She was aware of her behavior, but was unable to control it. Later in the afternoon when the effects of the anesthetic had diminished, she said to the nurse, "I behaved very badly when I was under the anesthetic, didn't I?" The nurse replied, "You certainly did." Mrs. Terrly burst into tears. She had not wanted to have her fears confirmed. What she had wanted was to be reassured that her behavior was not unusual. Had the nurse stopped to examine the intent of Mrs. Terrly's question, she might have replied in such a way that Mrs. Terrly would have been relieved.

Through the examination of the manner in which six patients reacted to illness, some of the causes of psychological stress have been reviewed. Another way to learn something about the psychological needs of patients during illness is to examine the reaction of patients during the different stages of illness. These are: the stage of onset, the stage of accepted illness, and the stage of convalescence. Some attention will also be given to the ways in which patients are expected to react and how they may affect the care that the patients receive.

What are some of the emotional reactions of the person who recognizes that he is ill?

The significant principle here is that anxiety alerts the person to danger and the amount of anxiety provoked in any situation of illness depends on the

[23] Stanley M. Kaplan, "Psychological Aspects of Cardiac Disease," *Psychosomatic Medicine*, XVIII, March, 1956, p. 233.

meaning of the illness or its effects to him. When the individual recognizes that his illness does not respond to home remedies or that he cannot explain its cause or effects to his satisfaction, his anxiety may act as a spur or stimulus to his seeking attention. In contrast, he may be so anxious that he denies that he is ill or attempts to avoid the fact that he is ill. He is too busy to see his doctor or his doctor is too busy to see him or he has an important meeting coming up. His denial may be so complete that he does not recognize that he is ill despite the fact that he is. This may be true even when the illness is obvious to his associates. Denial in some degree is a common psychological defense mechanism in the American culture.

Acceptance of illness requires of the person that he place himself in the hands of others. To do this he must return to an earlier mode of behaving, or regress. Inasmuch as he is able to do this, he will be able to follow orders and allow others to tend to his personal, emotional, and physical needs.

According to Barker et al.,[24] if the patient can tolerate being dependent on others, he regresses to a more childlike state that is characterized by four features.

1. He becomes self-centered. He sees events and people in relation to himself and existing for his benefit. He becomes demanding and less able to wait to have his needs and wants satisfied. Where he was once considerate of the needs of others, he now is concerned only with his own. Experienced nurses are well aware of this characteristic. One of the criteria by which a patient is judged to be recovering is evidence that he is less self-centered. For example, a previously self-centered patient is improving when he inquires about the well-being of a patient in the next bed, or when he suggests that his wife looks weary and that she should go home early.

2. His interest becomes circumscribed; that is, he is interested in what is happening to him at the present time. Things that were of interest to him before he became ill are of little concern to him. For example, when he is well he is an avid baseball fan; when he is ill he expresses little interest in the World Series. His interest is centered on himself and what is happening to him now.

3. He is dependent emotionally on those who care for him. He sees in the actions of those who care for him acceptance or rejection. When a new nurse is assigned to care for him he may interpret this to mean that the nurse who cared for him previously dislikes him. In addition, his feelings may be ambivalent; at one moment he feels that he is accepted and at another that he is rejected. Nurses and others who care for sick people should learn to recognize this tendency of the sick to be ambivalent and to take the patient's expression of feelings as part of his illness and to be neither elated nor downcast by them.

4. He becomes preoccupied with his bodily functions. He is concerned with

[24] R. G. Barker, et al., Adjustment to Physical Handicap and Illness, Rev. ed., Social Science Research Council, New York, 1953, pp. 239-42.

what he eats or does not eat, with whether the food is suitable for an invalid, with his bowel functions, with the amount of time he sleeps or does not, and so on.

Recognition of the value of and the characteristics of regression in the ill should be helpful to the nurse in accepting the patient and his behavior. Regression is helpful to the patient in his illness because it makes it possible for him to depend on others to do for him things which, when well, he could and would do for himself. Many of these involve activities that are of a personal nature. As he was growing up and became able to do these things for himself, this was accepted as evidence that he was maturing. Therefore, activities such as bathing and feeding himself have meanings that bear little relation to the actual activity. When, however, he is able to allow others to care for him, he can use his energy for recovery.

As his condition improves, he is expected to reassume responsibility for himself. In general, the belief is held that the sooner the patient reassumes his normal activities, the more rapid his recovery will be. However, he needs to understand that these activities are as much a part of his plan of therapy as are his medications or diet. The patient too often interprets being asked to bathe himself as the nurse's shifting some of her work to him because she is unwilling or too busy to care for him, rather than as an activity that contributes to his progress. He also needs to feel that the nurse is standing by to help him if and when he needs it.

With regression the patient frequently has feelings of anger. He may express his anger by being hostile to or rejecting of those who care for him. This may include his family as well as the nursing staff. If the nurse recognizes that the patient's behavior is part of his reaction to his illness, and knows that it serves a purpose, then she is better able to explore or to examine the total situation without herself becoming upset or hurt. Families frequently require some support in order for them to develop understanding of the situation. There is some evidence to support the observation that patients who express hostility during illness make more rapid recoveries than those who do not express hostility.

Some patients turn their anger inward and when they do they become depressed. Some degree of depression is probably associated with any serious illness and may indeed be a necessary stage in recovery. Inasmuch as it enables the patient to withdraw and conserve his energy, it is protective. Sutherland[25] found that patients having radical mastectomies almost always evidenced some depression for the first few days at home. In those instances where the family was accepting of the patient's withdrawal and increased dependency, the patient made a more rapid recovery than in those where the families were not accepting.

The depression that accompanies the loss of a part or of an ability that has

[25] Arthur Sutherland, "Psychological Impact of Cancer Surgery," *Public Health Report,* LXVII, November, 1952, pp. 1139-43.

been important to the patient may be accompanied by grief. Acceptance by the nursing staff of the fact that a patient not only does, but has the right to, mourn the loss of a part of himself, and that he may need help in expressing his grief, is fundamental to an adequate plan of care. The nurse may view the fact that a leg was gangrenous as a good reason for the patient to be glad to be rid of it. The patient views it differently. The leg was a part of himself and of his concept or image of himself. An adequate opportunity to express sorrow in an understanding and accepting environment lessens the need for feelings of self-pity. It is easier to do what one has to do when one feels that others are trying to understand one's point of view.

When the illness has been a serious threat to the individual's integrity, he is likely to be more or less confused. Though not all persons are able to express their feelings as directly as Mrs. Widow, who found her husband dead in bed beside her, this does not mean that they do not feel confused. Though Mrs. Widow had gone next door and asked for help, she could not remember going or how she got there. She kept repeating, "What did I do? How did I get to your house? I can't remember. I'm so confused. I do not know what to do." The thing she stated that was most helpful to her was that, after confirming the fact that her husband was dead, the neighbors assumed responsibility by calling the doctor, the relatives, and so on. They took the necessary responsibility and they appeared to have the situation under control. Sometimes confusion is not as evident as in the instance of Mrs. Widow and shows only when the patient is called upon to remember or to learn. It is likely, however, that it is more common than is generally appreciated. This is one of the reasons that instructions or explanation given to patients needs to be patiently repeated, sometimes over and over. Nurses, therefore, should not be surprised when patients do not remember instructions that have been given to them by themselves or by the physician.

As has been implied, patients may adapt to illness by attack (aggressive behavior) or by withdrawal (regression). Each method has its advantages and disadvantages and implications for nursing. During illness the patient needs his energy to recover. The patient who adapts by attack should be protected from circumstances that increase his feeling that he has to use aggressive behavior to have his needs met. This is often difficult for the nursing personnel (and others), because sick people are expected to follow orders and to appreciate the care that is offered to them. When the patient demands attention and does not appear to appreciate efforts made in his behalf, the nurses may feel frustrated and ineffectual. If the nurse understands that attack is one way of adapting to illness, she should have less need to feel that she is responsible for the patient's behavior. She may then find it easier to adapt the patient's care to his needs.

The patient who regresses during illness is also adapting. Through regression, he conserves his energy for recovery. He is more likely to be considered a "good patient" unless he regresses too far and becomes too dependent on those who provide his care. The problems in his care derive from the ability of those who care for him to accept him in his regressed state and to prevent the regression from going too far. This means that those who care for him must recognize when the patient no longer needs to conserve his energy and the time has come for him to assume responsibility for meeting his own needs and for making his own decisions. Especially when the patient has been seriously ill, this may take considerable time.

During the stage of convalescence the patient is expected to progress from illness to physical and emotional health. He must give up his dependent and self-centered behavior and fend for himself again. Lederer[26] states that there are many similarities between the dynamics of adolescence and illness. During this stage the patient goes from dependence to independence, and finally to interdependence. Particularly when the illness has been lengthy or the patient has been seriously ill, convalescence may be prolonged. Some patients find it difficult to give up being the center of attention and to assume responsibility for themselves again.

Illness may be unnecessarily prolonged if the patient has not been able to express his hostility against his attendants. This may be one of the reasons that the patient whose behavior is aggressive often makes a more prompt recovery than does his more passive roommate. Recovery may also be delayed if illness provides more satisfactions than does health. The many factors that contribute to the development of a preference for illness to health will not be discussed in detail. These are, however, defined as the secondary gains in illness. For some reason illness provides more satisfaction than health for certain persons. Mary Belle, who was previously described, and who continued to be an invalid despite correction of her cardiac disability, is one example.

There are, however, procedures that may be utilized to reduce the likelihood of this happening. The first is to encourage the patient to assume responsibility including making the decisions he is able to make. As this is done the patient should understand that, as he assumes responsibility, he helps himself to recover and that assistance is available, if and when he requires it. When to help the patient requires judgment in order that the patient not be assisted unnecessarily and thus be robbed of the feeling of accomplishment or, on the other hand, be pushed beyond his capacity to perform. The nurse also must be able to stand by and wait as the patient struggles. Through grappling with his problem he gains the strength to progress toward recovery.

Other practices have been useful in helping patients with long-term illnesses to keep the objective of returning to the community and an active life before them. Among these are: granting visiting privileges; permitting overnight hospital leaves; encouraging families and friends to take patients to community events; having patients wear their own clothing and, when at all possible wear daytime clothing during the day; encouraging listening to the radio and tele-

[26] Henry D. Lederer, "How the Sick View Their World," *Patients, Physicians and Illness*, ed. E. Gartley Jaco. The Free Press, Glencoe, Illinois, 1958, p. 253.

vision; and caring for patients at home when the home situation permits. For those with severe physical disabilities, the collapsible lightweight wheel chair has emancipated many from a life of imprisonment in one room or on one floor. Added to this, occupational therapy is valuable not only to develop weakened muscles, but to provide the convalescent with opportunities to gain satisfaction through the creation of useful products. It may also provide the person with a socially acceptable way of releasing tension. The man who is pounding leather as he prepares it for a billfold may be anticipating his wife's pleasure when he gives it to her as a gift. Or he may be thinking of the $5 he will receive when it is sold. With each blow of the hammer he may at the same time be releasing some of his anger at being ill or handicapped.

As the patient recovers, he may be encouraged to read or to be read to. Though reading may be done by the nurse, it may provide an opportunity for a relative or friend or volunteer to make a contribution to the patient's care. In the selection of reading material the patient's interests and well-being should be taken into account. The woman's page and fashions may be appropriate when the patient is a girl or woman, but are seldom of interest to a man. Games such as checkers or cribbage may also be useful in stimulating the patient's interest in recovery as well as in shortening the hours of the day. This is another area where members of the family or the patient's friends may be given an opportunity to be of service to the patient. Vocational counseling is of value in helping the person find a way to make a living and in nurturing the hope that there is something that he will be able to do that is useful.

Families and friends of handicapped persons or of those who have had a long illness and are being prepared to return to the community require instruction in how they should behave and what they should expect from the patient and what they should do for him. Families tend to react either by doing too much for the person and overprotecting him or by rejecting him. They may also need help and support the first few times they take the handicapped person out in public. They need some preparation for the fact that people are made uncomfortable by seeing those who are disabled and deformed. The day when most of these people were hidden from view is not very long past. Once the patient and his family get through the first painful adventures, they will begin to be less sensitive and will be surprised that people are generally helpful.

Because illness, particularly when the patient suffers some degree of incapacity or when hospitalization is required, is a crisis situation in the life of the patient and his family, it is likely to produce psychological stress which results in various types of discomfort one of which is some degree of anxiety. Despite popular opinion to the contrary, not all anxiety is bad or undesirable. Nor is it all preventable. However, much can be done in the practice of nursing to reduce the incidence of unnecessary anxiety and to provide the patient with needed support. To prevent and reduce unnecessary psychological stress the nurse not only needs to be aware of possible causes, but she must be able to recognize clues in the patient's behavior that indicate how the patient feels about himself and his illness.

What kinds of information will help the nurse identify the patient's emotional reaction to his illness?

According to Sartain,[27] emotion has four aspects. The first three are of the greatest significance here. The first is the personal emotional experience. This is what the person feels consciously, knows, and can describe verbally. The person, in describing his feeling, says, "I feel so happy that I could fly or cry, or "I feel so mad or angry or disappointed that I want to cry." He may say, "When I saw the expression on the face of the physician, I felt so frightened that I wanted to run and hide." The words used to describe emotions and the ability to describe feelings verbally vary from person to person. The nurse must therefore be alert to the significance not only of what the person says but of how and why he says it.

The second aspect of emotion is that it is also expressed through bodily changes. These changes are those associated with alerting the person to meet a danger and to restore the body to a resting state. They result from activation of the autonomic nervous system and the part of the hormonal system that enables the organism to respond to emergency situations. Examples include changes in blood pressure, blood sugar, heart and respiratory rates, and alterations in the activity of the alimentary canal. Physiological changes that may accompany disturbances such as anxiety include trembling or shaking, restlessness, sleep disturbances including insomnia—loss of appetite or anorexia, inability to concentrate, irritability, and symptoms indicating an imbalance in the autonomic nervous system. Increases in the pulse or respiratory rate and in the blood pressure are common, as are increased frequency of urination and disturbances in gastrointestinal activity. Peristalsis may be increased or decreased. As a result the patient may be nauseated, vomit, have diarrhea, suffer abdominal distention, or be constipated.

Skeletal muscle tension or relaxation also indicates something about the emotional state of the individual. The frightened or anxious individual tenses his muscles in preparation for flight or fight, even when neither course is open to him. To illustrate, Tom was an active 18-year-old who had been found on chest X ray to have a small, well-defined lesion in the lower lobe of his right lung. Surgery was performed promptly and the diseased tissue removed. Both he and his parents were badly frightened. Tom did not talk about his fears. However, as he lay against his pillows, his fists were clenched and muscular tension was obvious. Deep breathing, turning, and coughing were accompanied by more than the usual amount of pain and difficulty. His cough was unproductive, and the lung on the operated side was slow in re-expanding.

[27] Aaron Sartain, *et al., Psychology: Understanding Human Behavior,* 2nd ed., McGraw-Hill Book Co., Inc., New York, 1962, pp. 103-116.

Attempts at reassurance were of little help, until one morning when the surgeon came in and said, "The reports are back from the pathological laboratory. Your lung had a little harmless tumor in it. You are cured." The change in Tom was remarkable. He relaxed, assumed responsibility for his own care, and in other ways demonstrated that he was no longer frightened.

The third aspect of emotion is behavior that can be observed by others. These behaviors are expressive rather than coping. They are important in all relationships because expressive behavior is a significant part of nonverbal communication. They are especially useful to the nurse in understanding patients who are unable to talk much. Facial expression is one of the common sources of information about the emotional state of the individual. Some of the comments that follow illustrate the fact that people observe facial expression as a basis for evaluating the emotional state of the individual. Many more could, of course, be added. "He talks with his eyes." "You want to be careful when her eyes snap." "The boss is in a good mood today; he was smiling when he came in." "She looks as if something terrible has happened or as if she has lost her last friend." "Her face looks peaceful, as if she is a very happy person." Though clues to the emotional state of the individual may be obtained from examining the facial expression, more information is often required to assess how a patient is actually feeling. A person may smile when he feels like crying or he may pride himself on his "poker face." In some cultures, individuals learn to keep their faces immobile. These patients may suffer pain and other discomforts without any change of expression. When this is true, other means of estimating the person's degree of discomfort must be used.

Emotion may also be expressed through movements of the hands and body. In the instance of Tom, he expressed his fright by tensing his muscles and clenching his fists. Another patient may move about. In bed he twists and turns. Out of bed he paces the floor, wrings his hands, or shakes his fists. Other emotions are also expressed through bodily movement. Friendliness may be shown by the hand being extended. Joy or pleasure may be expressed by clapping the hands or by jumping up and down, and so on. Posture and step also reveal the feelings of the individual. When a person's posture is erect and his step is firm, he creates the impression that he is healthy and is feeling well toward himself and others. Conversely, when his shoulders sag, he drags his feet, and his movements are languid, he creates the impression of being dejected or depressed.

In the American culture, where a high value is placed on a healthy body and cleanliness, grooming and evidence of cleanliness are also clues to the emotional state of the individual. Uncombed and untidy hair, soiled and ragged clothing, dirty and poorly kept fingernails, run-over shoes, and other evidence of lack of attention to grooming and cleanliness—all may be interpreted as evidence that the individual has a low opinion of himself. Before arriving at a conclusion about the significance or any observation, however, one must also know what type of work the person does and what the expectations of the group with whom he identifies are. For example, a man who spends his working days greasing automobiles is likely to have a problem in keeping his nails clean. Dirty shoes worn by teenagers may be significant to the extent that this is part of the teenage uniform.

Vocal expressions of emotion may be through talking, crying, whistling, laughing, and screaming. In talking, the person's feeling is conveyed not only by what he says, but by whether what he says is usual for him and by his tone of voice. It is also helpful to know how the person usually expresses satisfaction or dissatisfaction. Sometimes the words used by the patient to express his emotion are offensive to the nurse. When this is true, the nurse should try to concentrate on what the patient is trying to communicate, rather than on the words themselves. When the patient is able to modify his behavior, limits can be set based on the patient's needs and those of the situation.

In general, laughter and expressions of humor are acceptable ways of expressing feeling in American culture. This may be related to the fact that laughter is often associated with a "good" emotion such as joy. The fact is that laughter may also hide sorrow or anxiety or even hostility. The patient who is always laughing and joking is usually much admired. A little thought given to the reasons behind his behavior might reveal that he is frightened or angry or both. Laughter is often used to relieve tension. Playwrights use a humorous situation to break tension in a serious drama. A wave of laughter may pass over a group when an embarrassing subject is discussed.

Though joy or gladness may be expressed by crying, crying is generally associated with "bad" feelings such as pain, sorrow, helplessness, and anger. Though adults have these feelings, for them to express them by crying is disapproved of. Moreover, when men, who are expected to be strong, cry, their behavior is regarded as being particularly inappropriate. Crying is for babies who are still dependent on their mothers and not for grown men and women who have long since reached adulthood. Nurses who find themselves with a crying adult may feel uncomfortable. They may be embarrassed because the patient is unable to control his behavior and feel that at the same time the discomfort which precipitated the crying should be relieved. They may also feel that they are in some way responsible for the fact that the patient is crying and for not being able to stop it. When the nurse can view the crying as a way in which the patient expresses emotion and a way to relieve the patient's feelings, she has a foundation for being helpful to the patient. Instead of concentrating her attention on trying to stop the crying, she may be able to concentrate on what the patient is trying to express by crying. She may then show that she is trying to understand the patient's situation by squeezing the patient's hand, by providing paper tissues, and by making comments directed toward the cause, such as, "You must be feeling upset or very strongly." After the patient has had an opportunity to relieve her feelings, she may be helped to regain her self-control by washing her face with cold water.

In addition, a woman may be helped to powder her face, apply lipstick, and the like.

Other ways in which patients express their emotions vocally are by shouting, screaming, moaning, and groaning. These behaviors, too, for much the same reasons as for crying, may be upsetting to nurses. They also are sometimes disturbing to other patients. When this behavior is continued and is upsetting to other patients, it may be necessary to isolate the patient in a soundproof room. In one hospital, isolation of Puerto Rican women who were in labor in a soundproof room was found to be necessary. When they reached a certain point in labor, they screamed. This screaming was very frightening to other patients. Before placing a patient in isolation one should be certain that the patient does not have a correctable reason for his behavior and that the reason for isolating the patient is for the good of other patients or in some way related to the welfare of the patient and not as punishment. When isolation is, or becomes necessary, the nurse has an obligation to identify and meet the needs of the patient. Someone ought to stay with the patient. Since the patient is shut off from others, he should know how to summon the nurse, and his calls should be answered promptly. Though the welfare of others may make isolation of a patient necessary, this procedure increases his need for nursing. Recent studies of the effects of isolation on healthy young men indicate the importance of environmental stimulation to healthy mental functioning. Soon after the subjects of study were separated from the external environment, they began to have hallucinations.[28]

Sometimes when the behavior of a patient is deemed to be unacceptable, he may be isolated by neglect rather than by physical isolation. For example, though Mr. Jonas was screaming as if he were in severe pain, no one was giving him any attention. The reason for his being neglected was that he was "just a neurotic with a low tolerance for pain." On investigation he was found to be hemorrhaging into his urinary bladder. The bladderwall had been eroded by a bladder stone. As he was paraplegic, he had what is called a neurogenic bladder; that is, it emptied spontaneously when it reached its capacity and its capacity was very small. As the bladder filled, painful muscle contractions were initiated. Blood clots blocked the urethra and prevented the bladder from emptying. As the bladder wall was stretched, the painful muscle spasms increased in frequency. Perhaps Mr. Jonas' tolerance for pain was minimal. Be that as it may, he was suffering and needed relief. Though his physician was delayed in seeing him by another emergency, when he did, he immediately scheduled Mr. Jonas for emergency surgery. Following the operation he was found to be a well-controlled, "good" patient. This is an excellent example of the danger of placing the patient whose behavior is disapproved into a category that justifies the disapproval. That some of this man's care was inhumane should not require saying. Moreover, conclusions about the cause

28 Woodburn Heron, "The Pathology of Boredom," *Scientific American*, CXCVI, January, 1957, pp. 52-56.

of a patient's behavior should not be made without thorough knowledge of the patient and situation. Stereotyping patients according to their behavior should be avoided.

There are many ways in which patients manifest their anxiety. A variety of behaviors characterized by action may be called a "flight into activity." The patient jokes and is the life of the ward. Talking relieves tension and serves much as whistling in the dark does. Pacing up and down the corridor and going from one activity to another serves a similar purpose. A careful listener may be rewarded with clues about the meaning of the patient's behavior. This may lead to the information that makes it possible to initiate action that helps to allay his fears. Knowing that someone understands and is interested in how he feels may be a great help.

One of the problems in planning care directed toward minimizing anxiety is that despite the presence of signs and symptoms, they do not in themselves indicate the cause of anxiety. Nor does the relief of anxiety always take precedence. The patient who is bleeding excessively will be anxious, but the problem that takes priority is the hemorrhage. At the time the most reassuring thing that can be done for the patient is to initiate prompt action to stop the bleeding and, if need be, to replace the blood. In the words of a patient who experienced this situation, "I turned on my light and Miss Junior came right away. She ran and got Miss Head Nurse who ran and got the doctor. The doctor came right away and I was in the operating room before I knew what was happening—and a good thing too. I owe my life to the fact that they were all on their toes."

It is not always possible to determine all the factors contributing to the anxiety or to relieve it entirely, if such a thing were desired. It is possible to recognize the fact that there are many factors in illness, its diagnosis, and treatment that are anxiety-provoking and to try to utilize this knowledge in modifying care, so that anxiety-provoking conditions are kept to a reasonable minimum. The nurse also should be alert to signs and symptoms that indicate that the patient is unduly anxious.

In individualizing care of patients, it is helpful to be able to recognize the pattern that the patient uses in establishing or avoiding relationships with others. In the American culture the mature adult is thought to be one who relates to others as an equal. That is, he can work interdependently or co-operatively with others. Each person in the relationship gives or takes as the situation demands. Not all adults, however, react on this level. Some interact by forming dependent relationships with others, some by dominating others, some by rebelling against others, and some by avoiding relationships with others.

In the past, and sometimes in the present, patients have been expected to place themselves in a dependent relationship to those who care for them. The trend is toward encouraging patients to make their own decisions, rather than to have decisions forced on them. In this view the patient is regarded as being the important element in whether or not he recovers; that is, the recovery of the patient depends on the patient. What the nurse or doctor does is to facilitate or assist him in the process. Since not all patients interact in the same manner, recognition of the patient's pattern should help to alert the nurse to some of the problems that may arise in his care. For example, the patient who characteristically rebels against others may have to be given time to talk himself into what he knows he must do. For this patient, pressure by another person may result in an increase in his resistance. When the pressure is too great, he may be forced to take a position from which he cannot retreat.

What can the nurse do to minimize psychological stress in her patients?

Florence Nightingale,[29] in *Notes on Nursing,* emphasizes the need for the nurse to recognize and relieve anxiety in the patient in the following statement:

Apprehension, uncertainty, waiting, expectation, fear of surprise, do a patient more harm than any expectation. Remember, he is face to face with his enemy all the time, internally wrestling with him, having long imaginary conversation with him. You are thinking of something else. Rid him of his adversary quickly, is the first rule of the sick.

Wertham,[30] a psychiatrist, in discussing his experiences as a patient makes the following comments about how the sick person can be helped. "Medical and surgical patients need psychological advice about how they should act, what their experiences mean; they need psychological preparation for what to expect; they need guidance, so that they can make the best of their possibilities."

He also lists the kinds of remarks that were antitherapeutic for him. Sometimes these comments were made in jest and sometimes to give information. The intention of those who made them was to reassure him. For example, he was told that thrombophlebitis, though fairly common in the legs, seldom affects the arms. To that time he had not considered the possibility of the disease affecting his arms. For some time thereafter, he was sure that he was developing thrombophlebitis in his arms. He would lie in bed and mentally examine his arms for indications of disease. Sometimes suggesting problems to the patient can be prevented by making certain what he wants to know when he asks a question, by asking another question or by saying, "I do not quite understand." The danger of increasing anxiety by giving the patient inappropriate information is one of the objections of physicians to nurses teaching patients.

[29] Florence Nightingale, *Notes on Nursing,* Harrison, London, 1859, p. 22.
[30] Frederic Wertham, "A Psychosomatic Study of Myself," *When Doctors Are Patients,* eds. Max Pinner and Benjamin Miller, W. W. Norton & Co., Inc., New York, 1952, p. 115.

The question "What can we do to relieve the patient's anxiety, and thus to reassure him?" suggests other questions. How docs one reassure another? What does reassurance mean? Is it accomplished by telling the other person that everything will be all right? Does one person stop worrying when another says, "Leave the worrying to me?" The dictionary defines "reassure" as a transitive verb meaning to restore to courage or confidence, also to re-establish. Its synonyms include to encourage, which in turn means to inspire with courage, hope, confidence, or resolution; to help forward as well as to animate, cheer, hearten, and inspire. It is also interesting to note that synonyms of encourage include console, comfort, solace, and sympathize with. How can the nurse through the practice of nursing assist the patient to regain his courage or confidence? The emphasis here is on the patient's regaining hope and confidence, not on the nurse's giving this to him. However, the nurse contributes to this both by how and what she does. Werthem[31] states that during an operation two factors contributed to decrease his general feeling of insecurity. One was the calm, deep, authoritative voice of the surgeon. The other was the soothing effect of the touch of a woman physician as she said something to him. Though he recognized that the friends who were with him were trying to reassure him by talking and joking, he did not find this behavior at all reassuring.

In a situation experienced by the writer, a patient who had undergone a bronchoscopy stated that he did not think that he could have withstood the procedure had the nurse not given him instructions during the procedure about what he should do and about the progress of the procedure. Here the talking was related directly to what the patient could expect from himself and from the situation and was not intended to distract his attention.

Reassurance of a patient is frequently difficult. Sometimes it is not achieved until the patient knows the outcome of his treatment. Though what is reassuring differs from one person to another, confidence that the situation is under control is often helpful. For some patients this is all that is necessary.

What are some of the things that nurses do that contribute to the patient's feeling that the situation is under control?

One of the ways to learn what kinds of actions support the patient's confidence is to listen to what he says. Some of the things that patients comment on as contributing to their confidence and security include: (1) having the ability to assess the situation as requiring prompt action and the initiation of such action; (2) appearing to know what to do; (3) taking over when the patient is overwhelmed, and knowing and doing the "right thing"; (4) being there when she is needed—a group of patients requested that a nurse not be transferred from night to day duty, because they could depend on her to be there when they needed her; this happened despite the nurse's dislike of working at

[31] *Ibid.*, p. 108.

night; (5) keeping the patient informed about what she is doing and why, when she can be expected, how long she will be away, and how much time she will be with him; (6) learning what the patient expects and correcting his misunderstandings and misconceptions as to what he can expect; and (7) maintaining uniformity in the performance of procedures that are frequently repeated in his care and appraising him of changes that are planned; patients are subjected to unnecessary anxiety when procedures are changed, because they tend to think the way that it has been done is the correct way; nurses should also inform themselves about the manner in which patients prefer to have procedures in their care performed before starting the patient's care; otherwise, patients develop the feeling that nurses do not know what they are doing or are incompetent; a not uncommon complaint on the part of patients is that each nurse has to be instructed about what the patient wants and how he wants it done; (8) encouraging the patient to help himself in ways that he is able, not because it helps the nurse, per se, but because this is a way he can help himself; (9) helping him to be aware of even small gains; (10) modifying her behavior in such a manner that the patient knows she is sensitive to and is concerned about his feelings; (11) taking care of his personal belongings, his flowers, and his physical environment; (12) sensing and giving attention to those things which are important to the patient; this may be any one of a thousand things ranging from tidying up his room before the doctor's visit to making certain that he gets a three-minute egg in the morning (if such a thing is possible); (13) keeping informed about changes in the therapeutic plan; this is not always easy; when, however, the patient's understanding differs from that of the nursing staff, an effort should be made to check with the physician.

Both the person and the circumstances under which the need for reassurance arises are determining factors in the type of behavior that is likely to be effective. Though some suggestions can be made for behavior that patients find reassuring, no recipe can be given that will always result in reassurance. Reassurance requires of the nurse real competence in the practice of nursing. By this is meant that the nurse knows what she is doing, why she does it, and how to do it. She cares for the patient with gentleness, carefulness, and thoroughness. She also cares for the patient and is concerned with the effect of her behavior on him. She gives appropriate attention to detail, not for the sake of the detail, but because it is important to the effect of what she is doing. She thinks about what she is doing, about its effect on the patient and how what she does can be improved. This and much more is important to encourage the patient in the feeling that he is valued as an individual human being, that his needs will be met, and that he is in safe hands. Acceptance involves a feeling that the patient is important and doing for and with the patient those things that are important to his welfare. It includes bathing, feeding, supporting, protecting, comforting, anticipating, relieving. It also includes allowing, encouraging, and supporting him in assuming responsibility for his own care as soon as he is able. It involves evaluating the meaning of his behavior and then acting appropriately.

To illustrate, a nurse answers Mr. Jason's call signal. She observes that he is irritable. She knows that irritability is common in sick people and that it indicates not what is wrong, but that something is wrong. It is a warning signal. Instead of feeling personally attacked, the nurse asks herself, "Why is Mr. Jason irritable? Is he receiving insulin in the treatment of his diabetes? If so, is he suffering from hypoglycemia? Is he having difficulty taking in or delivering oxygen to his body cells? Has he a low frustration level as a consequence of brain damage? Is he cold? Is he disappointed because his wife and family haven't been in to visit him? Has he had too many visitors? Is he troubled about something—the nature of his illness, its cost, or what is going to happen in relation to his job? Is he lonely? Has he been accustomed to consuming large amounts of alcohol so that he is beginning to show signs of its withdrawal? Did the patient in the next bed keep him awake all night? Is this the way he usually behaves under stress?" The nurse tries to determine the cause and then acts to relieve it. She gets a glass of orange juice, reapplies the oxygen tent, reduces her expectations for the patient, feeds him, gives him a glass of water, straightens his pillows, opens the window, calls his physician, listens to him, or calls the social worker or his minister or priest. What she does depends on her perception of the patient's need at the time. How she does it conveys to the patient whether or not she accepts him.

Another illustration is that of Mr. Xtus, who swears when he is in pain. The nurse notes the beads of perspiration on his brow and his clenched fists. She accepts Mr. Xtus, recognizes that his pain is severe and that he has to express its severity as he does. She reaches out and squeezes his hand to let him know that she appreciates his suffering, and says, "Your pain is bad, isn't it," changes his position and/or gets a pain-relieving drug, not because she approves of swearing, in fact she may disapprove very much, but because she examines his behavior and is concerned with its cause. Under other circumstances, Mr. Xtus' swearing may have other meanings. He may simply be in the habit of swearing or he may use it as an attention-getting device. The nurse may have to set limits by pointing out to him that his behavior is offensive to others and unnecessary. This requires some skill because she wants to convey to Mr. Xtus that because he is able to modify his behavior, he is expected to do so, and that she respects his dignity and rights and has faith in his ability to respect those of others. Furthermore, she may modify her care in some way so that his need to seek attention is reduced. For example, she may play checkers with him or arrange to have a Grey Lady visit him every afternoon. Through appropriate use of permissiveness and control the nurse conveys to each of these patients her acceptance of him and of his needs.

The nurse must also develop confidence in her capacity to meet the patient's needs. To do this she has to be aware of what causes her to become anxious. To return to Mr. Xtus, if the nurse is upset, that is, becomes anxious, when she hears a man swear, she may become so uncomfortable that she leaves him "to stew in his own juices" or until "he acts like a gentleman." If, however, she is aware of her own discomfort and still remains with Mr. Xtus, she may then be able to take the next step, which is to assess why he is behaving as he is. Her further action can then be directed toward meeting Mr. Xtus' needs, rather than her own. When she is successful in meeting the patient's needs, she also meets her own need for self-realization.

The contribution of physical care to the satisfaction of psychological needs of patients was emphasized in an earlier chapter. If the concepts that lower needs must be met before higher needs can be expressed is true, physical care is important to meeting psychological needs. Furthermore, the physical needs of the patient take the nurse to the patient. As a result of competent, kindly, and thoughtful care, the patient feels comforted and supported; some of his expectations for what nursing should provide are met.

Another skill in which the nurse needs to develop competency is the art of purposeful conversation. Though all conversation has a purpose, in conversations with patients the goals should be known. Basically conversation is for the purpose of furthering communication between two or more people. In the nurse-patient relationship conversation is used to further the nurse's relationship with the patient so that she can identify and satisfy the patient's needs.

Conversation with patients has many goals. It may be for the purpose of diversion, for companionship, for intellectual exchange, for sharing ideas, or for defending one's point of view. It may serve to relieve the patient's loneliness or to shorten a period of anticipation. As in other aspects of life, conversation may be used to gain or give information. It may be utilized to relieve feelings, to express feelings, to make plans. Since patients are people, they suffer from loneliness, frustration, and anger, as well as other emotions. They sometimes suffer psychological stress, and there are times when they are free or relatively free of it. The objective in nursing is to identify what the patient's need is at a particular time and then to try to provide a climate in which the need can be met.

The first step in purposeful conversation is to establish a goal that is valid and sincere. When a problem is known or suspected, the objective should be based on the desire to assist the patient rather than to identify the problem for the sake of knowing what the problem is.

Second, at one time or another people need to be reminded that conversation is a dialogue, not a monologue or a soliloquy, or even a debate. In the art of conversation, listening and hearing both the words and what they mean are important. This implies that the attention of the listener is concentrated on what the speaker is saying, how he is saying it, his facial expression, and what he does not say, rather than on how the listener will reply. Attention should be given to shifts in the person's conversation. This means, then, that the responder may need to take time to think out his reply after the person with whom he is conversing finishes speaking. To do this he must be able to keep the objective of the conversation in mind and to tolerate silence. Some of the world's most skillful conversationalists talk very little, but listen much. This is well illustrated by the taxi driver who, on discharging a passenger, said, "My, you are a good listener." During the hour's ride, the passenger had said little except, "Mm; not really; you like your work" and a few other similar comments. The only purpose of the listener's responding at all was to indicate that she was following what the driver was saying and was interested in it.

In addition to listening and hearing, conversation may be facilitated by asking open-ended questions and by asking the patient to clarify what he has said. In the use of open-ended questions, the questioner tries to avoid asking the question in a way that the answer is suggested. Statements such as, "I don't understand," "Could you clarify that?" or "You were saying," or even sounds like "Eh" or "Mmm" when said with a rising inflection can be used to indicate that one is interested and is following what the patient is saying and would like to hear more. The patient should be given time to respond. This means that the nurse must be able to stay with the patient and to remain silent until the patient responds.

The nurse may suspect that something is worrying the patient. She may also have clues as to the nature of what is troubling him. She must put these to the test. This can be done by repeating what the patient has said or what appears to be the intent of the patient's comment. For example, Miss Teen appeared to be upset when Miss Student tried to instruct her in how to inject her own insulin. Miss Student was surprised because up to this time Miss Teen had seemed eager to learn. Miss Student suspected that Miss Teen's hesitancy to inject the insulin might be related to something other than inserting the needle. To test her hypothesis she said, with a rising inflection, "You are troubled this morning"; then she waited. In a few moments Miss Teen started to cry. Between her sobs she told Miss Student that she had told her boy friend that she had diabetes and that he no longer wanted to "go steady."

Valuable as the capacity to tolerate silence is in encouraging people who are in trouble to talk about their problems, it has other uses as well. To make full use of silence in her relationship with patients, the nurse must regard it as a friend rather than an enemy. In the care of the seriously ill, conversation should be limited in order to conserve the patient's energy. Some seriously ill patients are calmed by having someone sitting quietly at their bedside. This may give a relative or close friend an opportunity to make a substantial contribution to the patient's welfare. A relative may need, however, some instruction in how to behave in the presence of the patient, and support and recognition of their contribution to the welfare of the patient from the nursing personnel. This is especially necessary when the patient is ill over a long period of time. For example, Mr. Klark was seriously ill in a hospital located some distance from his home. His wife was notified of his illness, and the suggestion was made that she arrange to come to the hospital as soon as possible. When she arrived, she was understandably distraught. The nurse, recognizing Mrs. Klark's emotional condition and that she had been riding on the bus all night, arranged for her to wash her face and hands and apply cosmetics. Then she suggested that after Mrs. Klark greeted her husband, she might sit quietly by his bed and, if she would like to do so, she might hold his hand. In this instance the nurse helped Mrs. Klark compose herself and then suggested how she might be helpful to her husband.

Another too frequently neglected practice of silence is what may be called friendly silence. Everyone feels good toward the other members of the group. All are comfortable and relaxed. This is the silence that says, "All is calm and serene. I am glad to be with you." With all the emphasis on togetherness and sociability, the fact that some persons need and desire an opportunity to be by themselves may be overlooked. Over the course of history the value and pain of solitude have been expressed in prose and poetry. Of modern writers few have expressed these more beautifully than Anne Morrow Lindbergh in *Gift From the Sea*. In essence she says that for life to have its full meaning and purpose, time must be set aside for contemplation in peace and quiet. To quote Mrs. Lindbergh, "Here there is time; time to be quiet; time to work without pressure; time to think; time to watch the heron, watching with frozen patience for his prey. . . . Time even not to talk."[32]

To summarize, a professional conversation is one of the tools used by the nurse to establish a therapeutic relationship with a patient. The goal of a particular conversation may be to identify what is troubling a patient so that, when possible, appropriate measures can be initiated to relieve him. Conversation may be used to gain or to impart information; to determine the patient's expectations; to determine what he knows and what he wants to know; or to learn something about his family, work, or living conditions, as a basis for planning future care. During recovery from an acute illness or during chronic illness, conversation may also provide needed diversion and recreation. Loneliness is one of the difficult problems in long-term illness. This is equally true whether the person is cared for at home or in the hospital. He longs for conversation with a sympathetic friend. A friendly listener may be the one bright spot in the person's day or week. Here again, attention to what the patient is saying, to what his interests are, and to encouraging him to expand his interest and to bring in a bit of outside world may be a rewarding experience for patient and nurse alike. Whatever the purpose of the conversation, its goals should be known. As in the use of other techniques in the care of the patient, the goals should be defined in terms of the needs of the patient. Conversation, like other skills, is learned and can be improved. This requires practice and evaluation of each conversation. What went well? Where did I get off the track? Why, What could have been done to keep on the track? What are my real goals? Why?

Throughout the chapter the goal, to establish a therapeutic or helping relationship with the patient, has been emphasized. The steps in the establish-

[32] Anne Morrow Lindbergh, *Gift from the Sea*, Pantheon, New York, 1955, p. 116.

ment of a significant relationship, as they have been stated by Schmahl,[33] follow. They are (1) "Awareness of one's own anxiety." In addition to this, the nurse must be willing to cope with it by moving slowly, waiting, and staying with it. (2) "Sustained physical thereness." The nurse must remain with the patient when he needs her. This is easier to do when giving physical care. The nurse should eventually develop the ability to stay with the patient when no physical care is required. (3) "Critical listening" and (4) "open-ended questions." As emphasized earlier in critical listening, attention is given not only to obvious meanings of the words that the patient uses, but to their hidden meanings. The use of open-ended questions has been discussed. (5) "Consensual validation." By consensual validation is meant the putting to the test hunches about the patient's feelings.

In this chapter some of the knowledge required by the nurse to meet the psychosocial needs of patients has been presented. Because of the rapidity with which knowledge in this area is growing, no single chapter can do more than summarize the more pertinent information. The hope is that students will become interested in exploring further resources.

Throughout the chapter emphasis has been placed on the fact that human behavior is the product of multiple factors. Each individual's behavior results from his reactions to and his interaction with his culture. His biological inheritance and structure are also a significant element in his behavior, for they determine his possibilities for development as well as his limits. A bird can fly. Man cannot, or could not until he invented the airplane. Sophia Moore is a grown woman, but she is less than 3 ft. tall. She is deeply depressed. She says, "I am a nobody. How can anyone who is small like me be anybody when to somebody one must be big?" Sophia's size is biologically based. Her self-concept is derived from the value placed on physical bigness in the culture into which she was born. In another culture she might have been made a queen or treated as a god. In another, where smallness was the rule, she would not have been the object of any special attention. Culture is both universal and unique to man. Though all men are of the same species and cultures have common characteristics, both men and culture run the gamut in relation to variety.

Illness is, however, a personal experience. How the person behaves during illness depends on how he behaves in other crisis situations in his life. Studies made of people who are ill reveal that not all persons react to illness in the same manner. This point is emphasized by the findings of Kaplan[34] who studied the psychological aspects of heart disease. Some of the factors that he found to influence the reaction of the individual included: (1) the personality of the patient before he became ill and his life situation, (2) the degree or extent of his physical incapacity, (3) the abruptness of the onset, (4) the degree of severity, (5) the duration of the illness, and (6) the relationship of

[33] Jane A. Schmahl, "The Price of Recovery," *American Journal of Nursing,* LVIII, January, 1958, p. 90.
[34] Kaplan, *Op. cit.,* p. 233.

the patient to his family and to his physician. Though the subjects for this study were patients having mitral commissurotomies, recent literature in the field indicates that these are factors which enter into the behavior of patients with other diagnoses. This supports the concept that it is the patient and not his diagnosis that is of first importance in his reaction to disease.

Failure to identify and interpret appropriately a patient's behavior may be a source of psychological stress to the patient and to the nurse. When the patient and the nurse have a common cultural heritage, their expectations and values are more likely to be in agreement than when they are from dissimilar backgrounds. When the behavior of the patient differs from that expected by the professional staff, they have a responsibility to accept the patient's behavior as having meaning and to adapt their own behavior appropriately. The burden should be on the professional person rather than on the patient. Application of knowledge of the psychosocial aspects of patient care should contribute to enhancement of the patient's feeling that he is accepted as an individual human being with dignity and rights. He should further feel that he is safe and protected and that he can depend on those who are responsible for his care to further his needs. Skillful use of the knowledge of the psychosocial needs of patients should add to the satisfaction the nurse derives from the practice of nursing.

REFERENCES

Books

Abdellah, Faye G., and Eugene Levine, *Effect of Nurse Staffing on Satisfactions with Nursing Care.* A study of how omissions in nursing services, as perceived by patients and personnel, are influenced by the number of nursing hours available, Hospital Monograph No. 4, American Hospital Association, Chicago, 1958.

Aldrich, C. Knight, *Psychiatry for the Family Physician*, Blakiston Division, McGraw-Hill Book Co., Inc., New York, 1955.

Allport, Floyd Henry, *Theories of Perception and the Concept of Structure*, Wiley Co., New York, 1955.

Apple, Dorrian (ed.), *Sociological Studies of Health and Sickness*, McGraw-Hill Book Co., Inc., New York, 1960.

Bauer, Julius, *The Person Behind the Disease*, Grune and Stratton, New York, 1956.

Bird, Brian, *Talking With Patients*, J. B. Lippincott Co., Philadelphia, 1955.

Garrett, Annette, *Interviewing*, Family Service Association of America, New York, 1959.

Ingle, Dwight J. (ed.), *Life and Disease*, Basic Books, Inc., New York, 1963.

King, Stanley H., *Perceptions of Illness and Medical Practice*, Russell Sage Foundation, New York, 1962.

Paul, Benjamin D. (ed.), *Health, Culture and Community*, Russell Sage Foundation, New York, 1955.

Philip, Solomon, *et al.* (ed.), *Sensory Deprivation*, Harvard University Press, Cambridge, Massachusetts, 1961.

Pinner, Max, and B. F. Miller (eds.), *When Doctors Are Patients*, W. W. Norton Co., New York, 1952.

Ruesch, Jurgen, and Gregory Bateson, *Communication: The Social Matrix of Psychiatry*, W. W. Norton and Co., Inc., New York, 1951.

Saunders, Lyle, *Cultural Differences and Medical Care*, Russell Sage Foundation, New York, 1954.

Schwartz, Doris, Barbara Henley, and Leonard Zeitz, *The Elderly Ambulatory Patient,* The Macmillan Company, New York, 1964.

Williams, J. Paul, *What Americans Believe and How They Worship,* Harper and Brothers, New York, 1952.

Articles

Alfano, Genrose, "What Rapport Means to Me," *Nursing Outlook,* III, June, 1955, p. 326.

Aasterud, Margaret, "Defenses Against Anxiety in the Nurse Patient Relationship," *Nursing Forum,* Summer, 1962, pp. 35-38.

Beecher, Henry K., "Nonspecific Forces Surrounding Disease and the Treatment of Disease," *Journal of the American Medical Association,* CLXXIX, February 10, 1962, pp. 437-40.

Ball, Geraldine, "Speaking Without Words," *American Journal of Nursing,* LX, May, 1960, pp. 692-93.

Bojar, Samuel, "The Psychotherapeutic Function of the General Hospital Nurse," *Nursing Outlook,* VI, March, 1958, pp. 151-53.

Cantril, Hadley, "A Study of Aspirations," *Scientific American,* February, 1963, pp. 41-45.

Cattell, Raymond B., "The Nature and Measurement of Anxiety," *Scientific American,* March, 1963, pp. 96-104.

Connally, Mary Grace, "What Acceptance Means to Patients," *American Journal of Nursing,* LX, December, 1960, pp. 1754-57.

Davis, Anne J., "The Skills of Communication," *American Journal of Nursing,* LXIII, January, 1963, pp. 66-70.

Eldred, Stanley J., "Improving Nurse-Patient Communication," *American Journal of Nursing,* LX, November, 1960, pp. 1600-2.

Engel, George, "A Unified Concept of Health and Disease," *Perspectives in Biology and Medicine,* III, Summer, 1960, p. 459.

Fantz, Robert L., "The Origin of Form Perception," *Scientific American,* May, 1961, p. 66.

Greenhill, M. H., "Interviewing with a Purpose," *American Journal of Nursing,* LVI, October, 1956, pp. 1259-62.

Harlow, Harry E., and Margaret K. Harlow, "Social Deprivation in Monkeys," *Scientific American,* November, 1962, pp. 136-46.

Hart, Betty L., and Anne W. Rohweder, "Support in Nursing," *American Journal of Nursing,* LIX, October, 1959, pp. 1398-1401.

Hess, Eckhard H., "Shadows and Depth Perception," *Scientific American,* March, 1961, p. 138.

Hewitt, Helon E., and Betty L. Pesznecker, "Major Blocks To Communicating With Patients," *American Journal of Nursing,* LXIV, No. 7, July, 1964, pp. 101-103.

Hulicka, Irene M., "Fostering Self-Respect In Aged Patients," *American Journal of Nursing,* XLIV, No. 3, March, 1963, p. 84-89.

Huges, Horace H., "No Eggs for Breakfast," *American Journal of Nursing,* LVII, April, 1957, pp. 470-72.

Hunter, John, "The Mark of Pain," *American Journal of Nursing,* LXI, October, 1961, p. 96.

Hyde, Robert S., and Norma E. Goggans, "When Nurses Have Guilt Feelings," *American Journal of Nursing,* LVIII, February, 1958, pp. 233-36.

Ingles, Thelma, "The Worst Patient on the Floor," *Nursing Outlook,* VI, February, 1958, pp. 99-100.

Ingles, Thelma, "Mrs. Belmont—A Good Patient," *Nursing Outlook,* VI, March, 1958, p. 163.

Jerome, Alberta, and Mabel Reid, "Ladies Who Listen," *Nursing Outlook,* V, April, 1957, p. 216-21.

Jourard, Sidney, M., "To Whom Can A Nurse Give Personalized Care," *American Journal of Nursing,* LXI, March, 1961, pp. 86-88.

Jourard, Sidney M., "How Well Do You Know Your Patients?" *American Journal of Nursing*, LIX, November, 1959, p. 1568-71.

Kaufman, Margaret A., and Dorothy E. Brown, "Pain Wears Many Faces," *American Journal of Nursing*, LXI, January, 1961, p. 48.

Koos, Earl, "Metropolis—What People Think of Their Medical Services," *Patients, Physicians and Illness*, The Free Press, Glencoe, Illinois, 1958, pp. 113-19.

Levine, D., "Anxiety About Illness," *Journal of Health and Human Behavior*, Spring, 1962.

Martin, Harry, and Arthur Prange, "The Stages of Illness—Psychosocial Approach," *Nursing Outlook*, X, March, 1962, pp. 168-71.

Mead, Beverly T., "Emotional Struggles in Adjusting to Old Age," *Postgraduate Medicine*, XXXI, February, 1962, p. 156.

Mead, Margaret, "Understanding Cultural Patterns," *Nursing Outlook*, IV, May, 1956, pp. 260-62.

Melzack, Ronald, "The Perception of Pain," *Scientific American*, CCIV, February, 1961, pp. 41-49.

Monteiro, Lois, "The Patient Had Difficulty Communicating," *American Journal of Nursing*, LXII, January, 1962, pp. 78-81.

Norris, Catherine M., "The Nurse and the Crying Patient," *American Journal of Nursing*, LVII, March, 1957, pp. 323-27.

Parsons, Talcott, "Definitions of Health and Illness in the Light of American Values and Social Structure," *Patients, Physicians, and Illness*, E. G. Jaco (ed.), The Free Press, Glencoe, Illinois, 1958, pp. 165-87.

Peplau, Hildegarde, "Loneliness," *American Journal of Nursing*, LV, December, 1955, pp. 1476-81.

Rapoport, Lydia, "Motivation in the Struggle for Health," *American Journal of Nursing*, LVII, November, 1957, pp. 1455-57.

Schmahl, Jane A., "The Price of Recovery," *American Journal of Nursing*, LVIII, January, 1958, pp. 88-90.

Schulman, Sam, "Basic Functional Roles in Nursing: Mother, Surrogate and Healer," *Patients, Physicians and Illness*, E. G. Jaco (ed.), The Free Press, Glenco, Illinois, 1958, p. 528.

Schwartz, Doris, "Hospital Ward, The Social Order," *The Atlantic Monthly*, CC, December, 1957, pp. 57-60.

Schwartz, Doris, "Uncooperative Patients?" *American Journal of Nursing*, LVIII, January, 1958, pp. 75-77.

Sesler, George C., "The Nurse and the Emotional Needs of the Patient," *The Canadian Nurse*, LIV, April, 1958, pp. 314-17.

Skipper, J. K., H. O. Mauksch, and D. Tagliacozzo, "Some Barriers to Communication Between Patients and Hospital Functionaries," *Nursing Forum*, II, No. I, 1963, pp. 15-23.

Skipper, James K., Daisy L. Tagliacozzo, and Hans O. Mauksch, "What Communication Means to Patients," *American Journal of Nursing*, LXIV, No. 4, April, 1964, p. 101-3.

Stevens, Leonard, "What Makes a Ward Climate Therapeutic," *American Journal of Nursing*, LXI, March, 1961, pp. 95-96.

Stevenson, Ian, "Explaining the Results of Examinations to Patients, Part I," *Postgraduate Medicine*, XXXI, June, 1962, p. 517.

Taren, James A., and Edgar A. Kahn, "The Surgical Relief of Intractable Pain," *Surgical Clinics of North America*, XLI, No. 5, October, 1961, p. 1159.

Turnbull, Colin M., "The Lesson of the Pygmee," *Scientific American*, January, 1963, pp. 28-37.

Wittreich, Warren J., "Visual Perception and Personality," *Scientific American*, April, 1959, p. 56.

Wolf, Stewart, "Disease as a Way of Life: Neural Integration in Systemic Pathology," *Perspective in Biology and Medicine*, IV, Spring, 1961, pp. 288-305.

7 : Nursing the Patient Having a Problem in Maintaining the Supply of Oxygen and/or in the Removal of Carbon Dioxide

> The only way of real advance in biology lies in taking as our starting point, not the separated parts of an organism and its environment, but the whole organism in its actual relation to environment, and defining the parts and activities in this whole in terms implying their existing relationships to the other parts and activities.[1]

In common with other living organisms, the survival of man depends on a continued supply of energy for the performance of work by his cells. Every manifestation of life is dependent on the liberation and utilization of free energy. Every increase in energy requires an increase in the supply of materials that can be converted to energy. Energy is obtained through the combination of oxygen with a limited variety of compounds—carbohydrates, fats, and proteins by the so-called oxidation-reduction reaction.

What are some of the circumstances or conditions in which oxygen supply may be threatened?

At body temperatures, the natural rate of oxidation is exceedingly slow. Enzymes are therefore required to catalyze or speed oxidation-reduction reactions. Survival is threatened by any condition interfering with the supply of oxygen or of carbon-containing compounds to the cells or with the processes involved in the release of energy by the cells. The child who is trapped in a discarded refrigerator dies because his supply of oxygen is limited. One of the reasons the child who drowns dies is because his air passages are blocked by water and ventilation is impeded. Since oxygen is required for the release of energy from its potential sources, cellular processes require not only oxygen, but compounds in which energy is stored. In shock, death is due to a failure of the circulation to supply cells with the oxygen and sources of energy. As a result cells are unable to continue metabolic activities that are essential to life. In cyanide poisoning oxidation-reduction reactions cease because cyanide poisons the enzymes catalyzing oxidation-reduction reactions. In all

[1] J. B. S. Haldane, *Respiration,* Yale University Press, New Haven, Connecticut, 1922.

the above disorders, death is due to the failure of the oxidation-reduction reactions by which cells release energy for the maintenance of their activities.

This chapter is devoted to the processes involved in providing cells with oxygen and with the elimination of carbon dioxide. The factors in the maintenance of a supply of carbon-containing compounds and the processes involved in their use will be discussed in a later chapter. Carbon dioxide is one of the products of oxidation-reduction reactions that is returned to the external environment. It participates in the regulation of the mechanisms for the supply of oxygen to cells and for its own elimination. All the processes involved in the delivery of oxygen to cells and the removal of carbon dioxide are known as respiration. Respiration is not really complete until oxygen is combined in the cell with the hydrogen ion to form water or with a compound containing carbon to form carbon dioxide. Respiration therefore includes:

1. Breathing or ventilation—transport of air from the atmosphere to the alveoli and back to the atmosphere. Ventilation takes place in two phases—inspiration and expiration.
2. Diffusion of oxygen and carbon dioxide from the alveoli to the blood and from the blood to the alveoli.
3. Transportation of oxygen and carbon dioxide by means of the blood and body fluids to and from cells.
4. Oxidation-reduction reactions in cells.
5. Regulation of all aspects of respiration—not only breathing, but all processes involved in supplying cells with oxygen and including those by which priority needs are met.

Knowledge of the importance of a continuous supply of oxygen to all cells has countless implications in the practice of nursing, which may be summarized as follows:

1. To prevent conditions in the external environment predisposing to a deficient supply of oxygen. For example, the nurse should support and promote community efforts to protect babies from smothering in plastic bags, or children from suffocation in discarded refrigerators.
2. To protect patients who are unable to protect themselves—for example, the unconscious patient who may be suffocated or drowned by his own secretions.
3. To protect patients from the effects of oxygen deficiency—local or general. The nurse must be able to recognize signs and symptoms indicating a lack of oxygen and to take appropriate steps to correct the situation.
4. To carry out measures to maintain ventilation or to increase the supply of oxygen available for absorption.

What are some of the factors influencing the quantity of oxygen required and the sensitivity of cells, tissues, and individuals to a lack of oxygen?

In order to obtain energy stored in foodstuffs, cells of all organisms require a continuous supply of oxygen. In the absence of oxygen cells die, just as they do when they are deprived of food. There is, however, considerable variability in sensitivity to low oxygen tension[2] among species, among individuals of the same species, as well as among tissues of the same individual. Moreover, a variety of conditions alter the requirements of a single individual for oxygen, as the need for oxygen is modified by exercise, body temperature, and metabolic rate. An increase in any of the above increases the demand for oxygen, while a decrease lessens the need for oxygen. Certain factors appear to influence the ability of the organism to withstand low oxygen tension. It is better tolerated by the fetus than by the adult, by immature cells than by mature cells, and by females than by males. The structural and physiological status of an individual is also a factor. For example, an individual whose circulatory system is able to compensate for a decrease in oxygen supply by increasing blood flow is better able to tolerate hypoxia than the one whose circulatory response is defective or lacking. For instance, Mrs. White, who has had an extensive sympathectomy, tolerates hypoxia poorly because she is unable to constrict the arterioles in a large part of her body. Her inability to constrict her arterioles in response to an increased need for oxygen prevents her from being able to maintain an adequate blood pressure in conditions calling for a greater supply of blood. Despite differences in sensitivity to low oxygen tension, all individuals have limits to their ability to adapt to and to survive deficiencies in the supply of oxygen. Moreover, since oxygen is not stored in appreciable quantities, the effects of an acute failure of supply can be observed almost immediately.

Tissues most sensitive to oxygen lack are the cerebral cortex, the myocardium, and the kidney. Although the cerebral cortex is highly sensitive to oxygen deprivation, it is probably the best protected by the circulation. In anoxia,[3] blood flow is rerouted to maintain blood flow to the cerebral cortex, sometimes at the expense of other organs. Irreparable damage to the cells of the cerebral cortex can result from failure to supply oxygen for as few as four or five minutes. Others parts of the central nervous system are better able to withstand anoxia. The medulla can function for as long as 20 to 30 minutes without oxygen. It is not unusual to see a patient whose brain has been temporarily deprived of its oxygen supply retain his ability to regulate vegeta-

[2] Oxygen tension is determined by the percentage composition of oxygen in the air and the pressure (usually atmospheric) under which it is confined. Low oxygen tension results from a reduction in the percentage composition of oxygen in the inspired air or a significant reduction in atmospheric pressure.

[3] Anoxia. A better term is hypoxia because it implies varying degrees of oxygen lack. Anoxia literally means an absolute lack of oxygen. However, anoxia continues to be used in the literature to describe different degrees of oxygen deficiency."

tive functions, but lose functions that are dependent on the cerebral cortex. For example, when the heart is started after prolonged cardiac arrest, cerebral cortical function may fail, or be markedly impaired, despite the return of vegetative functions. Mr. Peters experienced cardiac arrest associated with myocardial infarction. After some delay artificial respiration and cardiac massage were instituted and approximately an hour elapsed before cardiac function was re-established. Though Mr. Peters was able to eat, digest food, and breathe, he suffered serious mental deterioration. He gave little evidence of recognizing his wife or children and he had to be cared for like a young child. He was unable to assume any responsibility for his own care.

The myocardium and the kidney are also sensitive to a lack of oxygen. According to Davis,[4] the heart continues to contract for about five to ten minutes in the absence of oxygen, provided the individual is at rest. Exercise or activity decreases the length of time the heart will continue to contract in the absence of oxygen.

Unlike skeletal muscle, the myocardium is unable to accumulate more than a small oxygen debt before it ceases to function. Like the brain and the myocardium, the kidney is sensitive to anoxia. Renal shutdown is always a possibility in any condition associated with prolonged or severe anoxia, such as shock.

Other tissues such as bone and cartilage are able to withstand oxygen deprivation for longer periods of time. Because skeletal muscle is able to accumulate an oxygen debt, it can contract for a time despite a deficiency of oxygen. For muscle contraction to continue or the muscle be restored to its resting condition, oxygen must be provided to remove the lactate accumulated in the tissue during anaerobic catabolism. In biological systems, lactic acid appears to have only one possible fate, that is, reoxidation to pyruvic acid. All tissues, including those that are relatively insensitive to hypoxia and those that are able to function for a time anaerobically, must have oxygen to obtain the free energy from foodstuffs required to carry on their activities. Without it, they die.

How is the supply of oxygen to the tissues maintained?

Man's cells are similar to those of most other organisms inasmuch as they obtain oxygen from their fluid environment. Single-cell organisms and those consisting of relatively few cells obtain oxygen from the pool of fluid in which they are suspended. The fluid is, of course, in direct contact with the external environment, or atmosphere. In man the fluid bathing his cells is separated from the external environment by semipermeable membranes. Special structures are necessary to cleanse and bring air in contact with these membranes, as well as to distribute oxygen to the fluid environment of the cells. The process is finally complete when oxygen penetrates cells and enters into an

[4] Harry A. Davis, *Surgical Physiology*, Paul B. Hoeber, Inc., New York, 1957, p. 69.

oxidation-reduction reaction. The products of this reaction are heat, carbon dioxide, and water. Some of the heat is used as energy to perform the work of the cell. Most of the excess heat is eliminated by the skin. A small amount is lost through expired air. Most excess water is eliminated by the kidney. Carbon dioxide is eliminated by way of the same semipermeable membranes in the alveoli that serve as a site for the entrance of oxygen.

The source of oxygen is the air. Inspired air is composed of approximately 20.93 per cent oxygen, 79 per cent nitrogen, and 0.04 per cent carbon dioxide. Though the percentage composition of air is the same at all altitudes below 80,000 ft, the pressure under which air is confined decreases as elevation increases. At sea level atmospheric pressure is 760 mm of mercury, or 1 atmosphere. As elevation increases, atmospheric pressure decreases or becomes less than 760 mm of mercury. Atmospheric pressure is one of the significant factors in the exchange of gases in the lung.

Why atmospheric pressure is a factor in the exchange of gases in the lung is explained by the gas laws. They are:

Boyle's law

When the temperature of a gas remains constant, its pressure varies inversely with its volume. In other words, with increasing elevation above sea level, the volume or space in which the air is contained is enlarged, and as a result, pressure decreases. Movement of air into and out of the lung also illustrates Boyle's law. As the size (volume) of the lung is increased during inspiration, pressure within the lung decreases and air enters. Gases tend to move by diffusion from areas of greater concentration or pressure to areas of lesser concentration or pressure; the reverse happens during expiration.

Law of solubility of gases

As with other states of matter, gases vary in their solubility. Carbon dioxide is 20 times as soluble as oxygen. Other things being equal, however, gases go into solution in proportion to their partial pressures. If a mixture of gases is placed in contact with a liquid in a closed flask, each gas goes into solution until equilibrium is reached. To illustrate, if air is placed in a closed container with water, each constituent of the air will go into solution in proportion to its partial pressure.

Dalton's law, or the law of partial pressures

In a mixture of gases, each gas exerts its own pressure independently of the other gases. Each gas behaves as if it were alone. The total pressure of a mixture of gases is equal to the sum of the pressures of its components. For example, the pressure of air at sea level is 760 mm of mercury. The percentage composition of oxygen in dry air at sea level is 20.93. Its partial pressure is therefore 20.93 multiplied by 760, or about 159 mm of mercury. Air is approximately 79 per cent nitrogen. Its partial pressure is therefore about 600 mm of mercury. Together they add up to 759 mm of mercury.

The direction and rate of the movement of gases across the respiratory membranes are explained by Dalton's law of partial pressures and the law of solubility of gases. Since gases diffuse from areas of greater to lesser pressure and the partial pressure of oxygen is higher in the alveoli than it is in the blood, oxygen moves from the alveoli to the blood. The reverse is true for carbon dioxide. Moreover, the rate at which carbon dioxide is removed from the blood can be increased by increasing the rate and depth of respiration. When the alveoli are enlarged by deep breathing, their volume or capacity to hold air is increased. With an increase in volume, the partial pressure of carbon dioxide in the alveoli decreases—another illustration of Boyle's law. The difference in pressure or gradient between the partial pressure of carbon dioxide in the blood and that in the alveoli is raised. The capacity to alter the partial pressure of carbon dioxide in the alveolar air is of some importance in the regulation of acid-base balance of the body fluids and will be discussed more completely elsewhere.

Since atmospheric pressure varies inversely with the distance above sea level, the exchange of gases between the lung and the blood is affected by atmospheric pressure. The higher the elevation, the lower the atmospheric pressure, and the lower the partial pressure of each of its component gases. Despite a similar percentage composition of oxygen at sea level and at 18,000 ft., less oxygen is transferred across the alveolar membrane because its partial pressure is significantly lowered by elevation. Atmospheric pressure not only is important in maintaining oxygen supply, but is also a source of difficulty when a person rapidly changes from an atmosphere of high pressure to one that is markedly lower. Though people differ, a decrease of approximately 2 atmospheres is usually required to cause difficulty; that is, when the atmosphere to which an individual is exposed is rapidly halved, he is likely to experience a disorder variously known as Caisson disease, decompression sickness, or "the bends." For the manifestations of decompression sickness to appear, the person must have been in the region of relatively high atmospheric pressure long enough for the gases in the air to attain equilibrium between the air and his blood. The rapid reduction in the atmospheric pressure has two effects. The first results from the tendency of the volume of a gas to expand with a decrease in pressure—an illustration of Boyle's law. The air in the lung expands rapidly as the atmospheric pressure falls and first distends and then ruptures the lungs with the result that the air is drawn into the heart and large arteries. The second effect of a rapid drop in atmospheric pressure results from its effect on the solubility of gases. Since a gas, for example nitrogen, goes into and out of solution in proportion to its partial pressure, a decrease in atmospheric pressure causes a decrease in the solubility of the nitrogen in the blood. If the fall is precipitous, the gas comes out of solution in the form of bubbles. The effect is similar to that observed following the removal of a cap from a bottle of carbonated beverage such as ginger ale. The carbon dioxide which is confined in the liquid under pressure escapes from the liquid in the form of bubbles. The difference between the partial pressure of carbon dioxide in the ginger ale and in the air is so great that it escapes very rapidly from the liquid. On a hot day, if the bottle is shaken before it is opened, the gas and solution form foam and overflow the bottle. Were the gas to be released in a confined space, such as a blood vessel, the bubbles would fill the vessel and obstruct blood flow.

To illustrate what happens in man under similar circumstances, the experience of Mr. Gold, a miner, will be presented. Decompression sickness is not limited to miners, however, and it can develop during high-altitude flying, following deep-sea diving, or among submarine crews. Pilots of planes can prepare themselves for high-altitude flying by inhaling pure oxygen to remove nitrogen from their blood. Crew and passengers in planes are protected by the pressurizing of airplane cabins. Miners and others who work below the surface of the earth are protected by returning to the surface in decompression chambers. After working all day in a mine located well below the surface of the earth, nitrogen and oxygen dissolved in the blood of Mr. Gold are in equilibrium with the greater-than-sea-level partial pressure of nitrogen and oxygen in the air. When he returns to the surface of the earth quickly, the air in his lungs will expand rapidly causing distention of his lungs and possibly their rupture. The nitrogen and oxygen dissolved in his blood will come out of solution quickly. Bubbles of oxygen will cause him little trouble, because oxygen is utilized by his cells, but nitrogen is not utilized and blocks his blood vessels. To prevent decompression sickness, Mr. Gold and his fellow miners are moved slowly to the surface in a decompression chamber where the atmospheric pressure is slowly reduced to sea level. Persons who develop decompression sickness are treated by placing them in a decompression chamber and subjecting them to higher-than-atmospheric pressure. After their symptoms are relieved, they are gradually decompressed; that is, they are exposed to a gradually decreasing atmospheric pressure, and the nitrogen is removed from their blood without forming bubbles.

The signs and symptoms manifested by the person who experiences decompression sickness depend on which of his tissues are deprived of their blood supply. Nitrogen emboli can cause serious or even fatal damage when vessels supplying the brain or heart are obstructed. Pain in the bones and joints is common and accounts for the term "the bends." There are, of course, many other possible effects.

Another problem of importance to an ever-increasing number of people has its origin in the fact that atmospheric pressure diminishes as altitude increases. Despite individual differences, an altitude above sea level is finally reached where the partial pressure of oxygen is no longer adequate to maintain life. At one time this problem was largely confined to high, mountainous areas of the world. With high altitude and space travel, it is now frequently encountered. The effects of both acute and chronic oxygen deprivation are discussed later in the chapter. Much can be learned about the effects of continued oxygen deprivation and adaptation of man to it by reading the accounts of mountain climbers such as William O. Douglas.[5]

Under certain conditions the percentage of oxygen in the air may be reduced because it is utilized and not replaced or because of the dilution of oxygen with another gas. Two different types of situations may be responsible for the depletion of oxygen in the air. In one, an individual enters an airtight space. Examples include the child who is trapped in an old refrigerator or who pulls a lightweight plastic bag over his head, or a person who enters a room in which the oxygen content has been exhausted by a flame. In all the above instances a person is trapped in an oxygenless space. As soon as the oxygen supply is exhausted, he dies of suffocation. The second type of situation is which suffocation is possible is the administration of oxygen in a closed system, either by itself or in a mixture of gases. When the supply of oxygen is exhausted or its concentration is inadequate, hypoxia develops. This is a possibility that should be anticipated when inert gases such as helium or certain general anesthetics are administered. The use of some general anesthetics is limited by the fact that effective concentrations of the anesthetic limit oxygen supply too greatly. For example, for nitrous oxide to produce an adequate degree of relaxation for an abdominal operation, it must be present in a concentration of 90 per cent. Obviously, an oxygen concentration of 10 per cent is inadequate to the needs of the organism, and signs and symptoms of hypoxia would follow were the percentage composition of oxygen in the air reduced to this extent.

How is a lack of oxygen manifested by an individual?

Lack of oxygen may be either acute or chronic. The signs and symptoms accompanying the acute deprivation of oxygen resemble those of acute alcoholic intoxication, while those of chronic hypoxia are similar to those of fatigue. Symptoms that result from the effects of hypoxia on the nervous system include: headache, depression, apathy, slowness of thought, excitement that borders on panic, irritability, restlessness, loss of memory, defective judgment, emotional disturbances, poor muscular coordination, fatigue, stupor, and insomnia. When hypoxia is prolonged or is of marked degree, the person may suffer disturbances in seeing and hearing, or he may experience pain. Because of the numerous conditions that may be responsible for a lack of oxygen, nurses should be alert to the possibility of hypoxia when a patient exhibits one or more of the above signs and symptoms. Prompt action should be taken to correct the cause.

Hypoxia is accompanied by changes in the functioning of the nervous, circulatory, respiratory, and gastrointestinal systems. Since the nervous sys-

---

[5] William O. Douglas, *Beyond the High Himalayas,* Doubleday & Company, Inc., Garden City, New York, 1952, pp. 121-28.

tem regulates the activity of other organs, the effects of hypoxia can be either directly on the other organs, or through its effect on the nervous system. Inasmuch as alterations in function increase the supply of oxygen to cells, they are adaptive. In some instances they are maladaptive, as they increase the need for oxygen by increasing the activity of cells. For example, when a person panics and fights to escape from a space in which he is trapped, he uses more oxygen than he would if he were quiet. If he cannot escape quickly, the struggle is maladaptive, as it decreases his chances of survival.

Changes in the function of the circulatory system in hypoxia include tachycardia, which may be the earliest sign, especially in an anesthetized patient, a slight rise in blood pressure, and epistaxis. In advanced stages the heart rate and blood pressure fall and loss of consciousness also occurs. When the latter signs and symptoms appear in the patient suffering hypoxia, prognosis is grave.

As is to be expected in hypoxia, there is an attempt made to increase pulmonary ventilation. There is also a tendency toward periodic respiration, especially during sleep.

What conditions are prerequisite to the development of cyanosis?

Despite the importance ascribed to cyanosis, a condition in which the skin and mucous membranes are a dark blue or purplish color, a patient may be suffering from a severe degree of hypoxia and not be cyanotic. For cyanosis to be present, blood in the surface capillaries must contain a certain proportion of nonoxygenated hemoglobin or hemoglobin compounds such as methemoglobin or sulfhemoglobin. Some hemoglobin compounds such as carboxyhemoglobin (hemoglobin and carbon monoxide) do not cause cyanosis. Because carboxyhemoglobin is cherry-red in color, it gives the skin a pink tint. The patient is hypoxic, however, because the hemoglobin that is combined with carbon monoxide is not available to carry oxygen. With the exception of those conditions in which abnormal hemoglobin or its products are responsible for cyanosis, two conditions are required for cyanosis to be evident. Capillary blood must contain approximately 5 gm per 100 ml or more of unoxygenated hemoglobin, and the surface capillaries must be dilated and blood circulating through them.

According to Houssay,[6] four elements enter into the production of cyanosis. They are: (1) the level of hemoglobin in the blood; (2) the extent to which hemoglobin in the blood leaving the lungs is oxygenated; (3) the proportion of oxygenated arterial to venous blood when they are mixed, as when there is a right-to-left shunt in cardiac malformations; and (4) the extent to which oxygen is removed from the blood as it moves through the capillaries.

To illustrate, Mrs. Ash, who has a hemoglobin of 6 gm per 100 ml of blood (normal range for women is 12 to 15 gm per 100 ml), is not likely to be

[6] Bernardo A. Houssay, *et al.*, *Human Physiology*, 2nd ed., McGraw-Hill Book Company, Inc., New York, 1955, p. 309.

cyanotic, because her hemoglobin is fully oxygenated, but she is hypoxic. Cyanosis may also be present in the absence of hypoxia. Cyanosis without hypoxia occurs in persons with abnormally high hemoglobin levels, such as persons who are adapted to a high altitude. Persons may be hypoxic despite a high level of hemoglobin and a normal volume of oxygen per 100 ml of blood. Patients with polycythemia vera are, in effect, hypoxic even though the total quantity of oxygen carried per 100 ml of blood may be normal or high because arterial p o_2 is low and oxygen available to tissues is decreased. In these conditions, blood leaving the lung is not fully oxygenated. In disorders in which large portions of the lung are inactivated, poorly oxygenated hemoglobin will result in both cyanosis and hypoxia. The significance of cyanosis, therefore, depends on knowledge of the factors contributing to its development. In the care of sick people, other signs and symptoms indicating hypoxia should not be neglected because cyanosis is absent.

Because of the sensitivity of the gastrointestinal tract to conditions in the body, nausea and vomiting frequently occur in hypoxia.

From the preceding discussion, it should be clear that hypoxia has widespread effects. The most serious threat associated with a rapidly developing and acute hypoxia is to the central nervous system, particularly to the cerebral cortex.

What are some conditions that may cause sensations interpreted by the patient to be due to a lack of oxygen?

There are circumstances under which an individual may feel that he is not receiving enough oxygen when the supply is adequate. Certain conditions in the external environment predispose to sensations interpreted as a lack of oxygen. Probably the most common causes of discomfort are associated with the temperature, the humidity, and the movement of air. When the air is overheated and still, a person may feel that he is not obtaining sufficient oxygen. A feeling of suffocation is often a problem in a closed room ventilated by a poorly functioning air-conditioning system. Adding a fan may do much to improve comfort. Too great a movement of air, however, may cause chilling and should be avoided. When nothing can be done to lessen the movement of air, a properly placed screen may correct the condition by altering the flow of air.

What are some adaptations to slowly developing hypoxia?

When hypoxia develops slowly, the organism makes certain adaptations that enables it to survive, grow, and be productive. These adaptations have been studied in relation to acclimatization to high altitudes. As indicated earlier, atmospheric pressure decreases as altitude increases, with the result that the partial pressure of oxygen and other gases in the air also falls. At an altitude somewhere between 9,000 and 10,000 ft. most persons who are not acclimatized begin to show signs and symptoms of mountain sickness. Much higher altitudes can be tolerated by those who are adapted to high altitudes than by those who are not. Individuals differ in their susceptibility to mountain sickness so that signs and symptoms develop at a lower level for some than for others. Physical exercise or any other condition increasing oxygen requirements lowers the level at which signs and symptoms are manifested. Visitors to high mountains are advised to delay active sightseeing for a day or so, in order to avoid mountain sickness. Even then acclimatization will not be complete, as this may take days or weeks.

Signs and symptoms of mountain sickness are the result of oxygen want. Lack of oxygen to the centers in the brain leads to loss of memory, errors in judgment, headache, and dizziness. Nausea and vomiting occur as the oxygen tension falls. These, as well as other previously listed manifestations of oxygen deprivation, can be prevented by supplying oxygen under pressure. Within limits, and given time, man can adapt to altitudes of 10,000 ft. and higher.

Individuals who are born in, or have lived at, high altitudes for an extended period of time have made physiological adaptations which enable them to be more active than those not acclimatized. For example, there is an increase in their erythrocyte count and hemoglobin. Rises in the levels of hemoglobin and erythrocyte counts that occur soon after entering a region of high altitude are probably due to the contraction of the spleen. Elevation of the reticulocyte count indicates that the activity of the blood-producing elements in the bone marrow is stimulated, directly or indirectly, by the low oxygen tension in the blood. Persons living at high altitudes normally have higher hemoglobin levels than those living at sea level.

In addition to the increase in capacity of the blood to carry oxygen, changes in the composition of the alveolar gases and in the shape of the chest facilitate adaptation. According to Houssay,[7] partial pressure of carbon dioxide in the alveoli falls at high altitudes. This permits an increase in the alveolar oxygen tension and partly compensates for the low tension of oxygen in the atmosphere.

In individuals whose ancestors have lived at high altitudes for several generations, there is some evidence that the shape of the chest changes. For example, Indians living on the high plateaus of Peru have large chests in which the anterior-posterior diameter is greater than it is in persons living at lower levels. The visitor to this area cannot escape being impressed with two things. One is his own feeling of being short of breath with physical exertion; the other is the ease with which the natives perform heavy physical work.

How do structural facilities function in ventilation, or breathing?

As stated earlier, the first phase of respiration is ventilation, or breathing. During ventilation, air containing about 20 per cent oxygen is taken from the

[7] *Ibid.*, p. 292.

atmosphere, cleansed, warmed, humidified, and delivered to the alveoli, where it is exchanged for air containing a high concentration of carbon dioxide, some oxygen, and some water which is returned to the atmosphere. This cycle takes place some 14 to 18 times a minute throughout the lifetime of the individual. As with other vital functions, the rate varies with age, exercise, and other factors. Ventilation is the means by which air in the alveoli is renewed regularly making a constant supply of oxygen available and protecting the blood and cells from an undue accumulation of carbon dioxide and from contaminants in the external environment.

To achieve this regular interchange of air in the alveoli, structures are required to do the following:

1. Cleanse, warm, and moisten the air.
2. Provide a passageway for the air, that is, an airway.
3. Move the air through the airway and into and out of the alveoli.

There are many factors in illness and its treatment that decrease the efficiency of mechanisms utilized by the healthy individual to protect ventilation. Bed rest decreases ventilatory capacity. Narcotics, analgesics, and general anesthetics depress the mechanisms by which the patency of the tracheobronchial tree is maintained. They are also depressed in the unconscious state, whatever its cause. Most patients for whom bed rest is prescribed as part of therapy require some attention to ventilation. Although problems related to maintaining or re-establishing the patency of the airway are more frequent,

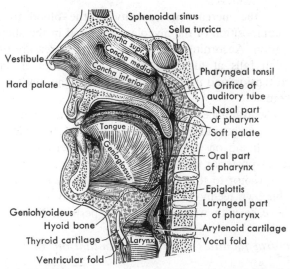

FIGURE 7—1. Sagittal section of the nose, mouth, pharynx, and larynx. (After Gray's *Anatomy*) (Adapted with permission of The Macmillan Company from *Anatomy and Physiology*, 14th ed., Fig. 292, p. 439, by Diana Clifford Kimber, Carolyn E. Gray, Caroline E. Stackpole, and Lutie C. Leavell. Copyright © The Macmillan Company 1961.)

disturbances in the mechanisms whereby air is moved into and out of the lung are not rare.

An understanding of the mechanisms that serve to protect the patency of the airway in health is necessary to the anticipation of conditions that are likely to threaten or disrupt them. It should also provide a basis for care directed toward the support or replacement of inefficient mechanisms until such time as the patient recovers sufficiently to meet his own need for oxygen.

The structures that form the airway can be seen in Figures 7-1 and 7-2. They are arbitrarily divided into the upper and lower respiratory tract. The upper division includes the larynx and the parts above it. The structures below the larynx form the lower respiratory tract. There is no barrier between the two divisions. Ventilation of the alveoli depends on all these structures being patent or unobstructed. The lower airway can be obstructed from within by foreign bodies, fluid, pus, or a tumor. It can be obstructed from within the wall of the airway by swelling, paralysis, or spasm of the vocal cords, and from the outside by hemorrhage, edema, or abscess.

The respiratory tract serves not only as a passageway for air but to condition it, so that the internal environment is protected from too rapid change in its constituents and from potentially harmful agents. The structure of the airway favors both these purposes. Figure 7-1 shows that the passageway is somewhat tortuous. Changes in the direction of the airway contribute to the cleansing of the air. As the air comes in contact with an obstruction, the

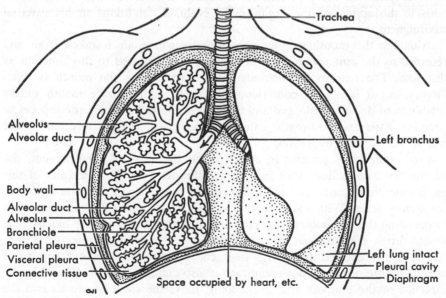

FIGURE 7—2. Lower respiratory tract, showing the lungs, with the right lung cut open to show the internal structure. (Adapted with permission of The Macmillan Company from College Zoology, 7th ed., Fig. 389, p. 537, by Robert W. Hegner and Karl A. Stiles. Copyright © The Macmillan Company 1959.)

direction of its flow is changed. Since the weight of air is less than that of particulate matter, its flow is impeded less than that of the heavier bodies. With deceleration, energy keeping the particles suspended is lost and the particles fall out of the moving stream of air. As a result, dusts and other contaminants in the air are caught by the sticky surface with which they come in contact. The structure of the nose and glottis is particularly adapted to cleansing the air. In both, air passes through a narrow passageway and the direction of its flow is deflected somewhat. Hair in the anterior nares is helpful in removing particulate matter. The most important factor in the cleansing of the air by the nose is what Guyton calls turbulent precipitation.[8] As the air passes through the nares it comes in contact with and is deflected by the turbinates and the septum. As indicated above, the movement of larger particles is slowed more than that of the air, and they are caught by the sticky mucous membranes.

The nose also contributes to the warming of the air. The mucous membrane covering the middle and inferior turbinates is richly supplied with blood vessels that dilate and increase the surface for warming the air. Some physicians discourage sleeping in a room with excessively low temperatures as this favors chronic engorgement of the nasal mucosa and predisposes to respiratory infections. Swelling of this tissue is responsible for obstruction of the nares in rhinitis. Irritation of the nasal mucosa initiates the reflex for sneezing and forcefully clears the nostrils of irritating materials. The mucosa lining the nares contains the receptor cells for the sense of smell and, as such, further adds to the ability of the organism to evaluate conditions in his external environment.

Although the mouth can serve as the site where air is taken from and returned to the atmosphere, it is not nearly as well suited to this function as the nose. The reasons are obvious. As a passageway, the mouth is satisfactory, but it is a poor conditioner of air. In addition, the mouth suffers readily from drying. Prolonged and unrelieved mouth breathing predisposes to parotitis. Patients who breathe entirely through their mouths lose pure water and are subject to dehydration.

Like other body cavities in contact with the external environment, the respiratory tract is lined with mucous membrane. Two characteristics of this membrane are of particular importance in the protection of the patency of the respiratory tract. With the exception of the vocal cords, the mucous membrane lining the respiratory tract contains goblet cells that secrete mucus. The mucus forms a continuous sheet throughout the respiratory tract. It is constantly being renewed and serves to catch any particulate matter coming in contact with it. The mucous membrane is also ciliated. The cilia sweep in the direction of the pharynx and, in so doing, move the sheet of mucus into the pharynx, where it is swallowed or expectorated. This is true in the nares as well as in lower structures. The mucous membrane of the nose and pharynx

[8] Arthur C. Guyton, *Textbook of Medical Physiology,* 2nd ed., W. B. Saunders Company, Philadelphia, 1961, p. 521.

may secrete as much as a quart of mucus a day. This accounts for much of the postnasal drip experienced by people who live in cold climates. In cold climates and in areas where the air is filled with soot or dust, secretion is likely to be increased. As long as the mucus is clear, the condition is probably physiological.

Removal of mucus from the tracheobronchial tree is facilitated by the changes in the diameter of the bronchi and their branches during inspiration and expiration. During inspiration, respiratory tubes lengthen and their diameter is decreased. There is some evidence that there are peristalticlike movements of the muscles in the bronchial tubes. The over-all direction of movement is toward the pharynx.

One of the most important mechanisms for the maintenance of the patency of the tracheobronchial tree is the cough reflex. Afferent nerve endings in the larynx, trachea, and bronchi are highly sensitive to irritants. Afferent impulses pass from these nerve endings by way of the vagus nerve to the medulla. Cough results from an integrated set of activities. These actions include: (1) the inspiration of a moderate amount of air; (2) closure of the glottis; and (3) the forceful expiration of air against the closed glottis. Forceful expiration which produces the cough is accomplished by contracting the abdominal muscles and pushing against the diaphragm and other expiratory muscles so that they contract forcefully. The cough occurs when the glottis opens and the air that has been confined under pressure is expelled explosively carrying with it mucus or other materials. Although the cough is generally beneficial, there are times when it may not be. A patient may be exhausted by a dry, nonproductive cough that continues over a period of time. Cough has also been implicated in the spread of infection throughout the lung. When coughing is an essential part of the patient's treatment, he should be instructed and helped to cough effectively.

In illness or as a result of some overwhelming condition in the external environment, the capacity of the natural mechanisms to maintain the patency of the airway may be threatened or disrupted. Some of the conditions under which this is most likely to occur have already been indicated. They include bed rest, drugs depressing to respiration, and unconsciousness. In general, conditions that predispose to obstruction of the tracheobronchial tree do so by inactivating or making ineffective one or more of the mechanisms by which it is cleansed, or by increasing the quantity of mucus or increasing its tenacity so that it is difficult to remove. Often a combination of factors contribute to the problem. To illustrate, Mrs. Fair, aged 45, underwent a cholecystectomy. In preparation for the operation she was given morphine sulfate, 10 mg (grains 1/6), and atropine sulfate, 0.4 mg (grains 1/150). The expected physiological responses to these drugs are:

1. Depression of the respiratory center by the morphine, which results in lessened respiratory excursion and may decrease the rate of respiration. Ventilation is, however, decreased without a decrease in rate.

2. Depression of the secretions of the glands in the respiratory tract due to the anticholinergic effects of atropine. This results in the formation of thick, tenacious mucus.

Both morphine and the anesthetic that Mrs. Fair received depress the action of cilia. Mrs. Fair's incision was high on the abdominal wall. To prevent pain, the area around the incision was splinted, and this resulted in shallow respirations. All these factors predispose to obstruction of the tracheobronchial tree and to the effects and complications discussed below.

Obstruction of a duct or tube leading to, or draining, an organ has three effects; *stasis* of secretions behind the obstruction, which predisposes *to infection* and *loss of function* of the part or organ. Which of these predominates depends on the organ and the extent of the obstruction. If the trachea is obstructed, air cannot reach the alveoli and asphyxia occurs rapidly. If, on the other hand, a main bronchus or one or more of its branches are obstructed, then the air is absorbed into the circulation from the affected lung or the portion of the lung that is collapsed. The condition resulting from the collapse of a lung or a portion thereof is known as atelectasis. Bacteria present in the area multiply and the patient develops pneumonia. Atelectasis is a possibility in any seriously ill patient including the one who is newly operated. Fever to 104° F. or higher with a corresponding increase in pulse and respiration in a patient who has recently experienced a general anesthetic or major surgery suggests the possibility of atelectasis. In addition, the patient usually has a productive cough with thick, tenacious sputum. Dyspnea and cyanosis are prominent when a large area of lung has collapsed. In order to prevent atelectasis, Mrs. Fair was moved from one side to the other and encouraged to deep-breathe and to cough every two hours. Despite preoperative instruction Mrs. Fair required considerable encouragement to cough effectively. In order to lessen the pain of coughing, the nurse supported Mrs. Fair's incision. As soon as she was able Mrs. Fair was taught to support her incision by placing her hands and arms across her upper abdomen for herself. Since standing and walking increase the depth of respiration and encourage productive coughing, Mrs. Fair was ambulated as soon as her surgeon prescribed it. The evening of the day she was operated on, she sat up with her feet hanging over the edge of the bed. The next day she was up and walking. Surgeons vary in the exact time they prescribe ambulation following various surgical procedures. There is seldom any delay, however, in mobilizing the patient in bed. One of the important aspects in nursing all patients who are confined to bed is attention to maintaining a clear airway.

In the preoperative period Mrs. Fair was instructed in how to deep-breathe and cough and why these were important to her convalescence. Instructions included explanation, diagrams, demonstrations, and supervised practice. Content selected to teach Mrs. Fair to cough was based on knowledge of coughing as an automatic act, which was previously described.

In addition to the mechanisms for clearing the tracheobronchial tree, the elasticity of the lung is a factor in the removal of secretions, particularly at the periphery. Any condition that is accompanied by a loss of elastic tissue favors the accumulation of secretions in the lung proper.

Despite the number and effectiveness of the mechanisms utilized to protect the alveoli from substances contaminating the air, particles less than 10 μ in diameter do pass through and line the alveolar walls. Ridding the alveoli of particulate matter depends on the action of phagocytes. To be effective, phagocytosis must be accomplished quickly.

To this point the discussion has centered on the protection of the alveoli from contaminants in the inspired air. They are also protected from foods and fluids that are ingested. They are protected despite the fact that the pharynx provides a common opening into both the esophagus and the larynx. In the healthy person, and barring some accident, inspiration and swallowing are so regulated and integrated that neither is air swallowed nor is food or fluid inhaled. Both breathing and swallowing are under the control of the nervous system. As food enters the pharynx, receptors are stimulated and impulses are transmitted to the medulla and lower pons. Centers in the brain stem initiate a series of automatic actions which progress in an orderly sequence with the result that one swallow differs very little from another. During swallowing the respiratory center is briefly inhibited so that swallowing may progress. The vocal folds are approximated so that the aperture in the larynx (glottis) is closed. The larynx is moved forward and the tongue moves back so that the epiglottis shields the glottis and food enters the esophagus rather than the larynx.

Injury to, or pressure on, the medulla, the pons, or the cranial nerves, 5 through 12, may disrupt the swallowing reflex and predispose to the aspiration of food or fluids into the tracheobronchial tree unless appropriate measures are taken. The aspiration of a large volume of fluid causes death by drowning. Lesser amounts may block a small unit in the lung and act as a focus for infection or aspiration pneumonia. Aspiration pneumonia is also a possibility when a patient is forced to ingest food or medications, and he resists by struggling. Under these circumstances the swallowing reflex may be inhibited and the material may be aspirated into the larynx rather than the esophagus.

Prevention of suffocation by aspiration of fluid or food by the patient who has partial or complete disruption in his swallowing reflex may be difficult. The patient who chokes when he is given food or fluids should be suspected of having difficulty in swallowing. If, when he attempts to swallow, fluids come back through his nose, he is having a problem and fluids should be discontinued until the swallowing reflex is re-established. Whenever there is any doubt about the ability of a patient to swallow, the physician should be notified promptly. When a patient has a problem with swallowing he should be placed in a position that favors fluid entering the esophagus or draining from the mouth. The back lying position, particularly when the head falls back, should be avoided. Depending on the extent of the difficulty the patient has with swallowing and other factors, he may be placed in a position with his head elevated and turned to one side; he may be horizontal, but lying on one side; he may be lying on his side with his head lower than the rest of his body; or he may be placed in a prone position with his head lower than his trunk and his head turned to the side. When secretions are abundant, regular suctioning of the mouth and pharynx may be necessary.

Obstruction to the flow of air may occur at any level of the respiratory tract. The consequences depend on the degree of obstruction and whether or not there is an alternate route through which air can pass. The causes of obstruction vary somewhat at different levels of the airway. For. example, obstruction of the nares does not interfere with the flow of air, because there is an alternate pathway, the mouth. It does lessen the extent to which the air is properly conditioned. Because of the richness of the blood supply of the middle and inferior turbinates and the narrowness of the passageway, vascular congestion quickly causes interference with breathing. Inflammations caused by viral and bacterial infections and allergic responses of the mucous membranes are always accompanied by vascular congestion. Congestion is sometimes aggravated by the overuse of nose drops containing a drug acting as a vasoconstrictor when it is applied locally. Constriction is followed by overdilatation and passive congestion of the nasal mucosa. Patients using drugs such as Neo-synephrine Hydrochloride[9] should be cautioned against their overuse, as it is likely to lead to a rebound congestion that is more severe than the original condition. The nares may also be obstructed by polyps or foreign bodies. Polyps are frequently associated with allergic rhinitis. The latter are more likely to be a problem in young children who introduce small objects such as peas, beans, or buttons into one or both nares.

Strictures or lesions in the pharynx most frequently obstruct the airway by blocking the glottis. One of the causes of death in diphtheria is obstruction of the airway by a pseudomembrane formed in the pharynx and/or larynx. Obstruction of the glottis is an ever-present danger to the unconscious patient whose reflexes are depressed and whose musculature is relaxed. If he is placed in bed on his back, there is danger that the base of his tongue and the other structures in his pharynx will sag against the glottis and block the opening. This can be prevented by a properly placed airway and/or by placing the unconscious patient on his side and maintaining him in this position until his reflexes and muscle tone have been restored. This simple precaution would have saved the life of Charles Brown, a healthy young man of 22. He had been given Pentothal Sodium[10] in preparation for a circumcision. After this minor procedure, he was returned to his room in an unconscious state. He was placed in bed on his back. Twenty minutes later, he was found dead from

---

[9] Trade name for phenylephrine hydrochloride, U.S.P.
[10] Trade name for thiopental sodium.

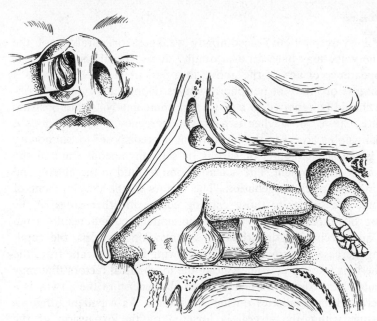

FIGURE 7–3. Nasal polyps, which obstruct the nasal passage. Shows the appearance of thce polyps when seen from the anterior view of the nose with retractors. (Adapted from "Anatomy of the Nose and Sinuses in Health and Diseases." Courtesy of *Pfizer Spectrum.*)

suffocation. The contents of his pharynx had obstructed his glottis. Any space-occupying mass in the pharynx may obstruct the glottis.

The glottis is the narrowest passageway in the upper airway. As such, it offers some resistance to the flow of air during inspiration. As indicated earlier, the sudden slowing of the flow of air contributes to the removal of particles by creating turbulence. The glottis offers even more resistance to the flow of air during expiration than it does during inspiration. The resulting turbulence is an important factor in the mixing of air in the respiratory tract and alveoli.

What are some of the causes of obstruction of the glottis?

There are a variety of sources of obstruction of the glottis. Some are extrinsic while others are intrinsic to the larynx. Any space-occupying mass in the neck or involving the vocal folds or other parts of the larynx may block the glottis. Neoplasms or hemorrhage into the neck usually does this by interrupting the passage of impulses over the recurrent laryngeal nerves. Passage of nerve impulses may be interrupted by injury to or severing of the recurrent laryngeal nerves during operation on the neck, such as thyroidectomy. The recurrent laryngeal nerves are motor to all of the muscles of the larynx except the cricothyroid. Severance of one nerve causes a paralysis of the vocal cords on one side with the result that the voice becomes bitonal. Disruption of both nerves results in suppression of phonation as well as causing serious disturbances in respiration. Hoarseness and respiratory stridor

397

(high-pitched, noisy respirations) accompany weakness or paralysis of the · vocal cords. The voice may have a nasal quality due to paralysis of the soft palate. The appearance of any of the above in a patient in whom there is a possibility of disease or injury of peripheral nerves or medullary centers controlling speech should be reported to a physician immediately. Acute obstruction of the glottis, larynx, or trachea is a grave emergency. Not only does it prevent air from gaining access to the alveoli, but it predisposes to pulmonary edema, which is the accumulation of serous or serosanguineous fluid in the alveoli, bronchioles, and bronchi. The accumulation of fluid in the alveoli and air passages further impairs oxygenation. The factors in the development of pulmonary edema are similar to those causing edema in other areas of the body. Following obstruction of the airway, pulmonary edema results from both chemical and mechanical disturbances. As hypoxia develops, the capillaries in the lung increase in permeability thus allowing fluid to escape from the capillaries in the lung into the alveoli. Among the mechanical factors that may contribute to pulmonary edema following severe obstruction of the airway is a suction effect created on capillaries during inspiration. As a patient attempts to inhale, pressure within the alveoli is lowered by the expansion of the thoracic cavity. When the airway is patent, air flows into the alveoli, thus maintaining pressure relationships between the alveoli and capillaries. When inspiration is blocked to a greater extent than expiration, pressure is lowered in the alveoli during inspiration and fluid exudes from the capillary to the alveoli. The situation may be further aggravated by interference with the outflow of blood from the left ventricle. Since blood flow to the right heart increases during inspiration, failure of the left ventricle to move blood into the circulation at as rapid a rate as it is presented to it results in a progressive accumulation of blood in the lungs. Pulmonary edema, whatever the cause or causes, is always a dangerous complication. A tracheotomy tray should be in readiness so that no time will be lost if a tracheostomy becomes necessary. Food and fluids should be withheld until the ability of the patient to swallow has been appraised.

When afferent fibers supplying the larynx are sectioned or there is a disturbance in their ability to transmit impulses, the larynx is insensitive to irritating particles that adhere to it. One unfortunate effect is the failure to initiate the cough reflex automatically when irritating materials come into contact with the larynx.

Occasionally the nurse cares for a patient who has a weakness or paralysis of one vocal cord that was caused by disease or injury to the centers in the brain that integrate breathing and swallowing. One such patient was Mrs. Oakson, who had been admitted to the hospital for a mitral commissurotomy —a procedure by which a narrowed mitral valve is enlarged. Some months earlier, she had a cerebrovascular accident which was believed to have been caused by an embolus, which originated from a thrombus in her left atria. According to Mrs. Oakson, despite good recovery her voice continued to be hoarse and nasal in quality. In addition, she noticed that she could not cough effectively. She was unable to close her glottis tightly and build up pressure behind it. She was therefore deprived of one of the most effective mechanisms for cleansing the tracheobronchial tree. After the mitral commissurotomy was performed, and despite real effort on her part, she was unable to clear her tracheobronchial tree of secretions. Bronchoscopy was required in order to remove secretions and to prevent atelectasis.

Tumors or edema of the vocal cords block the glottis. Hoarseness is common in both conditions. When a tumor is involved, the hoarseness is likely to be intermittent. With edema, hoarseness is likely to be progressive and, if the edema is marked, to be associated with respiratory obstruction.

What are some of the factors influencing the effect of obstruction of the bronchi?

The larynx narrows to form the trachea, which branches into the two bronchi. Each bronchus forms a series of branching tubes that finally terminate in the alveoli. Collectively these tubular structures form the airway. They may be obstructed at any level by accumulated secretions, blood, foreign bodies, or fluid. The effects of obstruction will depend on the nature of the obstructing agent, the level at which blocking occurs, and whether it is partial or complete. Obstruction of the trachea or larynx promptly causes asphyxia. Obstruction of a bronchus or one of its branches, when partial, may trap air in the lung and interfere with the drainage of secretions. When it is complete, the lung collapses as the air is absorbed. The major danger of a small airless region is that it is predisposed to infection because drainage is blocked. The consequences of a collapse of an entire lung are immediate, because the pressure relationships among the various structures in the thoracic cavity are disrupted. When a lung collapses because air cannot enter, the contents of the thoracic cavity may shift toward the side of decreased pressure (mediastinal shift) and the flow of air into the other lung is impaired. Furthermore the venous return to the heart is impaired by the alterations in pressure within the thoracic cavity. Prompt action to remove the obstructing body is imperative.

How do the structures of the various parts of the airway differ?

The walls of the larynx, trachea, bronchi, and its larger branches are strengthened with cartilage. In the trachea and bronchial tubes the rings of cartilage are incomplete dorsally, which permits some alteration in their size and shape during the various phases of breathing. At the point where the tubes are 1 mm or less in diameter, the cartilage disappears. These small tubes without cartilage in the walls are the bronchioles. As the cartilage decreases in the tubes, the smooth muscle and elastic tissue increases.

The smooth muscle in the tracheobronchial tree is innervated by the autonomic nervous system. Increased activity of the parasympathetic nervous system causes the muscles of the bronchioles to contract. With contraction, the bronchioles shorten and narrow. The sympathoadrenal system has the opposite effect. It causes the bronchioles to dilate and lengthen. The capacity to regulate the diameter of the bronchioles is a factor in regulation of the flow of air to the alveoli.

Constriction of the bronchioles, when appropriate in degree, is part of the system for the protection of the alveoli from noxious agents. For example, smoke reaching the bronchioles stimulates them to contract, thus limiting the quantity of smoke reaching the alveoli. When the response of the broncheolar musculature is appropriate to the stimulus, and appropriate in degree, it protects the alveoli from harmful contaminants in the air.

In contrast, when the bronchiolar musculature is hyperreactive, it may be the source of pathology. When, for example, hyperresponsive muscle contracts in response to inappropriate stimuli, its degree of contraction is too great, and/or the contraction is sustained for too long a period of time, there is likely to be some interference with ventilation. For example, in asthma and asthmalike diseases obstruction of the bronchioles interferes with ventilation. One of the factors in their obstruction is smooth-muscle spasm. Other elements increasing resistance to the flow of air in these disorders are edema of the mucosa due to increased capillary permeability and an increase in the secretion of mucus. All the above are in response to the release of serotonin and histamine by the injured cells. Since they interfere with expiration to a greater extent than with inspiration, air is trapped in the lungs and they are maintained in an inflated state. Irritation by highly irritating substances such as smoke provokes a similar type of inflammatory reaction.

The respiratory tract serves not only to deliver air to the respiratory alveoli, but to condition it so that it is protected from drying and other noxious conditions. Air, as it enters the airway, may be relatively clean or it may be laden with dust or microorganisms, or both. Despite the efficiency of the mechanisms for cleansing the air, particles may get beyond the glottis. When they are very small, they may even reach the alveoli. Thus bacteria or viruses may gain entrance to the body through the respiratory tract where they may set up an infectious process or gain entrance to the internal environment. The respiratory tract serves as the portal of entry for a large number of microorganisms. Microorganisms also escape into the atmosphere in discharge from the respiratory tract. Elements to be considered in the control of respiratory infections are treated in Chapter 4. The point should be made here, however, that appropriate measures should be utilized by the nurse to protect herself and others from respiratory discharges. The simplest measure is always to turn your head when someone coughs. Never allow anyone to cough in your face. Adequate ventilation so that fresh air dilutes the ward air is also helpful. Acute infections of the respiratory tract are by far the most frequent cause of acute disabling illness lasting only a few days.

Many of the manifestations resulting from the exposure of the respiratory tract to noxious agents are due to hyper- or hypoactivity of a protective mechanism. For example, the mucosa responds to irritation by an increase in the secretion of mucus. This reaction is beneficial inasmuch as it serves to dilute the irritant and to remove it from the body. It may, however, cause harm when the character or quantity of mucus is such that the mechanisms for its removal are overwhelmed. As mucus collects in the tubes forming the airway or in ducts draining into it, water is absorbed from the mucus and it becomes more difficult to remove. Unless drainage is maintained, a mucus plug obstructs the tube. With obstruction of the tube, the improperly drained area is liable to infection, and among other effects, the character of the drainage is altered. In infectious diseases of the lung, such as pneumonia, the exudate formed in the alveoli is discharged into the airway. Blood in the sputum, hemoptysis, results from bleeding into the alveoli or from the mucosa of the airway. The character of the discharge from the respiratory tract provides significant clues as to the nature of a patient's illness. Its color, odor, consistency, and amount should be observed and recorded.

Cough, as emphasized earlier, is a valuable mechanism for cleansing the lower respiratory tract. In disorders in which there is continued irritation of the larynx, trachea, and bronchi, its frequency is increased so that the person becomes aware that he is coughing. Like other symptoms, the circumstances under which the cough occurs modifies the importance the individual attaches to it. For example, many people who smoke dismiss a chronic cough as due to smoking. In contrast, most people perceive themselves to be ill when they have a cough which raises blood or purulent sputum, or when the cough is accompanied by evidence of an acute respiratory infection. Some of the observations that should be made about cough include the circumstances that attend its occurrence, its timing, whether or not it is productive, and its sound, that is, either wet or dry.

Other observations that provide information about the airway include the presence or absence of noticeable sound during breathing, changes in the voice, and laryngeal stridor. As air passes through fluids accumulated in the tracheobronchial tree, breath sounds are altered. They may or may not be audible to the ordinary listener. When they are heard on ausculation of the chest, they are known as râles. Air passing through fluid in the tracheobronchial tree produces what is known as a moist râle. Râles can sometimes be felt through the chest wall. The usual method of detecting râles is by listening through a stethoscope placed on the chest wall. Changes in the voice such as a nasal quality or hoarseness have been previously discussed. Since the character of the voice differs in healthy people, an observer who has not known a patient previously may have to depend on the judgment of the patient or a member of his family that his voice is or is not normal. Laryngeal stridor is always abnormal because it results from laryngeal spasm. It is characterized by a crowing or high-pitched sound on inspiration. The sound is sometimes compared to the blowing of the wind. Laryngeal stridor is usually accompanied by cyanosis. The most common condition in which laryngeal stridor occurs is croup in children, but it may also occur in tetany.

When an obstruction of the part of the airway for which there is no alternate route occurs suddenly, as in drowning or the blocking of the trachea or glottis by a foreign body, asphyxia develops in a matter of minutes. When it develops more slowly, as in an acute infectious process, signs and symptoms of oxygen want develop over a period of time. The urgency of the situation depends on the extent to which the patient is able to meet his own needs for oxygen. Accumulated secretions or any foreign body, whatever its size or source, must be removed. Even when they do not seriously interfere with ventilation, they block the ducts distal to the obstruction and predispose to infection. The usual method by which foreign bodies or secretions are extracted from the tracheobronchial tree is by bronchoscopy accompanied by bronchial aspiration.

*What is a bronchoscopy? What are the requirements of the
patient undergoing this procedure?*

Bronchoscopy is a procedure in which a flexible lighted tube is introduced into the trachea by way of the mouth, pharynx, glottis, and larynx. Like other scopes used in medicine, the bronchoscope contains a series of mirrors which are so located in the tube that the interior of the tracheobronchial tree can be directly visualized. The bronchoscope is used in diagnosis as well as in treatment. In diagnosis, the bronchoscope is useful in the examination of the larynx, trachea, and bronchi. Secretions and/or cells may be removed for study. In therapy it is used to remove foreign bodies, excessive secretions, or those that the patient cannot expel by his own efforts.

Bronchoscopy may therefore be performed as an emergency procedure or after a period of preparation. When relief of an acute obstruction is required to save the life of the individual, preparation is limited to the bare essentials. When bronchoscopy is planned for, the patient should be prepared for what to expect and for what will be expected of him. He should have answers to his questions. Bronchoscopy is not a pleasant procedure nor is it without danger. The patient may fear the implications of the procedure to diagnosis, most particularly to a diagnosis of cancer. Questions by the patient about the dangers of bronchoscopy or the possibility of cancer should be referred to the physician. Recognition by the nurse of the fact that the patient is worried may in itself be helpful. The patient should know that he will receive a medication, such as codeine and phenobarbital, which will help him to relax and to be less aware of his surroundings. The barbiturate also decreases the danger of a toxic reaction to the local anesthetic, as the barbiturates are antidotes to certain types of reaction to cocaine and its relatives. To lessen the concentration of bacteria in the mouth, special attention should be given to the care of the mouth the evening preceding and the morning of the day of bonchoscopy.

Removable bridges and dentures should, of course, be removed in preparation for the procedure.

In order to facilitate the passage of the bronchoscope, the patient is positioned so that the pharynx is brought into line with the glottis and trachea. A small, hard pillow is placed under the shoulders of the patient and the head is allowed to drop back. The eyes of the patient are covered with a folded towel, so that he will not have to watch the proceedings.

Before the bronchoscope is passed, the physician anesthetizes the pharynx and larynx with cocaine or one of its relatives. Since a topical anesthetic depresses the swallowing reflex, food and fluids are withheld for about eight hours before bronchoscopy is performed and for two or three hours after it is completed. It usually takes about this long for the swallowing reflex to return. When the patient is able to swallow his own saliva, he can safely be given fluids. Until the patient can swallow saliva, he should be encouraged to lie on his side and let it drain into an emesis basin.

During the performance of bronchoscopy, the nurse assists the physician as needed. She also directs her attention to the patient. Unless the physician acquaints the patient with the progress of the procedure, the nurse should do so. Mr. Roberts stated at the completion of bronchoscopy that he did not think he could have tolerated it if the nurse had not kept him informed about the progress of the procedure from start to finish.

Following bronchoscopy, the patient should be observed for indications that the swallowing reflex is re-established and for signs and symptoms signifying that cocaine has been absorbed. Cocaine stimulates the nervous system from above downward. Signs and symptoms that are associated with a moderate degree of absorption include an increase in the strength and rate of the pulse, elevation in blood pressure, increase in rate and depth of respirations, and increase in mental activities. The patient is active, talkative, and euphoric; that is, he has an exaggerated and often unrealistic sense of well-being. If the amount of drug absorbed is excessive, overstimulation is followed by depression of the nervous system, beginning with the higher centers and proceeding downward. Should symptoms of overactivity develop, the nurse should promptly administer a rapidly acting barbiturate, such as Seconal Sodium,[11] intramuscularly. In an extreme emergency the drug must be given intravenously by the physician. If there is no order, the nurse should obtain one promptly. The patient will also probably need some type of artificial respiration. Time is limited; unless prompt and appropriate action is taken, the patient dies from respiratory failure.

Although infrequent in occurrence, the trachea or a bronchus may be perforated during bronchoscopy. When this happens air and secretions escape into the mediastinum. Signs and symptoms depend on the size of the tear. They include minor to marked dyspnea, crepitus (crackling on pressure or

---

[11] Trade name for secobarbital sodium.

palpation) of tissues, and a puffing of the face and neck. The latter two are referred to as subcutaneous emphysema and are due to air escaping from the lung into the tissue. Any of the above signs or symptoms occurring should be reported promptly as this is a serious complication.

Another serious though infrequent complication is severe laryngeal edema. This blocks the airway and leads to respiratory embarrassment. The patient should always be observed for difficulty in breathing. Should it occur, the physician should be promptly notified. Preparation should be made for a tracheotomy should one be required.

Following bronchoscopy, the patient is likely to have a sore throat and to be hoarse. Administration of warm or cold liquid by mouth may lessen the degree of soreness. Some physicians prescribe warm saline gargles. As long as hoarseness continues, talking and smoking should be discouraged as they increase the irritation of the larynx. The patient may be given a pad of paper or a slate and pencil on which to write. The call light or bell should be within easy reach, and the patient should be instructed to call for the nurse when he needs her. The nurse should try to look in on the patient from time to time, and the call light or bell should be answered promptly.

In chronic condititions such as bronchiectasis or emphysema, the mechanisms for cleaning the tracheobronchial tree may be ineffective. Collections of secretions may then be removed by postural drainage. In postural drainage the patient is placed in a position so that the region to be drained is higher than the ducts through which the fluid is to pass to the outlet. Application is made of the well-known fact that, as a result of gravity, water runs downhill. For the postural drainage to accomplish its purpose the area to be drained must be known and the patient must be placed in (or assume) the appropriate position. Usually the disorders in which secretions accumulate are accompanied by bronchiolar spasm and thickening of secretions. In preparation for postural drainage a bronchiolar-dilating drug such as Isuprel® and a medical detergent such as Alevaire[12] to liquefy secretions may be inhaled about 10 to 15 minutes before postural drainage is initiated. When inhaled, Alevaire liquefies secretions and thereby facilitates their removal. Both types of drugs are converted to a fine mist in a nebulizer and inhaled.

After suitable preparation, the patient assumes the appropriate position, which is determined by the area of the lung to be drained. In the past, postural drainage was utilized to drain the posterior and lower lobes of the lung. Recently its use has been much extended to all parts of the lung. To increase the effectiveness of postural drainage the patient is instructed to perform two other procedures. One is to cough, a series of little rapid-fire coughs similar to clearing of the throat. The other is to tap the chest with the fingers of both hands beginning with the bottom of the ribs and continuing to the collarbone and back again. A member of the family can be taught the

---

[12] Trade name for tylaxapol.

chest-tapping routine and tap the posterior wall of the chest when the patient is in the prone or sitting position. Coughing and the chest-tapping techniques aid in loosening secretions by vibration.[13]

When postural drainage is prescribed, the patient assumes the appropriate position or series of positions. Postural drainage is frequently prescribed to drain posterior portions of the lower lobes. There are several methods which can be used in order to have the chest lower than the rest of the body. One method is to assist the patient to lie face down and crosswise on the bed. He is then assisted so that he hangs over the side of the bed at a 45-degree angle. Only his legs and thighs rest on the bed. His head and trunk are over the side. His arms rest on a pillow or low footstool on the floor. A basin should be placed at the patient's head to catch the drainage. From the nature of the position, it is obvious that it is unsuitable for very sick patients. All patients should be given assistance in attaining the position until they are able to get into the proper position and can do so without excessive fear. Some patients refuse to do postural drainage, because they are fearful of falling. In the beginning, the time should be limited to three minutes or even less. As the patient gains strength and confidence, he will be able to remain in the position for 20 to 30 minutes. Another method is to raise the knee gatch of the patient's bed and have him lie with his head and chest lower than the rest of the body. This position is particularly advantageous for elderly or debilitated patients who cannot tolerate lying over the side of the bed.

In addition to the situations cited above, what are some other causes of failure to adequately ventilate the lungs?

As emphasized, one of the essential factors in the maintenance of a supply of oxygen is a clear airway. In health the mechanisms for keeping it patent and for warming, moistening, and cleansing the air are usually adequate. In illness, they often are not. Any patient who is treated by bed rest is predisposed to obstruction of the tracheobronchial tree, primarily because of a reduction in the expansion of the chest. Expansion is limited by the resistance offered to the chest wall by the bed and by the loss of muscle power accompanying any decrease in activity. Distention of the abdomen by either gas or fluid exerts pressure on the diaphragm and prevents its descent during inspiration. Diseases involving areas in the nervous system regulating respiration or the muscles of respiration are also accompanied by a loss of muscle power. Drugs that depress the central nervous system—sedatives, narcotics, and general anesthetics—interfere with normal cleansing mechanisms by depressing the respiratory and cough centers and by paralyzing the cilia in the trachea and bronchi. In the unconscious state secretions are increased and the mechanisms for their removal are inhibited. Pain associated with breathing, whether

[13] See Albert Haas, *Essentials of Living with Pulmonary Emphysema,* Patient Publication Number 4, The Institute of Physical Medicine and Rehabilitation, New York University Medical Center, 1963.

due to disease involving the pleura or to surgical procedures in which the route of approach is through the chest wall or the upper abdomen, is accompanied by a protective inhibition of breathing. This is why the judicious use of narcotics in such patients is necessary in order to improve respiratory excursions. By prevention and relief of pain the patient can be encouraged to voluntarily increase the depth of inspiration and to cough. Infections, chemical irritants such as smoke, and allergic responses such as in asthma may increase secretions to such an extent that the normal physiological mechanisms for their removal are inadequate. There may be, in addition, some reduction in the adequacy of one or more mechanisms themselves. For example, spasm of the muscles of the bronchioles narrows their lumen and therefore increases the resistance to the removal of the secretions. The glottis may be blocked by soft tissues or foreign bodies including food in the hypopharynx, paralysis of the vocal cords, neoplasms, and swelling of the area that surrounds it.

There are few areas where the nurse can do more to protect and to assist the patient. To accomplish either of these, patients who are likely to have some problem in maintaining a clean airway must be identified. This requires that the nurse know what patients can be anticipated to have difficulty and that she recognize signs and symptoms indicating that pathology is developing—such as cough, wet-sounding respirations, and pain on breathing. When the signs and symptoms indicate that the patient is receiving an inadequate supply of oxygen, obstruction is either acute or extensive or both.

Prevention is, naturally, the most desirable objective. In the care of the bedfast and sick individual attention to a regular schedule of turning the patient from side to side, deep breathing, and coughing will usually do much to protect him from obstruction by secretions. When the patient can be up and walking this is of further assistance. When the patient has pain on coughing, splinting the affected area of the chest by supporting it with the hands or a binder may enable the patient to cough more deeply. Although pain-relieving medications do have an adverse effect when they are overused, they may also be a help when given about 15 minutes before the patient coughs or deep-breathes.

A patient may require assistance in removing secretions from his airway when (1) one or more of the mechanisms for their removal is inactivated; or (2) the quantity or character of the secretions makes their removal difficult or impossible. Often both factors play a part. For example, when in disease or its treatment swallowing mechanisms are inactivated, saliva collects in the hypopharynx. The patient should be placed in a position in which gravity facilitates drainage. The side-lying, prone, and Trendelenburg positions all facilitate drainage by gravity. When the patient lies on his back, his head should be turned to the side and his jaw moved forward and up. When the swallowing reflex continues to be depressed and secretions are abundant, they may have to be removed by suctioning. For it to be really effective, secretions must be removed from the hypopharynx and suctioning must also be performed frequently enough to prevent a large collection of fluid from accumulating.

When secretions accumulate in the tracheobronchial tree and natural methods are not successful in removing them, a catheter may be used to irritate the nerve endings in the larynx and stimulate coughing. This procedure is usually performed by the physician, and should not be done by the nurse unless she has received specialized instructions. Neither should the nurse who has not been instructed introduce a catheter into the tracheobronchial tree by way of the glottis for purposes of aspirating secretions. Either procedure is accompanied by the possibility of inducing laryngeal spasm and, with it, obstruction of the airway. Unless laryngeal spasm is promptly relieved the patient will suffocate. The precautions to be observed will be discussed under those that should be taken when tracheostomy is suctioned.

When the measures just described are insufficient to protect the patency of the airway, a tracheostomy may be performed. Particularly in the days when diphtheria was common, a crude kind of tracheostomy was part of the folk medicine of certain groups.[14] In tracheostomy an opening is made in the trachea by way of the neck. In scientific medicine a vertical slit is made in the anterior portion of the neck and a double-cannula airway is introduced. The incision in the trachea is usually below the first or second tracheal cartilage. The outer cannula is held in place by ties around the neck of the patient and the inner cannula is locked into the outer cannula. At one time tracheostomy was performed almost entirely as an emergency measure to relieve obstructions of the airway located in the pharynx and larynx. It is now employed to prevent or relieve hypoxia due to the accumulation of secretions in the lower tracheobronchial tree and to lessen the work of breathing as well as to bypass the naso-oral passage or the larynx.

Tracheostomy is utilized to prevent or to relieve hypoxia due to the accumulation of secretions in the tracheobronchial tree in patients suffering a wide variety of disorders. Among these are the weak and feeble, the critically ill, and those whose brains are injured or diseased. Among the latter are persons who have suffered head injuries, bulbar poliomyelitis, cerebrovascular accidents, or overdosage of drugs that depress the respiratory and cough centers in the brain. In these and other similar conditions secretions are formed more rapidly than they can be removed by natural mechanisms. The imbalance between the formation and removal of secretions may be due to an actual increase in secretion, or to a depression or failure of the cleansing mechanisms, or to both factors. In any event, secretions remain to block the airway and to prevent the passage of air to and from the alveoli. In the lung this predisposes to tracheobronchitis, atelectasis, and bronchopneumonia. The general and more immediately serious effect of one or more of these disturb-

14 Harriette Arnow, *The Dollmaker,* The Macmillan Company, New York, 1954, pp. 10-17.

ances is hypoxia. Since hypoxia is due to failure of the service facility to present adequate amounts of oxygen to the blood, the condition resulting from airway obstruction is sometimes called anoxic anoxia. In patients who have suffered head injury or some other disorder involving the brain, hypoxia is particularly dangerous as it worsens cerebral edema. Furthermore, obstruction of the airway not only causes anoxia, but it interferes with the elimination of carbon dioxide and predisposes to respiratory acidosis (discussed in Chapter 8).

In weak and feeble patients a tracheostomy may be instituted to reduce the work of breathing. This is accomplished primarily by lessening the volume of the anatomical dead air space by as much as 60 per cent. The anatomical dead air space extends from the nose and nasopharynx to the level in the respiratory tree where exchanges of oxygen and carbon dioxide take place. It holds a volume of approximately 150 ml of air. Although the air in the dead air space does not participate directly in the exchange of gases, it performs a valuable function. It dilutes the air entering and leaving the lung and thereby protects the alveoli from sudden change. It does, however, add to the work of breathing. The reduction in volume of air that is secured by the tracheostomy is therefore of considerable value. In a patient with an unstable chest wall ("flail chest" due to multiple fractures of the ribs), tracheostomy may also improve ventilation by reducing the work of breathing.

Tracheostomy is also performed to relieve obstruction of the larynx and upper trachea of either extrinsic or intrinsic origin. Though some of these were indicated earlier, they will be summarized here. The soft tissues in the pharynx are a frequent and often preventable cause of obstruction of the glottis. Hemorrhage into the pharynx or the soft tissues of the neck may be responsible for obstruction of the airway. In the first instance blood is aspirated into the airway. In the second, pressure is exerted externally on the trachea. Hemorrhage into the soft tissues causing pressure on the trachea is most frequently a complication following thyroidectomy and radical neck resection. Either surgical procedure may be responsible for obstruction of the glottis by paralyzing the vocal cords. Trauma to or severing of both recurrent laryngeal nerves may also be responsible. Collapse of one vocal cord does not cause complete obstruction of the glottis. It does, however, increase resistance to the passage of air. Edema involving the tissues of the neck or the larynx may also obstruct breathing.

A neoplasm having its origin in tissues within or without the respiratory tract may cause obstruction. Tumors may be located in the larynx, bronchi or in the mediastinum.

A tracheostomy may be temporary or permanent. In adults the most frequent reason for establishing a permanent tracheostomy is to maintain an airway following the removal of the larynx in the treatment of cancer of the larynx. With the loss of the larynx, the person loses, forever, his ability to speak normally. In conversations with patients who have experienced laryngectomy or are about to do so, the most terrifying aspect is the loss of the ability ever to speak again.

The reasons for the performance of a tracheostomy are summarized as follows:

1. It lessens the tracheopharyngeal dead air space and thereby reduces the work of breathing.
2. It bypasses the naso-oral passage and the larynx, establishing a new airway.
3. It provides easy access to the tracheobronchial tree and makes it easier to remove secretions.[11]
4. It may also be utilized with one of the various mechanical types of respirators now on the market to provide partial or total respiratory assistance to the patient. Nurses who are going to work with any type of mechanical respirator should learn how to operate the apparatus before they attempt to take care of the patient. Unless this equipment is properly used, the respirator is of no advantage to the patient and may actually be harmful.

The plan for the preparation of the patient who is facing a tracheostomy will depend on many factors. When the patient is conscious and time permits, the patient should know why it is required and what to expect, as well as what is expected of him. As with other surgical procedures, the physician has the responsibility for informing the patient about the nature of the procedure to be performed and why it is necessary. Often when a laryngectomy is to be performed, a person who has recovered from the procedure and has mastered esophageal speech will be asked to visit the patient preoperatively. Most cities have clubs made up of laryngectomized individuals who donate their time to helping others faced with this type of surgery. Many persons who have had laryngectomy are able to return to their former positions, and some very prominent positions are held by people who have recovered from this type of surgery.

The nurse has multiple responsibilities. These responsibilities differ some-what in detail, but not in principle, from those involved in the care of the patient who has any operative procedure. These are discussed in some detail in Chapter 15.

In both preoperative preparation and postoperative care the nurse should take into account the reason why the tracheostomy is performed and the way in which the physiology of the patient is altered. As implied earlier, the patient is unable to speak. In the patient who has an associated laryngectomy, loss of natural speech is permanent. Esophageal speech can be and is learned by many individuals, but it takes a strong desire coupled with time and effort. Those who have a temporary tracheostomy can speak by placing their fingers

[11] "Emergency Tracheotomy," *Medical Times,* LXXXVI, December, 1958, p. 1587.

over the tracheostomy tube. Sometimes when the patient is being prepared for the removal of the tracheostomy tube, the tube will be plugged for short periods of time before it is permanently removed to test the ability of the patient to breathe normally. When the patient is critically ill or he has a problem maintaining ventilation, closure of the tracheostomy tube is not recommended. Inability to speak or to cry out adds to the emotional stress of the patient. He fears that he will not be able to get help when he needs it. Particularly when the patient has a permanent loss of voice, he is likely to grieve because he will never be able to speak again. As a result of the loss of his voice he may fear that he will not be able to carry on his work or, equally as important, that he will become unacceptable to his family, friends, or co-workers. For these and other reasons discussed below, for the first few days following tracheostomy someone ought to be with the patient continuously.

To illustrate some of the problems experienced by the patient who is to have a tracheostomy, Mr. Frederickson will be described. Mr. Frederickson, who was in the process of making a decision of whether to have a laryngectomy for the removal of a malignant neoplasm, was able to express to his nurse the inner turmoil he felt at having to make this decision. Mr. Frederickson was 60 years old. Although he was nearly illiterate, he had a remarkable knowledge of the Bible, which he quoted frequently. He worked with his brother, who was a minister, as a lay minister. His nurse was a sensitive and perceptive woman who spent an entire morning listening to Mr. Frederickson debate with himself whether or not he should keep his voice and continue to do God's work as long as he lived or give up his voice and his work so that he might continue to live. At the end of the morning he agreed to wait to make his decision until a visitor from the laryngectomy club came in the afternoon to talk to him. Mr. Frederickson finally decided to have the laryngectomy. The decision was truly his. Following laryngectomy, Mr. Frederickson made a good recovery. He planned to learn esophageal speech as soon as possible.

A second physiological change is that the patient has been deprived of his mechanisms for conditioning environmental air. The air enters the tracheobronchial tree without having been filtered, warmed, and moistened. Moreover, objects (catheters) are introduced into the respiratory tract. The two problems that are most difficult to cope with in the care of the airway are achievement of an adequate degree of humidity of the air and maintenance of cleanliness of catheters introduced into the tracheostomy tube. Lack of moisture in the inspired air has two adverse effects. It dries the delicate mucous membrane lining of the respiratory tract, and the secretions become thick and viscous. Drying predisposes to the formation of encrustations of the trachea, which may be large enough to obstruct the trachea and to increase the difficulty of removing secretions. The most common site of tracheal encrustation is just beneath the tip of the tracheostomy tube and at the level of the coryna. Various methods are used to increase the humidity of the air. Cold steam or hot steam is added to the air to try to increase moisture content. Cold steam is formed by converting a liquid such as water into a fine mist by mechanical means. It has the advantage over hot steam of neither heating the air nor being a source of burns. To effectively elevate the moisture content of the air, the doors and windows should be kept closed. It is impossible to significantly elevate the moisture content of the air when windows and doors are open. Another method sometimes prescribed by the physician to combat the drying effect of the inspired air is to introduce 0.5 to 1 ml of sterile physiological saline solution into the tracheostomy tube at regular intervals. By this method water lost to the air by evaporation is replaced. Attention should also be paid to maintaining the fluid intake of the patient.

To limit the introduction of microorganisms into the tracheostomy tube a few elementary precautions should be taken. First, separate trays should be set up and plainly marked so that different catheters and rinsing solutions are available and *used* for suctioning the nose, mouth, and oropharynx and for suctioning the tracheostomy tube. The all-too-common practice of using the same catheter for suctioning the nose and oral cavities and the tracheostomy violates the most basic principles of microbiology.

Another grave omission often observed is failure of the person performing the suctioning of the tracheostomy to wash his hands. Although this procedure can never be a sterile one, utmost cleanliness is important. Techniques vary from institution to institution, but one of the basic principles is to keep the catheter as clean as possible. Thorough hand washing (sometimes with special solutions such as pHisoHex[15]), the wearing of rubber gloves, or the use of forceps in carrying out the procedure may be employed. The technique employed is probably not as important as are the recognition of the principle involved and consistency in carrying out a clean technique by those involved in the care of the patient.

Second, the procedure that is used should provide for keeping the equipment clean. A fresh sterile setup should be provided at least every eight hours. After suctioning, water or physiological saline should be drawn through the catheter to remove the secretions. Then it should be wiped clean with a sterile four-by-four sponge. Marchetta,[16] *et al.,* recommend that the catheter be wiped, with a sponge soaked in a small amount of Zephiran Chloride[17] and that it be detached from the suction apparatus and placed in a 1:10,000 dilution of benzalkonium solution. The reason for detaching the catheter is to prevent the tubing from being dragged out of the container. According to Marchetta, benzalkonium in the suggested dilution is effective in destroying bacteria and is at the same time nonirritating to the tracheal lining. In some hospitals, after use the catheter is rinsed, wiped dry, and stored in a bag or in a folded towel. The important point is that it not be draped on the suction machine or placed on a table top or some unclean surface. In an ideal technique a clean catheter

[15] Hexachlorophene soap.
[16] Frank C. Marchetta, Sirney Anthony, and Anna Aungst, "A Method of Tracheotomy Care," *A.M.A. Archives of Otolaryngology,* LXV, March, 1957, pp. 298-299.
[17] Trade name for benzalkonium chloride.

would be used each time the trachea was suctioned. With the introduction of inexpensive plastic catheters, the practice of discarding catheters may be feasible. Whatever the details of the method of handling the equipment used in suctioning, they should be based on the knowledge that the patient has been deprived of his own mechanisms for cleaning the air before it enters the tracheobronchial tree. The catheter is introduced into a region that in health is sterile. The lining of the trachea is not adapted to direct exposure to unconditioned air and can be injured by the catheter or the suctioning procedure.

Knowledge of the physiology of the trachea is also of significance in the care of the tracheostomy tubes. The physician is usually responsible for the changing of the outer cannula. The frequency with which the outer cannula is changed varies; it is usually dependent on the condition of the patient and whether or not the tube is patent. It may not be changed more frequently than every four to five days. The nurse is responsible for checking the ties on the outer cannula to be sure that they fit snugly around the neck of the patient and for having the necessary equipment ready for the physician. Though the nurse should check the ties, she should not remove them unless she has received instruction and the physician has delegated the responsibility to her. Should the cannula slip out of the trachea, the nurse may keep the trachea open with forceps or another dilating instrument to prevent suffocation.

In contrast to the outer cannula the nurse removes the inner cannula as necessary in order to clean it. When secretions are voluminous this may have to be done as often as every one-half to one hour. Procedures for cleaning the inner cannula vary. The procedure suggested by Marchetta,[18] and his co-workers is based on the following: (1) the inner cannula is coated with protein-containing mucus; (2) it is of silver or other metal;[19] and (3) is to be inserted into the outer cannula. They suggest the following:

1. The cannula should be placed in hydrogen peroxide and water to soften the mucus.
2. A soft brush and green soap and water should be used to cleanse the inside of the cannula. Some authorities suggest that pipe cleaners be used rather than a brush. When a brush is used there is a possibility that a bristle may remain in the cannula. As a precaution the cannula should be checked after it is cleansed for extraneous material.
3. The cannula should be scoured with silver polish.
4. The cannula should be rinsed thoroughly.
5. The cannula should be boiled for two minutes.
6. It should be cooled.
7. It should be reinserted.

Since the two parts of a tracheostomy tube are matched, one inner cannula cannot be substituted for another.

[18] *Ibid.,* p. 298.
[19] New materials such as plastic are now being used.

A third factor in the physiology of the respiratory tree having relevance in nursing is that secretions increase markedly during the first few hours after tracheostomy. The cilia are likely to be overwhelmed by the volume of secretion. The situation is aggravated by the fact that the newly tracheotomized patient is unable to cough efficiently. When the patient is able, he should be encouraged to cough. Before the patient attempts to cough, the suction apparatus should be in readiness. In preparation for coughing the patient is instructed to take a deep breath, and the tracheostomy tube is occluded as expiration begins. As secretions are raised, they should be removed by wiping the end of the tube with gauze and by suctioning the tube. Aspiration of secretions into the airway should, when possible, be avoided. Excessive coughing should be prevented, as this damages the ciliated epithelium of the respiratory tree. The combination of an increase in secretions and failure of mechanisms for ridding the tracheobronchial tree of them predisposes the patient to two dangers, encrustation of the trachea and tracheobronchitis. Tracheobronchitis further increases secretion and intensifies the destruction of the ciliated mucous membrane. Thus a vicious circle is initiated. Increased secretion overwhelms the cleansing mechanisms of the tracheobronchial tree and predisposes to encrustation and tracheobronchitis, which in turn further increase secretions. As indicated earlier, whenever secretions accumulate in the tracheobronchial tree, the patient is predisposed to ateleclasis and pneumonia.

To prevent the accumulation of secretions, suctioning is required. Whether the nurse does shallow or deep suctioning depends on the policy of the institution and of the physician attending the patient and on the skill and confidence of the nurse. To achieve the greatest benefit to the patient, the secretions in deeper structures must be regularly removed. When deep suctioning is performed, maximum consideration must be given to the fragility of the respiratory membrane. As emphasized earlier, attention must be paid to asepsis so that the patient is protected from the introduction of pathogenic microorganisms into the airway. Aspiration of the tracheobronchial tree must also take into consideration the fact that the airway is obstructed during suctioning and that hypoxia is intensified if the catheter is left in place too long.

How can tracheal suctioning be performed so that it is effective and trauma to the mucosa is minimized?

After studying the respiratory tree of tracheotomized persons who died and of rabbits that had been subjected to tracheotomy and suctioning, Plum and Dunning[20] devised a technique of deep suctioning that they state minimizes trauma to the mucous membrane. At the same time, it is effective in removing secretions. They state that suctioning, as it is all too frequently

[20] Fred Plum and Marcella F. Dunning, "Technics For Minimizing Trauma to the Tracheobronchial Tree After Tracheotomy," *New England Journal of Medicine*, CCLIV, February 2, 1956, pp. 193-99.

performed, serves as a crude biopsy technique. As do other authorities, they emphasize the importance of scrupulous cleanliness. They suggest that number 12 firm-rubber whistle-tip catheters be used and that 5 per cent sodium bicarbonate solution be employed as a lubricant. To prevent trauma to the wall of the trachea or bronchi as a result of the catheter's adhering to it, they place a Y tube in the suction line. The Y tube makes it possible to release the vacuum immediately by fingertip control. During insertion, the Y valve is left open. It is directed into the right or left bronchus by having the patient turn his head to the opposite side. The catheter is then withdrawn 1 to 2 cm to remove the tip from the mucous membrane before the suction is started by putting the finger over the Y valve. At any sign that the mucous membrane has been suctioned into the tube, the finger should be immediately removed from the Y valve to release the suction. As the tube is removed, it should be slowly rotated. When a Cuday catheter is used, it should not be rotated, as the hook on the end of the catheter traumatizes the mucosa. No aspiration should be longer than 15 seconds and the patient should be allowed to rest at least three minutes, unless secretions are so abundant that there is no choice but to remove them. A warning emphasized by Plum and Dunning is not to pinch the tube while suctioning, as this increases the negative pressure and the possibility of sucking the mucous membrane into the catheter.

In the words of John M. Lore,[21] the care of the patient following a tracheostomy is based on three principles: (1). "Keep moist." (2). Use "deep suction." (3) "Keep clean." Throughout this discussion, these three principles and ways of achieving them have been emphasized. These three principles take priority in achieving the purposes of the procedure. Unless the airway is kept open, the life of the patient is endangered from hypoxia. The patency of the airway is threatened by secretions, encrustations, and infection, which is predisposed to by the first two and intensifies both.

As indicated earlier, in the patient who is conscious, tracheostomy is a frightening procedure. Hypoxia, from whatever cause, is attended by feelings of anxiety which may be so great as to cause panic and intensify the degree of hypoxia by increasing activity. When the airway is kept clean, ventilation is improved and the feelings of anxiety are thereby reduced. Anxiety will be increased when the patient has reason to fear that he will not be able to get help when he needs it and therefore runs the risk of suffocation. Survival depends on a patent airway.

As soon as the patient *is able,* he should be taught to suction himself. Some patients ask to be taught. Others are reluctant to learn. Even when there is a policy to instruct patients as soon as possible, timing should take into account the readiness of the patient to learn and his physiological status. For example, Mrs. Cardinal, who had had a laryngectomy the day previously, asked to be taught to suction her own tracheostomy. The day following the operation she

[21] John M. Lore, "Tracheostomy," *A.M.A. Archives of Otolaryngology,* LXVIII, December, 1958, pp. 727-36.

found the noise of the air passing through mucus in her airway most irritating and frightening.

The nurse demonstrated the procedure and then helped Mrs. Cardinal suction herself. After several supervised practice periods, Mrs. Cardinal expressed confidence that she was able to carry on by herself. The nurse checked from time to time to be sure that Mrs. Cardinal was managing successfully and that the suction apparatus was in satisfactory working condition. Mrs. Cardinal learned to care for her tracheostomy very quickly. She was relieved by being able to control her own situation and expressed satisfaction with her ability to care for herself.

By way of contrast, Mr. Quill, an elderly and feeble man, refused to try to suction himself. In a conference with his physician, the decision was made not to insist that he try. Tracheostomy had been performed on Mr. Quill to lessen the work of breathing and to facilitate the removal of secretions. Because of widespread emphysema and his inability to clear his tracheobronchial tree of secretions, Mr. Quill was in a continuous state of hypoxia. He could not be expected to improve until the hypoxia was corrected. Nurses were to suction the airway for a few days with the hope that, as the physical status of Mr. Quill improved, he would possibly be able to assume some responsibility for himself. Because he had extensive emphysema and lack of motivation. to learn, efforts to teach him were not successful. His wife had recently died. Grief over the loss of his wife and changes in his living arrangements contributed to his lack of interest in living and in caring for himself. Therefore, it was decided that Mr. Quill required help with suctioning and that he should not be expected to perform the procedure for himself. His life situation was too overwhelming to permit him to act independently, and some degree of dependency was necessary for his recovery.

How does the structure of the lung enable it to function in ventilation?

In addition to a patent airway, two other interrelated structures, the lung and the thoracic cavity, enter into ventilation. The lungs are elastic distensible bodies that stretch as air enters and deflate as it leaves. They contain no muscles and are not attached at any point to the chest wall, yet they adhere to it closely and follow its motions faithfully. A number of factors account for the above. Because of their elasticity the lung and the chest wall each act like a spring. When they are expanded, their tendency to collapse is greater than their tendency to remain expanded. After expansion the lung and thorax tend to return to their resting state. Expansion is always opposed by the tendency to collapse. The characteristic of the lung enabling it to return to its resting state after it is stretched is known as elastic recoil, and the characteristic enabling it to expand is known as compliance. The wall of the thorax also exhibits these properties.

A diminution of elastic recoil or of compliance interferes with ventilation With a loss of elastic recoil, the lung remains partly expanded during expiration. The retained air adds to the volume of air that does not participate in ventilation; therefore, it adds to the dead space air by increasing the amount of residual air. It also adds to the difficulty of mixing inspired air with residual air. The disorder in which the air sacs in the lung are overinflated with air and their walls are disrupted is known as chronic emphysema. Walkup[22] defines emphysema as "an anatomic alteration of the lung characterized by an abnormal enlargement of the air space distal to the terminal, non respiratory bronchiole accompanied by destruction of the alveolar walls." As with other chronic progressive diseases, the progress of emphysema can frequently be delayed if it is detected early, and proper treatment is instituted. The frequency with which the diagnosis of emphysema is made has increased greatly in the last decade, and it can be expected to increase even more as the number of aged persons in our society increases.

Because of the loss of elastic tissue and changes in posture that accompany aging, emphysema is common in the aged. Though it reduces their respiratory reserve somewhat, when it is uncomplicated, emphysema in the aged is not of serious import.[23] When they are ill and bedfast, it does predispose them to respiratory complications. Moving and turning from side to side on a regular schedule of no less often than every two hours is imperative.

Compensatory emphysema is a physiological process following some conditions such as a lobectomy that reduce the lung parenchyma. Remaining or functioning portions of the lung tend to expand after a portion of the lung is removed by resection of the lung or destroyed by fibrosis. To a degree this type of emphysema is adaptive.

The most serious form of emphysema results from obstruction of the smaller bronchioles. Common etiological factors include bronchical asthma, chronic bronchitis, bronchiectasis, tuberculosis and other infections of the lungs, sarcoidosis, and pneumoconiosis.[24] The basic pathological change predisposing to emphysema is a narrowing of the airway, particularly of the smaller bronchioles, which may be caused by edema with exudate or by spasm of the bronchiolar musculature. Both are frequently factors. Because airways are wider during inspiration than expiration and the inspiratory muscles are more powerful than the expiratory muscles, air is trapped in the alveoli behind the partly obstructed bronchioles. Air is pulled into the alveoli during inspiration, but the forces of expiration are insufficient to drive it out. Because of small pores in alveolar walls, an alveolus whose bronchiole is blocked may receive air. The air trapped in the alveoli raises the intra-alveolar pressure, and with

[22] Harry E. Walkup, "The Dimensions of the Chronic Respiratory Disease Problem," *Supplement to American Journal of Public Health*, Part II, LIII, March, 1963, pp. 11-12.

[23] John H. Killough, "Protective Mechanisms of the Lungs' Pulmonary Disease; Pleural Disease," in William A. Sodeman, *Pathologic Physiology*, 3rd. ed., W. B. Saunders Company, Philadelphia, 1961, p. 6371.

[24] *Ibid.*, p. 635.

the rise, septa break down and the alveoli collapse. Dilated air sacs which do not collapse, that is, remain distended, during the entire respiratory cycle are called blebs. They reduce the surface available for the exchange of gases as well as decrease the area of the capillary bed in the lung. Blebs at the surface of the lung may rupture into the pleural space and establish a connection between the atmosphere and the pleural space which, if sufficient in size, can result in a spontaneous pneumothorax. In spontaneous pneumothorax there is a collapse of lung tissue due to the presence of atmospheric positive pressure in the pleural space where normally the pressure is subatmospheric or negative.

As a consequence of the physiological changes in obstructive emphysema the patient is predisposed to hypoxia, and shortness of breath is the earliest manifestation. Because emphysema interferes with the elimination of carbon dioxide as well as with the intake of oxygen, respiratory acidosis develops sooner or later. When the acidosis is severe, the medullary centers may be relatively insensitive to carbon dioxide, and the low oxygen tension in the blood serves as the stimulus to respiration. Unless the respiratory acidosis can be corrected, oxygen should be administered with extreme caution, as it may precipitate respiratory failure and result in the death of the patient. The correction of respiratory acidosis depends on improving ventilation, particularly the expiratory phase. Some type of mechanical respirator may be prescribed to improve ventilation. Oxygen may be ordered at only 1 to 2 l per minute, and when it is administered with intermittent positive pressure, the percentage of oxygen should not be over 40 per cent. Patients with emphysema who are receiving oxygen should be watched closely for signs of carbon dioxide narcosis. Patients who become restless or increasingly drowsy should be removed from oxygen and watched closely. If their signs improve without oxygen, this tends to support the conclusion that they are experiencing carbon dioxide narcosis. Above all, it is important for the nurse to understand that the patient's color will remain good, and if he is not removed from oxygen, he will go into progressive coma and die pink. He will not be cyanotic. The general objectives of therapy in emphysema are: (1) to eliminate inasfar as is possible existing infection and (2) to improve ventilation. To accomplish the first objective, to eliminate infection, antimicrobial drugs are administered orally or by intramuscular injection.

Accomplishment of the second objective, to improve ventilation, will be facilitated by the first. Removal of retained secretions and prevention of further accumulation are one of the essential factors in the improvement of ventilation. Some of the measures utilized to remove secretions have already been described. They are postural drainage, bronchiolar dilating drugs, medical detergents or wetting agents, and humidified air. In addition, attention should be paid to the intake of fluid by the patient. Dehydration aggravates the tendency to thick, tenacious secretions. Liquefying expectorants such as potassium iodide or ammonium chloride may be prescribed.

In the earlier stages of emphysema and before severe respiratory acidosis develops, oxygen or air may be administered under intermittent positive pressure. Oxygen is given by mask with a positive pressure machine. The mask is placed over the face during inspiration and removed during expiration. The administration of oxygen may improve the feeling of well-being of the patient by lessening the degree of hypoxia. When a positive pressure room is available, air, rather than oxygen, is used to ventilate the lungs. The patient may be taught to keep the bronchioles open by maintaining positive pressure during expiration by expiring against closed lips. Any method preventing the trapping of air in the lung at the end of expiration will improve ventilation.

As indicated previously, tracheostomy may be instituted to lessen the size of the dead air space and to facilitate the removal of secretions. In weak and tired patients, a respirator may be prescribed to improve the adequacy of ventilation.

Compliance or expansibility of the lung is decreased by a variety of disorders of the lung and of the structures of the chest wall. Diseases of the lung that reduce compliance are accompanied by one or more of the following changes: (1) destruction of lung tissue, as in tuberculosis with caseation necrosis and cavity formation; (2) fibrosis of the lung, as in tuberculosis with fibrosis; (3) pulmonary edema, as in congestive heart failure or associated with overloading a patient with a limited renal reserve with fluids; and (4) blocking of the alveoli with exudate, as in pneumococcic pneumonia. Although the pathology in each of the above is different, they all interfere with respiration by limiting the expansion of the lung.

Diseases or effects of disease limiting the expansion of the thoracic cage also have the effect of limiting the expansion of the lung. Kyphosis, severe scoliosis, fibrotic pleurisy, hydrothorax, paralyzed or fibrotic muscles—all limit in some manner the expansion of the lung and therefore decrease compliance. Some forms of therapy such as tight binders and bed rest decrease compliance; a person who lies in bed has a reduction in compliance on the side of his chest that lies next to the bed, which can and should be relieved by moving him or encouraging him to move from side to side.

In addition to a patent airway and the expansibility of the lung, the flow of air into and out of the lung is dependent on changes in the capacity of the thoracic cavity during breathing. Intrapleural pressure is normally less than atmospheric pressure; that is, intrapleural pressure is negative in relation to atmospheric pressure. Negative pressure is greatest during inspiration and least during expiration. Changes in intrapleural pressure are possible because the lungs are contained in a space or box that is too large for them. During growth the thoracic cage grows more rapidly than the lungs, with the result that the space containing the lungs is larger than the lungs are. The greater size of the thoracic cavity in relation to the size of the lung increases the elastic pull on the lung as well as the negative intrapleural pressure. Expansion of the lung during inspiration puts pulmonary tissue, including the elastic tissue of the bronchial tree, the blood vessels, and the air sacs, on a stretch.

As the lung is stretched, the elastic tissue offers resistance to further stretching and prevents the lung from being over expanded.

Another necessary condition in the maintenance of subatmospheric or negative pressure is that the intrapleural cavity is closed to the external environment. The chest wall is lined by serous membrane, the pleura, which continues and is reflected over the lung on the same side. Each pleura is similar to a sealed envelope with one side lining the chest and the other side reflected over the lung. The layer lining the chest is the parietal pleura. The layer covering the lung is the visceral pleura. The space between the two layers is comparable to the inside of the envelope and is known as the intrapleural space. It is actually a potential space as the pleura is separated only by a thin layer of fluid, which also holds the two layers together. The effect of the fluid can be demonstrated by placing the wet sides of two glass slides together. The water causes the slides to adhere to each other, and it takes considerable force to separate them. Without this fluid the lung would not follow the chest wall in breathing. The intrapleural fluid lessens the friction between the two layers and allows one layer to glide smoothly over the other.

During inspiration the chest is expanded in all directions. The length or vertical diameter is increased by the contraction and flattening of the diaphragm. Because the vertebrae are relatively fixed, most of the vertical increase is due to the elevation of the ribs and sternum and is in the anterior direction. Not all parts of the lung are expanded equally. Parts lying next to relatively fixed structures cannot expand unless other parts of the lung get out of the way. This effect can be demonstrated by inhaling while in a supine position and holding the breath while assuming the upright position. Breathing starts with inspiration. The same phenomena can be observed when a patient who has been lying in bed is ambulated. As he assumes the upright position, he takes a deep breath and, incidentally, often coughs.

In quiet breathing, expiration is largely passive. As the contraction of inspiratory muscles ceases, the chest wall and lung through its own weight and inherent elasticity tends to resume its former position. Air is forced out of the lungs by a lessening of the intrapleural negative pressure; that is, the pressure in the intrapleural space approaches that of the atmospheric pressure.

During inspiration negative pressure may reach 10 to 15 mm of mercury less than atmospheric pressure. During expiration muscles of expiration return the thorax to its resting position with a corresponding decrease in its size and a decrease in negative pressure. Intrapleural pressure is from 5 to 8 mm of mercury during expiration. Although the intrathoracic or intrapleural pressure is always less than atmospheric pressure, it approaches atmospheric pressure at the end of expiration.[25] As a result of lowering of intrathoracic pressure during inspiration, air is sucked into the airway to the alveoli. During

[25] The intrathoracic or intrapleural pressure should be distinguished from the intrapulmonary pressure. The first is the pressure within the space between the parietal and visceral pleural. The latter is the pressure in the alveoli. It is difficult to measure, but it varies rhythmically between being above and below atmospheric pressure.

expiration air is forced out of the lung. Expiration is largely due to the elastic rebound of the lungs.

Any disruption of the pleural membrane establishing a communication with the outside environment destroys the negative intrapleural pressure with the result that the lung collapses. Collapse should be expected, since the tendency of the lung to collapse is greater than the tendency for it to remain expanded. Collapse of the lung due to a collection of air in the intrapleural space is called pneumothorax. Collapse of the lung due to air entering the intrapleural space from the lung or large air passages is known as closed pneumothorax. The rupture of an emphysematous bleb or bulla is a common cause. Openings through the chest wall into the intrapleural space cause an open pneumothorax. Stab wounds of the chest extending through the chest wall and parietal pleura cause an open type of pneumothorax. In some types of injuries, air entering the pleural space during inspiration remains. This increases intrapleural pressure (decreases negative pressure) and leads to the development of tension pneumothorax, a dangerous condition which must be corrected if the life of the patient is to be saved.

According to Cherniack and Cherniack,[26] about 25 per cent of the deaths caused by traffic accidents are due to chest injuries. Most of these injuries are crushing or compression injuries. Occasionally there is a closed penetrating wound caused by a fractured rib, and only very rarely does an open penetrating wound occur. Open penetrating wounds are more likely to be caused by stabbing or gunshot.

When the chest wall becomes unstable, as following removal of ribs in thoracoplasty or in traumatic injuries causing fractured ribs, the patient may exhibit a type of breathing which is the opposite of normal and is therefore referred to as paradoxical. In paradoxical breathing the portion of the lung underlying the unstable area moves opposite to what is normally expected. Therefore, the involved area of the lung sucks in on inspiration and balloons out on expiration. If a large area of the lung is involved, a pool of unoxygenated air will be pushed from one lung to another by the abnormal respiratory movements.

An illustration of this type of breathing was demonstrated by Mrs. Anna Tree, who had three ribs removed prior to a pulmonary resection. When she returned to the recovery room she was awake, restless, and attempting to sit up in bed. When Miss Sutherland, the nursing student, took her vital signs, she noticed that Mrs. Tree's breathing was unusual, but she was not sure why. The surgeon came into the room at this point and Miss Sutherland mentioned her concern about the unusual breathing to him. He told her to place one hand on each side of Mrs. Tree's chest and to watch their movement. She noted that the operative side tended to move opposite to the unoperated side; that is, when the hand on the operated side was elevated by the chest wall, the

26 R. M. Cherniack and L. Cherniack, *Respiration in Health and Disease,* W. B. Saunders Company, Philadelphia, 1961, pp. 284-85.

Normal Respiration

Inspiration

O_2

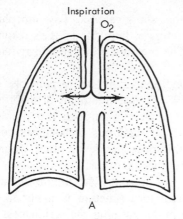

A

Expiration

CO_2

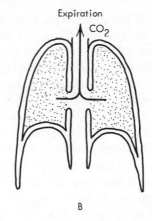

B

Paradoxical Motion

Inspiration

CO_2

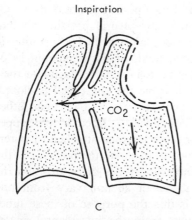

C

Expiration

CO_2

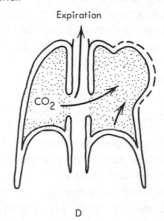

D

FIGURE 7—4. Normal respiration and paradoxical motion. (Adapted, with permission, from Julian Johnson and Charles K. Kirby: *Surgery of the Chest*; Edna Hill, illustrator. Chicago: Year Book Medical Publishers, Inc., 1954, p. 21.)

hand on the unoperated side was lowered. She asked if this was paradoxical breathing. (See Figure 7-4 for illustration of the difference between normal and paradoxical respiration.) The surgeon said it was, and reviewed with her what the treatment should be. Since the principle of treatment is to stabilize the chest wall, one of the following measures can be taken: (1) apply weights such as sandbags to the chest; or (2) apply a pressure binder to the chest. The latter is usually the most convenient as it allows the patient to move about more freely. In the absence of the physician, the nurse should turn the patient onto his operative side so that the mattress can offer some resistance to the unstable chest wall. The surgeon also called Miss Sutherland's attention to other characteristics of Mrs. Tree's respirations. They were short and rapid—40 per minute. He then suggested that she give Mrs. Tree morphine sulfate, 10 mg (gr 1/6), as needed. Fifteen minutes later Mrs. Tree's respirations were 28 and she was resting quietly. The pressure bandage had reduced the paradoxical motion considerably.

A variety of planned or accidental conditions may be responsible for pneumothorax. The route of approach in the surgical treatment of disorders of the lung, mediastinum, heart, and great vessels is through the thoracic cavity. As referred to earlier, a ruptured emphysematous bleb allows communication from the lung to the intrapleural space. Knife or other wounds penetrating the chest wall are not common, but they do occur.

Although emphasis has been on the effects of openings into the intrapleural cavity on the mechanics of respiration, circulatory function is likely to be severely disturbed as well. One of the factors determining the seriousness of the situation is the size of the opening into the thoracic cavity. Small openings may cause little difficulty when a patient is at rest. Large or multiple openings may very quickly cause asphyxia.

Treatment of the patient who has suffered an open pneumothorax is directed toward the re-establishment of negative intrapleural pressure so that the lung can be re-expanded and the expansion maintained. The opening in the chest wall must be closed, and the blood, fluid, or air remaining in or entering the pleural cavity after closure must be removed. To facilitate their removal, one or more tubes are inserted at the time the chest wall is closed. One tube is placed in the lower part of the cavity to remove blood and other fluids and a second tube may be, but is not always, placed in the upper intrapleural space to remove air. The tube or tubes are then attached to water-seal bottles. Suction may or may not be applied to facilitate the removal of the contents of the intrapleural cavity. The number and types of bottles and the devices used to obtain and regulate the degree of suction vary from one institution to another. The important point is that the purpose of these tubes and equipment is to *remove* foreign elements from the intrapleural space. Since intrapleural pressure is less than atmospheric pressure, precautions must be taken to prevent fluids or air in the tubing from being introduced into the intrapleural space. Unless certain precautions are observed, the tubing will act like the trachea when the pressure within the thoracic cavity is reduced. The first precaution taken is to place the tubing, connected to the catheter entering the chest, under water to prevent air from being aspirated into the pleural cavity. The second precaution is to always keep the bottle containing the water and draining the intrapleural space at a level lower than the chest, to prevent the water from running into the chest cavity. Should the bottle be elevated to or about the level of the chest, water will be suctioned into the intrapleural space. As long as the end of a chest tube is covered with water and the bottle into which it drains is kept below the level of the chest, and the system is intact and patent, air and fluid will be forced out of the intrapleural space with each inspiration. When the lung is fully expanded, no air or fluid remains.

To prevent the introduction of fluid or air into the pleural cavity, by raising the drainage bottles to or above the level of the chest, they may be taped to the floor. Taping the bottle to the floor should not be necessary if everyone, including the patient and his visitors, knows why the bottles are to be kept at a level lower than the chest. Since the chest bottles are of glass and may inadvertently be broken, one or two hemostats should be pinned or otherwise fastened to the top of the patient's bed or mattress where they are readily seen and are not likely to be removed. The patient, his relatives, and all personnel should be instructed to clamp the tube or tubes in case a bottle is broken.

In addition to making sure that the system draining the intrapleural space is intact and working, attention must be given to maintaining the patency of the tracheobronchial tree. Obstruction of the tracheobronchial tree is always possible because conditions interfering with the expansion of the lung also disturb the mechanisms for cleansing the tracheobronchial tree. All the previously discussed measures aiding in the cleansing of the airway should be instituted and carried out regularly at hourly or no less than two-hour intervals. When the patient is in the hospital for a day or more before the chest cavity is opened, he should be instructed in the how and why of the various procedures that will be utilized to promote the re-expansion of the lung. The patient who is admitted with a stab wound in his chest usually is treated as an emergency, and instruction is usually delayed until after closure of the wound.

Throughout the period of recovery the patient should be observed for signs of hypoxia, dyspnea, and infection. The drainage system should also be observed to be sure that all connections are tight and the system is in working order. The level of water in the bottle should be marked at the time the bottle is attached to the tubing connected with the catheter inserted into the intrapleural space, so that the quantity of drainage can be measured. Until the lung is fully re-expanded, the fluid in glass tubing connected to the chest tube and the end of which is submerged in water can be expected to fluctuate with respiration. When the fluid ceases to fluctuate, blood clotted in the tube may be responsible or the lung may be fully expanded. In order to prevent a blood clot from occluding the tube and interfering with drainage, the tubing may be milked or stripped at least every two hours. Before doing this the nurse should, however, check with the physician. When the nurse performs this procedure and it is not successful, then the surgeon should be notified. The extent to which the lung is expanded is checked by X ray. In some hospitals only physicians change the drainage bottles. In others, this responsibility is delegated to nursing. Some surgeons prefer that the drainage bottles not be changed unless the volume of drainage is unusually great and demands a new setup in order to (1) determine the amount of new drainage (i.e., bleeding), or (2) reduce the amount of negative pressure in the drainage bottle. When drainage bottles are changed, tubes should be clamped so that air cannot enter the pleural space and all equipment including the water should be sterile. Blood-containing fluids offer a fine media for the growth of bacteria.

The quality of nursing that a patient who has had an opening into his thoracic cavity receives influences for good or ill the rate at which he recovers and even if he recovers. This nursing should, inasmuch as the circumstances allow, do the following:

1. Prepare the patient for what to expect and for what is expected of him.
2. Maintain the integrity of the system for the removal of fluids and air from the intrapleural space.
3. Support the mechanisms for cleansing the tracheobronchial tree and for promoting the re-expansion of the lung.

In addition to air, collapse of the lung may be induced by collections of serous fluid (hydrothorax); blood (hemothorax); or pus (pyothorax, or empyema). Accumulation of serous fluids is commonly associated with pleural effusion due to infections involving the pleura. A frequent cause of pleurisy with effusion is tuberculosis, but it may also accompany neoplasms involving the lung or structures in the mediastinum. Whether or not accumulated fluid is removed from the pleural space will depend on the likelihood of its being absorbed and the degree to which the fluid causes respiratory embarrassment. Some surgeons are very reluctant to remove fluid unless it is causing respiratory embarrassment because of the danger of introducing pathogenic organisms during the procedure. An initial tap is done, however, to obtain specimens for culture and sensitivity to antimicrobial agents so that proper drugs may be ordered when necessary. Purulent material is usually removed, because it delays healing. As indicated elsewhere, pus acts as a foreign body and must be removed before healing can take place. When possible, the fluid is aspirated through a needle introduced into the thoracic cavity. The procedure is known as thoracentesis. Precautions are taken to prevent the introduction of air. [27]

Chronic empyema may require surgical intervention; that is, a thoracotomy may be performed. In this procedure a section of a rib is removed and a tube is inserted into the space containing pus. Often the tube is connected to a water-seal bottle and the pus drains into the drainage bottle. This type of water seal must be changed at least daily and sometimes more often if the amount of drainage is copious. If the chest wall is fixed and there is no danger of a pneumothorax developing, the drainage tube is often allowed to drain directly into a large chest dressing which is usually changed two to three times daily. Occasionally antimicrobial agents as well as enzymes that dissolve fibrinous and purulent materials are introduced into the empyema space, either through a needle or through the drainage tube.[28] If the drainage tube is used, it is clamped for a few hours after instillation of the drugs.

[27] Bertha Harmer and Virginia Henderson, *Textbook of the Principles and Practice of Nursing,* 5th ed., rev., The Macmillan Company, New York, 1955, pp. 805-10.
[28] Streptokinase-streptodornase (Varidase) is one preparation used for this purpose. It is available in forms suitable for buccal, and topical application as well as for intramuscular administration and injection into tubes.

The power by which the size of the chest is altered is provided by skeletal muscles. The most important muscles of respiration are the diaphragm and the intercostals. The nervous system initiates muscular activity and co-ordinates the various movements involved in breathing with circulation so that some degree of failure of one is compensated for by an increase in activity of the other. The effect of failure of respiratory function is illustrated by John Blue, who was dependent on a mechanical respirator to maintain ventilation. His pulse rate was consistently between 90 and 100 beats per minute. As his ventilation improved, his pulse rate fell toward normal. The integration of respiratory and circulatory function is protective, inasmuch as the effect of failure in one can to some extent be compensated for by in-creased activity of the other. These functions are dependent on the nervous system for stimulation as well as for the integration of breathing with the needs of the entire organism. When the need for oxygen is increased by exercise, fever, or a failure to maintain the supply of oxygen, the pulse rate rises.

There are a number of conditions which result in a reduction in muscle power. These include aging, debility and disease, and undernutrition. Of dis-eases of muscle, muscular dystrophy is the most common. In myasthenia gravis, as the name implies, there is grave or serious weakness of muscles. This results not from a failure of muscles, but from a defect in their stimula-iton. The transmission of impulses from the nerve ending to the muscle is defective. In poliomyelitis involving the respiratory centers in the brain, or the upper portion of the spinal cord, muscles fail from lack of stimulation. In poliomyelitis motor nerve cells are injured or destroyed thus depriving skeletal muscles of necessary stimulation.

How is breathing regulated?

The regulation and integration of the activities that are involved in breath-ing are highly complex and only partly understood. The rate of respiration is regulated so that there is a rhythmical change in the capacity of the thorax 15 to 16 times a minute. The depth is also regulated. At rest man breathes about 7 ll. of air per minute. During strenuous exercise rate and depth can be in-creased to as much as 20 ll. per minute.[29] In the healthy person oxygen supply is determined by the rate and depth of respiration.

The neural regulation of any activity and at any level can be described very simply as the action of a receptor and an effector with something in between. In breathing the effectors are the muscles of respiration. Receptors are pri-marily proprioceptors and interoceptors located in the alveoli, in the carotid and aortic bodies, and in centers in the brain stem. Exteroceptors sensitive to cold and pain also initiate impulses that cause alteration in breathing. The something in between the receptors and effectors includes afferent and efferent

[29] Wallace O. Fenn, "The Mechanism of Breathing," *Scientific American,* CCII, January, 1960, p. 138.

nerve pathways carrying impulses from receptors to centers in the brain stem and to the muscles of respiration. Afferent fibers arise primarily from the vagus nerve, though some sensory fibers in the phrenic nerve are involved.

Centers in the medulla and pons regulate respiration. There is no one center for respiration, but a group of interconnected centers. Though they have connections with the cerebral cortex, rhythmical breathing continues when these connections are destroyed. Animals decerebrated (connections between the cerebrum and lower centers destroyed) through the upper part of the pons maintain a normal type of respiration. Those in whom the structures in the brain stem are injured or seriously damaged by disease cannot maintain breathing without mechanical help. For example, the patient with the ascending spinal or bulbar type of poliomyelitis, or who has suffered trauma to these areas in the nervous system, requires mechanical help to continue breathing. According to Hardy,[30] there is a subsidiary respiratory center in the spinal cord which includes the motor cells located in the anterior horn of the cord. Anterior horn cells coordinate the action of respiratory muscles, but they do not coordinate respiration as a whole. Although higher centers can and do at times modify breathing, for the most part they have a minor effect.

Two principal types of stimuli play a role in initiating impulses resulting in breathing. The first of these is chemical. The second is the direct effect of stretching tissue of the lung. Stretching or tugging on other tissues, particularly the viscera, also causes changes in the rate and depth of respiration. Pain and emotional states such as fear are also accompanied by changes in breathing.

Three chemicals are natural stimulants to respiration. They are carbon dioxide, the hydrogen ion, and oxygen. Carbon dioxide and the hydrogen ion act by their presence in the respiratory center to stimulate the rate and depth of respiration. Oxygen acts, not by its presence, but by its absence. Minor deficits of oxygen are not believed to have an appreciable effect on breathing. Hypoxia has a depressing effect on respiratory centers. Authorities are not agreed as to whether severe hypoxia can be stimulating to the respiratory centers. Chemoreceptors in the aortic and carotid bodies are, however, sensitive to low oxygen tensions and initiate impulses resulting in the stimulation of respiration. Disagreement also exists as to whether carbon dioxide directly stimulates cells in the respiratory center or produces its effect by raising their hydrogen ion concentration. In any event, an elevation in the level of carbon dioxide or of hydrogen ions in the plasma is accompanied by an increase in the rate and depth of respiration. Conversely, a drop in the level of carbon dioxide or hydrogen ions in the blood plasma is accompanied by a decrease in respirations.

Breathing not only involves rate and depth and their integration with other bodily activities, but the coordination of inspiration and expiration so that the

[30] James D. Hardy, *Pathophysiology in Surgery,* The Williams and Wilkins Company, Baltimore, 1958, p. 470.

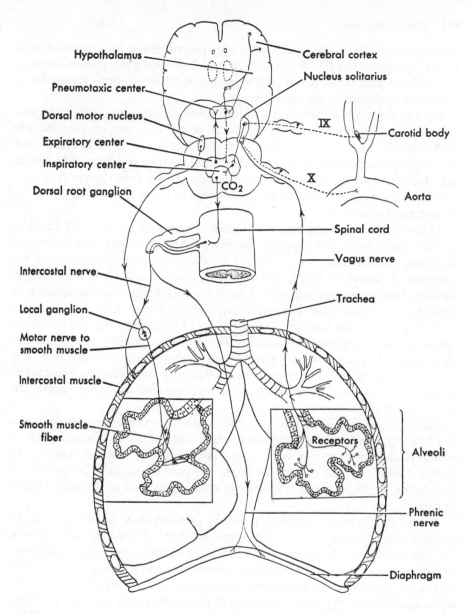

FIGURE 7—5. Nervous control of respiration. Arrows indicate the direction of the nerve impulse. (Adapted with permission of the Macmillan Company from *Anatomy and Physiology*, 14th ed., Fig. 304, p. 455, by Diana Clifford Kimber, Carolyn E. Gray, Caroline E. Stackpole, and Lutie C. Leavell. Copyright © The Macmillan Company 1961.)

act of breathing is in itself coordinated. The latter activity is what is usually referred to as the reflex control of breathing. Stretch receptors in the alveoli and the aortic and carotic bodies initiate impulses that are carried over vagal fibers to the inspiratory and expiratory centers in the brain stem. These reflexes are known as the stretch reflexes or the Hering-Breuer reflexes. These reflexes are inhibitory. In other words, they prevent either inspiration or expiration from going too far. As tissues are stretched during inspiration, impulses are initiated that result in the reflex inhibition of inspiration. Expiration is controlled in essentially the same manner.

By a combination of chemical and reflex control, rate and depth of respiration are regulated in relation to the needs of the cells for oxygen. Equally important, the pattern of breathing is modified in a variety of activities such as coughing and sneezing. Fear and other emotions may greatly modify breathing. Sudden exposure of the skin to cold such as in a cold shower is accompanied by a gasp and a holding of the breath. For short periods breathing can be controlled voluntarily.

In the regulation of respiration a number of activities are involved. In terms of the objectives of this chapter, the first activity is to regulate the act of breathing so that fresh air is brought to the respiratory membrane in the quantities required to supply the cells with oxygen and to remove carbon dioxide. The second, related to the first, is the coordination and integration of activities that protect the respiratory tree and the alveoli from foreign materials. The third is the coordination of the act of breathing with the metabolic needs of cells and with the circulation. Failure to accomplish one or more of these functions predisposes to hypoxia and to carbon dioxide retention. The most common sites of disturbances in regulation of breathing are the centers in the brain stem and at the myoneural junction (the site where nerve impulses are transmitted to the muscles).

Causes of depression and failure of the respiratory center include edema of the brain, pressure conus, depressant drugs, and infectious diseases such as poliomyelitis. An injury or disease that interferes with the function of, but does not inactivate, the cells of the medullary centers produces irregularity in the rhythm, depth, and rate of breathing. With inactivation of the cells, breathing ceases.

Edema of the brain occurs in a variety of conditions. Concussion of the brain as the result of a blow to the head is often followed by some edema. Any disorder markedly diminishing the flow of blood to the brain predisposes to brain edema. In hypertensive encephalopathy, edema results from the limitations on blood flow by markedly constricted arterioles. Capillary permeability is increased by hypoxia. Any disorder causing hypoxia sets into motion a vicious circle which, unless corrected, leads to death from depression of the respiratory and other vital centers.

In addition to edema of the brain, respiratory failure may be due to pressure conus. In pressure conus, the brain is pressed downward into the foramen magnum. Since the medulla oblongata is directly over the foramen magnum, pressure is exerted on the medulla and partly or completely cuts off its blood supply. Death as a consequence of respiratory failure occurs almost immediately. Pressure conus is one of the causes of death in the patient who has a head injury or a brain tumor causing a rise in intracranial pressure. In the patient who has increased intracranial pressure, removal of the cerebro-spinal fluid can precipitate pressure conus. With the reduction of the pressure in the spinal canal, the fluid in the cranial cavity rushes toward the area of reduced pressure, carrying the medulla with it, and causes the death of the patient. Patients who are predisposed to pressure conus should be regularly observed for signs of increasing intracranial pressure. The length of the interval between observations varies depending on the degree of increasing intracranial pressure and the possibility of its rising rapidly. The patient who is newly admitted after a head injury may be observed every 15 minutes for from four to eight hours. If, at the end of the designated time, he has no abnormal findings, the interval may be extended to one, two, or four hours. The observations, which include noting the character and rate of respiration, are listed in more detail in Chapter 13B.

To prevent pressure conus the patient who is predisposed is usually placed in the supine position. Since muscular activity causes some increase in intracranial pressure, the conscious patient should be instructed to lie quietly and to avoid sudden movements. He may be allowed one thin pillow, but he should not raise his head, nor should he feed himself. Activities which involve holding the breath after a deep inspiration, such as coughing and straining during defecation or urination, are particularly dangerous. Elevation of the intrathoracic pressure interferes with the venous return from the brain and thereby increases intracranial pressure. The importance of conscientious observation and the above regime in the prevention of respiratory failure in susceptible patients cannot be overemphasized.

One of the most common causes of depression of the respiratory centers in hospitalized patients is depressant drugs. These include general anesthetics, sedatives such as the barbiturates, and narcotics. In the therapeutic use of these agents, excessive respiratory depression can usually be prevented by limiting their dosage and by observing their effects. When depressant drugs such as the barbiturates are ingested for purposes of self-destruction, the patient may be in serious respiratory depression at the time he is admitted to the hospital; death, if it results, is due to respiratory arrest.

Although the depression of respiration is initiated by the effects of the drug on the respiratory center, it is intensified by two other related factors. With depression of the respiratory centers, ventilation becomes less adequate and some degree of hypoxia develops.[31] As the hypoxia of the brain increases, ventilation is further impaired and oxygenation of the blood becomes less and less effective. Moreover the depression of the breathing centers is accompanied by inhibition of the cough centers, as well as by the inactivation of cilia in the airway. Consequently, secretions accumulate in the airway and obstruct the passage of air, further decreasing ventilation. Therapy is based on two objectives, that is, to remove or decrease the concentration of the depressant drug, and to sustain breathing in order to improve the supply

[31] The effects of hypoxia have been previously discussed.

of oxygen to the brain and other tissues. To accomplish the first objective, drugs causing respiratory depression are discontinued, and an attempt is made to remove the accumulated drug from the body. When an artificial kidney is available, the drug may be removed by dialyzing the blood of the patient, or peritoneal dialysis may be employed.

The second objective is accomplished by the administration of oxygen, often under pressure, and by the use of mechanical devices which perform artificial respiration. Secretions must be removed from the tracheobronchial tree. The measures required will depend on the degree of depression. In the deeply depressed patient tracheobronchial suction may be required.

Any drug or disorder capable of lessening the effectiveness of ventilation by depressing the respiratory centers in the brain can also cause sufficient depression to stop breathing. In addition to the drugs listed above, curare causes respiratory failure by preventing the transmission of nerve impulses across the myoneural junction. Curare was originally utilized as a poison on the tips of arrows. It is utilized in modern medicine to increase muscular relaxation during some types of operative procedure. Other causes of respiratory failure not mentioned above are drowning and electric shock. Whatever its cause, cessation of breathing should always be treated as an emergency, and action should be taken immediately to re-establish breathing.

When breathing fails, life depends on the promptness with which ventilation is re-established. In fact, if resuscitation is to be successful, it must take precedence over all other procedures. Artificial respiration has as its goal the maintenance of breathing until the patient can perform this function himself. It should, therefore, be continued until natural breathing is re-established or until there is clear evidence that it cannot be.

Although there are a variety of methods used in artificial respiration, they all have three common objectives. These are: (1) to oxygenate the blood; (2) to remove carbon dioxide; and (3) to maintain the circulation. Three different types of artificial respiration are available to ventilate the lungs. They are classified as manual, mechanical, and mouth-to-mouth breathing. The method selected will depend on where the emergency occurs and the length of time that the patient can be expected to have a problem with breathing. For example, John Francis is rescued from a lake after being submerged for five minutes. Artificial respiration either by mouth-to-mouth breathing or by the manual method should be initiated as rapidly as possible. There is no time to wait and obtain special equipment. In contrast, Robin George, who is hospitalized with acute poliomyelitis, can be observed for manifestations of respiratory failure. A respirator may be in readiness outside his room to be used should his physician decide that it is necessary. Equipment is also available in the operating room to sustain respiratory function in Mr. Coombs, who stopped breathing during an operative procedure.

The manual methods of artificial respiration are of two types, the Schafer prone pressure method and the push-pull methods, one of which was introduced by a Danish physician, Dr. Holger. Although the Schafer method was in vogue for a number of years, it has been found to be the least effective of all the manual methods of artificial respiration.

In all the push-pull methods of artificial respiration the chest is compressed to cause expiration and then the body is lifted to increase the size of the chest and thus aid inspiration. Gordon, et al.,[23] found in all their studies that the hip-lift-back-pressure method provides the greatest amount of ventilation of the lungs. Furthermore it has the advantage of being easy to teach. It may, however, be difficult for small adults or children to perform. Gordon and his associates state that the arm-lift-back-pressure method is most applicable for general use. Because one method is not suitable in all instances, they emphasize that medical and other trained personnel should be competent in several methods. References describing the performance of the various methods are included at the end of the chapter.

The method that is said to be most efficient of all is mouth-to-mouth breathing. Despite the impression that mouth-to-mouth breathing is new, it is in fact very old. In movies and novels references are made to a doctor or midwife blowing "the breath of life" into the lungs of a newborn baby who fails to start to breathe. Mouth-to-mouth breathing fell from favor because of the belief that expired air would not contain enough oxygen to be of any value to the recipient. This is now known not to be true. Another factor probably influencing the rejection of mouth-to-mouth breathing was the acceptance of the germ theory in the causation of disease. One outcome of the germ theory was the concept that the secretions of one person were a potential source of danger to other persons. Since ideas are basis for action, a number of sanitary and hygienic measures are instilled in us to protect one person from the secretions of his fellows. For example, children are taught not to put anything in their mouth that has been in the mouth of another. Mothers teach their children not to allow casual acquaintances, or even close relatives, to kiss them on the lips. Thus by precept and by practice, the individual learns to avoid situations by which he may come in contact with the secretions of others. As a result, it is not unusual for a person to find it difficult if not impossible to place his mouth directly over that of another. For the person who finds it difficult to place his mouth over the mouth or nose of another person, some measure of protection, as well as feeling of being protected, can be afforded by placing a handkerchief or gauze over the face of the victim. When one is available, an S-shaped airway may be introduced into the mouth of the patient, over the tongue and back into the pharynx. Air is then expired by the operator into this tube. Such a tube should be kept with the emergency equipment on each hospital unit.

A number of points apply to all methods of artificial respiration. The first is

[32] Archer S. Gordon, Max S. Sadove, Frank Raymon, and A. C. Ivy, "Critical Survey of Manual Artificial Respiration," *Journal of the American Medical Association*, CXLVII, pp. 1444-53.

that time is a critical factor and delay can be fatal. Second, no method can be expected to be successful unless a clear airway is established and the procedure is performed properly. Before starting any procedure, foreign bodies and secretions in the mouth of the patient should be removed by inserting the fingers into the mouth and grasping the foreign body or wiping the secretions away. If materials are available and time allows, the fingers may be covered with gauze or a handkerchief. Suction can, of course, be used when it is available. Gravity may be utilized by placing the patient in a head-down position or turning the head to the side.

After foreign bodies and secretions have been removed, the airway should be established by fully extending the head of the patient and supporting the chin. Halfway measures are useless. The head may be turned from side to side to find the most favorable position. If these maneuvers are unsuccessful, the fingers should be flexed and placed behind the angles of the patient's mandible, and the patient's jaw should be moved forward as far as possible. Another method that may be used to move the mandible forward is to place the fingers under the chin of the patient and, with the thumb in his mouth, move the jaw forward.[33] After an open airway is established, the next step is to start ventilating the lungs.

In mouth-to-mouth respiration, the operator inhales deeply and blows the air forcibly into the nose or mouth of the patient. When air is blown into the mouth, the victim's nose must be closed, or vice versa. If an airway is used, be sure that it is in the posterior pharynx. As air is exhaled into the victim, his chest should rise. If it does not or there are rumblings of air in the stomach, the support to the jaw which holds the airway open should be improved. If this does not help, blow more forcefully. Placing a hand over the abdomen and pressing down slightly also seems to help. Unless the chest expands well, air is not being introduced into the lung in a sufficient amount. Expiration is allowed to take place naturally. Fishbein[34] recommends approximately 20 cycles per minute, but other authorities state that although as many as 20 may be required for optimum ventilation, 10 to 12 are probably adequate. When only one person is present, he should modify the rate so that he will be able to continue the procedure for an extended period of time.

To summarize the essentials of mouth-to-mouth respiration, the airway should be cleared and the lungs rhythmically inflated. Ventilation of the lungs must be continued for as long as the possibility of life exists.

In the hospital, equipment is available to blow air or oxygen into the lungs by way of a face mask or an endotracheal or tracheostomy tube. Although there are special machines for this purpose, an anesthesia machine with bag is often employed.

[33] Jay Jacoby, Carolyn H. Ziegler, Andrew Wooley, and Hugh Ray, "Treatment of Respiratory Emergencies," *Postgraduate Medicine*, XXV, 1959, pp. 373-75.
[34] Morris Fishbein, "Medical Progress 1958," *Postgraduate Medicine*, XXV, January, 1959, p. 111.

When there is a prolonged failure in breathing, other methods are used to maintain ventilatory function. These include tank and chest respirators and rocking beds. Tank and chest respirators operate on the same general principle. Ventilation is affected by alternating the pressure of the atmosphere surrounding the patient or his chest. Inspiration takes place as the pressure in the tank or jacket falls below atmospheric pressure. Expiration occurs as the pressure rises to or slightly above atmospheric pressure. Negative pressure is usually regulated between -10 and -20 cm of water, and the positive pressure rises to from 0 to $+5$ cm of water. The decision as to the pressures to be maintained is made by the physician and is based somewhat on the size of the patient. The nurse has the responsibility of checking the appropriate gauges, of making sure that all portholes are properly closed, and of reporting any problems in maintaining the desired range of pressures.

The nursing care of the patient in the respirator can be one of the most taxing experiences in nursing, particularly in the care of a seriously ill patient such as the one with acute poliomyelitis. This patient often regresses to a childlike state. He is apprehensive and demanding and dependent on the nurse not only to care for his every physical need, but to provide continuous emotional support. The needs of the patient may be so great that he demands that the nurse be present every moment. He becomes terrified when he is left alone for even a few minutes. When the respirator is opened, he complains that the nurse is unduly slow and has allowed the pressure in the tank to rise unnecessarily. When he is uncomfortable, he wants his position changed without delay. Should the nurse be successful in making him comfortable, he remains so for only a brief period of time.

The patient in the respirator for the first time frequently feels trapped—trapped by his illness and by a machine from which he is unable to escape. He may doubt that it can be depended upon to maintain his breathing. He may not be able to do a thing for himself. Try lying with a fly buzzing around your face, or with your nose itching, or your toe in a cramp, and then try to imagine the feeling that not being able to move a muscle would engender. The patient experiences hopelessness, often to the point of despair. He may also be angry —angry at everyone and everything. He directs his anger at those who are near him—the nurse and often the members of the family. If the nurse can remind herself that the patient is really angry with his fate and not with her as a person, she is usually better able to be helpful to him.

As implied, the nurse may also have negative as well as positive feelings as she cares for this patient. She may appreciate that the patient is very ill as well as the seriousness of his predicament. Yet she may be angry that he cannot be pleased and continues to complain. The nurse may also share some of the fears of the patient. Will the respirator continue to function properly? What will she do if it stops? Is the patient all right? How can she meet his demands? And so on and on. The apprehension or anxiety of the patient is communicable. Yet one of the things that he needs most is a nurse who is quietly confident that she can and will meet his needs. He also needs a nurse who can, as the acuteness of his illness subsides, encourage him by pointing out even small gains and by suggesting that he will be able to make a life for himself. The nurse may feel embarrassment at having to perform the most intimate procedures for the patient. He is unable to do anything including the brushing of a loose hair from his cheek. The nurse also feels pity at the patient's helplessness. When it begins to appear that the patient will be more or less dependent on the respirator for the rest of his life, she is likely to share the patient's feeling of hopelessness. Her depression may be intensified by the patient's dependence on her and by her seeming inability to satisfy his demands. For these and other reasons she too may feel anger. Because of her feelings she may feel guilty because the patient is sick and she is well or because she sometimes fails to be patient or to move quickly enough. Added to the emotional stress, nursing the patient in the respirator is hard physical work. In addition to the above, the nurse must be continuously alert to the condition of the patient and make sure that the machine is operating properly.

When a patient is to be placed in a respirator, he should, if he is conscious, be informed about the reason for the procedure. Patients, such as those with myasthenia gravis, who have been in the respirator earlier in their lives may actually welcome the help that it gives them in breathing.

The respirator should be ready at all times with a clean collar and pieces at the portholes. The mattress on the carriage or respirator bed should be covered with a cotton sheet. Three to five persons should be available to transfer the patient from his bed to the carriage. The carriage is pulled out and the respirator motor started before the patient is transferred into it. One person delivers the head through the collar at the head while the others stand at each side and lift the patient. To move him into position, the person at the head places one hand under the head of the patient and turns his face to one side. The other hand should be used to stretch the collar and to shield the nose and eyes of the patient. As soon as the patient is in position, the respirator should be closed. The collar should be adjusted so that it is comfortable around the neck. A towel may be placed around the patient's neck to prevent air from blowing out around the patient's face and to protect the neck from irritation.

After the patient is placed in the respirator, a problem may arise in regulating the rate and depth of respiration. In patients whose respiratory centers are still functioning, synchronizing the rate of the respirator to the rate of respiration maintained by the patient may be a problem. Although the patient is instructed to let the respirator do the work, he may find this difficult. It cannot be accomplished unless the rhythm of the breathing of the patient is regular. It is the physician who is responsible for prescribing the rate and depth of respiration, but the nurse is usually the one who is with the patient and who assists him in his adjustment.

In many patients who require assistance in maintaining breathing, secretions tend to accumulate in the airway. The methods used in this situation are similar to those previously described. The specific measures will depend on the severity of the problem.

One problem in the care of the patient in the respirator is that he can swallow only on expiration. As soon as he is given food or fluids by mouth, he should be taught to swallow only on expiration. Unlike a healthy person, the one in the respirator cannot inhibit inspiration when he swallows. Leafy foods such as lettuce should not be finely shredded, because a blast of air may carry a piece into the trachea. When fluids are offered through a straw, the head of the patient should be turned to the side, and the container, glass, or cup should be lower than his head. Otherwise the system acts as a siphon and the flow of fluid continues during inspiration as well as during expiration.

While the patient is in a tank respirator, he requires all of the care needed by any seriously ill patient. He must be moved, turned, and bathed, and his extremities put through the range of motion exercises. Unless there is a bubble oxygenator on the respirator, all care may have to be given through the portholes. One of the problems in caring for a patient in the respirator is maintaining negative pressure in the tank during inspiration. The portholes should be opened during expiration and the hands and arms introduced quickly. The sleeve of the porthole should fit snugly around the arms. Care should be taken when closing the portholes not to slam the covers as this disturbs many patients. As the dependence of the patient on the respirator diminishes, he may be taken out for some of his care. He should be continuously observed for signs and symptoms of hypoxia and returned should his condition warrant it.

Many patients who require respirator care recover sufficiently to maintain respiratory function independently. The period during which the patient is learning to live outside the respirator may also be a time of stress for him and for his attendants. If the patient has become very dependent on the respirator, he may lack confidence in his ability to maintain breathing without it. The nurse should encourage the patient to remain out of the respirator for increasing periods of time and she should try to bolster his confidence in himself. At the same time the patient should be protected from overfatigue. He should be observed for signs of developing hypoxia. In the past some persons who were believed to be psychologically dependent on the respirator were in fact physiologically dependent on it. Tests are now available to determine the degree of arterial oxygen saturation. Nurses should make careful observations of the behavior of the patient, so that nursing care and medical therapy can be planned to meet the needs of the patient. Moreover, the patient who is learning to breathe for himself should be confident that when he needs help he will get it.

The extensive discussion of considerations necessary in caring for a patient in a tank respirator is justified by the following facts: (1) Even in hospitals where mechanical cycling respirators are more commonly applied to tracheostomies to provide respiratory assistance, tank respirators are still available for emergency or supplementary use. When a tank respirator is needed, there is no time to obtain the information necessary for the safety and comfort of the patient. (2) Although any machine or device used to relieve a patient of impairment or arrest of respiration is attended by some anxiety in the patient, this problem seems to be intensified when the machine is a tank respirator. Because of the adverse effect of anxiety on respiratory function, it is imperative that the nurse know and do all in her power to alleviate or prevent anxiety in the patient with this type of problem.

Patients who require respirator care to maintain breathing usually have other serious threats to their lives and health. Since this chapter is devoted to the maintenance of oxygen supply to cells, these threats will not be discussed here.

In summary, the maintenance of breathing is essential in the total respiratory process. Breathing may fail temporarily or more or less permanently. In any event death ensues unless ventilation is promptly re-established and maintained. The essential features of any method include: (1) prompt action; (2) clearing of the airway; and (3) the use of the method that gets the air into and out of the lungs in sufficient volume to adequately ventilate the lungs.

What conditions are essential to the exchange of gases
in the lung?

As previously described, air must be regularly delivered to and removed from the respiratory membrane. The direction of movement of a gas across the respiratory membrane is determined by the difference in its partial pressure on the two sides of the membrane. Gases move from an area of higher to an area of lower pressure. Since the partial pressure of oxygen in the inspired air is higher than in the venous blood in the lung, oxygen moves from the alveoli into the blood. Since the tension of carbon dioxide in the blood is higher than in the inspired air, it moves from the blood to the alveoli.

How does the respiratory membrane affect the movement
of gases into and out of the blood?

Whereas the partial pressure of a gas on the two sides of a semipermeable membrane determines the rate and direction of movement, the permeability of the membrane regulates what is transferred across it. The respiratory membrane consists of the respiratory bronchiole, the alveolar ducts, and the alveoli as well as the corresponding capillaries, lymphatics, and connective tissues. The latter structures are included because of their intimate relationship with pulmonary membrane. The structure of the respiratory membrane is well suited to permit the free diffusion of gases between the air and the blood. It consists of an extremely thin layer of epithelium in the alveoli and of endothelium in the capillary. The total surface is enormous, as the alveolar membrane is variously estimated to present a surface of from 50 to 90 sq. M, and the capillaries surface area is estimated to be from 38 to 60 sq. M. The total alveolar surface is one half the size of a tennis court.

How do various disorders of the lung interfere with its function?

Aeration of the blood is protected by the fact that only a fraction of the pulmonary membrane is required to support most activities. Hypoxia due to a failure of diffusion does not occur unless there is an appreciable decrease in available pulmonary membrane or it is thickened; that is, the permeability of the membrane is diminished. Some of the disorders that are associated with a decrease in the area of pulmonary membrane have already been mentioned. They include emphysema, atelectasis, and pneumothorax. By thickening the membrane, pulmonary edema lessens its efficiency or permeability. In pneumonia consolidation of one or more lobes or of scattered areas reduces the area available for diffusion. Diseases such as tuberculosis predispose to tissue destruction and fibrosis. Surgical removal of a part or all of a lung lessens respiratory reserve, by diminishing the surface area available for the diffusion of gases.

How is ventilation of the alveoli protected?

Ventilation of the alveoli is protected and regulated by a number of conditions and elements. Dead space air prevents too rapid dilution of the alveolar air. Though all parts of the lung are not ventilated equally, the distribution of the air is facilitated by both structure and function. According to Fenn,[36] when the distance from the trachea to the alveoli is short, the tubes are narrower in diameter than they are when the distance is greater. The bronchioles contain muscle fibers which enable them to regulate air flow to alveoli. Pores in the walls of alveoli allow for the aeration of alveoli whose ducts are obstructed.

How does the pulmonary circulation differ from the arterial circulation?

Because of the relationship of the alveoli to the pulmonary circulation, alveolar pressure is believed to have important effects on the circulation of the blood through the lung. Unlike the systemic circulation, the pulmonary circulation is a low-pressure system. Whereas in the systemic circulation the capillaries are supported and surrounded by the tissue that they supply, pulmonary capillaries are surrounded by air and are supported by a thin network of elastic and reticulum cells. The pulmonary circulation carries all of the blood from the right to the left ventricle. It is a highly distensible system capable of holding the entire blood volume. It is affected not only by the beating of the heart, but by changes in the pressure within the thoracic cavity.

[36] *Op. cit.,* pp. 138-48.

Pulmonary circulation differs from arterial circulation in another way. In the systemic circulation, the hydrostatic pressure at the arteriolar end of the capillary is considerably higher than that of the colloid osmotic pressure of the blood proteins. This results in the transudation of fluid, water, and the substances dissolved in it into the interstitial space. This is discussed in more detail in Chapter 8.

Transudation in the pulmonary capillaries is avoided because the hydrostatic pressure of the blood is within a few millimeters of mercury of atmospheric pressure and is at least 20 to 25 mm lower than the colloid osmotic pressure (oncotic pressure) of the blood proteins. When the lungs are normally ventilated, air surrounding the capillaries creates a pressure that serves to counteract the effect of the hydrostatic pressure of the blood. Failure to aerate a lung or a portion thereof upsets the balance between the atomospheric pressure and the hydrostatic pressure in favor of the hydrostatic pressure and increases the possibility of pulmonary edema. The seriousness of the situation is increased by the fact that an increase in transudation is not followed by a comparable increase in tissue pressure. Hydrostatic pressure may be increased by any condition interfering with the flow of blood into the left auricle or increasing blood volume. It is an ever-present possibility in mitral valve disease, in failure of the left ventricle, and in high-volume anemias. It may occur in kidney failure, especially when there is sodium retention. Dyspnea is a common symptom in pulmonary edema and orthopnea is not uncommon. The responsibilities of the nurse in the prevention and treatment of the patient who is predisposed to or has pulmonary edema are discussed in Chapter 9.

As emphasized earlier, one of the significant factors in the diffusion of oxygen from the alveoli to the blood is differences in the pressure gradient between the atmosphere and the blood. One of the factors in maintaining this gradient is the regular renewal of alveolar air. Another is the high affinity of hemoglobin for oxygen. As venous blood circulates through the pulmonary capillaries, hemoglobin rapidly combines with oxygen in the plasma. Oxygen, however, diffuses through the respiratory membrane so rapidly that the oxygen pressure in the plasma is maintained at a level almost equal to that in the atmosphere.[37] Carbon dioxide passes through the respiratory membrane even more rapidly, as its rate is about 20 times that of oxygen. Despite the brief time that the blood remains in the pulmonary capillaries, the hemoglobin picks up a full complement of hemoglobin. The uptake of oxygen by hemoglobin is facilitated by the sudden drop in the level of carbon dioxide which increases the alkalinity of the blood. A decrease in hydrogen ion concentration increases the affinity of hemoglobin for oxygen, and a rise decreases it.

---

[37] George W. Wright, "Dyspnea and Allied Manifestations" in ed. T. R. Harrison, *Principles of Internal Medicine,* 4th ed., McGraw-Hill Book Company, Inc., New York, 1962, pp. 108-12.

*What factors influence the transfer of oxygen from the
blood to the cells?*

Oxyhemoglobin is carried through the arteries to the capillaries virtually
unchanged. In the tissues conditions change so that the dissociaton of oxyhemoglobin is facilitated. The partial pressure of oxygen in the tissues is low,
and oxygen moves from the plasma by way of the interstitial fluid to the cell.
The equilibrium between the oxygen dissolved in the plasma and the oxyhemoglobin is upset, and oxygen is released by the hemoglobin to restore the
balance. The decomposition of oxyhemoglobin is increased by elevation in the
temperature of the tissue and in the presence of carbon dioxide and acid
metabolites such as lactic acid. Depending on the degree of activity of a
tissue, the blood may lose from 20 per cent to almost all of its oxygen as it
passes through the capillaries.[38] The capacity to release oxygen from hemoglobin in relation to conditions in the tissue is adaptive, inasmuch as it reduces the burden on the circulatory system during exercise.

*What are some of the common causes of failure to
transport oxygen?*

Since hemoglobin is required for the transport of oxygen, any reduction in
its level or availability is accompanied by a decrease in the quantity of oxygen
delivered to the cells. Although there are some exceptions, 3 gm. of hemoglobin per 100 ml. of blood is generally required to sustain life.[39] The most
common cause of a deficiency of hemoglobin is anemia. In anemia there is a
decrease in the number of circulating erythrocytes as well as in the amount of
hemoglobin. Depending on the cause of the anemia, there may be a greater
decrease in one than in the other, but both are reduced. The principal effect of
anemia is a loss in the oxygen-carrying capacity of the blood. Most of the
signs and symptoms are due to hypoxia.

In addition to a deficient quantity of hemoglobin, hemoglobin though present in adequate quantities may be unavailable to carry oxygen. In carbon
monoxide poisoning, the level of hemoglobin is satisfactory, but varying
amounts of hemoglobin are unavailable to carry oxygen because it is in combination with carbon monoxide. Though carbon monoxide can be displaced
from hemoglobin, carboxyhemoglobin is a more stable compound than oxyhemoglobin. When carbon monoxide is inhaled, it is absorbed into the blood,
where it combines with the hemoglobin. The source of carbon monoxide is
incompletely oxidized carbon compounds. Poisoning, either accidental or in-
tentional, occurs when a person is exposed to gases formed in combustion.
For example, the Oriole family lived in a small house heated by a space

[38] Charles Herbert Best and Norman Burke Taylor (eds.), *The Physiological Basis
of Medical Practice,* 7th ed., The Williams & Wilkins Company, Baltimore, 1961, p.
458.
[39] Harry A. Davis, *Principles of Surgical Physiology,* Paul B. Hoeber Inc., New
York, 1957, p. 76.

heater. The weather was cold and the house was cold; so they kept a fire in the stove through the night. The windows were closed and insufficient oxygen was available for the complete combustion of the fuel. Therefore, carbon monoxide was formed rather than carbon dioxide. As it was formed, it was released into the surrounding air. Since carbon monoxide is odorless, the Oriole family had no warning that the air was poisoned. When the neighbors noticed that no one was about, they called the police, who discovered the family dead in their beds. Though the details differ, death which results from remaining in a closed automobile in which the motor has been left running is due to the same cause—carbon monoxide poisoning.

If one of the members of the Oriole family had awakened in time, their lives might have been saved by treatment with oxygen. This is one of the few situations in which oxygen may be administered in concentrations up to 100 per cent. The treatment of carbon monoxide poisoning with 100 per cent oxygen is based on the law of mass action. According to this law, the speed of a chemical reaction is proportional to the molecular concentrations of the reacting agents. The molecules of carbon monoxide and of oxygen both compete for hemoglobin molecules. The chances of oxygen combining with hemoglobin can be increased by increasing the amount of available oxygen.

At the tissue level, the availability of oxygen to the cells also depends on the adequacy of the blood flow. Therefore, any condition that decreases the output of blood by the heart or that increases resistance to the flow of blood will lessen the quantity of oxygen available to the tissue, that is, they cause ischemia. The harmful effect of diseases, such as atherosclerosis, that narrow the diameter of blood vessels is due to the fact that they interfere with the supply of blood to the tissues. Edema, either temporary or chronic, lessens blood supply by causing pressure on capillaries. Edema also interferes with the diffusion of oxygen delivered to the tissues. Any disturbances in oxygen supply to the tissue lessens the capacity to adapt to increased demands. The causes and effects of ischemia are discussed in more detail elsewhere.

Finally, for oxidation-reduction reactions to take place at body temperatures, enzymes are required to catalyze the necessary chemical reactions. These enzymes are sensitive to conditions in body tissues and are inactivated by certain poisons. Loss of homeostatic conditions—temperature, pH, water, and electrolytes—may inhibit the action of cellular enzymes. Poisons such as cyanide cause rapid and irreversible changes in cells because they inactivate the enzymes that enable the cells to utilize oxygen.

Whether or not cells receive enough oxygen depends, of course, on the degree to which the oxygen delivered to the cells meets the demands of the tissues. When the needs of the cells are in excess of the capacity of the organism to deliver oxygen, a condition of relative hypoxia exists. One of the limiting factors on strenuous exercise is the development of relative hypoxia. The needs of tissues for oxygen can be diminished by rest or by lowering of the body temperature. For patients who have some defect in their oxygen delivery mechanism, rest may be prescribed. Whether or not the patient actually achieves a state of rest depends in part on the skill of the nurse in modifying his social, psychological, and physical environment so that he achieves rest.

To recapitulate, the survival of all living organisms including man depends on a continuous supply of oxygen to the cells of the body and the removal of carbon dioxide which is formed in metabolism. In man oxygen is supplied to and carbon dioxide removed from the tissue by the coordinated functioning of the respiratory and circulatory systems. All cells require oxygen. Some cells, such as those in the nervous system, are highly sensitive to hypoxia.

Failure to supply oxygen in quantities required by the cells can therefore have its origin in the atmosphere, or in a failure in the respiratory, circulatory, or nervous systems. The causes of failure of oxygen supply may be summarized as follows:

1. Atmospheric
2. Failure of ventilation
    a. Obstruction of the airway
    { Mechanical
      Infections
      Allergy
      Neoplasms
    b. Paralysis of the muscles of respiration
    { Poliomyelitis
      Myasthenia gravis
      Injuries of the brain stem
      Muscle relaxants during
          anesthesia
    c. Loss of muscle tissue—muscular dystrophy
    d. Decreased compliance of lung
    e. Pneumothorax, hemothorax, pleural effusion
3. Loss of aereating surface in the lung
    a. Pulmonary edema
    b. Emphysema
    c. Pneumonia and other infections involving the lung
    d. Surgical removal of the lung
    e. Pneumothorax
    f. Atelectasis
4. Loss of oxygen-carrying power of the blood.
    a. Anemia
    b. Carbon monoxide poisoning
    c. Methemoglobinemia, sulfhemoglobinemia
    d. Other defects in hemoglobin
5. Insufficient blood delivered to the tissues—ischemia
    a. Generalized decrease in the output of the heart
    b. Localized ischemia
        (1) Atherosclerosis
        (2) Infarcts
        (3) Edema

6. Cellular utilization, anoxia
   a. Poisoning of respiratory enzymes
   b. Excessive demands of the tissues for oxygen[40]

The conditions and processes whereby oxygen is obtained from the atmosphere and made available to the cells have also been presented. The capacity to provide oxygen to the cells may be threatened at any point by the failure of one or more of these processes. When the condition develops slowly and is of long standing, the individual may be able to adapt by increasing the effectiveness of one of the processes or by decreasing his need for oxygen, or both. When the condition develops rapidly and is of marked degree, however, his survival is jeopardized. When the lack of oxygen is due to a failure of diffusion across the respiratory membrane, the addition of oxygen to the respired air may be lifesaving.

Oxygen therapy is prescribed by the physician in order to increase the supply of oxygen available to the cells. The prescription should include the method by which it is to be administered; the concentration to be maintained; and the duration of treatment. When inhalation therapists or oxygen technicians are employed, they are usually responsible for keeping the equipment in running order, for delivering equipment to the bedside of the patient, and for checking its operation throughout the procedure. The nurse prepares the patient physically and psychologically for the procedure, applies the required apparatus, supervises the care of the patient so that an effective concentration of oxygen is maintained, and attends to the personal, physical, and psychological needs of the patient. She instructs the patient, his visitors, and personnel in safety precautions and in the essential aspects of the treatment. The nurse also instructs the patient and his family in the performance of oxygen therapy at home. One of the more recent developments in the therapy of patients with chronic lung disease is the regular administration of oxygen under positive pressure. The patient is instructed to inhale oxygen under positive pressure three or four times a day. Because of the continuing contact of the nurse with the patient, most of the responsibility for oxygen therapy is borne by the nurse.

To fulfill her obligations, the nurse should have knowledge of the principles basic to effective and safe inhalation therapy and information about the different methods used to administer oxygen, as well as an understanding of the reasons that oxygen therapy is prescribed.

Oxygen therapy is frequently prescribed to combat arterial anoxia in pneumonia, pulmonary edema, or obstruction of the airway. It is also often prescribed for patients in congestive heart failure and following myocardial infarctions, as these patients usually have some degree of pulmonary edema as

---

[40] The formation of carbon dioxide and its elimination are intimately related to oxygen supply and use. Because of effects of carbon dioxide on cation-anion balance in the body, it is discussed in the following chapter.

well as failure of the peripheral circulation. In hot and humid weather, an oxygen tent has the additional value of providing a comfortable environment. Because of its availability oxygen is also utilized as a carrier gas in aerosol therapy.

As indicated earlier, the diffusion of oxygen and carbon dioxide across the respiratory membrane into the blood depends on: (1) the partial pressures of these gases in the respired air; (2) a patent airway; (3) the cyclical expansion and contraction of the chest; and (4) a diffusing surface adequate in extent and permeability. A deficiency in the supply of oxygen can therefore be the consequence of a low atmospheric or partial pressure of oxygen in the re-spired air, an obstructed airway, inadequate breathing, or a decrease in the quantity or permeability of the diffusing surface in the lung. Obviously, in-creasing the percentage composition of oxygen in the respired air will be of more value in some of these conditions than in others. For example, the addition of oxygen to the air is essential in the prevention of hypoxia in nonacclimatized persons at altitudes above 10,000 or 12,000 ft. A higher-than-normal concentration of oxygen is of little or no value unless the airway is patent and the patient is breathing. Increased concentrations of oxygen have their greatest value in the therapy of disorders in which the permeability of the diffusing membrane is decreased or the surface area is diminished. In the use of oxygen in therapy, the enrichment of the air with oxygen does not usually correct the cause of hypoxia, but it prevents its injurious effects.

Oxygen is administered by mask, catheter, tent, or canopy, or in a chamber or room. Each method has its advantages and disadvantages. For example, high concentrations of oxygen are most easily maintained by mask. Because the mask fits the face snugly, oxygen can also be administered under positive pressure by this means. Both the mask and the catheter require relatively simple equipment and allow the patient considerable freedom of movement. They offer little interference with personal care. The tent or canopy provides not only a satisfactory concentration of oxygen, but an air conditioner. The temperature and humidity of the air surrounding the patient can be main-tained at comfortable levels. In hot and humid weather, control of tempera-ture and humidity may make a valuable contribution to the well-being of the patient. Special rooms into which oxygen is piped are ideal inasmuch as the patient can be cared for in the same manner as he is in an ordinary room. The concentration of oxygen can be maintained at the desired level. Concentra-tions prescribed by the physician range from 45 to 100 per cent.

Some of the disadvantages of the different methods of administering oxygen can be minimized by appropriate nursing measures. The mask can cause irritation of the skin of the face, which can be minimized by adjusting the mask to the contours of the face and adjusting the straps so that the patient is comfortable. The straps should not be so loose that the mask moves about or so tight that the edges cut into the face. The mask should be removed every one and one-half to two hours and the face of the patient should be washed, dried, and dusted lightly with powder. Each time the mask is removed, necessary nursing procedures such as mouth care and fluids should be administered. The mask should be applied during exhalation. Some patients are very frightened about having anything applied over their face, and some are never able to adjust to the mask.

One of the methods most frequently selected for the administration of oxygen is by nasal catheter. The catheter is introduced by way of the nares into the naso- or oropharynx. Except for the level to which the catheter is introduced, the performance of the procedure is essentially the same. The nasal catheter has several disadvantages. Concentrations of oxygen above 50 per cent are difficult to secure. The catheter can be irritating to the nasal mucosa. To prevent injury to the mucosa, the catheter selected should fit comfortably and be lubricated with saline solution or a water-soluble lubricant before it is introduced. To maintain the patency of the catheter, it must be changed no less frequently than every eight hours. If nasal secretions are abundant, the catheter may have to be changed more frequently to maintain its patency. When it is reinserted after removal, the other nostril should be used. Occasionally, because of structural defect in the septum, only one nostril can be used.

After as large a catheter as can be introduced comfortably into the nares of the patient has been selected, it should be attached to the oxygen source and checked by placing the tip in a glass of water. Bubbling in the water indicates that the system is open. To determine the length of catheter to be introduced, using the catheter, measure the distance between the tip of the nose and the lobe of the ear. Mark the length of the catheter to be introduced with a small piece of tape. The direction of the natural droop of the catheter is then determined, by holding the taped portion of the catheter between the thumb and forefinger. The catheter is then rotated slowly until the tip hangs at its lowest level. The catheter is held in this position and slowly and gently inserted until the measured point reaches the entrance of the nostril. The position of the catheter should be observed through the mouth. The tip should lie just behind the uvula. The catheter should be taped firmly at the end of the nose and then carried across the cheek and taped at the temple. The catheter should be adjusted so that it lies on the inner floor of the nose, but does not loop in the nostril. It should not press against the skin of the nose, or obstruct the vision of the patient. (To prevent undue dilution of the oxygen by air, the patient should be instructed to breath only through his nose.) Because oxygen is dry, humidification of the air is essential.

The oxygen tent is another method frequently utilized for the administration of oxygen. The tent provides for a closed system in which the temperature, humidity, and oxygen concentration can be well controlled. It has several disadvantages. The patient is confined in the relatively small space of the tent. Unless the canopy is tucked in and the openings closed promptly after use, the oxygen concentration falls very rapidly.

Handbooks[41] are available that present in greater detail methods and types of equipment used in oxygen therapy, and the nurse may refer to these when questions arise. When she has access to a trained oxygen therapist, she can usually obtain desired information.

When oxygen is administered to the patient, it cannot be expected to be of benefit unless it reaches his alveoli in the desired concentration. All the equipment must be in working order, and a supply of oxygen must be available at all times. Appropriate measures must be instituted to maintain the concentration of oxygen in the respired air. Since oxygen therapy benefits the patient only if the oxygen can reach his alveoli, attention must be given to cleansing his airway. The patient should be moved, turned, and encouraged to deep-breathe and to cough. When these measures are ineffective, secretions have to be removed by suctioning. Tubing connecting the source of oxygen supply to the device by which oxygen is delivered to the patient should be checked to be sure that is is free from kinks and attached properly and tightly.

In many of the modern and well-equipped hospitals, nurses do not have to be concerned with the supply of oxygen as it is piped in from a central supply tank. In hospitals where oxygen is supplied in tanks and for patients receiving oxygen at home, the nurse carries a number of responsibilities. The nurse must check the pressure gauge to make certain that the tank contains oxygen under sufficient pressure to supply the patient with oxygen. Should the tank be allowed to empty, the concentration of oxygen in the inspired air will fall rapidly below that in the surrounding atmosphere. Precautions should also be taken to protect personnel and visitors from a falling tank. Tanks containing oxygen or other gases tend to be unstable, because they have a relatively narrow base in relation to their height. The danger of upsetting a tank can be lessened by placing it on a rack with a wide base or strapping it to the bed.

The maintenance of an adequate supply of oxygen and the safety of the patient depend on the application of knowledge of the physical and chemical characteristics of oxygen. It is a colorless, odorless, tasteless gas that is slightly heavier than air. It does not burn, but it supports combustion. The fact that it is colorless, odorless, and tasteless enables it to escape unnoticed into the surrounding atmosphere. Since oxygen is heavier than air, it tends to settle toward the bed or floor. This characteristic is most significant in the care of the patient in an oxygen tent. If the concentration of oxygen in the tent is to be maintained, the canopy must be smoothly tucked under the mattress. The part that goes over the thighs should be pulled toward the foot of the bed and tucked in at the sides and around the patient. Though instructions frequently state that a draw sheet should be utilized to secure the canopy over the thighs of the patient, according to the findings of a study made by Eileen Cronicun[42] this is not necessary. In fact, lower concentrations of oxygen

[41] *Linde Oxygen Therapy Handbook,* Linde Company Division of Union Carbide Corporation, New York City.
[42] Unpublished Master's Thesis.

were usually observed when a draw sheet was utilized to secure the canopy. When the draw sheet was tucked in tightly, patients felt restrained. They then raised their knees and dislodged not only the draw sheet, but the sides of the canopy. An important point in maintaining oxygen concentration was found to be keeping the canopy well tucked under the mattress. Since oxygen is heavier than air, the concentration of oxygen will be lowest near the lower part or floor of the tent. In fact, an effective concentration of oxygen can be maintained at the floor of a tent that has an open top.

Oxygen, as a gas, diffuses readily. Openings in the tent allow oxygen to escape and lower its concentration. Vents in the wall of the tent should be opened only when necessary to give care, and they should be closed completely after care is completed. The lower the opening, the more rapidly oxygen escapes.

Regardless of the method of application, the fact that oxygen supports combustion is an important consideration in the safety of the patient. Oxygen does not burn, but it lowers the kindling point of combustible materials, so that they burn, often with almost explosive rapidity. To illustrate, Frank Jay, a 58-year-old former carpenter, was in severe congestive heart failure. At the time he was placed in the oxygen tent, both he and the members of his family were instructed not to smoke. One evening when Mr. Jay's son came to visit him, Mr. Jay asked for a cigarette, which his son gave to him. Despite the fact that the canopy was made of rubber, it burned in a matter of moments. Although his face, hands, and scalp were burned, Mr. Jay was saved from death by an orderly who smothered the flames with a woolen blanket. To prevent this sort of accident, *No Smoking* signs should be prominently displayed. Relatives and friends, as well as the patient, should be helped to understand the importance of this prohibition. No open flame, whatever its source, is permissible. Patients such as Mr. Jay may be allowed to smoke once or twice daily, provided the supply of oxygen is discontinued for the duration of the period of smoking.

Sources of electric sparks, whether from static electricity or from faulty equipment, should be avoided. The call light of the patient should be replaced with one with a shockproof switch or with a hand bell. Because woolen blankets may be a source of static electricity, they should be replaced with cotton blankets. Static electricity is a particular problem in regions in which the humidity of the environment is low. Another precaution generally advised is to avoid the use of oil or alcohol when rubbing the back of the patient in an oxygen tent.

Should a procedure be performed that requires the use of electrical or thermal energy, the oxygen supply should be discontinued while it is in progress. For example, the oxygen supply should be discontinued during the taking of X rays at the bedside, and during the use of cautery and suction machines. Sometimes suctioning must be continued to keep the airway patent.

Because of the implications oxygen therapy has for many people, the patient may experience increased fear and anxiety as a result of his feeling unsafe, at the time the therapy is started. Furthermore most patients who are acutely hypoxic have some degree of anxiety. Before oxygen therapy is instituted, a simple statement to the effect that oxygen will improve his breathing should be made. While the equipment is being brought from the storeroom, the patient should be prepared by placing him in the desired position and making him as comfortable as possible. When oxygen is administered by tent, the motor should be turned on and the oxygen flow started before placing the patient in the tent. The flow of oxygen should be started before any device for administering oxygen is directly applied. Care should be taken to get the tent over the head and face of the patient without touching him. After oxygen therapy is instituted, the nurse should stay with the patient until she is sure that the equipment is operating properly and the patient is comfortable. Fifteen or twenty minutes spent with the patient at this time can do much to add to his feeling of safety. As with any seriously ill patient, he should be visited regularly for observation and care.

When oxygen is used more or less routinely in therapy, the patient should be prepared to expect it. For example, it often is prescribed in the postoperative treatment of patients undergoing a surgical procedure in which the route of approach is through the chest wall. Part of the preoperative preparation of the patient should be to inform him that oxygen therapy not only is possible, but is usual. If he wakes up in the oxygen tent, he will be less likely to be frightened.

Patients who are seriously ill at the time oxygen therapy is started may become dependent on it and be afraid to have it discontinued. The patient who is treated in a tent is more likely to have difficulty than patients treated by other techniques. Return to breathing ordinary air can usually be accomplished by gradually extending the time that the patient remains outside the canopy. The capacity of the patient to tolerate ordinary concentrations of oxygen can be checked by removing the canopy while he eats his meals or is bathed. The patient is returned to the tent if signs or symptoms indicating hypoxia appear. Some patients take very little time to become readjusted to breathing air; others require time and considerable support to make the transition. Among the advantages of discontinuing oxygen therapy during a period when the patient is receiving care is that it facilitates the giving of care. Furthermore, the patient is reassured by the presence of the nurse. He does not have to fear that he will have to wait to have the canopy replaced promptly should he require oxygen. The fact that the patient has been through a frightening experience should not be forgotten. He may require time, patience, and encouragement to regain confidence in his ability to maintain his own oxygen supply.

Oxygen administered by methods other than the oxygen tent threatens the safety of the patient by its effect on mucous membranes. Oxygen gas is dry, and when it comes in contact with the mucous membranes of the respiratory tract, it takes on moisture. Water is added to the oxygen gas by bubbling it through water. Although the oxygen gas introduced into the oxygen tent is dry, it is circulated in a closed system that contains the expired air of the patient. Therefore, moisture is readily available to moisturize the air. In fact, expired air contains more water than is required to maintain a suitable degree of humidity. Excess water is removed by circulating the air over ice or through a refrigeration unit. Steaming of the tent on the *inside* indicates some failure in this mechanism. Condensation on the *outside* occurs for the same reason that moisture accumulates on a pitcher of ice water on a hot, humid day. Cold air holds less moisture than hot air. When hot air is chilled rapidly, water precipitates as rain or as drops on a water glass.

Although oxygen poisoning does not occur very often in adults, it can occur when the patient inhales a high concentration for 24 hours or longer. Concentrations of 100 per cent can be inhaled for up to 24 hours without observable effects. With prolonged inhalation of high concentrations of oxygen, changes characteristic of irritation take place in the lung. Lung tissue becomes swollen. Treatment is to lessen the percentage concentration of oxygen inhaled. The condition can be prevented by reducing the percentage concentration of oxygen inhaled after 12 to 24 hours.

A point relating to the safety of the patient, though not directly affecting the effectiveness of oxygen therapy, is that all equipment should be clean when it is brought to the bedside of the patient. At the completion of oxygen therapy, all equipment that has been in contact with the patient, his secretions, or expired air should either be discarded or thoroughly washed and disinfected. For example, when disposable canopies are used, they should be removed and discarded. If they are saved, they should be washed in a detergent solution and dried. Though nurses are not always directly responsible for the cleanliness of the equipment, they should refuse to use it when it is unclean.

Whatever method is used for the administration of oxygen, attention to the comfort as well as the survival of the patient is essential. The care of the patient should be planned so that his hygienic needs are met. He should be bathed, moved, and turned, and have mouth and back care. An extra effort may have to be made to ensure an adequate fluid and food intake. Attention should be paid to the body alignment and the position of the patient in bed. A footboard serves not only to support the feet, but to lessen the weight of bed covering on the feet. Care directed toward increasing the comfort and relaxation of the patient is important, not only for the usual reasons, but because relaxation decreases the need for oxygen and thereby increases the effectiveness of oxygen therapy.

Finally, as in the care of any sick patient, observation is an important facet of care. Among the pertinent observations are included: (1) observations related to the degree to which the needs of the patient for oxygen are being met; (2) observation of the equipment; and (3) observation of safety precautions and identification of threats to the safety of the patient.

The nurse, therefore, has many responsibilities in the care of the patient under oxygen therapy. They include: (1) the preparation of the patient for what to expect; (2) care throughout the treatment that encourages his cooperation, lessens his fears, increases comfort and relaxation, and contributes to the benefits of the procedure; (3) attention to the details in the performance of oxygen therapy that increase the likelihood of the desired concentration of oxygen reaching the alveoli; (4) observations of the respiratory status of the patient, his reactions to oxygen therapy, and his general condition; (5) observation of the equipment and its functioning; (6) attention to the details that reduce the threats to the safety of the patient; (7) care directed toward keeping the airway clean and promoting the expansion of the lung; and (8) coordination of the care of the patient, so that his care is individualized.

How is the adequacy of respiratory function determined?

For the purposes of discussion, respiratory function can be considered as involving four general types of processes: (1) the movement of air to and from the respiratory membrane; (2) its diffusion across the respiratory membrane; (3) the transport of oxygen and carbon dioxide to and from the pulmonary circulation and the tissues; and (4) the utilization of oxygen by the cells.

With the development of thoracic surgery and the discoveries of the space age, interest in pulmonary function and ways of measuring it have been greatly stimulated. At one time, tests were limited to a determination of the vital capacity and to the clinical judgment of the physician. Methods are now available whereby function at the different levels can be measured with some degree of accuracy.

Some of the terms used to describe pulmonary function are defined below.

The *tidal volume* represents the volume of air moved in or out during one respiratory cycle. In the adult at rest, the tidal volume is approximately 500 ml of air. The *minute ventilation* can be obtained by multiplying the tidal volume by the number of times the person breathes per minute. If the patient can and does cooperate, a decrease in tidal volume is clinically significant. A normal volume may be found in patients with certain diseases of the lung, such as emphysema.

Inspiratory reserve volume is the maximum amount of air that can be inspired at the end of a tidal inspiration.

Expiratory reserve volume is the maximum quantity of air that can be expelled at the end of a tidal expiration.

The *residual volume* is the quantity of air remaining in the lung at the end of a maximum expiration.

The *vital capacity* is the largest volume of air that can be expelled after a maximum inspiration. At one time this was the only test of breathing that was available. Present knowledge indicates that, by itself, a normal vital capacity is not a very dependable indicator of pulmonary function. Its value can be increased by timing the length of expiration. This is known by the term *timed vital capacity.* The normal young person can expel at least 95 per cent of his vital capacity in three seconds. The findings in this test relate well with the maximum breathing capacity.[43] Patients with emphysema frequently have a normal untimed vital capacity, but an abnormal timed vital capacity.

The *total lung capacity* is the total volume of air found in the lung after a maximum inspiration. It equals the sum of the vital capacity and the residual air.

The maximum breathing capacity is the largest volume of air that can be breathed on command during a specified interval of time. The patient is instructed to breathe as rapidly and deeply as he can into a system that offers little resistance for a period of 15 seconds. The rate of breathing usually varies from 50 to 70 per minute. Whatever the unit of time, the result is converted to liters per minute. The normal value for men is from 80 to 120 ll per minute. For women it is somewhat less. This test gives more accurate information about an individual's pulmonary function than any single test. In some disorders of the lung the vital capacity is normal while the maximum breathing capacity is markedly diminished. The reverse may also be true. Though the accuracy of all the tests is influenced by the understanding and cooperation of the patient, cooperation is imperative to the performance of maximum breathing capacity

Although tests of ventilation may be determined under any degree of activity, they are usually obtained with the patient at rest. Physical activity, excitement, emotional upsets, or any condition increasing the need for oxygen will be accompanied by changes in ventilation. The patient who is to have his

[43] H. Corwin Hinshaw and L. Henry Garland, *Disease of the Chest,* 2nd ed., W. B. Saunders Company, Philadelphia, 1963, p. 100.

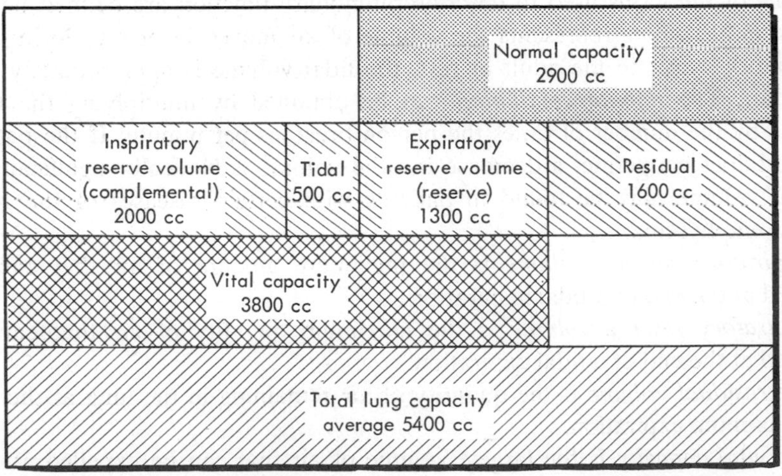

FIGURE 7—6. This diagram demonstrates the terms used to describe the various types of pulmonary volumes. (Adapted with permission of The Macmillan Company from *Textbook of Physiology,* p. 220, by Caroline E. Stackpole and Lutie C. Leavell. Copyright 1953 by The Macmillan Company.)

maximum breathing capacity measured should be prepared as if he were to have a test of basal metabolic rate. Though the details for the preparation of the patient vary somewhat in different institutions, they are essentially as follows:

1. No food is eaten after dinner or, at the latest, 9:00 P.M.
2. Breakfast and medications are withheld until after the test.
3. The patient is expected to retire early.
4. The patient is to stay in bed until after the test. Activities—morning care, shaving, showering, smoking, gum chewing—are prohibited.
5. Temperature, pulse, and respiration are then recorded before the test. An elevation in body temperature should be reported.
6. The patient should be transported to the respiratory laboratory in a wheel chair.
7. After the test has been completed, the patient should be served his breakfast and his usual schedule of activities should be restored.

The objective of the preparation of the patient is to send him to the laboratory in a relaxed state, so that the findings will have value. One of the reasons for performing the maximum breathing capacity is to determine whether or not the patient's respiratory reserve is sufficient for him to tolerate and benefit from the removal of a portion of his lung tissue. The patient requires information about what to expect and what is expected of him. The test may be performed with the patient in the sitting or standing position. He breathes into an instrument known as a spirometer. As the patient breathes into and out of the mouthpiece, changes in pressure in the floating drum cause it to move up and down. These excursions are recorded on the writing drum. From measurements of the size and number of respiratory cycles, the quantity of gas moved in each excursion or over a period of time can be calculated.

The nurse is usually responsible for the physical preparation of the patient for breathing tests. She is often responsible for explaining to the patient what to expect and what is expected of him.

A second type of test of pulmonary functional reserve is the exercise tolerance test. This test is performed in a variety of ways. The purpose is to determine the amount of exercise that the patient can take before he develops dyspnea. For example, if he can walk the length of a hallway or up one or two flights of stairs without experiencing dyspnea, he has a satisfactory respiratory reserve. If, on the other hand, he becomes dyspneic on walking a short distance or at rest, his reserve is probably unsatisfactory. His exercise tolerance can be measured more exactly by having him walk on a treadmill, pedal a stationary bicycle, or step up and down from a stair step. Ordinary exercise serves very well, however. Various methods are available to measure the volume of residual air. The test is usually performed by the inhalation of some gas such as helium and measurement of its dilution in the expired air.

Methods are available for determining the adequacy of diffusion of oxygen and carbon dioxide through the respiratory membrane as well as the degree of oxygen saturation of the blood. Carbon dioxide content can also be determined. The level of hemoglobin and the hematocrit provide information about the oxygen-carrying power of the blood. In chronic hypoxia, due to causes other than anemia, both are likely to be elevated. With a significant decrease in the level of hemoglobin in the blood, all the tissues are deprived of an adequate supply of oxygen.

The determination of the utilization of oxygen by the tissues is known as the basal metabolic rate. It is decreased in any condition in which the tissues are deprived of adequate supplies of oxygen- or caloric-containing compounds or of substances that regulate the rate of metabolism. Since temperature influences the rate of chemical reactions, the rate of metabolism is increased by fever and decreased by lowering the body temperature. The metabolic rate is elevated by exercise, ingestion of food, hyperthyroidism, and hyperthermia. It is also elevated in leukemia. Some examples of conditions in which the metabolic rate is diminished include starvation, inactivity, chronic hypoxia, hypothyroidism, and hypothermia.

The most common method used to determine the structural condition of the lung and its relationship to the other organs is X ray and/or fluoroscopy. X ray provides information about vital capacity as well. Chest X ray and photofluoroscopy are indispensable tools not only in diagnosis of diseases involving structures in the thoracic cavity, but in case finding. Though their most extensive use is in case finding, that is, in identifying persons who have lesions indicative of tuberculosis, they are proving to be of value in discovering other disease processes in the lung as well as in the heart and other structures in the mediastinum. When an abnormality is found, the patient is encouraged to see his physician for further study and diagnosis.

Despite the value of the various methods used to measure respiratory processes, the day-by-day evaluation of the status of the patient depends on the observation of the patient. Among these observations are included the characteristics of breathing. Normal breathing has certain characteristics that can be described. The breathing cycle occurs at regular intervals of from 14 to 16 per minute. During and immediately following strenuous exercise it may rise to as high as 24 cycles per minute, but it does not normally rise much beyond that. The depth of respiration is sufficient to move about 500 ml. of air during quiet respirations, but the quantity is increased during activity. One of the features of normal respiration is its effortless character. The individual is not consciously aware that he is breathing, and except when he has been exercising strenuously, the onlooker is not aware that he is making an effort. A simple description of normal breathing, then, is that it is rhythmical and effortless, and though the rate and depth do change, changes are within limits and are in response to a stimulus placing known extra demands on the organism.

Similar to other bodily functions, breathing may deviate from the normal. The rate and depth may be greater or less than normal. The rhythm may be abnormal, or breathing may become difficult or labored. Sources of disturbances in breathing include any condition that increases the need for oxygen or for the elimination of carbon dioxide. Since the functioning of respiratory and circulatory systems is integrated, disturbance in the function of either may cause alteration in breathing. Since the action of the muscles of respiration depends on stimulation from the nervous system, abnormalities of breathing may have their origin in the nervous system.

What prefixes are used to indicate abnormalities of breathing? Define each.

The same prefixes are used to indicate changes in the direction from normal as are used to describe deviations from the normal of other body functions. They include *a-, olig-, brady-, hypo-, hyper-, poly-, tachy-,* and *dys.* The prefix is added to the suffix, *-pnea,* which means to breathe. The term for normal or easy breathing is eupnea.

Tachypnea, hyperpnea, and polypnea are all terms that are loosely defined as rapid breathing. Tachypnea should be used when the rate of breathing is above 24 per minute, but the depth of respiration is not changed appreciably. In contrast, hyperpnea should be used when the depth of respiration is increased. The breathing of a well-trained athlete is a good example of the proper use of the term "hyperpnea." When he exercises, the depth of his respiration increases, but the rate rises very little. Polypnea should be used when the minute volume of breathing is markedly increased. The term "hyperventilation" is sometimes used as a synonym.

At the other end of the breathing range, apnea means a cessation of respiration. Continued apnea is, of course, incompatible with life. Apnea does occur in certain types of periodic breathing.

Bradypnea is used to characterize an excessively slow rate of breathing in which the rate is less than 10 cycles per minute. There is no appreciable change in the depth of respiration. A common cause of bradypnea is respiratory depression from excessive dosages of narcotics or sedatives.

Hypopnea is used to indicate a decrease in the depth of respiration that is out of proportion to the decrease in rate. Sleep is a condition in which hypopnea is physiological. Sedatives and narcotics may also be responsible for hypopnea.

What are the common types of periodic breathing? What mechanisms are involved in its development?

Two disturbances in breathing will be discussed in detail. They are periodic breathing and dyspnea. Periodic breathing occurs in a number of disease conditions. It is characterized by repeated cycles in which a person breathes deeply for a period of time and then breathes only slightly or not at all.

The most common type of periodic breathing is Cheyne-Stokes breathing. In Cheyne-Stokes respiration there is a slow waxing and waning of respirations with the cycle lasting from 45 seconds to three minutes. Although all the mechanisms for the development of Cheyne-Stokes respirations have not been explained, according to Guyton,[44] the condition must be initiated by some condition that under- or overstimulates respiration. For example, for some reason Mr. Oaks's breathing becomes more rapid and deeper than usual. With the increased rate and depth of respiration, the level of carbon dioxide in his blood falls. When, a few seconds later, arterial blood with a low tension of carbon dioxide reaches his brain, there is insufficient carbon dioxide to stimulate respiration, and his breathing wanes or ceases. During the period of hypopnea or apnea, the concentration of carbon dioxide in the blood plasma rises. When the level of plasma carbon dioxide is sufficiently elevated, breathing is reinitiated.

Although the mechanisms have not been clarified, Cheyne-Stokes respirations have been observed in aviators and mountain climbers at high altitudes and in patients with heart failure. Though the reasons for their occurrence have not been elucidated, they probably include one or a combination of the following: (1) a decrease in the sensitivity of the respiratory center to carbon dioxide; (2) a decrease in the carbon dioxide content of arterial blood; (3) oxygen deficiency; (4) a decrease in the flow of blood to the brain; and (5) a reflex increase in intracranial tension.[45]

Another type of periodic breathing is known as Biot's breathing. According to Guyton,[46] this type of breathing is frequently confused with Cheyne-Stokes breathing. Rather than waxing and waning, breaths come in couples, triples, quadruples, or some other number of cycles, with periods of apnea in between cycles of breathing. This type of breathing is characteristically associated with a disorder of the brain. It is seen in patients with very great increases in intracranial pressure, with contusion or compression of the brain tissues, or with destructive diseases of the brain. It is indicative of a very poor prognosis. Death usually follows soon after it appears.

The basic mechanism in the development of Biot's breathing is quite different from that of Cheyne-Stokes respiration, as the former is related to oscillations in the blood flow to the brain. High intracranial pressure compresses the arteries and cuts off the flow of blood to the brain. Lack of blood flow to the brain is followed by the initiation of reflexes which, if successful, elevate the pressure of the blood above that of the intracranial pressure. As the nutrition of the vasomotor center improves, impulses to maintain the high blood pressure diminish and the blood pressure falls. During the period when the blood

[44] *Op. cit.*, p. 564.
[45] John S. LaDue, "Cardiac Failure and Function Tests," in Sodeman, *Pathologic Physiology*, 3rd ed., W. B. Saunders Company, Philadelphia, 1961, p. 569.
[46] *Op. cit.*, p. 566.

pressure is rising, the individual breathes deeply. During the phase when it is falling, he stops breathing or is apneic.

How is dyspnea defined? What are some of the factors in its development?

A second commonly observed disturbance in breathing is dyspnea. Dyspnea is defined as difficult or painful breathing and as such is a subjective sensation. The patient who is dyspneic has a desire or hunger for air and is conscious of the need for increased respiratory effort. Some authorities do not exclude labored breathing from the definition, however. Rubin[47] quotes Christie as defining dyspnea as "a conscious or visible increase in respiratory effort." The latter definition covers the person who, though dyspneic when awake, is typically not conscious of having to make an increased respiratory effort when he is asleep. A person such as a well-trained athlete may be hyperpneic and yet not be dyspneic, as breathing, though increased in depth, is effortless. A person who is dyspneic may or may not have labored breathing which is obvious to the observer. To illustrate, Mary Willow flew from Lima to Cusco, Peru, which is at an elevation of about 12,000 ft. The hotel where Mary stayed had no elevator, and her room was on the second floor. Though she did not experience any difficulty as she walked up the stairs, after she arrived at her room, she felt short of breath. She did not have obviously labored breathing; but she felt short of breath, or dyspneic.

Mrs. Bird, who is described in the next chapter, has true dyspnea. She has congestive heart failure with marked edema of her lungs. She is conscious of the necessity for breathing, and her breathing appears labored. She has been experiencing air hunger and she makes an obvious effort to breathe.

What mechanism or mechanisms are responsible for the development of dyspnea?

According to Rubin,[48] whatever the nature of the disorder that predisposes to dyspnea, the immediate cause of increased effort in breathing is stimulation of the centers in the nervous system controlling respiration. Inasmuch as the respiratory centers are interconnected with the cerebral cortex, dyspnea may be initiated by impulses having their origin in the cerebral cortex or from the muscles of respiration. Since cells in the respiratory centers are sensitive to carbon dioxide and to hydrogen ions as well as to severe deficiencies in oxygen supply, a rise in the level of the first two or a fall in the latter may act as a stimulus in the development of dyspnea.

Guyton[49] summarizes the factors in the development of dyspnea as:

[47] Eli H. Rubin and Morris Rubin, *Thoracic Diseases,* W. B. Saunders Company, Philadelphia, 1961, p. 189.
[48] *Ibid.,* p. 190.
[49] Arthur C. Guyton, *Textbook of Medical Physiology,* 2nd ed., W. B. Saunders Company, Philadelphia, 1961, p. 578.

(1) "an actual abnormality of the respiratory gases in body fluids, especially hypercapnia,[50] but to a much less extent anoxia, (2) the amount of work that must be performed by respiratory muscles to provide adequate ventilation, and (3) the state of mind itself."

To relate the above to Engel's *Unified Concept of Disease,* previously discussed in Chapter 2, dyspnea may arise from a disturbance in the mental apparatus or from the direct effect of an injurious or potentially injurious agent on cells. In any given individual any one or all of the above factors may be operating.

Dyspnea is found in patients with a variety of disturbances in the pulmonary, circulatory, and nervous systems. Conditions associated with dyspnea include:

1. Pulmonary—conditions increasing the work of breathing or predisposing to carbon dioxide retention and to hypoxia, or to both
   a. Obstruction of the trachea and bronchi
   b. Loss of compliance of the lung, as in pulmonary edema from congestion, inflammation, or fibrosis of the lungs as seen in persons with far-advanced tuberculosis
   c. Following resection of the lung, particularly after pneumonectomy
   d. Limited movement of the chest and diaphragm
      (1) Emphysema—chest is almost fully expanded at end of expiration
      (2) Weakness or paralysis of muscles of respiration
      (3) Pneumothorax
2. Abnormalities in circulation
   a. Inadequate oxygenation of blood in lungs
   b. Increased blood in the pulmonary vascular tree
   c. Insufficient transport of oxygen
      (1) Severe anemia
      (2) Cardiac failure
3. Acidosis
   a. Respiratory acidosis (interference with elimination of carbon dioxide)
   b. Metabolic acidosis (accumulation of hydrogen ion)
4. State of mind—fear, anxiety

Persons differ greatly in their susceptibility to dyspnea. This is true even among those who have a serious reduction in their vital capacities. Persons whose dyspnea is on a psychic basis become short of breath when they are exposed to an anxiety-inducing situation. For one person dyspnea occurs only when he is in a crowd, or a closed room; for another, it develops when he enters an automobile or when he has to see his boss. The individual may or may not associate the anxiety-producing event with his dyspnea.

[50] Hypercapnia is the technical term for an elevated carbon dioxide in plasma.

Most, if not all, dyspneic persons who are conscious and alert suffer some psychic stress, for they know that breathing is essential to life. The diseases with which shortness of breath occurs are frequently of a serious nature. Most, if not all, patients are conscious of the implications of dyspnea. Moreover, dyspnea is accompanied by highly unpleasant sensations which in turn intensify the awareness of the patient of his precarious state. The degree to which altered biochemical conditions, that is, hypercapnia and hypoxia, and the psychic state influence the development of dyspnea in a given individual varies, but both are often present.

Despite some differences in the details, the following incident illustrates the influence of biochemical and psychic factors in dyspnea. Jim Warbler, aged 25, was acutely ill. His diagnosis was ascending spinal poliomyelitis. As the hours passed, his muscles of respiration became progressively weaker. To pull air into his lungs, he used his accessory muscles of respiration. As breathing became more difficult, Jim felt short of breath, and he could be seen to be using the muscles of his neck and upper thorax to breathe. Though he was placed in a tank-type respirator, he continued to complain of feeling that he was about to smother. Each time the portholes in the tank were open, he became frantic, and remained so, until they were tightly closed. At times Jim's behavior suggested that he was in a state of panic. The reasons underlying his behavior were physiological as well as psychological. Compared to normal respiration, the tank respirator is an inefficient instrument. Jim undoubtedly suffered from hypercapnia and relative hypoxia. He was acutely ill with a disease that deprived him of his capacity to meet his own need for oxygen and would probably leave him seriously handicapped. He had been discharged from the Army only a few months earlier and had just completed arrangements for his life work. Since the occupation that he had chosen was one requiring a strong and healthy body, the likelihood of his being able to carry out his plans seemed remote. Was it any wonder that in the first days after he was placed in the respirator, he was terrified? As Jim recovered, function returned to his muscles of respiration, and he was eventually able to maintain his own breathing without difficulty. During the period of acute illness, Jim's survival was threatened by his inability to ventilate his own lungs. His behavior was undoubtedly influenced by the meanings the entire situation had for him.

In patients whose dyspnea is associated with congestive heart failure, or emphysema, shortness of breath usually appears first in response to exercise. Mrs. Bird complained for some weeks that each time she walked upstairs, she had to stop and "catch her breath" on the landing before climbing to the top. She noticed that when she walked against the wind she became short of breath before she had walked very far. In individuals such as Mrs. Bird, dyspnea is protective, inasmuch as it decreases activity to the degree to which the pulmonary and circulatory system can supply oxygen to the tissues.

In planning the nursing of the patient who is dyspneic, several factors should be known. Certainly, the nature of the disorder responsible for the dyspnea influences the care required by the patient. When there is a significant defect in the ability of the patient to obtain oxygen or to eliminate carbon dioxide, his need for oxygen and for the elimination of carbon dioxide can be reduced by rest. The degree of rest required will vary with the nature and seriousness of the condition of the patient. In patients in congestive heart failure, such as Mrs. Bird, the sitting position often provides some relief, since the vital capacity is greater in the sitting than in the supine position. Although the reasons for the improved vital capacity are not completely known, it is probably due to the fact that the blood is pooled in the splanchnic areas and lower extremities.

In patients in whom dyspnea appears to be associated with an increase in a sensitivity of the vagal receptor mechanism, morphine sulfate may give relief by depressing this mechanism. Morphine sulfate is often prescribed for patients who are dyspneic in association with heart disease, as it not only lessens the dyspnea, but decreases awareness of the situation. Mrs. Bird's physician prescribed 10 mg (1/6 gr) of morphine sulfate for the relief of her dyspnea. Not only was her dyspnea improved, but she appeared to be less apprehensive. In contrast, morphine sulfate is contraindicated in patients whose dyspnea is associated with a depression of the respiratory center. For example, Jim Warbler was not given morphine. Neither was Mrs. Pine, who had asthma and an associated emphysema.

Orthopnea, which is usually associated with longstanding dyspnea, is made more difficult by the recumbent position. Orthopnea is usually associated with heart disease. Elevation of the diaphragm is believed to aggravate pre-existing pulmonary congestion and further decrease the vital capacity. Although the sitting position does not always completely relieve orthopnea, it is the position assumed by the patient, if he has a choice. Moreover, when orthopnea is severe, maximum relief is afforded by sitting forward slightly. The position can be attained by supporting the patient in the upright position and placing a tray table over his thighs to rest on. When a cardiac bed is available, the foot of the bed can be dropped, so that the bed essentially becomes a chair. A comfortable chair can be used in the same way. The chair or cardiac bed has at least two advantages. The legs and feet are in the dependent position, and a certain amount of fluid is in effect removed from the circulation and the position is more natural. Whatever type of bed or chair is utilized, the trunk and extremities of the patient should be well supported. When a patient is placed in a cardiac bed or chair, the feet should be supported on a footboard or footstool and should not be permitted to dangle. The objective of the position is to provide for the comfort of the patient and to ensure maximum rest.

In addition to orthopnea, another form of dyspnea is paroxysmal dyspnea. Though it is not a form of asthma, this condition is sometimes called cardiac asthma. Because of its tendency to occur at night, it is sometimes called paroxysmal nocturnal dyspnea. Although paroxysmal dyspnea develops in much the same manner as orthopnea, it differs from orthopnea inasmuch as it is accompanied by bronchiolar spasm. There is a wheezing type of respiration, which is probably due to an accumulation of exudate in the airway associated with a swelling of its mucous lining and bronchiolar spasm.

The circumstances under which an attack occurs are similar to the following. When Mr. Whipple, who has some degree of congestive heart failure, goes to bed at night, he lowers his headrest somewhat. Later he awakens, acutely short of breath and wheezing. He sits up, hanging his feet over the edge of the bed. After a short time his breathing improves and he coughs and removes the accumulated secretions.

One final alteration in breathing will be discussed, that is, hyperventilation, a condition in which both the depth and rate of breathing are increased. As is to be anticipated, hyperventilation increases the loss of carbon dioxide, and as a consequence respiratory alkalosis develops. The effects of hyperventilation can be corrected by holding the breath for a few moments or by rebreathing air in a paper bag. Hyperventilation occurs in healthy persons who are under stress or in a state of exhaustion and in the emotionally unstable, as well as in persons who have disorders in which the hydrogen ion content of the blood is raised. Hyperventilation, which occurs in metabolic acidosis, is known as Kussmaul breathing. It is physiological or compensatory inasmuch as the increase in the rate and depth of respiration is due to stimulation of the respiratory center by the hydrogen ion and for a time, at least, it facilitates cation-anion balance in the blood by increasing the elimination of carbon dioxide. (See Chapter 8 for a fuller discussion.)

As emphasized throughout the chapter, cell function depends on the continuous delivery of oxygen to the cells and the prompt removal of carbon dioxide. Carbon dioxide is not only a product of metabolism, but it regulates respiratory processes, both at the site of respiratory exchange in the lung and at the tissue level as well as by its effects on the respiratory center in the brain. The respiratory system is the site at which exchange of gases takes place between the internal and external environment. The two environments are separated by a semipermeable membrane, through which oxygen and carbon dioxide diffuse with great rapidity. In this chapter the importance of the exchange of gases—oxygen and carbon dioxide—to cell function has been stressed. The structure of the respiratory system is such that as air passes through it, the air is warmed, cleansed, and humidified. The organism is further protected from foreign material by an active phagocytic system that destroys particulate matter that reaches the alveoli.

The respiratory system is subject to a great variety of diseases. The general nature of these is no different from those found in other regions of the body. Their specific effects result from the nature of the function of the respiratory system and the part of the respiratory system that is involved. They are of infectious, chemical, hypersensitivity, neoplastic, degenerative, or traumatic origin. The upper and, to a lesser extent, the lower respiratory tracts are exposed to contaminants in the surrounding atmosphere. These include dust, smoke, bacteria, viruses, fungi, and other noxious agents. Exposure may be continuous or single, large or small. For example, exposure to smoke may be continuous or it may be an isolated event. The respiratory systems of persons who smoke heavily and who live in large cities are more or less continuously exposed to smoke and its products. Single or isolated exposures occur when individuals are in a smoke-filled room. Disorders of the respiratory system may be acute or chronic. According to reports by the U.S. National Health Survey, acute disorders of the respiratory system rank at the top as a cause of disabling illness involving one or more days in bed. The relationship of the various causes of acute disabling illness can be seen in Figure 7-7. Although

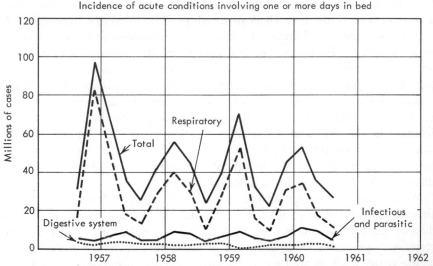

FIGURE 7–7. Acute Conditions and Disability. In the summer quarter of 1961, 26.5 million cases of acute conditions involving one or more days in bed were reported by the U.S. National Health Survey. Persons spent an average of 1.3 days in bed due to disability, and "currently employed" persons lost 1.2 days from work. The incidence of acute conditions and the persons' days of disability were generally greater than during the third quarter of 1960. (Adapted. Department of Health, Education and Welfare, Office of the Secretary, *Indicators*, April, 1962, p. 7.)

the incidence of respiratory diseases changes from year to year, it remains the most frequent cause of morbidity.

Within the last ten years increasing emphasis has been placed on chronic respiratory diseases as causes of morbidity and mortality. In the past, tuberculosis was the only major chronic disease of the respiratory system to receive much attention. Presently, malignant neoplasms of the respiratory system, chronic bronchitis, emphysema, bronchiectasis, and asthma–hay fever are known to be responsible for an increasing incidence of disability and mortality. According to the National Vital Statistics Division, Washington, D.C., whereas the death rate for all conditions rose 11.9 per cent between the years 1954–1959, the death rate from emphysema rose 158.0 per cent. The next highest increase was in malignant neoplasms of the trachea, bronchus, and lung, and specified as primary. The percentage increase was 54.1.

According to Walkup,[51] two respiratory diseases, emphysema and tuberculosis, account for a significant portion of disability benefits granted under the disability program of the Bureau of Old Age and Survivors Insurance. All of these disorders decrease respiratory reserve and, as such, limit the capacity of the individual to obtain oxygen from the air and to return carbon dioxide to it.

One aspect of respiratory disease that has not been discussed, because it does not have a direct bearing on respiratory function, is the fact that ducts from the paranasal sinuses and from the middle ear open into the nasal passages and nasopharynx. Furthermore, the mucous membrane lining these ducts and their related cavities is continuous with the mucous membrane lining the airway. Infections with swelling of the respiratory mucous membrane can interfere with drainage of the paranasal sinuses or middle ear by obstructing their respective ducts, or an infectious process can spread by way of a duct to one or more of the above structures. With the extension of an infection to the paranasal sinuses or to the middle ear, microorganisms multiply and abscess formation is likely. In addition to the signs and symptoms associated with a pyogenic process, there is pain in the area of the affected structure. Because of its proximity to the mastoid cells, infections of the middle ear may spread to the mastoid cells. Because of the proximity of the mastoid cells and the paranasal sinuses to the brain, infections in these structures predispose to meningitis and brain abscess. Middle-ear infections—otitis media—may also impair hearing. The drum membrane may rupture as a consequence of increased pressure. Subsequent scarring reduces its ability to respond to sound waves. The general factors in the therapy of infections are discussed in Chapter 4.

The focus of this chapter has been the importance to survival of supplying cells with oxygen, so that energy can be released to support the activities of the cell. Although oxygen is continuously present in the air, its partial pressure depends not only on its percentage composition but on atmospheric pressure. In the presence of an adequate partial pressure of oxygen in the air, delivery of oxygen to the cells depends on the coordinated functioning of the respiratory and circulatory systems. Integration and coordination of the functions of these two systems is effected by the nervous system. A number of activities are regulated: the act of breathing; modifications of breathing during swallowing, coughing, and sneezing; the rate and depth of respiration; the rate of circulation in relation to respiratory function; and the integration of respiratory and circulatory function in relation to the needs of the entire individual.

Disturbances in the function of respiration can occur at any level. Acute and chronic diseases that threaten respiratory function are common causes of disability and mortality. In the care of the acutely ill, one of the aspects of nursing care having a high priority is maintaining the supply of oxygen to the alveoli. Often the survival of the patient depends on the achievement of this objective.

The following summaries of diseases and/or conditions involving the respiratory system supplement the discussion in the text.

Summary of Diseases and/or Conditions Involving the Respiratory System

Diagnostic Category	Etiological Factors	Incubation Period and Nature of Onset	Severity of Illness and Course	Part of Respiratory Tract Involved and Response	Effect on Adequacy of Respiratory Function	Focus of Nursing	Major Medical Treatment
1. Infections: Common cold Acute rhinitis	Variety of viruses 1. Virus of Andrews 2. Enteroviruses 3. Adenoviruses 4. Myxoviruses	18–48 hours. Gradual onset with irritation, dryness, rawness, or tickling in the nasopharynx or nose. Highly contagious	Mild. Too sick to work but not enough to stay in bed	Nasal passages and related structures. Coryza, sneezing, nasal obstruction, thin watery discharge becomes thick and purulent and lasts for several days or weeks	Nasal congestion interferes with conditioning air	Isolation Rest Fluids Adequate diet Teach protection, prevention, and purpose and methods of treatment	Rest Medication for headache, nasal congestion, and elevated temperature Isolation Antibiotics have no effect on viruses and should not be used in primary infection Individual may be sensitized to the antibiotic
Sinusitis Paranasal	Bacterial infection secondary to allergic or viral rhinitis, obstruction which follows smoking, use of alcohol, and damp weather	Local pain and tenderness. Headache in morning when exudate has collected overnight. Sometimes have edema of overlying facial skin	Sinusitis usually subsides as primary infection runs its course. Can become serious with frank suppuration and abscess formation which can lead to osteomye-	Related sinuses—frontal, maxillary, ethmoid and sphenoid, and nasal passages. Nasal swelling and congestion. Drainage from sinuses into nasal pharynx. With repeated		Position—semi-Fowler's Control of pain Mouth care, especially if surgery with nasal packing Fluids encouraged	Re-establish drainage channels Surgery to correct structural defects, example: deviated septa Antibiotic therapy after causative organism has been identified Mucosa- and vessel-constrict-

Summary of Diseases and/or Conditions Involving the Respiratory System—Continued

Diagnostic Category	Etiological Factors	Incubation Period and Nature of Onset	Severity of Illness and Course	Part of Respiratory Tract Involved and Response	Effect on Adequacy of Respiratory Function	Focus of Nursing	Major Medical Treatment
			litis and spread of infection to the orbit, meninges, and brain	attacks there may be thickening of the sinus mucosa, continual partial obstruction, and chronic inflammation			ing medications Irrigation of sinuses
Tonsillitis Acute Chronic	Hemolytic 1. Streptococci 2. Staphylococci	Mild to severe sore throat. If chronic infection, becomes disseminated to other parts of the body, such as the joints, muscles, bursae, ear, and eye	Acute tonsillitis usually does not warrant hospitalization unless complications arise, such as pneumonia. Surgery is usually indicated in chronic tonsillitis	Tonsils and crypts Adenoids usually affected also Tonsils are inflamed and enlarged Ulcerations may be found in crypts	Obstruction to flow of air through the pharynx, usually not serious.	Bed rest Control of sore throat Throat irrigations Ice collar Control temperature Fluids encouraged Sponge bath	Tonsillitis usually treated by a tonsillectomy, after attack subsides Medication for pain, sore throat, and causative agent Antibiotics usually ordered after organism is identified and sensitivity studies are carried out
Pharyngitis (Chronic)	1. Sinusitis 2. Adenoiditis	Dryness, scratchiness, sense of	Can become severe infection	Mucous membranes of the	May have mild dis-	Alertness for streptoccal	Antibiotics Prevent superim-

Diagnostic Category	Etiological Factors	Incubation Period and Nature of Onset	Severity of Illness and Course	Part of Respiratory Tract Involved and Response	Effect on Adequacy of Respiratory Function	Focus of Nursing	Major Medical Treatment
	3. Allergic response to: a. Food b. Inhalants Smoke House dust	irritation with mild to severe soreness on swallowing	extending either upward to cause acute otitis media, rhinitis, or sinusitis or downward to cause laryngitis, tracheitis, bronchitis, or pneumonic	pharynx without infiltration or ulceration Mucosa becomes red with hypertrophy of superficial lymphoid nodules Dryness and crusting in nasopharynx May have hacking cough	turbances in transportation of incoming air	infections in those with a history of rheumatic fever Throat irrigations Easily swallowed diet Fluids encouraged	posed infection Throat irrigations Discovery and removal of etiological factor When lateral bands affected, 10% silver nitrate applied to reduce inflammation Nasal spray for dryness and crusting
Laryngitis inflammation	1. Filtrable viruses, sequelae of acute rhinitis 2. Pneumococci 3. Hemolytic streptococci 4. Hemolytic staphylococci 5. Other inflammation of the upper respiratory tract	First and most important symptom is hoarseness Cough and aching pain in larynx accompanied by hoarseness Fever usually the first day or two	May have epidemic character Edema of the larynx might necessitate tracheotomy Pharyngitis a common complication Cough may become choking and strangling.	Hyperemia of laryngeal mucosa Hoarseness, sore throat, sputum can become purulent Cough	Can lead to severe obstruction to incoming air—asphyxia	Isolation (not strict) Rest—especially to voice Anticipate needs Provide means of communication Fluids encouraged No opiates Diet limited to	Isolation Rest—limited use of voice Medication for causative agent Local treatment—silence Promote elimination—fluids Aspirin for elevated temperature Elixir of Pheno-

Summary of Diseases and/or Conditions Involving the Respiratory System—Continued

Diagnostic Category	Etiological Factors	Incubation Period and Nature of Onset	Severity of Illness and Course	Part of Respiratory Tract Involved and Response	Effect on Adequacy of Respiratory Function	Focus of Nursing	Major Medical Treatment
	6. Mouth breathing 7. Trauma—chronic a. Smoke b. Dust c. Voice abuse		Usually self-limiting within 10 days. However, without proper treatment and disuse of voice may lead to chronic situation			fluids in acute stages Room well ventilated, temperature 72° F. and humidity 50%	barbital or sodium bicarbonate for cough—NO OPIATES Throat sprays
Acute undifferentiated respiratory disease (includes "grippe" or "flu"—not influenza)	Adenoviruses (military populations)	4–7 days Gradual onset	More severe than common cold Frequently go to bed voluntarily	Pharynx and associated structures Lungs usually clear Sore throat, discomfort in chest Nasal discharge infrequent		Same as common cold	Symptomatic therapy Aspirin for relief of feverishness, headache, and malaise
Primary atypical pneumonia	Adenoviruses Eaton agent	12–14 days Insidious onset, may have minor respiratory symptoms for several	Acute illness usually lasts 1 week. Convalescence prolonged—6 weeks or more.	Lung—lower lobes most frequent Pulmonary lesions and infiltrates	Impairment of exchange of gases	See pneumonia	See pneumonia

Diagnostic Category	Etiological Factors	Incubation Period and Nature of Onset	Severity of Illness and Course	Part of Respiratory Tract Involved and Response	Effect on Adequacy of Respiratory Function	Focus of Nursing	Major Medical Treatment
		days	Return of strength slow	Cough, sputum (can become mucopurulent) Substernal discomfort Râles are audible			
Influenza (A used as example)	Viruses 1. Influenza A, B, and C 2. Sendai virus	18–36 hours to 3 days Sudden onset usually See last column	Sporadic infections are relatively mild; however, in epidemics some may be serious to critically ill Recovery ranges from 2–3 days to weeks depending on complications such as bacterial infections The most serious complication is staphylococcal pneumonia	Respiratory epithelium Response is often less than in common respiratory disease Sneezing, watery nasal discharge, or stuffy nose frequently occurs Productive cough usually develops along with substernal chest pain	Interference with conditioning of air	See common cold and care to minimize: Fever and chills Onset accompanied by severe frontal headache usually followed by fever and chills Stabbing retro-orbital pain Widespread myalgia especially in the legs Spasm of abdominal muscles, also	Vaccine for prevention (influenza A, A$_2$, and B) Chemotherapy reserved for secondary infections Bed rest Codeine for cough

467

Summary of Diseases and/or Conditions Involving the Respiratory System—Continued

Diagnostic Category	Etiological Factors	Incubation Period and Nature of Onset	Severity of Illness and Course	Part of Respiratory Tract Involved and Response	Effect on Adequacy of Respiratory Function	Focus of Nursing	Major Medical Treatment
						periarticular pain Prostration to some degree Most common secondary symptoms are anorexia, nausea, and constipation	
Chronic bronchitis	1. Irritants: smoke and other air pollutants 2. Pneumococcus 3. Staphylococcus	Insidious or may follow other respiratory diseases such as pneumonia and bronchial asthma Persistent cough and expectoration	Mild to severe depending on the development of other respiratory diseases, such as emphysema	Mucus secreting glands in mucosa of trachea and bronchi Hypersecretion of mucus, bronchial spasm, and bronchiolar fibrosis Chronic productive cough Sputum is ropy, white, and elastic Postnasal drip is frequent, choked-up feeling to dyspnea	Ventilation difficult because of the narrowing of the bronchial tree	Rest—isolation (limited exposure to others) Fluids encouraged Control of cough and expectorations	Promote cleansing airway with expectorants, steam inhalations, and proteolytic enzymes Antimicrobial therapy Intermittent positive pressure breathing may be necessary

Diagnostic Category	Etiological Factors	Incubation Period and Nature of Onset	Severity of Illness and Course	Part of Respiratory Tract Involved and Response	Effect on Adequacy of Respiratory Function	Focus of Nursing	Major Medical Treatment
Bronchiectasis	1. Bronchial obstruction 2. Infections such as bronchopneumonia which cause stagnant exudate 3. Atelectasis causes traction on bronchi	Symptoms can be intermittent or chronic depending on respiratory infections. Usually seen in lower lobes of the lung	Depends on superimposed infection and not necessarily degree of bronchial cilatation. Can become irreversible	Smooth muscle and elastic tissue of bronchial tubes Tubular or saccular dilatation of bronchial tube system. Patchy distribution or local. May lose ciliated epithelium which is replaced by fibrous tissue. Cough, mucopurulent sputum—large amounts in the morning and hemoptysis dyspnea. Postnasal drip, sinusitis	Loss of protective mechanisms. Difficulty in transportation of gases	Collection of sputum, postural drainage. Teach postural drainage Protection from other respiratory diseases. Control atmosphere (moist air) Position—ease of ventilation. Much emotional support—chronic recurring disease Teach patient to avoid infections by staying out of crowds, etc., especially in cold, damp	Antibacterial medication to control infection which is common diagnosis Postural drainage Bronchograph—extent of dilatation Tracheostomy—keep bronchial tree patent Aerosal to promote cough and expectoration Moist air—help liquefy tenacious sputum Resection of damaged bronchiectatic segments of the lung if disease is discovered early enough Chronic forms—treatment is mainly symp-

Summary of Diseases and/or Conditions Involving the Respiratory System—Continued

Diagnostic Category	Etiological Factors	Incubation Period and Nature of Onset	Severity of Illness and Course	Part of Respiratory Tract Involved and Response	Effect on Adequacy of Respiratory Function	Focus of Nursing	Major Medical Treatment
						weather	tomatic and supportive, as outlined above
Pneumonia	Infectious agents (70 types) 1. Pneumococcus 2. Staphylococcus 3. Hemolytic Streptococcus 4. Friedlander's bacillus 5. Other viruses, fungi, and parasites	Descending infection. Coryza may precede the onset of pneumonia for several days. Onset is usually abrupt with shaking, chills, fever, tachycardia, and the development of pleuritic pain and productive cough. Sputum is "rusty" or pinkish	Usually lasts 2 or 3 weeks with complete resolution Fatality with treatment is rare today in the middle-aged group Severe complications can arise: 1. Atelectasis 2. Plural effusion (empyema)	Entire lobe of lung (lobar) or patchy area throughout lung tissue (lobular or broncho-pneumonia) Lung consolidation in stages 1. Red hepatization (blood serum and cells pour into alveoli) 2. Gray hepatization, alveoli are packed with rbc's and fibrinous exudate 3. Resolution—by phagocytosis	Decrease in surface area of lung for the exchange of gases	Bed rest—respiratory isolation Fluid encouraged Collection of sputum Deep breathing and coughing Vital signs Mouth care Oxygen therapy Teach protection, prevention, and methods of treatment	Bed rest—respiratory isolation Antimicrobial therapy, depending on causative agent Medication for elevated temperature Sputum examined —gram stain and culture and sensitivity Blood studies and culture Oxygen therapy if necessary X rays—determine extent of lung consolidation and effects of treatment Fluid therapy Analgesics for chest

Diagnostic Category	Etiological Factors	Incubation Period and Nature of Onset	Severity of Illness and Course	Part of Respiratory Tract Involved and Response	Effect on Adequacy of Respiratory Function	Focus of Nursing	Major Medical Treatment
				Dyspnea, pleuritic pain, cough, sputum, râles			pain—no morphine (Cecil states it is used)
Pleural effusion		Usually secondary to some lesion outside the pleura. Example: (1) Inflammatory pleural effusion (pleurisy) is secondary to an inflammatory process of the lung. (2) Noninflammatory hydrothorax—clear, pale, straw-colored serous fluid—associated with healthy pleura. (3) Hemorrhagic hemothorax—frank blood—	Inflammatory transudate can become an exudate and progress to empyema (frank pus), severe constitutional symptoms—fever, night sweats, chills, anorexia	Pleura—clear transudate or exudate within the "pleural cavity." Dyspnea develops from compression. Chest pain produced—varies from dull to stabbing. Dry cough. Shift of mediastinum to unaffected side	Increase in negative pressure Decrease in distensibility of lung. Decreased vital capacity	95% of pleural effusion is tuberculous Use proper precautions Bed rest Fluids	1. Antimicrobial therapy if underlying cause is infection Many treat as primary tuberculous lesion for 3–6 months. Frequent X ray follow-up Antimicrobials may be instilled in the pleural cavity if nontuberculous 2. Removal of fluid if necessary by instituting water-sealed drainage or aspiration 3. With empyema usually surgical evacuation of

Summary of Diseases and/or Conditions Involving the Respiratory System—Continued

Diagnostic Category	Etiological Factors	Incubation Period and Nature of Onset	Severity of Illness and Course	Part of Respiratory Tract Involved and Response	Effect on Adequacy of Respiratory Function	Focus of Nursing	Major Medical Treatment
		traumatic penetration of chest wall					abscess is necessary 4. Analgesics for chest pain
Asthma	Bronchial obstruction due to (1) allergic reaction to inhaled antigens, (2) respiratory infection, and/or 1 and 2 together. Emotional disturbances. Some individuals have atopic tendency which is inherited. They should be protected from becoming sensitized to environmental and seasonal inhalants not	Episode may begin suddenly without warning and may last from minutes to several hours. Shortness of breath is usually accompanied by cough, wheezing, and respiratory effort. The person feels as if he is suffocating and exhibits fear	Episodes may be mild and controlled with medication or may persist with status asthmaticus which is resistant to treatment	Bronchial tubes: 1. Edema of mucosa 2. Hypertrophy of walls 3. Contraction of smooth muscle 4. Dilatation of blood vessels 5. Increase in secretion by mucous glands Response Expiratory dyspnea and wheezing Cough Overinflation of the lungs which can lead to emphysema	Disturbances in exchange of gases (ventilation). To maintain air exchange, great effort is required leading to fatigue	1. Observe situation and/or circumstances of episode 2. Position—ease of respiration 3. Medication given promptly for relief of attack 4. Rest 5. Oxygen therapy 6. Nonstimulating environment 7. No matter what the cause of the attack,	1. Bronchodilators—relief of bronchospasm by drugs such as aminophyllin, ephedrine, and epinephrine. Acute attack—epinephrine, 0.3 ml subcutaneous. May be followed by ephedrine, aminophyllin, etc. 2. Postural drainage 3. Expectorants—iodide compounds 4. Study of allergies—skin test, sensitivity, and

Diagnostic Category	Etiological Factors	Incubation Period and Nature of Onset	Severity of Illness and Course	Part of Respiratory Tract Involved and Response	Effect on Adequacy of Respiratory Function	Focus of Nursing	Major Medical Treatment
	harmful to nonatopic					treatment is necessary to neutralize the histamine release which is causing the symptoms	psychogenic causes 5. Oxygen therapy with intermittent, positive, pressure breathing 6. Antibiotics if superimposed infection 7. Limited use of sedation 8. Support general health 9. Adrenal cortical steroids—chronic episodes
Emphysema	1. Partial bronchial obstruction, ex.: chronic bronchitis, also atmospheric irritants—dusts and fumes 2. Loss of elasticity of pul-	Insidious. Shortness of breath upon raising without cough. Shortness of breath progresses to a point where a steady effort is required to ventilate the	Course of the disease may be rapid with ensuing death within a few years or the duration may be as long as 20–30 years depending on other super-	Air sacs become overdistended with air Productive cough Dyspnea Hyperinflation of chest—"barrel chest"	Poor distribution of gases throughout the lung Difficulty in expelling air Increase in residual lung vol-	1. Rest—conservation of energy 2. Teach breathing exercises, energy savers 3. Position—ease ventilation	1. Elimination of bronchial irritants—no smoking 2. Antibiotics to control infection 3. Bronchodilator drugs 4. Oxygen therapy should be used

Summary of Diseases and/or Conditions Involving the Respiratory System—Continued

Diagnostic Category	Etiological Factors	Incubation Period and Nature of Onset	Severity of Illness and Course	Part of Respiratory Tract Involved and Response	Effect on Adequacy of Respiratory Function	Focus of Nursing	Major Medical Treatment
	monary tissue —degenerative 3. Loss of pulmonary tissue (decrease in mass)	lungs during waking hours	imposed respiratory diseases		ume and decrease in maximal breathing capacity Decrease in arterial oxyhemoglobin saturation Respiratory failure may occur when normal gas exchange cannot be provided, resulting in carbon dioxide retention and unsaturated arterial blood Respiratory acidosis	4. Vital signs	with caution as patients with severe emphysema may have CO_2 narcosis and it is their lack of O_2 which is keeping them alive. Oxygen may be ordered at only 1–2 l per minute. Should not be over 40% oxygen when using intermittent positive pressure devices. Watch patient for signs of CO_2 narcosis 5. Breathing exercises—economy of ventilation 6. Treatment of cardiac complications

Diagnostic Category	Etiological Factors	Incubation Period and Nature of Onset	Severity of Illness and Course	Part of Respiratory Tract Involved and Response	Effect on Adequacy of Respiratory Function	Focus of Nursing	Major Medical Treatment
							7. Tracheostomy may be necessary with bronchial obstruction 8. Need some form of artificial respiration to help them eliminate CO_2. Also may need intermittent positive pressure devices, which will increase the inspiratory phase and deliver more oxygen across the alveolar membrane
Pneumothorax Open communication between	1. Bronchopleural fistula Tuberculosis Malignant disease Postoperative	Sudden large pneumothorax can be very serious with collapse of the lung on the	Absorption of the gases depends on the state of health of the pleura. Re-expansion	Gas in the pleural space shifts to the unaffected side. Collapse of lung tissue de-	Vital capacity decreases proportionately with amount of air in	1. Observe—stability of blood pressure. Productive character of	1. Medical emergency—air must be removed from pleural space to prevent mediastinal

Summary of Diseases and/or Conditions Involving the Respiratory System—Continued

Diagnostic Category	Etiological Factors	Incubation Period and Nature of Onset	Severity of Illness and Course	Part of Respiratory Tract Involved and Response	Effect on Adequacy of Respiratory Function	Focus of Nursing	Major Medical Treatment
pleural space and atmosphere Closed—not in communication with atmosphere	complication of lung resection Emphysema 2. Opening in thoracic wall (trauma) 3. Rupture of subpleural bleb 4. Artificial pneumothorax as therapy	affected side with exquisite chest pain and respiratory distress. A small pneumothorax may be asymptomatic. If spontaneous —usually have sudden sharp pain followed by dyspnea	of the lung may be prevented by fibrosed lung tissue or thickened visceral pleura	pending on amount of gas within pleural space, and this is dependent on the size of the pleural leak	pleural space Hypoxic hypercapnia may develop due to disturbances in exchange of gases	respiration. Chest pain. Increase in temperature 2. Care of patient with chest tubes and water-sealed drainage 3. Teach patient necessities of safety with tubes and purposes of treatment	shift and collapse of other lung, which would cause death 2. Removal of air from pleural cavity if necessary by instituting water-sealed drainage 3. Removal of fluid from pleural cavity if present by aspiration 4. Activity restricted until lung expands 5. Surgery may be indicated in the presence of a ruptured bulla that fails to close 6. Immediate closure of open wound

Diagnostic Category	Etiological Factors	Incubation Period and Nature of Onset	Severity of Illness and Course	Part of Respiratory Tract Involved and Response	Effect on Adequacy of Respiratory Function	Focus of Nursing	Major Medical Treatment
Atelectasis	1. Bronchial obstruction 2. External compression* 3. Failure of lung to expand at birth 4. Mucus, foreign body Reduced tone of respiratory muscles	May be sudden and/or gradual. If a lobe or entire lung collapses, person experiences anxiety, dyspnea, and tachypnea	Seen postoperatively due to mucus plugs. Mild to severe. Can lead to death from asphyxia. Also can lead to emphysema, spontaneous pneumothorax	Pulmonary alveoli. Collapse of alveoli. Dyspnea and tachypnea. Difficulty raising sputum	Prevents adequate exchange of respiratory gases	Coughing and deep breathing bedfast patients. Ambulation	7. Expansion of lung followed by X ray. Clear airway

* Reduced tone of respiratory muscles.

REFERENCES

Books

American Red Cross, *First Aid Textbook,* Prepared by The American National Red Cross for the Instruction of First Aid Classes. 4th ed. revised. Doubleday and Co., Inc., Garden City, New York, 1957.

Arnow, Harriette, *The Dollmaker,* The Macmillan Company, New York, 1954.

Banyai, Andres L. (ed.), *Nontuberculous Diseases of the Chest,* Charles C Thomas, Springfield, Illinois, 1954.

Best, Charles Herbert, and Norman Burke Taylor (ed.), *The Physiological Basis of Medical Practice,* 7th ed., The Williams and Wilkins Co., Baltimore, 1961.

Boies, L. R., *Fundamentals of Otolaryngology,* 3rd ed., W. B. Saunders Co., Philadelphia, 1959.

Cherniack, R. M., and L. Cherniack, *Respiration in Health and Disease,* W. B. Saunders Co., Philadelphia, 1961.

Comroe, Julius H., and Robert D. Dripps, *The Physiological Basis for Oxygen Therapy,* Chares C Thomas, Springfield, Illinois, 1950.

Davis, Harry A., *Principles of Surgical Physiology,* Paul B. Hoeber, Inc., New York, 1957.

Douglas, William O., *Beyond the High Himalayas,* Doubleday and Company, Inc., Garden City, New York, 1952.

Flitter, Hessel H., *An Introduction to Physics in Nursing,* 4th ed., The C. V. Mosby Co., St. Louis, 1962.

Harmer, Bertha, and Virginia Henderson, *Textbook of the Principles and Practices of Nursing,* 5th ed., The Macmillan Company, New York, 1955.

Hinshaw, H. Corwin, and L. Henry Garland, *Disease of the Chest,* W. B. Saunders Co., Philadelphia, 1956.

Introduction to Respiratory Diseases, National Tuberculosis Association, 1961.

Jenson, J. Trygve, *Introduction to Medical Physics,* J. B. Lippincott Co., Philadelphia, 1960.

Linde Oxygen Therapy Handbook, Linde Company, Division of Union Carbide Corporation, New York City.

Major, Ralph H., *Classic Descriptions of Disease,* Charles C Thomas, Springfield, Illinois, 1939, pp. 597-630, 635-40.

Manhattan Eye, Ear and Throat Hospital, *Nursing in Diseases of the Eye, Ear, Nose and Throat,* 10th ed., W. B. Saunders Co., Philadelphia, 1958.

Riley, Richard L., and Francis O'Grady, *Airborne Infection,* The Macmillan Company, New York, 1961.

Rubin, Eli, and Morris Rubin, *Thoracic Diseases,* W. B. Saunders Co., Philadelphia, 1961.

Sadove, Max, and James Cross, *The Recovery Room,* W. B. Saunders Co., Philadelphia, 1956.

Articles

Andrewes, Christopher Howard, "The Viruses of the Common Cold," *Scientific American,* CCIII, December, 1960, pp. 88-102.

Banyai, Andrew, "Chronic Bronchitis," *Geriatrics,* XVII, No. 1, January, 1962, pp. 5-14.

Baum, Gerald L., and Jan Schwarz, "Pulmonary Histoplasmosis," *New England Journal of Medicine,* CCLVIII, No. 14, April 3, 1958, pp. 677-84.

Bedell, George N., "Treatment of Pulmonary Emphysema," *Journal of the American Medical Association,* CLXIX, No. 15, April, 1959, pp. 1699-1702.

Bickerman, Hylan A., "Antitussives," *American Journal of Nursing,* LXIII, No. 4, April, 1963, pp. 61-64.

Boran, Hollis C., "Pulmonary Emphysema," *Medical Clinics of North America,* XLIII, No. 1, January, 1959, pp. 33-49.

Buechner, Howard A., and Morton Ziskind, "The Management of Respiratory Tract Emergencies," *Medical Clinics of North America,* XLVI, No. 2, March, 1962, pp. 437-56.

Burch, G. E., N. P. DePasquale, and A. L. Hyman, "Influence of Temperature and Oxygen Concentrations in Oxygen Tents," *Journal of the American Medical Association,* CLXXVI, June 24, 1961, pp. 1017-25.

Burrows, Benjamin, "Pulmonary and Respiratory Diseases in the Aged," *Postgraduate Medicine,* XXXI, No. 3, March, 1962, pp. 296-302.

Coates, E. Osborne, et al., "Oxygen Therapy," *Postgraduate Medicine,* XXIV, July, 1958, pp. 60-66.

Creighton, Helen, and William Coulter, "The Whys of a Pulmonary Function Test," *American Journal of Nursing,* LX, No. 12, December, 1960, pp. 1771-74.

Creighton, Helen, and J. Winthrop Peabody, Sr., "Inflammatory Diseases of the Pleura," *American Journal of Nursing,* LIX, No. 3, March, 1959, pp. 346-48.

Curtis, John K., Howard K. Rasmussen, and Edna Cree, "Clinical Evaluation of Pulmonary Function Tests," *Medical Clinics of North America,* XLIII, No. 1, January, 1959, pp. 17-25.

Dantzig, Senge B., et al., "A Mathematical Model of the Human External Respiratory System," *Perspectives in Biology and Medicine,* IV, Spring, 1961, pp. 324-76.

Davies, D. F., and A. H. Davies, "Lung Cancer—Cigarette Smoking as a Cause," *American Journal of Nursing,* LXI, No. 4, April, 1961, pp. 64-69.

Dickinson, Richard W., "Pulmonary Emphysema: Etiologic Factors and Clinical Forms," *Annuals of Internal Medicine,* LIII, No. 6, December 15, 1960, pp. 1105-19.

Eastman, Douglas, and Jean Maybrey, "Suction and Maintenance of an Airway," *American Journal of Nursing,* LIII, No. 5, May, 1953, pp. 552-53.

Ebert, Richard V., "Chronic Bronchitis and Pulmonary Emphysema," *Postgraduate Medicine,* XXIX, No. 4, April, 1961, pp. 341-45.

Fenn, Wallace, O., "The Mechanism of Breathing," *Scientific American,* CCII, No. 1, January, 1960, pp. 138-48.

Ferris, B. G., Jr., "Studies of Pulmonary Function," *New England Journal of Medicine,* CCLXII, March 17, 1960, pp. 557-62, and March 24, 1960, pp. 610-14.

Fishbein, Morris, "Medical Progress 1958," *Postgraduate Medicine,* XXV, January, 1959, pp. 107-12.

Frank, Nedd Robert, and Alice Mary Shedyah, "Laboratory Analysis of Pulmonary Function," *American Journal of Nursing,* LVI, August, 1956, pp. 1015-18.

Gardner, Warren, "Problems of Laryngectomees," *Journal of Chronic Diseases,* XIII, No. 3, March, 1961, pp. 253-60.

Gilmore, Stuart I., "Rehabilitation after Laryngectomy," *American Journal of Nursing,* LXI, No. 1, January, 1961, pp. 87-89.

Gordon, Archer S., et al., "Critical Survey of Manual Artificial Respiration," *The Journal of the American Medical Association,* CXLVII, December 8, 1951, pp. 1444-53.

Greene, Nicholas M., "Fatal Cardiovascular and Respiratory Failure Associated with Tracheotomy," *New England Journal of Medicine,* CCLXI, October 22, 1959, pp. 846-48.

Hadley, Florence, and Katherine J. Bordicks, "Respiratory Difficulty: Causes and Care," *American Journal of Nursing,* LXII, No. 10, October, 1962, pp. 64-67.

Hall, Wendell H., "The Specific Diagnosis and Treatment of the Pneumonias," *Medical Clinics of North America,* XLIII, No. 1, January, 1959, pp. 191-208.

Hammarsten, James F., and Stewart Wolf, "The Role of Emotions in Respiratory Disease," *Medical Clinics of North America,* XLIII, No. 1, January, 1959, pp. 113-25.

Harris, H. Williams, "What Do You Know About Coughing," *American Journal of Nursing,* LIII, No. 2, February, 1953, pp. 162-63.

Halinger, Paul H., Kenneth L. Johnston, and Mario D. Mansueto, "Cancer of the Larynx," *American Journal of Nursing,* LVII, No. 6, June, 1957, pp. 738-41.

Herbert, William M., "Crushing Injuries of the Chest," *American Journal of Nursing,* LIX, No. 5, May, 1959, pp. 678-81.

Horton, Gleen E., and A. L. Grerup, "Practical Pulmonary Function Testing for the Practicing Physician," *Geriatrics,* XIV, May, 1959, pp. 284-92.

Horton, Glenn, "Testing of Pulmonary Functions," *Geriatrics,* XVII, No. 2, February, 1962, pp. 73-81.

Hunter, Samuel, "Traumatic Hemopneumothorax," *Postgraduate Medicine,* XXIX, No. 4, April, 1961, pp. 374-80.

Jackson, G. G., *et al.,* "Susceptibility and Immunity to Common Upper Respiratory Viral Infections—The Common Cold," *Annals of Internal Medicine,* LIII, No. 4, October, 1960, pp. 719-37.

Jacoby, Jay, *et al.,* "Treatment of Respiratory Emergencies," *Postgraduate Medicine,* XXV, April, 1959, pp. 373-75.

Jimison, Carmin, "Nursing Care after Laryngectomy," *American Journal of Nursing,* LVII, No. 6, June, 1957, pp. 741-43.

Leithauser, Daniel J., "Early Ambulation," *American Journal of Nursing,* L, No. 4, April, 1950. pp. 203-6.

Leonhardt, Kurt O., "Resuscitation of the Moribund Asthmatic and Emphysematous Patient," *The New England Journal of Medicine,* CCLXIV, No. 14, April 20, 1961, pp. 785-90.

Linden, Maurice, E., "Some Psychological Aspects of Rescue Breathing," *American Journal of Nursing,* LX, No. 7, July, 1960, pp. 971-74.

Livingstone, Huberta M., "Nursing Care in Oxygen Therapy," *American Journal of Nursing,* LVII, No. 1, January, 1957, pp. 65-68.

Lore, John M., "Tracheostomy," *A.M.A. Archives of Otolaryngology,* LXVIII, December, 1958, pp. 727-36.

MacDonald, Frank M., "The Medical Management of Bronchiectasis," *Medical Clinics of North America,* XLIII, No. 1, January, 1959, 209-17.

MacVicer, Jean, "Exercises Before and After Thoracic Surgery," *American Journal of Nursing,* LXII, No. 1, January, 1962, pp. 61-62.

"The Major Pulmonary Diseases," *Medical Clinics of North America,* XLIII, No. 1, January. 1959, entire issue.

Marchetta, Frank C., Sidney Anthone, and Anna Aungst, "A Method of Tracheotomy Care," *A.M.A. Archives of Otolaryngology,* LXV, March, 1957, pp. 296-99.

Marks, Asher, *et al.,* "A New Ventilatory Assistor for Patients with Respiratory Acidosis," *The New England Journal of Medicine,* CCLXVIII, No. 2, January 10, 1963, pp. 61-67.

Marple, Charles D., "Cyanosis," *American Journal of Nursing,* LVIII, No. 2, February, 1958, pp. 222-25.

McClure, Eugenia, and Leighton L. Anderson, "Pulmonary Emphysema," *American Journal of Nursing,* LVII, No. 5, May, 1957, pp. 594-98.

McGrath, Dorothy, and Betty K. Kruger, "Chest Suction," *American Journal of Nursing,* LXII, No. 6, June, 1962, pp. 72-73.

Mitchell, Roger S., and Giles F. Filley, "Diffuse Obstructive Pulmonary Emphysema, a Poorly Understood Disorder," *Postgraduate Medicine,* XXIII, No. 2, February, 1958, pp. 156-63.

"Mouth-to-Mouth Artificial Respiration," *Nursing Outlook,* VII, September, 1959, p. 520.

Nelson, T. G., *et al.,* "Cricothyroidotomy," *American Journal of Nursing,* LXI, No. 1, November, 1961, pp. 74-76.

Noer, Rudolf, "The Management of Acute Chest Injuries," *Postgraduate Medicine,* XXIII, No. 4, April, 1958, pp. A40-A48.

Overholt, Richard, "Resection of Carotid Body for Asthma," *Journal of the American Medical Association,* CLXXX, No. 10, June 9, 1962, pp. 809-12.

Pecora, David V., and Diran Yegian, "Bacteriology of the Lower Respiratory Tract in Health and Chronic Diseases," *New England Journal of Medicine,* CCLVIII, January 9, 1958, pp. 71-74.

Plum, Fred, and Marcelle P. Dunning, "Techniques for Minimizing Trauma to the Tracheobronchial Tree after Tracheotomy," *The New England Journal of Medicine,* CCLIV, No. 5, February 2, 1956, pp. 193-200.

Rackemann, Francis M., "The Natural History of Hay Fever and Asthma," *The New England Journal of Medicine,* CCLXVIII, No. 8, February 21, 1963, pp. 415-19.

Reimann, Hobart, "Current Problems of the Pneumonias," *Annals of Internal Medicine,* LVI, No. 1, January, 1962, pp. 144-54.

Schaffer, Frank J., *et al.,* "Rehabilitation of Patients with Chronic Pulmonary Disease," *Medical Clinics of North America,* XLIII, No. 1, January, 1959, pp. 315-32.

Schlesinger, Eva M., "Nursing the Patient with a Crushed Chest," *American Journal of Nursing,* LIX, No. 5, May, 1959, pp. 682-84.

Shaffer, Joseph A., *et al.,* "Bronchial Asthma in Adults," *Journal of the American Medical Association,* CLXXIV, No. 14, December 3, 1960, pp. 1810-13.

Sloan, Herbert, and Mary Blackburn, "The Patient with Bronchiectasis," *American Journal of Nursing,* LV, No. 5, May, 1955, pp. 561-64.

Smith, Joanne R., and William S. Howland, "Endotracheal Tube as a Source of Infection," *Journal of the American Medical Association,* CLXIX, January 24, 1959, pp. 343-45.

Starzl, Thomas E., William H. Meyer, and John J. Farrell, "Prophylactic Tracheostomy in Aged and Poor Risk General Surgical Patients," *Journal of the American Medical Association,* CLXIX, February 14, 1959, pp. 691-95.

Steele, John D., "Those Mysterious Drainage Bottles," *American Journal of Nursing,* LV, No. 10, November, 1955, pp. 1358-59.

"Symposium on Bronchial and Pulmonary Disease," *The Medical Clinics of North America,* XXXVIII, July, 1954, entire issue.

Thomas, John M., and Elza B. Ulpis, "A Seasonal Hazard—Laryngotracheobronchitis," *American Journal of Nursing,* LXI, No. 3, March, 1961, pp. 52-54.

Totman, Laurence E., and Roger H. Lehman, "Tracheostomy Care," *American Journal of Nursing,* LXIV, No. 3, March, 1964, pp. 96-98.

United States Department of Health, Education, and Welfare, *Health, Education, and Welfare Indicators,* April, 1962, p. 7.

Valdivia, Enrique, "Mountain Sickness," *American Journal of Nursing,* LXI, August, 1961, pp. 77-78.

Wilson, Rodger H. L., and Seymour M. Farber, "Concepts and Misconceptions About Oxygen Therapy," *Postgraduate Medicine,* XXVII, February, 1960, pp. 158-64.

Zellos, S., "The Diagnosis and Treatment of Bronchial Adenoma," *Geriatrics,* XVIII, February, 1963, pp. 107-20.

8 : Nursing the Patient with a Disturbance in Fluid and Electrolyte Balance

When they went ashore the animals that took up land life carried with them a part of the sea in their bodies, a heritage which they passed on to their children and which even today links each land animal with its origin in the ancient sea. Fish, amphibian, and reptile, warm-blooded bird and mammal—each of us carries in our veins a salty stream in which the elements sodium, potassium, and calcium are combined in almost the same proportions as in sea water. This is our inheritance from the day, untold millions of years ago, when a remote ancestor, having progressed from the one-celled to the many-celled stage, first developed a circulatory system in which the fluid was merely the water of the sea. In the same way, our lime-hardened skeletons are the heritage from the calcium-rich ocean of Cambrian time. Even the protoplasm that streams within each cell of our bodies has the chemical structure impressed upon all living matter when the first simple creatures were brought forth in the ancient sea. And as life itself began in the sea, so each of us begins his individual life in a miniature ocean within his mother's womb, and in the stages of his embryonic development repeats the steps by which his race evolved, from gill-breathing inhabitants of a water world to creatures able to live on land.[1]

Just as a continuous supply of oxygen is necessary to life, health and life are dependent on the maintenance of the composition and distribution of body fluids. These fluids not only form the environment of the cells but also enter into their structure. In health, exchange between the internal and external environment is so regulated that (1) conditions favorable to the functioning of enzymes and hormones in cellular activities are preserved within the internal environment, (2) materials needed by the cells are supplied, (3) products of metabolism are removed from the cells, and, when in excess, are removed from the internal environment, and (4) waste products are removed.

In this chapter the discussion will be centered on (1) the constituents of the body fluids, (2) the function of each constituent, (3) the distribution and concentration of each constituent in the various fluid compartments, and (4) how each of these factors affects the volume, osmotic pressure, and hydrogen

[1] Rachel Carson, *The Sea Around Us,* Oxford University Press, New York, 1950, pp. 13-14.

ion concentration of body fluids. Most disturbances in fluid balance in the body are related to its volume, osmotic pressure, and hydrogen ion concentration. Most illnesses, acute or chronic, are accompanied by some local or general disturbance in the body fluids. One of the factors in recovery stems from the capacity of the individual to maintain or to restore the normal distribution and composition of body fluids. In order to anticipate and meet the needs of patients with understanding, the professional nurse requires some knowledge of the mechanisms of the body for maintaining the constancy of the internal environment and the manner in which these mechanisms are disrupted in illness.

Who is responsible for what in the maintenance of fluid and electrolyte balance in patients?

In the hospital the physician is usually responsible for the prescription of the amount, character, and route of administration of the patient's fluid intake. He shares with the nurse the responsibility for making observations to serve as a basis for decisions about the degree to which the fluid needs of the patient are being met and for future planning. The nurse is usually responsible for the administration of the fluids and for determining and meeting the related needs of patients.

To be helpful to patients, and to meet their needs for water and electrolytes, the nurse must, of course, be competent in all areas of nursing practice. In this chapter, however, the content will be limited to knowledge essential for: (1) the administration of fluids in a safe and effective manner, (2) "the ability to observe and report with clarity the signs and symptoms, and the deviations from normal behavior, which the patient presents," (3) "the ability to interpret the signs and symptoms which comprise the deviation from health and constitute nursing problems," and (4) "the analysis of nursing problems which will guide the nurse in carrying out nursing functions, and the selection of the necessary course of action which will help the patient attain the goal that is realistic for him, as she plans for total care."[2]

In the past, understanding of water and electrolyte balance has often been difficult. One of the reasons for this has been the confusing use of terminology. To prevent unnecessary confusion, a number of terms will be defined and, in some instances, discussed.

Electrolyte is a substance which, when dissolved in water, conducts an electric current. A characteristic of an electrolyte is that when it is dissolved in water, it dissociates into its component ions. The degree to which a dilute solution of a given electrolyte dissociates is constant, but it differs for each electrolyte.

[2] Faye G. Abdellah, *et al., Patient-Centered Approaches to Nursing,* The Macmillan Company, New York, 1960, p. 26.

Acids were once defined as compounds yielding hydrogen ions. They are now defined as *proton donors*.

Bases were once defined as compounds yielding hydroxyl ions. They are now defined as *proton acceptors*.

Ion is an electrically charged particle in solution. Examples are the hydrogen ion (H+) and the chloride ion (Cl−).

Ionization is the process whereby an electrolyte in solution dissociates into its component ions.

Cations are positively charged ions.

Anions are negatively charged ions.

Milliequivalent is one one-thousandth of an *equivalent weight*. An equivalent weight is the number of grams of an element that will combine with 8 gm or parts of oxygen or 1.008 gm of hydrogen. The equivalent weight of an element is obtained by dividing its atomic weight by its valence. For example, the atomic weight of oxygen is 16. It has a valence of 2. Its equivalent weight is therefore 8. In forming water, 2 atoms (parts) of hydrogen combine with 1 atom (part) of oxygen. In terms of equivalent weights, 2.016 gm of hydrogen combines with 16 gm of oxygen to yield 18.016 gm of water. To cite another example, 1 equivalent of potassium weighs 39.1 gm. This is the amount of potassium that will combine with 8 gm of oxygen. One equivalent of potassium (39.1 gm) combines with 1 equivalent of chlorine, which weighs 35.5 gm, to yield 74.6 gm of potassium chloride. Milliequivalents are used to express the concentration of electrolytes in body fluids, because the quantity of electrolytes found in a liter of body fluids is small.

Formerly, electrolytes in the blood were measured in milligrams per 100 ml of serum or plasma. The current trend in many hospitals and laboratories is toward reporting them in milliequivalents per liter. The reason for this change is that the milliequivalent provides information about the number of anions or cations available to combine with cations and anions. To illustrate, the level of sodium cations in the blood serum ranges from 137 to 147 (average 142) mEq per liter. This means there are approximately 142 sodium cations available to combine with 142 anions. The average level of chloride ions in blood serum is 103 mEq per liter. From this the deduction can be made that approximately 39 mEq of sodium are available to combine with other anions.

Buffer is a substance that protects a solution from changes in pH when an acid or base is added. It is sometimes referred to as a chemical sponge.

Buffer system is composed of a weak acid and a salt formed by neutralizing the weak acid with a strong base. There are a number of buffer systems in the blood—*oxyhemoglobin, reduced hemoglobin; sodium acid phosphate, bisodium phosphate; acid protein, B protein.*

Alkali reserve is a term used to refer to the sodium in the blood that is in combination with bicarbonate. It is called the alkali reserve because the sodium can be used to combine with other anions. The term is really a misnomer.

Osmotic pressure may be defined as the force created by particles in solution that attracts water across a membrane that is fully permeable to water. The direction of flow of the water is always from the less concentrated toward the more concentrated solution. Flow continues until the solution on the two sides of the membrane is of equal concentration. An increase in the osmotic pressure of the fluid in one fluid compartment in the body results in the movement of water into that compartment.

Hydrostatic pressure may be defined as the force exerted by a fluid against the wall of the chamber in which it is contained. Literally, it means the pressure created by the standing weight of water. Applied to the blood, it includes not only the pressure created by the weight of blood against the wall of the capillary, but the force with which the blood is propelled.

Osmolality is a term used to indicate the number of particles in a given space, rather than their size, molecular weight, or chemical constitution.

Filtration may be defined as the separation of a liquid from a solid by passing the liquid through a semipermeable membrane. The force responsible is gravity or weight.

Diffusion may be defined as the distribution of one substance throughout another by the movement of molecules.

Of what are body fluids composed?

Body fluids are composed of water with electrolytes and nonelectrolytes dissolved in it. The types and concentrations of electrolytes in body fluids resemble those of sea water. According to one popular theory of the origin of life, the first living creatures developed in the sea. Those that were successful in making the adaptation to living on land took some of the sea with them in the form of extracellular fluid. Land animals, including man, continue to surround their cells with fluids like those in the primeval sea. Undue loss of fluid is prevented by a watertight jacket—the skin. A special structure, the gastrointestinal tract, enables the organism to take from the external environment the materials required to replenish fluid constituents utilized by, or lost from, the body. The kidney, lung, and skin remove waste products and excesses in supply. All of these are regulated so they function with remarkable accuracy in maintaining the composition and concentration of this fluid. The seas of the world have no such means for protecting their composition and concentration. In the eons of their existence, water laden with minerals has been emptied into them by the rivers of the earth. Water is evaporated by the sun and wind with the result that minerals have become concentrated in the sea water.

As in the sea, the largest component of body fluids is water. In multicellular organisms body fluids are divided into two large compartments, the intracellular and the extracellular fluids. These two compartments are separated from each other by the semipermeable cell membrane. Water diffuses more or less freely across this membrane. The movement of solutes across the cell membrane is regulated so that each component in a fluid compartment is maintained within a limited range. Extracellular water is further divided into two compartments—the intravascular and the interstitial. Intravascular fluid is the fluid component of the blood. Interstitial fluid is that found in the spaces between blood vessels and surrounding cells. Most of the interstitial fluid is a transudate formed by the filtration of blood plasma through the capillary membrane. There are collections of extracellular fluids that are not simple transudates. They are formed by the secretory activity of cells. Examples include the cerebrospinal fluid, gastrointestinal secretions, bile, pancreatic secretions, etc. According to *Physician's Bulletin,*[3] these fluids comprise about 25 per cent of the total body water. All of the fluid compartments are interrelated. Recent studies have, however, demonstrated that water and electrolytes do not move as freely from some tissues as they do from others. Bone, cartilage, and other dense connective tissues contain electrolytes that are not freely exchangeable with other body components. Bone holds a volume of water about equal to the blood plasma.[4] Water in the interstitial spaces does not appear to be a simple solution of water and the electrolytes dissolved in it. It is held in the tissue spaces by a gellike substance, hyaluronic acid. Hyaluronic acid does not interfere with the capacity of the water to dissolve electrolytes or nonelectrolytes. It enters into the cement substance that binds cells together.[5]

The volume and distribution of water in the body vary with the age, sex, and weight of the individual. These differences are illustrated by the Martin family in Figure 8-1. The family is composed of five members—John Martin, aged 30; Mary Martin, aged 28; Billy, aged 9; Suzy, aged 8 weeks; and Mary Martin's mother, Mrs. Bird, aged 68. Because at all ages the intravascular fluid comprises about 5 per cent of the total body weight, the extracellular fluid, as shown in Figure 8-1, has not been divided into interstitial and intravascular compartments. The most marked difference in the distribution of water at the different age levels is in the amount of interstitial fluid. In the newborn baby, the proportion of body water in the interstitial fluid compartment is larger than at any period in life. From Figure 8-1 the reader will note that with advancing age there is a progressive decrease in the proportion of water in the interstitial space, as well as in the total volume of water in the body. Interstitial fluid accounts for 40 per cent of eight-week-old Suzy's weight, 30 per cent of Billy's weight, and only 20 per cent of the weight of the adults. Although not shown in Figure 8-1, the water content of the body falls

---

[3] "Clinical Application of Fluid and Electrolyte Balance," *Physician's Bulletin,* Eli Lilly and Company, Indianapolis, Indiana, XXVI, February, 1961, p. 6.
[4] *Ibid.*
[5] Charles Herbert Best and Norman Burke Taylor, *Physiological Basis of Medical Practice,* 7th ed., Williams & Wilkins Co., Baltimore, 1961, p. 21.

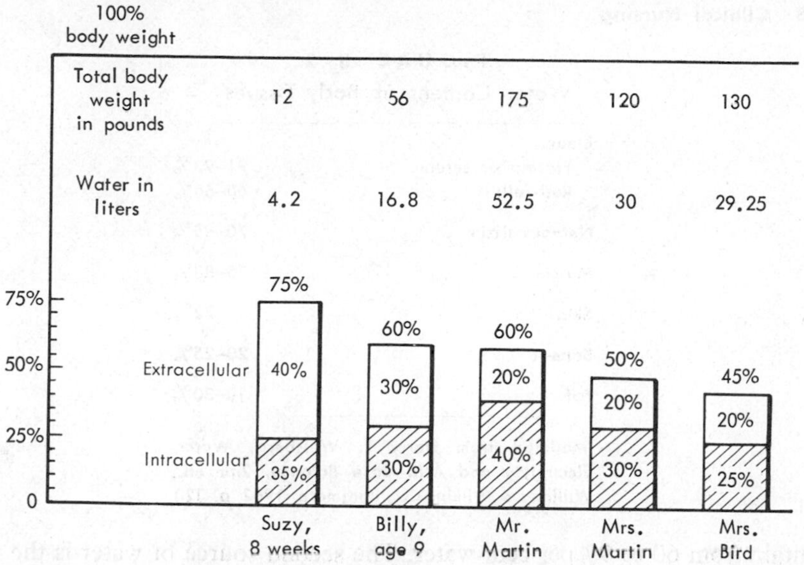

FIGURE 8—1. Volume and distribution of water in the body varies with age, sex, and weight of the individual, as seen in the Martin family.

sharply from birth to about four years of age and then levels off. Maturity, in respect to water and electrolytes, is reached at about 20 years of age. Thenceforth throughout life there is a slow decline in body water. This change is also demonstrated in Figure 8-1. Although water is responsible for 75 per cent of Suzy's weight, it accounts for only 45 per cent of her grandmother's weight. Objective evidence of the loss of water in older age groups is seen in the dry skin and hair of the aged. It is also seen in their flabby muscles and wrinkled skin. The degree of dryness of the skin should be taken into consideration when planning the number and type of baths for elderly people. Men, in particular, may be troubled by dry and itching skin. For the comfort of the patient, full baths may need to be limited to one or two a week. A mild soap should be selected. Rather than alcohol, a hand cream, or lotion, or other emollient should be used for back rubs and should be applied to other skin areas to reduce dryness. Mrs. Bird finds that her skin is excessively dry and applies an oily lotion to the skin of her legs and arms each day.

Tissues also vary in their water content. Enamel of the teeth is about 3 per cent water. Fat and bone are about 25 per cent water, while active tissues such as muscles, nerves, liver, and skin have a much higher water content. (See Figure 8-2.)

How is the supply of water replenished?

The maintenance of any homeostatic mechanism depends on a supply of required materials. Water is replenished in the body in two ways. One is by ingestion of fluids and food. Even solid foods such as meat and vegetables

FIGURE   8 - 2

Water Content of Body Tissues

Blood	
Plasma or serum	91–93%
Red cells	60–65%
Nervous tissue	70–85%
Muscle	75–80%
Skin	72%
Bone	20–25%
Fat	10–30%

(Modified from Harry F. Weisberg, *Water*, *Electrolyte and Acid Base Balance*, 2nd ed., Williams & Wilkins Co., Baltimore, 1962, p. 32.)

contain from 60 to 97 per cent water. The second source of water is the water of oxidation. One of the end products of oxidation-reduction reactions is water. (See Chapter 10.) Over 10 per cent of the daily requirement for water is derived from this second source. This is an important consideration in acute renal shutdown. The amount of water from metabolism must be calculated, if water intoxication is to be avoided. The point at which water is normally taken from the external environment into the internal environment is the gastrointestinal tract. Any condition disturbing the function of the gastrointestinal tract may interfere with the patient's intake of fluid, or result in a dependable indication of the need for water. Accurate measurement and recording of the patient's fluid intake, as well as losses, is essential when a disorder interferes with fluid intake. Rapid loss of weight is usually indicative of insufficient water intake.

Water is lost from the body in urine, feces, sweat, and expired air. The quantity lost in feces, sweat, and expired air is obligatory; that is, fluid is lost regardless of the fluid intake. This is not true of urine, as the kidney plays a primary role in the homeostasis of water and electrolytes in the extracellular fluids. In health, the kidney functions to maintain within limits: (1) the volume of water in extracellular fluid, (2) the concentration of electrolytes in extracellular fluid, (3) the osmotic pressure of extracellular fluid, and (4) the concentration of hydrogen ion in the extracellular fluid. The kidney is also the site for the excretion of the wastes of metabolism, particularly those of protein catabolism. Under certain abnormal conditions, the kidney produces vaso-excitatory substances or their precursors. At the present time this is thought to revolve around the juxtaglomerular apparatus and the renin-angiotensin system.

Although the kidneys are frequently referred to as organs of excretion, the above list of their functions indicates the inadequacy of this concept of renal function. The primary function of the kidneys is to regulate the volume and composition of the extracellular fluid; their excretory function is incidental to their regulatory function. The structure of the kidneys is such that it is admirably suited to its functions.

Describe the gross structure of the kidneys.

The kidneys are paired, somewhat flattened, bean-shaped organs, lying behind the peritoneum and situated one on each side of the vertebral column. The right kidney is slightly lower than the left as its upper pole lies on the twelfth rib; the left is over the eleventh and twelfth ribs. The combined weight of the two kidneys is approximately 300 gms (10 oz.) They are embedded in a mass of fat and loose areolar tissue.

All structures entering and leaving the kidney do so through the hilus, a longitudinal slit or gap occupying not quite a third of the medial border of the organ. Structures entering include the renal artery and nerves; those leaving include the renal veins, lymphatics, and ureters.

The kidney is invested by a tough capsule that is nearly indistensible and is loosely adherent to the underlying glandular tissue. The structures performing the functions of the kidney are arranged in lobes. In the human fetus and in animals such as the cow the lobes can be seen on the surface, but in the adult kidney, their fusion is so complete that they are no longer evident. From the exterior, the kidney appears to be a single structure. The outer portion of the

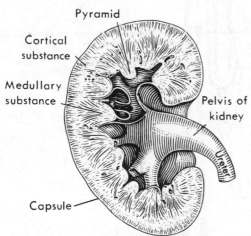

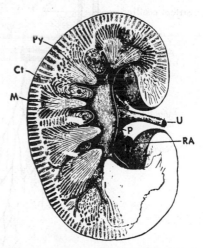

FIGURE 8–3. Diagrammatic longitudinal section of the human kidney. Each kidney is about 11.25 cm long, 5.0 to 7.5 cm broad, and 2.5 cm thick, and weighs about 135 gm. (Henel.) (Adapted with permission of The Macmillan Company from *Anatomy and Physiology*, 14th ed., Fig. 347, p. 592, by Diana Clifford Kimber, Carolyn E. Gray, Caroline E. Stackpole, and Lutie C. Leavell. Copyright © The Macmillan Company 1961.)

FIGURE 8–4. Longitudinal section of the kidney. Ct, the cortical substance; M, the medullary substance; Py, the pyramids; P, the pelvis of the kidney; U, the ureter; RA, the renal artery. (T. H. Huxley.) (Adapted with permission of The Macmillan Company from *Anatomy and Physiology*, 14th ed., Fig. 348, p. 592, by Diana Clifford Kimber, Carolyn E. Gray, Caroline E. Stackpole, and Lutie C. Leavell. Copyright © The Macmillan Company 1961.)

kidney is known as the cortex and the inner portion as the medulla. The cortex is reddish brown in color and dips down between adjacent renal pyramids. (See Figures 8-3 and 8-4.) These projections of the cortex are known as the columns of Bertini. The medulla varies in color from the reddish brown of the cortex to a grayish brown at the tips of the papillae. Its substance forms the renal pyramids. They appear to be striated; this is attributed to the parallel course of the loops of Henle and blood vessels.

Blood is supplied to the kidney by the renal artery, which has its source from the abdominal aorta. Occlusions of the aorta, whether due to thrombi or

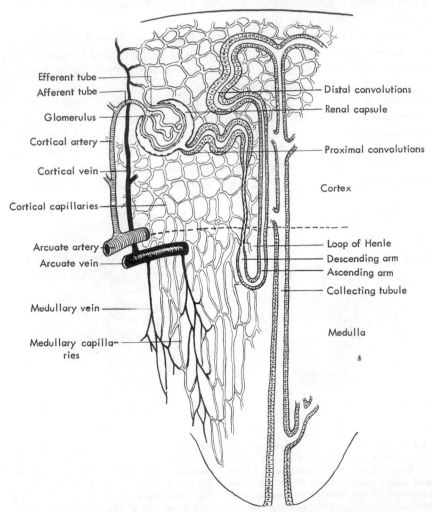

FIGURE 8–5. Nephron and its blood supply. Length of tubule approximately 35 to 40 mm, diameter about 0.02 mm; diameter of capsule about 0.2 mm. (Adapted with permission of The Macmillan Company from *Anatomy and Physiology*, 14th ed., Fig. 352, p. 596, by Diana Clifford Kimber, Carolyn E. Gray, Caroline E. Stackpole, and Lutie C. Leavell. Copyright © The Macmillan Company 1961.)

emboli, and located above the origin of the renal artery deprive the kidney of blood and predispose of renal failure. Just before or after the renal artery enters the hilus of the kidney, it divides into a series of branches. Abnormalities in the branching of a renal artery may obstruct a ureter and impede the drainage of urine from the renal pelvis. Since they pass between the lobes or pyramids, they are known as the interlobar arteries. At the base of the pyramids, the interlobar arteries divide to form a series of incomplete arches known as the arciform arteries. Arteries forming at right angles from arciform arteries run radially in cortical medullary rays toward the periphery of the kidney. (See Figure 8-5.) In general, the veins draining the kidney follow a pattern similar to that of the arteries. The details of glomerular and capillary circulation will be considered along with the morphology of the nephron. Possibly one of the most important points about the renal blood supply is that in health it receives about 25 per cent, or one quarter, of the cardiac output. This is despite the fact that it constitutes only approximately 0.4 per cent of the total body weight. More detailed discussions of the gross structure of the kidney may be found in any one of a number of anatomy textbooks.

How does the microscopic structure of the kidney enable it to regulate the volume and composition of the extracellular fluid?

The work of the kidney is performed by the nephron. In man there are a million or more nephrons in each kidney. They are all basically similar in structure and each one is presumed to be grossly similar to all others in function. Nephrons are located in the cortex. Those situated near the periphery of the kidney are called cortical nephrons. Those in the portion of the cortex adjacent to the medulla are called juxtamedullary nephrons. Classically a nephron is described as consisting of a renal or malpighian corpuscle (glomerulus and Bowman's capsule), proximal convoluted tubule, loop of Henle, and a distal convoluted tubule. Many nephrons empty their contents into a duct known as a collecting tubule. Until recently they were believed to be merely conduits to convey urine to the renal calyces. They are now known to be involved in many renal processes including concentrating urine, regulating acid-base balance, secreting potassium ions, and reabsorbing sodium ions in states associated with sodium depletion. Thus the collecting tubules have a significant role in the regulation of the internal environment of cells.

Several processes are involved in the formation of urine: filtration in the glomeruli, selective reabsorption, as well as secretion by the tubules and diffusion. Filtration in the glomeruli depends on the hydrostatic pressure created by the pumping action of the heart. The glomerular filtrate is actually an ultrafiltrate of the blood. It is similar in character to interstitial fluid found in other parts of the body. As an ultrafiltrate it does not contain red cells or colloidal materials such as protein. It does contain crystalloidal solutes such as electrolytes, glucose, urea, and other wastes of protein metabolism. The glomerular filtrate contains water and the substances dissolved in plasma water. The rate of glomerular filtration averages about 125 ml per minute in men and 110 ml in women.

Glomerular filtration rate can be measured by injecting a solute filtered by the glomeruli. Ideally such a substance should not be metabolized in the body or secreted or reabsorbed by the renal tubules. One such substance is inulin, a polysaccharide obtained from dahlia roots. Since inulin is neither reabsorbed nor secreted, the quantity found in the urine is equal to the amount filtered by the glomeruli. With knowledge of both the quantity and concentration of inulin in one minute's filtrate, the volume of plasma filtered, that is, the rate of glomerular filtration can be estimated. Suppose that the urinary excretion rate is 128 ml per minute; then the urine formed in one minute contains the amount of inulin found in 128 ml of plasma or glomerular filtrate. Since no single milliliter of plasma loses its entire complement of inulin (urea, creatinine) as it passes through the glomeruli, the results represent the volume of plasma required to provide the amount of a particular substance excreted by the kidney per minute.

Metabolites such as urea and creatinine are also employed in clearance tests. Since they are products of the metabolism of proteins, the patient should be kept quiet during the performance of the test. In calculating the results of the test, the fact that some urea diffuses back into the blood has to be taken into account.

In the tubules water and solutes are reabsorbed and solutes such as the hydrogen and potassium ions are also secreted into the urine. These processes are considered later in the chapter.

Inasmuch as the kidney regulates the volume and concentration of urine in relation to the quantity of water and solutes added to extracellular fluid from exogenous and endogenous sources, the quantity and composition of urine vary. With a large fluid intake, the kidney excretes a large volume of dilute urine; with a small fluid intake, it excretes a small volume of concentrated urine. When both salt and water intake are limited, the minimum volume of urine depends on the volume of nitrogenous wastes, principally urea, presented to the kidney for excretion and the kidney's capacity to concentrate urea. About 500 ml of water is required for this purpose. The capacity of the kidney to alter the concentration and volume of urine is adaptive. Within limits, it enables the body to survive water deprivation and/or loss and to rapidly eliminate excesses of intake. The extent to which the kidney is able to concentrate or dilute urine or specific substances in it is a useful test of renal function. The daily requirements, sources, organs of excretion, daily average excretion, and sources of excessive loss for water and electrolytes are summarized in Figure 8-6. Since all losses require replacement, accurate observation and reporting of the quantity lost by any avenue is important to the welfare of the patient.

FIGURE 8–6. Summary of Sources of and Factors Relating to Water and Electrolytes

Substance	Symbols	Daily Req.	Source of Intake	Organ of Excretion	Daily Avg. Excre.	Sources of Excessive Loss
Water	H·HO	1,500–3,000 ml	Fluids, 1,000 ml; Food, free water 1,000 ml; Water of oxidation, 300 ml	Skin; Kidney; Lung; Intestine	1,000–1,500 ml; 600–1,000 ml; 350 ml; 100 ml	Up to 8,000 ml of gastrointestinal secretions per day. Burn fluid; Renal failure; Sweating; Mouth breathing; Polyuria
Sodium	Na+	2–4 gm	Food and fluids including tap water	Kidney; Skin	2–4 gm	May be lost when excess loss of fluid from GI tract
Potassium	K+	3–4 gm	Abundant in food esp. fruit juices	Kidney		Polyuria associated with excessive catabolism of cells
Calcium	Ca++	800 mg	Milk, 2–3 glasses/day; dairy prod.; egg yolks	Intestine, as insoluble soaps; Urine		Renal failure; Inadequate intake of vitamin D; Hyperparathyroidism
Magnesium	Mg++	Not known—about 300 mg taken in/day		Intestine; Kidney	200 mg	
Chloride	Cl-		With sodium as sodium chloride	Kidney; Skin		Losses may be excessive when vomiting, if gastrointestinal tract suctioning continues
Bicarbonate	HCO3=		End product of metabolism	Lung		
Phosphate	HPO4=		With calcium. Intake adequate if intake of calcium is	Kidney; Possibly intestinal tract		See calcium
Sulfate	SO4=			Kidney		
Protein+		40–80 gm	Meat, milk, dairy products, eggs, lentils, legumes, etc.	End products of protein metabolism excreted by kidney, but not as protein		May be last via kidney, draining wounds, ulcers, burn
Hydrogen+	H+		Metabolism	Kidney		

Because some water is stored and because there are effective mechanisms for its renewal and conservation, the need for a continuous intake is not as urgent as is the need for intake of oxygen. Under favorable conditions an adult can live as long as ten days without water. The person who finds himself in a situation where there is an inadequate supply of fresh water can reduce water loss by shading himself from the sun and the wind, thereby reducing evaporation from the skin. He can reduce the amount of urea formed from the oxidation of tissue protein by remaining inactive. Under extreme conditions, such as those found in the desert, survival without water is limited to about two days. Children are more sensitive to water deprivation than are adults. They can survive only about five days without water. The younger the child, the more sensitive he is to water deprivation. Suzy Martin is much more sensitive to water deprivation than the other members of the family. This is true because infants have a relatively greater surface area, a higher metabolic rate, and their kidneys are less efficient in concentrating urine than they are in older children and adults. Suzy loses about twice as much fluid per gram of body weight through her skin as her father does. Any condition that interferes with Suzy's fluid intake, particularly when this is combined with an excessive loss of fluids, can produce serious effects within a few hours. With a relatively high metabolic rate, water is required to take up the heat produced in oxidation-reduction reactions and carry it to the surface of the body where it is eliminated. With the excessive loss of water, Suzy's temperature can be expected to rise. Since her kidney is unable to protect the volume of blood by concentrating urine, electrolytes become concentrated in the blood. Unless treatment is quickly instituted, the circulation fails, and with this death occurs.

Why is water well suited to its role in the body?

Water has a number of properties that make it well suited to its role in the body. It is chemically stable. It is a so-called universal solvent. This does not mean that all substances dissolve in it, but more do than in any other liquid. It has a high ionizing power. It also has a number of properties that make it well suited to its role in temperature regulation. These include its high specific heat, its high latent heat of evaporation, and its great capacity to conduct heat. Its specific heat is the highest for all liquids.

How does water function in the body?

Water functions in the body in many ways. As has been stated, it functions in temperature regulation by taking up large quantities of heat produced by cells and distributing it throughout the body. At the surface of the body, heat is lost to the atmosphere and the blood is cooled. Because of the large number of substances that are soluble in water, it serves as a vehicle for the transportation of substances to and from cells. In the lung, oxygen goes into solution as it enters the blood. Carbon dioxide is in solution in the blood before it escapes into the alveoli. The volume of blood is dependent on water. Products of metabolism are diluted by water and are thus prevented from injuring cells. End products of metabolism and excesses of intake dissolved in water are excreted by the kidney. Water is necessary to the physiochemical activities of the body. Digestion of food is accomplished by hydrolysis—the breakdown of molecules through the addition of water. The chemical processes within the cell take place in water. Storage of nutrients depends on water. For each gram of protein deposited in the body, 4 gms of water are needed. This is one of the reasons growing children require proportionately more water than do adults. Fat requires only 0.2 gm of water to store each gram.

Water as the principal solvent in the body regulates the osmolarity of body fluids. In other words, it determines the number of particles per unit of fluid. To illustrate, when 1 teaspoonful of salt is dissolved in a cup of water there are more particles of salt per milliliter of water than there are if the same teaspoonful of salt is dissolved in a gallon of water. When water is lost from the body in excess of that ingested, body fluids become concentrated and their osmolarity is increased. Because the osmotic effect is determined by the number of particles in solution, substances dissociating into ions have a greater osmotic effect than those that do not ionize. For example, when sodium chloride is dissolved in water, each molecule ionizes into two ions or particles. Each particle has nearly as much osmotic effect as the original molecule of sodium chloride. Conversely, when glucose is dissolved in water, its molecules do not ionize, but they remain as molecules. The number of particles in solution is, therefore, the same as the number of molecules of glucose. Consequently 1 mole of sodium chloride has approximately twice the osmotic effect as 1 mole of glucose.

Since the body does not tolerate differences in osmotic pressure between the fluid compartments, water is then shifted from the compartment in which the concentration of water is greatest to the one in which the concentration of electrolyte is greatest. For example, when extracellular fluid is hypertonic in relation to intracellular fluid, water moves from the cell into the interstitial fluid, thereby dehydrating the cell. When, on the other hand, the interstitial fluid is hypotonic in relation to the cellular fluid, water moves into the cell, causing it to swell. Responses of the body to increased concentration of body fluids, as well as the role of water in the regulation of hydrogen ions, will be discussed later. Since water and electrolytes function together, the causes and effects of deficits or excesses of both water and electrolytes will be considered together. Changes in the volume and distribution of one affect the other.

To summarize, water is essential to all body functions. It is the medium in which the physiochemical activities of the cell take place. In some bodily processes, such as hydrolysis, it is one of the reacting agents. In others, as in oxidation-reduction reactions, it may be a product. It is an essential element in the internal environment of the cell. It is the medium through or by which all substances are transported to and from the cell and external environment. Without it life is impossible.

In addition to water, what are the other components of body fluids?

Body fluids are composed not only of water, but of electrolytes that are dissolved in them. The electrolyte structure, which is described in Figure 8-7, has been modified from Gamble.[6] In each diagram, cations are to the left and anions to the right. The number of cations available to react with anions is equal. Extracellular fluid also contains small amounts of nonelectrolytes. Unless they are greatly increased, they do not affect the behavior of extracellular fluid.[7] Concentrations of each electrolyte are expressed in milliequivalents per liter.

Gamble was the first to draw attention to the similarities between the composition of sea water and extracellular fluid. Although there are marked similarities, there are also significant differences. One is that sea water contains a higher concentration of magnesium. This renders it unfit for human consumption. Another difference derives from the fact that extracellular fluid is part of a living system. As a result, it has a higher concentration of the bicarbonate anion and contains protein. The latter is not found in sea water.

Comparison of the composition of the fluids contained in the extracellular and intracellular compartments shows that the principal cation in extracellular fluid is sodium while that of the intracellular fluid is potassium. At one time scientists thought that sodium was not able to enter the cell or potassium to leave it. Evidence now indicates that sodium does enter the cell but that it is removed by a sodium or an electrolyte pump. The manner in which the pump acts to prevent sodium from accumulating in the cell is not clear. There is evidence, however, that energy is required. In conditions accompanied by starvation or semistarvation, sodium tends to replace potassium to the detriment of cellular activities. Improvement in a patient's condition may result from an increase in the intake of food. The principal anions in the intracellular and extracellular fluid can also be seen to differ. The principal anion in extracellular fluid is the chloride ion, while that in intracellular fluid is the phosphate ion. With the exception of the red blood cell, the quantity of chloride ion found within cells is believed to be small.

All the cations and anions entering into the composition of body fluids have important functions in the body. Healthy functioning of cells depends on the maintenance of the level of each electrolyte within its so-called normal range. Deviations outside this range in either a downward or upward direction can be anticipated to have adverse effects on bodily function. Some electrolytes,

---

[6] James L. Gamble, *Lane Medical Lectures: Companionship of Water and Electrolytes in the Organization of Body Fluids,* Stanford University Press, Stanford, California, 1951, p. 13.
[7] *Ibid.,* p. 12.

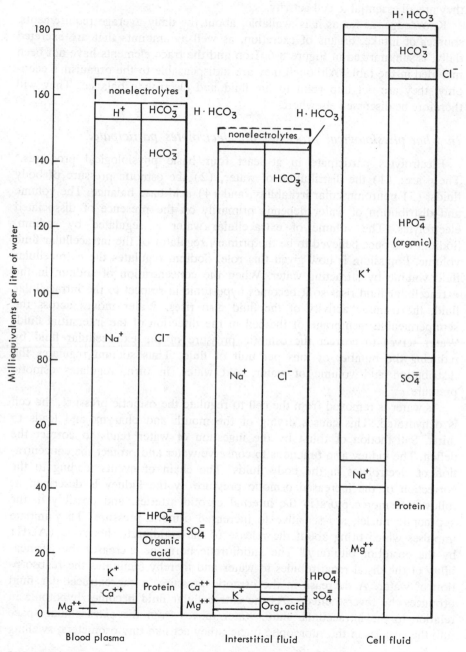

FIGURE 8—7. A comparison of the electrolyte composition of body fluids. (Adapted from James L. Gamble, *Companionship of Water and Electrolytes in the Organization of Body Fluids*, Stanford: Stanford University Press, 1951, p. 13. Reprinted by permission of the publishers.)

such as sodium, are present in relatively large amounts. Others, such as chromium, are found only in traces. Whether the quantity is large or small, they are all essential to cell activity.

Knowledge, as far as it is available, about the daily average requirements, sources of intake, organs of excretion, as well as amounts that are excreted daily, is summarized in Figure 8-6. Iron and the trace elements have not been included in the table. Although they are indispensable to the organism's economy, they are not important to the fluid and electrolyte balance. They will therefore be discussed elsewhere.

In what physiological processes do electrolytes participate?

Electrolytes participate in at least four basic physiological processes.[8] These are: (1) the distribution of water, (2) the osmotic pressure of body fluids, (3) neuromuscular irritability, and (4) acid-base balance. The volume and distribution of water depends primarily on the presence of dissociated electrolytes. The volume of extracellular water is regulated by sodium. Sodium was once believed to be the primary regulator of the intracellular fluid volume. Potassium is now given this role. Sodium regulates the extracellular fluid volume by attracting water. When the concentration of sodium in the extracellular fluid rises so it becomes hypertonic in respect to the intracellular fluid, the osmotic activity of the fluid also rises. Water moves across the semipermeable membrane of the cell in the direction of the interstitial fluid. Water serves to correct the osmotic pressure of the extracellular fluid by reducing the number of ions per unit of fluid. Thus sodium regulates the distribution and volume of water, and water, in turn, regulates osmotic pressure.

As water is removed from the cell to regulate the osmotic pressure, the cell is dehydrated. This causes drying of the mouth and pharynx and leads to thirst. Satisfaction of thirst by the ingestion of water tends to correct the deficit. The kidney also functions to conserve water and protect the concentration of electrolytes in the body fluids. The chain of events leading to the correction of the increased osmotic pressure by the kidney is described as follows: Osmoreceptors in the internal carotid arteries, and possibly in the supraoptic nuclei, are sensitive to increased osmotic pressure. They initiate impulses which bring about the release of the antidiuretic hormone (ADH) by the posterior pituitary.[9] The antidiuretic hormone increases the permeability of the distal renal tubules to water and thereby facilitates the reabsorption of water. A decrease in the osmotic pressure in the extracellular fluid produces the reverse effects. As the extracellular fluid becomes hypotonic in relation to the intracellular fluid, water moves from the extracellular space into the vesicles in the supraoptic nuclei; they act like tiny osometers, swelling

---

[8] Weisberg, *Op. cit.*, p. 66.
[9] There is some evidence that the antidiuretic hormone is formed by the hypothalamus and stored in the posterior pituitary gland.

when the extracellular fluid becomes hypotonic and shrinking when it becomes hypertonic. Swelling is thought to inhibit the secretion of the antidiuretic hormone; shrinking is presumed to stimulate its secretion. With a decrease in the level of ADH, the quantity of water reabsorbed is reduced and the volume excreted in the urine is increased. Conversely, augmentation of the secretion of ADH increases the reabsorption of water by the distal tubules and decreases the volume of water excreted in the urine.

Currently there is considerable discussion as to whether or not glomerular filtration is increased by water load; it seems most likely that it is *not* increased in the absence of increased solute excretion. The increased urine output is a reflection of distal tubular function, not of glomerular fitration.[10]

The kidney is likewise the site at which the quantity of sodium in the body is regulated. Some recent evidence suggests that the antidiuretic hormone may be responsible for the release of ACTH.[11] Since ACTH regulates the rate of production of the adrenal glucocorticoids, it may have an indirect effect on the reabsorption of sodium by the renal tubules. Perhaps the most important hormone to influence the reabsorption of sodium is aldosterone. The other adrenal cortical hormones may augment the effect of aldosterone. Adrenal cortical hormones increase the reabsorption of sodium by the kidney and the excretion of potassium. In the absence of sodium intake, the kidney is able to excrete a nearly sodium-free urine. Aldosterone, unlike the other adrenal cortical hormones, is secreted more or less independently of ACTH.

The regulation of water and electrolytes provides an excellent example of the functioning of a homeostatic mechanism. To summarize the processes involved in the homeostasis of water and electrolytes, we will return to Mr. Martin. On a hot, sunny Saturday afternoon he mowed the lawn. Because he was exercising and the day was warm, he perspired freely. Every now and then he stopped to mop his brow. By the time he had finished, his shirt and underwear were saturated. Evaporation of sweat enabled Mr. Martin to increase his heat loss. He was thereby able to keep his body temperature within physiological limits, despite an increase in heat production that accompanied his activity and the warmth of the day. His sweat was a hypotonic solution of water and electrolytes. In the hour Mr. Martin spent in mowing the lawn, let us suppose he lost a liter of water. As water was taken from the blood for the secretion of sweat, his blood plasma became concentrated, that is, the number of particles per unit of fluid in his intravascular compartment increased in proportion to those in his interstitial space. Water was attracted across his semipermeable capillary membranes by the increase in the osmolarity of the blood. The quantity of fluid added to the blood was not sufficient to restore its normal dilution. Osmoreceptors in the internal carotid arteries and the supra-

[10] Robert F. Pitts, *Physiology of the Kidney and Body Fluids,* Year Book Medical Publishers Incorporated, Chicago, 1963, p. 67 and 102-14.
[11] J. G. Hilton, "Adrenocorticotropic Action of Antidiuretic Hormone," *Circulation,* XXI, May, 1960, p. 1038.

optic nuclei were stimulated. This resulted in an increase in secretion of the antidiuretic hormone. Mr. Martin's kidney increased the reabsorption of water and the concentration of his urine. The wastes of protein metabolism were excreted in less water than usual. Since sodium is also lost in the sweat, a decreased serum sodium stimulates the secretion of aldosterone, which can be expected to have increased the reabsorption of sodium. As fluid moved from Mr. Martin's interstitial fluid to his blood, its osmotic pressure also increased. Water was attracted from the cells to correct the situation. As Mr. Martin entered the house, he shouted to his wife, "I'm thirsty. How about a pitcher of lemonade?" After his shower, he sat on the patio and drank lemonade and ate potato chips. Because he drank rapidly, his blood volume was temporarily elevated. The salt on the potato chips replaced the sodium chloride lost in sweating. Mr. Martin ingested more than enough water and salt to replace that lost by sweating. This condition lasted only briefly. After the volume, concentration, and distribution of his body fluids were restored to preexercise levels, the excess water and electrolytes were excreted by his kidney. Somewhere along the way his thirst was also quenched.

How is fluid transported from the intravascular to the interstitial compartment and back?

As was stated earlier, body fluids are separated into compartments by the semipermeable membranes surrounding cells and capillaries. These membranes serve as the points where exchange takes place between the organism and its external environment and between each cell and its fluid environment. The capillary is the site where the function of the circulatory system is accomplished. Four factors influence the movement of fluids across the capillary membrane. They are: (1) capillary permeability, (2) diffusion, (3) filtration pressure, and (4) the colloid osmotic pressure of the blood. More fluid moves from the intravascular to the interstitial compartment than returns by way of the capillary membrane. The lymphatic system functions to maintain the balance between the two compartments by returning the excess interstitial fluid to the blood. It also functions to return the protein that escapes through the capillary membrane to the blood.

The first element in the movement of fluid to and from capillaries is membrane permeability. In general, capillaries are freely permeable to electrolytes and nonelectrolytes and are less permeable or impermeable to blood proteins. The degree to which capillaries are permeable to proteins differs in various parts of the body. Those in the sinusoids of the liver, the heart, the lungs, and the gastrointestinal tract are quite permeable to protein. Those in the skin and skeletal muscles are much less permeable. Capillaries forming the glomeruli of the kidney are nearly impermeable to protein. The degree of capillary permeability influences the volume of water and the size of the molecules that can escape into the interstitial fluid compartment. For example, Mrs. Bird complains that on warm days her feet swell. One of the contributing factors is that, with an increase in the environmental temperature, peripheral blood vessels dilate to increase heat loss. As the capillaries dilate, permeability is increased and with it the volume of interstitial fluid is enlarged. A variety of physical and chemical agents increase capillary permeability. Some common examples include anoxia, some of the products of inflammation, bacterial toxins, and carbon dioxide. In any condition in which capillary membrane permeability is increased, the volume of fluid and the size of the molecules that move from the intravascular to the interstitial space can be expected to be increased. The cell membrane is less permeable to large molecules, such as glucose, than the capillary is.

Water and solutes move across the capillary membrane by diffusion, filtration, and osmosis. Permeability of the capillary membrane is a common limiting factor. Each of these forces affects the transfer of fluid into and out of the capillary. In general, diffusion of substances to which the capillary is freely permeable occurs along the entire length of the capillary and takes place in both directions. To illustrate, the capillary membrane is freely permeable to sodium ions. Therefore, sodium ions can be expected to pass into and out of the capillary without regard to direction. Any increase in the number of sodium ions in the blood plasma increases the chances of sodium ions coming in contact with the capillary membrane. This can be expected to result in an increase in the number of particles passing through the membrane. The same factors operate in the transfer of solutes and water back into the capillary. An increase in the concentration of a solute in either the blood plasma or the interstitial fluids can be anticipated to be followed by an increase in the rate at which it diffuses through the capillary membrane.

Whereas substances move into and out of the capillary by diffusion, the primary effect of filtration is to transfer fluid from the capillary to the interstitial space. The pressure of the blood in the capillary is responsible for filtration pressure. Three factors are of importance in determining capillary blood pressure: (1) the arterial blood pressure, (2) the rate of the flow of blood through the capillary, and (3) the venous pressure. Arterial blood pressure is created by such factors as the volume of blood, the force of the heart beat, the resistance of the arteries, and most particularly the arterioles, to the flow, and the viscosity of the blood. At the tissue level, capillary blood flow is regulated by arteriolar constriction or dilatation. Constriction of arterioles decreases blood flow into the capillaries, thereby decreasing filtration; dilatation increases blood flow and therefore filtration. Because the circulatory system is a closed system, the effect is an increase in blood pressure behind the constriction and a fall in the vessels distal to it.

Normally the hydrostatic pressure of the blood falls rather sharply from the arteriolar to the venous end of the capillary. This results in a corresponding decrease in the rate of filtration. The primary reason for the drop in hydrostatic pressure of the blood is that considerable energy is required to overcome the resistance offered by the capillary to the flow of blood. The effect of increasing resistance to the flow of a fluid on its movement can be demonstrated by placing water in a tuberculin syringe and in a 50-ml syringe. Water escapes from the tuberculin syringe very slowly because much of it comes in contact with the wall of the syringe and the wall offers resistance to the movement of the water. Water escapes very rapidly from the larger syringe because little of the water comes in contact with its wall. In other words, the smaller the lumen of a tube, the greater the surface to come in contact with the fluid contained in the tube and the greater the resistance to its movement.

Any condition that interferes with the flow of blood through a vein will increase the hydrostatic pressure of the blood in the capillary by increasing the volume of blood in the capillary. The effect is similar to that produced by placing a dam in a stream. The volume of fluid and therefore its weight behind the dam are increased. This will, of course, increase filtration of fluid from the capillary. The quantity of fluid that actually leaves the capillary by filtration is determined by the relationship of the hydrostatic pressure of the blood to the interstitial fluid pressure. The greater the hydrostatic pressure of the blood in relation to that of the interstitial fluid, the greater the net filtration pressure. The smaller the difference, the less it will be.

The force responsible for the transfer of fluids from the interstitial space into the capillary is created by the colloid osmotic pressure of the blood. Normally the concentration of protein is greater in the blood plasma than it is in interstitial fluid. In health, the level of protein in the blood plasma ranges from 6.5 to 8 gm per 100 ml. Of this, albumin comprises the largest fraction, with an average range of from 4.0 to 5.2 gm per 100 ml. Because it has the smallest molecules of the blood proteins, albumin's effect on the colloid osmotic pressure of the blood is greater than can be accounted for by its weight. The critical factor in osmotic pressure is the number of particles per unit of water and not the size of each particle. For example, if a particle the size of a grain of sand exerts approximately the same osmotic effect as one the size of a marble, then a cupful of osmotically active particles the size of a grain of sand will have many times the effect of a cupful of particles the size of marbles.

The extent to which osmotic pressure is effective in returning fluid to the capillary depends on a number of factors. One is the difference between the colloid osmotic pressure of the blood and that of the interstitial fluid. Anything that decreases the colloid osmotic pressure of the blood or increases that of the interstitial fluid will reduce the return of fluid to the capillary. The relationship of the hydrostatic pressure of the blood to its colloid osmotic pressure will also affect the rate of exchange between the capillary and the interstitial fluid. A rise in the hydrostatic pressure in relation to the colloid osmotic pressure of the blood will increase the quantity of fluid in the interstitial compartment.

Any condition that results in a serious loss of protein from the blood can be expected to interfere with the return of fluid from the interstitial fluid compartment to the blood. Examples of conditions in which blood protein levels fall include severe and prolonged starvation and continued loss of body fluids containing protein, such as in severe burns and in kidney disorders in which protein is lost in the urine. A blood albumin level of 2.0 gm or less is usually associated with an increase in the volume of interstitial fluid, that is, with edema. Restoration of the normal distribution of water depends on lessening the loss of protein from the body and raising the level of osmotically active substances in the blood. This is sometimes difficult to do. When the condition is severe, the patient may be given intravenous infusions of blood, plasma, or plasma expanders. If the patient is able to take food by mouth, he should be given appropriate assistance and encouraged to eat.

Return of interstitial fluid to capillaries is not usually complete. The lymphatic capillaries make a considerable contribution to maintaining the balance in the exchange between the capillaries and the interstitial fluid compartment by absorbing tissue fluid and to returning it to the blood stream via the lymphatic and thoracic ducts. Any obstruction to the flow of fluid in the lymphatics leads to the accumulation of interstitial fluid in the tissues. Following extensive injury to the soft tissues, scar tissue formed in healing may obstruct the lymph channels draining the area. In tropical regions, lymph channels may be obstructed by parasites. Affected parts may reach an enormous size. Lymphedema is a troublesome problem after extensive radical mastectomy. In this operation, the axillary lymph nodes are removed thereby interrupting flow of lymph. This results in swelling of the hand and arm on the affected side. The lymphatic system is an important mechanism in the maintenance of the distribution of body fluids. Anything that interferes with its capacity to function is reflected in the retention of fluid in the interstitial fluid compartment.

As stated earlier, sodium ions have little effect on the movement of fluids into and out of the capillary. Sodium is, however, responsible for about one half of the osmotic pressure of extracellular fluid with the result that it is an important factor in the movement of fluid between the intracellular and extracellular compartments. Any condition that results in the retention of sodium in the body will also be accompanied by the retention of water. Three common conditions in which there is sodium retention are congestive heart failure, renal failure, and an increase in the supply of adrenal cortical hormones. The nature of each of these conditions will be discussed later. Whatever the specific factor, any disorder that causes a retention of sodium in the extracellular fluids is accompanied by the retention of water and the expansion of the extracellular fluid volume. In persons whose mechanisms for eliminating sodium are defective or persons treated with a drug that increases the effectiveness of sodium-saving mechanisms, limitation of sodium intake can be expected to reduce water retention. For these reasons, sodium may be restricted in the therapy of heart and kidney diseases that are accompanied by edema formation or in patients who are treated with adrenal steroids. All salts containing sodium are interdicted, not just sodium chloride. Patients and those preparing their food should be taught to read the labels on prepared foods and medicines for evidence that sodium-containing salts have or have not been added. Foods, such as cured meats, to which salt has been added in preparation should ordinarily be avoided.

In health, a balance is maintained between the amount of fluid leaving and returning to the intravascular fluid compartment. The mechanisms involved in this exchange are summarized in Figure 8-8. Any condition that continues to

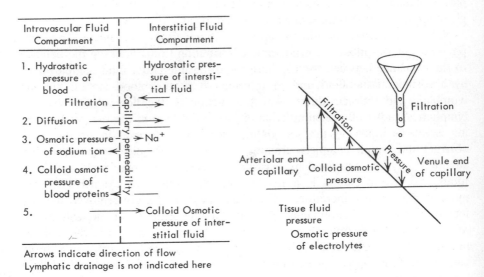

Arrows indicate direction of flow
Lymphatic drainage is not indicated here

FIGURE 8—8. The mechanisms by which fluids are exchanged between the intravascular and interstitial fluid compartments.

upset the equilibrium between the opposing forces can be expected to result in either a retention or a loss of extracellular fluid.

In most discussions of fluid and electrolyte balance more attention is given to the mechanisms for the regulation of the volume and concentration of extracellular fluid than to the intracellular fluid. (See Figure 8-8.) One reason for this is that intracellular fluid is difficult to obtain for study. Inasmuch as all body fluids are interrelated, indirect evidence of the state of intracellular fluids can be obtained from studies of extracellular fluids.

In addition to affecting the distribution of body fluids, certain ions regulate neuromuscular irritability. According to Weisberg,[12] elevated concentrations of sodium and potassium increase neuromuscular irritability, while decreased concentrations decrease it. The irritability of the myoneural junction is decreased by increased concentrations of calcium, magnesium, and hydrogen ions. It is increased by decreased levels of calcium. Potassium affects the

[12] *Op. cit.,* p. 67.

functioning of cardiac and skeletal muscle, and possibly smooth muscle. Increase in the intake of potassium often results in the improvement of patients with gastrointestinal distention. Alterations in the level of potassium in the blood in either direction have an adverse effect on the function of the heart with the result that the patient may die suddenly from heart failure.

Before considering the body's mechanisms for the control of the hydrogen ion, some of the common disturbances in water and electrolyte balance will be presented. Although this separation adds to the clarity of the presentation, the hydrogen ion is part of the electrolyte structure of body fluids. It does not function alone. Changes in the level of hydrogen ions affect the level, function, and regulation of both water and other ions.

Homeostasis of body fluids involves the maintenance of the composition and distribution of water and electrolytes among the three fluid compartments. Although the fluids in the intracellular, interstitial, and intravascular fluid compartments are interrelated, they differ in volume and composition. Physiological mechanisms function to regulate intake and output of electrolytes and water so that volume, osmotic pressure, and hydrogen ion concentration are maintained within so-called normal limits. As is to be expected, regulation involves a number of structures and functions. In health, disturbances in a homeostatic condition initiate a change which results in the correction of the situation.

The capacity to maintain the stability of body fluids is greatest during youth and early middle life and is least at the extremes of life. Many illnesses are accompanied by some disturbance in water and electrolyte balance. In some illnesses the disturbances are minor. In others the recovery of the patient may depend on the ability to correct disturbances and to restore and maintain the normal regulatory mechanisms. In these patients the regulation of fluid and electrolyte balance may be a major objective of the therapy. The constancy of the fluid environment of cells, as well as of the intracellular fluid, depends on: (1) the supply of required materials, (2) the regulation of intake, transportation, and storage, and (3) the elimination of one or more of the required materials. This may result from hypo-, hyper-, or disorganized function. A disturbance in the capacity of one organ to regulate one mechanism may set into action a chain of events leading to widespread and complicated disturbances.

Disturbances in body fluids are usually characterized by some change in volume, concentration, osmotic pressure, or hydrogen ion concentration. The specific effects on the patient will depend on factors such as whether the disturbance is local or general, how severe it is, and its effects on other components of the body fluid. Disturbances in a single component seldom occur. They are usually multiple and often complicated. Each substance entering into the composition of one of the fluid compartments has a significant function. Alterations in the level of any one component of body fluids outside the so-called normal range is likely to be attended by adverse effects.

The most frequent disturbances in fluid and electrolyte balance are those resulting from an excess or deficit of water or of sodium, potassium, calcium, or hydrogen ions. The effects of a disturbance on a particular person or patient will depend on: (1) the direction and degree of change, (2) the effects the disturbance has on the other components of the system, and (3) the effectiveness of the body's mechanisms for correcting or adapting to the disturbance. For example, as Mr. Martin mowed his lawn, he lost appreciable amounts of water and electrolytes in sweat, which is a hypotonic solution of sodium chloride. He also lost water in breathing. His mechanisms for adapting to these losses were efficient and he was able to maintain the stability of his extracellular fluids.

What are some of the causes of disturbances in fluid and electrolytes in illness?

In illness there are many causes of disturbances in fluid and electrolyte equilibrium. They fall into the following categories: (1) a simple deficit or excess of water and/or electrolytes—a lack of supply, (2) inability to ingest or to absorb water or electrolytes, (3) excessive losses through the normal avenues of escape—the skin, gastrointestinal tract, or kidney, (4) failure of the kidney to eliminate excesses of exogenous or endogenous origin, (5) loss of fluids through abnormal avenues or as the result of injury to tissues—surgery and other trauma, fistulae, burned tissues, blood loss, inflamed serous membranes, (6) disturbances in the transportation system, and (7) shifts of fluid from one compartment to another, as in ascites, edema, burns, acute gastric dilatation, and (8) disturbances in the regulation of water and electrolytes. The ultimate effect on the individual patient will be determined by how this change affects the volume, distribution, osmotic pressure, or hydrogen ion concentration of the fluid in each compartment.

What is the most frequent disturbance in water and electrolyte balance? What are some of its causes?

Probably the most frequent disturbance in water and electrolyte balance is a simple deficit of water. For some reason, output of water exceeds intake. This may simply be the result of an inadequate intake, or the output may be increased out of proportion to the intake. This leads to an increase in the concentration, and thereby an increase in the osmotic pressure, of the extracellular fluids. Water may be lost alone or in combination with electrolytes, such as sodium chloride. The loss of one may be greater than the loss of the other. Sweating causes proportionately greater loss of water than it does of sodium chloride. Diarrhea in the early stages has the same effect. In breathing, carbon dioxide, which is continuously replaced, and water are lost. Patients who breathe rapidly and deeply can be expected to require a larger intake of fluid than those who breathe normally. Water losses can be expected to be further increased in patients who breathe through their mouths. Often patients who have increased loss of water through respiration are those who have difficulty in replacing the water by their own efforts. Lethargic, comatose, or confused patients are likely to develop water deficits unless attention is paid to keeping up their fluid intake. Patients with fever lose water by sweating and during respiration. Correction of these losses requires a considerable increase in intake. To maintain the patient's fluid intake requires planning, patience, and effort.

What physiological changes result from a loss of extracellular fluid?

In any condition in which the loss of water from the body exceeds that of intake, water is lost from the extracellular fluid. As a result, the remaining extracellular fluid becomes hypertonic in relation to the intracellular fluid. According to the law of osmosis, water can be expected to move from the more dilute solution within the cell to the more concentrated extracellular fluid. This results in cellular dehydration. In the person who is conscious and competent the most prominent and reliable symptom is thirst. When water is available and the patient is able to ingest and absorb it, the condition is easily corrected by drinking water.

When the loss of water continues without a comparable loss of electrolytes, the amount of available intracellular fluid may be insufficient to correct the water deficit in the extracellular fluid. This results in an increase in the level of hemoglobin, nonprotein nitrogen, sodium, and other electrolytes in the blood. The hematocrit, that is, the proportion of red blood cells to the blood plasma, also rises. The kidney adapts by excreting a small volume of concentrated urine. In patients with adequate renal reserve, a urine output of less than 500 to 800 ml per 24 hours is indicative of an insufficient intake of water. As dehydration increases, skin and mucous membranes become dry and parched. The tongue becomes wrinkled and furry. Sordes, collections of dried secretions, shed cells, and other debris are formed in the mouth and on the lips. When fluid losses are great, water is taken from extracellular spaces, such as the eye globes, with the result that they become soft. In infants and young children, fever is to be expected. Irritability, muscle twitching, and eventually drowsiness and coma result as the brain becomes dehydrated.

To summarize, when any condition disturbs the balance between the intake and output of water so that more water is lost from the body than is replaced, the extracellular fluid becomes hypertonic in relation to the intracellular fluid. Since the body does not tolerate differences in osmotic pressure, intracellular fluid moves from the cell to the extracellular fluid. The increase in osmotic pressure also stimulates receptors which stimulate the sensation of thirst. As a result of decreased blood flow through the kidney and increased secretion of the antidiuretic hormone, the kidney secretes a small volume of concentrated urine. When the condition is allowed to persist, the body's mechanisms for adaptation fail. Circulatory collapse followed by death is the result.

For many patients, the prevention of a deficit of water involves little more than providing adequate amounts of water in a clean and palatable form. From a study reported by Walter,[13] the water offered to patients in carafes does not always meet the latter criteria. The water provided to patients was often as grossly contaminated with microorganisms as it was unpalatable, and possibly unsafe, for drinking. Two practices contributed to the contamination of the water. The carafes in which the water was served had narrow necks. This made thorough cleaning difficult. Ice used to chill the water was handled by hand rather than with the tongs provided for this purpose. The net result was that patients were served foul-smelling, potentially unsafe water.

Some patients require assistance with meeting their need for water. The nurse may have to help patients who, because of their age or the nature or degree of illness, are unable to meet their own need for water. The amount and type of assistance needed by patients varies greatly. The apathetic, the confused, or the very ill patient will require more attention than the patient who is alert and thirsty. The patient may be completely dependent on the nurse. When the patient is unable to drink unless water is placed in his mouth, a cup with a spout, a teaspoon, or drinking tube filled with water may be used. When water is placed in the mouth, care should be taken to adjust the patient's position so swallowing is favored and the danger of aspiration of fluid is minimized. The sitting position is, of course, most satisfactory. When a patient is in the supine position, his head should, if possible, be turned to the side. Those in mechanical respirators should be instructed to swallow during expiration. Another patient may only require that fluids be placed within easy reaching distance and an explanation of why a given fluid intake is desirable. Some patients will more willingly drink water that is iced. Others refuse to drink water, but will take other types of fluids such as ginger ale, broth, or tea. Whatever the problem, the nurse has a responsibility for identifying the needs of the patient, and, within the limits of the situation, for meeting them.

Attention should be given to the distribution of the patient's fluid intake over the ordinary waking hours. The patient should be observed for signs and symptoms indicating his need for water is being met. In addition to the absence of thirst, a urine output of at least 500 to 800 ml, lack of irritability, and moist, clean mucous membranes are all indications that the patient's fluid intake is adequate. Conversely, a urine output of less than 500 ml, irritability, and dry, cracked mucous membranes with sordes on the lips and in the mouth are indicative of an inadequate fluid intake. Signs and symptoms of an inadequate intake were previously enumerated. Day-to-day loss of a pound or more of weight indicates an insufficient intake of water.

Following surgical procedures involving the gastrointestinal tract and re-

[13] Carl D. Walter, et al., "Bacteriology of the Bedside Carafe," New England Journal of Medicine, CCLIX, December 18, 1958, p. 1198.

lated structures, and in acute illness, the patient may not tolerate fluids by mouth. Fluids must then be administered parenterally, usually by intravenous infusion. The dangers to which the patient is exposed are more numerous than when fluids are taken by mouth. Precautions should be taken to make certain the patient gets the correct solution, in the proper amounts, and at the rate prescribed. Attention should also be given to maintaining the sterility of the solution and of the equipment. Though all patients should be observed regularly throughout the period when fluids are being administered, observation is of special importance in those whose homeostatic mechanisms are inadequate or defective. When the rate at which fluids are to be administered is prescribed, some method should be used to simplify checking. For example, a marker may be placed on the bottle of solution indicating the number of drops per minute.

The patient who receives a blood transfusion is exposed to all the risks of patients receiving intravenous fluids. In addition, care must be taken to ensure that the patient is given blood that has been matched to his and to prevent air embolism. Most hospitals have policies for the identification of blood which, when followed, reduce to a minimum the danger of giving the patient the wrong type of blood. These policies should always be followed.

According to Tarail,[14] the possibility of air embolism during blood transfusion is not sufficiently appreciated. Although air embolism is possible in the administration of any intravenous injection, it is greatest when a Y setup is used. The point in the administration of blood when air embolism is most likely to occur is after the blood transfusion has been completed and the stopcock on the tubing leading to the saline bottle has been opened. The effect of this is illustrated in Figure 8-9. When clamps one and two are fully open and clamp three is only partly open, the pressure above clamp three is greater than atmospheric pressure. Below clamp three, the pressure is less than atmospheric pressure. Fluid can be expected to move from the area of greater to that of lesser pressure. As the pressure above clamp three is lessened, air is sucked through the blood bottle and into the tubing below clamp three, that is, air replaces the blood. To prevent air embolism, Tarail[15] suggests that when clamp three is opened, it should be opened wide and clamp two closed. This prevents air from entering the system via the blood bottle. Last, the rate of flow of fluid should be regulated by placing clamp one as close to the patient as is possible.

Another risk to the patient receiving parenteral fluids or blood transfusions is pulmonary edema. This danger is greatest in those receiving repeated blood transfusions, in elderly patients, and in persons who have a limited renal reserve. This hazard can be reduced by maintaining a slow rate of flow of blood or solution. The patient requires regular and frequent observation.

[14] Robert Tarail, "Practice of· Fluid Therapy," *Journal of the American Medical Association,* CLXXI, September 5, 1959, pp. 45-49.
[15] *Ibid.,* p. 46.

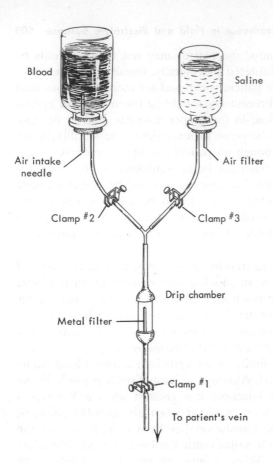

Blood

Saline

Air intake
needle

Air filter

Clamp #2

Clamp #3

FIGURE 8–9. Y-type blood transfusion administration set.

Drip chamber

Metal filter

Clamp #1

To patient's vein

Should the patient become short of breath, the flow of the blood or fluid should be discontinued and the physician notified.

Not only is the rate of flow of parenteral solutions a factor in the safety of the patient, but it affects his comfort and the stability of his fluid and electrolyte balance as well. Studies reported by Talbot,[16] indicate that fluids given over a 12- to 24-hour period contribute more to the patient's comfort and to the stability of his fluid and electrolyte balance than do fluids administered in a six-hour period. Patients had less thirst when fluids were distributed over a longer period. Talbot also found that fluid balance was the same whether fluids were given by mouth or by intravenous infusion.

The rate at which fluids can and should be administered varies with the condition of the patient and the concentration of the solution. According to Davis,[17] up to 600 ml of an isotonic solution can be safely administered in an hour. Under emergency situations the rate may be increased so the patient receives as much as 2,000 ml per hour. The patient must, however, be under

[16] N. B. Talbot, *et al.,* "Application of Homeostatic Principles to the Management of Nephritic Patients," *New England Journal of Medicine,* CCLV, October 4, 1956, p. 655.
[17] Harry A. Davis, *Principles of Surgical Physiology,* Paul B. Hoeber, Inc., 1957, p. 40.

constant supervision. Should the urinary output exceed 50 ml per hour, the rate of infusion should be decreased because the amount of solution the patient is receiving is too great. In elderly patients the rate of flow should be slower than in younger ones.[18] The concentration and the composition of the fluid also affect the rate at which it can be safely administered. Hypotonic and hypertonic solutions should be given at a slower rate than isotonic solutions. The rate for hypotonic solutions should be adjusted so not more than 250 to 400 ml is given per hour. Hypertonic solutions should not be administered at a rate faster than 200 ml per hour. The maximum rate of flow for glucose solutions is 0.5 gm per kilogram of body weight per hour. A more rapid rate results in glycosuria and the loss of potassium. When there is a question about the rate at which a solution should be administered, the nurse who is responsible for the care of the patient should consult with the patient's physician.

In the regulation of the flow of the solution both the number of drops per minute and the size of each drop are significant in the determination of the number of milliliters delivered per hour. Tarail[19] states that the Abbott set delivers about 20 drops to the milliliter. The Baxter set delivers 10. Micro sets are available that deliver 43 to 45 drops to the milliliter. After the rate of flow is adjusted, continued supervision is required. No matter how carefully the rate is set, it can be expected to change.

Continued observation of the patient is also necessary. Although parenteral injections are everyday procedures to hospital personnel, this is not necessarily true for patients. Patients receiving them are often very ill. Some patients receive intravenous injections because of serious illness. Patients with marginal renal or cardiac reserve are in danger of pulmonary edema or congestive heart failure. In some hospitals, patients are instructed to call the nurse when the solution stops running or when the bottle becomes nearly empty. Before a patient is asked to do this, the nurse should be sure the patient is emotionally and physically well enough to assume this responsibility. Moreover, the nurse should continue to observe the patient. Calls for help should be answered promptly. Should the patient give evidence of increased anxiety, the nurse should resume full responsibility for observing the fluid level. The importance of this to the sick patient is illustrated by an excerpt from a letter written by Mrs. Blonde, who wrote to a friend about her experience in a hospital during which she had a cholecystectomy. ". . . but to have to supervise every step of your own care when you feel rotten is, to say the very least, very disturbing. I had to be sure that I stayed awake to watch the I.V.'s, blood, etc., because sure as anything, if I dropped off to sleep, they would run dry, etc., etc. This happened even after I had discussed it with the head nurse and she had assured me that I could relax because they would watch it very closely." Whether Mrs. Blonde's physical safety was threatened is not known; certainly,

---

[18] *Ibid.*, p. 148.
[19] *Op. cit.*, p. 47.

she felt unsafe and neglected. Energy she should have been using for recovery was expended in protecting herself against possible injury. Relaxation, which she badly needed, was impossible to obtain.

Attention should also be given to the patient's general comfort. When the needle or cannula is inserted over a joint, the part should be supported by a padded board or splint. When necessary, the patient should be assisted in moving and turning. When a patient receiving intravenous fluids is ambulated, enough assistance should be available to give the patient the help he requires. He should be prepared for what to expect and what is expected of him. This may be an everyday procedure to the nurse, but this is not true for the patient.

As stated earlier, a deficit of water in the body is reflected in a decrease in the volume of extracellular fluid and a corresponding increase in its concentration. Unless the loss of fluid, including whole blood, is great or continued, the condition is corrected by an increased fluid intake and/or by dehydration of cells. The body's mechanisms for adapting to changes in the volume of extracellular fluid are such that the blood volume is kept constant. When however, the loss of water from the body is excessive, blood volume is also diminished. The seriousness of the situation depends on the extent to which the decrease in the volume of blood interferes with the nutrition of vital structures.

A function of the extracellular fluids is to serve as a vehicle for the transportation of materials to and from the cells of the body. An important element in the maintenance of the circulation is the relationship of the volume of blood to the capacity of the vascular chamber. When a disparity develops between the volume of circulating blood and the size of the vascular chamber, the condition is termed shock or peripheral circulatory failure. The outcome is a failure in tissue nutrition.

Shock is classified in many ways by different authorities. However, most agree that in shock a disproportion between the volume of blood and the capacity of the vascular chamber is the essential feature. This leads to an inadequate return of blood to the right side of the heart. Since the cardiac output is dependent on the venous return, there is a corresponding decrease in the quantity of blood delivered by the heart into the circulation. What happens at this point depends on the suddenness of the onset of shock and the degree of disparity between the size of the vascular chamber and the volume of blood. When the onset is sudden, the body may have no time to initiate mechanisms of adjustment. As a consequence, the brain is deprived of its blood supply and unconsciousness results. When the onset of shock is gradual, compensatory adjustments enable the body to maintain the cerebral circulation at a more or less normal level. Vasoconstriction in the less vital areas reduces the capacity (size) of the vascular chamber and thereby contributes to the maintenance of the blood pressure. The heart rate also increases. When the patient's compensatory mechanisms are effective, he may, for a time, be able to maintain his blood pressure within normal limits. If, however, the condition is allowed to continue, compensation will eventually fail and his blood pressure will fall. In some patients, the capacity to adapt to the loss of blood and fluid from the blood by vasoconstriction is considerable. Because a patient's blood pressure is within the normal limits, the nurse should not disregard other signs and symptoms of shock or evidence indicating shock is possible. When the patient is in the supine position, a fall in blood pressure may be a late finding. The patient who is losing appreciable quantities of blood may maintain his blood pressure for a time, only to have it suddenly fall to imperceptible levels. The exact level of blood pressure that is significant in an individual patient depends to some extent on his usual blood pressure. For example, some healthy people have systolic blood pressures around 100 mm of mercury. Obviously a blood pressure of this level does not indicate shock or impending shock. In another person whose blood pressure is usually 210 systolic, a blood pressure of 100 has quite a different meaning. In persons whose systolic blood pressures ordinarily range from 110 to 140, a blood pressure of 100 or less is significant. A systolic pressure of from 60 to 70 mm of mercury is necessary to maintain the coronary circulation. In addition to the level of the systolic pressure, a low pulse pressure is also indicative of shock. It is often less than 20 mm of mercury. Maintenance of the diastolic pressure is evidence of arteriolar constriction—a desirable compensatory mechanism under these circumstances.

As was stated earlier, manifestations of shock result from the compensatory mechanisms that are initiated and the effects of nutritional deprivation on vital structures such as the brain, kidney, heart, and liver. A sudden and massive hemorrhage may reduce the blood volume so rapidly that death occurs before corrective measures can be instituted. In addition to the previously discussed effects of shock on blood pressure, peripheral vasoconstriction results in pallor of the skin. The skin may be either cold and clammy or stiff and inelastic. The signs and symptoms associated with a lack of blood supply to the brain will be determined by the suddenness with which shock develops, as well as its severity. Fainting is likely to occur when shock develops suddenly. In the patient who is in a horizontal position, this may be manifested as a feeling of dizziness or faintness when he assumes an upright position. When shock develops over a period of several hours, apathy, lethargy, and confusion may be among the earlier signs. The patient may also be restless and abnormally alert. Many descriptions of the clinical picture of the person in shock emphasize the anxious or worried expression as a characteristic feature. Changes in the degree of alertness in either direction may be significant.

Kidney function is also affected in shock. Glomerular filtration depends on the pressure at which the blood is circulated through the glomerular capillaries. The average capillary pressure of blood in the glomeruli is much higher than in other capillaries. The kidney is able to maintain this pressure despite changes in the systemic blood pressure. Although the mechanisms by which this is accomplished are not completely understood, the afferent arterioles supplying the glomeruli dilate as the blood pressure falls and constrict as it rises. In this way they act much as a faucet on a water pipe. As with other adaptive mechanisms, there are limits to which the kidney is able to protect itself against a falling systemic blood pressure. Shock can, therefore, be expected to result in oliguria or anuria. Measurement of the urine output is important in the patient who is predisposed to shock. In the patient whose fluid intake is adequate, secretion of less than 25 ml of urine per hour is indicative of shock. Urine may be collected and measured hourly in patients in potential or actual shock. An output of less than 25 ml per hour should be reported promptly. The kidney may also suffer injury as a consequence of shock. The reason for this is not entirely clear. From the evidence, renal ischemia may be responsible. The ischemia may be the direct result of the low blood pressure. There is also the possibility that one of the body's compensatory mechanisms in shock is to shunt blood around the kidney. The kidney has a high rate of metabolism. This makes it susceptible to injury of the tubule cells when the blood supply is deficient. When the injury is severe and tubular necrosis occurs, the patient may die in renal failure. To obtain hourly specimens of urine an indwelling catheter is often required. Because this exposes the patient to the danger of an ascending urinary tract infection, some physicians do not use this method of checking the patient's status. They rely on other observations.

The prompt treatment of the patient in impending shock is imperative. Once the patient goes into irreversible shock, even intensive therapy is frequently without avail. Observation of the patient who is in danger of developing shock should be carried out conscientiously. Signs and symptoms such as low urine output, falling blood pressure, increasing pulse rate, restlessness, unexpected loss of blood, irritability, lethargy, worried expression, pallor, excessive weakness, or anything indicating all is not well should be reported promptly. In addition, the patient's care should be planned to eliminate from his environment those conditions that make effort on his part necessary, but do not contribute to his immediate welfare. Gentle handling of the patient and control of his environment so he is protected from unnecessary stimulation (loud and sudden noises, for example) should be the rule. Although the application of external heat is generally harmful because it favors vasodilation and sweating, the patient should be protected from undue heat loss. A room temperature of 68° to 70° F. is probably satisfactory. Elevation of the foot of the bed usually results in an increase in the blood pressure by improving the return of fluid from the lower extremities. Visitors should be limited to the immediate family. If at all possible, care should be planned so the patient has some periods of uninterrupted rest.

In planning the medical therapy of the patient in shock, the physician considers the factors responsible for the condition. When the primary feature is a decrease in the blood volume, the treatment is directed toward restoring the volume of blood. A common and well-known cause is the loss of whole blood. Blood volume can also be reduced by the loss of the fluid elements of the blood into the interstitial spaces or into or from body cavities. It can be reduced in severe dehydration such as develops when a person is lost in the desert. Examples of conditions in which fluid elements are lost from the blood include the patient who is burned, the patient with excessive losses of fluid into and from the gastrointestinal tract, the patient with kidney disease, or the patient who perspires excessively. In all these patients, the loss of fluid from the vascular compartment must be sufficiently in excess of intake to lower the blood volume. In these patients, treatment is directed toward replacing the deficient elements—water, electrolytes, blood proteins, and blood cells. Oxygen is frequently prescribed. The objective is to saturate the blood plasma circulating through the lung with oxygen. Use of oxygen in shock is usually irrational unless it can be used under pressure; in this circumstance the actual oxygen-carrying *capacity* of the plasma (not hemoglobin) can be significantly increased. Cyanosis in shock is due to *stasis* of blood, not to unsaturation of hemoglobin after passage through the pulmonary capillary bed.

In other patients, the primary factor in shock is the loss of vascular tone, and, as a consequence, an increase in the capacity of the vascular chamber. As a result of the loss of vascular tone, the blood vessels are unable to adapt to the volume of blood in order to maintain the blood pressure at a satisfactory level. Vascular tone is regulated by nervous and humoral factors. There is experimental evidence that a vasodilator material (VDM) is present in the blood in excess. Vascular tone may be lost as a result of surgical or chemical sympathectomy or spinal anesthesia. Emotional factors may lead to a temporary vasodilatation with syncope or fainting. Following extensive surgical sympathectomy, spinal anesthesia, spinal cord injury, and other similar conditions, the lower extremities may be wrapped with elastic bandages to prevent the pooling of blood when the patient assumes the upright position. Unless this is done, the patient may faint as a result of postural hypotension. Patients under treatment with antihypertensive drugs should be taught to assume the upright position in slow stages after they have been in a recumbent position. Spinal anesthesia and transection of the spinal cord also predispose to shock by interfering with the individual's ability to maintain vascular tone.

Shock in patients with serious conditions involving the viscera may be due in part to reflex vasodilatation and thus to an increase in the size of the vascular chamber. According to Dexter and Harrison,[20] this is a factor in the shock that accompanies conditions such as myocardial infarction and acute pancreatitis.

For patients in whom the primary problem is a loss of vascular tone, a vasoconstrictor drug such as Levophed bitartrate[21] or Aramine bitartrate[22] may

[20] Lewis Dexter and T. R. Harrison, "Circulatory Failure," *Principles of Internal Medicine,* ed. T. R. Harrison, 3rd ed., The Blakiston Division of The McGraw-Hill Book Co., Inc., New York, 1958, p. 116.
[21] Trade name for levarterenol bitartrate.
[22] Trade name for metaraminol bitartrate.

be prescribed. When levarterenol bitartrate is administered by intravenous injection, both the systolic and diastolic pressure rise and the pulse pressure usually increases.[23] Unless the administration of a large amount of fluid is contraindicated, 4 ml of the commercially prepared levarterenol bitartrate is diluted in 1,000 ml of 5 per cent glucose or 0.9 per cent sodium chloride. The rate of flow of the solution is then adjusted so the blood pressure is maintained within the desired range. All patients receiving levarterenol bitartrate should be under continuous supervision. The blood pressure should be carefully checked every 5 to 15 minutes, or at intervals specified by the physician, and the rate of flow of the solution adjusted as necessary. When a needle is introduced into a vein for the administration of the fluid, the surrounding area should be checked for evidence of leakage into the subcutaneous tissue. When a solution of levarterenol bitartrate infiltrates the tissue, it causes necrosis and sloughing. In patients in whom shock is primarily due to loss of blood volume, vasoconstrictor drugs are not very effective.

In myocardial failure the force of cardiac contraction may be insufficient to maintain the cardiac output. Although the signs and symptoms presented by the patient cannot be distinguished from those caused by failure of the peripheral circulation, they are due to the failure of the myocardium to pump enough blood into the arteries to maintain adequate cellular nutrition. Because the syndrome is due to the failure of the pumping action of the myocardium, it may be caused by any condition which fatigues or weakens the heart muscle. Thus in the healthy heart it may result from prolonged periods of tachycardia or in the diseased heart from myocardial ischemia. In the terminal phase of congestive heart failure, it is a common event. (See Chapter 9.) To the extent that the return flow of blood to the heart is reduced in peripheral circulatory failure, the nutrition of the heart muscle is also lessened. As its blood supply falls below its needs, myocardial contractility diminishes. With a lessening in the cardiac output the situation is further worsened. Peripheral circulatory stasis → reduced return of blood to heart → fall in arterial blood pressure → weakened cardiac contraction → lessened output → myocardial (and other tissue) ischemia.

In giving nursing care to patients with conditions predisposing to shock by decreasing vascular tone and thereby increasing the capacity of the vascular system, all the points previously emphasized are important. Conscientious observation of the patient with prompt reporting of symptoms and the initiation of appropriate emergency care is of prime importance in the prevention of irreversible shock. In some instances it may develop very quickly.

Since the capacity for adapting to stress is taxed in shock-inducing situations, the nurse has a responsibility for protecting the patient from unnecessary and controllable stimulation. She is usually responsible for the supervision of therapeutic procedures directed toward correcting the basic pathologi-

[23] Louis S. Goodman and Alfred Gilman, *The Pharmacological Basis of Therapeutics*, 2nd ed., The Macmillan Company, New York, 1956, p. 501.

cal physiology. Sometimes the causative factor is clear-cut. Frequently it is not. The patient may have both an inadequate blood volume and an increased capacity of the vascular system. In the prevention of irreversible shock, treatment is directed toward restoring the blood volume, increasing the vascular tone, and supporting the nutrition of the tissues. When the patient has a correctable condition, such as hemorrhage, the condition must also be controlled. In the case of hemorrhage, bleeding must be stopped and the blood volume restored.

One precaution in the care of the patient in impending shock that has not been previously emphasized relates to the use of narcotics and sedatives. Unless the patient is in real pain, they should not be used. Restlessness is not always an indication of pain, as it usually indicates a lack of oxgen to the brain. Shock may actually be worsened by sedative drugs, such as the barbiturates, because they may increase vasodilation. The patient who has severe pain and requires morphine should have it administered intravenously. When morphine is given subcutaneously to the patient in shock, it may not be absorbed. When the patient's condition improves, the morphine is then absorbed. If he has had several injections, he may then suffer from morphine poisoning. The restless patient is often relieved by the administration of oxygen, rather than narcotics.

Shock or peripheral vascular failure is a very common condition. It is a frequent precursor of death. In severe and sudden injuries, the body may have no opportunity to initiate compensatory mechanisms to protect vital structures from a loss of blood supply. In disease or injury in which the onset is gradual, compensatory mechanisms are activated to protect vital structures from nutritional deprivation. These mechanisms serve to maintain an appropriate ratio between the blood volume and the capacity of the blood vessels. Compensation is easiest when the patient is in a horizontal position. Signs and symptoms of impending shock may not be evident unless the patient is in the upright position. Signs and symptoms have their origin in the compensatory adjustments made by the cardiovascular system and in the failure of nutrition of vital structures. Knowledge of the basic pathophysiology of shock should help the nurse to understand and fulfill her role in the care of patients.

*What are some of the causes and effects of excess water
in the body?*

Water may be found in the body in excess as well as in deficit. With an excess of water there is a change in the volume of water in one or more of the fluid compartments. This then alters the osmotic pressure relationship between the intracellular and the extracellular fluid compartments. Since materials from the external environment enter and leave the body by way of the extracellular fluid, an excess of water is usually first reflected in a change in the extracellular fluid volume. Neither the healthy nor the sick will ordinarily drink themselves into water intoxication, but they may occasionally be persuaded to do so. In the sick, the usual source is water administered by intravenous or rectal injections. In longstanding disorders, the water of oxidation may contribute to the total quantity of water in the body. Water intoxication need not develop if attention is given to the patient's reaction to drinking fluids and some thought is given to the observation that the patient's fluid intake is in excess of his total fluid output. The patient's weight also provides evidence for or against the storage of water. A gain in weight by a patient who is ingesting a limited amount of food should create more than a suspicion that water intake is exceeding its loss. For each pound of weight gained, about a pint of fluid is retained. Tarail[24] states that, in the absence of food intake, a patient should be expected to lose about 14 oz a day. To obtain an accurate weight, the patient should be weighed at the same time each day and with the same amount of clothing. When at all possible, the patient should be weighed in the morning before breakfast and after having emptied his bladder. If he is able to stand on a scale, the simplest way is to remove all clothing except a hospital gown, and have the patient step onto a paper towel that has been placed on the scale. If he is weighed on a bed scale, the same amount of covering can be used each day or it can be weighed each time and subtracted from the total. Of course, the scale should be balanced before the weight is taken. Accurate weighing of the patient contributes data which, when added to other facts, can be used to judge the patient's response to therapy. It is probably the best single measure of the state of the patient's fluid intake. Improperly done, the weight obtained is worthless. It may even be the basis for making harmful changes in therapy. To state this another way, the value of the information obtained by weighing a patient depends, as do the data in any scientific investigation, on the care with which the variables are controlled.

Whereas a deficit of water results in the hypertonicity of extracellular fluids and an increase in osmotic pressure, an excess of water results in hypotonicity. This reduces the osmotic pressure of the extracellular fluid by decreasing the number of particles per unit of water. As a consequence of the loss of osmotic pressure, water moves from the extracellular fluid into the cell causing the cell to swell. The symptoms presented by the patient have their origin in disturbed cerebral function. They include disturbed thought and behavior. If the condition is allowed to continue, coma and death will follow.

As has been previously emphasized, thirst is a reliable indicator of the need for water. For a variety of reasons, the quantity of water ingested may be insufficient or in excess of the needs of the individual. In health, the kidney does a remarkably efficient job of removing or conserving water. Under most circumstances, water intoxication is not likely unless the renal mechanisms for the elimination of water fail. The fault may be in the kidney itself, or in the overproduction of the antidiuretic hormone, or the result of an impairment in

[24] *Op. cit.,* p. 48.

the circulation of blood through the kidney. The first few days after surgical procedure,[25] or following a serious injury, patients are susceptible to overloading with water. This is the reason accurate recording of intake, output, and weight is important during this period.

Prevention and treatment of water intoxication include the limitation of the patient's water intake, so that water is not allowed to accumulate in the body. In patients with acute renal failure, this may mean the patient receives as little as 300 to 500 ml of fluid in 24 hours. Careful observation and recording of the patient's intake, output, and weight provide information about the patient upon which his needs for fluid can be based. Urine may be collected and measured hourly as well as for 24 hours. Since specific gravity of urine is determined by the capacity of the kidney to concentrate urine, each specimen of urine may be tested for specific gravity.

What are some of the causes of the loss of sodium from the body?

Since the extracellular fluid volume depends on an adequate level of sodium in the body, a reduction in sodium will be attended by a decreased volume of extracellular fluid. Many conditions are associated with a loss of sodium from the body. They include in particular those conditions in which gastrointestinal secretions are lost in excessive quantities and over a period of time. Short illnesses in which there is vomiting or diarrhea cause more significant losses of water than of sodium ions. Patients having gastrointestinal drainage or those with fluid drainage from an ileostomy or fistula lose some sodium. Other conditions also responsible for sodium loss include: (1) excessive sweating, (2) renal insufficiency in which salt is not reabsorbed, (3) the overuse of diuretics, and (4) the overconscientious restriction of salt in the diet. Sodium loss is also a problem in adrenal insufficiency, because the body's mechanism for conserving sodium is defective.

What causes the symptoms that result from too little sodium in the body?

Since sodium is necessary for the maintenance of the volume of blood and interstitial fluid, untoward symptoms result from too little extracellular fluid. When the condition develops acutely, the symptoms are those of circulatory collapse. There is a low plasma volume, a high hematocrit, hypotension, thready pulse, tachycardia, and collapsed neck veins. Because of the loss of interstitial fluid, there is a loss of tissue turgor. The skin becomes sticky; that is, when it is picked up between the fingers, it tends to stick together and to remain standing rather than returning quickly to the original position. The tongue becomes shrunken and wrinkled. In advanced cases, the eyeballs

[25] D. A. K. Black, "Symptoms and Signs of Disorders of Body Fluids," *Journal of Chronic Diseases*, XI, March, 1960, pp. 340-47.

become soft and the eyes appear to be set deep in their sockets. When sodium deficits develop slowly, as might be the case in the patient on a restricted diet, particularly during hot weather, manifestations are less dramatic. They may include cramps, fainting on assuming the upright position as the result of postural hypotension, or simply general lethargy. The onset of hot weather, with the attendant increase in perspiration, may precipitate a sodium deficit in patients who have been on a prolonged regime of diuretics and salt restriction. The nurse supervising the care of these patients, in either the hospital or the home, should be alert to this possibility and should not too quickly dismiss the patient's complaints of fatigue or loss of energy, or of feeling faint on arising in the morning, as being due to spring fever. What the patient needs is not sulfur and molasses, but an increase in his salt intake. Therefore, his symptoms should be reported to his physician.

Sodium deficits require replacement of both sodium and water. Fluids may be administered by mouth or by intravenous injection. The salt content of oral fluids may be increased by giving them in the form of bouillon or soup. If fruit juices are administered, they should have salt added to them. When the loss of sodium is proportionately greater than the loss of chloride, sodium alone may be administered. Intravenous fluids containing sodium bicarbonate and sometimes sodium lactate may also be used. Control of the rate of administration is important. Too rapid administration leads to an increased loss of electrolytes, and thus defeats the purpose of the treatment. In patients who have prolonged gastric or intestinal suction, physiological saline solution should be used to irrigate the tube to prevent the loss of sodium and chloride ions.

Sodium excess

As is to be expected, an increase in the retention of sodium in the body results in the retention of water and an increase in the extracellular fluid volume. This produces a generalized edema. The most immediate and serious results are edema of the lung and an overloading of the circulatory system. Generalized edema occurs when the body's homeostatic mechanisms for eliminating excess sodium break down. As stated previously, the kidney regulates the level of the sodium ion in extracellular fluid. Kidney function depends on an adequate blood flow and the presence of aldosterone. The level of aldosterone depends on the relationship of the quantity secreted by the adrenal cortex and the rate at which it is destroyed by the liver. Therefore, sodium excess becomes a problem in: (1) renal failure accompanied by salt retention; (2) disorders in which circulation of blood through the kidney is inadequate, such as congestive heart failure; (3) cirrhosis of the liver; (4) disorders characterized by overproduction of aldosterone by the adrenal cortex; and (5) patients who are treated with large doses of adrenal corticoids. In all these conditions there is sodium retention and with it an increase in the volume of extracellular fluid.

Prevention and treatment of sodium excess is directed toward correction of the condition causing sodium retention, combined with the restriction of sodium intake. The degree to which salt intake is reduced varies. In some patients, all that is required is to eliminate the use of salt in cooking. In others, all salts of sodium are prohibited. This includes sodium as bicarbonate, lactate, or benzoate. These patients should be taught to read the labels on foods and medicines and to reject those to which any sodium salt has been added. In the patient with congestive heart failure, restoration of the normal force of the heart beat by digitalis, coupled with a restricted salt intake and diuretics to increase water and salt elimination, may be accompanied by remarkable changes in the patient. For example, Mrs. Martin, who suffered from a severe degree of cardiac insufficiency, lost 50 lb.—25 ll of fluid—during her first week in the hospital. She entered the hospital short of breath to the point of orthopnea, cyanotic, nauseated, and looking very ill. Within a week she was no longer orthopneic at rest. Her color and appetite were also improved.

Although an excess of sodium ion in the extracellular fluid predisposes to edema by holding water, it is not the only factor in edema (edema is the abnormal retention of fluid in the interstitial spaces or in serous cavities). It results when the balance between the quantity of fluid entering the interstitial space is greater than that leaving it. In severe and generalized edema, the volume of blood may also be increased. The physiological factors having a role in the movement of fluids across the capillary membrane are listed below. In the summary that follows, some of the disorders that predispose to the development of edema have been enumerated. From this summary the conclusion that, in edema, more than one mechanism is frequently involved is valid.

Physiological Factors	*Increase in Interstitial Fluid Volume (Edema)*
1. Capillary permeability ↑	a. Inflammation—increases capillary permeability b. Acute nephritis c. Burns
2. Hydrostatic pressure in the capillary ↑	a. Local venous obstruction, as in the use of constricting bandages or casts, pressing on vein, swelling, varicose veins, etc. b. Generalized increase in venous pressure, as in congestive heart failure
3. Colloid osmotic pressure of blood proteins (decrease in ↓ blood proteins)	a. Nephrosis b. Starvation c. Burns d. Chronic diarrhea e. Acute nephritis, but not a usual cause

Physiological Factors

4. Sodium retention ↑

5. Lymphatic drainage ↓

Increase in Interstitial Fluid Volume (Edema)

a. Congestive heart failure
b. Salt-saving nephritis
c. Increase in level of adrenal cortical hormones (Endogenous)
                      (Exogenous)
   (1) Aldosterone
   (2) Desoxycorticosterone
   (3) Cortisone, hydrocortisone, etc.
d. Following trauma
   (1) Surgical procedures
   (2) Burns
   (3) Fractures

Lymphatic obstruction
Cancerous lymph nodes, removal of lymph nodes, elephantiasis such as follows parasitic invasion of lymph channels

What are some of the factors influencing the location of edema? How does its location influence its effects?

The location of edema depends on the nature of the cause and whether it is localized or generalized. Generally, edema appears first in tissues that are poorly protected against the effects of hydrostatic pressure, such as the skin and subcutaneous tissues, and in dependent parts of the body. As a consequence, edema is found in the feet and ankles of those who are up and about and in the buttocks and sacrum of the bedridden. The influence of gravity on the distribution of edema fluid can sometimes be observed in the patient who has marked generalized edema. In the morning, after the patient spends the night on a lowered headrest, the eyelids may be so swollen that the patient has difficulty in opening his eyes. Later in the day, and after he has been sitting upright, the swelling is much less marked. Edema of the lungs is a possibility in patients with limited cardiac or renal reserve, or in conditions accompanied by capillary injury such as infections involving the lung. When the hydrostatic pressure of the blood in the pulmonary capillaries rises so it is equal to, or exceeds, the colloid osmotic pressure of the blood, transudation of fluid into the lung tissue takes place. Pulmonary edema is always a serious condition. Manifestations depend on the extent to which the hydrostatic pressure is increased and the rapidity with which the condition develops. In milder cases, the patient can be expected to have moist râles and shortness of breath. In severe cases, the alveoli may fill with fluid causing ventilation to fail. Essentially, the patient drowns in his own fluids. In patients who are predisposed to pulmonary edema, the possibility of this catastrophe can be reduced by modifying fluid intake in relation to the output. Intravenous infusions and blood transfusions should be regulated so the rate of flow is slow enough so the blood volume will not be suddenly increased. Throughout the procedure, the patient should be observed for shortness of breath and an increase in pulse or respiratory rate. The urine output should also be measured hourly so the status of the patient's output in relation to his intake will be known. Should there be any indication that excessive fluid is being retained or that pulmonary edema is developing, the flow of the solution should be stopped or slowed to a minimum rate and the physician called immediately.

Edema in tissues other than the lung interferes with their nutrition by limiting the flow of blood to them. This renders the tissue more vulnerable to injury. In the bedfast patient with edema of the sacrum and buttocks, special attention to these areas is required to prevent the development of decubiti. Prevention of decubiti is especially difficult when the patient is orthopneic as a result of pulmonary edema. In orthopnea, the patient's breathing is so difficult that he is comfortable only when he sits leaning forward, if even then. Because he is short of breath and miserable, he resists changes in position. Continued pressure on edematous tissue leads to tissue breakdown. Prevention taxes the best efforts of the nurse. Small shifts in position, the use of an alternating pressure mattress, or a sheepskin pelt under the buttocks of the patient may be helpful in the prevention of decubiti.

Patients with generalized edema are often seriously undernourished. When measures are initiated that are successful in eliminating edema fluid, the patient generally becomes thin or even emaciated. Improvement of the patient, therefore, depends not only on the elimination of edematous fluid, but on improvement of his nutritional state. In some patients, edema lessens as the patient's nutrition is rectified. The feeding of the patient is therefore an important aspect of his nursing care.

The edema or swelling following injury is discussed elsewhere. This is also true for the effects of edema in specialized organs such as the brain. The effect of edema fluid in any structure is that it limits the blood flow to the part, thereby interfering with its nutrition.

A variety of terms are used to describe the location of edema fluid. A severe and generalized edema is called anasarca. Accumulations of fluid in the peritoneal cavity is called ascites. In the pleural cavity, it is called hydrothorax, and an accumulation in the pericardial sac is known as hydropericardium. In all these conditions the fluid occupies space in a body cavity normally occupied by an organ or system and thereby interferes with its function. The clinical effects depend on the site and quantity of the edema fluid.

To summarize, the factors that enter into the development of edema and its effects will be reviewed in relation to Mrs. Bird, who was admitted to the hospital in congestive heart failure. Mrs. Bird has been selected because multiple factors appeared to play a role in the development of edema in her case (heart disease). For many years, Mrs. Bird had essential hypertension. For the last few months she had noticed that her ankles had been swelling and that she became short of breath when she walked up a flight of stairs or walked rapidly. On medical examination she was found to have cardiac insufficiency on the basis of longstanding essential hypertension.

All the factors responsible for the development of edema in the patient with cardiac insufficiency are not understood. Authorities appear to agree that, as a result of a decrease in the force of the heart beat, blood flow to the kidney is diminished. Applied to Mrs. Bird, this would mean her heart was no longer able to fully overcome the resistance to the flow of blood by her constricted arteries. Blood flow to her tissues, including her kidneys, was diminished. The heart was unable to move as much blood into the circulation as was delivered to it. This predisposed to increased venous hydrostatic pressure. As a consequence, she retained salt and water. The condition may have been aggravated by an increase in the production of aldosterone by the adrenal cortex and possibly by a rise in the production of the antidiuretic hormone by the posterior pituitary. As a consequence, the volume of her extracellular fluid rose. As the blood volume enlarged, the hydrostatic pressure of the blood rose. With the elevation in hydrostatic pressure, filtration of fluid from the capillary to the interstitial space exceeded that removed from it. This, combined with the inability of the kidney to remove the necessary amount of water and salt, resulted in edema. In cardiac edema, the interstitial fluid is hypotonic. The reason for this is not known.

In the treatment of Mrs. Bird, the physician had two principal objectives. One was to correct the condition causing the edema. The other was to support the body's physiological mechanisms for the elimination of salt and water. The first objective was directed toward augmenting the strength of cardiac contraction. This was achieved by digitalizing Mrs. Bird with Digitoxin, U.S.P. Digitalization was maintained by a daily dose of 0.2 mg of Digitoxin, U.S.P. To support her physiological mechanisms for the regulation of sodium and water, she was placed on a low-sodium diet and her daily water intake was limited to 1,200 ml. To this was added chlormerodrin, 18.3 mg orally, and acetazolamide U.S.P. 250 mg. Both these drugs act to increase the excretion of salt and water by the kidney.

The objectives on which the nursing care of Mrs. Bird was based included: (1) making pertinent observations as the basis for modifications in the medical regime and the nursing care of Mrs. Bird, (2) reducing the work of the heart by meeting Mrs. Bird's physical and emotional needs, (3) preventing the breakdown of edematous tissue, (4) carrying out those aspects of the medical regime that are the responsibility of the nurse so that the therapy is effective, and (5) as Mrs. Bird recovers, participating in a program to prepare her to return home and to activity.

The observation of Mrs. Bird was directed toward gathering information about how she was responding to her illness and to the therapy, and how she regarded her illness. Her nurse was interested in what Mrs. Bird expected in relation to her illness, hospitalization, nursing, and medical care. Since Mrs. Bird was obviously ill and apprehensive when she was admitted, she was given complete physical care. Every effort was made to reassure Mrs. Bird that her needs would be met promptly and to prepare her for what to expect. Her environment was controlled so all unnecessary stimuli were eliminated. Planned periods of rest were provided. Visitors were restricted to the members of her immediate family. Arrangements were made for the hospital chaplain to visit her each day. As her general condition improved, as evidenced by the fact that (1) she felt better, (2) she had a marked diuresis— she excreted 25 ll of urine and lost 50 lb. during the first week of hospitalization, (3) she could breathe comfortably in a recumbent position, and (4) her appetite improved, her activity was increased and she was given some responsibility for performing activities of daily living. With each increase in activity, the nurse checked her pulse and noted her respirations. Had her pulse rate risen more than 10 beats per minute, or continued to rise, the nurse would have reduced her activity for the time being. She also explained to Mrs. Bird that the reason for her increased activity was that she was improving. As Mrs. Bird improved, her daughter was also included in discussions of planning for Mrs. Bird's convalescence after her discharge from the hospital. Further and more detailed discussion of the care of the patient in congestive heart failure may be found in Chapter 9.

What are the functions of potassium in the body?

When compared to sodium, the level of potassium in the extracellular fluid is low. Nonetheless, cells are sensitive to deviations of potassium outside the normal range. As stated earlier, potassium, as the most abundant cation in the intracellular fluid, plays an important role in the maintenance of the volume of fluid within the cell. It participates in the regulation of neuromuscular irritability and in the maintenance of the hydrogen ion concentration in the blood. Because of the difficulties involved in testing the level of potassium in the cell, the state of potassium balance is inferred from its level in the blood potassium. The blood plasma level may or may not give an accurate picture. It may be normal or even elevated in the presence of an excess of potassium in the body. This is most likely to be true in conditions in which the cells are deprived of an adequate supply of oxygen, that is, in tissue anoxia, or when fluids and electrolytes are lost in excessive quantities. Common examples include diabetic acidosis and gastrointestinal disorders associated with the continued loss of secretions. For example, Mary Kay was admitted to the emergency room with a tentative diagnosis of acute appendicitis. On examination, her urine was found to contain glucose, acetone, and diacetic acid. Further investigation revealed that she was in diabetic acidosis. For some time she had been drinking large amounts of water (polydipsia) and voiding large quantities of urine (polyuria). Her blood sugar was 700 mg per 100 ml of blood plasma, and her carbon dioxide-combining power was 10 volumes per cent. The level of potassium in her blood was within normal limits. To correct her severe dehydration she was given 10,000 ml of fluid intravenously in a period of about ten hours. Unfortunately for Mary Kay, her illness developed before knowledge was available that a potassium deficit may not be manifested until fluid deficits are corrected. Despite the fact that metabolism of glucose was re-established by insulin therapy and her dehydration corrected, she died suddenly from cardiac failure. Just preceding her death, her respirations became shallow, her pulse weak and rapid, and her color ashen. Though the cause of her sudden death was not known at the time, death was undoubtedly due to the effect of hypokalemia—too little potassium in her blood.

The body's mechanisms for conserving potassium are not as effective as they are for sodium. Some potassium continues to be lost in the urine, even in the absence of its intake. As a consequence, most patients with medical or surgical disorders suffer some depletion of potassium. Certain measures used in the therapy of the patient aggravate its loss. These include enemas, mercurial diuretics, and the adrenocortical steroids. Patients who have been in the habit of taking drastic cathartics or enemas may be suffering from a deficiency of potassium at the time they are admitted to the hospital.

Low levels of potassium are associated with evidences of failure of cardiac, skeletal, and possibly smooth muscle. The sensitivity of the heart muscle to digitalis is increased,[26] and symptoms of toxicity may occur at dosages that are ordinarily therapeutic. For this reason, patients who suffer from digitalis toxicity may be given a salt of potassium, such as potassium chloride. Symptoms of a potassium deficit include tachycardia, cardiac arrhythmias, hypotension, muscle weakness, tetany, and abdominal distention.

The treatment is to replace the potassium that has been lost. Fruit juices, especially unstrained orange juice, bouillon, and meat broths, are rich in potassium. As soon as the patient eats a varied diet, potassium is promptly restored. When the patient is unable to take fluids by mouth, potassium may be given by intravenous infusion. Especially in patients who have a limited renal reserve, care should be taken to limit the rate of flow, so blood levels do not become excessive. The patient who is receiving intravenous injections containing potassium requires conscientious supervision. He should be observed for signs and symptoms indicating hyperkalemia—level of potassium in blood above upper limit of normal. The symptoms include paresthesias, which may be of the scalp rather than of the extremities, muscle weakness, and cardiac arrythmias. Death may result from cardiac failure.

What are two of the disorders in which hyperkalemia occurs? What measures may be employed in the control of the level of potassium?

Two disorders in which hyperkalemia most commonly occurs are acute renal failure and adrenal insufficiency. In adrenal insufficiency, hyperkalemia

[26] Goodman and Gilman, *Op. cit.,* p. 690.

can be controlled by the administration of the adrenal cortical hormones. In patients with acute renal failure, the control of the level of potassium in the blood may be more difficult. When the failure is of short duration, this may be accomplished by eliminating all potassium intake and maintaining the patient at complete bed rest. Since most foods contain some potassium, the diet may be limited to glucose and vegetable oil, neither of which contains potassium. Elimination of potassium by the gastrointestinal tract may be increased by the ingestion of nonpotassium cation exchange resins. Unfortunately many patients do not tolerate these very well.

Some patients, such as Mrs. Murray, respond to conservative therapy. She suffered an acute renal shutdown as the result of transfusion with about 400 ml of incompatible blood. At the time she was admitted to Hospital X for possible hemodialysis, she was completely anuric, and had been for two days. Blood studies and electrocardiogram indicated she had some elevation of potassium, but was not in any immediate danger. She was placed on strict bed rest, ice chips not to exceed 200 ml in 24 hours, and a diet composed of glucose and Crisco, daily weight, daily electrocardiogram, and daily blood specimens for potassium, sodium, and urea. A polyethylene catheter was introduced into the saphenous vein. It was to be kept patent with a 10 per cent solution of glucose. A micro set was used in order to minimize the quantity of solution required. An indwelling catheter was introduced, so all urine excreted could be collected. Fortunately for Mrs. Murray, on the fifth day following the onset of anuria, she started to excrete urine. Since the ability to concentrate urine does not return as rapidly as the ability to excrete water, the urine had a low specific gravity. Despite a marked increase in the volume of urine, Mrs. Murray's blood potassium and urea did not begin to fall for a few days. During the initial period of diuresis, Mrs. Murray was carefully observed for indications of electrolyte imbalance. Either hypo- or hypernatremia may occur. Neither developed. Sometimes diuresis is so great that the patient requires a large fluid intake. Fortunately for Mrs. Murray, her kidney function was restored rapidly enough so that hemodialysis was not required.

Mrs. Murray's nursing care was directed toward trying to make it possible for her to achieve a maximum amount of rest. Since activity increases the rate of metabolism, she was given complete care. She was turned and rubbed every two hours and encouraged to lie quietly. Because of the nature of her diet, and limitations on her fluid intake, she was given special mouth care every four hours. The ice chips were divided over the 24-hour period. Because the rate of flow of the intravenous solution was important, this was noted at hourly or more frequent intervals. Strict control of fluid intake so it does not exceed output is one of the most important aspects of the patient's care. Unless this is done, the patient may die from the effects of overhydration. Inasmuch as Mrs. Murray was from out of town, she had no visitors except her husband and the hospital chaplain. Both Mr. and Mrs. Murray were concerned about the possible outcome of her illness. Nurses and doctors were aware of this, and of the fact that they could not be sure either. They encouraged Mrs. Murray's hope and were sympathetic to her feelings of uncertainty. Through attention to meeting her immediate needs, they were able to minimize her discomfort and to convey to her that everyone was concerned about her welfare.

Not all patients in acute renal failure are as fortunate as Mrs. Murray. Recovery of the kidney may be slow and the levels of potassium in the blood may be elevated to the point of toxicity. In this event, the level of potassium and the nonprotein nitrogenous wastes in the blood may be lowered by hemo- or peritoneal dialysis. These procedures have other uses as well. One or the other may be utilized to remove ingested poisons such as barbiturates, salicylates, bromides, and others. Neither is ordinarily used in the treatment of chronic renal failure unless there is some promise that the patient will receive more than temporary benefit.

Hemodialysis of blood involves the use of the artificial kidney. The artificial kidney is based on the principle that a substance present in different concentrations on two sides of a semipermeable membrane moves from the side of the greater to that of the lesser concentration. If the process is continued, the concentration of the substance will eventually be equalized on the two sides of the membrane. This device can perform most of the kidney's functions. It can remove the wastes of protein metabolism and restore acid-base balance, primarily by removing sodium and hydrogen ions. It can also remove other electrolytes, such as potassium. It cannot take part in regulating physiological processes such as blood pressure.[27]

In the artificial kidney, blood is circulated through cellophane tubing that is similar to sausage casing. It is permeable to ions and molecules of small size and impermeable to large molecules such as protein, some viruses, and bacteria. The latter characteristics simplify the procedure, because ordinary non-sterile tap water can be used to bathe the tubing through which the blood is circulated. The tubing is placed on a device suspended in a tank of water to which is added sufficient glucose and electrolytes to make it isotonic with normal blood plasma. When the purpose of the procedure is to reduce the level of potassium or magnesium or some other constituent in the blood, none or limited quantities of the substances to be removed are added to the water bath.

In order to maintain the patient's blood volume, and at the same time fill the dialyzing membrane, about 1,200 to 1,500 ml of blood are required to prime the system. To prevent the blood from clotting, heparin is added. A cannula is placed in either the radial artery or the saphenous artery for the purpose of removing blood from the patient. Another is placed in a vein, usually the brachial, to return the blood to the patient. When the level of urea and electrolytes in the water bath approaches that of the blood, the fluid in the bath is changed. The procedure is terminated when the components of the

[27] John P. Merrill, "The Artificial Kidney," *Scientific American*, CCV, July, 1961, pp. 56-64.

blood are restored to normal or near normal levels. Because of the nature of the procedure and the seriousness of the patient's condition, the patient is attended throughout by one or more physicians. With the use of monitoring devices, this may not be necessary. Greater responsibility for continued supervision of the patient is assigned to the nurse.

In the performance of her role, the nurse should be guided by the fact that all material and equipment with which the blood comes in contact must be kept sterile. Provisions should be made for the taking of blood samples. Much of the physician's time will be taken with the operation of the equipment and the evaluation of the effectiveness of the procedure and its effect on the patient. The procedure may take up to six hours. The patient is sick. Frequently he is seriously ill. The patient and his family often regard the artificial kidney as a "last ditch" effort to save him. This belief may be true. The procedure also requires that the patient be on his back, though the backrest may be elevated somewhat. The nurse's initial responsibility is to take the patient's blood pressure continuously and to report it to the physician. Since the level of the blood pressure depends on the relationship of the amount of blood removed from the patient to circulate through the machine to that returning to the patient, the physician uses this information to regulate blood flow. After the blood pressure is stabilized, it is taken every 15 minutes throughout the procedure. To lessen the patient's discomfort from being in one position, the nurse should initiate measures to increase his comfort. This may be done by placing the hand under the small of the back and rubbing it, by placing a small pillow or roll in the hollow of the back, and by slightly raising the backrest of the bed. After the procedure is under way, passive exercise of the extremities may be instituted. Even slight changes in position lessen muscle tension and contribute to comfort. Since fluids by mouth are limited, the patient should have mouth care. The nurse should also observe the patient for indications that he is or is not responding to the treatment. She should also remind physicians and nurses that the patient is present so that conversation either includes him or is limited to that required for the progress of the procedure. The family should not be neglected. At the very least, they should be informed periodically about the condition of the patient. The latter is particularly important when the procedure is being performed for the first time.

The general principles, objectives, and uses of peritoneal dialysis are similar to those of the artificial kidney. Isotonic solutions of electrolytes are introduced into and removed from the peritoneal cavity. As the fluid bathes the peritoneal membrane, substances to which the membrane is permeable diffuse into it. Although they diffuse in both directions, the net transfer is in the direction of lower concentration. This effect is the same as with the artificial kidney. Peritoneal dialysis has the advantage of not requiring the use of blood. Peritoneal dialysis can also be carried on more or less continuously and the concentration of substances normally removed by the kidney maintained within physiological levels. Because the peritoneal cavity is entered, there is the danger of infection of the peritoneum with resulting peritonitis.

Patients treated by peritoneal dialysis require competent nursing care with careful attention given to their physiological and emotional needs, and moving and turning to prevent pulmonary complications and decubiti. Inasmuch as is possible, extremities should be put through normal range of motion at least daily. Muscle strain should be relieved by shifting the patient's position and by raising and lowering the headrest of the bed. If the patient is conscious, he should be encouraged to cough and deep-breathe. Special mouth care is required because oral intake is limited. When monitoring devices are applied, such as continuous recordings of the blood pressure and the electrocardiogram, the nurse should check to see that they are properly applied and working. In the case of blood pressure, the nurse should report significant changes in either directon.

What are the functions of calcium in the body?

Calcium is an indispensable mineral in the body. Although it has little effect on the shift of fluids in the body, it has many important functions. Although about 99 per cent of it is found in the bone, it is also found in all body cells and fluids. In addition to the formation of bone, it functions in the (1) regulation of neuromuscular irritability, (2) coagulation of the blood, (3) regulation of the irritability of the heart muscle, and (4) formation of milk.

Calcium exists in the blood in two forms. One form is bound to the serum protein and is nondiffusible. The other is for the most part ionized and is diffusible. The level of calcium in the blood serum is regulated in relation to the level of the phosphate ion, and the product of the two is kept constant. With an increase in one, the level of the other can be expected to decrease. The level of calcium in the blood is regulated by the parathyroid hormone. Exactly how this is accomplished is in doubt. According to Best and Taylor,[28] the parathyroid hormone acts on both the kidney and bone. It also acts to increase absorption of calcium from the intestine.

As with other elements of body fluids, calcium may be present in deficit or in excess. Deficits of calcium may be in the total quantity or in the proportion that is in ionized form. In alkalosis, the proportion of calcium in the ionized form diminishes, whereas it rises in acidosis. A condition called tetany results when the level of calcium in the blood is low. Tetany may develop when the quantity of calcium in the blood is within normal limits, but the amount of calcium in the ionized form is diminished. For example, tetany develops in susceptible persons who overbreathe or hyperventilate.Tetany is seen in infants and very young children with rickets, as a result of a lack of calcium and/or vitamin D. In adults, tetany may follow injury or removal of the parathyroid glands during thyroid surgery or following the removal of an adenoma of the parathyroid gland. In the absence of the parathyroid hormone, the level of calcium in the serum falls. In advanced renal disease, the kidney loses its

[28] *Op. cit.,* p. 1059.

ability to conserve calcium. As a consequence, it is lost from the blood. Whatever the cause, a decrease in the level of calcium in the blood is followed by a heightening in neuromuscular irritability. With an increase in muscular irritability, the hands and feet assume a characteristic position which is referred to as carpopedal spasm. In infants, spasms of the glottis may interfere with breathing. In patients whose blood level of calcium remains just above the critical point, tapping over the facial nerve in front of the ear causes a twitching of the muscles of the face. Muscle spasm is accompanied by considerable pain and discomfort which can be relieved by the intravenous administration of calcium gluconate.

How does the organism regulate the concentration of hydrogen ions?

One of the truly remarkable features of the body fluids is that despite continuous additions of metabolites from cells and food in health, their pH is maintained at a constant level. As with other homeostatic conditions, the body has a number of mechanisms for regulating the concentration of hydrogen ions. These include: (1) the dilution of the products of metabolism by a large volume of fluid, (2) the removal of the hydrogen ion by buffering, and (3) the elimination of hydrogen ions, as well as other cations and anions, by the lung and kidney.

The dilution of strong acids and alkalies by a large volume of water is one of the most effective means of diminishing their effect. The principle is utilized in first aid when dilution is used to minimize the effects of a strong acid or alkali on tissue. A tissue or structure exposed to either of these is flooded with a large volume of running water. In other words, a teaspoonful of concentrated sulfuric acid in contact with the skin or mucous membrane produces serious tissue injury. Diluted by 10 gal of water, it has little, if any, effect. In the living organism, the extracellular fluid dilutes the strong acids produced by the cells in the process of metabolism and thereby prevents them from injuring tissues.

A second mechanism utilized by the body to control the level of the hydrogen ion is the elimination of carbon dioxide by the lung. This serves two purposes. In addition to helping regulate the level of the hydrogen ion, it also serves to keep the level of cations equal to anions without the loss of water. This mechanism is, in fact, the most rapid method the body has for adjusting the level of anions in the blood plasma. It will be described in detail in the discussion of buffering.

How do buffer systems work?

A third mechanism for the protection of a solution against changes in hydrogen ion concentration is buffering. A buffer can be described as a chemical sponge. It can take up or release hydrogen ions as the circumstances demand. In this way it protects the fluid against changes in pH. Each buffer system is a solution of a weak acid and one of its salts, formed by neutralizing the acid with a strong base. The acid and salt are maintained in a definite relationship to each other. There are a number of so-called buffer systems in the body. They include: (1) carbonic acid and sodium bicarbonate, (2) monosodium or potassium phosphate and disodium or dipotassium phosphate, (3) oxyhemoglobin and reduced hemoglobin, each in relation to its potassium salt, and (4) acid proteinate and alkaline proteinate. They all function in essentially the same manner. A pertinent point here is that in nature the strong take from the weak. In the presence of a strong acid, the following events take place:

1. The cation from the salt of the weak acid and the strong base (sodium or potassium, for example) combines with
2. the anion (chloride, sulfate, phosphate, acetate, etc.) from the strong acid, and
3. the hydrogen ion from the strong acid (hydrochloric, phosphoric, lactic, acetoacetic) combines with
4. the anion from salt of the weak acid to form
5. a weak acid and a salt.

The weak acid ionizes less completely than the strong acid that it replaces, that is, it does not release hydrogen ions as readily as the stronger acid. Hydrogen ions are therefore removed from the solution. To state the above simply, as the result of buffering, the strong acid is replaced by a weak acid and a neutral salt. In a weak acid, a larger proportion of the substance remains in the molecular form and fewer hydrogen ions are released than in a strong acid.

To further clarify, and to apply the manner in which buffer systems function in the body, the carbonic acid–sodium bicarbonate system is described below. This system plays an important role in the protection of the extracellular fluid from changes in the hydrogen ion concentration. Carbonic acid is a weak acid. Sodium bicarbonate ($NaHCo_3$) is a salt formed by the neutralization of carbonic acid (H_2CO_3) with sodium hydroxide ($NaOH$), a strong base. In health, 1 part of carbonic acid is maintained in the blood to every 20 parts of sodium bicarbonate.

When an acid stronger than carbonic acid is formed in, or ingested into, the body, it ionizes to the hydrogen ion and the appropriate anion. The anion combines with the sodium ion to form a salt. The hydrogen ion unites with the bicarbonate anion to form the weak carbonic acid. For example, $(H^+ + Cl^-) + (Na^+ + HCO_3) = NaCl + H_2CO_3$.

By what mechanism is a suitable level of the bicarbonate anion maintained in the blood plasma?

The mechanism for maintaining a suitable level of the bicarbonate anion in the blood plasma involves the excretion of carbon dioxide by the lung. The level of the bicarbonate anion in the blood is regulated by the quantity of carbon dioxide dissolved in the blood. The more carbon dioxide dissolved in the blood, the higher the level of the bicarbonate anion, and vice versa. The level of carbon dioxide in the blood, in turn, depends on the partial pressure of carbon dioxide in the alveoli. Therefore, the partial pressure of carbon dioxide in the alveoli regulates the level of the bicarbonate anion in the blood. The way in which this functions in the body is described below. When the level of chloride, sulfate, phosphate, or organic acid anions increases, the number of sodium cations (alkali reserve) available to combine with bicarbonate anions decreases. This is followed by an increase in the concentration of carbon dioxide and of hydrogen ions in the respiratory center. As a result, the depth and rate of respiration are increased. With an increase in the depth of respiration, the capacity of the alveoli is increased. With the enlargement of the alveoli, the partial pressure of the carbon dioxide is lessened.[29] As stated earlier, the level of bicarbonate ion in the blood is regulated by the partial pressure of carbon dioxide in the alveolar air. As the partial pressure of the carbon dioxide in the alveolar air decreases, carbon dioxide moves from the blood to the alveoli. As the level of carbon dioxide in the blood plasma drops, carbonic acid in the presence of carbonic anhydrase decomposes to carbon dioxide and water. This results in a lowering of the level of the bicarbonate and the hydrogen ions in the blood plasma.[30]

With the removal of carbon dioxide and the hydrogen ion from the respiratory center, the process is reversed. Respiration diminishes in rate and depth. The partial pressure of carbon dioxide in the alveoli increases. This is followed by an increase in the level of carbon dioxide in the blood. Finally this is reflected by an increase in the bicarbonate ion in the blood. Through the process just described, the body controls the hydrogen ion and adjusts the anion level so anions are kept equal to cations without the loss of water.

As previously stated, the immediate source of the bicarbonate ion in the blood plasma is sodium bicarbonate ($NaHCO_3$) and hydrogen carbonate (H_2CO_3). A small amount of hydrogen carbonate ionizes when dissolved in water to form hydrogen and bicarbonate ions, that is, carbonic acid. The quantity present in the molecular form, that is, as hydrogen carbonate, can be increased by adding more of the bicarbonate ion in the form of sodium bicarbonate. Conversely, the amount of hydrogen carbonate that ionizes can be increased by decreasing the level of sodium bicarbonate in the blood. This results from what is known as the common ion effect. Additions of sodium bicarbonate to the blood decrease the number of hydrogen ions in the blood by decreasing the ionization of hydrogen carbonate. The same effect can be produced by inhaling carbon dioxide or by holding one's breath.

Just as increases in the level of other anions result in a lowering of the level

---

[29] The pressure of a gas within a container is inversely proportional to the size of the chamber.

[30] [(HCO_3^-) in the presence of carbonic anhydrase $CO_2 + (OH^-)$] the (OH^-) combines with the H^+ (from whatever acid that is present) to form HOH, or water.

of the bicarbonate ion, a depression in the level of other anions is compensated for by an increase in the bicarbonate ion. A fall in the level of the chloride ion in the blood is compensated for by an increase in the bicarbonate ion. Although the levels of the chloride and other anions in the blood plasma are subject to change, there do not appear to be as active mechanisms for their upward or downward adjustment as there are with bicarbonate. Through the active adjustment of bicarbonate anions, anions are kept equal to cations.

To return to Mr. Martin for a moment, though the day was hot, he hurried as he mowed the lawn. This required a considerable expenditure of energy. In the process of obtaining the energy, he formed and released into his extracellular fluid a considerable volume of organic and inorganic acids. More specifically, hydrogen ions and the corresponding anions were added to his extracellular fluid. To adjust the level of anions to that of the cations, principally sodium, in his blood, some of the bicarbonate anion in his blood was eliminated by the lungs as carbon dioxide. In the process, hydrogen ions were converted to water and therefore had no effect on the acid-base equilibrium of Mr. Martin's extracellular fluid. The anions from the acids that were stronger than carbonic acid combined with sodium to form salts. This resulted in a reduction in Mr. Martin's alkali reserve, that is, in the quantity of sodium ion in the form of sodium bicarbonate in the blood. With a reduction in the bicarbonate in the blood, the capacity of the blood to carry carbon dioxide is diminished. Carbon dioxide and hydrogen ions accumulated in Mr. Martin's cells, including his respiratory center. His respirations increased in rate and depth. With the increase in the size of the alveoli, the partial pressure of carbon dioxide in his alveolar air fell. The tension of carbon dioxide in the blood was higher than in the alveolar air. Carbon dioxide therefore diffused from the blood to the alveoli to equalize the pressure on the two sides of the membrane. With a lowering of the tension of carbon dioxide in the blood, carbon dioxide and hydrogen ions were removed from the respiratory center. The depth and rate of his respirations diminished. The partial pressure of carbon dioxide in his alveolar air rose and, as a consequence, the level of carbon dioxide and the carbonic acid in his blood plasma also rose.

What is the role of the kidney in regulating the concentration of the hydrogen ion in the blood plasma?

By regulating the level of carbon dioxide in the blood plasma, the lung plays an important role in acid-base equilibrium. However, neither the buffer system nor the lung is able to completely control the hydrogen ion concentration. The kidney plays a significant part in this by selectively reabsorbing or rejecting both cations and anions. Its role in the maintenance of the concentration of sodium and potassium in body fluids has previously been discussed. The kidney utilizes three mechanisms to control the hydrogen ion. First, the tubule cells secrete the hydrogen ions. Second, the kidney forms ammonia, which combines with a hydrogen ion to form the ammonium ion. Each molecule of ammonia thus removes and eliminates one hydrogen ion. Since ammonium ions can replace sodium or other cations in the urine, they are part of the mechanism for the excretion of "strong" anions without losing necessary cations. Third, the kidney converts bisodium phosphate to monosodium phosphate. By all of these mechanisms, the kidney eliminates the hydrogen ion. The second and third mechanisms enable the kidney to conserve the sodium ion as well. The functions of the various parts of the nephron and the processes utilized by the kidney in the excretion of the hydrogen ion and the conservation of the sodium ion are summarized in Figures 8-10 and 8-11.

In the presence of an excess of sodium ions in the blood, these mechanisms may not be used.

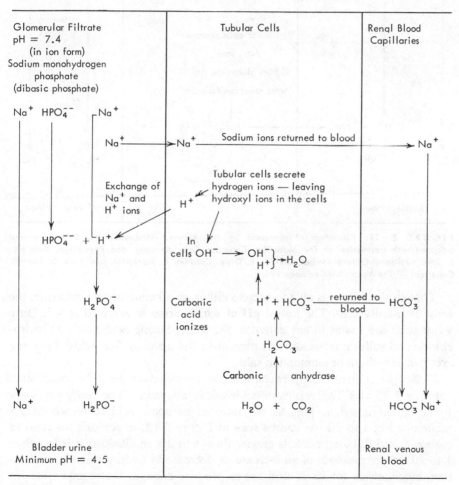

FIGURE 8–10. Mechanism by which urine becomes acidified by changing the dibasic phosphate to monobasic or dihydrogen phosphate. (Modified from Davenport and adapted with permission of The Macmillan Company from *Anatomy and Physiology*, 14th ed., p. 597, by Diana Clifford Kimber, Carolyn E. Gray, Caroline E. Stackpole, and Lutie C. Leavell. Copyright © The Macmillan Company 1961.)

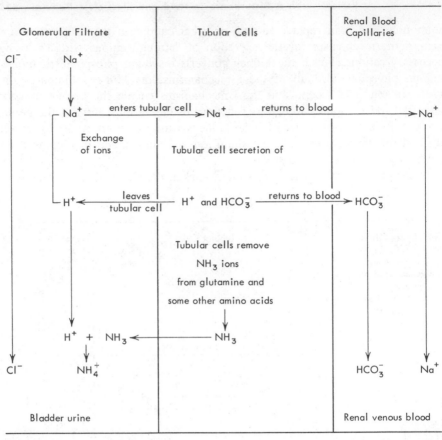

FIGURE 8—11. Formation of ammonia by the kidney. (Modified from Davenport and adapted with permission of The Macmillan Company from *Anatomy and Physiology,* 14th ed., p. 598, by Diana Clifford Kimber, Carolyn E. Gray, Caroline E. Stackpole, and Lutie C. Leavell. Copyright © The Macmillan Company 1961.)

Though the kidney is able to excrete either an alkaline or an acid urine, the urine is usually acid. The lowest pH at which urine is excreted is 4.5. Only weak acids are found to any extent in the urine. Strong acids, such as hydrochloric and sulfuric acids, are not present in the urine as free acids. They are excreted as sodium or ammonium salts.

Failure to control the hydrogen ion concentration so the pH is maintained between 7.35 and 7.45 results in acidemia or alkalemia. The condition is said to be compensated as long as the ratio of carbonic acid to bicarbonate is maintained at 1 to 20. As can be seen in Figure 8-12, in acidosis the ratio of carbonic acid to bicarbonate is greater than 1 to 20; in alkalosis it is less than 1 to 20. In the presence of an increase or decrease in hydrogen ion concentration, mechanisms for its control act to produce changes that compensate for alterations and restore the ratio of carbonic acid to bicarbonate.

These mechanisms include the taking up or release of hydrogen ions by the buffer systems, increase or decrease in ventilation by the lung, and elimination

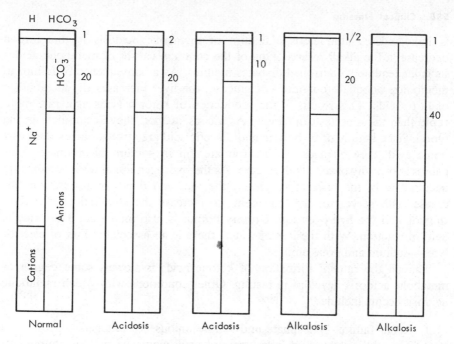

FIGURE 8—12. Possible changes in H-HCO₃ to HCO₃ in acidosis and alkalosis.

or conservation of hydrogen and bicarbonate ions by the kidney. A decrease in ventilation reduces the elimination of carbon dioxide and favors the formation of carbonic acid. An increase in the rate and depth of respiration has the reverse effect.

As with the respiratory mechanisms for the control of the hydrogen ion concentrations of the blood, the kidney intensifies its normal mechanisms for controlling the level of the hydrogen ion. When the level of the bicarbonate ion in the blood is excessive, reabsorption of bicarbonate is decreased and the quantity in the urine is increased. An increase in the production of hydrogen ions is followed by a rise in the rate at which tubular cells secrete them. The kidney also excretes monosodium phosphate and the hydrogen ion and conserves sodium by eliminating the phosphate ion in the monosodium form and other anions as ammonium salts. All these mechanisms serve to restore the hydrogen ion concentration so the pH of the blood is maintained within levels compatible with life.

Depending on their origin, deviations in the concentration of the hydrogen ion are classified as metabolic or respiratory.

What are some of the important causes of metabolic acidosis?

Metabolic acidosis

In metabolic acidosis the ratio of carbonic acid to bicarbonate is increased by a reduction in the quantity of sodium available to combine with bicarbonate; the quantity of sodium in combination with anions other than bicarbonate

537

is increased. A characteristic feature of metabolic acidosis is therefore a decrease in the alkali reserve. One of the common causes of metabolic acidosis is inadequately controlled diabetes mellitus. As a consequence of failure to metabolize adequate quantities of glucose, the liver increases the metabolism of fatty acids. This results in the production of ketonic acids at a rate more rapid than the muscles can handle. As a consequence, they accumulate in the blood. Since beta hydroxybutyric and diacetic acid are stronger acids than carbonic acid, they displace the bicarbonate ion in sodium bicarbonate. This causes a lowering of the alkali reserve. As the hydrogen ion and carbon dioxide accumulate in the respiratory center, the rate and depth of respirations increase. This serves for the time being to increase the elimination of carbon dioxide and the hydrogen ion. Urinary output is also increased. The urine is acid in reaction. With the loss of water, there is an associated loss of electrolytes—sodium and potassium.

Though the rate of formation of ketone acids is slower, some degree of metabolic acidosis develops in fasting. Other conditions with which metabolic acidosis occurs include:

1. Renal failure—phosphate and sulfate anions are retained.
2. The administration of large doses of acidifying salts such as ammonium chloride.
3. Excessive exercise.
4. Anoxia.
5. Severe diarrhea in which the loss of sodium ions exceeds that of chloride ions.

Whatever the underlying cause, hyperpnea of the type known as Kussmaul breathing is the outstanding symptom. As carbon dioxide accumulates in the tissue, it increases capillary dilatation. As a result, flushing of the skin is common. In severe or prolonged acidosis, the kidney mechanisms for conserving sodium and water and for excreting the hydrogen ion fail. As a result, water, sodium, and potassium are lost in excess of intake and the pH of body fluids falls. The situation is frequently aggravated by the loss of fluid by vomiting. As a consequence, tissue turgor diminishes. The skin and mucous membrane become dry. Even the eyeballs may lose fluid with a reduction in their tension. With the loss of fluid and the decrease in pH, restlessness, abdominal pain, and eventually coma develop. Unless the condition is corrected, death results from renal or respiratory failure.

Treatment of metabolic acidosis is directed toward two objectives. The first is to correct the underlying cause. The second is to restore the water, electrolytes, and nutrients that have been lost from the body. In the instance of Mary Kay, she was given insulin and glucose to enable her to metabolize glucose and to decrease the formation of ketone acids. In this way the underlying cause of her acidosis was attacked. At the same time, she received fluids containing sodium chloride, and sodium lactate. At the present time, she would also have been given some form of potassium. Since the lactate ion is metabolized, the sodium ion becomes available to combine with the bicarbonate ion. The sodium ion thus enlarges the alkali reserve. In the beginning, the fluids are likely to be administered parenterally. After the patient is able to tolerate fluids by mouth, they may be given in the form of bouillon, orange juice, or water containing sodium chloride and sodium bicarbonate.

The functions of the nurse include making pertinent observations, protecting the patient from injury, performing therapeutic procedures, and providing for the comfort and well-being of the patient. Significant observations include his general behavior. Is he conscious, drowsy, or stuporous? Is he quiet or restless? What is the character of his breathing? His color? Is his skin dry or moist? Particularly in acidosis associated with uncontrolled diabetes mellitus the urine reflects the state of glucose metabolism. Because the urine is subjected to regular and frequent analysis, an indwelling catheter is sometimes inserted so that urine can be obtained for half-hourly or hourly analyses. In addition to notation and recording of the rate of urine formation, it is tested for glucose, acetone, diacetic acid, specific gravity, and reaction. Samples of blood may also be checked at regular intervals for glucose, sodium, potassium, chlorides, carbon dioxide or carbon dioxide-combining power, and acetone. Hemoconcentration of the blood is present when the hematocrit reading or the level of hemoglobin in the blood is elevated. The performance of these diagnostic tests involves venipuncture. The patient is likely to require some reassurance as to why repeated venipuncture is necessary.

The commonly used therapeutic measures have been indicated. The nurse's responsibilities in each of these have been discussed elsewhere. After fluids are started by mouth, attention should be given to make certain the patient gets and ingests them. The patient in acidosis has a tendency to gastric dilatation. When this occurs, the fluid ingested remains in the stomach. Later the patient vomits—often a large quantity of fluid. A feeling of fullness in the epigastric region is the common warning symptom accompanying gastric retention.

When the patient is restless and less than fully conscious, more than usual attention to his safety is required. Side rails may be placed on the bed to lessen the danger of his falling out of bed. If he is very restless, these should be padded. Other precautions in his care do not differ materially from those for any patient, who is not fully responsible. They have been discussed elsewhere.

As in the care of any other patient, the nurse should be alert to the need of the patient for comfort and support. This, too, has been emphasized earlier and will not be repeated. During the period when the patient is not fully conscious, the nurse should assume responsibility for reminding everyone involved in the care of the patient that he is present and able to hear.

In addition to acidosis of metabolic origin, acidosis may result from a failure of the body to control the level of carbonic acid in the extracellular fluid. This type is known as respiratory acidosis, because the body's mechanism for controlling carbonic acid is respiratory. In respiratory acidosis, the level of carbonic acid in the blood plasma is increased, and the ratio of carbonic acid to bicarbonate is increased. This results in an increase in the hydrogen ion concentration in the blood. Respiratory acidosis occurs in a wide range of conditions in which there is an inadequate exchange of gases in the lungs with the retention of carbon dioxide in the blood. Inadequate exchange of gases in the lung is predisposed to by anything that depresses the respiratory center in the medulla or that decreases the aerating surface in the lung. Narcotics, such as morphine and meperdine hydrochloride, general anesthetics, and barbiturates all predispose to respiratory acidosis inasmuch as they depress the respiratory center. Diseases, such as poliomyelitis, and injuries that involve the respiratory center can be expected to do so as well. Emphysema, bronchiectasis and pneumonia predispose to respiratory acidosis by decreasing the aerating surface in the lung.

As in metabolic acidosis, the kidney's mechanisms for maintaining the level of the hydrogen ions are utilized. The buffers also help. As the blood level of carbonic acid rises, chloride moves into the red cell, leaving sodium available to form sodium bicarbonate and hence tending to restore the carbonic acid to bicarbonate ratio to 1 to 20.

In the prevention and treatment of respiratory acidosis therapy is directed toward correcting the cause. Narcotics should be given only as frequently and in the amounts required to relieve pain. When a patient is receiving narcotic drugs he should be encouraged to perform deep-breathing exercises at regular intervals. In the patient with emphysema a tracheostomy is sometimes performed to reduce the dead air space and to facilitate the removal of secretions. The patient who is suffering from respiratory paralysis is placed in a respirator. In patients who have a decreased aerating surface in the lung, acidosis results from interference with the elimination of carbon dioxide and from the failure to absorb oxygen. Since anoxia increases the degree of acidosis, the administration of oxygen would appear to be indicated. However, it may have disastrous effects in patients with severe emphysema. The theory, here, is that the relative lack of oxygen serves as a respiratory stimulant. When this stimulus is removed by the administration of oxygen, respiration ceases. This also presupposes that the respiratory center is relatively insensitive to carbon dioxide and hydrogen ion.

What are some of the usual causes of alkalosis?

In certain disorders the level of the hydrogen ion may be decreased below the normal level. This results in alkalosis. Like acidosis, alkalosis may be of metabolic or respiratory origin. In metabolic alkalosis, the bicarbonate anion is increased in relation to carbonic acid. This results in an increase in the ratio of bicarbonate to carbonic acid; there are more than 20 parts of bicarbonate ions to 1 part of carbonic acid. Another way this is stated is that there is a relative increase of fixed cations in relation to fixed anions. Metabolic alkalosis is most commonly associated with disorders in which there is an undue loss of the chloride ion or excessive intake of sodium bicarbonate. Continued vomiting and gastric suction are the most frequent causes of chloride depletion. Loss of chlorides from the patient on gastric suction is intensified by vigorous irrigation of the nasogastric tube. For this reason, some physicians limit irrigation or ask that isotonic saline solution be used. Fluid intake is generally limited for the same reason in the patient having gastric suction. Chloride depletion also occurs in patients who are given mercurial diuretics frequently. Loss of potassium from the body is accompanied by loss of chloride.

The ingestion of excessive quantities of sodium bicarbonate is most likely to be observed in persons who treat themselves for indigestion and who have a limited renal reserve. Everyone, especially persons in older age groups, should be cautioned against this practice.

The chararacteristic symptom of alkalosis is shallow breathing. This is often the first sign that alkalosis is developing in the patient who is losing gastric secretions. This results from the body's attempt to raise the level of carbonic acid in the blood. In shallow breathing the capacity of the alveoli is diminished, and the concentration of carbon dioxide in the alveolar air is raised. This serves to raise the level of carbonic acid in the blood. The kidney also responds by excreting sodium bicarbonate in the urine and by depressing the mechanisms for the excretion of the hydrogen ion. Less hydrogen ion is secreted by the tubules. The formation of ammonia is suppressed. Phosphates are excreted as disodium rather than monosodium salts. Lactic acid and ketone acid anions are reabsorbed. They help to displace the bicarbonate ion in the plasma. The urine excreted is alkaline in reaction. Thus, the body, through the initiation of compensatory mechanisms, attempts to maintain the pH of the blood within normal limits.

Treatment in alkalosis is based on the same general principles as in acidosis. It is directed toward the correction of the cause and the support of the body's compensatory mechanisms. Several authorities emphasize that in alkalosis, potassium is lost and the condition cannot be treated successfully without repairing the deficit of potassium. In addition to replacement of chlorides, attention should be given to improving the patient's nutrition.

Respiratory alkalosis occurs less frequently than do other disturbances in hydrogen ion concentration. It results when the concentration of carbonic acid in the blood is decreased in proportion to the bicarbonate anion. The most common cause is an increase in the rate and depth of respirations in the absence of an increase in the hydrogen ion or of carbon dioxide. Respiratory alkalosis is an example of a disorder arising from the inappropriate use of a physiological mechanism. This condition is most commonly seen in the nervous patient who overbreathes. Because the hydrogen ion concentration of the blood plasma is diminished, the level of ionized calcium in the blood is also lessened. As a consequence, these persons frequently have symptoms and signs of tetany. Treatment is directed toward correcting the underlying cause of the condition. Tetany can be corrected by any measure that elevates the level of carbon dioxide in the alveoli and therefore in the blood plasma. This can be done by holding the breath, by rebreathing expired air, or by inhaling carbon dioxide.

Summary

Disturbances in the acid-base balance or in the hydrogen ion concentration of extracellular fluids produce alterations in the ratio of carbonic acid to the bicarbonate ion in the blood plasma. In disorders of metabolic origin, the change is primarily in the level of the bicarbonate anion. In acidosis the bicarbonate anion is decreased. In alkalosis it is increased. In disorders of respiratory origin, the site of the disorder is in the carbonic acid fraction. In acidosis it is increased. In alkalosis it is decreased in relation to the bicarbonate ion.

The manifestations observed in these conditions depend in part on the nature of the condition responsible for the disorder, as well as on the effect the acidosis and alkalosis have on the loss of water and other electrolytes. The characteristic symptom is a change in the rate and depth of respiration. In acidosis, ventilation is increased by an increase in the rate and depth of respiration. In alkalosis, breathing becomes shallow. As indicated previously, changes in rate and depth of respiration are physiological mechanisms by which the organism attempts to correct the shift in hydrogen ion concentration.

Treatment is directed toward removing the cause and supporting the body's mechanisms for correcting the disturbance. This includes not only providing the patients with the water and electrolytes that have been lost, but also restoring his nutritional state.

The essential factors in the regulation of water and electrolytes are summarized below. The volume, distribution, and concentration of water and electrolytes in the various fluid compartments result from a carefully regulated balance between intake and output. An increase in intake or output results in the initiation of mechanisms that very quickly correct any change. Continued deficits in supply or failure in any of the mechanisms by which fluid and electrolyte balance is regulated result in a loss of homeostasis and disturbed cellular function.

From the preceding discussion, the reader should be well aware that disturbances in fluid and electrolyte balance result in disturbances in volume, osmotic pressure, and the hydrogen ion concentration of body fluids. Although fluid and electrolyte balance does not become a serious problem in every sick person, there is always some disturbance. It becomes a problem when the illness persists or when the patient's mechanisms for adjusting to the situation are inadequate. When this happens, a diagnosis of the nature and extent of the problem becomes necessary.

The physician carries the responsibility for making the medical diagnosis and for establishing the plan of therapy. The nurse assists in the collection of the data on which the diagnosis is based, she participates in and supervises therapeutic measures, and she provides comfort and support for the patient. For all patients, and most particularly those who have a chronic condition, she assists in their instruction. She may carry more or less responsibility for assisting them in their adjustment after dismissal from the hospital.

The characteristic signs and symptoms of alterations in volume, osmotic pressure, and hydrogen ion concentration have been previously discussed. They are summarized, not in relation to a specific condition, but in general terms. They include changes in (1) the patient's mental state and behavior, particularly increasing apathy or lethargy and weakness, (2) the skin—either increasing or decreasing turgor as well as dryness, (3) the mucous membranes—dryness in the mouth and sordes, (4) the urine output—polyuria or oliguria, (5) the concentration of urine, specific gravity—lowered, elevated, or fixed in the region of 1.010, (6) respiration—increased or decreased in rate or depth, (7) thirst—increased or absent, and (8) the blood—increase or decrease in the level of electrolytes and the nonprotein nitrogenous wastes as expressed by the blood urea, urea nitrogen, or nonprotein nitrogen. Any or all elements in the blood may be increased when additions to the blood exceed losses or when the addition of water falls below its output. The level of any substance in the blood will be decreased when losses exceed supply or the addition of water is greater than its loss. For example, in renal failure the nitrogenous wastes as well as electrolytes such as potassium and sodium tend to rise in the blood. In salt-wasting nephritis, the level of sodium cations may fall because the kidney's mechanisms for conserving sodium are defective. When water intake is insufficient, the hematocrit, hemoglobin, blood proteins, and electrolytes, as well as nitrogenous wastes, tend to rise.

In conditions in which the body mechanisms are likely to need assistance in maintaining or restoring the normal character of the extracellular fluids, the blood and urine may be examined to determine the level of the various constituents. In complicated cases where the results may give misleading information, other body fluids such as gastric juice may be analyzed.

Some examinations of blood include the following:

1. *Hematocrit.* The blood is treated with an anticoagulant and then centrifuged. The cells are packed in the bottom of the tube. The average range for packed cells is from 41 to 48 per cent. Increases in the hematocrit are associated with a loss of extracellular fluid. In severe burns it may be as high as 75 per cent.

2. *Hemoglobin.* With a loss of extracellular fluid, the hemoglobin is increased in concentration. In patients whose hemoglobin is usually

within the average range, 14 to 16 gm per 100 ml of blood, the level may rise to 18 or 20 gm.

3. *Levels of electrolytes in the blood plasma.* These may rise or fall.
4. *Carbon dioxide content.* The measurement of carbon dioxide, carbonic acid, and bicarbonate of the plasma collected under oil is called carbon dioxide content. It is reported in volumes per cent.
5. *Carbon dioxide-combining power.* Plasma is equilibrated with air and then the carbon dioxide content is determined.
6. *The pH of the plasma* may be determined to differentiate between respiratory acidosis and metabolic alkalosis.

Examinations of the urine also provide valuable information about the status of the patient's fluid and electrolyte disturbances. They include:

1. Urine volume.
2. Specific gravity. With a healthy kidney the specific gravity decreases as the fluid intake increases. A fixed specific gravity of about 1.010 indicates severe renal failure. So-called concentration tests may be performed to determine the capacity of the kidney to alter the specific gravity.
3. pH of the urine. Normally acid, but may vary from 4.5 to 8.5 depending on the nature of the food and chemicals ingested.
4. Presence of electrolytes in abnormal amounts or types. For example, an absence of the sodium ion in the urine usually indicates a deficit of sodium in the body. The presence of the ketonic acids in appreciable amounts is indicative of acidosis in which the metabolism of fat is excessive.

Some of the ways in which data are obtained whereby the status of the patient's fluid and electrolyte balance can be estimated have been presented. These include a knowledge of the patient, his history, his disorder, observation of him and his behavior, and the chemical examinations of his blood and other body fluids. In short-term illnesses in patients whose health is essentially good, attention to the patient's desire for water is a satisfactory guide to his fluid intake. In patients who are suffering from serious or long-term illness or whose capacity to adapt is limited, the problem of evaluating fluid and electrolyte status may be difficult and require many procedures.

The objectives of medical therapy will depend on the nature of the patient's disturbance. In general they will be:

1. To maintain the volume of blood.
   a. Too little endangers the nutrition of the brain, kidney, and heart.
   b. Too much overburdens the heart and circulation and predisposes to pulmonary edema.

2. To replace past and current losses of water and electrolytes.
3. To provide an intake of water of sufficient volume for the kidney to excrete nitrogenous wastes.
4. To supply water and electrolytes in such amounts that dehydration or water logging of tissues and acidosis or alkalosis are prevented or corrected.

The nursing objectives include:

1. To observe each patient for signs and symptoms that indicate his physiological status.
2. To carry out the necessary procedures in a safe and effective manner.
3. To care for the patient in such a manner that he is protected from unnecessary discomfort and feels safe, protected, and cared for.

In the preceding pages emphasis has been placed on the regulation of water and electrolytes. In the section that follows, disorders of the kidney which are likely to lead to renal failure are summarized.

Obviously disturbances in water and electrolyte balance can result from disorders in gastrointestinal, respiratory, circulatory, or renal function. The first three are discussed in detail in other chapters and will not be further considered here. Like other organs, the kidney is subject to a variety of diseases which, depending on their extent and nature, reduce renal reserve or result in renal failure. Because one half of one kidney contains enough tissue to perform the functions of the kidney, there may be considerable kidney damage before evidence of renal failure develops. When one kidney is healthy, the other one can be safely removed. The manifestations accompanying renal disease depend on the nature of the cause and the extent to which renal function is impaired. For example, bacterial infections of the kidney are accompanied by signs and symptoms of infection. Whether or not renal failure occurs depends on the extent to which nephrons are destroyed by the infectious process or by the healing process. Disorders of the glomeruli usually render them more permeable to constituents of the blood. In nephroses, profuse amounts of protein are lost into the urine because the glomerular capillaries become permeable to protein. Because large quantities of protein are lost in the urine, blood level falls. Many of the other manifestations observed in the nephrotic patient are due to the effects of the low blood protein. In acute glomerular nephritis, the kidney is hyperemic; some glomeruli rupture, and blood escapes into the urine. Prolonged ischemia of the kidneys or agents toxic to the kidneys may cause tubular necrosis. Whatever the cause, tubular necrosis results in acute renal failure and is manifested by oliguria or anuria and rapidly developing azotemia.

Some of the more common disorders leading to a loss in the renal reserve are summarized on the following pages.

Disorders of the Kidney Which Are Common Causes of Renal Failure

Classification	Etiology	Nature of Onset	Severity and Course of Illness	Structures Involved, Primary Disease
I. Bilateral inflammatory diseases of the kidney				
A. Glomerulonephritis				
1. Acute	Most frequently associated with infections due to group A beta hemolytic Streptococcus. Not a bacterial infection, but an obscure antigen-antibody reaction damaging the glomeruli. Most common in childhood and young adults, but may occur at any age	Classically an abrupt onset occurring a few days to three weeks after an attack of pharyngitis or scarletina	Evidence of healing occurs within three weeks. Most patients go on to complete recovery. A few die during the acute phase of the disease or progress into the subacute or chronic phase of the disease	Diffuse exudation and proliferative inflammation of the kidneys
2. Chronic glomerulonephritis	Failure of kidneys to heal following an attack of acute glomerulonephritis	Following a latent phase which may persist for as long as 20–30 years or even longer. Patient develops evidence of renal failure		Few signs and symptoms of renal insufficiency develop until renal function diminishes below 20 per cent or less of normal

Major Manifestations

1. Puffy eyes, swelling of feet and ankles
2. Albuminuria
3. Hematuria. Urine may be smoky
4. Oliguria
5. Hypertension. Some degree is a common occurrence. When severe may precipitate cardiac failure or cerebral manifestations

Major Medical or Surgical Therapy

1. Treatment of infection with group A streptococci by penicillin. Penicillin is of no value unless streptococci are present
2. Bed rest until gross hematuria, edema, and hypertension have disappeared
3. Nutrition. With evidence of impaired renal function and obliguria, intake of protein, sodium, and potassium is restricted

Major Manifestations	Major Medical or Surgical Therapy
6. Headache	4. Fluid intake. In presence of oliguria, intake may be restricted. If nausea and vomiting, intake may be more liberal
7. Malaise	
8. Anorexia	5. Antihypertensive therapy. When hypertension and headaches are severe, drugs such as hydralazine hydrochloride, reserpine, or a combination of the two may be administered parenterally
9. May be moderate to severe aching in lumbar regions	
10. About one half of hospitalized patients have normal renal function. Others have some degree of retention of nitrogenous wastes	
11. In renal failure hyperkalemia (elevated blood potassium)	6. Antiuremia therapy

Onset of renal failure

	Latent phase—none
1. Nocturia	
2. Elevated blood urea—nitrogen	
3. Anemia	
4. Weakness	
5. Hypertension	
6. Electrolyte abnormalities	

Nephrotic syndrome or phase—occurs sometime before death in one half of patients

1. Heavy loss of protein in urine	
2. Hypoalbuminemia	
3. Hypercholesterolemia	
4. Edema	

Advanced and terminal glomerulonephritis
See discussion of renal failure

See discussion of chronic renal failure

Acute pyelonephritis

1. Sudden rise of body temperature to 102° to 105° F.	1. Attempt to sterilize the urine. (Difficult to do.) Drugs employed:
2. Shaking chills	a. Mandealmine*
3. Aching pains in one of costovertebral areas or flanks	b. Nitrofuratcin
4. Symptoms of inflammation of the bladder (a) Frequency of urination (b) burning pain on urination (dysuria) (c) Passage of cloudy and occasionally blood-tinged urine	c. Methionine (an acidifying agent that inhibits the growth of bacteria)
	d. Streptomycin (not used alone because streptomycin-resistant bacteria emerge rapidly)
5. Tenderness in region of the kidney	e. Other antibiotics such as tetracycline (Chloramphenicol)
	f. Sulfanilamides

547

Disorders of the Kidney Which Are Common Causes of Renal Failure—Continued

Classification	Etiology	Nature of Onset	Severity and Course of Illness	Structures Involved, Primary Disease
B. Pyelonephritis. Term refers to bacterial infections of the kidney. May be:				

1. Acute	Usually caused by gram-negative enteric bacilli. Frequently follows urinary-tract infections. A small number caused by gram-positive *Streptococcus*, *enterococcus*, and *Staphylococcus*. Infection may reach the kidney via the blood or by way of the urinary tract
	
	Predisposing factors:
	1. About one-half of cases —not known
	2. Obstruction—prostatic hypertrophy cicatricial tissue anomailes
	3. Age and sex
	  a. A comparatively high incidence before 18 months of age. More common in female than in male infants
	  b. Much more common in females 18–40 yrs. than in males
		Sudden		Lesion(s)—diffuse
				1. Inflammation of the renal pelvis and calyces
				2. Infection of renal substance, medulla, cortex, with the formation of minute abscesses
				3. Healing with the formation of scar tissue

548

Classification	Etiology	Nature of Onset	Severity and Course of Illness	Structures Involved, Primary Disease
	c. Instrumentation of the urinary tract including catheterization d. Autonomic disturbances of bladder function e. Diabetes mellitus 4. Indwelling (Foley) Catheter			
2. Chronic pyelonephritis, one of the most common forms of chronic renal disease	Results from the effects of scar tissue formed in the healing of an earlier bacterial infection of the kidney	Over half of the persons with chronic pyelonephritis have a history of having had attacks of acute urinary-tract infections Usually onset is insidious and the progress of the disease is often slow		
II. The nephrotic syndrome	1. Idiopathic 2. A phase of glomerulonephritis			In some textbooks of pathology this disease is referred to as a disease of the tubules. It is a disease in which the glomeruli are affected in such a manner that massive quantities of protein are lost in the urine
III. Diseases of the arterioles (nephroscleroses) A. Benign B. Malignant				

Disorders of the Kidney Which Are Common Causes of Renal Failure—Continued

Major Manifestations	Major Medical or Surgical Therapy
6. Laboratory tests (a) Polymorphonuclear leukocytosis (b) Many leuko-cytes in the urine (c) Bacteria in the urine	2. Maintain water intake to keep urine dilute 3. Relieve or remove obstructing lesions

1. Usually no symptoms of infection
2. Symptoms common to chronic illness
   Fatigue
   Headache (may be related to hypertension)
   Poor appetite
   Weight loss
3. Symptoms associated with failing renal function
   Polyuria
   Thirst
4. Signs of renal failure
   Impaired capacity to concentrate urine
   Elevated blood urea nitrogen
	1. Eliminate urinary-tract infections by drug therapy and by the removal of obstructing lesions

Primary manifestation: 1. Profuse proteinuria secondary to loss of proteins 2. Hyperlipemia 3. Hypoalbuminemia 4. Generalized edema Other signs and symptoms depend on the cause	Idiopathic 1. ACTH and adrenal steroids. Treatment continued for six months or longer. 2. A nutritious diet containing adequate amounts of protein. Should be sufficient to cover amounts lost in urine

* Trade name for methenamine mandelate.

Many of the details about the above disorders have not been included in the summary. Among them are the particular hazards to which each exposes the patient. In the essay that follows, the role of the nurse in anticipating and identifying evidence of developing cardiac failure or of hypertensive encephalopathy in the child or young adult with acute glomerular nephritis is outlined. Although acute glomerular nephritis is more common among children, it can and does occur in young adults.

Patients suffering from acute glomerular nephritis:
Apologia for vigilance[31]

Every year, especially in the springtime, nurses who are serving in medical units of children's hospitals or in the pediatric department of general hospitals care for patients suffering from acute glomerular nephritis. Some years there are more children than others, but always there are several. Usually, they are from four to seven years old. While sometimes a child is very sick, often the patients are not much bothered by their symptoms. More than 95 times out of a hundred they recover completely, often after little in the way of specific treatment. But of the four or five for whom this is not the happy outcome, two or three may die quite promptly. These children usually die of heart failure or hypertensive encephalopathy, which develops rapidly indeed, but not as a rule without a few signs to herald its coming. Lack of treatment, available but not instituted because the approaching demand for it was not recognized in time by those present, may be the cause for much sadness, as well as for resentment, anger, and guilt. And the child's life is lost to society.

The significant point in the above may be found in the inference that the progression of symptoms in the child usually gives some clues to the prepared observer. The observer who is prepared both to recognize and comprehend their meaning may use these clues to the patient's advantage. A hospital unit which admits acutely sick children may be expected to have one or more professional nurses there at all hours, even though physicians may not always be at hand. These nurses should be the prepared observers, able to evaluate what they see in the sick child on the basis, not just of their general knowledge of children, but of an understanding of what changes are induced in the body by acute glomerular nephritis and in what manner these changes may quickly embarrass the essential welfare of the patient. Nurses who can go this far will not often fail to take the next step to benefit the child—that of acting on the orders already available and procuring the physician promptly to meet the critical medical needs of the child.

Although most children recover from acute glomerular nephritis without evident permanent injury to the kidneys, the changes that occur incident to the damaging inflammation are considerable, and the effects at the time may be severe. The sequence often starts a week or two after sore throat caused by

[31] This portion of the chapter was contributed by Esther H. Read, R.N., pp. 551-555.

infection with group A beta hemolytic *Streptococcus,* type 12. Presumably, the *Streptococcus* toxin releases an antigen from the kidney. This circulates and reaches the plasma cells where antibody to it is formed. This, returning by the circulation to the kidney, unites with the fixed kidney antigen to produce the nephritis.

In the glomerulus, the endothelial cells proliferate and swell, and blood entering by way of the afferent vessel is obstructed. With increase of capillary permeability incident to inflammation, blood cells, both red and white, and albumin escape into Bowman's capsule and thence to the tubules which, although not accused by name, are nevertheless involved in the disease. Their cells swell and contain fatty deposits. The interstitial cells of the kidney as well become somewhat edematous so that, as a whole, the kidney is ischemic and thereby handicapped.

Generalized vasospasm is a characteristic of this type of nephritis, and awareness of this fact contributes to understanding of some of the symptoms. Normally there is a narrowing of the afferent vessel as it enters the glomerulus, a device which assures a good head of pressure to assist filtration; but when the vessels are all in spasm, as in this type of nephritis, the blood delivered to the kidney may be reduced in amount. Vasospasm increases peripheral resistance. Even the amount of blood that enters comes at the expense of increased effort by the heart. The arterial pressure rises, and unless the child has a weakened heart anyway, the pulse rate may be expected to slow somewhat because of pressure on the receptors in the carotid sinus with resultant discharge of impulses to vasomotor centers. If the vasospasm is extremely severe, the heart muscle itself may suffer hypoxia and fail under the strain of the effort, in a weakened state, of pumping a large volume of blood, increased as a result of sodium and water retention, out into vessels narrowed by spasm. Cerebral anemia may result from inadequate supply to the brain as a result of the vascular spasm alone or assisted by heart failure. The child may be drowsy, or have headache, dimness of vision, or convulsions.

Children with acute glomerular nephritis do not usually look very edematous, but, if weighed, show an increase which suggest that there is a good deal of water retention consequent to the sodium reabsorption that occurs. If the child is in heart failure, not only will the edema be more marked than otherwise, but failure further jeopardizes his welfare; for no organ, the heart included, is receiving the nutrition it needs.

Much of the pathophysiology is revealed by physical examination and laboratory tests, but the reports of these come late to the child's record. Concern here is for comprehension of what the sick child himself can demonstrate to his nurse of his needs for her attention and understanding care.

Usually he is of an age to talk readily. Children of four, five, and six years suffer severely in hospital from homesickness, and especially from conscious, expressed need for their mothers. Nurses cannot by any means satisfy this, but they can mitigate suffering a little by expressing kindly sympathy for the child in his unhappiness and by showing their readiness to let him talk about his mother. With a little skill they can help him to build verbal bridges to his home. It is not, as a rule, helpful to a sick child to try to divert him when he is mournful, even though one can do it. He is put in the position of having to do his mourning alone, which is sad for him and lessens, rather than strengthens, his nurse's relationship with him.

In pediatric nursing one has often to do without verbal communication because the patients are too little to talk. When, however, a nurse has an acutely sick child who is old enough to be articulate, she is unwise indeed if she does not use every opportunity to demonstrate to him both by word and action her interest, her liking, and her desire to know all about him. The child should learn that his nurse wants to know about him and to take care of him however he feels—sick, lonely, or, as he invariably replies to the casual inquirer, "fine." The relentless amuser, who cannot see a child sitting forlornly in bed without feeling constrained to try to cheer him up and play with him, may not be his most helpful nurse. He may not confide in her the things she would like to know, for she has not shown him that she likes him when he is unhappy; she seems always to want to change him.

The prepared nurse, faced with the responsibilty for care and professional nursing observation of a child newly sick with acute glomerular nephritis, will value her understanding of children for many reasons, one of which is that it contributes to the excellence of her nursing care. This is, however, but a part of all she needs to know, and she may do well to review whatever relevant knowledge she has from all fields and consider the application of it to her patient.

With inflammation present in the glomeruli, she expects to see evidence of blood in the urine. With sodium retention she expects the amount passed daily to be diminished. In order to become aware of whether or not the oliguria is becoming more severe, signaling less efficient glomerular filtration and increased water retention, she realizes the need for accuracy and completeness in the recording of fluid intake and output and not only sees that this is accomplished, but keeps informed herself of the relationships. If the blood pressure is elevated or the child is gaining weight, if he looks paler or more puffy than before, she stops and observes his breathing. Two checks may be necessary before she can assure herself that this ever-useful indicator of cardiac embarrassment (increase in respiratory rate without increase in patient activity) is not a source of concern for her about the patient at this time. She has been led to make this observation by knowing that vasospasm has increased the peripheral load for the heart and may be severe enough to result in some hypoxia to the myocardium, which, emptying the chambers of the heart incompletely with each stroke, initiates the whole sequence of adjustments made by the body to compensate for the lessening efficiency of the heart muscle. Of these, increasing respiratory rate is one.

When, however, she does observe that the child is breathing faster, she has something to do. First, it is to help the patient to the position of comfort and to provide him with the pillow supports he needs so that he requires no exertion to maintain it. Then she will count the pulse, note the quality, measure the blood pressure, and procure the means of administering oxygen to assist the failing efforts of the heart. It may be that the blood pressure is rising and that she already has orders provided for medication to relax vascular spasm. In this event, she is prepared to treat the child further at once. But when there is no medical order to act upon, the nurse will do well to gain a little more information from her patient in the next two or three minutes before calling his physician. The prepared nurse will have this sequence pass through her mind: vasospasm → hypertension → cerebral anemia → cerebral hypoxia → cerebral symptoms. Then, she will say to herself: Does he have any? Here is the place where one *does* try to capture the attention of the child, whatever his mood, but with an objective grimmer than that simply of diversion. By showing him a small picture of a familiar object, or reviewing the illustrations of a picture book he knows well, a fair guess can be made as to whether the child's vision is still clear. A far better judgment can be made at the same time as to his mental alertness, for if the child and his nurse are already good friends, he will try to respond to her, however ill he feels. By his response he will reveal the absence or extent of his drowsiness. It may be that after a sudden light tap or from a moment's close observation she will see muscle twitching—twitching that may presage a convulsion soon to follow. So, within a minute or two, his nurse will have added useful information to that she already has to give the doctor when she proceeds immediately to notify him of the changes in the condition of the patient and to request his presence.

If, in the absence of a physician to note rapidly advancing symptoms, there is no nurse prepared to recognize and act upon significant changes, the child who goes quickly into heart failure may die. When his needs are promptly recognized and successfully treated, his recovery from this emergency is quick and complete. The same is essentially true of hypertensive encephalopathy, although there is no one who would like to say that convulsions and cerebral hypoxia are conditions that one wants to see occurring often in any child.

Sometimes, when everyone has been alert and all have given their best knowledge and skill to care and treatment, a child with acute glomerular nephritis will die. At the present time, this cannot be avoided. In this paper an effort has been made to indicate some, though not by any means all, of the pathological changes that take place in this disease. These are changes which produce symptoms with accompanying physical signs that a nurse can recognize. Recognizing the signs and relating them to a disease process of which she has an understanding permits her to make judgments that are useful. It is at this point that she becomes free to do professional nursing.

The sick child whose parents have loaned him to the hospital for care has been entrusted by them to the doctors and nurses only because they believe that specialized care may, for a little time, be better for him than their own. If their confidence is not to have been falsely placed, not only the doctor but also the nurses, with whom the child surely will find less comfort than with his mother when he is sick, must be able to offer something that is even more important for him at the moment than her presence. This is, from nurses, intelligent vigilance based on a knowledge of emergencies that can arise due to the stress of the child's disease on his body. Confidence that they are fulfilling their entire responsibility can be felt by nurses only when they (as well as doctors for whom this is to be assumed) accept the thesis that all aspects of the care of the sick child are subjects for their attention and concern: "No Trespassing" signs have no proper place in pediatrics. All that each nurse knows about children, whether it is normal growth and development, normal or pathophysiology, techniques and skills of bedside nursing, or psychology, will be of value only when integrated and used to further the objective of all who are devoted to the hospital care of sick children. This objective is fairly met when a child is returned home, well on the road to health, with, as far as can be managed, few lasting scars sustained from his hazardous journey.

Although many of the consequences of renal failure have been stated or implied in the discussion of water and electrolyte balance, they merit discussion and emphasis here. Renal failure may develop suddenly from prolonged ischemia of the kidney or from the effect of nephrotoxic agents. More commonly, it develops slowly over the course of months and years from the effects of ischemia secondary to disease of the arterioles or arteries supplying them, from infection of kidney tissue, or from other causes. Whatever the cause or causative factors of renal failure in a given patient, the presenting signs and symptoms are due to the effect on all the organ systems of the body of the *inability of the kidney to maintain the composition and volume of body fluids.* The eventual prognosis of the patient depends on the cause as well as the ability to prevent hyperkalemia, hypertensive encephalopathy, and congestive heart failure, all of which may complicate renal failure. When the degree of injury to the kidney is such that too little renal tissue remains to perform the functions of the kidney, many patients can still be helped to lead a reasonably comfortable existence for a time by proper medical management.

The syndrome resulting from functional failure of the kidney is known as uremia or azotemia. The term "uremia" is the older and means, literally, urine in the blood. The term azotemia has a more limited meaning inasmuch as it refers to the presence of excessive quantities of nitrogenous compounds in the blood. The manifestations of uremia are due to the effects of the failure of the kidney to regulate the volume and composition of body fluids on total bodily functioning.

In contrast to the rapidly developing threat to life that characterizes acute renal failure, the manifestations accompanying chronic renal failure are that the patient may be only aware that he tires more easily than formerly and that he has some degree of muscular weakness. He seeks medical attention because he does not feel well, and he may not have felt healthy or energetic for some time. Other systemic effects of chronic renal failure include increased susceptibility to infection and delayed wound healing. In children growth and development may be retarded.

Among the most disagreeable effects of the uremic syndrome are those on the alimentary tract, as the patient experiences anorexia, nausea, and vomiting. These symptoms may be so severe that they are precipitated by the smell, sight, or even thought of food. When they are marked, they lead to marked emaciation as a consequence of failure to ingest sufficient food to meet the caloric needs of the tissues. Every effort should be made to encourage the patient to try to eat. Some patients desire special foods and will try to eat if they are provided with them. Particularly in advanced stages of the uremic syndrome, the breath has an ammoniacal or uriniferous odor; it limits the ability of the patient to taste food. Some patients find food with a definite taste more acceptable than bland ones. For example, Mr. Thomas, who was in the terminal phase of the uremic syndrome, requested canned clams. He could taste them because they have a strong and pungent taste.

In the later stages of uremia, ulcerations along the gastrointestinal tract are common. In the mouth they are associated with stomatitis (inflammation of the soft tissues of the mouth). Ulcerations in the stomach or more distal portions of the alimentary canal may lead to gastrointestinal bleeding. Although mouth care should be given regularly, the tissues should be treated with gentleness. Vomitus as well as feces should be observed for blood.

As the uremic syndrome develops, functioning of the nervous system is altered. In the early stages, the patient may be irritable. Later as the disorder progresses, he becomes apathetic, drowsy, and eventually comatose. Muscular weakness and twitching, neuralgic or neuritic pains, headache and dizziness may be observed. In patients in whom there is some degree of hypertensive encephalopathy, failing vision or even blindness occurs.

Effects on the respiratory systems are due to congestive heart failure, and in advanced renal failure to pulmonary edema, as well as to metabolic acidoses. Dyspnea occurs as a result of the first two; Kussmaul breathing as a result of the acidosis.

Many of the manifestations referrable to the circulatory system are due to the hypertension accompanying renal disease. Some are, however, due to the effects of the failure of the kidney to regulate the composition and volume of the blood. The effects of hyperkalemia on the contractility of the myocardium have been previously discussed. In addition, purpura develops as a result of increased capillary fragility and alteration in the clotting mechanism. A marked and progressive anemia develops as a consequence of hemolysis and failure of hematopoiesis. Uremic pericarditis causes precordial pain and a friction rub.

Changes in the skeleton include osteomalacia in the adult and rickets in children.

The skin is also affected. One of the earliest symptoms is pruritus. The pruritus may be intense, leading to extensive self-inflected excoriations of the skin. Later after the level of nonprotein nitrogenous substances in the blood becomes very high, urea frost can be seen on the skin. The white crystals are more easily seen in areas where perspiration is most abundant, such as around the mouth. They can and should be removed by bathing.

Because the composition and volume of body fluids depend on the adequate renal function, the uremic patient often presents many problems including: (1) malnutrition, (2) anemia, (3) water and electrolyte imbalance, (4) hypertensive vascular disease, and (5) circulatory failure. The principles underlying the treatment of each of the above are discussed elsewhere.

In nursing the patient who is in some phase of renal failure, attention should be given to the maintenance of his physiological status as well as to his general comfort. Inasmuch as his physiological status can be supported, his feelings of well-being will be improved. Eventually the patient becomes dependent on others to meet most if not all of his needs. He should be observed for evidence of changes in his condition, and his care should be modified as necessary.

REFERENCES

Books

Abbott Laboratories, *Fluid and Electrolytes,* Abbott Laboratories, North Chicago, Illinois, 1960.

Abbott Laboratories, *Parenteral Administration,* Abbott Laboratories, North Chicago, Illinois, 1959.

Ainsworth-Davis, J. C., *Essentials of Urology,* Charles C Thomas Co., Springfield, Illinois, 1950.

Allen, J. Garrott, *et al.* (eds.), *Surgery,* J. B. Lippincott Co., Philadelphia, 1957, pp. 97-117.

Best, Charles H., and Norman B. Taylor, *The Living Body,* 4th ed., Henry Holt and Co., New York, 1958.

Black, D. A. K., Editor *Renal Disease,* Revised Reprint, Blackwell Scientific Publications, Oxford, 1963.

Bland, John H., *Clinical Recognition and Management of Disturbances of Fluid Balance,* 2nd ed., W. B. Saunders Co., Philadelphia, 1956.

Brooks, Stewart, *Basic Facts of Body Water and Ions,* Springer Publishing Co., Inc., New York, 1960.

Colby, Fletcher H., *Essential Urology,* 4th ed., The Williams and Wilkins Co., Baltimore, 1961.

Harmer, Bertha, and Virginia Henderson, *Textbook of the Principles and Practice of Nursing,* 5th ed., The Macmillan Company, New York, 1955, pp. 1050-59.

Lakeside Laboratories, *Of Water, Salt and Life,* Lakeside Laboratories, Inc., Milwaukee, 1956.

Pitts, Robert F., *Physiology of the Kidney and Body Fluids,* Year Book Medical Publishers, Inc., Chicago, 1963.

Snively, William D., *Sea Within,* J. B. Lippincott Co., Philadelphia, 1960.

Statland, Harry, *Fluid and Electrolytes in Practice,* 2nd ed., J. B. Lippincott Co., Philadelphia, 1957.

Articles

Abbott, W. E., "Nutrition, Body Fluids, Shock and Burns," *Surgery, Gynecology and Obstetrics,* CXVI, February, 1963, pp. 141-46.

Amos, William H., "The Life of a Sand Dune," *Scientific American,* CCI, July, 1959, pp. 91-99.

Ansell, Julian S., "Nephrectomy and Nephrostomy," *American Journal of Nursing,* LVIII, October, 1958, pp. 1394-96.

Barnes, Roger W., and Varner S. Johns, "Medical Considerations in Surgical Renal Disease," *Medical Clinics of North America,* XLIII, No. 4, July, 1959, pp. 1177-94.

Barnes, Roger W., and Angus Purdey, "Prostatic Tumors," *American Journal of Nursing,* LVI, August, 1956, pp. 982-87.

Black, D. A. K., "Symptoms and Signs in Disorders of Body Fluid," *Journal of Chronic Diseases,* XI, March, 1960, pp. 340-47.

Bonsnes, R. W., "Postoperative and Parenteral Nutrition," *Surgical Clinics of North America,* XXXVII, April, 1957, pp. 307-20.

Brooke, Clement E., and Constantine S. Anast, "Oral Fluid and Electrolytes," *Journal of the American Medical Association,* CLXXIX, March 10, 1962, p. 792.

Burnell, James M., Richard R. Paton, and Belding H. Scribner, "The Problem of Sodium and Water Needs of Patients," *Journal of Chronic Diseases,* XI, March, 1960, pp. 189-97.

Christensen, H. N., "Control of Hydrogen Ion," *New England Journal of Medicine,* CCXLVII, July 31, 1952, pp. 174-75.

Clarke, B. G., and Sumner Joress, "Quantitative Bacteriuria After Use of Indwelling Catheters," *Journal of the American Medical Association,* CLXXIV, No. 12, November 19, 1960, p. 1593.

"Clinical Application of Fluid and Electrolyte Balance," *Physician's Bulletin,* XXVI, February, 1961.

Colston, J. A. Campbell, "Radical Perineal Prostatectomy for Early Cancer," *Journal of the American Medical Association,* CLXIX, No. 7, February 14, 1959, pp. 700-3

Comarr, A. Estin, A. Karchak, and R. Snelson, "An Improved Bladder Training Device," *The Journal of Urology,* XC, No. 3, September, 1963, pp. 335-7.

"Commonly Mismanaged Urologic Problems," *Medical Clinics of North America,* XLIII, November, 1959, p. 6.

Corcoran, A. C., "Renal Failure," *American Journal of Nursing,* LVI, June, 1956, pp. 768-75.

Cox, Claire, "Incidence of Bacteriuria with Indwelling Catheter in Normal Bladders," *Journal of the American Medical Association,* CLXXVIII, December 2, 1961, p. 919.

Creery, C. Donald, "Ileac Diversion of the Urine," *American Journal of Nursing,* LIX, April, 1959, pp. 530-33.

Culp, David A., "Acute Urinary Retention," *Postgraduate Medicine,* XXXI, March, 1962, p. 252.

Danowski, T. S., "Electrolytes and Nutrition," *Postgraduate Medicine,* XXIII, April, 1958, pp. 372-76.

Davis, David M., "Manifestations and Findings in Urologic Disease," *Medical Clinics of North America,* XLVI, May, 1962, p. 795.

Desautels, Robert E., and I. Hartwell Harrison, "The Mismanagement of Urethral Catheter," *Medical Clinics of North America,* XLIII, No. 6, November, 1959, pp. 1573-84.

Dick, Vernon S., "Carcinoma of the Prostate Gland with Metastases," *Surgical Clinics of North America,* XLII, June, 1962, pp. 771-77.

Dunning, M. F., and F. Plum, "Potassium Depletion by Enemas," *American Journal of Medicine,* XX, May, 1956, pp. 789-92.

Ewert, Earl, "Evaluation of the Symptoms Resulting from Bladder Neck Obstruction in the Adult Male," *Surgical Clinics of North America,* XLII, June, 1962, pp. 765-70.

Farr, Hallon W., "Fluid and Electrolyte Balance with Special Reference to the Gastro-intestinal Tract," *American Journal of Nursing,* LIV, July, 1954, pp. 827-31.

Gallagher, J. C., and David Seligson, "Significance of Abnormally Low Blood Urea Levels," *New England Journal of Medicine,* CCLXVI, March 8, 1962, pp. 492-95.

"Genitourinary Conditions," Special Issue, *Postgraduate Medicine,* XXXIII, No. 5, May, 1963.

Gibson, John G., and Carl W. Walter, "The Development of Blood Component Therapy at the Peter Brent Brigham Hospital," *Medical Clinics of North America,* XLIV, September, 1960, pp. 1413-23.

Grayhack, John T., "Hormonal Treatment of Prostatic Cancer," *Surgical Clinics of North America,* XXXIX, No. 1, February, 1959, pp. 13-27.

Greisman, Sheldon E., "The Physiological Basis for Vasopressor Therapy during Shock," *Annals of Internal Medicine,* L, May, 1959, pp. 1092-1109.

Hand, John R., "Infections of the Urinary Tract," *American Journal of Nursing,* LVII, August, 1957, p. 1008.

Hart, Elizabeth L., and Margaret J. Mager, "Collecting Urine Specimens," *American Journal of Nursing,* LVII, October, 1957, pp. 1323-24.

Heap, Beth, "Sodium Restricted Diets," *American Journal of Nursing,* LX, February, 1960, pp. 206-9.

Howard, John M., "Fluid Replacement in Shock and Hemorrhage," *Journal of the American Medical Association,* CLXXIII, June 4, 1960, p. 516.

"Hypertonic Sodium for 'Irreversible' Oligaemic Shock," *Lancet,* I, No. 7280, March 9, 1963, pp. 539-40.

Kark, Robert M., "Office and Bedside Examination of Patients Suspected of Having a Renal Disorder," *Medical Clinics of North America,* XLVI, No. 3, May, 1962, p. 785.

Kessler, Edward, "The Relation of Potassium to Alkalosis and Acidosis," *American Practitioner and Digest of Treatment,* X, March, 1959, pp. 425-28.

Lauer, D. John, "Salt in Heat Sickness," *American Journal of Nursing,* LIII, August, 1953, pp. 938-39.

Lich, Robert, *et al.,* "A Clinical Evaluation of the Urethral Catheter," *Journal of the American Medical Association,* CLXXX, June 9, 1962, p. 183.

Lowe, Charles U., "Principles of Parenteral Fluid Therapy," *American Journal of Nursing,* LIII, August, 1953, pp. 963-65.

Maclean, M. Moira, Helen Creighton, and Leonard B. Berman, "Hemodialysis and the Artificial Kidney," *American Journal of Nursing,* LVIII, December, 1958, pp. 1672-74.

Manitius, Andrzej, *et al.,* "On the Mechanism of Impairment of Renal Concentrating Ability in Hypercalcemia," *Journal of Clinical Investigation,* XXIX, April, 1960, pp. 693-97.

Merrill, Arthur J., "Nutrition in Chronic Renal Failure," *Journal of the American Medical Association,* CLXXIII, June 25, 1960, pp. 905-11.

Merrill, John B., "The Artificial Kidney," *Scientific American,* CCV, July, 1961, pp. 56-64.

Mossholder, Irene, "When the Patient Has a Radical Retro-pubic Prostatectomy," *American Journal of Nursing,* LXII, July, 1962, pp. 101-4.

Mudge, G. H., "Introduction to a Symposium on Electrolyte Metabolism," *American Journal of Medicine,* XV, December, 1953, pp. 761-64.

Nelson, Alice C., "Why Won't Stevie Drink?" *American Journal of Nursing,* LXI, July, 1961, pp. 44-48.

Newman, Gustave, and Claude R. Nichols, "Sexual Activities and Attitudes in Older Persons," *Journal of the American Medical Association,* CLXXIII, No. 1, May 7, 1960, p. 33.

Obermeyer, William B., "Crotch Care," *American Journal of Nursing,* LVII, May, 1957, p. 618.

O'Connor, Vincent J., "Early Recognition of Prostatic Disease," *Surgical Clinics of North America,* XXXVIII, January, 1958, pp. 279-84.

Prout, Harry C., "The Modern Concept of Surgical Shock," *American Journal of Nursing,* LVIII, January, 1958, pp. 78-79.

Reams, Gerald B., and Elmad Powel, "Postoperative Catheterization—Yes or No?" *American Journal of Nursing,* LX, No. 3, March, 1960, p. 371.

Reidenburg, Marcus, "The Role of Bone in Electrolyte Metabolism," *Archives of Internal Medicine,* CVII, April, 1961, pp. 578-81.

Reiss, Eric, *et al.,* "Fluid and Electrolyte Balance in Burns," *Journal of the American Medical Association,* CLII, August 1, 1953, pp. 1309-13.

Relman, A. S., "What Are Acids and Bases?" *American Journal of Medicine,* XVII, October, 1954, pp. 435-37.

Robertson, James, *Young Children in Hospitals,* Basic Books, Inc., New York, 1958.

Robertson, J. David, "The Membrane of the Living Cell," *Scientific American,* CCVI, April, 1962, pp. 64-72.

Rosenthal, Sanford, "Wound Shock," *Scientific American,* CIC, December, 1958, pp. 115-24.

Rubin, Mitchell I., "Disturbances of the Kidney," in Waldo Nelson, (ed.), *Textbook of Pediatrics,* 7th ed., W. B. Saunders Co., Philadelphia, 1959.

Schilling, John, "A New Approach to Fluid Therapy of the Severely Burned Patients: The Use of Urea as an Electrolyte Substitute," *Annals of Surgery,* CL, October, 1959, pp. 756-67.

Schmid-Nielson, Knul, "Physiology of the Camel," *Scientific American,* CCI, December, 1959, pp. 140-51.

Schwartz, William B., and Adolf Polak, "Electrolyte Disorders in Chronic Renal Disease," *Journal of Chronic Disease,* XI, March, 1960, pp. 319-39.

Sheiner, Ben, and Bernard D. Pinck, "Promethazine Drip in the Postoperative Management of Supra Pubic Prostatectomy," *Journal of the American Medical Association,* CLXXI, No. 15, December 5, 1959, pp. 1955-56.

Snively, William D., and Barbara Brown, "In the Balance," *American Journal of Nursing,* LVIII, January, 1958, pp. 55-57.

Solomon, Arthur K., "Pumps in the Living Cell," *Scientific American,* CCVII, August, 1962, pp. 100-8.

Spencer, Richard, "Potassium Metabolism and Gastrointestinal Function: A Review," *American Journal of Digestive Disease,* IV, February, 1959, pp. 145-58.

Symposium, "Absorption of Water and Electrolytes from the Gastrointestinal Tract: An Experimental Approach," *The American Journal of Digestive Diseases,* VII, January, 1962, pp. 1-68.

Symposium, "Water and Electrolyte Metabolism," *Journal of Chronic Diseases,* XI, March, 1960, pp. 187-98.

Tarail, Robert, "Practice of Fluid Therapy," *Journal of the American Medical Association,* CLXXI, September 5, 1959, pp. 45-49.

Thomas, William C., *et al.,* "Diagnostic Considerations in Hypercalcemia," *New England Journal of Medicine,* CCLX, March, 1959, pp. 591-96.

Twiss, Mary R., and Morton H. Maxwell, "Peritoneal Dialysis," *American Journal of Nursing,* LIX, November, 1959, pp. 1560-63.

Vertes, Victor, "Electrolyte-Free Liquid Formula Diet," *Journal of the American Medical Association,* CLXXII, April 23, 1960, pp. 1893-97.

Walker, James E. C., and Roe E. Wells, "Heat and Water Exchange in the Respiratory Tract," *American Journal of Medicine,* XXX, February, 1961, pp. 259-67.

Walsh, Michael A., *et al.,* "Neo-Bladder," *American Journal of Nursing,* LXIII, No. 4, April, 1963, pp. 107-10.

Weil, Paul G., "Blood Transfusions in Geriatric Practice," *Geriatrics,* XIV, October, 1959, pp. 631-33.

Weisberg, Harry F., "A Better Understanding of Anion-Cation ('Acid-Base') Balance," *Surgical Clinics of North America,* XXXIX, February, 1959, pp. 93-119.

Winters, Robert, and Ralph Dell, "Clinical Physiology of Metabolic Acidosis," *Postgraduate Medicine,* XXXI, February, 1962, pp. 161-68.

Wolf, Edith S., "The Nurse and Fluid Therapy," *American Journal of Nursing,* LIV, July, 1954, pp. 831-33.

Zinsser, Hans H., "Urinary Calculi," *Journal of the American Medical Association,* CLXXIV, No. 16, December 17, 1960, p. 2062.

9 : Nursing the Patient Having a Problem with Some Aspects of Transporting Material to and from Cells

It is proved by the structure of the heart that the blood is continuously transferred through the lungs into the aorta, as by two clacks of a water bellows to raise water. It is proved by the ligature that there is a passage of blood from the arteries to the veins. It is therefore demonstrated that the continuous movement of the blood in a circle is brought about by the beat of the heart. Is this for the sake of nutrition, or the better preservation of the blood and members by the infusion of heat, the blood in turn being cooled by heating the members and heated by the heart?[1]

Emphasis has been placed on the fact that survival, growth, reproduction, and productivity depend on a continued supply of the materials required by cells to support their chemical activities. Waste products must be removed from the cells and eliminated so the physical and chemical conditions of the fluid environment of cells are maintained within limits favorable to cell processes. Excesses of supply must be stored or eliminated. Products produced by one group of cells, such as hormones, require some means of distribution if they are to influence the activity of other cells. In earlier chapters, discussion has centered around how the organism acquires needed materials from its external environment and around the mechanisms involved in maintaining the constancy of the internal environment within limits.

References have been made to the importance of transportation to each of the above. Unless required substances can be taken into the internal environment and distributed to the cells, life ceases. This chapter is devoted to the factors important to the transportation of materials from one part of the body to another, and to the causes and consequences of failure of transportation.

In man, cells are bathed in a fluid that is separated from the external environment by semipermeable membranes. To meet the needs of the cells, materials must be transported to and from these membranes. This is accomplished by a system of tubes arranged in what is essentially a closed circuit. Some of these tubes are thick-walled structures serving as distensible and

[1] William Harvey, quoted in "Lives in Science," *A Scientific American Book,* Simon and Schuster, New York, 1953, p. 189.

elastic conduits conveying blood from the heart to the tissues or from the tissues back to the heart. After tubes (arteries) leave the heart and approach the tissues, they branch into smaller and smaller vessels. Finally, they form microscopic structures (capillaries) that are only one endothelial cell in thickness. It is in the capillary that the function of transportation is accomplished. In the capillary materials are taken into the internal environment, or returned to the external environment. Materials are exchanged between the internal and external environment, as well as between the blood and the interstitial fluid.

The circuit is filled with a modifiable medium of exchange, the blood. Some of the substances transported in the blood are in solution. Others are as formed elements. Still others are in chemical or physical combination with formed elements.

What factors aid in the movement of blood?

The major factor in the movement of blood is the force of contraction of the heart. Other factors that contribute to keeping the circuit filled and to a continuous flow of blood to tissues include: (1) the distensibility and elasticity of the arteries; (2) the resistance offered by the walls of arteries, particularly small arteries, to the flow of blood; and (3) the viscosity of the blood. Return flow of blood through the veins is supported by the contraction of skeletal muscles and valves which prevent backflow in veins carrying blood against gravity. Because of their contribution to the forward movement of blood in veins, skeletal muscles are sometimes referred to as secondary hearts. Lessening of pressure in the thoracic cavity during inspiration as well as reduction of pressure within the heart following systole also aids in the return of blood to the heart.

One of the remarkable features of circulatory function is that, in health, blood is moved into and out of all of the tissues of the body, so the needs of cells in varying states of activity are met.[2] Moreover, function can be adapted in relation to the activity of the entire organism or to a localized area of tissue. At the same time, blood flow is regulated so that vital structures, such as the brain, heart, and kidney, are nourished despite greatly increased demands by other parts of the body. Respiration and circulatory functions are regulated in relation to each other, so that their function is complementary. The mechanisms for the regulation of circulatory function will be discussed in more detail later.

Like other tissues in the body, the structures comprising the transportation system are susceptible to conditions in the internal environment. They are dependent for continued function on the quantity and quality of blood circulated through them. They are also subject to disease and injury. Malfunction

---

[2] Factors in the movement of substances to and from the blood and the cell are discussed in Chapter 8.

may result from disturbances in the mental apparatus (see Chapter 2) or from direct injury to cells. Injury, beyond that induced by the initiating factor, may result from excessive response of damaged tissues. For example, deformations of the heart valves as a result of rheumatic fever can be increased by the formation of excessive quantities of scar tissue. Conversely, scarring and its undesirable sequelae can be reduced, if the severity of the exudative and proliferative phases of the disease can be lessened.

What are the general causes of failure of transportation?

Although the effects of failure in function will be discussed later in the chapter, the causes of failure of transportation may generally be summarized as: (1) inadequate quantity or quality of the blood; (2) insufficient power to move blood into the arteries; (3) failure to return blood to the heart; (4) obstruction, intrinsic or extrinsic, to the flow of blood; (5) overdilatation of the tubular structures—local or general; (6) disturbances in the volume of circulating fluid; and (7) disturbances arising from defects in regulation of one or more parts of the transportation system.

What are some of the factors influencing the nature of the manifestations following disease or injury of the transportation system?

Manifestations resulting from disease or injury to the transportation system depend on the degree to which the needs of the tissues are met and the specific tissues affected. As long as an activity of a person is within the adaptive capacity of his circulatory system, there may be no symptoms and few, if any, observable signs indicating failure of transportation. The affected tissues may receive sufficient blood of high enough quality to function at rest or during mild or even moderate activity. Examples include the instance of Frank Sparrow, who has arteriosclerosis obliterans of the arteries of his lower extremities. Blood flow is impeded, but not completely obstructed. He can walk from his house to the corner—about a short city block—without discomfort. When he tries to walk further, he develops a cramplike pain in the calf of his leg. For some weeks, Mrs. Bird (the grandmother in Chapter 8), who had a diagnosis of congestive heart failure, found she became short of breath when she walked up a flight of stairs or walked against the wind. Enid Elm's hemoglobin was 7 gm per 100 ml of blood. She was comfortable only when resting. She became short of breath when climbing stairs or ran for a bus. Although each of these individuals had a disorder limiting the functional capacity of some part of their circulatory system, the blood supplied to the tissues of each of them was adequate in quantity and quality when they were at rest or exercising moderately. It was not sufficient, however, to enable them to increase their activity.

Many of the manifestations of failure in transportation result from a lack in the supply of oxygen and nutrients and from an accumulation of carbon dioxide and other metabolites in the affected tissues. Effects of failure will also be influenced by whether the disturbance involves the entire individual or is limited to a localized area of tissue. Disorders involving the heart or blood frequently affect the function of the body as a whole. Signs and symptoms are likely to be the result of disturbances in the functions of organs particularly sensitive to oxygen want or carbon dioxide excess. Sooner or later all tissues —organs and systems—will be affected. Lesions involving blood vessels may have either local or general effects. In some diseases of blood vessels, such as atherosclerosis, the disorder may be more or less generalized, but its effects are more marked in some organs than in others, as in the brain, kidney, heart, and lower extremities. Whatever the causative factor or factors, the effects of failure in transportation result from inadequate nourishment of cells. Survival of the affected cells is possible when the failure is relative, but death of cells or of the entire organism quickly follows complete failure. It is important to note that any disturbance, whatever its origin, involving circulatory function can be expected to arouse some degree of anxiety in the patient. This anxiety is often a factor in the magnitude of the response of the patient to his illness.

Knowledge of the factors necessary for the maintenance of a satisfactory blood supply to all tissues of the body, as well as of some of the causes and effects of failure, is essential in the practice of nursing. Some of the causes of failure are the result of the general effect of illness or its therapy on the circulatory system. Others are the consequence of disease or injury of some part of the circulatory system itself. Often the manifestations are due to multiple factors. As an illustration, Mr. Frank has generalized atherosclerosis. Because neither his heart nor his arteries are able to adapt to an increase in activity, bed rest has been prescribed. A decrease in activity is accompanied by venous stasis, thus predisposing to the formation of thrombi in the veins. Pressure, particularly over bony prominences, impedes arterial circulation and leads to tissue injury because it limits the blood supply to the affected part.

Diseases involving the cardiovascular system rank first as a cause of death. They are also important causes of morbidity and disability. They are found among people in all age groups and in all walks of life. With the exception of the second decade of life, their incidence rises from birth to death. From the community point of view, the most serious form of disease is the one that kills or maims persons in the productive years of life.

What are some of the objectives toward which the nursing of patients should be planned?

Because of differences in the function of the various structures in transportation, each will be presented separately. No part, however, functions alone. Each part is dependent on all others, if tissues are to be adequately nourished.

Nursing care as it relates to a disturbance in transportation should be planned to achieve one or more of the following objectives:

1. To lessen the activity of a part or of the whole individual so the discrepancy between supply and demand is minimized.
2. To strengthen or improve the functioning capacity of the diseased organ or organs.
3. To supply needed materials for cellular activity.
4. To assist the patient to as full a recovery as his condition permits.
5. To provide an environment that affords the patient physical and emotional comfort and support.
6. To protect the patient from disturbances or conditions in his internal or external environment which will place added stress on his already defective transportation system.

In the following pages, the consequences of failure of the heart, arteries, veins, capillaries, and blood to function within physiological limits will be discussed. Implications for nursing care will be indicated.

What is the ultimate test of cardiac function?

Anyone who reads the daily newspaper knows the heart is an important source of mortality, morbidity, and disability. What may not be sufficiently appreciated is that, in health, the heart is a powerful organ with a considerable degree of reserve power. According to authorities such as Paul Dudley White, the heart, rather than being injured by, benefits from physical exercise. This is apparently true of the diseased heart as well as the healthy heart. In health, the heart is capable of adapting the quantity of its output of blood to the quantity of blood delivered to it by the veins. Stated simply and directly, cardiac output equals cardiac intake. The ultimate test of cardiac function is the capacity or power of the heart to move as much blood into the arteries as is delivered to it by the veins. This implies that when the volume of blood delivered to the heart is increased, cardiac output is also increased. After a stroke or two, a new balance is struck between intake and output and there is no gain in the quantity of blood remaining in the heart at the end of systole.

Cite evidence to support the statement that the heart has a remarkable reserve power.

The remarkable power of the heart is illustrated by the fact that the heart of an adult weighing 70 kg pumps about 60 ml per stroke, or about 5 liters of blood, each minute, at rest, and up to 120 to 150 ml per stroke, or 20 or 25 liters each minute, during exercise. In a well-trained athlete, the cardiac output may be as high as 35 liters per minute.[3] An important characteristic of a healthy heart is its ability to adjust its output to the needs of the tissues.

[3] Carl J. Wiggers, "The Heart," *Scientific American*, CXCVI, May, 1957, p. 75.

How does the structure of the heart facilitate its function?

In structure, the heart is a double pump, each side of which has two chambers—an atrium and a ventricle. The two sides of the heart are separated from each other by a muscular septum which prevents the mixing of arterial and venous blood. Openings in the septum may be due to failure to close the foramen ovale [4] or to failure to close either the interventricular or interauricular septum in the developing embryo. Septal defects, especially those in the ventricular septum which allow for mixing of arterial and venous blood, are one of the more serious congenital anomalies of the heart. Interseptal defects, when combined with other anomalies such as pulmonic stenosis or right ventricular hypertrophy, are a cause of cyanotic heart disease as in the so-called "blue baby."

[4] The foramen ovale is an opening in the interatrial septum that connects the right and left atria in the fetal heart.

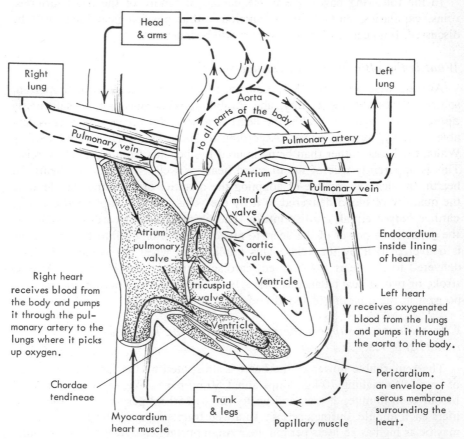

FIGURE 9—1. A diagram of the human heart, the veins and arteries entering and leaving it, and the route of the blood through the heart and to parts of the body indicated by arrows. (Modified from *Your Heart and How It Works.* Courtesy of American Heart Association, 1963.)

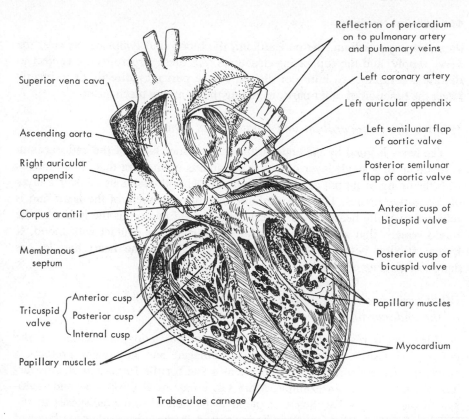

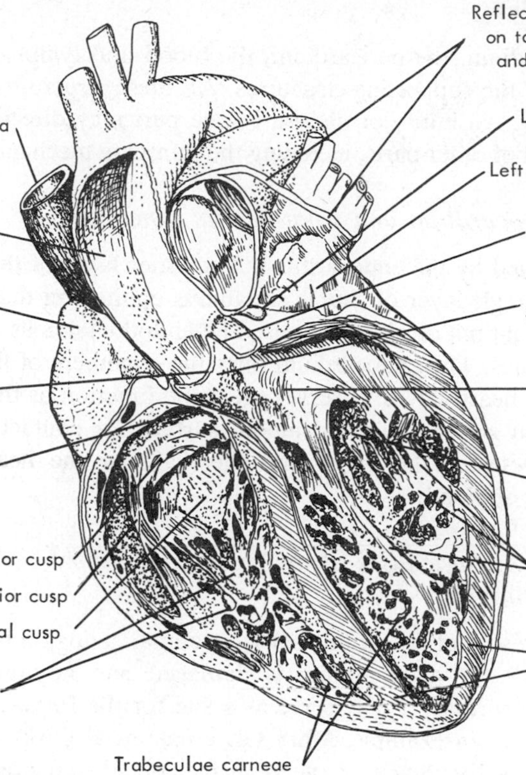
Reflection of pericardium on to pulmonary artery and pulmonary veins
Superior vena cava
Left coronary artery
Left auricular appendix
Ascending aorta
Left semilunar flap of aortic valve
Right auricular appendix
Posterior semilunar flap of aortic valve
Corpus arantii
Anterior cusp of bicuspid valve
Membranous septum
Posterior cusp of bicuspid valve
Tricuspid valve
Anterior cusp
Posterior cusp
Internal cusp
Papillary muscles
Myocardium
Papillary muscles
Trabeculae carneae

FIGURE 9–2. The heart seen from the front. (Toldt.) What is the function of the right heart? The left heart? Why are valves needed? (Adapted with permission of The Macmillan Company from *Anatomy and Physiology*, 14th ed., Fig. 221, p. 311, by Diana Clifford Kimber, Carolyn E. Gray, Caroline E. Stackpole, and Lutie C. Leavell. Copyright © The Macmillan Company, 1961.)

The right side of the heart receives blood from the systemic circulation and ejects blood into the pulmonary or lesser circulation. The left side of the heart receives blood from the pulmonary circulation and pumps blood into the systemic circulation. With the exception of the small amount of blood circulated through the bronchial arteries, the right side pumps the same quantity of blood as the left. The bronchial veins empty into the pulmonary veins and thus drain into the left rather than the right atrium. The myocardium of the right ventricle is not as thick as the left ventricle because it pumps blood into a relatively low-pressure system while the left ventricle pumps blood into a high-pressure system. In health, the ventricle provides the main force in the movement of blood, while the atrium acts primarily as a reservoir. In disease of the heart, the atria may account for as much as 30 per cent of the propulsive power of the heart.

As indicated above, the heart is a rhythmically contracting organ that regularly ejects the blood received from the venous circulation into the arteries. In Figures 9-1 and 9-2 the layers and other essential structures of the heart are depicted. The essential structures of the heart include the endocardium, the myocardium, the pericardium, the blood and lymphatic vessels, the nerve supply, and the supporting structures. All these structures are subject to disease and injury. An injury or disease in one part may directly or indirectly affect the function of other parts, including the pumping mechanism.

What is the endocardium and what are its functions?

The heart is lined by the endocardium. The inner layer of the endocardium is made up of a single layer of simple squamous epithelium that is continuous with the lining or intima of blood vessels. The endothelial cells lie over a layer of connective tissues. The endocardium lines the chambers of the heart and is reflected over the heart valves. It serves the same function as the intima of the blood vessels, that is, it provides a smooth surface for contact with blood. It lessens friction between the blood and the walls of the heart and lessens danger of clotting of blood.

What are some of the causes of and results of injury of the endocardium?

When, as a result of infection, stasis, trauma, aging, infarction, or the collagen diseases,[5] the endocardium is damaged and no longer presents a nearly frictionless surface, it may serve as a site for the formation of intracardiac thrombosis. As an example, Mary Olive has atrial fibrillation and stenosis[6] of the mitral valve. Stasis of blood in the left atrium predisposes to the clotting of blood. Thrombi have been formed in the auricular appendages of her left auricle. As another example, Mr. Frank Carp has a serious myocardial infarction.[7] The area of ischemia extends through the myocardium and into the endocardium of his left ventricle. Necrosis of endothelial' cells roughened the endocardium and predisposed to the formation of a thrombus.[8] Whenever a thrombus is present in any part of the vascular system, there is always a possibility that before the thrombus is organized, a piece will be

[5] The collagen diseases are a group of disorders or syndromes involving connective tissue. They are grouped together because they have certain histological features in common, such as widespread inflammatory injury of the connective tissue and the deposition of a fibrinoid material in the ground substance. Each collagen disease presents a distinct clinical picture, but they have general manifestations as well as local lesions in a variety of organs including the joints, heart, blood vessels, skin, muscle, and supporting reticulum of other organs. The involvement of one or more organs should be expected, since some type of connective tissue is found in all parts of the body. The specific clinical manifestations of the collagen diseases will depend on the location of lesions and the rate at which they develop. Many of these disorders respond favorably for a time to therapy with the adrenal corticosteroids. Included among the collagen diseases are systemic lupus erythematosus, dermatomyositis, and polyarteritis. (A. McGehee Harvey, "Diseases of Connective Tissue," in Cecil-Loeb, *Textbook of Medicine*, 11th ed., edited by Paul B. Beeson and Walsh McDermott, eds., W. B. Saunders Company, Philadelphia, 1963, pp. 469-91.

[6] Stenosis is a condition in which an opening or tubular structure is narrowed or constricted.

[7] Death of an area of heart muscle as a result of obstruction of the blood supply to it.

[8] Because the thrombus is attached to the wall of the heart, it is called a mural (wall) thrombus.

dislodged and become an embolus and be carried forward in the circulation until it obstructs an artery. The site of obstruction will depend on whether the embolus originates in the right or left side of the heart and on the size of the clot. An embolus originating in the left side of the heart will block an artery in the systemic circulation. The blood supply to any organ supplied by the systemic circulation may be partly or entirely obstructed. Emboli originating in the right side obstruct the pulmonary circulation. Besides obstructing arterial blood flow, thrombi or emboli may serve as sites of infection.

How does the structure of the heart valves contribute to the forward movement of blood?

In addition to predisposing to intracardiac thromboses, disease or injury of the endocardium often results in deformity of one or more of the valves of the heart and, as a consequence, interference with valvular function. The effects of injury to the valves can best be understood in the light of their structure and function. Valves in the heart help to keep the blood moving in one direction through the vascular circuit. They and their attachments are so shaped and arranged that pressure in one (forward) direction causes the valve to open, and pressure in the other or (backward) direction causes the valve to close. The valves between the auricles and ventricles are prevented from inverting during systole by the chordae tendineae and the papillary muscles. See Figures 9-1, 9-2, 9-3, and 9-4. During closure there is a consid-

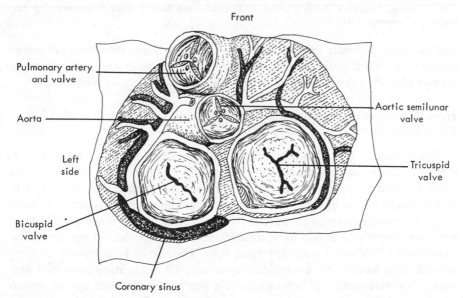

FIGURE 9–3. Valves of the heart as seen from above, atria removed. (Adapted with permission of The Macmillan Company from *Anatomy and Physiology*, 14th ed., Fig. 224, p. 313, by Diana Clifford Kimber, Carolyn E. Gray, Caroline E. Stackpole, and Lutie C. Leavell. Copyright © The Macmillan Company, 1961.)

erable degree of overlapping of the valve leaflets, which helps prevent the backward flow of blood. The semilunar valves, which lie between the ventricles and the pulmonary arteries and the aorta, are cup-shaped, with the bowl of the cup toward the pulmonary artery or aorta. As the artery fills so do the cusps (cups). The filling of the cusps brings the edges of the valve into contact. Unlike the auricular ventricular valves, there is no overlapping of the edges of the valvular cusps. During diastole the pressure of blood in the artery

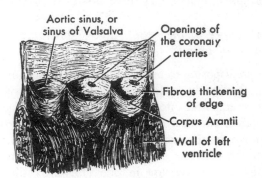

FIGURE 9—4. Aortic valve. The artery has been cut open to show the aortic semilunar valve. The sinuses of Valsalva are three pouches or slight dilations which are located between the semilunar valves and the wall of the aorta. These sinuses are also found on the pulmonary artery between the semilunar valves and the wall of the artery. Note the openings of the coronary arteries and the cup shape of the aortic semilunar valves. (Adapted with permission of The Macmillan Company from *Anatomy and Physiology*, 14th ed., Fig. 225, p. 314, by Diana Clifford Kimber, Carolyn E. Gray, Caroline E. Stackpole, and Lutie C. Leavell. Copyright © The Macmillan Company, 1961.)

and the cusps is greater than the pressure within the heart; the valves are maintained in a closed position. During systole, the pressure within the heart is greater than the pressure in the arteries and the valves are opened.

How does disease or injury alter the functioning of the heart valves?

When, as a result of injury or disease, the valve leaflets, or cusps, are damaged, the valve may no longer close tightly or open fully. Failure of the valve to close an opening between the atrium and ventricle or the ventricle and its artery allows blood to flow in a backward direction. Failure of a valve to open normally impedes the forward movement of blood. When a valve does not close properly, it is said to be insufficient or incompetent. In lay terms, the valve "leaks." When it does not open fully, because it is narrowed or constricted, it is said to be stenosed. Valves may be both insufficient and stenosed. The seriousness of deformities of a heart valve depends on the degree of "leakiness" or obstruction and on its location. For example, when the aortic semilunar valve is incompetent, blood leaks back into the heart during diastole. The return of arterial blood to the left ventricle has two serious effects. The heart has to move "leaked blood" back into the aorta, as well as the blood delivered to the heart by the veins, and it has difficulty in meeting its own nutritional needs. Maximum blood flow through the coronary arteries takes place at the end of systole and beginning of diastole. Coronary artery blood flow, especially to the left ventricle, depends on the pressure of the blood in the ascending aorta at the beginning of diastole. The contracting ventricle obstructs the lumen of its own blood vessels and limits the flow of blood to the myocardium during systole. Therefore, any condition resulting in a lowering of the pressure of the blood in the ascending aorta during diastole lessens the quantity of blood circulated to the myocardium. To recapitulate, a leaking aortic valve allows blood to fall back into the heart as soon as diastole begins. Blood, therefore, moves not only forward into the circulation, but backward into the ventricle, with the result that the pressure of the blood in the ascending aorta falls abruptly. As a consequence, there is a loss in the force required to move blood through the coronary arteries. Each time the heart contracts, it is called upon to move the blood that returns to it from the aorta during diastole as well as the blood that continues in the normal circuit. Despite the increase in the demands made upon it for work, the capacity of the heart to nourish itself is diminished rather than increased. The heart is called upon to perform increased work despite a decrease in supply of oxygen and nutrients.

What is a heart murmur?

In addition to the effect of stenosis or insufficiency on the forward move-ment of the blood, deformation of the valves increases the turbulence of the blood as it passes through the opening guarded by the heart valve. These changes in turbulence result in alterations in the heart sounds caused by the flow of blood from one chamber to another in the heart. These abnormal sounds are called murmurs. Contrary to popular opinion, murmurs do not always indicate serious disease of the heart. Factors such as the time they occur in the cardiac cycle and the conditions under which they are heard aid the physician in making a decision about their significance. Unfortunately, persons have been invalided by themselves or their parents after they learned of the presence of a heart murmur. When a patient or a parent appears to be concerned about a heart murmur, this information should be brought to the attention of the physician.

What are some of the causes of valvular deformity?

Valvular deformity may be the direct result of a developmental defect or the effect of the injury caused by hypersensitivity reactions, infections, or other types of inflammatory processes which cause cellular necrosis and stim-ulate fibrous tissue proliferation. Frequently the degree of deformity is increased by the scar tissue formed in the process of healing. The latter illustrates Claude Bernard's thesis and more recently Selye's that processes set in motion by disease or injury may cause further and sometimes greater damage than the initiating factor. As an example, in rheumatic fever, scar tissue formed in healing the affected valves may increase the degree of valvular deformity. Damage to cells stimulates the formation of scar tissue. The scar tissue which is formed contracts as it matures and deforms the affected valves so the opening is narrowed (stenosed), or does not close properly (incompetent), or both. In addition to the above, over a period of years calcium may be deposited in the already deformed valve, thus adding to its rigidity.

Finally, valvular or other cardiac deformities involving the endocardium predispose to infection of the abnormal tissues. The most common organism infecting the defective heart valves is the *Streptococcus viridans,* which causes subacute bacterial endocarditis. The major manifestations of this condition result from: (1) infection; (2) embolic phenomena; and (3) failure of the heart as a pump. Minor surgical procedures such as dental extraction or tonsillectomy may be followed by subacute bacterial endocarditis in persons who have old rheumatic or congenital heart lesions. Persons with valvular heart lesions should be advised to see their physicians for a course of antibiotic or chemotherapy before undergoing any form of surgical therapy.

The effects of injury to the endocardium and valves which have been discussed can be summarized as:

1. Predisposition to intracardiac thrombosis.
2. Obstruction to the movement of blood from one chamber to another or from a ventricle to the great arteries.
3. Regurgitation of blood into the chamber from whence it came.
4. Predisposition to infection of the deformed valve.

These conditions predispose to failure of the heart as a pump chiefly by increasing the work performed by the heart and/or by decreasing cardiac nutrition. In general stenosis leads to failure of the chamber behind the narrowed valve and insufficiency leads to failure of the chamber both preceding and following the insufficient valve. Some disorders, such as rheumatic fever, not only injure the endocardium but also cause direct injury to the muscle and pericardial layers as well.

How can deformities of the heart valves be prevented?

Fundamentally, the prevention of valvular deformity depends on the prevention of a number of disorders, including rheumatic fever, developmental cardiac defects, atherosclerosis, syphilis, bacterial endocarditis, and trauma. With the exception of trauma and possibly of congenital anomalies, prevention of valvular deformities depends on the prevention of some other disorder. Whatever the nature of the cause, deformities of the heart valve place an added burden on the pumping mechanism of the heart by their mechanical effects. Because rheumatic fever is relatively common and is the most frequent cause of heart disease among the young it will be discussed here in some detail. The elements in the prevention of rheumatic fever as well as of heart damage after the disease is in progress will both be presented.

To illustrate the factors in the development of, as well as the problems accompanying, rheumatic fever, Henry Crabtree will be presented. At this time Henry is a 16-year-old boy. He is tall and slender. He lives with his mother and five siblings in a four-room flat in Northeastern Central City. His father is living, but lives apart from the family. He maintains some contact with the children, though he does not see them regularly. The family is supported by Aid to Dependent Children (ADC). When Henry completed the eighth grade at 15 years of age he dropped out of school. Henry has only two interests, sports and automobiles. He hopes to become, as is an older brother, a professional basketball player. A year previous to his present admission he was hospitalized for eight weeks and treated for rheumatic fever. Two or three weeks previous to his first attack of rheumatic fever, Henry had a sore throat and fever from which he appeared to recover completely. The day before his first admission to the hospital he had a fever of 38.9° C. (102° F.) and severe pain in his knee joints. When he was discharged, he was instructed to return to the clinic at monthly intervals to have his progress checked and to receive a supply of oral penicillin. He kept his clinic appointments each month for three months, after which he failed to return. A year after his initial attack he was readmitted to the hospital for the treatment of an acute attack of rheumatic fever. This time there was noticeable damage to his heart.

What are the characteristic features of rheumatic fever?

The name rheumatic fever is derived from the manifestations resulting from inflammation of the joints. Pathology is neither limited to the joints nor is inflammation of the joints its most serious effect, for multiple areas of focal inflammation are found in the heart and blood vessels, as well. The most serious effects are those on the heart. The areas of focal inflammation are widely scattered throughout the body and have a special predilection for connective tissues. Small blood vessels are extensively involved. Lesions found in the myocardium of the heart are known as the Aschoff body or nodule. Actually, lesions similar to the Aschoff body occur wherever the connective-tissue components are found. Moreover, similar lesions are found in other diseases in which there is injury to the collagen fibers.

Although authorities are not certain of the specific etiology of rheumatic fever, they are generally agreed that it follows infections by the group A hemolytic *Streptococcus*. As such, it is similar to acute glomerulonephritis, which follows an infection by a nephrotoxic *Streptococcus*. Recent evidence indicates that the myocardium and the streptococcus contain a common antigen. Antibody formed in response to the streptococcal antigen also reacts against the myocardial antigen. It has been demonstrated that the streptococci are not in the lesions of rheumatic fever, and may or may not be recoverable from the nose and throat at the time of the onset of the disease. Even when streptococci are found and eradicated by antimicrobial therapy, the course of rheumatic fever is not altered.

What is the incidence of rheumatic fever?

The exact incidence is not known and estimates vary. However, about 3 per cent of individuals having streptococcal infections develop rheumatic fever. From 30 to 50 per cent of individuals experiencing one attack of rheumatic fever have one or more recurrences of the disease. Although the incidence of both streptococcal disease and rheumatic fever is believed to be declining, rheumatic fever remains an important disease among children and adolescents. Henry illustrates a number of factors which appear to affect the incidence of rheumatic fever. He falls within the age group in which it is most common. Though rheumatic fever may occur at any age, its onset is highest between the ages of 5 and 15. Henry was 15 at the time of his first known attack. Socioeconomic conditions appear to influence the likelihood of developing rheumatic fever, as the incidence seems to be higher among those who live under overcrowded conditions. Overcrowding is important because it increases the opportunities for the transmission of infectious agents. Henry shares a small bedroom with three brothers. Because they sleep in the same room, the intensity and duration of exposure to any infection acquired by one person to others is increased. Since several people live in four rooms, there is little possibility of isolating the sick from the well. When income is limited, the nutritional status of the children may be less good than when more money is available. Susceptibility to rheumatic fever may possibly be increased by inadequate nutrition during early life.[9] Though Henry was slender, he was thought to be reasonably well nourished at the time of his admission. Heredity appears to be another factor predisposing to rheumatic fever, as several siblings in the same family sometimes develop the disease. A history of rheumatic fever in the family of the affected child is not uncommon. The nature of the hereditary factor is not known, but it is believed to be related to the tendency to develop rheumatic fever and not to susceptibility to streptococcal disease. There was no known history of rheumatic fever in Henry's family. One further factor appearing to predispose to rheumatic fever is climate. The incidence of the disease is believed to be higher in colder than in warmer climates. A variety of factors, therefore, predispose to rheumatic fever. Some, such as age, overcrowding, diet deficient in essential nutrients, and climate, probably do so by increasing the possibility of streptococcal infections. Infection by the group A hemolytic Streptococcus is directly or indirectly required

9 Alvin F. Coburn, "The Pathogenesis of Rheumatic Fever—A Concept," *Perspectives in Biology and Medicine*, VI, Summer, 1963, p. 495.

to trigger the response. Second, there must be some type of genetic defect which makes the child susceptible. Third, a diet deficient in essential nutrients early in life may increase the likelihood of the susceptible child developing rheumatic fever.

What are the clinical manifestations of rheumatic fever?

The following points about the nature of rheumatic fever are useful in anticipating its clinical manifestations. It is a febrile disease. Furthermore rheumatic fever is not limited to a single organ. Rather, focal inflammatory lesions are distributed throughout the body in the mesenchymal connective tissues. According to Coburn,[10] one of the earliest lesions in rheumatic fever is swelling of the vascular endothelium. With each attack the lining of the arterial tree suffers physical and chemical injury. Signs and symptoms vary in intensity and range. Some individuals who have heart damage characteristic of rheumatic fever have not had a known attack of the disease, while others experience a classical picture of the disease.

Henry experienced an almost textbook picture of the disease in both attacks. He had several of the so-called major manifestations which included fever, pain in his joints, and evidence of cardiac involvement. He did not have abdominal pain nor did he have skin manifestations, chorea, or epistaxis (nose bleeds). As in most febrile disorders he had anorexia, weight loss, fatigability, and weakness. His erythrocyte sedimentation rate was markedly elevated. Elevation of the sedimentation rate is characteristic of rheumatic fever, as it occurs in almost all instances. The degree to which it is elevated is an index of the activity of the disease. The leukocyte count is usually elevated to from 15,000 to 30,000 during the acute phase of the disease, but it may be normal. Henry's leukocyte count was elevated. As he improved, his sedimentation rate fell toward normal and his leukocyte count became normal.

As is not infrequently observed, particularly among older children and adults, Henry had polyarthritis. Joint pain is less common among young children, though it may occur in a mild form and be dismissed as growing pains. The degree of pain varies from a vague pain to the exquisite pain associated with acutely inflamed and swollen joints. Although the degree of pain experienced by Henry was moderate, in some patients it is so severe that actions resulting in jarring of the bed or any movement of the bed are unbearable. Among the characteristic features of the arthritis associated with rheumatic fever is that it tends to involve one joint or area at a time and to be migratory, that is, to move from one joint to another. It involves large and small joints and heals without causing crippling of the joints.

When the joints are painful, measures should be instituted to protect the patient from unnecessary discomfort. Jarring of the patient should be avoided. Bed coverings should be supported, so that the joints are protected from their

[10] *Ibid.*, p. 507.

weight. Since the joints are not likely to be deformed by the disease process, the extremities should be supported in the position the patient finds to be most comfortable. When handling the affected extremity, care should be taken to minimize movement of the joint. To do this, the extremity should be supported both above and below the joint. Measures prescribed by the physician such as local applications of heat may give the patient a measure of relief. They should be carried out conscientiously. Other measures prescribed to modify the inflammatory response minimize the discomfort to the patient.

As should be expected in view of the widespread involvement of connective and vascular tissues, lesions of the skin and subcutaneous tissues develop in some patients with rheumatic fever. About 25 per cent of children have a skin lesion known as erythema marginatum or circinatum. The lesions are red and roughly circular in shape. Since adjacent lesions tend to coalesce, they form larger lesions with an irregular outline. They are usually flat (macular), though some may be slightly raised (papular). They are not usually the cause of discomfort, though they may occasionally be accompanied by itching.

Another skin lesion, erythema nodosum, is believed to be a manifestation of acute rheumatic fever. It does not occur as frequently as erythema marginatum, and it sometimes develops when other rheumatic manifestations are minimal or lacking. The lesions are dull red nodules occurring most frequently on the extensor surfaces of the extremities. Unlike the lesions of erythema marginatum, those of erythema nodosum are exquisitely tender to touch and discomfort is increased with movement. Affected extremities should be protected from the weight of the bedding by the use of cradles. Gentleness should be an outstanding characteristic when extremities are moved.

Subcutaneous nodules are firm, insensitive lesions occurring over bony prominences of the various joints and tendons of the extremities. They are more frequently observed in patients with a serious form of rheumatic fever and who have severe heart damage.

Chorea, or, as it is frequently called by lay persons, St. Vitus's dance, is a disorder characterized by marked involuntary contractions of the skeletal muscles. Though it is not easily described, one of the outstanding features of movement in chorea is its purposelessness. At the onset of chorea, the child may appear to be awkward and careless. He spills his food when he tries to eat, drops his schoolbooks and other objects. As the manifestations become more severe, the purposeless movements made by the child may be ascribed to nervousness. Later they may become so severe as to be incapacitating. Chorea results from the involvement of the nervous system. It may be the sole manifestation of rheumatic fever. It generally occurs late.

Just as the degree and range of the possible manifestations in rheumatic fever are highly variable, the nature of the course and the outcome of an attack are also variable. Though few die during the first attack, some have a fulminating form of the disease and die within a few days or weeks. Some recover in as few as three or four weeks, while others such as Henry (he was ill for eight weeks) are ill for more extended periods of time. Some individuals improve, but some degree of activity persists for weeks or months, or for the lifetime of the individual. Although some recover fully from the first attack and never have another, one attack predisposes to recurrences of the disease. As in the instance of Henry, the extent of cardiac damage during the first attack of rheumatic fever is frequently minimal, but with each subsequent attack the degree and permanence of cardiac damage increases. At the time Henry was discharged from the hospital after his second attack of rheumatic fever he had mitral and aortic stenosis.

What can be said about the long-term prognosis for Henry and others with a similar history?

A statement of prognosis is a prediction of probable outcome which is based on past experience. Fundamentally, Henry's prognosis depends on the nature and degree of involvement of his heart. Certainly his prognosis was better after his first attack of rheumatic fever and becomes poorer with each subsequent attack, inasmuch as the extent and degree of cardiac damage are likely to be increased. Most of the patients who have severe cardiac involvement die within ten years in congestive heart failure. In addition, patients with deformed heart valves are predisposed to the formation of intracardiac thrombosis and to bacterial endocarditis—usually of the subacute type.

On what premises is treatment of rheumatic fever based?

Rheumatic fever is an acute febrile disease which may cause a period of extended illness. Though focal inflammatory lesions can and do occur throughout the body and may be responsible for discomfort or even temporary disability, the lesions in the heart are the ones most likely to cause permanent injury and death. Treatment is therefore directed toward the alleviation of the symptoms and the prevention of cardiac damage. An important aspect of prevention is the prevention of recurrences.

In the traditional and conservative management of rheumatic fever the physician prescribes bed rest for as long as the disease is active. Currently some clinicians are modifying this practice and allowing greater amounts of activity than in the past. When rest is prescribed, as it often is, the nurse has the responsibility for creating an environment in which the patient can rest. In order to achieve rest for the patient, the cooperation of the patient and his family are essential.

Henry was treated by bed rest. During the first two weeks of his illness he was encouraged to lie quietly and to have all activities of daily living performed for him. He was fed, given mouth care, turned, and bathed. He was allowed to be up once a day to go to the bathroom. Otherwise he was to remain quietly in bed. Since his knees and later his wrists and elbows were acutely inflamed, he was glad to lie still. Later, as he recovered, the maintenance of bed rest became more difficult to achieve.

As soon as Henry began to improve, recreational activities were planned to occupy his time. Since Henry was interested only in sports and in automobiles, this was taken into consideration in planning. Provisions were made for him to listen to football and hockey games on the radio. Since his intellectual achievements and interests were limited, reading material was selected with his interests in mind. His nurse tried to encourage him to consider returning to school in order to obtain specialized training, but his real interest was in becoming a professional basketball player. Although a visiting teacher was available and arrangements were made for her to visit Henry, he was unwilling to consider a study program at this time. Because of the prospects for an extended period of illness, recreational, occupational, and educational facilities should be available to the patient with rheumatic fever. Through their appropriate use, the morale of the patient can be maintained and the child or adolescent prevented from falling too far behind in school. When indicated, they may also help the patient to select a new or modified occupation.

In addition to bed rest (or modified activity) drugs are prescribed to eradicate the *Streptococcus* and to relieve the symptoms and effects of the disease. The drug employed to eliminate the *Streptococcus* is penicillin. The preparation and dosage of penicillin are prescribed by the physician. The drug should be administered as prescribed in order to maintain a satisfactory level at all times. In addition to therapy to eliminate the *Streptococcus,* the patient should be protected against exposure to persons with respiratory infections.

Two different types of drugs, the salicylates and corticosteroids, are prescribed singly or in combination to relieve the symptoms of rheumatic fever and to decrease the tissue response. Again the physician makes the decision as to the drug to be employed. The corticosteroids bring about the relief of signs and symptoms more quickly than the salicylates; they are more likely to be prescribed when there is a significant degree of carditis.

Exactly how the salicylates or the corticosteroids act is not known, but they are believed to alter the tissue response to the abnormal process. They do not, however, accelerate the rate at which the patient recovers from rheumatic fever. When the above drugs are administered in adequate dosages, not only do the signs and symptoms associated with the disease disappear, but the blood changes tend to return to normal. The erythrocyte sedimentation rate and the leukocyte count drop. If, however, treatment is prematurely discontinued, signs and symptoms and the changes in the blood characteristic of rheumatic fever reappear. Since the length of the course of the disease is unpredictable, the physician sometimes has difficulty in being certain as to whether the improvement of the patient is due to the suppressive therapy or to the elimination of the cause of the inflammatory reaction. Therefore, at the time drug therapy is being discontinued, the patient should be under observation, so that therapy can be re-established, if indications of rheumatic activity reappear.

A problem may arise following the relief of the patient's symptoms, because the patient feels well. As Henry improved, he rejected the idea that he was ill. He felt well and therefore he was certain that he must be well. He interpreted the taking of medicine and continued attendance at the clinic as a sign of weakness. Henry's feelings are not unusual. In some instances, it is possible through education of the patient and his parents to make and ensure a plan for continued treatment.

As in other long-term illnesses, the education of the patient and/or family members in the nature and effects of rheumatic fever is imperative if they are to assume responsibility for treatment of the current attack and prevent recurrences. When the home situation allows, patients may be discharged from the hospital after the acute manifestations are relieved. Even when the patient is "cured," antimicrobial therapy in the form of penicillin is prescribed. This therapy may be continued for from one to five years or as long as the child is in school. Responsibility for the continuance of treatment is borne by the patient or a family member. Regular medical supervision is also necessary, not only for renewal of the required prescriptions, but to maintain the interest of the patient in continuing his therapy.

In addition to caring for the patient during the acute phase of his illness, the nurse has many opportunities to serve the patient. Often it is a nurse who instructs the parents and/or the patient in the reasons continued medical supervision is necessary and in the need for his medication. The nurse may also uncover areas of misunderstanding or reasons for the failure of the patient to follow instructions. The visiting or public health nurse may visit the patient's home to determine whether home care is a reasonable possibility and to help the person who is responsible to carry out the prescribed regime. She may act as a liaison between the patient and his physician. Because the continued use of penicillin and other drugs is expensive, the patient may be able to obtain them from the state or city health department. The nurse should know what the resources are in the area where she is practicing and know how to assist the patient in securing aid when this is necessary. Since the physician is responsible for prescribing the extent of the patient's activity, the nurse should know what his plans are for the patient. There is usually no reason, however, for her not to discuss with the physician the possibility of a service such as a visiting teacher, if the condition of the patient seems to warrant it. The physician, as well as the nurse, is desirous not only of preventing recurrences of the disease, but of minimizing as much as possible undesirable effects of the disease.

What forms of surgical therapy are available to the patient with deformities of the heart valves?

Until recently, once the valves of a patient's heart were deformed nothing could be done to restore normal or nearly normal function. During the last decade or two, surgical procedures have been developed by which stenosed and incompetent valves are opened and repaired or valvular prostheses are introduced to replace damaged ones. In some patients these operations are highly successful. In others they are less so. Some of the factors appearing to influence the outcome of surgery include the extent of damage to the heart muscle, whether or not the disease process is inactive, and how early in life and the extent to which the person was invalided by his disease. Some individuals who are "cured" by surgical correction of defects in the heart remain invalids, because for them invalidism is a way of life. Individuals whose cardiac disability occurred early in life and continued for many years are more likely to have a problem in adjusting to the responsibilities of a healthy life than those whose defect is corrected early or whose cardiac disability developed later in life. In some persons, heart damage is so great that the operation comes too late to be of real benefit. In others, the disease appears to be quiescent, but is reactivated following surgical therapy. The expectation that surgical treatment of cardiac defects will benefit the patient is, of course, realized in many patients.

Patients undergoing cardiac surgery have needs relating to the following:

1. The fact of a surgical procedure.
2. The fact that the route of approach is through the chest wall.
3. The fact that the heart is the organ involved and it has suffered previous injury.

The first two points are discussed in the chapter on the preoperative and postoperative needs of patients. The care of the patient undergoing cardiac surgery will not be discussed in detail. The remarks that follow apply to patients who have surgery on the heart and are not limited to those who have surgery to correct a defective heart valve. The writer believes that patients undergoing cardiac surgery require care by nurses who are experienced and who have specialized preparation. In the words of Thung and Dammann,[11] "The best postoperative care requires that the patient be placed in a special unit, equipped with the necessary instruments for monitoring, a complete supply of the needed medications and well trained, experienced, and well-motivated personnel." Books and journal articles devoted to the problems of patients undergoing cardiac surgery are included in the References.

As in other types of surgery, the preoperative preparation of the patient for cardiac surgery is as important to his recovery as other phases of therapy. The patient is usually admitted to the hospital a few days previous to the date of operation for the purpose of performing diagnostic procedures requiring hospitalization and for improving his health status. Attention is paid to:

1. Acquainting the patient with the personnel who are to be responsible for his care and hopefully enhancing his confidence in their competence

[11] Nalda Thung and J. Francis Dammann, "Postoperative Care After Heart Surgery," *The Heart Bulletin,* XII, September-October, 1963, p. 87.

and interest in his welfare. They prepare him for what to expect and for what is expected of him.

2. Improving his nutritional status. Patients who have been in chronic heart failure and have been eating poorly and/or have impaired liver function require improvement in their intake of protein, glucose, and vitamins, including vitamin K.

3. Correcting fluid and electrolyte imbalances, including elimination of edema. Because diuretics may cause electrolyte imbalances, they are usually discontinued about two days before surgery is anticipated.

4. Eliminating infections in the respiratory tract. Because respiratory infections increase the risk of cardiac surgery, the patient should be protected from persons who have infections.

5. Improving cardiac functioning, when this is required.

During the postoperative period the patient is exposed to all of the possible surgical complications. Though the patient is often able to tolerate one or more complications, the poorer his condition, the more severe the complication, and the more numerous their number, the greater the hazard to the patient. To state it positively, the patient who is in good physical condition, who develops few complications which, when they do occur, are spaced at intervals, and in whom complications are not allowed to become severe is not likely to be seriously affected by one or more complications. Therefore, one of the most important aspects of the postoperative care of the patient who has undergone cardiac surgery is observation of vital functions by means of monitoring devices as well as the more usual methods.

Action taken in the care of the patient who has undergone cardiac surgery should be based on observations tempered by knowledge of the causes and effects of complications. Since monitoring equipment is not infallible, clinical judgment developed by study and thoughtful experience is indispensable. The earlier threats to the well-being of the patient are discovered, the greater his chances for survival.

The complications of cardiac surgery are similar to those associated with other types of surgery, but their import is more immediately serious. Among the most common and important complications is respiratory insufficiency, that is, the inability to transport the quantity of oxygen required by the cells and/or to remove the carbon dioxide formed in metabolism. Unless respiratory insufficiency is detected early and the resulting hypoxia and hypercapnia are corrected promptly, there will be a deterioration in essential body functions leading to the death of the patient. Respiratory insufficiency may be due to impaired ventilation, to pulmonary or cardiac failure, or to an increase in the demands made by the cells for oxygen. The causes of impaired ventilation and pulmonary failure are discussed in Chapter 7. The causes and effects of cardiac failure are considered in this chapter. Any condition leading to the increased use of oxygen by the cells, such as exercise or elevated body temperature, will increase their need for oxygen and predispose to or intensify hypoxia and hypercapnia. In the immediate postoperative period following cardiac surgery, much of the care provided for the patient is directed toward the prevention of respiratory insufficiency and the earliest possible detection of evidence that it is developing.

The general principles applying to the care of any patient undergoing surgical therapy apply to the patient having heart surgery. Because the heart is directly involved, the need for attention to the details of care during all phases of surgery cannot, however, be overemphasized. Certainly the patient undergoing heart surgery deserves to have his chances for recovery improved by being cared for by nurses who as a result of education and experience are prepared to meet his needs. Just as surgeons who perform cardiac surgery undergo a period of specialized training, it is no less important that nurses do likewise.

How does the pericardium interfere with cardiac function?

The outer covering of the heart, or pericardium, may also be a source of interference with the action of the heart as a pump. The pericardium is an inelastic sac or envelope reflected over the heart and lining the cavity. The layer lying next to the heart, the visceral layer, adheres closely to the heart. The outer portion of the sac is known as the parietal layer. The inner and outer surfaces of the pericardial sac are separated by serous fluid. The pericardium has a number of important functions. It helps to anchor the heart and to lessen the friction between the heart and its environment. Because the pericardium does not stretch, it prevents overdilatation of the heart during diastole.

The pericardium may be injured by trauma, infection, or neoplasms with the result that fluid, blood, or pus collects in the pericardial sac. As the fluid accumulates, it occupies space in the pericardial sac and reduces the capacity of the heart during diastole. Since the blood is circulated in a closed system, the lessening of the capacity of the heart to receive blood has at least two detrimental effects on the entire system. Because the heart can only deliver into the arterial system the blood that it receives during diastole, cardiac output falls. Tissues throughout the body suffer from the effects of undernutrition. When cardiac output is markedly diminished, the coronary circulation cannot be maintained, and the heart dies in fibrillation.[12] A second major effect is due to interference with the venous return. Because of the limitations on the quantity of blood that the heart can accommodate during diastole, blood tends to accumulate in the veins causing passive congestion of organs such as the liver. The situation is similar to that resulting from placing a dam in a river. The dam or obstruction impedes the forward flow of water. When water is added to the channel behind the dam, it floods the land in the

---

[12] Multiple and ineffective contractions of individual muscle fibers rather than the more or less synchronous contraction of the entire myocardium.

surrounding area. Similarly, the limitations on the capacity of the heart during diastole act to impede the forward movement of blood from the veins into the heart with the result that it accumulates in the veins. The effects of venous congestion are discussed later in the chapter.

Because of the location of the pericardium, disease of other organs in the thoracic cavity may spread to it. For example, the pericardium may be infected by the Mycobacterium of tuberculosis as well as the pneumococcus. Disease of the pericardium may also extend to and injure the myocardium, coronary vessels, and the nerves supplying the heart. In the process of healing, bands or sheets of fibrous tissue, with or without calcification, may encompass the heart and lead to slow cardiac failure. Because they act as a splint, they limit the degree to which the heart can expand or dilate just as a splint or cast encasing a limb limits the degree to which blood can enter it. The effects are similar to those produced by the distention of the pericardial sac with fluid, but they are likely to develop more slowly. Furthermore, the myocardium and other structures of the heart may be damaged by the infectious process causing the pericarditis, as well as by lack of use. The myocardium is similar to other muscles. It responds to a decrease in work by atrophy and to an increase by hypertrophy. The fact that the myocardium atrophies in the presence of constrictive pericarditis is an important consideration in its surgical treatment. Sometimes the constrictive bands can be removed successfully by cardiac decortication. The procedure may have to be discontinued because the myocardium may have been so weakened by disease and the consequent scarring, and by lack of use, that on the removal of the fibrous tissue splint, the heart dilates excessively. When damage to the heart muscle is not too great, the patient may be greatly benefited by resection of the pericardium. Treatment of constrictive pericarditis is also directed toward relieving venous congestion and improving the general status of the patient.

What part of the heart accomplishes its primary function?

From the standpoint of function, the essential part of the heart is the myocardium. This is true because it provides the power that keeps blood moving through the circuit. Like all other tissues, the myocardium is dependent on a continuous blood supply. Since it does not tolerate an oxygen debt to the same extent skeletal muscle does, the myocardium is more susceptible to hypoxia than skeletal muscle. Death of cells occurs when oxygen deprivation continues longer than 30 minutes.

How does the structure of the myocardium contribute to its effectiveness as a pump?

The function of the myocardium can be simply stated as the ejection into the arteries of the blood delivered to it by the venous circulation. A number of factors contribute to the effectiveness of the myocardium as a pump. One is the arrangement of the muscle fibers. Layers of muscle fibers are wrapped around the heart in spiral and circular directions. This arrangement has a number of mechanical advantages. As the ventricles contract, blood is not only pushed, but it is literally wrung out of the heart much as water is wrung out of a cloth. Since the muscle fibers extend around the heart, both ventricles contract at the same time and move the same quantity of blood. The effectiveness of ventricular contraction is further increased by the fact that during contraction, the septum stiffens and acts as a fulcrum to which muscle fibers are attached.

Any disorder that deprives the myocardium of its blood supply, either in whole or in part, or injures it, may decrease its efficiency as a pump. Before discussing the possible consequences, of failure of the myocardium as a pump however, some of the structural and functional characteristics of myocardial cells will be reviewed. Two developments have contributed much to an understanding of the structure of myocardial cells. They are the electron microscope and a technique for separating individual living mammalian myocardial cells. In the past the myocardium was usually described as a single multinucleated cell. As a result of his studies with individual heart cells, Harary[13] confirmed earlier reports that nuclei in the myocardium are surrounded by a membrane. The myocardium is, therefore, composed of many cells.

*What are the properties of the myocardial cells that are
particularly important to function?*

Like other muscle cells, those of the myocardium are contractile. When stimulated, they shorten and thicken. Following contraction they lengthen. They are also similar to skeletal muscle in that they obey the all-or-none law; that is, when they contract they do so to the fullest extent possible. Although this might be interpreted to mean the force of cardiac contraction should always be the same, it does not, as another factor also influences the force of myocardial contraction. The force of contraction is a function of the length of the fiber at the end of diastole. Within physiological limits, the longer the muscle fiber is at the end of diastole (or at the beginning of systole), the more forceful the contraction of the heart (Starling's law of the heart.) It can be demonstrated by stretching a rubber or elastic band. When the band is stretched and released, the force with which it returns to its original form depends on the degree to which it was stretched. Within the limits of its extensibility, the more it is stretched, the more forcibly it contracts. With a small amount of stretching, the contraction of the band is weak. When the degree of stretching approaches the limits of its extensibility, the force of contraction is great. It too demonstrates the all-or-none law inasmuch as the rubber band contracts fully or not all.

---

[13] Isaac Harary, "Heart Cells in Vitro," *Scientific American,* CCVI, May, 1962, p. 148.

How does lengthening of the myocardial fibers affect their capacity to do work?

A healthy heart can adapt to an increase in venous return without much increase in the diastolic fiber length. Within a stroke or two the heart is able to eject as much blood into the circulation as is delivered to it by the veins. When, as a result of disease, this is no longer possible, muscle fibers lengthen. For a time this lengthening, and with it dilatation of the chambers of the heart, may enable the heart to meet the needs of all cells including its own, without signs of embarrassment. The healthy, and often the diseased, heart has a reserve power that enables it to maintain an appropriate balance between intake and output. This reserve power lies in the difference between the degree to which the muscle fiber must lengthen to eject as much blood into the circulation as is delivered to it and the extent to which it can lengthen and function physiologically. The longer the diastolic fiber length, the more forceful the contraction, but the less the cardiac reserve. When the point is reached that further lengthening of the muscle fibers during diastole results in inefficient function, cardiac reserve has been lost. At this point the heart is no longer able to adapt to an increase in venous return or to increase output in relation to the requirements of cells. The individual is no longer able to increase his activity above resting levels without manifestations associated with failure of the heart as a pump. Eventually he may be unable to meet the needs of his cells at rest.

How does the heart adapt to an increase in the demands made upon it?

The capacity of the heart muscle to lengthen (dilate) is one of the ways in which the heart adapts to an increase in work. This, combined with an increase in heart rate, enables the heart to move the increased volume of blood delivered to it as a result of an increase in activity. Adaptation fails, sooner or later, as do other adaptive mechanisms when a condition exists that makes continued adaptation necessary or directly injures the myocardium.

As might be expected, the size of an individual's heart is roughly proportional to the size of his body. Contrary to popular opinion, physical exercise is necessary to a healthy heart. As stated earlier, the heart responds to "lack of use" by atrophy, as do other tissues. Likewise, the heart muscle adapts to a continued increase in work load by hypertrophy. Associated with hypertrophy of the myocardium is dilatation of one or more chambers of the heart. Authorities are not agreed as to whether hypertrophy precedes dilatation of the heart or dilatation precedes hypertrophy. The hypertrophied heart is larger than the healthy heart. Hypertrophy is physiological inasmuch as it occurs in response to an increased work load. Hypertrophy enables the heart to move blood against an increased resistance and at the same time to maintain the normal equilibrium between intake and output. Like other adaptive mechanisms, hypertrophy has certain limitations. One important limitation is that as muscle mass increases, the blood supply does not increase to a comparable degree. In the healthy heart a capillary is said to be available to supply each muscle fiber. Even when this ratio is maintained in the hypertrophied heart, the quantity of blood delivered to the tissue is reduced in relation to its mass. A larger fiber receives no more blood than the former smaller fiber. Blood supply is therefore not increased in proportion to the quantity of tissue to be nourished. Undernutrition may be further aggravated by vascular disease which limits blood flow to the myocardium.

Summary

For the most part, the healthy heart adapts to changes in the demands made on it by altering its rate of contraction and by adapting the force of contraction to the quantity of venous blood returned to it. Essentially the function of the heart as a pump is satisfactory as long as: (1) the myocardium is able to eject as much blood into the circulation as is delivered to it without a gain in residual blood at the end of systole, and (2) it can meet the needs of the tissues under different degrees of activity. When activity is increased, there should be no increase of residual blood in the heart. Neither should there be evidence of marked or unexpected increase in the heart or respiratory rate. Although some rise in the pulse and respiratory rates does occur during physical activity, this should not be out of proportion to the degree of activity and should be within physiological limits. The pulse rate should also return to normal within a reasonable period of time. The return to normal usually occurs in two stages. Within a short period of time after exercise ceases, the pulse rate drops sharply toward, but not to, pre-exercise level. It then declines slowly. The healthy heart can also adapt to a regular program of physical exercise. In well-trained athletes, the resting pulse rates are lower than average, but the output per beat is greater.[14]

What are the causes of failure of the pumping mechanism of the heart?

Pruitt[15] summarizes the causes of failure in the pumping mechanism under three general headings: (1) failure to fill, (2) overloading, and (3) deterioration in functional capacity. Each of these will be discussed briefly.

Failure of the heart to fill depends on three factors. There must be a sufficient volume of blood in the circulation in relation to the size of the vascular chamber to provide for an adequate venous return. For the heart to move blood into the arteries, it must receive blood from the veins, and it can

[14] Arthur C. Guyton, *Textbook of Medical Physiology,* 2nd ed., W. B. Saunders Company, Philadelphia, 1961, p. 320.
[15] Raymond D. Pruitt, "The Origins of Cardiac Failure," *The Heart Bulletin,* VII, January-February, 1958, pp. 8-20.

only eject the quantity of blood that is delivered to it. The most common cause of an inadequate venous return is shock. Shock results from any disorder causing a disproportion between the circulating blood volume and the capacity of the vascular chamber. The blood volume may fall as a result of hemorrhage or from the excessive loss of fluid into the tissues such as occurs in burns. Or the volume of blood may be within physiological limits, but generalized dilatation of the blood vessels may enlarge the capacity of the vascular system so much that the quantity of blood returned to the heart is insufficient to maintain an adequate output. The result in either instance is ischemia of the tissues. If it is severe or continued, death may result. The reader is referred to Chapter 8 for a more detailed discussion of shock.

A second cause of inadequate ventricular filling is obstruction to the inflow of blood. The most common cause is mitral stenosis. Sometimes the stenosis is so severe that the opening is no larger than a broom straw. Such marked narrowing of the mitral valve seriously limits the quantity of blood that can enter the left ventricle. As previously indicated, constrictive pericarditis, by limiting diastole, interferes with the filling of the heart. Like any other pump, the heart can only eject into the arteries the quantity of blood that enters into it.

A third factor that may limit the intake of blood is a reduction in the length of diastole or of the interval during which the heart fills. Blood enters the heart only during diastole. When ventricular rates are excessively high, the length of diastole is shortened to a greater extent than systole. Consequently, the period for filling is relatively shorter than the period for the ejection of blood. An extreme example may be seen in auricular fibrillation when the volume of blood entering the heart during diastole may be so little that, despite ventricular contraction, there is no pulse. Excessively high ventricular rates may, when continued, lead to heart failure.

In contrast to failure due to inadequate ventricular filling, the myocardium may fail because too much blood is delivered to it or the resistance which it must overcome in moving the blood into the arteries is excessive. When the myocardium fails because too much blood is returned to it, the condition is called high-output failure. According to Pruitt,[16] high-output failure is of two types. In the first, a large volume of blood is received by the heart and is ejected into the circulation. Common examples include thyrotoxicosis, fever, and anemia. In these disorders the organism adapts to an increased need for oxygen and nutrients or to failure to carry oxygen by increasing the blood volume. Because an elevation in the blood volume increases the work performed by the heart, disorders accompanied by increased blood volume will, if continued, and particularly in the presence of pre-existing disease of the heart, precipitate failure of the heart.

In the second type of high-output failure, the heart also expels an increased volume of blood into the arteries, but some of the blood returns to the heart

16 *Ibid.,* p. 19.

during diastole. The increased volume of blood ejected by the heart results from a failure to maintain the forward movement of blood in the circuit. Common causes of regurgitation of blood include mitral and aortic insufficiency, uncomplicated patent ductus arteriosus,[17] and arteriovenous shunts.[18] The effects of aortic regurgitation can be felt in the pulse. During systole the pulse is full and bounding. As diastole begins the artery collapses quickly. The pulse associated with aortic regurgitation is the so-called water-hammer or Corrigan's pulse.

The second type of ventricular overloading Pruitt[19] calls high-resistance failure. The site of the resistance may be any place between the outlet of the ventricle and the peripheral arterioles. An example of the first is aortic stenosis, and of the latter, the arteriolar sclerosis associated with hypertension, or aortic stenosis, such as is seen in coarctation of the aorta.[20] In all of the above and similar conditions, the ventricle must move the blood with sufficient force to overcome the resistance offered by the narrowed channels. The amount of energy required is well illustrated by coarctation of the aorta. Above the point of narrowing, the systolic blood pressure may be 200 mm of mercury or more. Below, it may be 100 mm or less.

The third general cause of heart failure is incompetence of the ventricle as a result of disease of the myocardium. Pruitt[21] classifies myocardial diseases as: (1) degenerative diseases, (2) inflammatory diseases, (3) metabolic diseases of the myocardium, and (4) disturbances in the rhythm of the heart.

The most common cause of failure of the heart due to degeneration of the heart muscle is coronary sclerosis complicated by myocardial infarction. Because of the importance of this disorder, it will be discussed in more detail later in the chapter.

Inflammatory diseases affecting the myocardium include rheumatic carditis, diphtheria, infectious mononucleosis, and lupus erythematosus. Diphtheritic myocarditis is infrequent in the United States, and could be eliminated by immunization.

A number of metabolic disorders are accompanied by weakening of the myocardium. These disorders cause biochemical or biophysical changes that interfere with the utilization of nutrients. These include thyrotoxicosis, hypothyroidism, beriberi, anemia, and shock. Most of the above can be prevented or cured by early and effective treatment of the precipitating abnormality. Some, such as hypothyroidism (myxedema heart), require therapy through-

---

[17] In the fetal circulation, the pulmonary artery and the aorta are connected by the ductus arteriosus. Shortly after birth the ductus closes and becomes a fibrous cord or band. Occasionally the ductus arteriosus remains open or patent, thus the term "patent ductus."

[18] In an arteriovenous shunt there is a direct connection between an artery and a vein.

[19] Pruitt, *Op. cit.,* p. 18.

[20] In coarctation of the aorta, the aorta is markedly narrowed at some point after it leaves the heart. The condition is usually of congenital origin.

[21] *Op. cit.,* p. 19.

out the lifetime of the individual. In hypothyroidism the thyroid hormone is required for the remainder of the life of the individual.

Disturbances in the rhythm of the heart, either by excessively high or low heart rates, predispose to myocardial weakening by interfering with the capacity of the heart to maintain its own nutrition. These are discussed later in the chapter.

With advancing years, even in the absence of demonstrable lesions in the heart, there is a reduction in the myocardial reserve and with it a decrease in the capacity of the myocardium to cope with the various handicaps placed on it. For example, one of the reasons that elderly persons tolerate a rapid or large increase in blood volume less well than younger persons is that their cardiac reserve is less adequate. Although the degree to which myocardial reserve is diminished differs among elderly persons, any elderly person who is receiving a blood transfusion or one or more intravenous infusions should be observed for evidence indicating that his heart is or is not tolerating the increase in blood volume. (See Chapter 8.) The patient should be observed for evidence of circulatory distress or developing pulmonary edema.

Should either occur, the rate of flow of the fluid should be reduced to the minimum required to keep the needle open and the physician should be called immediately. According to Resnik and Harrison,[22] occasionally an elderly person who dies in congestive heart failure is seen at autopsy with no significant cardiac lesions other than hypertrophy and dilatation. Apparently, in these patients, their hearts become so weakened as a result of senile changes that they die of senile heart disease.

Summary

In the preceding paragraphs, the causes of heart failure have been summarized in relation to the effect the causative factor has on the pumping action of the heart. According to this classification, the heart may fail because it receives too little or too much blood or must pump the blood against too great resistance. It may also fail because the muscle degenerates as the result of injury caused by a variety of diseases. Although not the result of disease, the adaptive capacity of the heart diminishes with advancing age. This lessens the capacity of the heart to cope with any additional burden. Eventually, when the heart fails, it is unable to supply the tissues with the blood required to support their activities. What happens then depends on the completeness of failure and the rate at which failure develops. Like other chronic illnesses, heart failure is frequently, though not invariably, the result of the interaction of multiple factors.

In the patient whose cardiac reserve is seriously reduced, any condition making demands on the heart for increased circulation of blood may precipi-

[22] William H. Resnick and T. R. Harrison, "Diseases of the Heart," in T. R. Harrison, *Principles of Internal Medicine,* 4th ed., The Blakiston Division, McGraw-Hill Book Company, Inc., New York, 1962, p. 1378.

tate heart failure. Thus infection, particularly when it is accompanied by a fever or a cough, may precipitate congestive heart failure. Emotional stress, excessive activity, the ingestion of excessive amounts of salt, anemia, and the onset of hyperthyroidism may do likewise. The list is not exhaustive. Any disorder that increases the demands made on the heart can be responsible.

The estimated deaths from specific diseases of the heart and blood vessels are summarized in the following chart. In this chart diseases are categorized according to structures involved. It can be noted that coronary artery disease far exceeds other diseases of the heart as a cause of death.

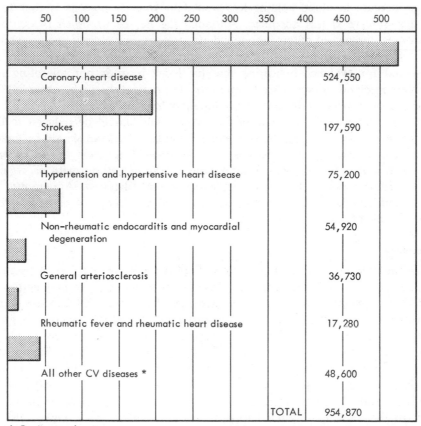

50	100	150	200	250	300	350	400	450	500	

Coronary heart disease — 524,550

Strokes — 197,590

Hypertension and hypertensive heart disease — 75,200

Non-rheumatic endocarditis and myocardial degeneration — 54,920

General arteriosclerosis — 36,730

Rheumatic fever and rheumatic heart disease — 17,280

All other CV diseases * — 48,600

TOTAL — 954,870

* Cardiovascular diseases

FIGURE 9 – 5. Estimated number of deaths caused by specific diseases of the cardiovascular system (heart and blood vessels). (Adapted. National Office of Vital Statistics, 1962.)

To what degree may the pumping mechanism of the heart fail?

Terminology used to describe the degree of heart failure includes cardiac arrest or standstill, acute heart failure, and chronic heart failure or cardiac decompensation. In cardiac arrest or standstill, the heart stops beating with the result that the circulation of blood ceases. In acute and chronic heart failure, the myocardium contracts, but the mechanical efficiency of the heart as a pump is below that required to meet the oxygen and nutritional requirements of the tissues under varying degrees of activity and to prevent an increase of residual blood in the ventricle at the end of systole. Acute and chronic heart failure differ in the suddenness with which failure develops. There are also differences in the manifestations which the patient exhibits.

What is cardiac arrest, its causes, and consequences?

As the term "cardiac arrest" or "standstill" implies, myocardial contraction ceases and with it the circulation of the blood. Unless the heart beat is restarted in approximately four minutes, permanent damage to the higher centers in the brain is likely. As emphasized in other chapters, time, therefore, is of the essence. Cardiac arrest may be caused by any condition resulting in ventricular fibrillation, overactivity of some of the vagal reflexes, or heart block resulting from disease of the bundle of His. Perhaps the most common cause of ventricular fibrillation is myocardial infarction. Electrocution is, however, a not infrequent cause. As an example of the latter, six-year-old Bobby went out to explore the damage done by a windstorm; he stepped on a broken high-tension wire. The high-voltage electric current caused his ventricles to fibrillate. Since the fibrillating ventricle is unable to eject the blood from the heart with sufficient force to maintain its own blood supply, the myocardium quickly deteriorated. By the time Bobby was discovered, he was dead.

Cardiac arrest occasionally occurs in the anesthetized patient. For example, Mrs. Thatcher was undergoing a cholecystectomy. As a result of the handling of her abdominal organs and stretching of the peritoneum or mesentery, vagal reflexes which stopped her heart were initiated. Under these circumstances, the condition was detected immediately, and personnel and equipment were available to attempt restoration of heart action and circulation. Depending on the circumstances, the chest may be opened and the heart massaged directly or external cardiac massage may be initiated. Application of electric current may also cause the heart to resume a regular beat. Because of its limited value, thumping the chest wall with the fist is perhaps a more common event in television than in the real life situation. External cardiac massage was successful in restarting Mrs. Thatcher's heart.

After an acute insult such as a myocardial infarction, the heart may continue to contract, but its efficiency as a pump is diminished. Sometimes sympathetic reflexes, initiated automatically, compensate for much of the failure, with the result that signs and symptoms of heart failure are minimal. The sequence of events is usually as follows: As the output of the heart falls, the pressure of the blood in the aorta and carotid artery falls. Pressure receptors are stimulated with the result that the sympathetic nervous system is activated. This increases the force of myocardial contraction and constricts peripheral blood vessels.[23] Constriction of the peripheral blood vessels, most particularly the veins, in turn, improves venous return by diminishing the quantity of blood held in them.

When cardiac output is low, renal function may be diminished. The quantity of fluid excreted by the kidney becomes lessened and the blood volume becomes enlarged. This mechanism may, within limits, further compensate for the decrease in cardiac output. Again, within limits, an increase in blood delivered to the heart is followed by more forceful contraction. This is often true of the failing, as well as of the normal, heart.

What are some of the characteristic features of chronic heart failure?

When injury to the heart takes place slowly, the manifestations of heart failure develop gradually over a period of days, weeks, or months. Blood flow to tissues is diminished and congestion of fluid in the tissues is an outstanding feature.

Some of the signs and symptoms evidenced are due to lack of nutrition of the tissues, while others result from congestion of blood in the lungs or extrapulmonary tissues or both. The latter interferes with function by occupying space and by limiting blood flow through the affected tissues. Although all tissues are affected when the heart fails, the effects on the function of vital organs such as the kidney, lung, brain, liver, and the heart itself are for obvious reasons the most serious.

Mrs. Bird, who was introduced in Chapter 8, illustrates the course of events in chronic heart failure. Multiple factors contributed to her loss of myocardial reserve. Aging, with its attendant loss of muscle tissue, essential hypertension, and atherosclerosis, of which the latter two increased the resistances against which the blood had to be moved, contributed to a loss of cardiac reserve. The hypertension, accompanied by arteriosclerosis, diminished the quantity of blood circulated to the heart muscle. Over a period of time, hypertrophy and dilatation of her heart occurred. The growth of new capillaries lagged behind the increase in the mass of myocardium. This further added to the discrepancy between the quantity of blood delivered to her myocardium and its nutritional requirements. Mrs. Bird was unable to augment the supply of blood to her myocardium in proportion to the increase in work load. Eventually her heart was not able to adapt the quantity of blood delivered into her circulation to the needs of her tissues during activity. In fact, stimuli, such as exercise or excitement, that call forth an increase in cardiac output in persons with a healthy heart actually were followed by a decrease in output of Mrs. Bird's heart. A fall in cardiac output when activity is increased is frequent in

[23] Guyton, *Op. cit.*, p. 467.

patients with congestive heart failure.[24] At rest Mrs. Bird's heart was able to eject as much blood into her circulation as was delivered to it. When she exercised, her heart was no longer strong enough to eject as much blood as was returned to it, and the quantity of blood remaining in the heart at the end of systole increased. As time passed, she found she required several pillows at night to avoid feeling short of breath. Activities such as walking to the corner store or up a flight of stairs caused her heart to pound (palpitation) and shortness of breath. At night she noted her feet were swollen and in the morning she had difficulty in putting on her shoes. Despite a loss in appetite, or anorexia, she also had a marked gain in weight. Eventually, shortness of breath was present at rest, even when she was in the sitting position. By this time, blood flow to all of Mrs. Bird's tissues was diminished.

Although congestion of fluid in the tissues is a major manifestation of chronic or congestive heart failure, authorities are not agreed about the mechanisms responsible for it. Two principal theories—the forward theory and the backward theory—are advanced to explain the course of events leading to the retention of excess fluid. Neither completely accounts for all of the manifestations of congestive heart failure. Since the blood is contained in a closed circuit, both forward and backward failure must be involved. The major argument is over which comes first. Some of the signs and symptoms are due to impairment of the nutrition of the tissues resulting from the failure in blood supply. Others are due to failure to remove blood from the tissues.

The premise on which the theory of forward failure is based is that, as the heart fails, its output falls, and causes a relative ischemia of the tissues. According to Guyton,[25] this low cardiac output has a profound effect on renal function. The kidney responds to diminished blood flow by a reduction in glomerular filtration. Renal blood flow is further decreased by the activation of sympathetic reflexes which cause a marked constriction of afferent renal arterioles. Although it has been suggested that one of the factors in edema formation in congestive heart failure is an increase in the secretion of aldosterone, chronically elevated levels of aldosterone do not lead to edema, even though the total circulating blood volume may be increased. Blood volume may possibly be further increased by the release of the antidiuretic hormone by an ischemic posterior hypophysis. There is recent evidence that a humoral extra-adrenal, extrarenal factor may be implicated in the development of edema in heart failure. Its source and type are unknown.[26] According to the forward theory of failure, therefore, the increase in the blood volume and the congestion of tissues result primarily from the inability of the heart to eject as much blood into the circulation as needed by the tissues to

[24] Eugene A. Stead, "Pathological Physiology of Heart Failure," in Paul B. Beeson and Walsh McDermott (eds.), Cecil-Loeb, *Textbook of Medicine*, W. B. Saunders Company, Philadelphia, 11th ed., 1963, p. 619.

[25] *Op. cit.*, pp. 468-69.

[26] An Extra-adrenal Factor Essential For Chronic Renal Sodium Retention in Presence of Increased Sodium-Retaining Hormone," *Circulation Research*, XIV, January, 1964, pp. 17-31.

maintain their function. A number of hypotheses have been proposed to explain the increase in the volume of extracellular fluid and congestion of tissues accompanying chronic heart failure. Currently more factors than the response of the kidney and its regulatory agencies to ischemia are thought to be involved.

Explain the backward theory of congestive heart failure

The second theory used to explain the congestion of the tissues with fluid is called the backward theory. According to this theory, congestion of the tissues is primarily due to a failure of the ventricles to eject as much blood into the circulation as is delivered to them. Output may or may not be reduced below normal limits. Because output is less than input, blood accumulates in the heart. The increase of residual blood in the heart causes the myocardial fibers to stretch. For a time the increase in residual blood may stimulate the myocardium to contract more forcibly. This is to be expected unless some condition, such as dilatation, exists that weakens the heart muscle. According to the law of the heart, lengthening of the myocardial fibers results in increased force of contraction. Eventually, however, the residual blood in the ventricles becomes so great that the heart is overdilated. Despite an increased expenditure of energy, the heart is no longer effective as a pump. As blood accumulates in the heart, the intra-atrial pressure rises and offers resistance to the incoming or venous blood. The increase in venous pressure is reflected by elevation of pressure in the great veins as well as in the venous tributaries. As the pressure of blood within the veins, that is, the venous hydrostatic pressure, rises, the tissues drained by these veins become congested with blood and fluid.

Although neither theory completely explains the development of edema in congestive heart failure, they are both helpful in explaining the effects of heart failure. Although both sides of the heart are often involved in heart failure, at least in the beginning, one side may fail while the other is competent as a pump. Pure left-sided failure is more frequent than pure right-sided failure. Failure of the left side preceded that of the right in the instance of Mrs. Bird. In left-sided heart failure, congestion of the lungs is a prominent finding. In right-sided heart failure, the congestion is in the systemic circulation.

What changes are responsible for the signs and symptoms in congestive heart failure?

Signs and symptoms in congestive heart failure arise from the failure of the heart to adequately nourish and oxygenate the tissues and from the accumulation of blood and fluid in the various tissues and organs in the body. In the early stages of congestive (chronic) heart failure, the most outstanding symptom is shortness of breath during ordinary activities. The reader will remember that Mrs. Bird's first symptom was shortness of breath when she walked to the store or up a flight of stairs. With the elapse of time the amount of activity required to precipitate the sensation of breathlessness becomes less and less. Apprehension usually accompanies shortness of breath because anything interfering with respiration threatens survival. Despite the presence of fatigue and lack of energy, patients seldom complain of these effects.

What are the signs and symptoms associated with pulmonary congestion?

The signs and symptoms accompanying pulmonary congestion due to left-sided heart failure are similar to those resulting from congestion of the lung from any cause. With the congestion of blood in the lung, pulmonary edema develops. Both the slowing of the flow of blood through the lung and the pulmonary edema predispose to hypoxia and hypercarbia. Many of the manifestations observed in congestive heart failure are due to failure to adequately oxygenate the blood and to remove carbon dioxide from it. Some of the manifestations commonly observed are due to the congestion of the lung tissue itself.

As indicated, one of the early and most distressing symptoms in congestive heart failure is dyspnea. Although the symptom dyspnea was discussed in some detail in Chapter 7 it, along with other disturbances in breathing, will be reviewed in relation to heart disease. Although dyspnea in heart disease is associated with pulmonary congestion, its severity is not always in direct proportion to the degree of congestion. Why this is true has not been explained to the satisfaction of all who are interested in this problem.

Because dyspnea can be induced in a healthy person by a variety of physical (strenuous exercise) and emotional factors (fear, excitement, or other strong emotions), some believe it results when one or a number of factors in combination are sufficiently powerful. As a result of a series of experiments Wasserman and his associates,[27] concluded that dyspnea results from the "summated effects of a number of physiologic stimuli to respiration." (See Chapter 7.) Further, a single stimulus may be so great that dyspnea occurs. Under other circumstances, a number of less powerful stimuli may combine to produce it. In the healthy or nondyspneic person, a balance is maintained between the impulses stimulating respiration and those inhibiting it. According to the above authors,[28] in dyspnea, there is a powerful stimulus to inspiration and in some instances an accompanying reduction in respiratory inhibition.

In the patient in congestive heart failure, the lungs become engorged with blood with the result that the lung becomes inelastic and edematous. This causes a reduction of the vital capacity. The patient, may, however, be relatively free of dyspnea at rest. During activity, because his ventilatory minute

---

[27] A. J. Wasserman, H. P. Mauck, Jr., and J. L. Patterson, Jr., "Dyspnea," *Heart Bulletin,* XI, January-February, 1962, pp. 1-3 and 20.
[28] *Ibid.,* p. 3.

volume of air rises, he becomes dyspneic. The activity may be physical exercise, but it may also be excitement or anger. As previously emphasized, some patients experience dyspnea with less engorgement of their lungs than others do. Dyspnea is made worse by conditions that reduce vital capacity or the effective ventilating surface of the lung such as hydrothorax, pulmonary infarcts, and ascites.

When dyspnea or breathlessness becomes so severe that the patient cannot lie in a recumbent position, the patient is said to be orthopneic. Orthopnea can often be relieved by elevating the trunk in relation to the rest of the body. Though there is some increase in the vital capacity when the trunk is raised, some authorities do not feel this completely explains the beneficial effect of the upright position. A variety of methods may be used to secure the desired result. The patient may sit in Fowler's position in bed; the head of the bed may be elevated; or he may be more comfortable sitting in a chair. Whether he sits in bed or a chair, the patient often seeks relief by sitting forward. When the most comfortable position is found, the patient should be adequately supported with pillows. An over-the-bed table may be placed so the patient can rest on it as he leans forward. As previously emphasized, the patient should be supported in a comfortable position and in good alignment by the supports. Also, his position should be changed regularly.

Both dyspnea and orthopnea are causes of and result from apprehension. For this reason every effort should be made to assure the patient that his needs will be met and that he can trust his safety to those responsible for his care. Because morphine sulfate depresses the higher centers in the brain, it is sometimes prescribed to alleviate anxiety. This is one of the few instances in which morphine sulfate is administered for relief of a symptom other than pain.

The importance of the relief of dyspnea and orthopnea is illustrated by Mrs. Oriole, a young woman in severe congestive failure associated with mitral stenosis and rheumatic heart disease. She was markedly orthopneic. Relief was not achieved by the orthopneic position. Her basal metabolic rate was found to be +100 per cent. This young woman, whose heart was unable to perform as an efficient pump, was actually "working hard." The pathophysiology in the instance of Mrs. Oriole is an illustration of a positive feedback (a vicious circle). One event—failure of her myocardium—led to congestion of her lungs and the development of orthopnea. As her need for breathing increased, she required more energy to maintain breathing. As the work required to breathe increased, strain on her weakened myocardium was increased. One event initiated a second which either directly or indirectly intensified the first. Unless the chain is broken, and in this instance the strength of the myocardium is increased, death results.

Another form of dyspnea is known as paroxysmal nocturnal dyspnea or cardiac asthma. It is most frequently observed in patients who have a disorder that places a burden on the left ventricle. Since it usually occurs after the patient has been asleep and is therefore seen most frequently at night, it is referred to as nocturnal. Nocturnal dyspnea may develop in patients who do not have dyspnea when they are up and about and who may even be able to work. The recumbent position predisposes to or precipitates dyspnea because blood tends to accumulate in the lungs in this position. In the patient who already has some impingement on his vital capacity, a few hundred milliliters of blood added to that already present in the lung may be sufficient to cause dyspnea. During an attack of paroxysmal dyspnea the patient is awakened from sleep. He either sits upright, hangs his feet over the edge of the bed, or stands upright. He may be ashen in color and sweating profusely. Since there is often some bronchial constriction, he may be wheezing. He is usually frightened.

Other signs and symptoms that occur include periodic or Cheyne-Stokes respiration and cyanosis. They are both discussed in Chapter 7.

Cough with clear or blood-tinged sputum may accompany pulmonary edema. Though cough is an important mechanism in maintaining a clear airway, it requires a considerable expenditure of energy and may interfere with sleep.

Although blood-tinged sputum is not uncommon in left heart failure, larger amounts may appear. Hemoptysis may result from a sudden increase in pulmonary venous pressure which leads to the rupture of a pulmonary vessel or to an infarction in the lung. Although it is not usually dangerous *it may be*, and any quantity of blood in the sputum is likely to frighten the patient.

Needless to say, appreciable amounts of blood in the sputum are likely to terrify the patient as well as other persons in his environment. Blood issuing from the lung is bright pink or red and foamy in appearance. Foaming is due to air passing through it. When blood appears in the sputum for the first time or is present in considerable quantity, the physician should be notified. The quantity of blood should be estimated or measured and described accurately. The patient should be encouraged to lie quietly in whatever position he finds is comfortable. Because morphine sulfate allays apprehension, the physician may prescribe it. When at all possible the nurse should remain with the patient in order to increase his feeling of safety and to determine the extent of his bleeding.

To recapitulate, besides interfering with the oxygenation of the blood and the removal of carbon dioxide, pulmonary congestion is responsible for a number of other effects. It causes several disturbances in breathing, the most common of which are dyspnea and orthopnea. Cough with clear or blood-tinged sputum is not infrequent.

In addition to disturbances in breathing, pulmonary congestion places an added burden on the right ventricle by increasing the resistance against which it has to move the blood. Eventually, unless the left-sided heart failure is corrected, the right heart fails. Failure of the right side of the heart may be secondary to diseases of the lung which cause an increase in resistance to the flow of blood through the lung. Diseases such as emphysema, therefore, predispose to failure of the right heart.

What are some of the possible factors in the development of generalized edema in congestive heart failure?

Sooner or later patients in chronic congestive heart failure develop generalized systemic edema. In the beginning the principal evidence of edema may be a gain in weight as a patient can be expected to store at least 10 to 20 lbs. (5 to 10 l) of fluid before pitting edema occurs. Usually by the time a patient has dyspnea at rest he has stored at least 30 lbs. of fluid.

The cause of edema in heart failure has never been adequately explained. As stated earlier, one implied factor includes the evalation of the hydrostatic pressure of the blood in the capillaries as a result of increased venous pressure. Factors in this increase include augmented tone of veins and resistance to incoming blood by an overdilated ventricle. A second factor is the retention of salt and water by the kidney. An extra-adrenal and extrarenal humoral agent may be implicated. Why edema occurs has not been agreed upon. With the retention of salt and water, the blood volume increases and the quantity of protein in the blood is also elevated. During the day, the fluid is deposited in tissues below the level of the heart. At night it tends to be more generally distributed. The patient notices that his ankles swell during the day and that his shoes are tight. By morning the swelling disappears. As the disorder progresses, the edema is continuous. The patient may also complain of a feeling of heaviness, but not of pain. In general, edema appears where capillary pressure is high and tissue pressure is low. Later, when the patient becomes bedfast, sacral edema as well as edema of the genitalia may be manifested. When edema is severe, the skin becomes tightly stretched and shiny in appearance. Because it has difficulty in maintaining its nutrition, it breaks down and fluids drain from it. Cellulitis may result from infection. When the legs are very distended with fluid, needles or small tubes may be introduced into the subcutaneous tissue to drain off some of the fluid.

Although accumulation of fluid in the parts below the heart is less dangerous to the patient than pulmonary edema, it does create problems for the patient. For the reasons cited above, a patient in congestive failure is a candidate for decubiti unless special care is given. In the severely orthopneic patient the problem is commonly aggravated by resistance to moving and turning. Mr. Ash illustrates how quickly and extensively the skin may break down. He was severely orthopneic. About seven o'clock in the evening, when back care was given, the skin of his buttocks was edematous, but intact. In the morning, 12 hours later, the skin on the cheeks of both buttocks was denuded and bleeding. See Chapter 3.

Generalized edema may mask a serious state of undernourishment. In the children physical and even mental development may be seriously retarded.

Undernutrition and edema go hand in hand with chronic illness whatever the cause. When the patient responds to therapy, the true state of his nutrition becomes evident. It is not uncommon for these patients to appear to be nothing more than skin and bones following the removal of edema fluid. In some patients improvement of their nutritional status may be required before efforts to relieve their edema are successful.

Symptoms indicating involvement of the gastrointestinal tract are common. Anorexia, nausea, and vomiting are common. The patient frequently complains of indigestion. Especially in acute heart failure, these may be the predominant symptoms. The reasons for the symptoms have not been completely identified. The gastrointestinal tract is highly sensitive to disturbances in homeostasis. Both the heart and the gastrointestinal tract are supplied by branches of the vagus nerve. Reflexes arising in one organ may affect the function of the other through intermedullary connections between the heart and the stomach. Congestion of the viscera is also a possibility. In advanced heart failure, metabolism of the brain may be sufficiently disturbed to cause reflex vomiting. At times the origin of the gastrointestinal symptoms may create a problem in differential diagnosis for the physician. Mr. Sparrow illustrates this point. He sought medical attention with complaints suggestive of cholecystitis. The diagnosis of cholecystitis was confirmed and he was admitted to the hospital. A nurse noted and reported to his physician that at times his pulse was irregular. An electrocardiogram indicated some myocardial injury. In this instance the patient had both cholecystitis and heart damage. Knowledge of the status of his heart was an important consideration in making the decision about whether surgical therapy was to be undertaken. Furthermore, it influenced the selection of the surgical procedure to be performed as well as his care before, during, and after surgery.

Swelling of the liver (hepatomegaly) and abdominal pain are frequent. Because only about a fourth of the blood supply of the liver is arterial, under the most favorable circumstances it borders on hypoxia. In congestive heart failure, hypoxia leads to necrosis of the hepatic cells surrounding central veins. There may also be swelling of the liver due to edema. In addition to abdominal pain, some patients experience jaundice.

Hypoglycemia occurs in severe congestive heart failure. This may be due to inadequate storage of glycogen in the liver and increased breakdown of glucose to lactic acid in the presence of hypoxia.

Distention and pulsation of the neck veins may be observed. Distention is especially marked when the patient is in the recumbent position.

Cerebral symptoms do not usually become marked until the patient has dyspnea at rest. Although the principal factor in their development may be insufficient oxygenation and nutrition of the brain, other elements enter into their development. Early symptoms are irritability, restlessness, and difficulty in fixing attention. They may also include personality changes, mild delirium, and mental depression. In terminal stages stupor and coma occur.

One symptom specific to the heart is palpitation—consciousness of the beating of the heart. The two common physiological changes predisposing to palpitation are an increase in cardiac output and a change in the rhythm of the heart. The causes may be physiological or pathological. For example, Mrs. Oaks, a middle-aged and somewhat obese housewife, ran around the block, or tried to. By the time she returned to her home, she was dyspneic and her heart was pounding. A few nights later, she had difficulty in going to sleep. One of the factors making sleep difficult was the pounding of her heart. She had had a stimulating evening playing bridge and an argument with her husband over how the last hand should have been bid. In both instances the response is physiological. In the first the stimulus is exercise. In the second it is a psychological incident.

Mrs. Oaks's neighbor, Mrs. Maple, was severely anemic. Since increase in blood volume is one of the mechanisms of adaptation to anemia, one of her most worrisome symptoms was palpitation. Correction of the anemia eliminated the cause and relieved the palpitation. Palpitation may also be observed in thyrotoxicosis and fever as well as in psychological disorders. Consciousness of the heart beating associated with changes in rhythm will be discussed with the arrhythmias.

What are some of the differences in the distribution of fluids and electrolytes in acute and chronic heart failure?

Patients in longstanding and chronic heart failure differ from those with acute heart failure inasmuch as they have disturbances in the concentrations of electrolytes, while the latter do not. Characteristically, whenever edema develops, there is sodium retention. The level of sodium per unit of blood plasma will depend on whether water and sodium are equally retained or water is retained in excess of sodium. In the latter event, the concentration of sodium in the plasma will be low. In longstanding and intractable heart failure, diuretics become ineffective.

The making of a medical diagnosis of heart disease is the responsibility of the physician. The symptoms usually observed in patients with congestive heart failure have already been described in some detail. In the early stages of failure, the physician must evaluate each symptom in light of the age of the individual, his weight in relation to height, and emotional status, as well as the presence of some other disease that may account for a symptom or group of symptoms. Through objective observation and reporting, the nurse can often add to the information obtained by the physician. For example, she can note any conditions seeming to precipitate or relieve a given symptom and the patient's reaction to it.

Diagnostic procedures specific to the heart include the electrocardiogram, X ray of the heart, and the circulation time. The electrocardiogram is discussed in another section of the chapter. From X ray or fluoroscopy of the heart and chest, the physician obtains information about the size and position of the heart and the great vessels. Evidence of congestion of the lungs can also be obtained.

The circulation time can be defined as the time it takes one particle to travel from one point in the circulation to another. Circulation time can be estimated by injecting a substance and then measuring the time required for it to reach a specific receptor. In one method either *dehydrocholic acid, U.S.P.* (Decholin[29]) or ether is injected into a vein in the arm. When dehydrocholic acid, U.S.P. is injected, the time elapsing after administration until the person can taste it—it has a bitter taste—is measured. The normal time is from 8 to 17 seconds. This is known as the arm-to-tongue circulation time. The arm-to-tongue circulation time is increased in left heart failure. Both Mrs. Bird and Mrs. Oriole had an increase in arm-to-tongue circulation time. When ether is used, the patient smells it when it reaches the lung. Normally the arm-to-lung time is from 4 to 8 seconds. Arm-to-lung time is increased in right heart failure. For experimental work more accurate measures are now available in the form of dyes and radioisotopes.

Most patients in congestive heart failure have some increase in venous pressure. The procedure used to determine the venous pressure is essentially a venipuncture followed by the attachment of a glass tube or manometer to a needle introduced into the antecubital vein. To achieve an accurate result, the arm should be elevated to the level of the right atrium. Harrison[30] states that the normal venous pressure in the antecubital vein is from 70 to 140 mm of water. Expressed in centimeters, this is 7 to 14.

As in all medical diagnosis, the history and physical examination are important. Sometimes the patient fails to give the physician pertinent information. The nurse, as she gains information, is responsible for relaying it to the proper persons.

Patients in full-blown congestive heart failure offer few problems in the diagnosis of a failing heart. Early diagnosis of impending failure may be more difficult, but it may make it possible to institute a regime to protect the heart from added injury. As a case finder, the nurse should encourage patients to seek medical advice early.

To summarize, when the heart fails as a pump, the manifestations of failure depend on the degree of failure and rate at which it fails. In all degrees of heart failure many of the effects are directly or indirectly due to an inadequate supply of oxygen or to the accumulation of carbon dioxide. In cardiac arrest death or incapacitating brain damage occurs unless the circulation is re-established within approximately four minutes. In acute heart failure the manifestations depend on the efficiency of the person's mechanisms for adapting to cardiac inefficiency and in many instances they are adequate. When adaptation is inadequate, the manifestations of heart failure are due to the effects of

[29] Trade name.
[30] *Op. cit.,* 4th ed., p. 1944.

failure of the heart to meet the needs of the tissues for oxygen and nutrition and to the retention of salt and water. In acute heart failure generalized edema is not usually marked. Pulmonary engorgement and edema are likely, however. When severe, they are life-threatening.

In chronic heart failure, signs and symptoms develop gradually over a period of time. They, too, result from failure of the heart to adequately nourish and oxygenate the tissues and from the increase in the volume of extracellular fluid. Generalized edema is marked and many of the accompanying signs and symptoms are due to it. There is also some degree of pulmonary congestion.

*Toward what objectives is the therapy in chronic heart
failure directed? How is it accomplished?*

Therapy of the patient in heart failure depends on the degree and suddenness with which his heart fails. Since the most common cause of acute heart failure is myocardial infarction, the treatment of the patient in acute heart failure will be discussed with this most important disorder. The objective of treatment of the patient in chronic or congestive heart failure is to restore the capacity of the heart to adapt or respond efficiently to the demands placed on it, that is, to restore the pumping mechanism of the heart so that as much blood is propelled into the circulation as enters the heart during diastole and there is no increase in residual blood at the end of systole. The re-establishment of the efficiency of the heart as a pump requires a two-pronged attack. One is to increase the force or strength of contraction of the myocardium. The other is to reduce the demands made on the myocardium until the efficiency of the pumping mechanism has been restored. Later the reserve power of the heart muscle will have to be evaluated and plans made with the patient and his family regarding any modifications of his living and working habits.

At the time a patient, such as Mrs. Bird or Mrs. Oriole, seeks medical attention, he is often seriously, if not critically, ill. Health and life depend on restoring the pumping mechanism to as full efficiency as possible. Both aspects of treatment are carried out simultaneously. The physician prescribes a cardiac glucoside—usually a preparation of digitalis—to strengthen the force of cardiac contraction; a regime of rest and activity to limit the demands made on the failing heart; and diuretics combined with sodium restriction to reduce the volume of fluid in the body and thus lessen the burden on the weakened heart.

Digitalis contains an active principle in the form of a glucoside that has a number of important effects on the heart muscle. In congestive heart failure it increases the strength of ventricular contraction with the result that the volume of residual blood is reduced at the end of systole, that is, it increases the efficiency of the pumping mechanism of the heart. It has a second action that is modified by the level of potassium in the body. In the presence of normal amounts of potassium, it lessens the responsiveness of the conduction system of the heart. This has its greatest value in the patient who has auricular fibrillation. In auricular fibrillation the ventricle is bombarded by numerous impulses. Despite its failure to respond to all of them, diastole is sometimes so short that the heart receives little blood. Energy expended in the succeeding systole is largely wasted. Reduction in the number of impulses reaching the ventricles has the obvious advantage of reducing the number of wasteful contractions. Although digitalis occasionally restores the normal atrial contraction, it does not usually do so. For example, when Mrs. Bird was admitted to the hospital, her atria were fibrillating. Her pulse rate was completely irregular and averaged about 100 beats per minute. Her ventricular rate when counted by stethoscope was about 140; she had a pulse deficit of about 40. (The pulse deficit is defined as the difference between the number of ventricular contractions and pulse beat.) After Mrs. Bird was digitalized, her atria continued to fibrillate, but her pulse rate averaged between 65 and 75 beats per minute. The pulse deficit disappeared.

Digitalis increases the irritability of the heart muscle whether the level of potassium is normal or low, but the effect is more marked in the presence of low potassium levels. The mechanism seems to be related to the effect on intracardiac calcium concentration. Potassium levels can also be effectively lowered by intravenous administration of glucose in water. Increased myocardial irritability may be manifested by premature beats and an increase in the pulse rate. The latter condition is known as pulsus bigeminus. Since there is an extra contraction interspersed between the normal contraction, the pulse rate is increased, but is not irregular. Although all alterations in the rate and rhythm of the pulse are important and should be reported, this is particularly important for the patient taking digitalis. To prevent the possibility of digitalis-induced arrhythmias, potassium chloride is frequently administered to patients who are under regular and prolonged therapy with diuretics, as they predispose to potassium depletion. Inadequate food intake, whether due to anorexia or to poor food habits, also adds to the likelihood of potassium deficiency.

The specific preparation of digitalis prescribed by the physician will depend on his personal preference and the acuteness of the patient's symptoms. When the patient's life is endangered by marked pulmonary edema, the physician is likely to prescribe a rapidly acting preparation to be administered intravenously. For example, when Mrs. Oriole was admitted to the hospital, her lungs were engorged and her vital capacity was seriously reduced. Her physician prescribed and administered intravenously Lanatoside C, 1.6 mg N.F. (Cedilanid[31]). Later she was placed on Digitoxin U.S.P., administered orally.

At the time Mrs. Bird sought medical attention her condition was less urgent. Her physician, therefore, digitalized her slowly. Many physicians pre-

[31] Trade name.

fer this method as there is less likelihood of digitalis intoxication. He ordered Digitoxin U.S.P., 0.6 mg, to be followed in six hours by another 0.6 mg. The dosage was then reduced to 0.2 mg every six hours, to be continued until beneficial effects or early toxic effects were observed. Thereafter, 0.1 mg was sufficient to maintain the digitalis effect.

Both patients were given a relatively large initial dosage of digitalis. A smaller dosage was required to maintain its effect. Since digitalis is absorbed more rapidly than it is destroyed and excreted from the body, it tends to accumulate. Consequently sufficient digitalis is administered over a period of 24 to 48 hours to produce the desired action. This procedure is known as digitalization. Thereafter, only enough digitalis is administered to replace that which is destroyed or eliminated. The quantity of drug required is referred to as the maintenance dosage.

Among the responsibilities of the nurse in the care of patients under digitalis therapy is the administration of the drug at the times and in the quantities prescribed by the physician. Perhaps even more important is the observation of the effects—desired as well as undesired—on the patient and the reporting and/or possible adjustment of the dosage according to pertinent observations. There is a common misconception that all patients require the same dosage, but this is not true. Moreover, a given patient may vary from time to time in his susceptibility to digitalis.

Few descriptions of the effects of digitalis have improved on the one left by William Withering, who first introduced the drug about the time of the American Revolution. He said: "Let the medicine . . . be continued until it either acts on the kidneys, the stomach, the pulse, or the bowels; let it be stopped upon the first appearance of any of these effects."

In the past literature of nursing and in its practice, great emphasis has been and is being placed on a pulse rate of 60 as an absolute criterion for the administration of digitalis. There has been a tendency to neglect other and more significant observations of developing toxicity. The pulse rate is a good guide to adequacy of digitalization *only* in patients with atrial fibrillation. In patients with sinus rhythm, a slowing pulse indicates either restoration of cardiac compensation or complete heart block. Harrison[32] states the gastrointestinal symptoms—anorexia, nausea, and vomiting developing in this order are most common evidence of digitalis toxicity. Diarrhea is not common, although it can occur. These are followed by cardiac arrhythmias, premature beat, bigeminal rhythm, and atrial tachycardia. Excessive slowing of the pulse is not even mentioned. A less common toxic effect is a disturbance in color vision. Visual abnormalities can include all types of color vision disturbances (yellow is most common). Central nervous system excitation is an unusual but possible effect (digitalis madness).

Observations indicating the heart is responding favorably to digitalis include slowing of the pulse to 75 or 80 beats per minute, diminishing pulse

[32] *Op. cit.,* p. 1388.

deficit, greater force of cardiac contraction, and increase in the output of urine. As the mechanical efficiency of the heart improves, the patient's general status improves. He is less dyspneic and apprehensive. The backrest can be lowered. His appetite is better. His morale is improved. He sleeps better. With the loss of fluid he loses weight. In some patients loss of edema fluid may be so great that the skin hangs in loose folds and they appear emaciated. The safety of the patient often depends on the accuracy of observation of the effects of digitalis on the patient. Adjustments in dosage depend on the effects of the drug. Most of these observations can be made by an informed and interested nurse.

The nurse has another responsibility to the patient who is treated with digitalis. All patients who are receiving digitalis must take it for prolonged periods of time, and most of them must take it for as long as they live. As in other situations where the patient and his family are responsible for continued treatment, the nurse can be helpful to him by ascertaining what he knows and what he wants to know. Certainly the patient should know how and where to obtain the drug he needs and how many tablets or pills he should take each day. He should be instructed about the meaning of, and what to do about, loss of appetite, nausea or vomiting. Patients on a regime of diuretics usually are instructed to take potassium chloride, 1 gm three times a day. Since carbohydrate increases the loss of potassium, the patient should be advised to avoid carbohydrate "binges," that is, the eating of excessive amounts of candies or pastries. In elderly patients living alone and with a limited income, carbohydrate in the form of bread may form the basic part of the diet. Patients do not always follow directions. In one instance observed by the writer, 77-year-old Mr. Henry adjusted his dosage of digitalis according to how he felt. When he felt well, he omitted it. When he had a bad day, he took an extra tablet or two. The reasons for this behavior were not explored. Superficially they may relate to the fact that many people judge the state of their health by how they feel; medicines are to be taken when they do not feel well. Since the effects of omitting a dose or two of digitalis are not felt immediately, some time may elapse before the patient feels sick. By that time, he may be in serious trouble.

Why are diuretics prescribed in the therapy of heart failure?

As indicated above, diuretics are widely used in the therapy of congestive heart failure. They may increase the effectiveness of digitalis and, by increasing the elimination of salt and water, reduce the burden on the weakened heart. Digitalis has a diuretic effect inasmuch as it improves the circulation of the kidneys and thereby improves their function.

The true diuretics used in the treatment of congestive heart failure are those that suppress the reabsorption of salt and water by the kidney. In the past the mercurial diuretics were used for this purpose. Today their use is generally limited to patients with massive edema or who fail to respond to newer diuretics. One disadvantage of most preparations of mercurial diuretics is that they must be administered intramuscularly.

According to Harrison,[33] the most generally useful group of diuretics is the chlorothiazide group. They, like the mercurials, block the reabsorption of the chloride, sodium, and potassium ions in the proximal tubules. "Whither goes sodium chloride, thither goes water." Continued and frequent use of these drugs may lead to the previously mentioned potassium depletion. When combined with a low-sodium intake, they may also cause a sodium deficiency. See Chapter 8 for further details.

Harrison[34] suggests chlorothiazide U.S.P. (Diuril[35]) be administered in dosages of from 250 to 500 mg two to four times daily for five consecutive days each week. Potassium chloride is administered at the same time to prevent potassium deficiency.

One of the mechanisms implicated in the retention of salt and water is the oversecretion of aldosterone. It is believed to act principally in the distal tubule. To counteract the action of aldosternone an antagonist, spironolactone (Aldactone), has been developed. So far the results of its use in cardiac failure have been disappointing.

The nurse has the usual responsibilities when administering drugs with a diuretic effect. Not only should the urine output be measured, but the weight of the patient should be accurately checked. Particularly pertinent to nurses working with patients in outpatient clinics and at home is the observation of patients for signs and symptoms of electrolyte depletion.

In addition to measures utilized to facilitate the excretion of sodium, its retention can be further diminished by decreasing its intake. In areas where the drinking water has a high sodium content bottled water may be necessary. The quantity of salt allowed in the diet varies greatly. At one extreme is the limitation of intake to from 200 to 400 mg of sodium. At the other, the patient is instructed not to add any salt to his food at the table. A very low sodium intake is usually prescribed for the patient who has marked edema and is continued only during the acute phase of the illness. Mrs. Oriole is a good example. To achieve a sodium content of between 200 and 400 mg, all medicines containing sodium salts and foods naturally high in sodium, as well as those prepared with sodium salts, are restricted. Sodium is the offending agent and not the chloride anion. Therefore, Mrs. Oriole should not be given sodium bicarbonate nor should she be given breads, cakes, or pastries leavened with it. There is at least one brand of baking powder prepared with a potassium rather than a sodium salt. Foods prepared with salts of sodium should be avoided. The patient should be taught to look at the label on food. If it contains a sodium salt, it should not be used. Other foods limited during a period when sodium intake is markedly restricted include milk and celery. Continued marked reduction in sodium is not the rule.

[33] *Ibid.*, p. 1389.
[34] *Ibid.*, p. 1389.
[35] Trade name.

At one time water intake was markedly restricted. Presently, the trend is toward moderate or no restriction. Some physicians allow the patient as much water as he wishes. Others limit intake to as little as 800 ml a day. A prescription of from 1,500 to 2,000 ml is common. Whatever the prescription, the nurse has the responsibility for carrying it out and for bringing problems to the attention of the physician. When fluid intake is markedly restricted, a plan should be made to distribute it over the 24-hour period. The use of a small glass filled with chipped ice and just enough water to fill the spaces makes it easier to extend a limited quantity of water over the day.

When a patient has acute pulmonary edema, blood volume and consequently pulmonary engorgement may be reduced by venesection. Usually about 300 or 400 ml of blood can be removed without causing a fall in blood pressure. The patient and his family may require reassurance about why the removal of blood is therapeutic.

The volume of blood circulating through the lungs can be temporarily reduced by applying tourniquets to the extremities, so that blood enters but does not leave the area below the tourniquet. The blood pressure cuff is safer than ordinary tourniquets as the degree of pressure can be controlled. Ordinary tourniquets are frequently applied too tightly with the result that the tissues become ischemic. Tourniquets should be inflated to a level between the diastolic and systolic blood pressure. The pulses in the arteries should be palpated regularly, to be sure that blood is gaining access to the parts below the tourniquets. Tourniquets may be applied to all four extremities or to three extremities with the fourth free. In the latter instance, they are rotated according to a regular pattern, so each extremity is free one fourth of the time. The pattern should be established when the treatment is initiated, so that the circulation to each extremity is regularly released. Usually tourniquets are applied to three extremities and then rotated every 10 to 15 minutes. With this pattern, the tourniquet remains on each extremity about 30 to 45 minutes. When the tourniquets are discontinued, they should be removed, one at a time. Otherwise a large amount of fluid may gain entry into the circulation with a recurrence of pulmonary congestion. Following the removal of tourniquets, the patient may show some transient hyperpnea, because of the release of carbon dioxide into the blood. During the period in which the tourniquets are in place, the patient should be observed for manifestations of shock. The sudden reduction of venous return to the lung predisposes to shock, by lessening the volume of blood delivered to the left ventricle. Since cardiac output depends on cardiac intake, circulation cannot be maintained unless intake is adequate. Evidence indicating the development of shock should, of course, be brought immediately to the attention of the physician.

Other measures utilized to reduce the demands placed on the heart include the administration of oxygen, sedatives, and bed or chair rest. When oxygenation of the blood is impaired, oxygen therapy may also improve the quality of blood circulated to the heart muscle. In hot weather, oxygen administered by tent has the further advantage of providing an air-conditioned unit.

During the period in which the patient is acutely ill, sedatives may add greatly to the patient's comfort. Morphine sulfate or Pantopium hydrochloride may be prescribed by the physician to allay the apprehension and to relieve dyspnea. When narcotics are used, they may be prescribed for bedtime in order to help the patient sleep well. Overuse with its attendant danger of habituation should be avoided. One of the meprobamate tranquilizing drugs or small doses of phenobarbital may be ordered for the daytime. Care must be taken not to oversedate the patient as this renders him less able to cooperate with measures required to prevent thrombophlebitis.

Although the discussion of rest and its antithesis, activity, is included here, much of the discussion applies equally well to any situation in which rest and activity are modified. Despite the fact that rest is probably one of the oldest forms of medical therapy, its use in the treatment of heart disease is of relatively modern origin. For the last 10 to 20 years, there has been some critical examination of the effects of bed rest and a considerable change in thought about the value of bed rest in the treatment of diseases of the heart as well as of other diseases.

What does the term "bedrest" mean?

Despite the frequency with which "rest" and "bedrest" are prescribed, there is little agreement about what either term means. Sometimes little or no thought is given to whether rest in the true sense is likely to be achieved or is even possible. For example, about a year previous to her admission Mrs. Oriole's physician told her that she must get "more rest." Mrs. Oriole had three healthy preschool children. The oldest was four and the youngest was about a year old. Her husband worked long hours in a gas station to enable him to support his family and to pay his wife's medical bills. Neither Mr. nor Mrs. Oriole had any near relatives. Mrs. Oriole needed some help to analyze her situation and to find ways to get the rest she needed. Another example is that of Franz Timothy. When he visited his physician, the suggestion was made that he "get some rest." He went home and told his wife he needed a rest and that they would start for California (or Maine) the next morning. Mr. Timothy interpreted the term rest as a change in activity. Another patient, Mrs. Clover, informed her family after she received the same general prescription that her doctor wanted her to go to bed for a week. In the latter two instances, both persons interpreted the term "rest" differently. In one instance rest was a change. In the other, it meant a withdrawal from most, if not all, activity.

Interpretation of the term "bedrest" by physicians and nurses varies just as greatly. At one extreme, it means the patient is to be as completely immobilized as is possible. At the other, it means he is merely confined to his bed and can do anything in or from his bed. In the first instance the patient is fed, bathed, turned, and given any other care he requires. He may be instructed that the only voluntary activity he may perform is to turn on his light signal. In the latter instance, the patient may be responsible for much of his own personal care and may actually expend as much energy as he would were he up and about, or more. Although the physician has the responsibility for prescribing the amount of activity for a patient, the nurse interprets the prescription to the patient and tries to provide the kind of environment that makes its achievement possible. Therefore, the nurse has a responsibility to determine how much activity the physician's prescription actually allows. To ensure consistency in interpretation of prescriptions for rest and activity, some hospital, medical, and nursing staffs have defined or classified degrees of activity. This is often done in hospitals where patients are treated for tuberculosis or heart disease. For example, patients in class I are to be maintained on complete bed rest. They are to be fed, bathed twice a week, shaved, turned, and have all possible activities performed for them. They are allowed to use a bedside commode once daily. Patients in class II may in addition to the activities in class I feed themselves, wash their own face and hands, and go to the bathroom twice a day. Patients in higher classes are permitted more and more activity. Exactly what is allowed in a particular class is not important. What is important is that patient and personnel alike understand the limitation and the reason for it. Reasonable consistency in practice should increase the security of the patient and the likelihood of his receiving care suited to his needs.

In addition to widely differing interpretations of what bed rest means, true rest is more than a matter of limited physical activity. This is implied by the common definition of rest, that is, to take repose by lying down, particularly by going to sleep. Synonyms for the noun "rest" include calm, calmness, ease, pause, peace, peacefulness, repose, and tranquillity. There are others, but these words convey the broad meaning of the term. What rest is not is clarified by some of its antonyms: agitation, commotion, disquiet, disturbance, excitement, restlessness, tumult, unrest, and work. Bed rest does not necessarily include or exclude any of the above states. All the states indicated by the antonyms involve more than the expenditure of physical energy.

A prescription for rest therefore involves more than limitation of physical activity. There are many elements in sickness and all it entails that interfere with true rest, or a tranquil or peaceful state. Though many of these have been indicated in earlier chapters, a few will be repeated here. Boredom, loneliness, and worry about the possible outcome of the illness and the effect this will have on family, job, and future plans probably plague most patients. A high percentage of patients who suffer myocardial infarctions are in the prime of life when job and family obligations are great. In some patients, the dependent state precipitates intense anxiety. Anxiety may be aggravated by the insistence that the patient's life depends on immediate and complete conformity to the medical regime. Physical discomfort, resulting from pain and unpleasant diagnostic procedures, adds its bit to the failure to achieve repose.

Even when a patient lies still in bed, he may not be in a state of rest. Tension may be betrayed by a worried or uneasy expression on his face, evidence of muscle tension, a higher than normal pulse rate or blood pressure, or an irritable reaction. True rest implies a state in which the individual is physically, emotionally, mentally, and socially at ease.

The elements that are necessary in assisting the patient to rest have been indicated in earlier chapters. Basic is always the acceptance of the patient as a human being having dignity and worth. Attention to his physical comfort and personal needs and wishes makes a significant contribution. Regulation of his environment, both social and physical, so he is protected from unnecessary stresses is essential. Answering his questions or providing him with the assistance he requires to get them answered will help to remove one important source of disquiet among patients.

The objective toward which rest is directed in the therapy of the patient in heart failure is to reduce the need for the heart to adapt to varying volumes of venous return. In general the dorsal recumbent position is most restful. Immediately after one goes to bed, the blood pressure falls slightly and the work performed by skeletal muscles is diminished. With a reduction in the activity of skeletal muscles venous return to the heart is decreased. Obviously a reduction in blood presented to the heart lessens its work. The dorsal recumbent position has a serious disadvantage for the patient in, or in danger of, congestive heart failure. When he assumes the recumbent position, fluid in tissues below the level of the heart returns to the blood and increases the blood volume. This, in turn, increases the quantity of blood returned to the heart and with it the need to increase the cardiac output. Should the output of the right ventricle exceed that of the left by even a very small amount, this results in pulmonary congestion.[36] With pulmonary congestion there is a decrease in vital capacity.

Continued bed rest in the recumbent position has other adverse effects on pulmonary and circulatory function. After a week or so in the recumbent position the capacity to adapt circulation to the erect position is limited. In the healthy person a change from the prone to the upright position is accompanied by peripheral vasoconstriction and a slight rise in blood pressure. These changes protect the brain from an inadequate blood supply as a consequence of the effect of gravity on the blood in vessels below the heart. In the person who has been inactive in bed for a period of time, assumption of the upright position is accompanied by orthostatic (standing) hypotension, tachycardia, and possibly syncope (fainting). The usual explanation is that these effects are largely due to a loss of tone in the muscles and veins of the legs. To prevent fainting, the patient should assume the upright position gradually. First the head of the bed is raised. After the patient has had an opportunity to adapt to this position he can shift his legs over the edge of the bed and

[36] S. A. Levine, "The Myth of Strict Bed Rest in the Treatment of Heart Disease," *American Heart Journal*, XLII, September, 1951, p. 406.

"dangle." During this time he should be encouraged to flex and extend his ankles and swing his legs back and forth. At this time his pulse should be checked. If there is a marked tachycardia, this is a sign to go slow. Before finally assisting the patient to his feet, the nurse should be sure she has enough help to support him should it be needed. Once the patient gains his balance, he should be assisted to walk or be returned to bed. Unnecessary motionless standing should be avoided. Contraction of the muscles of the legs is essential to maintaining the venous return against gravity.

In addition to the wasting of muscle with the accompanying loss of nitrogen, bed rest and inactivity have other adverse effects. Calcium is absorbed from the bones and thereby predisposes to osteoporosis and renal lithiasis. Stasis of blood in the veins combined with chemical changes in the blood predisposes to thrombophlebitis. Gastrointestinal function is impaired. Few if any physiological and metabolic functions escape adverse effects. Altered psychological functioning as well as mental depression is the rule.

The recumbent position is associated with a low expenditure of energy, but many routine activities require more work when performed in bed. Moreover, when these activities are performed in bed, they are more likely to be accompanied by what is known as the Valsalva maneuver. To perform the Valsalva maneuver, the person takes a deep breath, closes his glottis, and expires forcibly against the closed glottis, using both the muscles of expiration and the abdominal muscles. This exercise markedly raises the intrathoracic pressure. From the description, the reader will recognize the similarity between the Valsalva maneuver and straining or bearing down at stool. In addition to requiring a considerable expenditure of energy, the Valsalva maneuver places an additional burden on the heart. During the period of forced expiration, pressure within the thoracic cavity is elevated,[36] and this interferes with blood entering the large veins. At the termination of the procedure, a large volume of blood rushes in and is delivered to the heart. In the already failing heart, cardiac arrest may be precipitated. To prevent the Valsalva maneuver, patients should be cautioned against holding their breath and straining. When they are active, they should make a conscious effort to breath normally.

To reduce the hazards of bedrest, many physicians modify it to some extent. Patients are generally kept in bed only as long as is absolutely necessary. During the time the patient is confined to bed, the extremities should be put through the normal range of motion several times a day. Elastic bandages are applied from the toes to the groin to support the veins and to prevent the pooling of blood in them. They should be applied with firm, even pressure, so that they give support without obstructing the venous circulation. They should be removed and reapplied at least every 24 hours. They should be removed and reapplied at any time they become loose or are creating uneven pressure at any point. Active exercises, especially of the legs, should be encouraged. A

[36] "Bed Rest and Chair Rest in Cardiovascular Disease," *Heart Bulletin*, III, September-October, 1954, pp. 97-100.

footboard should be placed in position to support the patient's feet and extremities in good alignment. The patient should be encouraged to press his feet against the board. This exercise is of value in preventing loss of muscle tone and in promoting the circulation in the lower extremities.

Because less energy is required to use a commode or bathroom stool than a bedpan most physicians prefer to have the patient assisted out of bed for defecation. When the patient goes to the bathroom, he should be taken in a wheel chair until such time as he is up and walking.

Despite studies demonstrating the superiority of chair rest to bedrest, the practice is not widespread. It minimizes most of the adverse effects of bedrest including the common postmyocardial infarction depression. Perhaps chair rest would be prescribed more frequently if physicians were sure everyone—nurses, patients, family and friends—understood and acted on the knowledge that these patients are seriously ill. Chair rest does not mean they are not ill. They require all the care needed by any sick patient. The chair should be comfortable and provide adequate support for the back, head, and extremities. Ideally it should allow for changes in position.

In some hospitals so-called cardiac beds are available. They are designed in such a manner that a bed can be converted to a chair. The head of the bed becomes the back of the chair, the center the seat, and the foot is dropped down so that the lower legs and feet hang over the edge. Unless care is taken to adjust the bed properly, the seat may slant downward, causing the patient to slip forward. An adjustable footboard is also required to provide a firm surface for the support of the feet. Pillows and an overbed table are required to support the arms. Since the depth of the seat may be too great for the patient, supports at the back may be required to keep the patient in a comfortable position.

In the immediately preceding paragraphs, discussion has been centered on the values and limitations of rest in the therapy of the patient with an impairment of cardiac function. As indicated, activity is also important to recovery. Although the physician prescribes the degree of activity, the nurse will be better able to interpret the prescription to the patient if she understands the reason for it. One of the factors regulating metabolism in cells is the physical stress placed on them. Physical inactivity is accompanied by wastage of cellular substance and loss of strength.

In popular as well as professional literature, Dr. Paul Dudley White is frequently quoted as stating that physical exercise is important not only to the healthy heart, but to the diseased one as well. The critical aspect in the patient with a diseased heart is to avoid those activities placing an excessive strain on the heart. The most dangerous are those characterized by a sudden and great increase in work, as increased muscular activity is followed by a marked increase in volume of the venous return. For example, the patient should avoid running for a bus or assisting with pushing a car out of the mud or snow. Extremes of heat and cold should also be avoided as they place an extra burden on the heart. As patients are recovering from congestive heart failure or a myocardial infarction, they should be taught not only what they should not do, but even more important what they will be able to do. As the value of activity to the health of the heart is coming to be appreciated, more emphasis is being placed on what the patient can do rather than what he cannot do.

When a person with heart disease is obese, weight reduction is usually advised. The importance of loss of weight can be interpreted in graphic terms. A person who is 50 lb overweight is carrying the equivalent of a 50-lb sack of flour around with him all the time. Moreover, his already impaired heart must move blood through the adipose tissue. One figure cited is that each pound of fat contains seven tenths of a mile of capillaries. In 50 lb, there are, therefore, 35 miles of capillaries.

Because the degree to which the functional capacity of the heart is impaired varies among individuals, various systems of classification have been developed. The one cited below was developed by *The Criteria Committee of the New York Heart Association,* fifth edition. The classifications listed below are therapeutic classes. Functional classes (I-I) have been defined. They reflect the patient's ability; therapeutic classes are an indication of what he should do.

Class A. Patients with cardiac disease whose physical activity need not be restricted.
Class B. Patients with cardiac disease whose ordinary physical activity need not be restricted, but who should be advised against severe or competitive physical sports.
Class C. Patients with cardiac disease whose ordinary physical activity should be moderately restricted and whose strenuous efforts should be discontinued.
Class D. Patients with cardiac disease whose ordinary physical activity should be markedly restricted.
Class E. Patients with cardiac disease who should be at complete rest, confined to bed or chair.

Over the last 15 or 20 years studies, such as the one performed in the work classification unit at Bellevue Hospital, have demonstrated that many patients with heart disease can continue to be productive.[37] Studies have also been made of the energy requirements for various activities.[38] Whether or not a person who has recovered from acute cardiovascular disease will be able to perform a particular job depends on many factors other than the amount of energy it requires. These include his work experience, emotional status, temperament, and dexterity. Some patients do not require any change in work.

[37] "Cardiac Work Classification Unit," *Heart Bulletin,* II, September-October, 1953, pp. 99-100.
[38] Edward E. Gordon, "Rehabilitation of the Cardiac Patient," *Heart Bulletin,* VII, November-December, 1958, pp. 108-10.

Sometimes the patient can continue in the same job, but he needs to alter the way in which he approaches his work or the manner in which it is performed.

An example of the latter is the housewife who suffers from heart disease. Considerable work has been done in recent years by the American Heart Association to help the housewife with heart disease evaluate her methods of housekeeping and to plan her house and work so that unnecessary work is eliminated and the work she does is performed as easily as possible. In some communities, classes sponsored by the local heart association are taught for housewives. They and their husbands can learn how to evaluate and improve housekeeping methods.

Rehabilitation services are available to patients with heart disease through the Office of Vocational Rehabilitation or the American Heart Association. The first can usually be contacted through the state health department, and the latter through the local heart association. At least as important as the rehabilitation of adults is that of children with heart disease. Career planning considering the limitations of the child is important. Emphasis on what the child may do is an essential aspect of helping him realize a productive life.

Exactly what each person who has heart disease will be able to do is related to him as an individual. The consensus at the present time is that many patients can do something worthwhile. Perhaps the greatest deterrent is fear and misinformation about the effects of exercise on the heart. The first step with each patient is to help him to develop a healthy and optimistic attitude. Most people in the American society want to be productive and want an opportunity to do something constructive. One of the standards by which they judge their productiveness is that they are economically self-supporting. The stress arising from continued inactivity and dependency may be as great as or greater than that involved in useful work.

Families also need help in interpretation both of the patient's limitations and of his strengths. Nurses can often reinforce the recommendations of the physician and assist the patient and his family members to make reasonably realistic plans. This is as important when the family tends to overprotect the patient as when they push him too hard. It is difficult to remember when the life of a loved one appears to be threatened "that there is a breadth to life as well as a length. There is no area in a straight line."

The patient in congestive heart failure is subject to certain hazards, some of which can be prevented, minimized, or at least delayed. Eventually, most patients who have experienced heart failure no longer respond to therapeutic measures; congestive failure becomes intractable and the patient dies. Death may be due to the failure of the heart as a pump or to a complication arising from the effects of heart disease and/or its treatment. For example, pulmonary infarction is not an infrequent complication in both acute and chronic heart disease. The source of the embolus is usually a thrombus in the veins of the legs. As stated earlier, passive and active leg exercises, regularly performed, supporting bandages, and footboards are preventive measures.

The heart may also be the source of emboli. Thrombi in the left heart may form emboli that occlude cerebral or renal arteries or arteries supplying the lower extremities. Signs and symptoms depend on the structures deprived of their blood supply.

To sum up: In the preceding pages some of the causes, effects, and types of failure of the heart as a pump have been reviewed. Congestive heart failure is a common medical problem. It can result from any disorder which places an abnormal burden on the heart, lessens its nutrition, or interferes with the metabolic machinery of the myocardium. When the pumping mechanism of the heart is unable to adapt its output to the needs of the tissues, all tissues suffer. In the beginning the patient experiences symptoms when he performs activities that he was formerly able to do easily. Eventually the manifestations of disturbed cerebral, respiratory, renal, gastrointestinal, and liver function as well as disturbances of other structures become evident. One of the important objectives of therapy is to reduce the load placed on the pumping mechanism of the heart until the myocardium recovers some degree of cardiac reserve.

What factors enter into the regulation of cardiac function?

Heart muscle is similar to other muscle in that it is irritable or excitable; it is capable of responding to stimuli. It differs from skeletal muscle inasmuch as its refractory period (the period of recovery following contraction when it will not respond to stimuli) is relatively long. The prolonged refractory period protects the heart muscle from remaining in a continuous state of contraction and thereby interrupting the circulation.

One of the most important characteristics of heart muscle is its capacity to contract independently from the nervous system. Unlike the muscles of respiration and other skeletal muscles, the heart continues to contract even when it is removed from the body. The mammalian heart does not continue to function for more than 30 minutes unless provisions are made to supply it with oxygen. When oxygen is supplied, the heart can be kept contracting for several hours. In vitro studies (made in a test tube) using mammalian myocardial cells show that they contract in the tissue culture fluid. Amphibian hearts beat for 24 or more hours provided they are perfused with frog Ringer's solution. In the past the property of automaticity, that is, the capacity to initiate their own contraction, was thought to be the property of all myocardial cells. Recent studies made by Harary[39] indicate that there are two types of heart cells. One type, which he calls leading cells, beat spontaneously. The other, or following cells, beat only on contact with a leading cell.

The property of automaticity and rhythmicity facilitates survival when there is a failure of conduction of impulses from regulatory centers to the muscle of the ventricle. Normally the lead cells scattered throughout the myocardium follow the lead of higher regulatory centers. When for some

[39] *Op. cit.,* p. 148.

reason one or more groups of cells become abnormally irritable, they may initiate ectopic beats and create abnormalities of rhythm. Whether or not these are of a minor or serious import depends on the cause and the effect they have on the heart rate. When the connection between the higher and lower lead cells is disrupted, the latter may take over and maintain the heart beat. The resulting rate is slower than the normal rate.

Before presenting disorders in the rate and rhythm of the heart, however, the system for the regulation of the heart will be discussed. The function of the heart is regulated in relation to the activity of the body as a whole. Circulatory and respiratory functioning are also synchronized. The various components of the circulatory system are regulated in relation to each other.

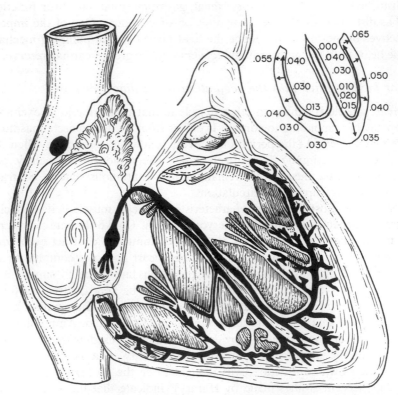

FIGURE 9–6. Diagram of the atrioventricular bundle of His. The atrioventricular (A-V) node can be seen near the opening of the coronary sinus in the right atrium. At the upper end of the ventricular septum the bundle divides. The two branches run down in the ventricular septum and give off many smaller branches to the papillary muscles and to the muscular walls of the ventricles. Bundle indicated in red. Part of the sinoatrial (S-A) node is seen in red between the base of the superior vena cava and the right auricular appendix. The tip of the left ventricular chamber is not shown. The figures in the small inset indicate the time in seconds taken for the nerve impulses to reach the areas indicated. (Adapted with permission of The Macmillan Company from *Anatomy and Physiology*, 14th ed., Fig. 261, p. 368, by Diana Clifford Kimber, Carolyn E. Gray, Caroline E. Stackpole, and Lutie C. Leavell. Copyright © The Macmillan Company, 1961.)

Heart rate and blood pressure are adjusted in relation to each other. The coordination of heart rate and blood pressure is stated in Marey's law: as the heart rate rises, reflexes are initiated to decrease the blood pressure. As the blood pressure rises, the heart rate slows. When either the pulse rate or the blood pressure rises, the other falls. Integration of the activity of the heart with the activity of the body as a whole is under the control of the autonomic nervous system. Stimulation of the sympathoadrenal system increases the rate of the heart and also dilates the coronary arteries. Stimulation of the vagus nerve slows the heart. The heart is also responsive to the hormonal and chemical conditions in the body.

Within the heart itself are specialized cells that have as their function the conduction of impulses over the entire heart. (See Figures 9-6 and 9-7.) Because atria and ventricles are separated by fibrous connective tissue, impulses do not spread directly from one to another as they do in smaller animals such as the frog. In the healthy heart the contraction is initiated in the sinoauricular node. In Figure 9-6 it can be seen to lie just under the superior vena cava. From the sinoauricular node the impulse spreads over the atria and to the auriculoventricular node. As the impulse passes over the atria, contraction begins. After a slight delay, the impulse passes from the auriculoventricular node over the bundle of His and the branching Purkinje system to the muscle fibers of the ventricles. Although all the cells in the conducting system including the lead cells in the myocardium are capable of initiating myocardial contraction, in health they do not. The gradient or irritability of

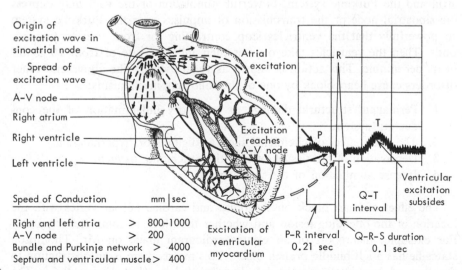

FIGURE 9—7. Diagram showing the conduction system of the heart. Impulses are initiated at the S-A node. As the wave of excitation travels through the conduction system, its relation to a tracing of a normal electrocardiogram is shown. (Adapted with permission of The Macmillan Company from *Textbook of Physiology,* 14th ed., Fig. 73, p. 187, by Caroline E. Stackpole and Lutie C. Leavell. Copyright 1953 by The Macmillan Company.)

cells of the regulating system diminishes from the sinoauricular node downward. To be more specific, in health the cells of the sinoauricular node initiate from 70 to 80 impulses per minute, while the lead cells in the ventricles initiate about 35 impulses per minute. Because the higher leading cells initiate impulses more rapidly than those in the myocardium and the refractory period of the myocardium is relatively long, the impulses arising from the sinoauricular node control rate and rhythm.

What are some of the causes and effects of heart block?

As a result of disease, the passage of impulses over the conduction system may be impeded or completely blocked or obstructed. The most frequent causes of complete heart block are coronary arteriosclerosis and carditis (inflammation of the heart) associated with rheumatic fever and diphtheria. Digitalis poisoning may also be responsible. Hyperkalemia (excessive level of potassium in the blood) may precipitate heart block. When complete heart block is associated with hyperkalemia, myocardial irritability is decreased, the rate is usually slow, the duration of systole is prolonged, and the heart is in imminent danger of stopping in diastole.

Heart block may be induced by powerful stimulation of the vagus nerve. The parasympathetic nervous system, by way of the vagi, provides few fibers to the ventricles. It sends most of its fibers to the atria. The effect of stimulation of the vagi is to slow the heart by decreasing the rhythm of the sinoauricular node and by decreasing the excitability of the fibers lying between the atria and the Purkinje system. Powerful stimulation of the vagi may depress the sinoatrial node or the transmission of impulses over the Purkinje system so powerfully that the ventricles stop contracting for from four to ten seconds. Then the ventricles take over at their inherent rate of from 10 to 35 beats per minute. This action is known as vagal escape. The above and other disorders cause heart block by one of the following mechanisms:

1. Permanent structural damage or transitory inflammation of the conducting system.
2. The toxic effect of chemicals such as digitalis or hyperkalemia.
3. Deprivation of the tissues of nutrition, including oxygen.
4. Intense stimulation of the vagus nerve.[40]

The effect of heart block on the pulse and cardiac output varies with the location of the offending lesion and whether the block is complete or partial. For example, the report of an electrocardiogram made on Mr. Thompson states he has a left bundle branch block. This means there is an obstruction to the flow of impulses over the left bundle of His. (See Figure 9-6.) The

[40] Calvin F. Kay, "Clinical Principles," Cecil-Loeb, *Textbook of Medicine*, 11th ed., Paul B. Beeson and Walsh McDermott (eds.), W. B. Saunders Company, Philadelphia, 1963, p. 738.

blocking was caused by a myocardial infarction. The underlying disorder is coronary atherosclerosis and is not uncommon among the elderly. Because only one branch of the bundle of His is interrupted and the muscle fibers are in continuous sheets around the heart, the major way bundle branch block can be detected is by electrocardiogram. Left bundle branch block can, however, be detected by auscultation. (There is a paradoxical splitting of the second heart sound.) There is no detectable alteration of the pulse rate or rhythm of the pulse.

In partial heart block; the effect on the pulse rate and rhythm depends on the rate at which impulses are initiated by the sinoauricular node (and other irritable sites) and the extent to which impulses reach the ventricles. For example, if every other impulse fails to reach the ventricles, then the auricles will contract twice for every contraction of the ventricles. This is known as a two-to-one block. The pulse will be regular in rate and rhythm. In other instances, the auricles may contract three times to every two times the ventricles beat—a three-to-two block—the rhythm is regular inasmuch as the same pattern recurs. It is abnormal, as the length of time elapsing between the contractions following the blocked impulse or preceding the next regular contraction is greater than normal. The force of each contraction varies with the length of the interval between beats. The greater the interval, the more time the heart has to fill during diastole and the more forceful the contraction during systole. When the patient is aware of the forceful contraction, he may interpret this as the heart skipping a beat. He is not likely to be aware of the missed beats.

In instances of complete heart block in which the flow of impulses from the atrioventricular node to the ventricle is interrupted and an irritable focus is established in one of the ventricles, the usual heart rate is about 35 beats per minute. It may, however, be as low as 15 or 20. Death occurs after complete heart block unless an irritable focus in one of the ventricles takes over promptly. Sometimes life can be saved after cardiac arrest by applying electrical impulses to the chest wall until the natural pacemakers take over. Even more recently a technique for applying external cardiac massage so circulation is maintained until the heart resumes contracting has been introduced. Both procedures require knowledge and training. Neither should be light-heartedly undertaken. References on external cardiac massage, including those questioning its practice by nurses, are included in the References.

For patients who are unable to maintain a heart rate adequate to their needs, an artificial pacemaker may be applied more or less permanently. Electrodes are introduced into the myocardium and connected to a transistorized battery located in the peritoneal cavity. Since the connecting wires are placed under the skin, none of the device is exposed. Patients are taught to count their pulse and to report to their physicians when the rate changes.

After the ventricles establish their own rate in heart block, the rate of contraction may be adequate not only for survival, but also for comfort at rest or even during activity. Although the heart rate is slowed, the output at each contraction is increased. The body adapts its metabolic rate to the quantity of materials delivered to its cells. Some patients are able to lead active lives if they avoid overexertion. Others, particularly those with excessively slow rates, have difficulty in adapting. They experience dizziness and dyspnea on exertion and have attacks of syncope (fainting). Until the heart rate becomes established at a sufficiently rapid rate, they may also have convulsive seizures. The point should be emphasized, however, that complete heart block by itself may be completely asymptomatic and require no treatment (e.g., congenital or post-diphtheritic chronic heart block) and the patient may lead a normal, active life. Symptoms occur and treatment is indicated when (1) the rhythm is irregular (asystole or runs or irregular rhythm), or (2) the rate is excessively slow.

When the patient continues to have frequent attacks of syncope, drugs increasing the irritability of the heart muscle may be injected subcutaneously. One such drug is epinephrine, 0.5 to 1 ml of epinephrine, 1:1,000 solution. Since its effects last only one to two hours, its action can be prolonged by giving it in oil. Other drugs that may be useful in the treatment of the patient with chronic heart block include ephedrine sulfate, 20 to 30 mg three times daily. It has the advantage of oral administration. In general, sympathomimetic agents are useful. Atropine is useful in some patients as it lessens the effect of the vagus nerve by depressing the effector substance responding to vagal stimulation. The nurse has the obvious responsibility of making certain that the patient gets his medications regularly, that his questions about them are answered by herself or his physician, and that he and his family understand why they should be continued—if they are to be—after his discharge from the hospital.

As with all patients, the nurse has a responsibility for the safety of the patient. Until heart block is stabilized, he is subject to syncope. To help lessen its likelihood, he should be taught to avoid sudden and rapid movement and straining. Changes in position, especially from the prone to upright, should be made slowly. Both to reassure the patient and to protect him from injury, the nurse should plan to have someone present when he gets out of bed.

Since any disorder in which the heart is involved carries with it the implication of the possibility of sudden death, most patients will also experience feelings of being unsafe. Attention should therefore be directed toward trying to increase the patient's feeling that, inasmuch as is possible, his needs will be met.

*In addition to heart block, what are other disturbances in
the rate and rhythm of the heart?*

In addition to the obstruction of impulses over the conduction system, other disturbances in the rhythm of the heart may arise because of hyperirritability of leading cells some place in the heart. According to Harary,[41] the cells that control and regulate the contraction of the myocardium are those that are initiating impulses at the most rapid rate. When cells other than those in the sinoatrial node become hyperirritable, they regulate the rate and rhythm of the heart. Theoretically, any group of cells can, therefore, regulate the beating of the heart. The site at which impulses originate can be identified by an electrocardiogram.

In what conditions does tachycardia occur?

The most frequent change in the rate of the heart is an increase, or tachycardia. Although an irritable focus in any part of the heart may be responsible for an acceleration in rate, the usual site is the sinoatrial node. When an increase in rate is initiated by the sinoatrial node, the condition is called sinus tachycardia. An acceleration of the heart rate is a normal response to any condition in which the metabolic needs of cells are increased or in which there is some defect in the processes involved in supplying cells with needed substances. Conversely, the pulse rate tends to fall when the condition initiating the rise is relieved. Like other homeostatic responses, a rise in the pulse rate is physiological as long as it is initiated by an appropriate stimulus, is maintained within limits, and continues only as long as needed. The pulse rate can be expected to rise during exercise, with the ingestion of food, and as a result of excitement, fear, or anxiety. Tachycardia usually accompanies diseases in which there is fever or a rise in the metabolic rate, such as hyperthyroidism. In patients who have been ill for some time, particularly when they have been on bed rest, tachycardia associated with exercise may be excessive and the pulse rate slow to return to resting levels. Nurses should, therefore, check the pulse rate of patients whose activity is being increased. Should tachycardia occur or be sustained, the activity of the patient should be decreased and then increased more slowly.

As stated above, the heart rate may be accelerated by fear and anxiety. Conversely, an increase in the heart rate may also be responsible for anxiety, particularly when the patient is conscious of the increase in rate and when it is accompanied by pounding. For example, Mrs. Almond is a tense woman who suffers from periodic attacks of tachycardia accompanied by palpitation and a "smothery" feeling. As far as she knows there is no relationship between the onset of an attack and any particular activity. Despite repeated reassurance on the part of her physician that she has a healthy heart, she continues to have what she calls "spells." During an attack she responds well to kindly and firm reassurance that she is not having a heart attack and to recognition of her obvious discomfort. Mrs. Almond's heart is believed to be responding to an impulse originating in her mental apparatus and affecting her heart by way of the accelerator nerves of the sympathetic nervous system. Her physician ex-

[41] *Op. cit.*, p. 150.

plains Mrs. Almond's symptoms to her by saying her nervous system is playing tricks on her. It is behaving as if she were in danger despite the lack of any
obvious danger in her external environment. Because Mrs. Almond's attacks
are infrequent and are of short duration, she is treated by supportive reassurance. In patients who are incapacitated, psychotherapy may be advised.

What are the common types of disturbance in the rhythm of the heart?

Although there are a number of disturbances in the rhythm of the heart,
only three types are of common occurrence. These are sinus arrhythmia,
premature beat, and auricular fibrillation. Sinus arrhythmia occurs in most
healthy children and adolescents. During inspiration the pulse rate speeds up;
during expiration it slows down. In a healthy young person, these changes in
the rhythm of the pulse are of no significance. Knowledge of this fact should
be useful to nurses working in schools. When a child's pulse speeds up as he
inhales and slows during exhalation, there is no cause for concern.

Premature beats are also a common phenomenon. They may arise from an
irritable focus in the atria, in junctional tissues, or in the ventricles. Though
they are more common in persons who have structural disease of the heart,
they are not infrequent in healthy persons. Why they occur in the healthy
heart frequently cannot be determined. Sometimes they can be shown to be
related to such factors as emotional stress, or the excessive use of coffee, tea,
or tobacco. Some individuals have attacks of premature beats during minor
infections, such as the common cold.

As indicated by its name, a premature beat is one that occurs before the
next contraction is due. It is ordinarily followed by an abnormally long interval. The normal contraction does not occur because the heart is in the refractory period at the time the normal impulse is initiated. The contraction
following the premature beat is stronger than those occurring at normal intervals. The patient may be conscious of the disturbance in rhythm.

Sometimes the premature beats may come in groups and regular rhythm is
restored by exercise. Some times, premature beats occur regularly between
normal beats and do not thereby cause a disturbance in rhythm, though they
do double the heart rate. This is known as a bigeminal rhythm. Its usual cause
is digitalis toxicity.

The treatment of premature contractions depends on their cause. When
they occur infrequently and there is no evidence of organic heart disease, no
treatment is usually necessary. When the physician believes excessive use of
coffee, tea, or tobacco may be a contributing factor, their influence can be
tested by eliminating them temporarily. In tense and anxious patients premature beats can sometimes be abolished by a mild sedative or tranquilizer.
When they occur in patients receiving digitalis, the digitalis should be discontinued for a few days. According to Harrison and Resnik,[42] a meal high in

---

[42] *Op. cit.,* 4th ed., p. 1398.

carbohydrate may precipitate premature beats in patients receiving digitalis. This is apparently related to a low level of potassium in the blood. When this is true, the premature beats disappear when the patient is given potassium chloride, 3 to 6 gm daily in divided doses. When patients being treated with digitalis develop irregularities in pulse, they should be recorded and reported to the patient's physician before another dose is administered. As stated previously, the carbohydrate content of the diet should also be reviewed. Particularly around holidays such as Thanksgiving and Christmas, patients should be cautioned to avoid eating a large quantity of sweets.

To recapitulate, premature beats are contractions of the heart arising from an abnormal focus in the heart that initiates a contraction before a normal one is due. The condition, though more frequently associated with structural changes in the heart, also occurs in persons who have no evidence of heart disease. The effects on the individual depend on the frequency with which premature beats occur and the extent to which they interfere with his capacity to function. In persons with organic heart disease, an increase in the heart rate due to premature beats may lead to a decrease in cardiac efficiency and predispose to failure. The needs of the patient will depend on the causative factors as well as his cardiac status.

Describe auricular fibrillation. What are its effects?

The most common cardiac arrhythmia to require therapy is auricular fibrillation. In this condition the muscle fibers of the auricles contract independently of each other with the result that the surface of the auricles appears to quiver. Authorities do not agree as to what causes fibrillation. An old theory states fibrillation is due to the circular movement of contraction over the muscle of the atria. An impulse starts at one point and continues in a circular fashion over the same tissue. A newer theory gaining acceptance is that auricular fibrillation, like other cardiac arrhythmias, arises from areas of abnormal irritability.

Whatever mechanism is responsible, auricular fibrillation has a number of adverse effects on cardiac function. Fibrillation of muscle renders it ineffective as a source of power. The most serious effect is that the conduction system is bombarded with impulses. They are both frequent and irregular. Not all these impulses result in myocardial contraction. Many of them fail to stimulate contraction because the conducting system or the myocardium is in the absolute refractory period at the time of their arrival. Even so, the myocardium does respond to many of them with the result that the pulse is rapid and totally irregular. Both the strength of contraction and distance between beats vary from one beat to another. There is no predictable pattern of rhythm.

When the interval between beats is very short, ventricular contraction may be too feeble to force open the aortic semilunar valves and drive blood into the arteries. The energy expended in each ineffective contraction is wasted. This places an additional burden on the heart. One measure of the extent to which ventricular contractions are ineffective is the pulse deficit. The pulse deficit is most accurately determined by the simultaneous counting of the ventricular and pulse rates. One person counts the ventricular rate using a stethoscope. Another counts the pulse at the wrist. When two people are not available, it can be approximated by counting first one and then another. Because of the highly irregular pulse, the pulse and the apical rate should be counted for at least a minute. The determination of the pulse deficit is often delegated to the nurse. The results are used to evaluate the extent to which the heart is wasteful of its energy and, perhaps most significantly, to evaluate the effectiveness of treatment.

When auricular fibrillation continues over a period of time, congestive heart failure is likely to be precipitated. Treatment is therefore usually instituted to restore the normal rhythm or to lessen the effect of the abnormal one. Despite the seeming appropriateness of directing therapy toward correcting the fibrillation, this is not always possible or even desirable. Stasis of blood in fibrillating atria predisposes to mural thrombosis which may be dislodged if effective contraction is restored. When auricular fibrillation is newly established, the likelihood of mural thrombosis is minimal. Quinidine sulfate, U.S.P., B.P. may be prescribed because it lengthens the effective refractory period of cardiac muscle. It is not used when the patient is in congestive heart failure, because it decreases the force of cardiac contraction.

When quinidine sulfate, U.S.P., B.P. is prescribed for a patient, the directions left by the physician should be followed explicitly. It is a potentially dangerous drug,[43] because a considerable number of individuals are hypersensitive to it. Since it is an alkaloid of cinchona, it may also cause symptoms of cinchonism, or quinine poisoning. Because of the possibility of a dangerous hypersensitivity, the patient is given a test dose to determine his reactions to quinidine sulfate. He should be observed for tinnitus, vertigo, disturbances in vision, headache, confusion, skin rashes, nausea and vomiting, diarrhea, and abdominal cramps. The more severe manifestations of hypersensitivity are similar to those described earlier under acute anaphylactic reactions (see Chapter 4). Attacks of fainting as a result of ventricular standstill may also occur in patients taking quinidine sulfate U.S.P., B.P. Any patient being treated with quinidine sulfate should, therefore, be subject to careful and regular observation. Should any manifestation of hypersensitivity or toxicity be evidenced or an adverse change in the rhythm of the heart appear, the drug should be discontinued and the physician notified. The use of quinidine sulfate is not limited to the treatment of auricular fibrillation. It may be prescribed for patients with other disorders, in which there is hyperirritability of the heart muscle such as premature systole.

Digitalis is the most common drug to be employed in the therapy of auricular fibrillation. It does not usually abolish the fibrillation, but it slows the

[43] Louis S. Goodman and Alfred Gilman, *The Pharmacological Basis of Therapeutics,* 2nd ed., The Macmillan Co., New York, 1955, p. 717.

heart and lessens the pulse deficit. Its action and use are discussed with congestive heart failure.

What is the significance of ventricular fibrillation?

One cardiac arrhythmia, ventricular fibrillation, is incompatible with life because the ventricles are incapable of maintaining the circulation. Unless action is taken immediately and is effective in restoring ventricular contraction, death follows within a few minutes. Some of the causes of ventricular fibrillation are myocardial infarction, electrocution, and chilling of the heart. Ventricular fibrillation is one of the hazards of hypothermia. At a certain point in the warming or cooling of the heart, the myocardium becomes hyper-irritable and there is danger of fibrillation. Because of the possibility of ventricular fibrillation, patients must be continuously observed during hypothermia.

In addition to conditions previously mentioned such as alterations in the level of potassium ions a number of disorders predisposes to alterations in the rate and rhythm of the heart. In hyperthyroidism, the heart rate is increased as is the irritability of the myocardium. Output is increased and, when hyperthyroidism continues over a period of time, predisposes to high-output failure of the heart. These patients are sensitive to epinephrine, and ventricular fibrillation can result from its use.

The heart muscle is also very sensitive to the physical and chemical conditions of extracellular fluids. As stated earlier, myocardial function cannot be maintained for more than 30 minutes in the absence of oxygen. Sodium and calcium ions have marked effects on the action of the myocardium. See Chapter 8 for a discussion of the effects of the various electrolytes on function.

Summary

There are a number of other arrhythmias having their origin in hyperirritable foci in the lead cells of the heart. Since they are of less frequent occurrence, they are not discussed here. Essentially disturbances in conduction and in the function of pacemakers have one or more of the following effects. They alter the rate and/or rhythm of the heart. Serious disturbances in rate and rhythm of the heart may decrease the mechanical efficiency of the heart and lead eventually to a loss in cardiac reserve. When a patient has a mild type of arrhythmia, he may suffer needlessly unless he can be helped to understand there is no objective cause for concern.

What kinds of information can the physician obtain from an electrocardiogram?

A physician can often establish the nature and significance of an arrhythmia from a study of the patient and the character of his heart beat and pulse.

When he wishes to have additional information, he has an electrocardiogram performed (ECG). An electrocardiogram is a graphic record of the electrical activity of the heart. An electrocardiograph is a device that receives the electrical impulses as they vary during the cardiac cycle and transforms them into a graphic record.[44] This machine not only records changes in electrical activity, but it also makes the film so a given distance on it is equal to a known time interval. From the information obtained during an electrocardiogram it is possible to determine not only alterations in electrical activity, but changes in the timing of each phase in the cardiac cycle.

Similar to other diagnostic devices, an electrocardiogram has uses and limitations. It is useful in detecting alterations in irritability or excitability of the various parts of the heart, interference with conduction of electrical impulses over the heart, and areas of injury to the heart muscle. In the absence of some change in electrical activity, the electrocardiogram can be expected to be normal. A patient may have a normal electrocardiogram in the presence of heart disease. A patient might develop a myocardial infarction two days after a normal electrocardiogram.

A physician who has special training usually reads or interprets electrocardiograms. Nurses are, however, often interested in knowing what the record means. The electrocardiogram is made up of three components or waves. These are the P wave, the QRS wave, and the T wave (see Figure 9-7). The QRS wave really consists of three waves, the Q wave, the R wave, and the S wave. The P wave is caused by the electrical activity as the wave of contraction passes over the atria. The QRS wave or complex is the result of the electrical changes that take place in the ventricle during contraction. Both the P wave and the QRS waves result from depolarization of cells. The T wave occurs during the period in which the ventricles relax and recover from contraction, and the electrical activity of the heart is repolarized. Factors such as the height, shape, and timing of each wave are considered in the interpretation of an electrocardiogram. For example, in auricular fibrillation, the P wave is greatly altered. As the result of therapy with digitalis, the T wave becomes negative.

Although the nurse does not have the specialized knowledge required to interpret an electrocardiogram, she is frequently called on to prepare the patient who has not experienced the procedure before. The unknown is a common source of anxiety. In addition, any possibility of disease of the heart is anxiety-provoking in most people. Persons unfamiliar with electrocardiograms sometimes interpret the procedure as involving the passage of electrical currents from the machine to themselves, rather than the reverse. When the patient is conscious and able to communicate, the nurse has a responsibility to find out what the patient knows and thinks he knows and to correct frightening misconceptions.

[44] Albert A. Kattus, Jr., and E. Raymond Borun, in Best and Taylor, *The Physiological Basis of Medical Practice,* The Williams & Wilkins Company, Baltimore, 7th ed., 1961, p. 169.

To do this the nurse must know that the electrical activity is generated by the heart and transmitted to the surface of the body by blood and other tissues. Electrodes are applied to the patient and connected to wires or leads attached to the positive and negative terminals of the electrocardiograph. Lead I is recorded by connecting the negative terminal of the electrocardiograph to the right wrist and the positive terminal to the left arm. Lead II is attached so the electrode on the left leg connects with the positive terminal and the right wrist is connected to the negative lead. Lead III is recorded with the left ankle attached to the positive terminal and the left wrist is attached to the negative terminal of the machine. Sometimes a fourth electrode is applied to the anterior chest wall in order to study the various arrhythmias and the polarization and depolarization of the heart. Because the electrodes must adhere tightly to the skin, they are applied with a kind of jelly. This may cause a smarting sensation, but it does not damage the skin. Because the jelly is irritating, the nurse must remember to wash the patient's skin at the termination of the procedure.

What are the effects of failure in the coronary circulation?

Another way in which the heart may break down or fail is in its ability to maintain its own nutrition and oxygenation. Although the quantity varies with activity, an average of about 225 ml of blood flows through the coronary arteries each minute. The blood is carried to the myocardium by the right and left coronary arteries. Despite some individual differences, the left coronary artery supplies mainly the left ventricle, and the right coronary artery supplies the right ventricle. There are relatively few connections between the main coronary arteries. There are, however, many among the smaller branches.

As in other organs in the body, blood flow depends on the level of the blood pressure and the patency of the arteries. Although obstruction is by far the most frequent cause of ischemia of the heart muscle, any disorder resulting in a pathologically low blood pressure will be followed by myocardial ischemia. One of the threats to life in the patient in peripheral circulatory failure or shock is myocardial ischemia. As discussed earlier, a second, though less common, cause of failure to maintain the blood under a sufficient head of pressure is incompetency of the aortic semilunar valves. Aortic insufficiency may be the result of injury to the valves as the result of rheumatic fever or syphilis. An aneurysm of the ascending aorta may also be responsible. At one time all aneurysms of the aorta were believed to be due to syphilis. Arteriosclerosis may, however, also be responsible.

The most frequent cause of myocardial ischemia is disease of the coronary artery, due to coronary atherosclerosis. The importance of coronary artery disease as a cause of morbidity and mortality is emphasized by Dawber and Kannel,[45] who state that it accounts for two thirds of all heart disease in the

[45] Thomas R. Dawber and William B. Kannel, "Susceptibility to Coronary Artery Disease," *Modern Concepts of Cardiovascular Disease*, XXX, July, 1961, p. 671.

United States. According to Wright,[46] a million or more persons per year suffer myocardial infarctions. The exact number is not known because many cases are not recognized. Myocardial infarction is also the leading cause of death as well as a major cause of disability among those between the ages of 45 and 60 years of age. Some authorities now describe coronary heart disease as reaching near epidemic proportions. Awareness of its incidence is not confined to those in the health fields. One middle-aged man has encouraged his wife to return to school and prepare herself as a teacher, so that she will be prepared to support the family should this become necessary.

Among the misconceptions about coronary atherosclerosis is that it is a new disease. It is not, as evidence of it has been identified in the arteries of Egyptian mummies. Neither is this disorder confined to human beings. It occurs in dogs and other animals as well.

What causes atherosclerosis?

The simplest answer is that the cause is not known. From what has been learned about it, atherosclerosis will probably be demonstrated to be due to the interaction of diverse genetic and environmental factors when together their total effect is sufficient to produce the disease. At the present time a number of factors have been identified as being frequently associated with coronary atherosclerosis. For some of these, it is not known whether they are coincidental, causative, or dependent on other conditions within the individual. As with other chronic diseases, no single causative factor is likely to be identified as the sole necessary element. Some of these etiological agents may be controlled so that the onset of the disease is delayed. Currently a large amount of money, effort, and time is being spent in an effort to learn more about the causes and, hopefully, the prevention of coronary artery disease as well as the other effects due to atherosclerosis. Theories about etiological agents are being extensively and intensively explored. These studies range from those in which normally herbivorous animals such as the rabbit are fed diets high in fat to those in which the effect of the saturated and unsaturated fatty acids on blood fats in man is determined. Not only are individuals studied, but entire populations are studied to determine the nature of their living habits. The value of comparisons between two groups of people depends upon accurate knowledge and evaluation of the ways in which the population of the two groups are alike and different. The fact that the incidence of atherosclerosis is low in one group and high in another may be easy to establish. The significance of any one factor in its development is much more difficult to estimate.

When discussing the many factors contributing to the development of atherosclerosis, scientists sometimes say, somewhat facetiously, that the best

[46] Irving S. Wright, "Summary, Prevention and Control of Heart Disease," *American Journal of Public Health,* L, March, 1960, pp. 31-34.

protection against atherosclerosis is to have parents and grandparents who were resistant to it and to be a female. Both heredity and the female sex hormones offer protection. A number of environmental factors are also believed to influence its occurrence. Knowledge of these is important because they are subject to modification or control. These include emotional stress, insufficient exercise, smoking, excess carbohydrates and fats in the diet, and protein deficiency. There is a body of epidemiological and experimental evidence to support the theory that a high intake of fat accelerates the development of atherosclerosis. Some authorities believe fats composed of saturated fatty acids are the most serious offenders. Some unsaturated fatty acids, at least for a period of time, have a blood lipid lowering effect. In persons who have diseases such as diabetes mellitus, hypothyroidism and essential hypertension, atherosclerosis develops at an earlier age than in those who are free of these conditions. From these findings the conclusion that atherosclerosis develops as the consequence of the interaction of a number of factors seems sound.

Since the incidence of atherosclerosis including that occurring in the coronary arteries tends to rise with age, some authorities have in the past related it to the aging process. Evidence against this theory is that the disorder occurs in all age groups. It has been observed in the arteries of newborn infants. Atheromatous plaques have been demonstrated in the coronary arteries of young men dying in battle or as the result of an accident. Some persons who die in their eighties and nineties do not have any evidence of it. According to a *Special Research Report* of the American Heart Association, however, by middle age most Americans have some degree of coronary atherosclerosis.

Problems in the prevention of atherosclerosis and its sequellae relate to a number of factors. Atherosclerotic changes may be present for a long period of time without causing any demonstrable effect. Despite the presence of pathology individuals are frequently free of signs and symptoms of coronary disease. They are believed to be healthy by themselves and by others. Presently no method is available to identify those who have coronary artery disease, but who are apparently healthy, until blood flow is sufficiently impeded to impair the nutrition to the myocardium. A number of studies are under way that may provide information which will help the physician to identify those who are predisposed to coronary disease.

Not until the characteristic clinical manifestations of coronary artery atherosclerosis appear are affected individuals aware of it. Clinical evidence may occur in the twenties and thirties, though this is not common. After the age 40 in men and approximately 15 years later in women, the incidence of overt coronary heart diseases rises. With the exception of women who are diabetic or hypertensive, coronary artery disease is unusual in women before the menopause. Following the menopause women lose their protection.

Because the etiology of atherosclerosis is uncertain, prevention consists of controlling the factors that are associated with it. According to the current hypothesis, control of atherosclerosis is predicated on long-term change in food, exercise, smoking, working, and living habits. If one word were to be used to summarize all of the above, it would be moderation. There is not at this time, and may possibly never be, any magic substance that will prevent the formation of atheroma in the coronary or other arteries of all people. There are, however, measures known to be effective in preventing some heart attacks. Possibly, the prevention of heart attacks is even more important than their cure, since a sizable proportion die during their first attack. It has been demonstrated that a heavy smoker who stops smoking can decrease the risk of having a heart attack. The possibility of a heart attack is also lessened by weight reduction in the obese. The maintenance of a desirable weight by diet and exercise is necessary. Hypertension, which predisposes to both congestive heart failure and to atherosclerosis, can be controlled by drugs. *The American Heart*[47] quotes Warren as saying that the death rate from hypertension and related heart disease has fallen 44 per cent between 1950 and 1960. This drop is attributed to be largely due to the availability of drugs to control hypertension. Thus through the control of conditions contributing to the development of coronary artery disease, its incidence can be reduced.

Since the incidence of atherosclerosis is higher in populations in which the level of cholesterol in the blood is high than it is in populations where the average level is low, some authorities suggest that the total intake of lipids in the diet should be controlled. Dale[48] recommends that fats comprise no more than 25 to 30 per cent of the food intake. Since this quantity exceeds that ingested by some groups such as Italians and Spanish, it is judged to be compatible with health.

There is some disagreement about the relative importance of the type of fat ingested to the development of atherosclerosis. Some authorities are of the opinion that more than half of the fat should be in the form of unsaturated fatty acids. Others are of the opinion that the most important consideration is the total consumption of fats. Since the liver synthesizes cholesterol, there will always be some cholesterol in the blood, whatever the intake of fat or cholesterol-containing substances. Although agents such as the estrogens have a cholesterol lowering effect upon the blood, and heparin lowers the total blood lipids their use is limited to those who have a greater than average predisposition to atherosclerosis. Many men find estrogens unacceptable because of their feminizing effect. New chemicals are being developed with the hope that they will depress the level of lipids in the blood, without, at the same time, causing feminization.

To recapitulate, factors in the development of coronary heart disease are being studied intensively at the present time. Studies are also under way to try to develop tests whereby persons who are predisposed to the disease or

[47] *Op. cit.,* p. 3.
[48] Sebion C. Dale, "Dietary Fat, Blood Cholesterol, and Atherogenesis," *Heart Bulletin,* XV, September-October, 1961, pp. 87-88.

who are in its early stages may be identified. These persons may then be advised to undertake a regime designed to prevent or delay the onset of coronary heart disease. Though an individual cannot alter his heredity or body build, he can control the amount and type of food that he eats, the amount of exercise that he takes, whether or not he smokes, and the way he approaches the problems in his life.

Not only is there uncertainty about etiology and prevention of atherosclerosis, but not very much is known about the formation of atheromatous plaques. According to Mann,[49] three hypotheses are currently suggested to explain their development. He summarizes them as:

"1. Diet
     Stress   } Lipemia → Atherosclerosis → Clinical Event.
     High Blood Pressure
 2. Thrombosis → Atheroscelrosis → Clinical Event.
 3. Ground Substance Damage → Atherosclerosis → Clinical Event."

He states that the first is by far the most popular. According to the second hypothesis, the first event is the formation of a thrombus on the wall of the artery. This is followed by the formation of the atheromatous plaque and eventually the clinical event. The third hypothesis postulates some injury in the wall of the artery. Although the focal nature of atherosclerosis supports this theory, there is little other evidence in its favor.

In keeping with the first hypothesis, the formation of atheromatous plaques progresses somewhat as follows. After an indefinite period of lipemia plaques form in the subintimal tissue of one or more arteries. These plaques which are a yellowish color are formed of cholesterol, other lipids and of macrophages. Authorities are not agreed as to how the cholesterol gets into the intima. One theory is that it enters the intima directly from the blood. The other is that it is formed in the intima itself. According to the infiltration theory,[50] fatty particles flow constantly to and from the tissues forming the walls of the blood vessels. For some reason the rate of outflow does not keep up with the rate of inflow. Fatty particles accumulate at the junction of the media and the intima of the coronary arteries. One hypothesis offered to explain the site at which lipids are deposited is that the structures are congenitally defective. In the beginning, the accumulated lipids resemble those of the blood. As time goes on their character changes, and the proportion of cholesterol to other substances changes. The lipids, especially cholesterol and fatty acids, act as irritants or foreign bodies. They cause degeneration of the wall of the artery. This is accompanied by low grade inflammation, and eventually

    9 George V. Mann, "Current Trends in the Study of Atherosclerosis," *Heart Bulletin,* IX, March-April, 1960, pp. 21-23.
    50 Henry Kruse, Chairman, "Committee on Cultural, Societal, Familial, Psychological, and Genetic Influences," *Supplement to American Journal of Public Health,* L, October, 1960, p. 97.

the area may undergo calcification. The entire process results in the formation of raised areas (plaques) in the lumen of the artery, which in small arteries may be sufficient to cause obstruction. A second source of obstruction is that a roughened area may serve as a focus for the formation of a thrombus which then obstructs the artery. Hemorrhage into the atheroma may also precipitate the formation of a thrombus.

In addition to patchy changes in the walls of the blood vessels themselves, there is evidence that the factors contributing to their development also increase the coagulability of the blood and decrease fibrinolysis.[51] As a consequence of atherosclerosis, tissues may be partially or completely deprived of their blood supply. When the walls of arteries are weakened, aneurysms may form. In those vessels where thinning of the arterial wall is marked, the vessel may rupture and hemorrhage occur. Depending upon whether or not the blood supply to the tissue is gradually or suddenly decreased, the resulting ischemia that follows may not be accompanied by necrosis of the tissue supplied by the diseased artery. When the ischemia comes about slowly, the tissue atrophies and is accompanied by a decrease in its ability to function. For example, as a consequence of atherosclerosis of the coronary arteries, the blood supply to the heart muscle may decrease. As a result of a gradually diminishing blood supply, the capacity of the heart to move as much blood into the circulation as the tissues require diminishes. Relative ischemia of the lower extremities renders them vulnerable to trauma or other injuries that would normally be of little or no consequence. Atrophy of the brain is accompanied by a variety of changes including alterations in personality. The consequences may be serious when it occurs in individuals in responsible positions. The implications of ischemia were discussed previously in the chapter and were discussed in greater detail in earlier chapters.

Sudden obstruction of an artery is accompanied by tissue necrosis, such as occurs in myocardial infarction. The specific manifestations presented by the patient will, of course, depend upon the organ that is deprived of its blood supply and the extent of the collateral circulation in the region. The heart, the brain and the lower extremities are the most commonly affected organs.

In atherosclerosis, the abdominal aorta is the common site for the formation of aneurysms (an outward bulging of the wall). They are often small and are of no significance. When they are large, they may serve as a site for the formation of a thrombus or of rupture. With the occlusion of the abdominal aorta, the supply of blood to the lower extremities is diminished or shut off. If the occlusion occurs at the level of the renal arteries, renal failure develops rapidly. When occlusion develops gradually, the patient, usually a man, complains of cramping pains in the calf of his leg or in his feet on walking which is relieved with rest. Over a period of time, the distance that he is able to walk becomes shorter.

[51] William Dock, "Arteriosclerosis," in Harrison, *Principles of Internal Medicine,* 4th ed., 1962; *Op. cit.,* p. 1362.

The majority of infarcts in the brain are caused by a thrombus which develops on an atherosclerotic plaque. However, arteries in the brain are thinner walled than those in other parts of the body and are therefore susceptible to rupture when they become atherosclerotic. This is especially true when hypertension is also present. According to Hopps (*Op. cit.,* 110), hemorrhage into the brain is more serious than is thrombosis. Not only is a part of the brain deprived of its blood supply, but the blood escaping from the blood vessel damages the brain tissue. It also increases intracranial pressure directly or by increasing the osmotic particles in the area. The needs of patients experiencing these effects for nursing will be discussed in Chapter 13B.

Summary

Although authorities do not agree as to how the changes that lead to the development of atherosclerosis come about, two factors seem to be of importance. One relates to the changes taking place in the walls of arteries and the other to the tendency of blood to form clots or thrombi within blood vessels. The arteries in which atherosclerosis develops early or produces a serious degree of dysfunction are known. Atherosclerosis is found most frequently in the vessels in which there is a large amount of elastic tissue in the media. These include the aorta and its major branches, the larger arteries of the brain, and the coronary arteries. The changes developing in the proximal aorta occur relatively early in life and rarely cause any serious difficulty. The changes in the branches of the aorta, or in its distal portions, as well as those that occur in the arteries supplying the brain and heart, may have serious effects.

What complications are associated with coronary artery disease?

The preceding discussion applies equally well to atherosclerosis in any important artery in the body. Because the coronary arteries supply the heart muscle, atherosclerosis in these vessels creates problems related to the heart. Coronary artery disease carries with it the possibility of three complications: sudden death due to cardiac arrest or ventricular fibrillation, myocardial infarction, and angina pectoris. Not by any means all persons who have atheroma in their coronary arteries develop any of these. These conditions all result from the effects on the heart muscle of an inadequate supply of blood, that is, ischemia of the heart muscle. When there is death of myocardial cells, and the person survives, healing by fibrosis occurs. Ischemia of myocardial cells followed by fibrosis probably occurs more frequently than is generally appreciated, as hearts examined at autopsy of persons who have not had heart attacks are found to have areas of scarring. In addition to the possible loss of myocardial cells, ischemia of some parts of the heart may set up abnormal electrical changes which may be responsible in part for some of its effects.

What is the outstanding symptom in ischemic heart disease?

The major manifestation of ischemic heart disease is pain due to a deficiency of oxygen to the myocardium. Blood supply may be impaired or it may be completely blocked so that no blood reaches the muscle. Either partial or total blocking of the coronary arteries may be the cause of sudden death. The clinical picture differs depending on whether or not the heart muscle is partially or permanently and completely deprived of its blood supply and the extent to which it is ischemic. The condition in which blood supply is deficient, but not entirely lacking, is known as angina pectoris. Since in angina pectoris the capacity of the coronary arteries to adapt the supply of oxygen to the needs of the myocardium under varying degrees of activity is deficient, signs and symptoms are precipitated by physical or emotional stress. In contrast, when the blood supply is blocked signs and symptoms may or may not be precipitated by activity, but they are not relieved by rest. Though coronary atherosclerosis is the usual cause of these conditions, there are others. Furthermore, coronary atheroma may be present in the absence of either. Neither condition develops until the blood supply is sufficiently compromised to cause hypoxia of the heart muscle.

The term "angina pectoris" when translated literally means sore throat of the chest. Sprague[52] calls it the cry of the myocardium suffering from anoxia. Doyle[53] describes it as: "A discomfort or pain, occurring across both sides of the anterior chest wall or located centrally in the sternal region, brought on by effort, e.g., exercise, emotion, exposure to cold and wind. It may radiate to the left arm or both arms, the shoulders, the neck or jaw." The words used by different patients to describe the pain vary, for example, tight, heavy, pressing, burning, crushing, and numbing. This pain is usually promptly relieved by rest or nitroglycerine. Because of the severity of the pain most patients try to avoid activities that precipitate it.

With progressive occlusion of the coronary arteries, the blood supply is further impaired and angina is precipitated with less and less activity, or myocardial infarction occurs. The results are not always unfavorable, however. In many individuals, despite marked impingement on the lumen of coronary arteries, the blood supply to the heart muscle may be protected by the development of the collateral blood vessels as well as the recanalization of obstructed ones.

Toward what objectives is the therapy in angina pectoris directed?

The medical management of the patient who experiences angina pectoris is directed toward two objectives. One is to help the patient learn to regulate his

[52] Howard B. Sprague, "Coronary Heart Disease," *The Heart Bulletin,* I, September-October, 1952, pp. 73-75.
[53] Joseph T. Doyle, "Committee on Criteria for Diagnosis of Disease and Clinical Evaluation." Supplement to *American Journal of Public Health,* L, October, 1960, p. 21.

life so that his heart is protected from periods of anoxia. The other is to improve the blood supply to the myocardium. The patient who is obese is encouraged to reduce his weight. Circumstances causing nervous tension or emotional stress should be identified and avoided when possible. Although many physicians advise patients who smoke to stop, and some refuse to treat them if they will not, others encourage them to smoke sparingly, if they must smoke. Studies indicate that the death rate from coronary artery disease is significantly higher among those who smoke than among those who do not.[54]

The most frequently prescribed drug in the treatment of angina pectoris is nitroglycerine. It is equally useful in the prevention of pain induced by exercise or emotion. One patient wrote a newspaper columnist physician to thank him for making this fact known to her. She commented that she found the use of nitroglycerine to prevent pain even more beneficial than to provide relief. By relaxing the blood vessels, alcoholic beverages in small amounts are often helpful in the prevention of anginal attacks. Alcohol is particularly useful when taken at night to prevent nocturnal angina.[55]

The nurse can frequently be helpful to the patient in identifying those aspects of his life that require modification and in learning to follow the medical regime. The combination of a diagnosis of disease of the heart, the pain, and the knowledge that sudden death is a possibility is frightening to even the most stoic. Some patients fear taking any medication lest they become habituated to it. The modification of important aspects of life is not easy. Someone to talk to and to suggest possible alternatives may be helpful.

How does myocardial infarction differ from angina pectoris?

When blood flow is obstructed by coronary atherosclerosis so that no blood reaches the myocardium, myocardial infarction occurs. Mr. Anderson illustrates many of the characteristics of this disorder.

One morning shortly after eight o'clock, Mr. Anderson, a 60-year-old, native-born American, was admitted to Community Hospital. After arriving at work, he had collapsed. He stated that he had severe crushing pain in his chest radiating to his left shoulder. He might have employed any of the terms used to describe the pain of angina to characterize his pain. The pain differs from that of angina, however, inasmuch as it is a steady pain and is not relieved by rest or nitroglycerine. It frequently develops when the patient is at rest or some time following a meal or an activity. Mr. Anderson located the pain by placing his hand over his sternum and then moving it over his upper chest. The location of his pain is identical with that observed in angina pectoris. It might have radiated to the right shoulder and down either arm. The ancients noted the frequency with which pain radiated from the region of the heart down the left arm to the ring finger. According to legend, they believed that the left ring finger was directly connected to the heart, and this

---

[54] Howard B. Sprague, "What I Tell My Patients About Smoking," *Modern Concepts of Cardiovascular Disease*, XXXIII, October, 1964, pp. 881-4.
[55] Sprague, *Op. cit.*, p. 74.

belief is said to be the reason for placing the wedding ring on the left ring finger, thus securing constancy of affections.

What are the facts that have been presented about Mr. Anderson that are related to myocardial infarction?

As a male between the ages of 45 and 64, Mr. Anderson is in the age group in which the incidence of coronary arteriosclerotic heart disease is highest. In this age group, it causes about 85 per cent of the deaths due to heart disease and about two fifths of all deaths. In the decade just preceding, it caused about 80 per cent of the deaths due to heart disease. After 65 years of age, there is a moderate decline in the death rate from coronary arteriosclerosis.[56]

In addition to being predisposed by age to myocardial infarction, Mr. Anderson was also hypertensive. For a number of years his blood pressure had fluctuated between 150/90 and 200/100. He had taken medications to lower his blood pressure for the past two years. Since the problems of the patient who is hypertensive are to be discussed later, they will not be presented here. Two of his brothers died following myocardial infarction. Whether this was a coincidence or indicated a common genetic defect or the effect of a common environment is not known. Any of the above could be true. Certainly knowledge that his brothers had died after "heart attacks" could be expected to increase Mr. Anderson's anxiety during his illness.

Mr. Anderson was of average height, large-boned, and muscular. Though he was a big man he did not appear to be fat. His body type was that described by the term "mesomorph." Some authorities claim that the incidence of coronary heart disease is highest among this group.

Mr. Anderson's food intake was similar to that of other Americans of modest income. His wife stated that despite a preference for meat, he ate some of most other foods. His preference in meat was for beef that was well marbled with fat. For the past two or three years, his salt intake had been restricted. He had smoked up to two packages of cigarettes a day until his high blood pressure had been discovered. For a time he stopped smoking entirely. Recently, he had been seen smoking occasionally.

At one time his work required quite a bit of physical exercise. For the past ten years he had a sedentary job. Mr. Anderson's supervisor described him as a good and careful worker who arrived at work on time and did a full day's work. Though he bowled occasionally in the wintertime, and mowed the lawn in the summer, he got very little physical exercise. Despite his intentions to exercise regularly, he seldom walked when he could ride. He was too tired or there was not time to walk.

From this superficial survey of the life of Mr. Anderson, many of the factors that appear to be associated with coronary heart disease are seen to be a part of his life. They include a possible genetic predisposition to the disease,

[56] Metropolitan Life Insurance Company, *Statistical Bulletin*, XLII, March, 1961, p. 6.

body build, food and working habits, hypertension, lack of physical exercise, and smoking. These and other factors are presumed to have acted over time to lead to changes in his coronary arteries that were eventually manifested as a myocardial infarction.

Despite the fact that the onset appeared to be sudden, Mr. Anderson had had previous attacks of discomfort and mild pain in his chest. He had dismissed them by ascribing them to indigestion or to something that he had eaten. His reaction was by no means unusual. Neither is it unusual for patients to have attacks of pain before a myocardial infarction. According to Beamish and Storrie,[57] the reported incidence of warning symptoms is from 30 to 50 per cent. They also indicate that evidence is accumulating indicating that the incidence of sudden death and myocardial infarction can be prevented by the prompt administration of anticoagulant drugs. If this is true, it becomes important for men and women who have premonitory pain to report this pain to their physicians immediately. Characteristically, this warning pain occurs in a person who has been in good or relatively good health. He finds that he cannot walk very far before he has pain. He also has chest pain at night when he is at rest. If he takes nitroglycerine, the pain is relieved; but it takes increasingly larger doses to be effective. Nurses working in industry or elsewhere and in the community are not infrequently consulted by patients or their families. When an apparently healthy man or woman recites the above history, he should be encouraged to see his physician promptly for diagnosis. Should a myocardial infarction be impending, there is a possibility that it can be prevented. Should future studies demonstrate that myocardial infarction can be prevented, then the role of the nurse as a case finder and in public education will become increasingly important.

To return to Mr. Anderson, immediately after he collapsed in severe pain, the plant physician was called and Mr. Anderson was moved in a wheel chair to the plant infirmary. The physician prescribed morphine sulfate, gr ¼ (15 mg), to be given subcutaneously. Practice varies as to which particular analgesic is prescribed and the route selected for administration. Prompt relief of pain is important, as pain intensifies shock, which is always present in some degree in clinical myocardial infarction. Many physicians prefer that the drug be administered intravenously as no time is lost during the absorption of the drug and the full dosage can be expected to be effective. As a consequence of peripheral circulatory failure in shock, absorption from subcutaneous tissues may be so poor that the patient gets little or no relief. Later, as the circulation improves, the drug is absorbed. When repeated, but poorly absorbed, dosages are given, the patient may suffer from toxic effects. Although morphine was administered subcutaneously to Mr. Anderson, he experienced relief from his pain.

Besides pain, which was the predominant symptom at the onset of Mr.

[57] R. E. Beamish and V. Marie Storrie, "Impending Myocardial Infarction," *The Heart Bulletin*, X, May-June, 1961, pp. 41-44.

Anderson's illness, he also felt weak. Beads of perspiration stood out on his brow and his skin was an ashen gray in color. He complained of feeling short of breath. Shortly after his admission to the infirmary, his blood pressure dropped to 110/70. Some drop in blood pressure is common. Though Mr. Anderson was nauseated, he did not vomit. Both nausea and vomiting are also frequent symptoms. After an electrocardiogram confirmed the plant physician's diagnosis that Mr. Anderson had suffered a myocardial infarction, preparations were made to transfer him by ambulance to Community Hospital. Some physicians advise against moving seriously ill patients or those who are in profound shock.[58] During the period that follows the onset of clinical manifestations of myocardial infarction the patient is in danger of ventricular fibrillation and shock. Neither the heart nor the peripheral circulation can be depended on to respond favorably to increased demands made by moving or being transported to another location. Even minor stimuli can and often do worsen the patient's condition. The patient should therefore be protected in so far as possible from all emotional and physical stimuli. Despite the seeming importance of getting the patient to the hospital where he can be treated, the transfer should be made without hurry or a feeling of great urgency. There should be no fast driving over rough roads with the siren screaming. The atmosphere surrounding the patient should in so far as possible be one of calm and gentleness. Many modern ambulances are now equipped with oxygen and other lifesaving devices. These can be used as indicated. Attention should be directed to the patient and his responses.

In order to prepare Mr. Anderson for the move, the plant physician told Mr. Anderson that he should be transferred to Community Hospital where they had the facilities to care for him. Mr. Anderson asked that his wife be notified and that they try not to "scare her to death." Transfer was made promptly. Since the hospital had been called, emergency room personnel were expecting Mr. Anderson. At the time of his arrival, he had some, but not marked, chest pain. He was sweating profusely and his skin was cold to touch. His skin was ashen gray in color. His blood pressure had fallen to 100/80. Before he was transferred to a hospital bed for care, an electrocardiogram was made. This showed that Mr. Anderson had had a posterior myocardial infarct.

What is the possible sequence of events leading to myocardial infarction of Mr. Anderson's heart?

As emphasized previously, myocardial infarction usually is associated with coronary atherosclerosis. The sequence of events leading to the obstruction of the coronary arteries are discussed on pages 631-632. After a coronary artery is obstructed by a thrombus, cells in the myocardium die. Depending on the

[58] Milton Plotz, "Treatment of Acute Myocardial Infarction," *Heart Bulletin*, VII, May-June, 1958, p. 58.

size and location of the occluded vessel, the area of necrosis may extend to, and include, the endocardium and pericardium. Another consequence of arterial obstruction is an uneven distribution of blood to the myocardium. According to Beck,[59] this disturbance in the distribution of blood results in electrical changes; the electrical changes are responsible for the heart attack.

With the insult to the heart, the sympathetic nervous system is activated. When sympathetic reflexes are effective, arteries and veins in the peripheral circulation constrict, and blood pressure and circulation are maintained within reasonable limits. When the myocardial infarction is large or the mechanisms for adapting the diameter of the blood vessels are defective, then cardiac shock develops. As stated earlier, at the onset of symptoms, Mr. Anderson presented evidence of shock, and by the time of his admission to Community Hospital, he was in profound shock. If Mr. Anderson was to survive, the competency of his peripheral circulation had to be restored as soon as possible. Otherwise, tissue hypoxia, including hypoxia of the myocardium, with progressive deterioration of cell function occurs. Restoration of the circulation to the tissues, therefore, has a high priority in the management of any patient who has recently experienced a myocardial infarction. The improvement of the circulation is essential to the recovery of the heart and to the prevention of injury to other tissues.

In order to protect Mr. Anderson's heart from any unnecessary demands, Mr. Anderson's physician prescribed strict bed rest for him for 48 hours. This meant that Mr. Anderson was to do nothing for himself. He was to be washed, turned, and fed. His food intake was limited to fruit juices. Intake of water, including the intravenous solution, was not to exceed 1,500 ml. The only voluntary activity that he was permitted was to turn on his light or to ask his nurse for assistance. Insofar as was possible, his external environment was to be regulated so he was protected from all psychological, social, and physical stimuli. Visitors were restricted to the members of his immediate family. They were encouraged to sit quietly in his room or to sit on the sun porch.

As frequently occurs following a serious myocardial infarction, Mr. Anderson had pulmonary edema and was dyspneic. The head of his bed was therefore elevated, to lessen the dyspnea and therefore to promote rest. Morphine sulfate, 15 mg (gr ¼), was prescribed to relieve pain.

Despite the relief of his pain and despite bed rest, Mr. Anderson's blood pressure did not rise to a safe level. Therefore a vasopressor (blood pressure-raising) drug was prescribed. A variety of preparations are available. One of the most potent of these drugs is norepinephrine (Levarterenol or Levophed). It causes constriction of all blood vessels, except the coronaries, which it dilates.[60] It also increases the force of cardiac contraction and stroke vol-

---

[59] Claude S. Beck, "Coronary Artery Disease," *Heart Bulletin*, VII, March-April, 1958, pp. 22-24.

[60] Clarence M. Agress, "Heart Shock in Myocardial Infarction," *Heart Bulletin*, XI, March-April, 1962, pp. 25-28.

ume, as well as cardiac irritability. It diminishes renal blood flow. It must be administered intravenously, as it causes a slough when it infiltrates the tissues. It is rapidly destroyed and must therefore be administered continuously. Because of the problems involved in keeping a needle patent and to lessen the possibility of tissue infiltration, a cannula or catheter may be introduced into the vein rather than a needle. Because of the potency of norepinephrine, continuous observation is required.

There are a number of other preparations of vasopressor agents with similar, but not identical, effects. In general they are less potent than norepinephrine. Some of them have more sustained effects. Some do not injure the tissues with which they come in contact and can be administered by intramuscular or subcutaneous injection. Some do not increase the irritability of the heart muscle. Before supervising the administration of a vasopressor drug to any patient, the nurse should acquaint herself with the facts about the prescribed drug. The drug prescribed by the physician will depend on the condition of the patient and the physician's experience with and preference for a particular preparation.

Metaraminal (Aramine), 200 mg per liter of 5 per cent glucose in water, was prescribed for Mr. Anderson. In nonhypertensive patients, the critical level for the systolic blood pressure is 100 mm of mercury. In the hypertensive patient, it is somewhat higher. Following the administration of Metaraminal Mr. Anderson's blood pressure rose as expected.

Any patient who is receiving a potent vasopressor agent should be continuously attended by a competent nurse. The nurse has two general responsibilities: to lessen the demands made on the patient to respond to his environment and to observe the effects of the treatment—both therapeutic and toxic. Within the limits prescribed by the physician, she modifies the therapeutic regime. Vasopressor agents may fail to raise the blood pressure, or they may elevate it too much. Although the blood pressure rises, there may not be a comparable increase in tissue nutrition. In the absence of the latter they may be of no benefit to the patient. When they are administered in intravenous fluids, the rate of flow of the solution should be under constant surveillance. When the rate of flow is too slow, blood will clot in the needle or cannula. When it is too rapid, toxic doses of the drug may be delivered. In addition, the already feeble heart may be overburdened and the capacity of blood vessels to deliver blood restricted.

Even when the blood pressure is restored to physiological levels, the patient may still be in shock. The most sensitive index of shock is urine output. It should be at least 30 ml per hour.[61] In the mid-afternoon, Mr. Anderson voided 500 ml of urine. This, along with the stability of his systolic blood pressure at 120 mm of mercury, indicated that the shock had been relieved. His condition, however, continued to be critical.

A fourth measure prescribed for Mr. Anderson was the administration of

[61] Agress, *Op. cit.*, p. 28.

oxygen by tent. The presence of pulmonary edema was the most important indication for oxygen as congestion of the lung decreases its efficiency in oxygenating the blood. Attention to maintaining the concentration of oxygen in the tent at a therapeutic level was imperative. (See Chapter 7.) As sometimes happens, the administration of oxygen to Mr. Anderson was accompanied by some relief of pain. In addition to providing Mr. Anderson with a high concentration of oxygen, the tent made it possible to control the environmental temperature. Since the day was hot and humid, temperature control was of considerable benefit to him.

At no time should the fact that the patient is an individual human being be lost from sight. Despite the need for prompt and effective treatment, there is no place for hurry in the presence of the patient. The implications of the pain can be expected to provoke anxiety in the patient. The patient should not be permitted to suffer. If the prescription left by the physician for relief of pain is ineffective, he should be notified. Shifting from an independent, active state to a dependent, inactive one is a source of further anxiety and feeling of frustration. The very fact that strict bed rest is prescribed and every effort is made to enforce it tends to reinforce the patient's belief that he is seriously ill.

Mr. Anderson had been an active man. He found it frustrating to allow his nurse to feed him like a baby. The nurse tried to indicate that she recognized how he felt. After a day or so, arrangements were made for his wife to assist him with his evening meal. This also gave Mrs. Anderson a tangible way she could be of assistance to her husband.

At least a responsible member of the family should know that the patient is critically ill. Mrs. Anderson was so informed by the physician. Though he tried not to be too pessimistic, he did indicate the uncertainty of the outcome. Relatives of patients frequently require support and sympathetic understanding during this period.

For the first 24 to 48 hours, nursing care and medical therapy are both planned to eliminate, insofar as is possible, any demands on the patient to adapt to his environment. Care is also directed toward relieving shock and restoring the adequacy of circulation to his tissues. These objectives take precedence over all others, and unless they are accomplished, the patient will not recover. The length of time that the patient is kept on strict bed rest depends on many factors. For example, the patient who has been in definite shock is likely to be maintained on strict bed rest longer than the one who has not. Some physicians are more conservative than others.

After approximately two days, the regime of the patient who has recovered from the shock phase of the illness changes. Rest continues to be important, but bed rest is no longer essential provided certain precautions are observed and rest is achieved. Medical authorities directly and by implication emphasize the importance of competent nursing to the achievement of basal rest.[62]

[62] John LaDue, "Cardiac Failure and Function Tests," in Sodeman, *Pathologic Physiology,* 3rd ed., W. B. Saunders and Company, Philadelphia, 1961, pp. 574.

When a patient is allowed out of bed, he should be assisted in getting out of bed to the chair by two people. The chair should be placed beside the bed. One person should stand on each side of the person and assist him to a sitting position with his feet hanging over the edge of the bed. He should then be helped to a standing position, turned, and supported as he sits in the chair. He should not be allowed to walk until walking is prescribed by his physician. After he sits, his position should be checked to determine whether or not the chair is supporting him. If he is short, a footstool of the proper height should be placed under his feet. A chair of the proper depth should be selected, or if one is not available, a cushion should be placed behind his back so he is supported. Pressure against the calves of the legs is to be avoided. Chair rest carries with it one hazard; that is, the patient, his family, and even hospital personnel may assume that because he is up in a chair, he is no longer sick. Nothing could be further from the truth.

After two or three days the patient is usually allowed to use a bedside commode. He should be instructed not to strain or bear down during defecation (the Valsalva maneuver). To facilitate defecation, the physician may prescribe the patient's favorite laxative, provided it does not cause griping, or one of the stool softeners. The patient is soon allowed to feed himself and to comb his hair. Shaving himself may be delayed for a time. During this period the patient should be protected from unnecessary and preventable stress— physical as well as emotional.

What effects can be observed as a result of the absorption of the products of tissue necrosis?

Usually the pain which marks the onset of myocardial infarction disappears after a variable period of time. It does not usually last, however, more than 24 to 48 hours. Sometimes the acute pain disappears and is replaced by a dull ache that persists for a few hours to a day or so. Signs and symptoms that relate to tissue necrosis include: leukocytosis, fever, and an elevated sedimen-

Sign or Symptom	Period When it is Likely to be Abnormal	Usual Finding	Mr. Anderson
Pain	Variable to 48 hours	Steady Unremitting	18 hours
Leukocytosis	Begins a few hours after onset of pain. Usually returns to normal after the acute stress is over— 1 to 2 days	12,000 to 18,000	18,150 the evening of the first day
Sedimentation rate	Rate of elevation slower than leukocytes, lasts 3 to 4 weeks		42 mm per hour fifth day
Serum glutamic oxalacetic transaminase (SGOT) (8 to 40 units)	Usually begins to rise in 6 to 12 hours and reaches a peak within 24 to 48 hours. Subsides to normal in 3 to 4 days		146 units first day

tation rate. As the membrane around the myocardial cells becomes more permeable than normal or the cells disintegrate cellular enzymes are released into the blood with the result that their level is elevated.

In addition to the changes in the electrocardiogram, the intensity of the signs and symptoms presented by the patient is of value to the physician in predicting extent of injury to the heart. When any of them continue for longer than the expected period of time, this may indicate a new insult to the heart or the development of a complication. The expected changes, as well as the findings as they occurred in Mr. Anderson, are summarized on previous page.

From the history, clinical course, and laboratory findings, the physician concluded that Mr. Anderson had experienced a major myocardial infarct.

As myocardial cells degenerate, substances released in the area stimulate fibrosis, and a scar is formed. This scar is essentially the same as one formed in any part of the body. It serves as a patch to bridge the area of necrosis. Like scar tissue in other parts of the body, it does not perform the function of parenchymal tissue. Cardiac reserve is, therefore, decreased to the extent that muscle cells are lost. During the period of necrosis and until the scar is fully mature, the area of necrosis is weak. It is, therefore, liable to rupture or to an aneurysm. During systole the weakened area in the wall of a ventricle may give way rather than resist distention with the result that the heart does not empty completely. Furthermore when the myocardial reserve is sufficiently reduced by the loss of cells, the heart will no longer be able to adapt the circulation to the needs of the organism. Consequently, congestive heart failure may develop. Throughout the period of recovery, disturbances in the rate and rhythm of the heart continue to be a possibility.

One of the most serious problems during the convalescence of the patient is the possibility of intravascular clotting or thrombosis. Most, if not all, patients have more than one atheromatous plaque in their coronary arteries. Atheromatous plaques in arteries in other sites such as the brain or extremities may also serve as foci for the formation of blood clots. When necrosis extends to and includes the endocardium, the area is roughened and serves as a possible site for the formation of a mural thrombus. Whether or not there is an increase in the tendency of the blood to clot before the formation of the initial thrombus has been neither proven nor disproven. After a myocardial infarction, the possibility of intravascular clotting is increased. The tendency to thrombosis is intensified by the inactivity of the patient.

The implications of the diagnosis and the nature of the required treatment may also result in psychological complications. As emphasized earlier, the highest incidence of coronary heart disease is among men, and they are usually men, who are in the most productive years of their lives. They usually have families dependent on them for support. Moreover, among the implications of myocardial infarction are sudden death, the possibility of a life of invalidism, or at least major adjustments in life. These are all sources of psychological stress. Bed rest and inactivity are also accompanied by physiological and metabolic changes which are part of the total effect. Finally, the patient cannot help but be affected by the reaction of his family, friends, and business associates.

What aspect of any illness is of paramount significance varies with each individual patient. Few, if any, escape some feeling of depression. Even the patient who makes a great show of taking his situation lightly experiences some degree of depression. The patient may be making or appear to be making good recovery and be exceptionally cheerful, and yet be depressed. One patient typifies this point. He was boisterous and appeared to be carefree. About ten days after his admission, he was unusually quiet as the nurse bathed him. Finally he looked up at her and said, "I beat it [death] this time, didn't I? It was a close call, wasn't it?" His usual behavior was a front to cover his true feelings.

Summary

As discussed in the preceding pages, the most frequent threats to Mr. Anderson's life during the first 24 to 48 hours included ventricular fibrillation and arrest, pulmonary edema, extension of infarction, and shock. Other ventricular arrhythmias are also of serious import. The length of the period of acute illness varies. In a few hours a patient may be feeling well and be trying to assure himself and members of his family that nothing really happened or it was just an attack of indigestion. In some patients pulmonary edema and/or shock continues for several days or until the patient dies. Nursing care during this period is directed toward preventing any increase in the shock or pulmonary edema and supporting efforts for their relief.

What are some of the later effects of myocardial infarction?

As the heart muscle degenerates, rupture of the heart is a possibility. The danger is greatest from the ninth to fourteenth day. According to Harrison,[63] the danger is greatest in patients over 70 and the rupture is particularly common in older women. When the heart ruptures, blood escapes into the pericardial sac and prevents the heart from filling. Death occurs suddenly. To lessen the possibility of rupture of the heart, Mr. Anderson should be instructed to avoid straining and sudden movements. He should be assisted out of bed and with activities likely to increase venous return.

Two types of measures were utilized to prevent the formation of thromboses and the possibility of embolism. Mr. Anderson's physician ordered an anticoagulant agent, and stasis of blood in the extremities was minimized. Physicians vary in their opinion as to when an anticoagulant should be started and the preparation to be used. For coumarin compounds or phenindione to be used with safety, facilities need to be available to accurately check the patient's prothrombin time. When the patient continues on anticoagulant drug

[63] *Op. cit.,* 4th ed., p. 1453.

therapy over an extended period of time, he must continue to have his pro-thrombin time checked at regular intervals. The patient must understand and accept the importance of regular testing. Both inconvenience and expense are involved. Adequate medical supervision is also important. Before anticoag-ulant therapy is started, the patient's prothrombin time is determined. Shortly after Mr. Anderson was admitted, blood was drawn for the determination of his prothrombin time.

The specific anticoagulant preparation selected by the physician depends on the rapidity with which action is desired as well as other factors. Heparin acts immediately by depressing the conversion of fibrinogen to fibrin and prevents the agglutination of blood platelets. Neither heparin nor other anticoagulants dissolve already formed blood clots. The formation of new clots is prevented. Heparin is administered intravenously or subcutaneously with a small quan-tity of procaine, and the anticoagulant effect is controlled by clotting times.

Derivatives of coumarin or phenindione are generally prescribed for long-term anticoagulant effects. Since they depress the formation of prothrombin, their action is delayed and their effect persists over a longer period of time than that of heparin. The dosage for each patient has to be adjusted in relation to the effect of the drug on his prothrombin time. The objective of the therapy is to prolong the prothrombin time enough to decrease its tendency to clot and at the same time protect the patient from the danger of spontaneous hemorrhage or hemorrhage resulting from minor injuries. Similar to other bodily functions, there are limits within which the clotting of the blood can safely be extended. Mr. Anderson's preanticoagulant therapy prothrombin time was 15 seconds. The objective was to raise it to between 25 and 35 seconds. Prothrombin time within this range decreases the tendency to intra-vascular clotting without exposing the patient to unnecessary danger of hemorrhage.

The drug prescribed for Mr. Anderson was warfarin (coumadin). It was administered by mouth. Daily prothrombin times were performed. On the third day his prothrombin time was 66 seconds. The next day it was up to 75 seconds, and the fifth day 145 seconds. On each of these days the control was 15 seconds. On the fifth day the physician prescribed vitamin K, a precursor of prothrombin. The next day Mr. Anderson's prothrombin time had returned to 33 seconds. The possibility of hemorrhage was decreased to a correspond-ing degree.

The nurse has a number of responsibilities in the care of the patient on anticoagulant therapy. Until the dosage has been established, daily pro-thrombin times must be taken and recorded. When the prescribed drug is administered daily, the nurse should check the prothrombin time before administering it. Vitamin K should be readily available so it can be given promptly should it be required. The patient should be observed for evidence of bleeding. Hematuria and bleeding from the gastrointestinal tract, as well as from small injuries, may occur. When Mr. Anderson's prothrombin time was

145 seconds, the small injury caused by the venipuncture resulted in bleeding from the site. Pressure over the area was continued for ten minutes before the bleeding stopped. Should bleeding take place, the physician should be notified. With proper checking of the prothrombin time and adjustment in the dosage of the anticoagulant drug, the danger to the patient is minimized. Without adequate supervision, the patient may be exposed to serious harm. Supervision must be continued as long as anticoagulant therapy is continued. The nurse has a responsibility to ascertain whether or not the patient understands what procedure he should follow, and why. The patient should also understand why he should not alter the prescribed dosage.

The following instance illustrates the possible consequences of inadequate care of a patient under continued anticoagulant therapy. The patient, a 30-year-old woman, had mitral stenosis following rheumatic fever. After experiencing a cerebral vascular accident caused by an embolus originating from a thrombus in her left atrium, she was placed on anticoagulant therapy. She took the drug faithfully, but her prothrombin time was not determined for several months. One afternoon at work she commenced to bleed from a number of mucous surfaces. For a time her life was in danger. Treatment with vitamin K reduced the prothrombin time to safe limits, and she recovered. By the time treatment was instituted, however, she had lost considerable blood and had bled into her pleural and peritoneal cavities.

Nursing measures to prevent venous stasis have been emphasized elsewhere. Because of their importance, they will be summarized, however. As soon as emergency or lifesaving procedures have been carried out, attention should be given to the improvement of venous circulation from the lower extremities. Some physicians prescribe elastic bandages from toe to groin to support the walls of the veins. Passive exercises of the legs should be instituted as soon as feasible unless interdicted by the physician. These have previously been described. Getting the patient out of bed and into the chair also aids in improving venous flow from the legs. The importance of the prevention of pressure against the popliteal space or against the calf of the leg has also been indicated. This should not be neglected.

Congestive heart failure is a possibility. The care required by the patient who develops this complication has been discussed. When digitalis is prescribed, and it usually is, observation of the patient for toxic effects, especially cardiac arrhythmias, should be noted and reported promptly.

A disabling disorder, the shoulder-hand syndrome, develops occasionally. It is characterized by pain and tenderness in the shoulder. It is followed by pain redness and tenderness in the hand. Occasionally, the small muscles in the hand atrophy. According to Harrison,[64] the condition occurs in 5 to 10 per cent of patients and may develop within a year following a myocardial infarction.

Hiccoughs, when they occur, indicate a poor prognosis. Why this is true is

64 *Ibid.*, p. 1454.

not known. Continued hiccoughs in the otherwise healthy person are fatiguing. Perhaps fatigue is a factor in the unfavorable prognosis.

The diet prescribed for Mr. Anderson was low in salt, controlled in fat, and restricted to 1,800 calories. Salt was restricted to lessen the tendency to edema formation and because there may be a relationship between salt intake and hypertension. Fat was to be restricted in amount and type. Instead of the usual 40 to 45 per cent of the diet in the form of fat, the total was not to exceed 35 per cent. A larger proportion than is ingested by the average American was to be in the form of vegetable oils. Vegetable oils contain a higher percentage of unsaturated fatty acids than animal fats. The purpose of decreasing the intake of fat is to lower the level of lipids in the blood. Although there is no definite proof that altering the kind and quantity of fat ingested decreases the incidence of coronary artery disease, a number of studies suggest that it may. Although Mr. Anderson was not overweight, calories were limited to decrease the likelihood of a gain in weight.

An essential part of the care of a patient is to prepare him to return to as full activity as the condition of his heart allows. Many patients can return to full or nearly full activity. The trend toward emphasizing what the patient can or will be able to do helps some patients move from attention on what he has lost to what he has and is able to do. Mr. Anderson had been performing a type of work that required a modest expenditure of energy. His work was also performed at a steady, but moderate, rate. Neither his safety nor the safety of others would be endangered were he to return to his job. His physician advised him to take a ten-minute rest period every two hours. Since he has an understanding employer, he thinks that this can be arranged. He has hospitalization insurance. This lessens his worry about expenses. His family is grown and his wife is employed. Financial worries are at a minimum. He hopes that he will be able to work until he is 65, when he will be eligible for full social security benefits.

Not all patients have as favorable a situation as Mr. Anderson. Some, such as Mr. Strongboy, have many problems. He is only 35 years of age. He has been divorced and has no one dependent on him. Neither does he have any one on whom he can depend. Though he has worked since he was 14 years of age, he has gone from one job to another and he has not established seniority in his work. Neither does he have savings nor income insurance. His doctor has told him that he should think of doing some type of work other than truck driving. He lacks either the education or the experience required for most sedentary jobs. He expressed little interest when the subject of training for a suitable type of work was introduced. At one point he suggested the possibility of a job as dispatcher in the office of the firm where he was employed. Though referral to a sheltered workshop for cardiac patients was suggested to him, he was not interested. On discharge from the hospital, he planned to go to a hotel for men where rates were low. Because of all the factors involved,

Mr. Strongboy's future did not appear to be very promising. He had neither the background nor the interest to profit from retraining.

Summary

In the preceding pages the ways in which the heart may fail have been discussed along with the implications of each of these to the needs of the patient for nursing. The causes of heart failure are summarized below in the words of Carl Wiggers:[65] (1) Failure of the pacemakers, including the main pacemaker—the sinoauricular node; (2) too many pacemakers; (3) a break-down in the system for the conduction of impulses over the heart muscle; (4) loss of the power of contraction; (5) obstruction of the coronary arteries; and (6) defective heart valves—they may either leak or be narrowed—stenosed. In an individual patient more than one factor is frequently involved. Whether or not a specific disorder of cardiac functioning leads to the failure of the heart as a pump depends on (1) the extent to which the condition deprives the myocardium of adequate nutrition; (2) the degree to which the heart must utilize its reserve to maintain the circulation; (3) the capacity of myocardial lead cells to initiate contraction under emergency conditions; and (4) the degree to which disorders disrupt the normal rate and rhythm of the heart.

The responsibilities of the nurse as they relate to disease of the heart include:

1. Participating in programs of prevention of conditions that predispose to disease of the heart.
2. Acting as a case finder in detecting individuals who have heart disease.
3. Participating in programs of education of the public and employers so that those who have or have had heart disease and who want to be and are able to be are employed.
4. Providing competent nursing of the person sick with heart disease, including his fullest rehabilitation.
5. Supporting programs of research into the cause and treatment of heart disease.

This chapter has not included a discussion of congenital malformations of the heart. Usually congenital malformations are manifested in childhood. In general they affect the circulation by some defect in the one-way circuit or by an obstruction to the flow of blood. Either one or both of these place an added burden on the myocardium and, depending on the nature and location of the lesion, result in a mixing of arterial and venous blood. Since an adequate circulation of the blood is essential not only to survival, but to normal growth and development, serious congenital defects of the heart and great vessels are usually accompanied by failure of the child to grow and to mature normally. Furthermore, defective structures appear to be more prone to infec-

[65] *Op. cit.*, p. 87.

tion by microorganisms than do normal ones. Persons with congenital heart malformations are, therefore, prone to bacterial endocarditis.

As indicated in the introduction to the chapter, the blood vessels together with the heart form a closed circuit through which blood is circulated. The heart, aided by skeletal muscles, furnishes the power by which the blood is propelled through the system. Ways in which the heart may fail and the effects of failure have been discussed in some detail. Some of the causes and consequences of failure of blood vessel function have also been presented. Further, some reference is made to some aspect of circulation in most chapters. Emphasis in this area is justified as many nursing activities are directed toward preserving the circulation or protecting the individual or some part of him from a defect in his circulation. With the steady increase in the number of aged in the population, the proportion of persons with disorders in circulation is also increasing.

Where is the function of the circulatory system accomplished?

Stress has been on the importance of the continuous movement of blood through the circuit. Nothing would be accomplished by this movement, however, were it not for the capillaries where exhange takes place between the interstitial fluid and the blood. In a very real sense, the capillaries are the site where the ultimate function of the circulatory system is accomplished.

How does the structure of the blood vessels enable them to perform their function?

The structure of the blood vessels varies with their location in the circuit and with their function. With the exception of the capillaries, blood vessels are composed of three layers, or coats. The outer layer, or tunica adventitia, is largely areolar connective tissue. The middle layer, or tunica media, contains varying proportions of elastic and muscular tissue. The inner, or tunica intima, is also composed of three layers: a layer of elastic tissue lying next to the media, a thin layer of connective tissue, and finally a layer of endothelial cells. Differences in structure are significant not only to their function, but to the pathophysiology accompanying disease. The walls of the large arteries, such as the aorta and the pulmonary artery, are thick and contain a large amount of elastic tissue, but relatively little muscle. In medium-sized and small arteries conditions are reversed. As arteries decrease in size, the amount of elastic tissue also decreases and their walls contain relatively more muscle. The arterioles are largely muscle.

The highly elastic structure of the aorta enables it to distend as the blood is ejected into it during systole. As a consequence, the aorta is capable of storing about half the blood it receives from the heart during systole. During diastole the elastic tissue shortens as the blood flows out into the circuit. With the decrease in the volume of blood in the aorta, the potential (stored) energy built up as the elastic tissue in its wall is stretched is released as kinetic (moving) energy. This energy aids the forward movement of the blood. The familiar example of the rubber band can be used to illustrate the above changes. An elastic band is stretched. As it is stretched, potential energy accumulates. When the band is released, it returns to its prestretched form and at the same time releases kinetic energy. The kinetic energy may be used to move a part in a model airplane or for some other purpose. When it is released by the wall of a blood vessel, it propels the blood in the vessel forward.

The elasticity of the aorta is a factor in the continuous flow of blood through the arteries, and it helps to protect the smaller vessels from the full force of systolic contraction of the heart. Were the aorta a rigid tube, the blood pressure would be higher at the end of systole and lower during diastole. This is essentially what happens when the aorta becomes sclerosed. With aging, there is a loss of elastic tissue, and the wall of the aorta becomes increasingly rigid. As the wall of the aorta increases in rigidity, the systolic blood pressure rises. The diastolic blood pressure does not always fall, though it may. Sometimes the aorta increases in size as it becomes sclerosed. The increase in capacity tends to compensate for the loss of elasticity. Arteriosclerosis, characterized by a loss of elastic tissue in the intima and media of the aorta, starts at a relatively early age. Evidence of this can be seen at the age of 20 or thereabouts. Changes in the media of other arteries also take place with aging. They lead to tortuosity and stiffening of the vessel wall. Arteriosclerosis is not the same disorder as atherosclerosis, which was discussed earlier.

The structure of the artery is also a factor in the limitation of bleeding after tissue continuity is disrupted. When an artery is cut, elastic tissue shortens and retracts the artery a little beneath its sheath. At the same time the muscle contracts somewhat and narrows the opening in the artery. "Self-sealing" is completed by the formation of a blood clot in the end of the artery.

Arterioles, in contrast to larger arteries, are largely muscle. They are therefore capable of adapting the diameter of their lumen to the volume of blood in the body and to the localized needs of tissues. Changes in the walls of muscular arteries affect not only the diameter of their lumen, but the hemodynamics of the circulation. The outflow from the arterioles affects not only the volume and velocity of blood flowing through the capillaries but the pressure of the blood in the larger arteries. Whereas the measure of the force with which the blood is ejected into the arteries is the systolic blood pressure, the measure of the degree of constriction of arterioles (peripheral resistance) is the level of the diastolic blood pressure. There may also be an increase in the cardiac output. Other factors in the regulation of the arterial blood pressure as well as theories to explain essential hypertension will be presented later.

As indicated above, the function of the circulatory system is accomplished in the capillaries. Other parts serve to propel and convey blood to and from the capillaries where the exchange takes place between the blood and the interstitial fluid surrounding cells. Capillaries are composed of a single layer of endothelial cells that are continuous with the lining cells of the arteries and veins. The capillaries and the arterioles together form the microcirculation. Some capillaries are thoroughfare channels, while others are true capillaries. The thoroughfare channels enable the body to shift blood around a part. The factors involved in the exchange between the blood in the capillaries and the interstitial fluid are discussed in Chapter 8. According to Zweifach,[66] the distance from a capillary to a cell is never greater than 0.005 inch. The total length of capillaries is 60,000 miles, or an average of 400 miles per pound of body weight. The potential capacity of the capillaries is large enough to hold all the blood in the body. In health the arterioles and precapillary sphincters regulate the flow of blood through the capillaries so they are not all open at one time. When tissue is observed under the microscope, capillary channels can be seen to open and close at different times. When tissues are active, the number of functioning capillaries is greater than when they are at rest. This is another way in which the body is able to adapt function to the needs of the body. In peripheral circulatory failure, the ability to regulate the number of functioning capillaries is lost with the result that the potential capacity of the vascular system exceeds the blood volume. The volume of blood returned to the heart drops and as a consequence the cardiac output drops. Blood pressure falls and the affected person is in shock. Unless the disturbance is corrected promptly, life ceases.

How are veins similar to and different from arteries?

The veins, like the arteries, are composed of three layers. The walls of the veins tend to be thinner than those of the arteries and the media is not as well developed. They contain less muscle and elastic tissue than the media of the arteries. Because of the thinness of their walls, veins have a tendency to collapse when they are cut. They are also easily collapsed by pressure. Since the relatively thick walls of arteries resist collapse, blood continues to enter tissues in which veins have been obstructed by pressure. This leads to swelling, which, if it is allowed to continue, will eventually limit the inflow of blood. Some veins, especially those in which the blood is moved against gravity, are provided with valves. These valves are important to keeping the blood moving forward in the vascular circuit. When the valves in the veins are congenitally defective or are destroyed by disease, stasis of blood in the affected vein results.

In comparison with that in the arteries, the pressure of blood in the veins is low. To a great extent, the pressure of blood in the peripheral veins is determined by the pressure in the right atrium, and the pressure in the right atrium

[66] Benjamin W. Zweifach, "The Microcirculation of the Blood," *Scientific American,* CC, January, 1959, p. 54.

is largely determined by the efficiency of the heart as a pump. Total blood volume affects the amount of blood available to return to the heart. Within limits the veins are capable of adapting to a decrease in blood volume by constricting. The veins have a large potential capacity for blood, and this is also a factor in shock.

The return of blood from the lower extremities is facilitated by the contraction of skeletal muscles. They are sometimes referred to as a venous pump. Prolonged motionless standing or sitting with pressure against the popliteal space results in a rise in venous pressure in the legs and feet. Fainting may occur in susceptible individuals following as little as ten minutes of motionless standing. Continued sitting such as on long bus or automobile trips predisposes to edema of the feet and legs. There have been some instances reported in the literature of elderly persons developing convulsions as a result of shifts in the distribution of body fluids during extended bus or automobile travel. Preventive measures include getting out of the car or bus at hourly or two-hour intervals and walking about. Exercises such as flexing and extending the foot at the ankle, and setting the quadriceps muscles while sitting, are also beneficial. Many older persons would be well advised to break extended journeys by spending the night in a hotel or motel.

Similar to other service facilities, blood vessels are subject to regulation. Through regulation the over-all needs of the body are met, priority is given to areas with high metabolic requirements, and special needs of local areas of tissue are met. The nervous system has an important role in the regulation of the diameter of arteries and veins, but there is little evidence that it directly regulates the capillaries. The capillary circulation is believed to be regulated primarily by local conditions in the tissues. Through the regulation of the caliber of arteries and veins and the force and rate of the heart, blood is delivered to and removed from the capillaries.

Many of the circumstances when sympathetic nervous system regulation is important have been previously discussed. They include the maintenance of normal blood pressure in persons who have sustained blood loss or in whom the cardiac output is low. Sympathetic reflexes prevent cerebral hypotension when shifting from the supine to the standing position. Sympathetic reflexes are also involved when blood is shifted from one area to another.

Both the sympathetic and parasympathetic nervous system participate in the regulation of the coordination of cardiac and vascular functioning. For example, an increase in the volume of blood delivered to the right atrium stimulates receptors in the vena cava and results in an increase in the heart rate. Conversely, an increase in the pressure of blood in the aorta initiates a reflex slowing the heart.

Not all the elements in the local regulation of blood flow are known. Some of the possibilities include a lack of essential nutrients and oxygen or the liberation of a substance by the ischemic tissue that is responsible for arteriolar and capillary dilatation. The hormones epinephrine and norepinephrine cause contraction of all blood vessels except the coronary arteries. Acetylcholine causes muscle cells to relax. In the process of metabolism, chemicals are formed which, when they come in contact with the precapillary sphincter, cause it to relax. In the local regulation of the blood supply, the processes are self-correcting. When the condition initiating the response is corrected, conditions tend to return to the prestimulus state. For example, blood vessels dilate in area in response to exercise of the muscles. As a result of the increased blood flow, ischemia is corrected and products that directly dilate the blood vessels are removed. With the elimination of conditions initiating dilatation, the blood vessels automatically constrict.

Tissues are also protected from the effects of arterial obstruction by the collateral circulation, that is, the circulation around and connecting smaller branches of the main circulation. The collateral circulation offers the greatest protection when an obstruction develops slowly. New capillaries can develop in the tissues and larger vessels can be recanalized, but the body requires from one to six months to increase the vascularity of tissues. If the loss of blood supply is not so great that the basal needs of the tissues cannot be met and if the tissues are protected from increased demands, the affected part (arm, leg, heart) can sometimes be saved until an adequate circulation is established.

What are the causes and effects of diseases of the blood vessels?

Not unlike other organs, blood vessels are subject to abnormalities of structure and function. Diseases of blood vessels, including those of the heart, kidney, and brain, stand at the head of the list as causes of mortality. Equally important, if not more, they cause a high incidence of morbidity. The most important of the vascular diseases are widespread diseases. Some localized defects occurring in blood vessels, such as a single aneurysm of an artery supplying the brain or an aneurysm of the aorta, threaten disaster to the whole individual. Disorders characterized by structural changes are said to be organic, while those in which there is a disturbance in function in the absence of a structural change are said to be functional. Functional disorders may in time lead to structural changes in the walls of affected blood vessels. When a disease of the blood vessel results in obstruction of its lumen, it is known as an occlusive vascular disease.

Areas in the walls of arteries and veins may be weakened by congenital defects, injury, or disease. Such vessels are subject to dilatation and thinning of the wall. Abnormal dilatations of arteries are known as aneurysms; those of veins, as varicosities. Although both types of disorders impede the flow of blood and pressure against the wall of the affected vessel increases the degree of dilatation, there are significant differences between the two disorders.

What is an aneurysm?

An aneurysm is a saclike dilatation occurring in the wall of a blood vessel and is due to a weakness in its structure. Common sites of arterial aneurysms include the circle of Willis and the aorta. Those in the circle of Willis are due to congenital defects in the walls of the arteries. Aortic aneurysms may be due to syphilis, arteriosclerosis, or trauma. In syphilis, the spirochete invades the media and weakens the wall of the artery. Whatever its cause or site, the wall of an aneurysm is weak and, therefore, predisposed to rupture. To prevent rupture, the patient should be instructed to avoid all activities that result in an increase in blood pressure, such as straining during defecation, coughing, lifting heavy objects, or having strenuous activity. When an aneurysm is believed to be very thin-walled, strict bed rest may be prescribed for the patient.

The signs and symptoms accompanying an aneurysm will, of course, be affected by its location. An aneurysm in the ascending aorta predisposes to congestive heart failure as well as to the formation of thrombi in the vessels. Rupture of an aortic aneurysm is a cause of sudden death. Rupture of an aneurysm in an artery forming the circle of Willis (they are frequently multiple) releases blood into the cerebrospinal fluid. Meningeal signs such as stiff neck occur as well as evidence of increased intracranial pressure. The outcome varies. Some patients die suddenly. Others recover, but have other aneurysms rupture at later times.

Various surgical methods have been developed to reinforce or replace the weakened wall of the aorta or other arteries in which an aneurysm has developed. In the preoperative preparation of the patient the major objective is to prevent any increase, particularly sudden increase, in pressure against the wall of the weakened vessel. Earlier discussion on achieving rest is pertinent here. In the postoperative care, prevention of strain on the operated area and prevention of clotting of blood in the operated or other vessels are major objectives.

Principles basic to the achievement of both these objectives have been discussed earlier. Certain aspects of care will depend on the route of approach to the aneurysm. For example, was it through the chest or abdominal wall? It is most important that each person be considered as an individual. Repair of an aneurysm is a major procedure and if located in the circle of Willis or aorta is attended with the possibility that the patient will not survive the operation. To the extent to which the patient understands or imagines the degree of risk to which he is exposed, the nature of the disorder and the therapy are sources of anxiety.

What are some of the effects of localized dilatations of veins?

Dilated veins or varicosities, particularly those located in the esophagus, may also rupture and cause serious, and not infrequently fatal, hemorrhage. Intracutaneous varicosities in the skin of the lower extremities may also rupture and bleed. Bleeding is limited because the vessels are small and the tissue offers counterpressure against the wall of the bleeding vessel. The epithelium over the area is thin. Trauma due to bumping may break the skin and result in profuse bleeding. Discoloration of the skin may be a cause of emotional distress, however. The anatomy of the intracutaneous vessels may, when they are dilated, be responsible for further distress. The veins draining the intracutaneous tissue are characterized by a central vein with numerous spiderlike feeder veins. Increased pressure within these veins leading to their dilatation results in a spiderlike lesion, which understandably enough is called a spider angioma. They are unsightly, but relatively harmless.

A second site where varicosities occur is the greater and lesser saphenous veins draining the lower extremities. As they dilate, pressure of blood against their walls increases causing further dilatation. The veins not only increase in diameter, but they elongate and become tortuous. Veins lying in the subcutaneous tissue are visible and unsightly. A patient may have one type of varicosity or both. According to Cooper,[67] uncomplicated varicose veins actually cause few symptoms and are rarely incapacitating. The usual symptoms are a feeling of heaviness and fullness in the legs and a stinging sensation along the course of the veins after the person has been standing for some time. There may be mild edema in the region of the ankle and mild stasis dermatitis. Ulceration of the skin is almost entirely limited to the person who has a combination of varicosities and deep venous insufficiency.[68] In the uncomplicated form, varicosities are largely hereditary, but they may also follow thrombophlebitis in which the inflammatory process destroys the valves in the veins. Varicosities occur more frequently in women than in men. They become worse during menstrual periods and with each succeeding pregnancy. Rapid weight gain and occupations requiring prolonged motionless standing are associated with enlargement of varicosities.

According to Cooper,[69] the usual reason for treating uncomplicated varicosities is cosmetic. The treatment of intracutaneous varicosities is unsatisfactory. The most satisfactory treatment of large tortuous veins is by stripping. Injection and ligation are accompanied by a high percentage of recurrence. In patients who have deep vein insufficiency, stripping the veins does not return the patient completely to normal. The legs may look better, but the patient should still wear elastic stockings and elevate the legs regularly. The new type of elastic stocking is relatively expensive but not unattractive.

How is the status of venous function determined?

Blood flow in the veins and the competency of the valves in preventing the backflow of blood into the subcutaneous veins or in veins connecting superficial and deep veins can be determined. To test the competency of the deep veins to carry blood, the physician occludes the superficial veins with a tourniquet at the level of the knee or thigh. The patient then walks. The normal pumping action of the muscles against the walls of the veins should cause the

---

[67] F. W. Cooper, "Varicose Veins," *Heart Bulletin*, IX, May-June, 1960, pp. 57-58.
[68] *Ibid.*, p. 57.
[69] *Ibid.*, p. 58.

varices to empty. If they do not, this indicates that the valves in a large perforating vein are incompetent.

Competency of the subcutaneous veins is determined by first draining veins of the leg by elevating it and then applying a tourniquet. The leg is then lowered. If the veins fill slowly, this indicates that the valves from the perforating veins are competent. If it fills rapidly, they are incompetent. If, after the tourniquet is removed, the veins fill rapidly, the valves in the saphenous veins are incompetent. A physician performs these tests, but the nurse should be able to assist the patient and physician with the tests and be prepared to answer the patient's questions.

What are some of the causes and effects of arteriovenous fistulae?

As a result of defective development or trauma, direct connections between arteries and veins may exist or be formed. A common effect of the abnormal opening is that arterial blood is circulated directly to the affected vein.[70] The effects depend somewhat on the location of the fistula and the age of the individual at the time it is formed. For example, John Sparrow, aged 30, developed a fistula between his aorta and inferior vena cava as a result of a gunshot wound in the abdomen. For a time he was reasonably well. As a consequence of a chronic overloading of his heart by recirculated blood, his heart eventually failed as a pump. Such an abnormal connection between a distal artery and vein would not have as serious an effect.

What is meant by the term "peripheral vascular disease" and what are some of its causes and consequences?

Disease of blood vessels in the periphery, especially those supplying the extremities, is known as peripheral vascular disease. These diseases may be either functional or organic. Any disorder in the function of blood vessels implies some disturbance in the capacity to deliver blood to the tissues or to remove it. So-called functional disturbances of arteries may be limited to certain structures, or they may be generalized. An example of the first is Raynaud's disease and of the second hypertension. In Raynaud's disease the blood vessels of the hands and/or feet respond to cold or emotion by vasospasm. The degree of spasm may be so great that no blood enters the affected areas during the height of the attack. Hypertension is a very important disease and will be discussed later.

The most common cause of peripheral arterial disease is atherosclerosis. The pathogenesis of this disease is the same in all arteries and it has been fully discussed previously. When the disease involves vessels supplying the extremities, manifestations due to an inadequate blood supply can be observed. One

[70] In keeping with the well-known fact, fluids move from areas of high to those of low pressure.

further point is of some significance in nursing. Diseased as well as normal arteries (arterioles) respond to conditions in the environment. Therefore, the patient who has atherosclerosis of arteries supplying the extremities responds to cold by constriction and to warmth by vasodilatation. Other factors such as food, smoking, emotional states, and exercise may also influence the degree of arterial constriction or dilatation. Furthermore, though some disorders affect either arteries or veins, others affect both.

The signs and symptoms associated with disturbances in circulation to the peripheral tissues have been listed by Allen, Barker, and Hines.[71] They include: (1) pain, (2) color changes of the skin or nails, (3) ulceration or gangrene, scleroderma, and impairment of the growth of the nails, (4) size of the extremities altered by either an increase or decrease, (5) abnormality of temperature of the extremities—either abnormally cold or abnormally warm, and (6) enlarged or abnormal pulsations of veins.

There are some other significant signs and symptoms as well, such as color changes and eczema of the skin that accompany chronic venous stasis, impaired arterial pulsation, and unusual changes with elevation or dependency of the extremity. Because of abnormalities in the flow of blood in aneurysms or in arteriovenous fistulae, murmurs may be heard. A sound that can be felt as a vibration is called a thrill. In peripheral vascular disease most of the signs and symptoms result from vasodilatation or some type of disorder decreasing the diameter of the blood vessels such as vasospasm. Both cause an alteration in the volume of blood delivered to the tissues and a failure in the capacity to adapt blood supply to tissue needs.

The objective in the nursing of the patient whose tissues have an insufficient supply of blood that takes first priority is (1) to protect these tissues from injury. Other objectives include: (2) to prevent and relieve symptoms, (3) to participate in the program of education for the patient, so he learns how, and is motivated, to prevent injury to affected tissues, (4) to carry out the part of the therapeutic regime that is expected to promote the development of the collateral circulation.

Measures to protect the affected tissues depend in part on the nature of the disorder. For example, Ann Blue has Raynaud's syndrome. Despite the discomfort associated with an attack, Raynaud's disease is almost always a harmless disorder. Miss Blue seems to have a mild form of the disease, and at this time there is no evidence that it is progressive. She has no difficulty unless her hands are exposed to cold, and attacks can be prevented by protecting her hands from the cold. By wearing warm mittens during cold weather and avoiding getting chilled, she keeps from having difficulty. Gangrene is unusual in Raynaud's syndrome, though superficial ulcers and scleroderma do sometimes occur. From what is known about Miss Blue, there is little reason to suppose that she will develop either complication.

[71] Edgar V. Allen, Nelson W. Barker, and Edgar A. Hines, *Peripheral Vascular Diseases,* 3rd ed., W. B. Saunders Company, Philadelphia, 1962, pp. 5-41.

*How do the problems of occlusive vascular disease differ
from those seen in Raynaud's disease? Why?*

Unlike Raynaud's disease, occlusive arterial disease is generally of serious import. Mr. Marker illustrates some of the problems associated with the disease. At the moment he is sitting on the edge of his bed with his left leg hanging over the edge. His right leg was amputated two years ago. There is an ulcer on his right index finger, the result of a cigarette burn. Since burning himself, he has stopped smoking. He had continued to smoke, despite the explanation given to Mr. Marker by his physician that cigarette smoking was a possible factor in causation and undoubtedly aggravated his condition. He is now faced with the possibility of having to have his left leg amputated. He is not an old man; he is only 29 years of age.

Mr. Marker has a form of occlusive peripheral vascular disease that in the past was, and still is, identified by some physicians as Buerger's disease or thromboangiitis obliterans. Some physicians doubt that Buerger's disease is a distinct clinical entity; they believe it to be peripheral atherosclerosis occurring in young men. One distinction made between peripheral atherosclerosis and thromboangiitis obliterans is the age at which it occurs. Thromboangiitis usually develops before the age of 45 to 50 years and atherosclerosis after 45 years of age. Many of the pathological features of thromboangiitis obliterans are similar, if not identical to, those of peripheral atherosclerosis. The age of the patient does influence the manner in which he responds to his illness, and many of the problems that he faces. In arterial occlusion, the manifestations are due to tissue ischemia.[72] In meeting needs of Mr. Marker for nursing two points are of greatest significance. One is that the need of the tissues of his extremities is greater than the capacity of his body to supply blood. The other relates to the fact that he is presently suffering pain.

Several factors may enter into the causation of his pain. In ulceration and gangrene pain is common; pain may be a forerunner of ulceration and is called the pretropic pain of ischemia. It is constant and severe. It interferes with the ability to sleep. The pain is less severe when the affected extremity is dependent. Thus Mr. Marker secured some relief by having his foot over the edge of the bed. Heat, if not too great and if it does not elevate the metabolic rate to a greater extent than it does the blood supply, may help to relieve the pain. Pain is aggravated by elevation of the extremity and by cold.

A second possible cause of pain in occlusive arterial disease is ischemic neuritis. The pain may be burning, throbbing, shooting, or tearing. It may be severe and extensive. It may fluctuate in severity, the patient having paroxysms when the pain is worse than it is at other times. Acute inflammation of the arteries and veins may cause a mild pain or a dull ache. It is usually manifested as tenderness on pressure.

For some time previous to his admission to the hospital Mr. Marker had

[72] Eugene A. Stead, in Harrison, *Op. cit.,* 4th ed., p. 1370.

had pain in the calf of his leg after he walked for a block or so. He had noted that the distance he could walk in comfort had become progressively less and that the pain was cramplike in character. It was relieved by rest. Pain associated with exercise is believed to be caused by insufficient supply of blood—ischemia—to the contracting muscle.

Another cause of pain in peripheral vascular disorders is sudden arterial occlusion. Occlusion may be due to either a thrombus or an embolism that causes complete acute obstruction. Pain occurs at rest and is sudden and severe. The cause of the pain has not been completely explained. It may be due in part to, or intensified by, spasm of associated collateral vessels. Surprisingly, in some instances pain is slight or even absent in patients with major arterial embolism. A possible explanation is that the peripheral nerves are rendered functionless by acute ischemia. The affected extremity is also pale and cold, further indicating severe ischemia. There is usually a sharp line of demarcation between the ischemic and normal tissue. Within a short time after onset, there is a loss of sensory as well as of motor function. The patient notes that he is unable to move his fingers or toes. The skin become insensitive to pain and touch. The extremity should, therefore, be protected from pressure. It is easily injured by heat, both because a rise in the temperature of tissues increases their metabolic needs and because the mechanism for cooling the tissue is defective or lacking. Pulses in the arteries distal to the site of obstruction are absent or weak when tested by palpation or by oscillometry. Unless the circulation is re-established promptly, the extremity will become gangrenous and require amputation. Accurate observation and prompt reporting are imperative. The part should be in a dependent position. When a lower extremity is involved, this is accomplished by elevating the head of the bed on blocks. Cold may be applied to the affected extremity to reduce the rate of metabolism. Measures such as sympathetic block may be performed to dilate the collateral blood vessels. The tendency of thrombi to propagate, that is, continue to grow, is combated by the use of anticoagulants. Heparin is frequently chosen because of its immediate effects and limited length of action.

When the clot is large, it is usually surgically removed. Thrombectomy or embolectomy must be performed as soon as possible and while the tissues are still viable (living). According to Julian and Dye,[73] an embolectomy should be performed within eight hours of the onset of symptoms. Postoperatively attention should be given to the prevention of stasis of blood in the operated extremity. An anticoagulant is also prescribed to lessen the danger of thrombosis in the operated vessels and in other blood vessels as well.

Several elements contribute to the pain associated with occlusive arterial disease. For a patient such as Mr. Marker pain becomes the focus of his attention. That this should be true is not surprising, since his pain was severe

[73] Ormand C. Julian and William S. Dye, "Peripheral Vascular Surgery," in Harkens, et al. *Surgery, Principles and Practice*, 2nd ed., J. B. Lippincott Company, Philadelphia, 1961, p. 1081.

and unrelenting and was more severe at night. Constant pain combined with a loss of sleep is damaging to the morale. Even when Mr. Marker secured some relief from his pain, he was depressed by the thought, "How can a man without legs possibly support himself, let alone his family?" When whiskey and aspirin did not give Mr. Marker relief, his physician prescribed meperidine hydrochloride (Demerol). According to Barker,[74] when pain at rest is severe, the use of narcotics is justified. The nurse has essentially the same responsibilities she has any time she administers a narcotic. Does the patient have pain? What is its nature? Where is it located? How does the patient describe it? Does the pain require a narcotic or can it be relieved by some other measure? Is the pain relieved after the drug is administered? How long does its effect last? Is there anything that the nurse can do to increase the effectiveness of the analgesic narcotic?

In addition to pain, Mr. Marker also had other signs and symptoms indicating ischemia. His feet were cold to touch. There were marked changes in color on change in position. The feet were a dusky-red color on dependency and pale on elevation. The nails on his toes were unusually thick and brittle for a man as young as Mr. Marker.

The problem of preventing the breakdown of tissue until Mr. Marker is able to develop a collateral circulation is urgent. Even the slightest trauma or the mildest irritating chemical may be sufficient to upset the balance between the supply of food and the needs of the tissues. Viability of the tissue is protected by decreasing the local metabolic needs of the tissue and by increasing the blood flow to the ischemic part. Careful nursing is essential to the accomplishment of both objectives.

When Mr. Marker was admitted to the hospital, his physician prescribed bed rest in a constant-temperature room. A cradle was placed over his foot to prevent the bed covering from causing pressure. In order to minimize the danger of traumatizing his toes or foot, a cradle the width of the bed was selected. The bed linen was inspected to be certain that there were no patches or seams. Because Mr. Marker moved about freely and frequently, there was little danger of pressure from a part remaining in one position. In less active patients, attention should be given to regular changes in the position of the extremity and the use of devices to evenly distribute the pressure.

Heat in the form of hot-water bottles or heating pads should not be used. No chemical lotion, or other agent unless specifically prescribed by the physician, should be applied to the skin. Before cutting the patient's nails, the nurse should acquaint herself with the policy of the hospital. In some hospitals a physician's prescription is required before the toenails are cut. In others nails are cut by a chiropodist. Before the nails are cut, the feet should be soaked in warm, not hot, soapy water for ten minutes to soften the nails. Before the foot is placed in water for bathing, the temperature of the water should be checked with the hand. The water should be warm, not hot or cold. A temperature

[74] *Op. cit.*, p. 753.

between 85° and 95° F. is suggested as acceptable. The nails should be cut straight across and not too close to the flesh. Should any injury, no matter how slight, be inflicted, it should be immediately brought to the attention of the physician. As Mr. Marker's foot was dry and scaly, lanolin was applied. Care was taken when drying his foot to pat gently with a soft towel, rather than to rub. Attention was paid to drying between the toes. Skin that is continuously moist softens and becomes macerated and is thereby predisposed to infection. Lamb's wool was placed between the toes to absorb moisture. In patients whose feet tend to be moist, powder is used.

Not only is the nurse responsible for trying to identify and remove possible sources of injury to the patient's feet, but the cooperation and assistance of the patient are essential. Furthermore, even when the treatment of the hospitalized patient is successful, a regime similar to that followed in the hospital is essential if the tissues in the extremities are to be maintained in a reasonably healthy condition. The patient must know how to care for his extremities, especially his feet, and understand why this care is important. He must also be helped to understand that although doctors and nurses will do their best to assist him, the main responsibility in the control of his disorder is his. The patient should therefore be given written as well as verbal instructions and demonstrations of the care of the feet. He should have an opportunity to practice the essential procedures under supervision. These instructions are appropriate for all patients who have peripheral occlusive vascular disease, including those who also have diabetes mellitus.

The prevention of ulceration and gangrene is easier than the cure. Almost all ulceration and gangrene of ischemic extremities can be charged to chemical, mechanical, or thermal injury, or to local bacterial infection of tissues. Injury need not be severe. Often minor injuries, especially when neglected, lead to ulceration and gangrene. The injury does not have to disrupt the skin. From the experience of the writer, an elderly man comes to mind who developed gangrene of his foot after he had kicked a cow in an effort to get her to move a leg. Later in the evening he noted soreness and redness in the great toe of the same foot. A week later he was admitted to the hospital. The toe was gangrenous.

Points to be emphasized in the care of the feet include:

1. Cleanliness
   DO
   A. Wash no less frequently than every other day in warm soapy water.
   B. Dry thoroughly between the toes with a soft cloth. Use a patting or mopping action.
   C. Take care not to bruise the feet or break the skin.
   D. Powder the feet if they have a tendency to perspire.
   E. Lubricate the feet with an ointment consisting of 50 parts lanolin and 50 parts petroleum jelly if they are dry.

2. Shoes
   A. Never go barefoot. Always wear shoes when out of bed.
   B. Wear well-built shoes of soft leather.
   C. Wear shoes with a broad toe and a sensible heel. They should give the feet adequate support.
   D. Never wear new shoes more than one-half day at a time.
   E. Never wear shoes with exposed nails, defects in the lining, or any other roughened surfaces that will come in contact with the feet. Have defective shoes repaired before wearing.
3. Hose
   A. Wear seamless hose without holes, darns, or patches.
   B. Wear clean stockings daily. (Cotton stockings are preferred as they can be boiled when washed.)
   C. Be sure to buy hose sufficiently long. Too short stockings are as harmful as too short shoes.
   D. Lamb's wool should be worn between the toes.
4. Toenails
   A. If you go to a chiropodist, tell him that you have a reduction in blood flow to your feet.
   B. Before cutting toenails, soak feet in warm, soapy water.
   C. Cut the toenails straight across and not too short, i.e., not too close to the flesh.
   D. Place cotton wicks under the corners of the great toenails if there is a tendency to ingrown toenails.
5. Corns and calluses
   A. Do not cut corns and calluses.
   B. Do not use medicated corn plasters.
   C. Have corns and calluses taken care of by a doctor or a chiropodist who understands your condition.
6. Cold and heat
   A. In cold weather wear adequate foot covering to protect the feet from excessive cold. Wear loose, thick, warm socks. Do not stay out in the cold for long periods of time. Cold contracts your blood vessels and lessens the supply of blood to your feet.
   B. Do not place hot-water bottles, heating pads, or other heating devices near to or on the feet or legs. Do not use any form of heat without the advice of your physician.
   C. Do not place the feet in an oven, on a heating stove, or on a radiator.
   D. If your feet are cold, warm them by wearing woolen bed socks or wrap them in a warm blanket.
   E. Remember that your feet are sensitive to both heat and cold and that both should be avoided!
7. Rest and elevation of the feet
   A. Sit down and elevate your feet on a footstool at least once every

two hours. (Many industrial concerns allow rest periods, usually 15 minutes, for their employees. This time could be used for elevating your feet on a footstool or a chair. This is most important for the older diabetic patient who has arteriosclerosis.)

B. Do not cross your knees when you sit.

8. Injury—any injury, however slight, may become ulcerous or gangrenous if treatment is delayed.

A. Take care not to injure your feet. Avoid crowded places.

B. A pillow may be used to prevent pressure on the feet by bed covering.

C. Do not delay in consulting your physician should any redness, blistering, swelling, or pain develop.

D. When tissue is cut or bruised, the part should be covered with a clean bandage and kept moist with a solution of equal parts of boric and alcohol solution.

E. Do not use strong antiseptics such as iodine, Lysol, carbolic acid, and bichloride of mercury. No medicine should be placed on your feet, unless prescribed by your physician.

F. Avoid sunburn and bathing in cold water or at beaches where there is a possibility of injuring the feet.

9. Athlete's foot

A deficient supply of blood to the feet predisposes to athlete's foot. It starts out with burning and itching between the toes. You should report these symptoms to your physician so treatment can be started immediately.

Too much emphasis cannot be placed on the importance of the care of the feet of the patient who has occlusive peripheral vascular disease. Attention should be centered not only on the measures outlined above, but on identification of conditions in the environment that predispose to injury. Any condition that increases metabolism in tissues with an inadequate blood supply may thereby upset the balance between supply and demand and result in ulceration and gangrene.

When a break in the skin occurs or an ulcer is present, the area should be protected from infection and the patient should be kept at bed rest. No weight bearing should be permitted. As repeatedly emphasized, when the blood supply decreases, resistance to infection also diminishes. With the development of infection, tissue demands are increased. If the continuity of the skin is disrupted, the area should be covered with a clean, sterile dressing. Since adhesive tape is irritating to the skin of some people, some other method of anchoring the dressing in place is advisable. If a bandage is used, care should be taken to apply it evenly without pressure at any point. Physicians differ in their opinions about the value of locally applied antibiotics. An antibiotic active against the infecting microorganism is usually administered systemically.

What measures may be employed to improve the blood
flow in peripheral vascular disease?

The second objective in therapy of occlusive peripheral vascular disease is to improve the blood flow. Measures used to increase blood flow include heat, abstinence from tobacco, position, and sympathectomy. Heat is usually applied in the form of a light cradle over the extremities. Mr. Marker was placed in a warm room in which the temperature was maintained at 80° F. At this temperature there is generalized vasodilatation. The humidity was controlled so 80° F. was not uncomfortable. By maintenance of a warm environmental temperature, the stimulus to vasoconstriction was eliminated. The cradle placed over Mr. Marker's leg was also a heat cradle in which the temperature was thermostatically controlled at 88° F. When this type of cradle is not available, and a light bulb is used as a source of heat, no more than a 25-watt bulb should be used and a thermometer hung in the cradle to check the temperature. The thermometer should be placed where there is little likelihood of the patient bumping it. In any type of cradle, the source of heat should be shielded in order to prevent the patient from inadvertently coming in contact with it. The temperature inside the cradle should not exceed 90° F. The objective is to induce maximum vasodilatation without stimulating metabolism. Should the warm environmental temperature increase the patient's pain, as it sometimes does, the heat should be discontinued and the physician notified. Under these circumstances, the rise in the temperature of the tissue increases its metabolism without a comparable increase in the supply of blood, because a sufficient degree of vasodilatation does not occur.

For many years cigarette smoking has been known to cause vasoconstriction. An interesting observation has been made that when persons who are accustomed to smoking just go through the motions of smoking, their peripheral blood vessels constrict. Any influence causing even temporary vasoconstriction may have an adverse effect on already ischemic tissues. The possibility also exists that in some individuals, the blood vessels are allergic to tobacco. Occasionally a man who stops smoking after an episode characterized by ischemia of peripheral tissues then resumes smoking only to have an exacerbation of the previously quiescent disease. Whether or not tobacco directly enters into the etiology of occlusive peripheral vascular disease, it intensifies its harmful effects by causing vasoconstriction.

People vary in the difficulty that they have in breaking the habit of smoking. Some do it relatively easily; others find it difficult or are unwilling to try. For a person to be successful, he must really want to stop smoking and feel that the discomforts experienced are worth tolerating. The nurse can be helpful to the patient by letting him know that she recognizes how he feels. Some physicians handle the problem of the patient who finds breaking the habit very difficult by suggesting to the patient that he limit himself to one cigarette after each meal and possibly one at bedtime. Others refuse to treat the patient unless he ceases to smoke. In the latter instance, the nurse may find that a patient smokes but tries to conceal his actions. She is then faced with several problems. Her sympathies may be with the patient, but she is committed to carry out the medical regime. The patient has a right to decide to follow or not to follow instructions, provided he is in condition to make a rational judgment. Does the patient fully understand what is at stake? If the patient is confined to bed, surreptitious smoking increases the danger of fire. When a nurse is confronted with this problem, she should try to convey to the patient her appreciation of the difficulty he is experiencing. When appropriate she should attempt to reinforce the physician's explanation of why smoking is contraindicated. She should also bring the problem to the attention of his physician, not because the patient has been bad or disobedient, but because the physician needs to know just as he needs to know of any failure of the patient to respond to therapy.

Position can also be used to improve blood flow. By hanging his foot over the edge of his bed Mr. Marker secured some relief of his pain. Gravity causes blood, as well as other fluids, to run downhill. A comparable effect might have been obtained for Mr. Marker by elevating the head of his bed on 6-in. blocks.

An electrically operated oscillating (Sanders) bed is used in some hospitals to alternately fill and drain the vessels of the lower extremities. Its use is more or less limited to patients who have ischemia with pain at rest, that is, the pain associated with ischemic neuropathy, and with minor noninfected ulcers or gangrenous lesions. This bed is designed on the same principle as a seesaw. The springs are attached at the center to a fulcrum, so when one end of the bed is elevated the other is depressed. The rate at which the bed oscillates can be adjusted. According to Horwitz,[75] the maximum increase in blood flow to the toes can be achieved by holding the foot of the bed in the down position for five minutes with the feet at a 20-degree angle from the horizontal. The bed should then be elevated to at least a five-degree angle above the horizontal for a few seconds to drain the veins. The length of the cycle and the extent to which the bed is lowered and raised in relation to the horizontal are prescribed by the physician. The length of the cycle in a given situation may be modified by individual physicians and the needs of patients. Barker[76] states that the bed should be adjusted so that pallor occurs at the end of the up cycle and the color returns while the feet are in the down, or dependent, position. The patient should have an explanation of why the bed is used and what it is expected to accomplish. Some patients require

[75] Orville Horwitz, "Peripheral Vascular Disease," in Michael C. Wohl, *Long-Term Illness,* W. B. Saunders Company, Philadelphia, 1959, p. 160.
[76] Nelson W. Barker, "Chronic Occlusive Diseases of the Peripheral Arteries," *Heart Bulletin,* VIII, July-August, 1959, p. 78.

time to adjust to the motion and to having their heads dependent part of the time. Symptoms such as dizziness, headache, and nausea are believed in many instances to be largely of psychic origin, but they cause the patient considerable discomfort. Patients should be assured that these effects are not uncommon and that they usually disappear as the patient becomes adjusted to the bed. A little time spent with the patient, particularly when he is on the bed for the first time, is usually very helpful. A new and frightening experience can be made easier by having an experienced person whom you trust nearby.

A third method of using position to improve blood flow to the extremities is the Buerger or Buerger-Allen exercises. In these exercises gravity is used to alternately fill and empty the blood vessels. The legs are alternately elevated and lowered with a period of rest between cycles. According to Horwitz,[77] the time that the legs are in the down position should exceed the time they are in the up position by at least three to one. Some physicians prefer to use the color of the legs as the criterion for determining the length of time in each position. Under these circumstances the legs are kept in the down position until they are red and in the up position until they are blanched or pale. The patient then rests in a horizontal position for a few moments before again placing his legs in the down position. To take the down position, the patient can dangle or hang his legs over the edge of the bed. A well-padded chair or an over-the-bed table may be placed in the bed to support the legs when they are in the up position. Whatever is used as a support must be well padded, and the patient should be cautioned not to bump a foot against it even then. When the patient goes home, he is usually instructed to carry on the exercises. He can use a method similar to the hospital's or he can support his legs on the end of a sofa or on the wall. The greater the degree of elevation of the legs, the shorter should be the duration of the up position.

Drugs are also utilized to improve the flow of blood to the extremities by lessening vasospasm and thereby improving the collateral circulation. Vasodilator drugs are effective to the degree to which vasospasm is present. The patient who has little or no vasospasm cannot be expected to get much benefit from them. Prolonged action is also required. Short-acting vasodilators, such as nitroglycerine, are not very helpful. One of the most effective in inducing relaxation of the peripheral vessels is ethyl alcohol, but its use is limited by the tendency of patients to develop addiction to alcohol. Some patients object to its use on moral grounds. When some form of ethyl alcohol is prescribed, the nurse should observe the patient for indications of developing addiction. When request is made for alcohol with increasing frequency, this should be brought to the attention of the physician. The vasodilatory effects of alcohol last about four hours. Sometimes the patient solves the problem of supply by having his favorite brand brought in by a visitor. This is a problem that is seldom easy to handle. The patient secures relief from the alcohol. The fact that he is adding another to his already serious problems may not seem very

[77] *Op. cit.*, p. 160.

important to him at the time. Because of the very real possibility of the patient becoming an alcoholic, some physicians rarely prescribe alcohol.

Many other drugs have been tried to improve blood flow by decreasing vasospasm. These include papaverine hydrochloride, U.S.P., B.P. Its most frequent use has been to relieve vasospasm that accompanies embolism. Unlike most of the alkaloids of opium, it is not habit-forming. Some patients are benefitted by Aminophyllin U.S.P., B.P., (theophylline and ethylenediamine) orally, 0.1 to 0.3 gm three times a day. Among the newer drugs are a number that lessen the activity of the sympathetic nervous system. These drugs are known as adrenolytic, sympatholytic, and ganglionic blocking agents. In effect they produce a chemical sympathectomy. The adrenolytic drugs are perhaps better described by the term "adrenergic blocking agents." They combine with the effector substance in the cells. The cell is then unable to respond to the chemical mediator released on stimulation of the sympathetic nervous system. The result of the action of adrenergic blocking agents on blood vessels is dilatation. Among a number of drugs available, one of the most widely used is tolazoline hydrochloride U.S.P. (Priscoline hydrochloride).[78] One of its advantages is that it has a directly dilating effect on the walls of small blood vessels.[79] It increases the heart rate. Toxic effects include tachycardia, angina, flushing of the skin, peculiar sensations of the skin such as needles-and-pins sensations, and evidence of overactivity of the parasympathetic nervous system, increase in gastric acidity, and nausea. Should toxic symptoms develop, the physician should be notified. In patients who have a high degree of vasospasm and who respond to adrenergic blocking agents or to blocking of the sympathetic nervous system by procaine, sympathectomy may be useful.

When treatment is unsuccessful in preventing gangrene, then amputation becomes necessary. Fortunately, this is required much less frequently than in the past. Most patients view amputation of even a finger or a toe as a mutilating operation. They face the procedure with reluctance and are likely to suffer from a grief reaction afterwards. This is no less true in the patient who has an amputation as a result of gangrene than in the one who loses a part in an accident.

In addition to the occlusion of arteries by a disease process such as atherosclerosis, arteries may be occluded by bodies or emboli floating free in the blood stream. Though fat and air may be responsible, a blood clot or thrombus is the most frequent occurrence. The usual sites for the formation of thrombi are the heart and the large veins, usually the deep veins, in the leg. In the heart the two most frequent causes are atrial fibrillation and myocardial infarction accompanied by mural thrombosis. In atrial fibrillation blood tends to stand in the atrial appendages. Thrombosis of the deep veins of the leg is

[78] Trade name.
[79] Ruth D. Musser and Joseph G. Bird, *Modern Pharamacology and Therapeutics,* 2nd ed., The Macmillan Company, New York, 1961.

associated with prolonged bed rest, childbirth, and systemic infections, and may occur following operation. A portion of the blood clot is dislodged and is carried by the blood until it reaches an artery through which it cannot pass, with the result that it occludes or obstructs the artery. The effect is frequently intensified by widespread vasospasm. The spasm of the arteries may be so great that no blood circulates to the tissues in the affected area. Thus an organic factor, a blood clot, may induce a functional response, vasospasm, that is as or even more injurious than the clot by itself.

When the blood clot originates in the venous system, it travels to the heart and from there to the pulmonary artery. When the embolus is large or the combination of the embolus and vasospasm prevents blood from entering the lung, death occurs suddenly. When blood flow is maintained to most of the lung, the area deprived of its blood supply undergoes necrosis with the development of a pulmonary infarction. Symptoms are the result of the infarct.

Diagnostic tests used to study the status of blood vessels are of two general types. In one type, the effects of various procedures on function are determined. In the other, measures are used to determine the location and extent of structural change. A variety of methods are used to determine the functional status of the vascular system. Essentially all tests of function involve exposing the individual or a part of his body to a physiological stimulus and then observing his response directly or by means of an instrument.

A rough test of the capacity of an artery or group of arteries to meet the demands of tissues for nutrients and oxygen is whether or not pain and tenderness in the muscle are associated with activity. This may be determined by asking the person how far he can walk before he has pain. It can be determined more exactly by having the person step up and down on a stair step at a predetermined rate. The result is known as the claudication time.

A second method used to determine the adequacy of blood flow is to test the ability of the artery to maintain blood flow against gravity. In a man such as Mr. Marker with pain at rest, this test provides the physician with valuable information about the degree of failure of his arterial circulation. If pallor develops when the extremity is elevated, this indicates that there is a marked degree of arterial insufficiency. When the extremity is placed in a horizontal or dependent position, a slow rate of filling further indicates arterial insufficiency. Some physicians regard this test as among the most useful in estimating the degree of arterial insufficiency.

In peripheral occlusive vascular disease the physician may wish to determine the response of the blood vessels to physiological stimuli and the degree to which vasospasm is responsible for the signs and symptoms. To determine the degree of vasospasm some method is used to remove the effect of the sympathetic nervous system. Methods include exposing the patient to a warm environment or blocking the sympathetic ganglia or the peripheral nerve supply of the area. The effect of drugs such as alcohol or nicotine (smoking) may also be studied. The changes in blood flow may be determined by measuring the skin temperature, or by the use of instruments such as an oscillometer or a plethysmograph. The oscillometer is a manometer attached to the cuff used to measure the blood pressure. It is employed in peripheral occlusive vascular disease to determine the point of pressure at which circulation through the deep vessels to the thigh or calf ceases. Essentially the same test may be performed by pressing superficial arteries with the fingers and estimating the amount of pressure required to obliterate the pulse. Neither test provides exact information. The oscillometer is most useful in demonstrating differences between the circulation to the two extremities. The plethysmograph is a more sensitive instrument than the oscillometer. It measures the actual amount of blood entering the tissue.

Skin temperature is determined by a thermometer or thermocouple held in place in contact with the skin. Except when the temperature of the skin on one extremity differs markedly from that of another, the results may not be very valuable. Conditions such as exposure to cold or heat, exercise, the ingestion of food, and the emotional state of the person all influence skin temperature. In an attempt to minimize these factors the test is performed in a warm room with the patient at rest. Other conditions prescribed by the physician should be carefully met. The patient should be apprised of the procedure to be followed and the reasons for what is done.

In addition to determination of the degree to which spasm is present in blood vessels, the assessment of the patient may include the degree to which local or generalized vasospasm can be induced by exposure to cold. The test is usually performed by having the patient plunge his hand and forearm into a container of ice water. Depending on whether the local or general effects are of interest, the hands are checked for pallor and the other color changes characteristic of Raynaud's syndrome or the blood pressure is taken. The latter is known as the cold pressor test. Persons who have a greater-than-average rise in blood pressure are known as hyperreactors.

How is the structural status of blood vessels determined?

The location and extent of lesions in blood vessels may be studied by angiiography or arteriography. The specific method used in the performance of each test depends on the location of the artery under study. In all these studies a radiopaque substance is injected into the artery. Following this the area is X-rayed. Specific directions for the preparation and aftercare of the patient are given by the patient's physician or the physician performing the procedure.

All diagnostic tests are part of the total evaluation of the effect that a particular disease condition has on the patient. The nurse who cares for the patient has the continuing responsibility to assist in the preparation of the patient for what lies ahead, to assist with or to perform certain diagnostic procedures, and to provide aftercare for the patient. Sometimes a specific regime is required. Often, however, the care required relates more to the outcome of the test than it does to the test itself. When a period of time must elapse between the time the test is performed and the outcome is known, the patient and his family are likely to experience anxiety. Not all patients are relieved by a negative report. Was the test performed properly? What causes the symptoms? When the outcome is unfavorable, the patient is sometimes faced with an uncertain future. The nurse must be prepared to give the patient and his family emotional support and help him (them) learn to carry out the medical regime required.

Many problems of the patient who has an occlusive vascular disease are similar to those experienced by patients with other chronic diseases. Prevention of or delay in the progress of peripheral vascular disease often requires that the patient be willing to modify habits of eating, exercise, and smoking. Treatment and the prevention of serious complications make these measures imperative. Besides the patient must learn and practice the measures required to protect affected tissues. As in other chronic illnesses, much of the responsibility for continued therapy depends on the patient and his family. Unless they are willing and prepared to carry out the prescribed therapeutic regime, it is likely to fail. The nurse has a responsibility to assist the patient to learn to assume the day-by-day management of his disease and its complications.

Finally, as in other types of illness, the therapeutic regime may fail to effect improvement. Instead of getting better, the condition of the patient worsens. The patient still has needs, and something can be done to improve his comfort and well-being. Goals in nursing should be adapted to the needs and status of the patient.

Without the continuous movement of blood throughout the vascular circuit, life ceases. Some of the causes and effects of failure of the heart as a pump (source of power) and of occlusion of the vascular system have previously been delineated and related to the nursing needs of patients. Another crucial factor in circulatory function is the maintenance, within limits, of the pressure of the blood within the blood vessels. The effects of hypotension, or low blood pressure, have been discussed in other relationships and will not be further examined. In the following discussion some of the causes and effects of excessive blood pressure will be considered.

What is the normal range for the blood pressure and how does it vary during the lifetime of the individual?

As indicated in an earlier discussion of homeostatic mechanisms, the capacity to regulate the level of the blood pressure within physiological limits is essential to survival. Despite differences in the pressure of the blood in all parts of the vascular system, there is a normal range of pressure for each part. Arterial pressure is greater than venous pressure, but both have a normal range. In the following discussion, unless otherwise specified, references are to arterial blood pressure. Similar to other homeostatic mechanisms, the blood pressure is not regulated at the exact level, but fluctuates within limits. It varies among individuals as well as in the same person under different conditions. The level of the blood pressure is altered by changes in position, exercise, rest, emotional status, and age. It is slightly higher when the individual is in the sitting or upright position than when he is in the recumbent position. It is higher during exercise than at rest. It often drops during sleep. Emotional states, discomfort, a distended bladder, pain—all have an effect on the blood pressure, particularly on the level of the systolic pressure. Fear, anxiety, and apprehension may influence the level of the blood pressure. In some individuals, they may cause a marked rise.

Age is a significant factor in the level of the arterial blood pressure as it rises gradually from birth to maturity. In many persons it continues to rise throughout the life span. In the healthy newborn infant the arterial blood pressure is approximately 55 mm of mercury systolic and 40 mm of mercury diastolic. Blood pressure rises rapidly during the first few days of life, and by the tenth day the systolic pressure is around 78 mm of mercury. Blood pressure then rises gradually until maturity. The average healthy young adult has a blood pressure of about 120 systolic and 80 diastolic. The normal range, however, extends from 90 to 140 mm of mercury systolic and 60 to 90 mm of mercury diastolic. Moia[80] states that a blood pressure of 150 mm of mercury systolic and 90 mm of mercury diastolic is widely accepted as the upper limit of normal. Goldblatt[81] sets 140/90 as the upper limit of normal for persons at the age of 40. Despite more or less general agreement as to the physiological range for arterial blood pressure, there is no exact level below or above which the arterial blood pressure is normal or abnormal. People vary greatly in the capacity of their blood vessels to tolerate pressures above established "normal" limits. The age of the individual at which the elevation occurs is also of some significance. For example, a blood pressure of 160/100 is more significant in a girl of 15 than in a woman of 60.

Another factor making the problem of determining the upper limit of normal difficult is that, in many persons, the arterial blood pressure tends to continue to rise over the entire life span. This is particularly true of the systolic pressure. A blood pressure of 140/90 or higher is found in 40 per cent of individuals between the ages of 45 and 49 years of age and in 60 per cent of those between 60 and 64 years of age. Goldblatt[82] states that in the United States, at least 50 per cent of persons who are over 50 years of age have hypertension, and in at least 25 per cent of all persons above 50 years of age, it plays some part in their deaths. Statistical studies indicate that even a

---

[80] Blas Moia, "The Range of Normal Blood Pressure," *Cardiology*, IV, 1959, section 12-3, p. 8.
[81] Harry Goldblatt, "Mechanism of Hypertension in Cardiology," *Cardiology*, IV, 1959, section 12-30, p. 36.
[82] *Ibid.*, pp. 12-30.

small elevation in blood pressure shortens life expectancy.[83] These statistics have predictive value when applied to a group, but are of less value in anticipating the effect of elevation of the blood pressure in a specific individual. Some persons live to an advanced age despite a considerable elevation in arterial blood pressure. For example, Mrs. Timmins lived to age 88. For some time before her death, her blood pressure was 180/110, and it had been elevated for many years. Despite a marked degree of hypertension and the lack of specific therapy, she had always been well and active. In fact, she appeared to be in better health than many of her younger neighbors. For some reason her blood vessels were able to tolerate the increase in pressure without suffering a serious degree of vascular injury. One of the medical problems receiving attention is the finding of some method which will enable the physician to predict which patients with hypertension are most likely to develop progressive vascular disease.

The lower limit of normal is as difficult to define as the upper. Unlike the person whose blood pressure is at or above the upper limit of normal, the one whose blood pressure is below the norm, but who is otherwise healthy, has a better-than-average life expectancy. A systolic blood pressure of 90 to 100, in the absence of evidence of disease, is not usually regarded as evidence of pathology. In a sick patient a fall in the arterial blood pressure should always be questioned. The level at which blood pressure becomes abnormally low depends on the usual blood pressure. For example, Mrs. Timmins' blood pressure at rest was 190/110. A sudden fall to 120/70, though within the normal range for a healthy person, probably would indicate hypotension. Another patient's blood pressure is usually about 120/70. A blood pressure of 90/50 indicates some degree of hypotension. In the patient who has untreated adrenal insufficiency, blood pressure is usually low. A systolic blood pressure of 90 to 100 is not unusual. Unless the patient is under some kind of stress, emergency treatment is not usually required to elevate the blood pressure. In the patient who has adrenal insufficiency, even what appears to be a minor drop in the blood pressure should be considered as cause for concern and brought to the attention of the physician. In general, a marked or continuing fall in the level of the blood pressure should be regarded as abnormal and measures should be instituted to stabilize or elevate it. Patients who are being treated with hypotensive agents may be an exception. They should, however, be observed for the effects of their therapy. As a general rule, even in these patients, treatment is regulated in order to prevent sudden and marked lowering of the blood pressure. Since the pressure of the blood in the blood vessels is one of the factors in maintaining tissue nutrition, a sharp fall may result in relative ischemia of the tissues. Among the factors to be considered in evaluating the significance of one blood pressure reading are knowledge of the level compatible with the maintenance of a sufficient degree of hydrostatic pressure

[83] Metropolitan Life Insurance Company, *Statistical Bulletin*, XLI, August, 1960, p. 6.

to maintain tissue nutrition, the height of pressure that arteries are likely to tolerate, and the usual blood pressure of the patient.

As with other homeostatic mechanisms, the maintenance of blood pressure within limits requires a number of structures that are regulated not only individually, but in relation to each other. These components of the vascular system that affect the level of the blood pressure include: (1) the viscosity of the blood, (2) the total volume of the blood, (3) the rebound of the elastic material in the arterial wall during ventricular diastole, (4) the total peripheral resistance, and (5) the force with which the heart pumps blood into the arteries. Blood pressure remains stable as long as alterations in one or more factors are effectively opposed by changes in others. For example, a reduction in cardiac output will not result in a fall in the blood pressure if at the same time peripheral resistance is increased. The reverse is also true. When the cardiac output rises, the arterial blood pressure remains stable provided peripheral resistance diminishes; cardiac output also rises in the absence of a compensatory decrease in peripheral resistance. A reduction in peripheral resistance will likewise be accompanied by a fall in blood pressure unless there is a compensatory rise in cardiac output. Among the factors affecting arterial blood pressure, changes in peripheral resistance have the most profound effect. Relatively large changes in blood volume, blood viscosity, or arterial elasticity are required before the level of the blood pressure is altered appreciably.

What are the mechanisms for the regulation of the blood pressure? How does each mechanism function?

Although there may be other mechanisms regulating the level of the arterial blood pressure, Guyton[84] lists three: (1) the capillary fluid shift mechanism, (2) the sympathoadrenal, and (3) the kidney. Humoral agents including certain hormones should be added to the above classification since they have a regulatory effect on blood vessels as well as the kidney. The extent to which the kidney affects blood pressure in health is the subject of considerable debate.

How does the capillary fluid shift mechanism function in the regulation of blood pressure?

Each of the factors in the maintenance of blood pressure will be examined briefly. The capillary fluid shift mechanism effectively regulates the arterial blood pressure by altering the blood volume. When the arterial blood pressure rises, hydrostatic pressure within the capillaries is elevated and fluid is rapidly transferred into the interstitial space. As the blood volume diminishes, the interstitial fluid volume is enlarged, and blood pressure is prevented from rising excessively. Under some circumstances, such as in the seriously burned

[84] *Op. cit.,* p. 414.

patient, loss of fluid into the interstitial space in noninjured, as well as burned, areas may be sufficient to cause hypotension. The reverse process may also take place. With a decrease in the volume of blood, the pressure of blood in the capillaries falls. Fluid then moves from the interstitial space into the capillary and the blood volume is restored. As blood volume increases, arterial blood pressure is elevated. This mechanism is very important in the protection of the individual against the effects of rapid changes in the blood volume. It may also be a source of danger. A marked increase in blood volume, particularly when combined with an inadequate renal reserve, predisposes to pulmonary edema which can be severe enough to cause death. (See Chapter 8.) A rapid increase in blood volume also places a burden on the heart and predisposes to high-output failure. Within limits the capillary fluid shift mechanism protects the blood volume and the blood pressure by rapidly removing or adding fluid to the blood.

What are the factors contributing to peripheral resistance?

Before discussion of the roles played by the sympathetic nervous system and the kidney in the regulation of the blood pressure, the nature of and factors in peripheral resistance will be presented.

Peripheral resistance can be simply defined as the force opposing the movement of blood. The most important single factor in peripheral resistance is the arterioles and the small arteries because they have highly muscular walls and small lumens. Even small changes in the diameter of the arterioles has a marked effect on peripheral arterial resistance. Guyton[85] states that by reducing the diameter of an arteriole by one half, its resistance is increased as much as 16 times, while a fourfold decrease in arteriolar diameter can increase resistance as much as 256 times. As the lumen of the arteriole diminishes in size, a larger proportion of the blood passing through it comes in contact with the arteriolar wall which offers resistance to the movement of the blood. As arteriolar resistance or arterial peripheral resistance rises, the diastolic blood pressure is elevated. Usually, but not invariably, the systolic blood pressure also rises with the result that the pulse pressure remains within normal limits.

Although most of the peripheral resistance is due to the opposition offered by small arteries and arterioles to the flow of blood, all blood vessels offer some degree of resistance. A loss of tone in any part of the peripheral vascular bed predisposes to a drop in the blood pressure. From information gained through the use of monitoring equipment, one of the earliest changes in shock is an increase in venous pressure resulting from a loss of muscle tone in the veins. Peripheral resistance involves two different factors, the mechanisms regulating the tone of the vascular musculature and the responsiveness of the arterial musculature to stimulation. As long as the degree of stimulation and the responsiveness of the blood vessels are within physiological limits, periph-

[85] *Ibid.,* p. 365.

eral resistance as reflected by the blood pressure should also be within its normal range. Uncompensated abnormalities in either aspect of peripheral resistance, that is, over- or underregulation of hypo- or hyperresponsiveness of the vascular musculature, can be presumed to result in abnormal alterations in the level of the blood pressure.

The mechanisms regulating peripheral resistance include the sympathetic nervous system and humoral substances which affect vascular tone. Some of the humoral agents are secreted by the endocrine glands, some are formed by the ischemic kidney, and others are formed and act locally. Though a humoral vasodilator with widespread action has been postulated, its presence has not been proved. Certain products of metabolism, such as carbon dioxide, as well as substances released by injured cells dilate capillaries. These substances are of particular importance in regulating blood flow to the needs of localized tissue areas. As a consequence of a variety of regulatory mechanisms, large organisms with well-developed circulatory systems are capable of adapting peripheral resistance, and as a result blood flows, so that the needs of its cells are met. Under conditions of rest and moderate activity, tissues regulate their own blood supply in accordance with their needs. Under emergency situations or when activity is greatly increased, blood flow can be modified in relation to the needs of the entire individual or to those of a particular or of a specialized tissue.

What is the role of the sympathetic nervous system in the regulation of blood pressure?

The nervous system, principally the sympathetic nervous system, regulates the smooth muscle in blood vessels causing either vasoconstriction or vasodilatation. As a result of activation of the sympathetic nervous system, there may be generalized vasoconstriction of blood vessels, or those in certain regions of the body may be constricted or dilated. Apparently depending on the degree and type of stimulation, activation of the sympathetic nervous system may result in vasoconstriction or vasodilatation. Although the effect may be general, it may also enable the body to shift blood from one region to another. As an illustration, constriction of the renal arteries limits blood flow through the kidney. Since approximately 1,200 ml of blood flows through the kidneys each minute, a reduction to 200 ml will make available 1,000 ml to circulate to more immediately vital organs such as the brain and heart.[86] Because the nervous system acts rapidly, it enables the individual to react quickly and as a whole to changes in the environment and to protect the function of vital organs. Although adjustments in the blood pressure are made rapidly by the nervous system, they are not sustained for a long period of time.

Regulation of the caliber of blood vessels by the nervous system involves

---

[86] Robert F. Pitts, *Physiology of the Kidney and Body Fluids,* The Year Book Publishers, Inc., Chicago, 1963, p. 136.

higher as well as lower centers.[87] Centers for the regulation of the diameter of blood vessels are located in the cerebral cortex, the hypothalamus, and the medulla. These centers not only regulate the sending of messages to blood vessels in the periphery, usually by way of the sympathetic nervous system, but they have an inhibitory effect on each other. Impulses arriving in these centers have their origin in receptors located in various parts of the body. Some are located within the vascular system while others are outside it. Among those situated within the vascular system are receptors in the arch of the aorta and in the carotid sinus; they are stimulated by increases in the pressure of the blood. Although they are called baro- or mechanoreceptors, they are actually stimulated by stretching or dilatation of the aorta or carotid sinus. Receptors located outside the vascular system which may initiate impulses resulting in a change in the caliber of blood vessels include those of sight, sound, hearing, heat, cold, touch, and pain. Biochemical changes, such as changes in the pH of body fluids, may stimulate vasomotor centers in the nervous system resulting in changes in the caliber of blood vessels. Because man reacts to symbols or the meaning events have for him, these too may act as stimuli and result in alterations in peripheral resistance and therefore in the level of blood pressure.

With a few exceptions, such as the coronary arteries, the sympathetic nervous system regulates both vasconstriction and vasodilatation. Vasoconstriction results from an increase in sympathetic activity. Vasodilatation in many regions of the body results from a lessening of sympathetic tone. In some organs such as the coronary arteries and the skeletal muscles, the sympathetic nervous system actively dilates blood vessels. This is its only effect on the coronary arteries.

Although the regulation of caliber of blood vessels by the nervous system facilitates adaptation to the environment, the sympathetic nervous system can be removed and the individual will survive. His capacity to respond to stresses such as changing his position from the recumbent to the upright and to hemorrhage is, of course, reduced. Because increase in the activity of the sympathetic nervous system increases peripheral resistance, it may be a factor in hypertension. Some authorities suggest that although the capacity to constrict blood vessels quickly once facilitated survival, in a protected society such as ours, it may be a handicap.

In regulating peripheral resistance, the action of the sympathetic nervous system is supported by hormones secreted by the adrenal medulla, norepinephrine and epinephrine. Norepinephrine exerts a vasoconstrictor effect, while epinephrine increases the force of cardiac contraction. Both hormones lead to an elevation in blood pressure through their actions on the heart and blood vessels.[88] These hormones probably have little effect on the blood pressure

[87] See Best and Taylor, *Op. cit.*, 7th ed., p. 258.
[88] Harold A. Harper, *Review of Physiological Chemistry,* 8th ed., Lange Medical Publications, Los Altos, California, 1961.

during ordinary activity, but augment the effect of the sympathetic nervous system during stress.

What is the role of the kidney in the regulation of the blood pressure?

A number of factors have contributed to the belief that the kidney has one or more roles in the regulation of the blood pressure. Exactly what its role(s) is (are) has not been proved. Such questions as whether the kidney regulates blood flow through itself are a subject of great interest and of great controversy. The fact that there is some relationship between decreased blood flow through the kidney and the level of arterial blood pressure has been established clinically and experimentally. The classical experiment of Goldblatt demonstrates that obstruction to the flow of blood through the kidney is followed by an elevation in the arterial blood pressure. In the preparation of a Goldblatt kidney, clamps are applied to the renal arteries to limit blood flow to the kidney. After a few weeks the systemic blood pressure rises above the preclamp level, and the blood pressure in the arteries distal to the clamp, that is, within the kidney, also rises. Diseases in which there is a diminished flow of blood through the kidney such as acute glomerulonephritis and chronic pyelonephritis are accompanied by hypertension.

What are some of the hypotheses proposed to explain the role of the kidney in the regulation of the blood pressure?

A number of hypotheses have been suggested to explain the apparent role of the kidney in the regulation of the arterial blood pressure. Currently there is evidence that the kidney may affect blood pressure in three different ways: (1) under certain circumstances the kidney releases an enzyme which reacts with a component in the plasma to form a pressor substance, (2) the healthy kidneys either destroy a pressor substance found in the blood or they release a depressor factor, and (3) they produce a substance that sensitizes the arterioles to circulating pressor materials.[89]

Of the three possible roles of the kidney in the regulation of the blood pressure, most is known about the first. Almost 100 years ago it was learned that a substance extracted from the kidney had a pressor or blood pressure-elevating effect. Because of its origin, the material was named renin. Renin has been purified. It is released by a hypoxic kidney into the blood, where it interacts with a serum protein, an alpha-2-globulin which is formed in the liver to form a weak pressor substance called angiotensin I. Angiotensin I is converted by an enzyme found in the blood plasma to angiotensin II, a highly active pressor material. Angiotensin is destroyed by an enzyme angiotensinase, which is present in the blood plasma and in many organs including the kidney, intestine, and liver. There is considerable doubt among scientists as to

[89] Pitts, *Op. cit.,* p. 140.

whether the renin-angiotensin system functions in the regulation of blood flow through the kidney in health. Its action may well be limited to situations in which blood supply to the kidney is threatened. Whether or not this system plays a role in the development of human hypertension is also a subject of controversy.

How is the term "hypertension" defined?

A so-called normal blood pressure results when the various components within the vascular system are functioning within limits and the regulatory mechanisms are capable of effecting appropriate adjustments among them. That the body is not always able to make appropriate adjustments is attested to by the frequency with which blood pressure falls below or exceeds the levels required to maintain blood supply to the tissues. When the level of the blood pressure exceeds physiological limits, the condition is referred to as hypertension or arterial hypertension. Depending on which component is elevated, it is called systolic or diastolic hypertension. When both the systolic and diastolic blood pressures are elevated, it is called systolic-diastolic hypertension. An abnormal elevation in the arterial blood pressure, or hypertension, is a finding associated with an abnormality of function and sometimes of structure, but it is not a disease per se any more than pain or fever is. Some authorities distinguish between hypertension and hypertensive disease. They employ the word "hypertension" to denote the elevation of the blood pressure in the absence of demonstrable changes in the vascular system, and "hypertensive disease" to indicate the presence of vascular disease.

What are the causes of hypertension?

Abnormal elevations in the blood pressure may be of known or unknown origin. In about 10 per cent of persons with hypertension, the elevation of the blood pressure is secondary to some known disorder. In approximately 90 per cent the cause is not known and the disorder is classified as essential hypertension.

Among the disorders known to cause hypertension are:

1. Systolic hypertension
   A. Increased stroke volume of the heart
      (1) Anemia
      (2) Thyrotoxicosis
   B. Aortic rigidity (atherosclerosis the most common cause)
2. Diastolic and systolic hypertension
   A. Disorders of the central nervous system
      (1) Diseases of the brain stem and spinal cord (poliomyelitis and tabes dorsalis)

       (2) Increased intracranial pressure
         (a) Neoplasms
         (b) Inflammatory lesions
  B. Disorders of adrenal and chromaffin tissues
     (1) Pheochromocytoma
     (2) Cushing's syndrome
     (3) Primary aldosteronism
  C. Disorders of the kidney (usually in those disorders in which the blood supply is impaired or there is injury to the parenchyma)
     (1) Acute and chronic glomerulonephritis
     (2) Pyelonephritis
     (3) Disorders impairing the blood supply to the kidney
         (a) Acute renal ischemia
         (b) Lesions obstructing the renal artery (embolic, thrombotic, etc.)
     (4) Urinary-tract obstruction
  D. Toxemia of pregnancy (not discussed)
  E. Coarctation of the aorta

In anemia and thyrotoxicosis the abnormal elevation in the systolic blood pressure is due to an increase in cardiac output. In either disorder, blood pressure can be restored to normal by correcting the underlying disorder.

Systolic hypertension due to aortic rigidity is a very common finding among older individuals. By itself it does not usually seriously affect the life of the individual. The elevation in the blood pressure is permanent.

Disorders in the nervous system that impinge on the blood supply of the brain, particularly when they develop rapidly, are usually accompanied by an increase in blood pressure. As the blood pressure rises, there is often a decrease in the pulse rate. The rise in the blood pressure results from the initiation of mechanisms for the maintenance of cerebral blood flow. As such they are protective. A rise in blood pressure in a patient with a lesion likely to threaten the blood supply of the brain, such as an acute inflammatory process, a head injury, or a neoplasm, should always be regarded as indicating the possibility of cerebral ischemia. (See Chapter 13 B.)

Hypertension may be due to disorders involving either the medulla or the cortex of the adrenal gland. Hypertension associated with hypersecretion of the adrenal medulla is usually due to a tumor of the medulla or chromaffin tissue known as a pheochromocytoma. The pheochromocytoma secretes both epinephrine and norepinephrine. Epinephrine affects the blood pressure primarily by increasing the force of cardiac contraction, and norepinephine, by increasing peripheral resistance by its vasoconstrictor effect. In addition to hypertension, there are usually other manifestations indicating excessive secretion of epinephrine including palpitation, nausea and vomiting, sweating, anxiety, dyspnea, pounding headache, paresthesia, vertigo, and glycosuria.

One patient observed by the writer had periodic attacks of anxiety so severe that she was diagnosed as being in an acute anxiety state. Pheochromocytoma causes one of the curable types of hypertension, since it can be excised surgically. Although the blood pressure may be elevated continuously, periodic attacks of hypertension are common. Hypertension due to pheochromocytoma can frequently be established by the patient's response to phentolamine hydrochloride (Regitine), an adrenergic blocking agent. Following the administration of phentolamine hydrochloride, the blood pressure should drop appreciably, as the drug prevents the effector substance in the arteriole from responding to norepinephrine. In hypertension due to other causes than pheochromocytoma, lowering of the blood pressure to a significant degree does not occur.

Both Cushing's syndrome and primary aldosteronism are disorders of the adrenal cortex. Cushing's syndrome results from a neoplasm or hyperplasia of the adrenal cortex. Aldosteronism results from a neoplasm. One possible factor in hypertension in these disorders is that excessive quantities of the adrenal cortical hormones, most particularly the mineralocorticoids, desoxycorticosterone, and aldosterone, enhance arteriolar responsiveness. Not only does hypertension accompany disorders accompanied by hypersecretion by the adrenal cortex, but it may be precipitated by desoxycorticosterone administered in the treatment of disease. When desoxycorticosterone was first introduced in the treatment of Addison's disease (chronic adrenal insufficiency), several patients died from complications induced by the effects of rapidly developing hypertension. Persons who have adrenal insufficiency characteristically have low blood pressures.

Not all the relationships of the adrenal steroids to vascular reactivity are known. They act conditionally; that is, their effects depend on the presence of the sodium ion. The reactivity of smooth muscle is affected by the balance of ions within the cells as well as in the intracellular fluid. The adrenal cortical hormones affect this balance among ions. Correction of the cause of excess secretion of adrenal cortical hormones is often followed by a restoration of the level of the blood pressure to normal.

In the discussion of the possible role of the kidney in the regulation of arterial blood pressure, the point was made that hypertension is common in any disorder in which the blood supply to the kidney is impaired. It is also found in disorders in which the parenchyma is diseased. In some instances in which only one kidney is diseased and it is removed surgically, the blood pressure returns to normal. When both kidneys are diseased, hypertension continues.

Finally, a known and curable cause of hypertension is coarctation of the aorta. In this disorder, at some point along the aorta a constricting band reduces the size of its lumen. In some instances, the channel may be so small that a broom straw may scarcely be able to pass through the occluded portion. These patients are hypertensive in the blood vessels above the site of constriction. They are usually hypotensive in those below the constriction. When the site of narrowing can be removed surgically, the blood pressure returns to physiological limits after the obstruction is removed.

What is the most common form of diastolic and systolic hypertension in the United States?

By far the most frequent type of diastolic and systolic hypertension in the United States is essential hypertension, that is, hypertension of unknown cause. About 90 per cent of persons with hypertension have this type. About 5 per cent of the population have essential or primary hypertension. Despite an elevation of the diastolic and usually, though not invariably, the systolic blood pressure, the specific cause for this is not known. The constriction of the arterioles and small arteries is believed to be about equally distributed throughout the body. Schroeder[90] states that three hypotheses have been suggested to account for this vasoconstriction. They are:

1. Sympathetic vasoconstrictor nerves are hyperactive.
2. There is a vasoconstrictor substance in the blood which acts directly on smooth muscle of the blood vessels.
3. The smooth muscle becomes "sensitized" to normally acting sympathetic nerves or to constrictor substances.

Whether the cause of hypertension is primary or secondary to a specific disease, a rise in the blood pressure causes vascular damage in proportion to the degree of elevation.[91] Although it is generally true that the higher the blood pressure, the greater the damage to blood vessels, the susceptibility of different individuals to the effects of hypertension varies greatly. Some people tolerate markedly elevated blood pressures for a long time without much evidence of vascular damage. Why this is true is not known. As indicated in the discussion of coronary artery disease, hypertension accelerates the rate at which atherosclerosis and arteriolar sclerosis develop.

The serious consequences of hypertension arise from its effects on the heart, the kidney, and the brain. As the peripheral arterioles narrow, peripheral resistance rises. The heart muscle undergoes work hypertrophy, and for a period of time at least, blood flow to the tissues is maintained within physiological limits. Eventually, for reasons already explained, the heart muscle may fail as a pump. Congestive heart failure eventually occurs in about 25 per cent of persons with hypertension. Myocardial infarction also occurs at an earlier age in hypertensive than in normotensive persons.

That the kidney is involved in essential hypertension is demonstrated by

[90] Henry A. Schroeder, "Biochemical Aspects of Hypertension," *Cardiology*, IV, 1959, pp. 12-20, 12-29.
[91] John H. Moyer, "Blood Pressure Regulation in the Treatment of Hypertension," *American Journal of Cardiology*, IX, June, 1962, p. 821.

scars found in the kidneys of some persons dying as a consequence of one of the complications of hypertension. In the most rapidly progressive and serious phase of hypertension, changes in the structure of the kidney are invariably found.

Involvement of the blood vessels supplying the brain results in hypertensive headache, hypertensive encephalopathy, and cerebral thrombosis or hemorrhage. Not all persons with hypertension develop any of the cerebral complications. The reason for the headache is not known. It is usually in the occipital region and awakens the patient in the morning and disappears as the day progresses. Caffeine often gives relief.

According to Sommers *et al*,[92] hypertensive encephalopathy is a more advanced stage of hypertensive headache. In this stage, decreased tone of the arterioles in the brain allows the relatively high pressures to be transmitted to the capillary bed. With the increased blood pressure, transudation of fluid is increased and the brain becomes edematous. The consequences of cerebral edema and increased intracranial pressure are discussed in detail in Chapter 13 B.

According to the authors cited above, cerebral blood flow and metabolism in the tissues of the brain of most patients who are hypertensive are normal. Hypertension does, however, predispose to the earlier development of cerebrovascular changes than in persons whose blood pressures are within normal limits. The result of cerebral hemorrhage due to rupture of a cerebral artery, or to the occlusion of an artery supplying the brain by a thrombus, is known as a stroke or cerebrovascular accident. The manifestations experienced by the patient will depend on the location and extent to which the brain is deprived of its blood supply. Hemiplegia is a common sequela though it is not inevitable.

The blood vessels in the retina of the eye are also affected. Since they can be observed directly by ophthalmoscopic examination, information about the degree of vasoconstriction and the structural alterations in the arterioles and other vessels can be obtained by direct observation. Papilledema or swelling of the optic disc can also be observed when retinoscopy (the examination of the retina of the eye through an ophthalmoscope) is to be performed by the physician; the patient should be informed that it is a painless procedure. A drop of a cycloplegic is usually placed in each eye to paralyze the iris and the ciliary muscle. The pupils dilate and do not react to light. After the pupils are dilated, the patient will usually experience some blurring of near vision such as when attempting to read. With short-acting cycloplegics blurring is present for only a short period of time. With long-acting ones, such as atropine, the effect may last for a day or more. In patients with glaucoma, a disorder characterized by elevated intraocular pressure, cycloplegics are not used, be-

[92] Sheldon C. Sommers, Robert J. McLaughlin, and Robert L. McAuley, "Pathology of Diastolic Hypertension as Generalized Vascular Disease," *American Journal of Cardiology*, IX, May, 1962, p. 653.

cause dilatation of the pupil is accompanied by a decrease in the degree of the angle of Schlemm. Drainage of fluid from the globe is thereby decreased and the intraocular pressure is raised. With the elevation in the intraocular pressure, blood flow to the tissues of the eye is diminished and damage to the eye increases. In susceptible patients, the injury may be sufficient to cause blindness. In preparation for a retinoscopic examination the room should be darkened. During the examination the patient who is able to cooperate will be asked to look at a fixed point and not to move his eye. As implied above, retinoscopy is a widely used procedure to determine the condition of the retina and its blood vessels as well as of the optic disc. In addition to information about conditions within the eyeball itself, deductions can be made about the state of the blood vessels throughout the body as well as pressure conditions within the cranial cavity.

For the sake of emphasis, some of the essential points about the nature and effects of essential hypertension are repeated below. Although a specific cause cannot be identified in essential hypertension, the elevation in the blood pressure is believed to be due to an imbalance between sympathomimetic activity and the responsiveness of small arteries and arterioles to stimulation. With greater vasoconstriction, peripheral resistance is increased and with it the diastolic blood pressure. Some authorities suggest that the initiating event in essential hypertension is an increase in cardiac output. In response to the increase in cardiac output, small arteries and arterioles constrict to protect the capillaries from excessive pressure. Eventually arteriolar constriction becomes the prominent feature. There is also the possibility that arteriolar constriction precedes other changes. In the past some authorities believed that the elevation of the blood pressure followed rather than preceded vascular damage. Presently, however, vascular injury is more generally believed to follow the elevation of the blood pressure. In accordance with this hypothesis, arteriolar hypertrophy is the result of more or less continued contraction of arteriolar musculature. Whatever the sequence of events, arteriolar sclerosis and atherosclerosis develop at an earlier age in hypertensive than in nonhypertensive persons.

Until vascular damage occurs, other than for the elevation in the blood pressure, there are often no other manifestations of the disturbance. As a result many persons are discovered to be hypertensive at the time they are examined for insurance policies or for some other purpose. Other cases are not discovered until some vascular catastrophe occurs. Although the organs most frequently involved in the complications of hypertension are the heart, the kidney, and the brain, hypertension is nevertheless a generalized disturbance in which there is excessive constriction of the small arteries and arterioles throughout the body. These changes can be directly observed in the retina of the eye. Once complications have occurred, many of the needs of the patient for nursing will be determined by the nature of the complication.

As implied by the previous discussion, hypertension predisposes to vascular damage and with it serious complications involving the heart, kidney, and brain. Despite the frequency with which these conditions are associated, hypertension does not invariably injure blood vessels. There is also a difference among individuals as to the length of time their blood vessels will tolerate hypertension before evidence of vascular injury occurs. As stated earlier, some physicians classify patients whose blood pressures are elevated, but who do not have evidence of vascular injury, as hypertensives and those with vascular injury as having hypertensive disease. Therefore hypertension may be classified according to the phase or stage of the disease. These various phases include prehypertension, labile, benign, and malignant hypertension. Not all persons go through all phases or progress from one to another.

In the person who is in the prehypertensive phase, the arterial blood pressure is within the normal range most of the time. His blood pressure may be at the upper end of the normal range, however. He differs from nonhypertensive individuals, because he hyperreacts to vasoconstricting stimuli by manifesting a greater or more sustained rise in his blood pressure than do normotensive persons. Studies of the effect of the cold pressor test on schoolchildren indicate that although all children have some rise in blood pressure during the test, some hyperreact to the test by elevating their blood pressures to higher-than-expected levels. The cold pressor test is performed by determining the resting blood pressure; then the person being tested plunges his arm into a container of iced water. Since cold initiates impulses resulting in increased peripheral vasoconstriction, blood pressure rises. A rise in the diastolic blood pressure has predictive value in terms of later development of essential hypertension. According to Hines[93] a rise in the level of the diastolic pressure during the cold pressor test predicts the development of sustained hypertension in more than 50 per cent of individuals.

Recently reported studies of the effect of emotional stress on blood pressure indicate that in some persons, elevations in the blood pressure are sustained for a longer period of time than they are in others. Not all persons whose blood vessels hyperreact do, however, develop hypertension. If methods could be developed to identify those persons who are most likely to become hypertensive, that is, who are truly prehypertensive, perhaps preventive measures could be instituted to delay the onset and progress of the disease.

Some persons have what is known as labile hypertension at the time they come to medical attention. The word "labile" is derived from the Latin word *labilis meaning* "likely to slip." When used as an adjective to describe a disease or state, labile means unstable. Therefore labile hypertension is unstable; that is, the blood pressure is subject to fluctuation. During periods of stress, the blood pressure may be markedly elevated; when the individual is at rest or relaxed, it may be at or near normal levels. It is not at all unusual for a patient to be admitted to the hospital with a diastolic blood pressure of 110 or

[93] Edgar A. Hines, "The Significance of Vascular Hyperreaction As Measured By The Cold-Pressor Test, *The American Heart Journal*, XIX, 1940, pp. 408-16.

more and a systolic blood pressure of 180 or more and after a period of rest to find that his blood pressure has fallen to normal, or nearly normal, levels. These individuals have labile hypertension. Labile hypertension is an important finding inasmuch as it is frequently followed by permanent hypertension. According to Moia,[94] permanent hypertension develops three to five times more frequently in an individual with labile hypertension than in one whose blood vessels do not overrespond. Persons who are in this phase of hypertension may in some instances be able to delay the development of hypertensive disease by appropriate changes in their habits of living.

When patients are admitted to the hospital for the treatment of hypertension, they are usually in the benign or malignant phase of the disease. Formerly benign and malignant hypertension were believed to be two different diseases. Currently malignant hypertension is usually regarded as an accelerated form of hypertension. In the terminal stage of benign hypertension, it may become malignant.

When the terms "benign" and "malignant" are used as adjectives to describe the character of a disease, their true meaning should be remembered. The word benign means kindly. A benign person is kindly. Used to describe the character of a disease, it means that it is relatively harmless. It does not mean that under some circumstances it will not cause harm, however. Benign diseases, including benign hypertension, usually progress slowly. Benign hypertension is defined by Goldblatt[95] as "persistently elevated blood pressure of unknown origin not accompanied by significant renal excretory functional disturbance." In contrast to benign disease, malignant disease endangers the life of the individual, often within a relatively short period of time. At one time a patient with malignant hypertension did not usually survive for more than a year. Because of the availability and use of drugs that are effective in lowering the blood pressure, prognosis in malignant hypertension has improved. The definition of malignant hypertension which follows indicates why the prognosis is guarded.

Malignant hypertension, as defined by the Medical Advisory Board of the Council for High Blood Pressure of the American Heart Association, is as follows: "A clinical phase, rarely occurring, de novo, more often appearing after a primary or secondary hypertension, characterized by diastolic hypertension and by accelerated and progressive renal damage, usually (but not necessarily) accompanied by papilledema, often by retinal hemorrhage and 'exudate' and giving rise to death from uremia, unless the course is terminated along the way by complicating brain or heart damage."

What are some of the factors contributing to the development of essential hypertension?

As in other chronic disorders involving a failure in a homeostatic mechanism, hypertension probably results from the interaction of a number of fac-

---

[94] Moia, *Op. cit.*, p. 12-7.
[95] *Op. cit.*, pp. 12-31.

tors. Hypertension develops when a combination of necessary and sufficient conditions is present. One factor appearing to predispose to essential hypertension is heredity. The incidence of hypertension is higher among offspring of hypertensive parents or grandparents than among those whose parents or grandparents are normotensive. In persons who are predisposed to hypertension by heredity, elevations in the diastolic and systolic blood pressures can be induced by chilling, frustration, anger, and anxiety. According to Merrill,[96] even the anticipation of a pleasant event may be accompanied by a rise in arterial blood pressure. Although exactly how heredity predisposes to hypertension has not been settled, one hypothesis is that it determines the responsiveness of the smooth muscle in the small arteries and arterioles to sympathomimetic agents.

Among other factors seeming to predispose to hypertension, or to aggravate it, are sex, obesity, race, body build, and personality. Hypertension is somewhat more common among women than men, but women tolerate it better. Women who are hypertensive are likely to be obese, but men do not differ in weight and stature from the ordinary population. Essential hypertension has a higher incidence and develops at an earlier age among Negroes living in the United States and in Panama than it does in Caucasians and Indians. Negroes also have a higher incidence of the disease in the accelerated or malignant form. Authorities have somewhat different views on the relationship of personality to the development of essential hypertension. Perera[97] states that despite efforts to relate personality to the development of essential hypertension, it is doubtful that there is a specific personality pattern characteristic of this disorder. Merrill[98] states that the majority of patients with hypertension have disorders of personality which may be made worse by environmental or emotional stress. Fluctuations in blood pressure of these patients can be correlated with changes in the emotional state in the individual.

Cardon[99] agrees that efforts to describe a personality pattern exclusively and always present in patients with hypertension have not been successful. He lists a number of characteristics which have been observed by different investigators. They are: "(1) neurotic traits, (2) excessive dependency needs, (3) poorly handled feelings of hostility, (4) difficulties in inter-personal relationships, (5) excessive rigidity, and (6) easily injured or afraid of injuring others." Other writers describe the hypertensive person as being excessively anxious. All the above characteristics may be observed in normotensive persons. Furthermore, not all hypertensive persons manifest these traits. Another observation that may prove to be of some significance is that persons whose hypertension is associated with a specific cause show the same behavior as

[96] *Op. cit.,* p. 1350.
[97] Perera, *Op. cit.,* p. 715.
[98] Merrill, *Op. cit.,* p. 1356.
[99] Philippe V. Cardon, "Psychic Factors in Hypertension," *Cardiology,* IV, 1959, pp. 12-9 to 12-14.

those with essential hypertension. Moreover, emotional tension, which is common among these persons, is relieved by surgical or chemical treatment that is effective in restoring them to a normotensive state. The behavior of hypertensive individuals may in some instances be due to the disease, rather than the cause of it.

The possibility that the kidney is responsible for hypertension has been extensively debated for many years. Evidence cited in support of the kidney's role includes the fact that the incidence of hypertension is higher among women than among men. Since the incidence of pyelonephritis is also higher among women, a possible relationship is suggested. Diseases of the kidney, particularly those in which the blood supply is impaired or the parenchyma is diseased, are accompanied by hypertension. The ischemic kidney is known to produce a pressor substance or a precursor to a pressor agent. Against the hypothesis is the fact that although some persons with hypertension do have kidney disease, by no means do all.

Summary

At the present time the specific factors in the etiology of essential hypertension are not known. The factors contributing to the disorder appear to be due to an imbalance between sympathomimetic activity and vascular responsiveness.[100] There is disagreement among authorities, however, about the degree to which each of these factors is responsible. Though there are specific disorders in which hypertension is associated with increased sympathomimetic activity or with increased vascular responsiveness, in most persons with hypertension the specific cause of the hypertension cannot be identified. Whatever its role in the genesis of hypertension, an increase in sympathomimetic activity aggravates pre-existing hypertension. This fact has many implications for nursing.

As a consequence of constriction of small arteries and arterioles, peripheral resistance is increased; the diastolic pressure is increased. Essential hypertension induces pathology by increasing the work of the myocardium and accelerating the rate at which atherosclerosis develops. Despite its generally deleterious effects, some individuals are able to tolerate hypertension for many years.

Although knowledge of specific causation is lacking, much can be done to slow the progress of hypertension and to prevent the development of its complications. The fact that an individual's blood pressure is or is not within the normal range is easily determined. The procedure has become so common and is so generally accepted that at least one mail order catalogue offers: "Sphygmomanometer takes your blood pressure. No fuss, no bother, no office visits when you want a reading. Directions are also given for its use and the

[100] John H. Moyer, "Etiology of Hypertension," *American Journal of Cardiology,* IX, May, 1962, pp. 651-52.

cost only $19.95." A blood pressure determination is a part of almost all screening as well as diagnostic examinations.

When the blood pressure is found to be elevated, the physician tries to establish the etiology. When a specific condition associated with hypertension is found that can be cured, the blood pressure can usually be expected to return to normal levels after treatment of the disorder. In patients who have incurable disorders or essential hypertension, the same degree of specificity in treatment is not available. In general, controlling and delaying the progress of the disorder, not curing it, are the principal objectives. Merrill[101] emphasizes the importance of remembering that a patient and not just an elevated blood pressure is being treated.

There is as much disagreement among physicians as to how and who should be treated for hypertension as there is about which factor or factors is/are responsible for its development. Different physicians hold opposing views and all shades of opinion in between. Most physicians agree that the patient in the accelerated phase of the disease should be treated. Because the patient in the accelerated phase has a high diastolic pressure and rapidly progressing lesions in the retina and kidney, he should be treated with any measure that is successful in lowering blood pressure. Methods used in the therapy of hypertension include superficial or intensive psychotherapy, diet, drugs, surgery, and modifications in the mode of life. The principal objective of all these forms of therapy is to lower the blood pressure by lessening vasoconstriction. After the blood pressure is lowered, a regime is established in an effort to maintain it within normal or nearly normal limits. This objective is based on growing evidence that elevation of the blood pressure has a damaging effect on blood vessels.

Among all the types of therapy, psychotherapy is most commonly used. For most patients psychotherapy is in the form of constructive physician- and/or nurse-patient relationship. In some instances patients do undergo intensive psychotherapy. According to Merrill,[102] the results are at least as good as those of other forms of treatment. Knowledge is not yet available as to whether treated patients continue over time to remain normotensive. Once intensive psychotherapy is initiated the patient must continue treatment as long as indicated, since there is the possibility the hypertension will be exaggerated for a time after therapy is initiated. For the patient to benefit, he must continue under treatment through this period and until the therapy is completed.

Superficial psychotherapy is administered by the patient's own physician and by others in his environment. Writers describing the characteristics of the manner of the physician use words such as quiet and calm manner, confidence, patience, and enthusiasm to indicate a helpful approach to the patient. These characteristics would seem to be no less important to the nurse.

101 Merrill, *Op. cit.,* p. 1356.
102 *Ibid.,* p. 1356.

As in other chronic disorders, one of the important objectives of therapy is to help the patient learn to cope with his disease. This objective could be stated as, "to assist the patient in the identification of situations in his life causing him to constrict his blood vessels and to then help him to learn to handle these situations so that they do not result in vasoconstriction." The attitudes of the patient toward his life, work, home, religion, members of his family, the neighbors, his co-workers, and other persons all affect the level of his blood pressure. Each patient may be expected to react to different aspects of life differently; a factor that is a cause of stress in one individual may not be in another. What the hypertensive patient should be helped to do is to identify those things that cause him to constrict his blood vessels and then try to modify his reaction or change the situation. Sometimes this is relatively easy. For example, Martha Brown, whose blood pressure was 190/120, found that as she approached a red traffic light, she became tense and angry. She acted as if the red light were a personal affront. By starting ten minutes earlier than usual in the morning and making a conscious effort to relax her muscles when a light turned red as she approached, she was able to remove this one stimulus to vasoconstriction. Other problems required other approaches. For example, her desk at work was near that of a woman who irritated her excessively. One solution was, of course, to resign or to request to move into another office. Since neither of these choices was practical, Miss Brown decided, insofar as she could, to ignore the woman's remarks and to try to find the reason for her own excessive reactions to her. Another cause of stress to Miss Brown was the fact that because her invalid mother lived with her, she felt she could not take a vacation. Miss Brown recognized that, despite her protestations to the contrary, she resented not being able to take a vacation. As a result she decided to talk to her married sister about the possibility of the sister caring for their mother while Miss Brown spent two weeks at a vacation resort and of relieving her one week end each month. With regular relief from the responsibility for her mother, her resentment diminished and her day-to-day relationship with her mother improved. The level of her blood pressure also fell. The nurse and the physician, by their manner and interest, helped Miss Brown to identify the circumstances in her life contributing to her hypertension. They were also able to suggest possible alternatives available to her. They encouraged her to continue to try to modify her behavior and approach to the troublesome aspects of her life. They could not, however, alter the circumstances in Miss Brown's environment; only Miss Brown could do that. They could and did provide her with support when she needed it.

In addition to the problems the patient brings with him at the time the diagnosis is established, the fact of hypertension is often fear-provoking. Recently the writer was with Mrs. Willow when her physician told her her blood pressure was normal. After the physician left, Mrs. Willow turned and said, "In that case, I do not have to worry about a stroke and becoming paralyzed." Mrs. Willow's son responded in a similar manner when his mother told him her blood pressure was normal. The possibility of a stroke is not an uncommon fear among hypertensive persons. A stroke and paralysis are, of course, not inevitable. They can also occur in the absence of hypertension. Should the patient express this fear to the nurse, she should try to convey to the patient her acceptance of his feeling. She should also bring to the attention of the physician the fact that the patient is afraid that he will have a stroke and be paralyzed.

When a hypertensive patient is hospitalized for diagnosis and treatment, the nurse should try to control the physical and psychosocial environment of the patient so that the stressful situations are kept to a minimum. According to Janis[103] most patients find distressing procedures easier to bear if they do not have to know about them too far in advance. Then they should be told only the necessary details. Relating all the possible sources of stress is, obviously, impossible. Two having particular pertinence are the exact level of the blood pressure and inappropriate remarks made in the presence of the patient.

In many hospitals and physicians' offices only the physician tells the patient what the level of his blood pressure is. Patients react differently to this practice. Some patients accept the statement that the nurse is not permitted to tell him. Other patients are distressed by the refusal of the nurse to provide them with the desired information. In this event, the nurse should relay the desires of the patient to the physician. She should, also, try to convey to the patient her understanding of his feelings, but in this matter she must defer to the wishes of his physician. There are several reasons for the desire of the physician to control the information given to the patient. A single blood pressure reading apart from others is not highly significant. There is also some virtue in all the information about the patient and his progress coming from one source. Most patients know or soon learn what the hospital policies are in respect to their care. Sometimes they ask the nurse for information she cannot give them to test her. They may be reassured by the suggestion of the nurse to ask their physicians. Since people are individuals, the nurse should try to evaluate the effect of withholding information from the patient. When it appears to lead to an increase in anxiety, this should be discussed with the physician.

Patients may also be subjected to unnecessary stress by hearing thoughtless or tactless remarks or by hearing "their case" discussed, as if they were not present. Physicians state in their writings that patients need stability, reassurance, and confidence. Yet the advantages and disadvantages of various hypotheses about cause and treatment may be discussed in detail in the presence of the patient. When this happens, the nurse has a responsibility to remind the physician or physicians, tactfully to be sure, but firmly, of the presence of the patient. Nurses should also exercise care in what they say to, and in the presence of, the patient.

[103] Irving L. Janis, *Psychological Stress,* John Wiley and Sons, New York, 1958, pp. 386-87.

The patient with hypertension is affected by the same general causes of stress as other patients in the hospital environment. Noise, confusion, lack of knowledge of what to expect, discourtesy, visitors, unfamiliar routines, lack of routine, uncertainty about diagnosis, lack of confidence in persons providing care, concern about family—all are among the many possible sources of distress to the patient. Although causes of unnecessary stress should be identified and eliminated for all patients, this is particularly important for the patient who is hypertensive.

For most persons with essential hypertension, control is a life time endeavor. In a broad sense, hypertension can be compared to diabetes mellitus and other chronic disorders. Much can be done to delay its progress and prevent complications, but few persons are cured. Control involves developing a way of life that lessens the tendency to constrict blood vessels. Moderation should be the watchword. Excesses of all types should be avoided. This includes excesses of eating, smoking, and working. For the patient who is free of complications, exercises such as walking, swimming, calisthenics, golf, bicycle riding, and fishing are generally recommended. The form of exercise selected should be based on the desires of the patient. Exercise should be a pleasure, not a punishment. Moreover, it should be undertaken in the spirit of attaining relaxation and not for the purpose of excelling. Once impairment of cardiovascular function is evidenced, physical exercise should be carefully regulated. During periods when the blood pressure rises to critical levels bed rest may be prescribed for a week or two.[104]

In addition to exercise, persons with essential hypertension require regular periods of rest and relaxation. In the early stages of the disease, the person should plan to spend eight hours in bed and, if possible, to relax after each meal. He must be aware of nervous tension and practice consciously relaxing his muscles. One suggestion sometimes made to a patient who is learning to relax is to consciously tense the muscles of a part of his body such as an arm and hand. After it is forcefully contracted, he then consciously lets it become limp. Telling most patients that they must relax frequently is of little value. They need specific help and encouragement in learning how to relax. The physician may also prescribe a mild sedative such as phenobarbital or one of the newer tranquilizing drugs to make relaxation easier.

For persons with a mild and nonprogressive type of hypertension, superficial psychotherapy with attention to the mode of living of the patient may be all that is required in therapy. Patients with more severe types, however, require other forms of therapy. Among these is diet. All hypertensive persons should limit their caloric intake to the quantity required to maintain normal weight and strength. Excess calories should be avoided as well as other excesses. Weight reduction should be carried out in all patients who are overweight. In any program of weight reduction an important goal is for the patient to develop habits of eating compatible with the desired weight.

---

[104] Charles K. Friedberg, *Diseases of the Heart,* 2nd ed., W. B. Saunders Company, Philadelphia, 1956, p. 934.

In addition to the restriction of calories to the quantity required to maintain normal weight and strength, sodium intake may also be restricted. This is based on the observation that salt plus the adrenal mineralocorticoids can result in hypertension. In early hypertension, salt intake is not usually greatly restricted. Particularly in the later stages it may be. In the rice-fruit diet of Kempner[105] the sodium content may be as low as 150 mg a day. This diet consists of rice, raw and canned fruits and juices, which may be sweetened, but to which no salt may be added, and sweeteners such as honey and syrups. For the rice diet to be successful, it must be continued for from four to six weeks. Because of its monotonous character, some patients refuse to continue it for the required time, although some do. Physicians also vary in their enthusiasm for this diet. Many state that most patients will not continue it for any length of time. Some, also, emphasize its inadequacies, one of which is for protein; it contains only from 15 to 30 gm of protein a day. Though vitamin deficiencies can be prevented by the daily administration of vitamin pills and capsules, the pills are usually a source of sodium. In the selection of the degree of salt restriction most physicians try to follow the dictum of Griffiths,[106] who is of the opinion that diet should be a source of pleasure and not another source of stress. Emphasis should be on what to eat rather than on what not to eat. Flavoring agents that do not contain salts of sodium may be used as desired. The patient requires the same general instructions as any patient on a sodium-restricted diet.

Patients whose sodium intake is limited over a long period of time, especially when restriction is combined with sodium-depleting diuretics, are in danger of excessive salt depletion. Although evidence of sodium deficiency may occur at any time, it is most likely to be precipitated by conditions accompanied by increased secretion of sweat. For example, with the advent of hot weather the patient develops one or more of the following manifestations: marked weakness, nausea, vomiting, and collapse. The physician should be notified promptly. Therapy is to correct the sodium deficiency by increasing salt intake.

What types of drugs have hypotensive effects and how do they act?

Drugs having hypotensive effects have been available for some time. There are a variety of new potent hypotensive drugs which can be used alone or in combination to lower the blood pressure to any desired level. Besides lowering the resting blood pressure, an effective drug should lower the blood pressure during exercise and, ideally, during stress situations. The drug should not have undesirable side effects nor should it interfere with the intellectual or physical working capacity of the patient when it is administered in therapeutic

[105] Proudfit and Robinson, *Op. cit.,* 12th ed., p. 520.
[106] George C. Griffiths, "The General Approach to the Treatment of Patient with Diastolic Hypertension," *American Journal of Cardiology,* IX, June, 1962, pp. 822-29.

doses. In some patients it is not possible to lower the blood pressure to a sufficient degree and at the same time avoid all side effects. When the blood pressure must be lowered, the patient may, therefore, have to tolerate the side effects of the drug, if he is to be adequately treated.

One of the most important groups of drugs used in the treatment of hypertension is the saluretics (sodium-excreting diuretics). Either mercurial diuretics or thiazide preparations may be prescribed for this purpose. At present, the trend is to use the thiazide preparations first and to reserve the mercurials for patients in whom the thiazide preparations are no longer effective. In addition to increasing the elimination of sodium, thiazide diuretics are antihypertensive. This action is probably independent of their saluretic effect. The thiazides also potentiate the action of the antihypertensive drugs with the result that they can be prescribed in lower dosages and their side effects can be minimized. Therefore, the thiazide diuretics are often prescribed with a hypotensive drug. One possible side effect of some of the newer diuretics such as the thiazides is that in some people they cause "photosensitivity reactions." Persons who are taking one of these preparations should observe areas of skin exposed to the sun for reddening or other symptoms indicating skin irritation. Should sensitivity of the skin to sunlight develop, the physician should be notified. The local lesions may be treated with topical medications. Usually the offending medication is discontinued and another drug substituted. The skin should be protected from the rays of the sun and sensitized persons should be warned not to use sun or ultraviolet lamps.[107]

How do hypotensive agents act?

Chemicals classified as hypotensive agents act by a number of mechanisms. Some, such as alpha methyldopa (Aldomet), interfere with the synthesis of catecholamines (epinephrine and norepinephrine). Some, such as reserpine, guanethidine, and bretylium, are catechol amine depleters. Some, such as guanethidine and bretylium, are also sympatholytic agents. Though used extensively in the past, the ganglionic blocking agents are no longer used to any extent. Sedatives such as phenobarbital or one of the tranquilizing agents may also be prescribed for their relaxing effect and to diminish the degree to which the individual responds to stress.

In the following table some information about drugs currently being prescribed for their hypotensive effects is summarized.

For some hypotensive drugs therapeutic and toxic dosages overlap. Most of them are highly potent drugs. Most of them cause undesirable side effects which may make their use difficult in a particular patient. The patient, therefore, requires careful observation. For example, rauwolfia compounds sometimes cause mental depression. Any patient who is receiving one of these

---

[107] Morton Fuchs, "The Pharmacology and Clinical Use of Diuretics in the Treatment of Hypertension," *American Journal of Cardiology,* IX, June, 1962, pp. 825-29.

Types of Action	Forms	Action and Results of Action	Side Effects and Undesirable Aspects
Catecholamine depleters	Reserpine (rauwolfia) Guanethidine Bretylium tosylate	They deplete the store of catecholamines in the brain, myocardium, and vessel walls	Mental depression should be carefully watched for. May occur months or even a year after drug therapy is initiated
	See below for further information about the latter 2 drugs		
Sympatholytic agents	Bretylium tosylate	Lower peripheral resistance. Exact mode of action not known	Absorption unpredictable. Many patients develop tolerance. No parasympathetic depression, but diarrhea common presumably because of lack of sympathetic damping effect on the parasympathetics
	Guanethidine. Used in combination with saluretics. Preferred to bretylium. Effective in small dosage. Effects prolonged	Supposedly block the postganglionic transmission of norepinephrine to the vascular receptors. The drug interferes with the release of the chemical mediators at the myoneural junction. As indicated above, also depletes the store of peripheral catecholamines. Little or no tolerance developed	Postural hypotension. Worse in the morning and improves in the day. A few patients develop diarrhea. See above
Decarboxylase inhibitors	Alphamethyldopa (Aldomet[1]). Used in combination with the saluretics	Diminish the in vivo production of catecholamines (norepinephrine) through competitive inhibition with the decarboxylase, an enzyme catalyzing the conversion of dopa to dopamine. Not known whether its hypotensive effect is due to its interference with the synthesis of norepinephrine	Not always effective and it is not always possible to predict if it will be effective Some patients develop a tolerance to it Postural hypotension in some patients Drowsiness in initial phases of treatment May be depression and psychiatric complaints such as feelings of unreality Some physicians consider it to be superior to other antihypertensive agents

1 Trade name.

preparations should be carefully observed for evidence of depression. Since it may not occur immediately, but may be delayed for as much as a year, observation over an extended period of time is required.

Some drugs, such as the sympatholytic and ganglionic blocking agents as well as the decarboxylase inhibitors, cause postural hypotension. Patients who complain of dizziness or feel faint when they assume the upright position should be taught to rise slowly, in order to prevent syncope (fainting). Until it is known whether or not the patient manifests this side effect, he should be assisted out of bed. If the patient develops postural hypotension, the physician should be acquainted with this fact.

Diarrhea is a troublesome side effect of some of the sympatholytic agents. The problem is less severe with guanethidine than with bretylium tosylate.

During the initial phase of treatment, the decorboxylase inhibitors cause drowsiness in about one third of patients. Patients receiving Alpha Methyl Dopa (dihydroxyphenalaline) or another similar preparation should be warned not to drive a car during the time when drowsiness is present. Fortunately, this effect usually disappears after a period of time. Patients may also develop a mild depression and psychiatric complaints such as a feeling of unreality. When these side effects develop, they should be reported to the physician. Usually they are not severe enough to be handicapping to the patient.

To lessen the possibility of side effects, a number of drugs may be given in combination. In the hospital, the problem faced by the patient is "swallowing all those pills." When the patient receives a large number of pills, attention should be given to the possibility of distributing them more frequently, but in smaller numbers at one time. When he is at home, he is responsible for selecting, counting, and evaluating their effects. At times he may feel like a walking pharmacy without a pharmacist. In a report of a study of elderly patients taking drugs at home, Schwartz[108] enumerates some of the problems they encounter as well as some procedures found to be helpful. Among the types of errors made by patients were the following: "(1) a medicine was taken by the patient, but not ordered by the physician; (2) a medicine was ordered by the physician, but not taken by the patient; or (3) a medicine ordered by the physician was taken but in incorrect doses or at the wrong time (when time was a significant factor) or with a total lack of understanding of its purpose." Schwartz,[109] in discussing the role of the nurse in helping the newly discharged or ambulatory patient, states that the nurse must understand the regimen prescribed by the physician. She must also determine the extent to which the patient understands his part in his therapy as well as how he proposes to carry it out. She suggests that nurses ask themselves the following questions: "What evidence do I have that my patients understand any better

---

[108] Doris Schwartz, "Medication Errors Made by Aged Patients," *American Journal of Nursing*, LXII, August, 1962, pp. 51-53.

[109] *Ibid.*, p. 52.

or act any differently? How can I find out what they think and do? Would medication calendars or other visual aids be useful? Are there unexplored ways of reminding patients?" What Schwartz is asking, is how effective is our instruction of patients? Do we really know? How can it be made more effective? As long as we accept what we do without question, we cannot know whether it is effective or not. Neither will better approaches be developed.

Depending on the seriousness of the patient's illness and other factors, treatment may or may not require that he be hospitalized. Eventually, however, he will have to assume the major responsibility for the management of his disease. Unless the patient is hospitalized, he and his family must carry out the therapeutic regime. He must make periodic visits to his physician so that his progress can be checked and the regime modified as required by his condition. The assumption of responsibility by the patient at home can often be facilitated by one or more visits by a public health or visiting nurse. Even when the patient is given detailed instructions while he is in the hospital, or in the office of the physician, he is likely to have some problems at home. The visiting nurse can help him to resolve his difficulties and to increase his confidence in his own competence. Family members also require preparation and assistance in learning what to do and in acquiring the necessary knowledge and skill.

In order to illustrate some of the problems encountered by the patient after discharge, let us consider Mrs. Pine, who has been in the hospital for the treatment of rapidly progressive essential hypertension. She is a 59-year-old widow whose income is barely sufficient for her to meet her essential needs. Although her chronological age is less than that of the patients studied by Schwartz, what reason is there to believe she will find coping with a complicated medical regimen easy? Since hypertension is accompanied by injury to the vascular system, Mrs. Pine may be older than her age in years. Further in common with many other persons, she is frightened by the diagnosis "high blood pressure." Added to the manifestations indicating a high degree of anxiety before her diagnosis was established is the anxiety engendered by the implications of hypertension and a relatively expensive and complicated regimen. Although both her physician and nurse reviewed her therapeutic regimen with her and she had some practice in taking her own blood pressure, what assurance did either of them have that she would be able to follow the following medical regime?

1. Phenobarbital 30 mg at eight in the morning, one in the afternoon, and eight at night.
2. Reserpine, 0.5 mg daily. Since this is supplied in 0.25 mg tablets, she was to take two tablets.
3. Hydrochlorothiazide, U.S.P. (Esidrix[110]) 25 mg after breakfast and 25 mg after lunch each day.
4. Multivitamin capsules, two daily.

[110] Trade name.

5. Digitoxin 0.1 mg daily.
6. A low-sodium diet. No salt was to be added to her food during preparation, and foods in which salt was used in their preparation were to be eliminated.
7. She was to spend ten hours in bed each night.
8. She was to take her own blood pressure each morning and to notify her physician should her blood pressure fall below 150/70.

Before Mrs. Pine left the hospital, all the details of her regime were presented to her in some detail. With the exception of taking her own blood pressure twice, she had no practice in selecting the drugs to be taken or in planning her menu. When she obtained the drugs at the pharmacy, she was shocked at their cost. She was bewildered by their number. She wondered whether they were really necessary and how she would manage to keep track of all of them. After she arrived home, she was visited by Mrs. Always, who knew the exact remedy to control high blood pressure. Mrs. Always was so convincing that Mrs. Pine was sorely tempted to try her prescription: dried spinach powder dissolved in sea water and the elimination of tomatoes from her diet. Fortunately, Miss Visiting Nurse arrived the next day and went over her plans with her. Between them they worked out a plan for the medicine schedule that made the treatment program somewhat less burdensome. Meal plans were made. Mrs. Pine took her own blood pressure and then Miss V. N. checked it for accuracy. Mrs. Pine also had an opportunity to ask Miss V. N. about the effectiveness of spinach powder in the treatment of high blood pressure. As Miss V. N. left she promised to return the next day to see how Mrs. Pine was progressing.

In patients in whom the preceding methods of treatment are unsuccessful, sympathectomy may be done. Because the drugs that are now available are highly effective, sympathectomy is seldom performed. The procedure involves either the resection of preganglionic vasoconstrictor fillers or the removal of some or all of the sympathetic ganglia. In general the less extensive operations are performed in preference to the more extensive procedures. The surgeon tries to remove enough of the sympathetic nervous system to effectively lower the blood pressure without severe postural hypotension resulting. Care of the patient after sympathectomy relates to the fact of surgery and the possibility of postural hypotension.

What complication is unique to hypertension?

The complication of hypertension which is unique to the disorder is hypertensive encephalopathy. Encephalopathy is not limited to hypertension of any specific etiology, as it is very frequent in patients with acute renal disease, such as acute glomerulonephritis. It also occurs in toxemia of pregnancy (a serious complication in pregnancy) and in rapidly progressive malignant hypertension. Signs and symptoms include rapidly rising blood pressure, visual disturbances progressing to blindness, papilledema, vomiting, coma, stertorous breathing, psychosis, and convulsions. Since the damage to the brain is not permanent, the patient may recover from hypertensive encephalopathy, provided he does not die in acute heart failure. Many of the patients with this condition are children or young adults. In caring for patients who are predisposed to hypertensive encephalopathy, the nurse should check the blood pressure of the patient not only regularly as prescribed by the physician, but at any time the condition of the patient appears to be worsening. Should the blood pressure be found to be rising, the physician should be notified and treatment initiated immediately. Unless the nurse is alert and acts promptly, the patient may die needlessly, as there are chemical means available to lower the blood pressure.

In children and some young adults, vasospasm may be lessened by the intramuscular injection of a 50 per cent solution of magnesium sulfate; 0.2 mg is administered per kilogram of body weight. It may be repeated every four hours to keep the blood pressure within a reasonable level. Later, when the most critical period is past, up to 30 ml of a 50 per cent solution may be administered orally two to three times a day. The child should be observed for increasing somnolence and respiratory difficulties. Some physicians prescribe large dosages of protoveratrine A and B or reserpine. U.S.P., B.P. (Serpasil[111]).

Summary

Hypertension is a commonly occurring condition affecting a high percentage of persons over 40 years of age. Its frequency increases with age. Though systolic hypertension occurs, the most serious type is associated with an elevation of the diastolic blood pressure. Diastolic hypertension may be of specific or nonspecific cause. The latter is known as essential, or primary, hypertension. Despite differences in causation, there are many similarities among hypertensive persons. The mechanism or mechanisms initiating and perpetuating diastolic hypertension appear to be related to some imbalance between sympathomimetic activity and vascular responsiveness. Authorities disagree as to the significance of each factor in causation. They also disagree about the harmful effects of the elevation of the blood pressure on vascular integrity. Although hypertension does not kill directly, complications involving the heart, brain, retina, and kidney cripple and kill a large number of persons prematurely.

Therapy is directed toward helping the person adjust his life and habits of living so that he protects his blood vessels from overconstriction. Moderation in all aspects of life is recommended for persons suffering any degree of hypertension. For those persons with moderate and severe hypertension,

[111] Trade name.

therapy with drugs and diet is added to directly or indirectly lessen the degree of vasoconstriction.

Hypertension is similar to other chronic diseases as continued control is necessary. The burden of the therapeutic regime is eventually borne by the patient and his family. The nurse has a responsibility to help the patient consider his alternatives and to provide him with needed support and instruction.

As in other disorders requiring some degree of modification in the life of the individual, not all persons respond as physicians and nurses would like them to do. Some persons become so anxious that their entire attention is centered on their illness and themselves. There are others who have no wish to alter their way of living in order to gain a few more months or years of life. Steinbeck[112] describes both types of adjustment to illness. In his statement that he prefers quality to quantity, Steinbeck makes his feelings about modifying his life quite clear. It is also clear that he has a rationale for making his choice. When the patient selects a course contrary to that prescribed by the physician, the nurse may feel that she or the physician has been inadequate or failed in some respect. Neither is necessarily true. The patient does have a right to choose among the possible alternatives and to have his choice respected.

Although not all the answers to the problems created by essential hypertension have been found, there is optimism that in time they will be. Furthermore nothing slows progress more than blind acceptance of the *status quo*.

What are some of the causes and effects of pulmonary hypertension?

In the preceding section hypertension occurring in systemic arteries has been considered. Hypertension, however, occurs not only in the systemic arteries, but in the pulmonary arteries as well. Because of differences in the character of the pulmonary and systemic arterial beds, the causes and consequences of pulmonary hypertension differ from those of systemic hypertension. The term applied to pulmonary hypertension is pulmonary heart disease or cor pulmonale—cor meaning heart and pulmonale lung. Spain[113] prefers the term "pulmonary hypertensive heart disease." He defines chronic cor pulmonale as "that form of hypertrophy of the right side of the heart (with or without congestive failure) that develops secondary to diseases of the lung, pulmonary blood vessels, chest cage or primary pulmonary hypertension." Some authorities also include in this classification pulmonary hypertension which is secondary to mitral stenosis and certain forms of congenital heart disease.

According to Harrison *et al.*,[114] pulmonary hypertension resulting from

---

[112] John Steinbeck, *Travels with Charley*, Bantam Book, New York, 1963, pp. 19-20.
[113] David M. Spain, "Pathology of Chronic Cor Pulmonale," *Cardiology*, IV, 1959, pp. 13-3.
[114] Harrison *et al., Op. cit.,* p. 1537.

disease of the lungs is one of the most frequent causes of congestive heart failure in the United States, and it has an even higher incidence in Great Britain. Its frequency appears to be related to the incidence of longstanding chronic bronchitis associated with emphysema. With an increase in the occurrence of these two conditions, the incidence of cor pulmonale is also expected to rise.

The causes and effects of pulmonary hypertension differ from those of systemic hypertension. Whereas blood is circulated through the systemic arteries under a relatively high blood pressure, the pulmonary circulation is a relatively low-pressure system. Three factors are responsible for the low pressure: (1) the walls of the pulmonary arteries contain relatively little muscle; (2) they are highly distensible; and (3) there is a large reserve of vessels. Were it to be fully dilated, the pulmonary vascular bed would be capable of holding the entire blood volume. Mechanical and other functional factors are therefore more important in controlling pressure in the pulmonary arterial system than in the systemic circulation. Either increased blood flow or resistance to blood flow may result in pulmonary hypertension. Both factors may be contributing. The effects of these two factors on pulmonary blood pressure are explained by the following physical principle. When blood or other fluid flows through a cylindrical tube in layers (laminar flow), the volume of fluid passing per unit of time is directly proportional to the differences in pressure at the two ends of the tube and is inversely proportional to the resistance to flow factors hindering flow. In terms of this principle, pulmonary hypertension may result from any condition in which more blood is ejected by the right ventricle into the pulmonary vascular bed than is removed from it by the left ventricle or from disorders increasing resistance to the flow of blood through the pulmonary vascular bed.

In addition to other effects of right heart failure, the problems created by pulmonary hypertension result primarily from the effect of an increase of blood and fluid in the lung on the capacity to oxygenate the blood and to remove carbon dioxide. Increased bronchial secretions which are associated with pulmonary congestion that interferes with oxygenating the blood often complicate the problem. The outcome of a patient with pulmonary hypertension depends on the factors in causation as well as the degree of loss of cardiac reserve.

The nursing care problems which have been discussed elsewhere relate to the needs of a patient: (1) in congestive heart failure, (2) who is anoxic (hypoxic), (3) who has hypercapnia (problem eliminating carbon dioxide), (4) who has increased bronchial secretions, and (5) who is an individual human being.

Summary

Cor pulmonale (right ventricular hypertrophy and congestive heart failure) is rising in incidence, and it is expected to continue to rise. It is associated with disorders in functions of the heart and lungs that increase blood flow or resistance to circulation through the pulmonary circulation. The effects differ from those of systemic hypertension because the pulmonary circulation is a low-pressure system. In addition to the systemic effects of failure of the right ventricle as a pump, congestion of blood in the pulmonary circulation predisposes to hypoxia and hypercapnia, which are worsened by the fact that the bronchiolar tree responds by increasing secretions. This is a very fine example of how function of one system affects that of another. Prevention depends on the elimination of conditions predisposing to disorders such as emphysema.

Finally, for the function of the circulatory system to be achieved without acceleration of the rate at which the blood vessels deteriorate, the pressure of the blood must be maintained within certain limits. Blood pressure results from a variety of factors regulated so that pressure in the system is maintained within limits and the needs of cells are met, not only during rest, but in activity. Systemic and pulmonary hypertension differ in causes and effects, but both are significant causes of disease, disability, and death.

A third element in transportation is the blood. Whereas the heart and blood vessels provide the power and the channels through which blood circulates, as well as the site of exchange between the blood and the interstitial fluids, blood is the vehicle by which materials are distributed. In addition to its significance in the transportation of substances between the cells and the external environment, the blood has a number of other functions. Blood flow is so regulated that homeostasis of body fluids is maintained. The blood participates in the maintenance of its volume and composition by regulating the functioning of organs such as the bone marrow, endocrine glands, liver, and spleen. A self-sealing mechanism protects against the loss of blood after the disruption of the wall of a blood vessel. The blood also plays a significant role in the defense system of the body. Many functions of the blood and results of their failure are discussed in detail in other areas. Other than for a brief or summarizing review, most of the content presented in the succeeding pages will relate to the erythrocytes and thrombocytes.

Although the functions of the heart, blood vessels, and blood are interdependent, they are often classified as two different systems. The heart and blood vessels comprise the circulatory system, and the blood is part of the hematopoietic system. The hematopoietic system includes not only the circulating blood, but the red bone marrow, the lymph nodes, the spleen, and the reticuloendothelial cells, which are scattered throughout the body. One of the important sites in which reticuloendothelial cells is found is the liver. With the obvious exception of the circulating blood, the structures listed above are sites where blood cells are formed or destroyed or both. Some, such as the spleen, serve as reservoirs for the storage of blood. The liver not only forms red blood cells in the embryo, but it stores some of the materials required for the formation and maturation of blood cells. It synthesizes blood proteins, which are essential components of blood plasma and are necessary to maintaining an effective osmotic pressure of the blood.

A number of terms used in the discussion are defined below:

Anemia is used to denote a reduction in the number of erythrocytes or in the quantity of hemoglobin or both.

Hematopoiesis means the formation of blood.

Agranulocytosis means without granulocytes. The term agranulocytopenia is preferable, as granulocytes are reduced in number, rather than absent.

Aniocytosis means marked variations in the size of cells.

Poikilocytosis means abnormalities in the shape of cells.

The blood is a highly complex fluid in which the blood cells are suspended. The fluid or plasma comprises about 54 per cent of the total blood volume and the cells about 46 per cent, but these figures are subject to some variation. In women the percentage of cells is somewhat lower than in men, the average being about 42 per cent. The proportion of cells to the total volume of blood is determined by centrifuging whole blood. The cells settle to the bottom of the tube, and the length of the column of cells or fluid can be measured. The result is reported as a whole number, such as 42 or 48. The number indicates the percentage of the blood that is cells and is called a hematocrit. For example, Mr. Bok's hematocrit is 47. This means that his blood cells comprise 47 per cent of his total blood volume. The other 53 per cent is plasma. Following blood loss, blood volume may be maintained by an increase in the blood plasma, and the hematocrit falls below the lower limits of normal. After the loss of water from the body, such as following severe burns or excessive diaphoresis (sweating), the hematocrit rises. The proportion of cells to blood plasma is increased.

What are the functions of the blood plasma?

The plasma and its constituents are examined in detail in Chapter 8, and the discussion of them will therefore be limited. The plasma is an essential part of the blood. Its high water content (it is over 90 per cent water) enables the plasma to dissolve and carry in solution a large variety of organic and inorganic substances between the cells and the external environment. It also contains the blood proteins—albumin, globulin, and fibrinogen—as well as internal secretions, antibodies, and a variety of enzymes. Water in the plasma and other body fluids participates in the regulation of body temperature.

What are the types of blood cells?

The cells in the blood are of three types, the erythrocytes, or red corpuscles; the leukocytes, or white blood corpuscles; and the thrombocytes, or blood platelets. The leukocytes are part of the system of defense of the body. They are discussed in Chapter 5.

The number of each of the various types of cells in the blood is due to a balance between the production and destruction of cells. Since the number of cells per unit of blood is regulated automatically, and the cells are maintained within well-defined limits, this is another example of a homeostatic mechanism. Similar to other homeostatic mechanisms, the equilibrium between blood cell production and destruction may be unbalanced with a loss of homeostasis. The effects will, of course, depend on the type of cell involved and in some instances the cause of the failure. Because of the liquid nature of the blood, cells and plasma may also be lost more rapidly than they can be replaced. When the loss of blood is rapid, circulation is threatened by the loss of blood volume as well as by the loss of cells.

Not all changes in the level of blood cells indicate a failure in homeostasis. In fact, a failure to alter the number of cells would point to such a failure. For example, the number of leukocytes rises above normal levels in response to certain threats to the organism. This is true in acute appendicitis or in an acute infection caused by one of the pyogenic cocci. The total number of leukocytes is expected to be elevated. The polymorphonuclear leukocytes, particularly the neutrophils, are responsible for the rise. Inasmuch as the increase in cells represents an appropriate response to a stimulus—threat of injury to cells—it is homeostatic. This conclusion is further supported by the fact that the cells involved are defensive in nature and their number returns to normal levels once the threatening agent is removed. Although the number of cells is increased and many of the cells are not fully mature, they are in a normal stage of development. The cells are released into the circulation before they are fully mature. The number of erythrocytes may also be increased above the so-called normal range in response to a chronic deficiency of oxygen such as in congenital heart disease or at high altitudes. A failure of the organism to increase the number of blood cells in response to an appropriate stimulus is indicative of a failure in a homeostatic mechanism.

In blood dyscrasias, that is, in disorders of the blood, the number and/or character of one or more of the blood cells is abnormal. Moreover, the alteration in the number cannot be explained as a normal response to a threat to the organism. For example, in leukemia both the number and character of white blood cells are abnormal. Except in late stages of the disease, the number is usually markedly increased and the cells are both abnormal and immature. In sickle cell anemia, the erythrocytes contain an abnormal hemoglobin and are abnormal in shape, that is, they are sickle-shaped. Under certain conditions they undergo increased destruction with the result that their number falls to below normal levels. Cells may be poorly or abnormally constructed, so they are too fragile or too resistant to destruction. In familial hemolytic anemia, erythrocytes are abnormally fragile. They are therefore subject to increased destruction. In hemophilia the victim may bleed to death because his thrombocytes are abnormally resistant.

The disorders in function resulting from the blood dyscrasias include the following:

1. Failure to maintain the constancy of the fluid environment of cells. (See Chapter 8.)
2. Failure to transport substances required by the cells for metabolism or to remove the products of metabolism.
3. Failure to successfully combat the agents of infection. (See Chapter 4.)
4. Failure of the self-sealing mechanism.

Possible etiological factors in blood dyscrasias include: genetic abnormalities, neoplasia of the bone marrow, deficiency of materials required to form the various constituents of the blood, failure of the bone marrow, infection, blood loss—acute or chronic—and allergic responses of the bone marrow. As with other tissues, the causes of some abnormalities have not been explained. The effects associated with each disturbance are related to the function of the particular component involved and the rapidity with which the condition develops.

The needs of the patient with a disorder involving the blood will be affected by the nature and effects of the disturbance as well as its possible outcome. The person with the disorder is no less important than is his disease.

What are the functions of erythrocytes? What are some of the effects of abnormalities of erythrocytes?

With the preceding discussion as a background, the role of erythrocytes in the body economy and the cause and effects of abnormalities will be explored. The erythrocyte is a biconcave disc with an average diameter of about 7.2 μ and a thickness of about 2.2 μ at its thickest part and of 1 μ or less in its center. It is sometimes described as a bag which is capable of great change in shape as it passes through capillaries. Though the erythrocyte lacks a nucleus, it carries out metabolic functions. For this reason, Best and Taylor[115] state that it is a living, but specialized, cell.

The average number of erythrocytes in a healthy man is approximately 5,000,000 cells per cubic millimeter of blood with a range of $\pm$ 600,000. In women the figure is slightly lower, with the average being about 4,500,000. The range in women is also slightly smaller than in men as it is about $\pm$ 500,-000. Hemoglobin content also varies with sex and from individual to individual. The average for men is about 16 gm per 100 ml of blood. For women, it is about 14 gm.

The erythrocyte has several important functions. First, it transports hemoglobin and, by means of it, conveys oxygen from the lung to the tissues. Second, the erythrocyte contains large quantities of carbonic acid. As a consequence the transport of carbon dioxide from the tissues to the lung is facilitated. A third function of the erthythrocyte is the buffering effect of the hemoglobin and the electrolytes contained in the cell. According to Guy-

115 *Op. cit.,* 7th ed., p. 10.

ton,[116] the erythrocyte is responsible for about 70 per cent of the buffering action of whole blood.

The sites in which erythrocytes are formed change from embryonic to adult life. In the first weeks of fetal life erythrocytes are formed in the primitive yolk sac. Later the liver serves as the principal site for their formation, though they are also formed in the spleen and lymph nodes. As the fetus matures, the site of formation of erythrocytes shifts to the bone marrow, and by the time of birth, it is the main site of erythrocyte production. The bone marrow continues to be the site of formation throughout the remainder of the life span. Up until the time of adolescence, the bone marrow in the shaft of long bones functions in erythrocyte production. After about the age of 20, it becomes quite fatty and produces no more erythrocytes, and red cell production takes place primarily in the flat bones such as the vertebrae, skull, sternum, and ribs. Because the productive bone marrow gradually lessens in amount throughout the life span, a mild anemia is not infrequent in the aged. In emergency situations in which large numbers of red cells are required, bone marrow that has stopped producing cells may become productive.

In the formation of erythrocytes, two factors are of significance, the cell itself and the hemoglobin in the cell. Many complex processes are involved in the formation of both. Many substances must be available and a number of enzymes are required to catalyze the reactions involved in the formation and maturation of the cell and its hemoglobin. In the process of development the cell goes through a number of stages. The reticulum cell in the bone marrow forms a primordial cell known as a hemocytoblast. This cell is nucleated and it does not contain hemoglobin. In the next stage, the synthesis of hemoglobin is begun. As the cell develops, the nucleus shrinks in size, and the quantity of hemoglobin increases. The cell at the stage in which the nucleus disappears and a full complement of hemoglobin is present is known as a normoblast. Most cells contain no nuclear material at the time they enter the circulating blood. They are fully mature erythrocytes. A few cells containing fine strands of basophilic material do find their way into the blood, however. They are known as reticulocytes. Normally, they comprise about 2 percent of the total circulating erythrocytes. Following hemorrhage or the treatment of anemia they may account for 10 per cent or more of the total number of erythrocytes. Because they are less mature forms of erythrocytes, the presence of an increased proportion of reticulocytes to mature erythrocytes following treatment of anemia is taken as an indication of a rise in red cell production or erythropoiesis.

Failure of the bone marrow to produce erythrocytes in adequate numbers results in anemia. This failure may be due to a congenital defect in which the bone marrow fails to develop or may be the result of injury to the hematopoietic (blood-producing) tissues at some time following birth. In either instance, hematopoietic (blood-forming) tissues may be absent or insufficient in

[116] *Op. cit.*, p. 145.

quantity. Red bone marrow is either entirely or partly replaced by fatty or yellow marrow. In the absence of any evidence of hematopoietic activity, the bone marrow is said to be aplastic. Bone marrow showing less than normal activity is hypoplastic. In the absence of red cell-producing tissue, all types of blood corpuscles, erythrocytes, granulocytes, and thrombocytes will be decreased in number. The patient will have not only anemia, but granulocytopenia and thrombopenia as well. The consequences will depend on the cause of the condition. In a patient in whom there is an acute depression of the bone marrow, survival may depend on whether or not he can be protected from infection and hemorrhage until his bone marrow recovers from injury.

What are some of the causes of aplasia and hypoplasia on the bone marrow?

There are many possible causes of aplasia or hypoplasia of the bone marrow. Bone marrow may fail as a terminal event in leukemia or as a result of metastasis of malignant neoplasms from other parts of the body. The bone marrow is highly sensitive to a variety of chemical and physical agents. Wintrobe[117] divides these agents into two groups: (1) those which inevitably cause aplasia or hypoplasia of the bone marrow if they are given in sufficient dosage and (2) those causing bone marrow injury in some persons and not in others and which are therefore thought to be due to an idiosyncrasy. Among the agents falling in the first category are those utilized in the therapy of malignant neoplasms. They include all forms of ionizing radiation, nitrogen and sulfur mustards, triethylenemelamine (TEM), urethan, and the antimetabolites such as folic acid compounds. Aromatic fat solvents such as benzene (benzol) are used in many industries and are toxic to the bone marrow. Unless adequate precautions are taken to protect those using these agents, sufficient quantities may be inhaled to cause hypoplasia or aplasia of the bone marrow.

Among agents in the second group are a large group of chemicals including a number of drugs. Aplasia or hypoplasia of the bone marrow occurs occasionally in individuals after exposure to one of a number of drugs or other chemical agents such as insecticides. Among the drugs most frequently associated with aplastic or hypoplastic bone marrow are the arsenicals used in the treatment of syphilis, the antithyroid drugs, antihistamines, trinitrotoluene, and preparations of gold. Insecticides have also been implicated. Before prescribing a drug reported to be associated with the development of hypoplasia or aplasia of bone marrow, it is imperative that the physician weigh the possibility of danger to the patient against the possible good. Moreover, the greater the possibility of injury, the greater the need for accurate observation and follow-up of the patient. The nurse has a further obligation to participate in public education to prevent needless or overexposure to drugs or insecti-

[117] Harrison, *Op. cit.,* 4th ed., p. 1324.

cides. Children, as well as other members of the family, should be protected from the careless handling and use of drugs.

In addition to healthy hemopoietic cells in the bone marrow, blood production depends on an adequate supply of materials needed for the formation, maturation, and release of cells. In general these do not differ from those required by other cells. They include amino acids to form the stroma of the red cell as well as for the globin portion of the hemoglobin. Besides the usual requirements for materials in cell formation, iron is an essential part of the hemoglobin molecule.

Hemoglobin is formed, therefore, only to the extent that iron is available. In the presence of iron deficiency, each erythrocyte receives less than a full quantity of hemoglobin and is smaller than normal, or microcytic. Since the hemoglobin is usually decreased out of proportion to the number of erythrocytes, the color index is less than normal and the cells are pale in color. The term "hypochromic," which means too little color, is used to describe this characteristic of the blood. In anemias due to iron deficiency the blood is characterized by a greater decrease in hemoglobin than in erythrocytes, small or microcytic cells, low color index, and hypochromia.

What are the sources of iron?

Sources of iron include organ and lean meats, egg yolk, and shellfish. Certain fruits and vegetables are good sources provided they are eaten fairly frequently. The fruits include apricots, peaches, prunes, grapes, and raisins. Among vegetable sources of iron are green leafy vegetables, whole-grain cereals, enriched cereals, and dark molasses.[118]

Absorption of iron from the gastrointestinal tract is regulated, and once iron is absorbed, there is no mechanism for its elimination. Somewhat over one half of the iron in the body is in the hemoglobin. About 10 percent is in the form of myoglobin. The remainder is stored in the liver, kidneys, spleen, and bone marrow.[119] Iron deficiency may result from an inadequate intake or absorption or from the loss of blood, particularly chronic blood loss. In the United States, deficiency due to inadequate intake of iron is possibly less common than it once was. Enrichment of cereals and flours with iron is primarily responsible.

Attention to infant nutrition and the early addition of iron-containing foods have lessened the incidence of iron-deficiency anemias in young children. In the past and in the present among children reared in families with limited income, anemia was and is frequently found in the child of a year or 18 months of age. Ronny Little illustrates how a limited diet leads to anemia. Ronny, a slender, pale child of 18 months, was admitted to the hospital acutely ill from a respiratory infection. On examination he was found to be

[118] Fairfax T. Proudfit and Corinne H. Robinson, *Normal and Therapeutic Nutrition,* 12th ed., The Macmillan Company, New York, 1961, pp. 99-100.
[119] *Ibid.,* p. 97.

anemic. Investigation of his dietary showed that except for orange juice, his food intake was limited to milk and a limited amount of a refined cereal. Since the iron content of milk is low, Ronny's intake of iron was insufficient to meet his needs. To prevent iron deficiency, mothers are advised to introduce egg yolk and other iron-containing foods into the dietary of the infant early. One of the problems in the nursing of Ronny was to enlarge his food intake to include egg yolk, liver, and meat and to help his mother understand why these foods were important. Mrs. Little also needed some assistance in selecting an adequate dietary and in budgeting a limited income to cover essential needs.

At the beginning of the century iron-deficiency anemias due to an inadequate intake of iron were common in the United States. Today they are more likely to be associated with chronic blood loss. One common factor predisposing to loss of blood are ulcerative lesions—whether benign or malignant—of the gastrointestinal tract. Even when the quantity lost at one time is small, a blood loss continued over time leads to development of anemia. In disorders involving the gastrointestinal tract, food intake is likely to be limited by a poor appetite or nausea. Vomiting and/or diarrhea may further aggravate the problem by removing ingested food from the alimentary canal before absorption can take place. Another source of anemia due to blood loss is the female reproductive tract. Lesions involving the lining of the uterus and cervix and excessive menstruation are common factors. In areas where hookworm disease is endemic and going barefoot is practiced, anemia due to blood loss also occurs. In the iron-deficiency anemias, the erythrocytes are of smaller-than-normal size. The number of red cells may be at normal, or nearly normal, levels, however. The number may be less than average. The cells are of small size, or microcytic, as a result of insufficient iron to form hemoglobin and the anemia is called a microcytic anemia. In iron-deficiency anemias therapy is directed toward two objectives, to determine the cause and to correct the deficiency of iron. In the accomplishment of the latter objective, the simplest and least expensive salts of iron, such as ferrous sulfate, are said to be as effective as more complicated and expensive preparations. Some patients develop diarrhea when iron therapy is initiated. Should diarrhea occur, the drug should be temporarily discontinued and then restarted in small dosage. As the patient develops tolerance for iron, the dosage can be increased. Since iron is incompletely absorbed from the gastrointestinal tract, much of it is excreted in the stool and the stool is black in color. The patient should be told to expect this so he will not be frightened. Persons whose dietary has been poor in iron should also be encouraged to increase the intake of iron-containing foods in their diets. This is not always easy to accomplish. Habit, limited income, misconceptions about the effects of certain foods, and lack of energy associated with ill health often interfere with any appreciable change in the dietary. In the elderly, loneliness and eating alone add to the problem of securing an adequate intake of food.

Other minerals such as copper and cobalt have been demonstrated to be essential in hematopoiesis in experimental animals. Cobalt is a component of vitamin B_{12}. Since the required quantity of these substances is small, the possibility of a deficiency in man is remote.

A third factor or group of factors in the production of blood is the B vitamins. Many years ago Castle postulated that some substance in the diet was essential to the maturation of erythrocytes. He called it the extrinsic factor. Later the extrinsic factor was identified as vitamin B_{12} (or cyanocobalamin). Vitamin B_{12} is required for the growth of all cells in the body. A deficiency of vitamin B_{12} is accompanied by the depression of growth in all the cells in the body. Because erythrocyte-forming tissues grow and proliferate rapidly, the production of red cells is markedly inhibited. A lack of vitamin B_{12} has two effects on red cell production. The rate of production is slowed, and the cells that are formed are abnormal. The cells are larger than normal and they are also abnormal in construction. The cell membrane is poorly formed and very fragile with the result that the cell is more easily destroyed than healthy cells. One characteristic of anemias associated with marked deficiency of vitamin B_{12} is a lemon-yellow color of the skin caused by increased destruction of erythrocytes. The stroma of the red cell is also thought to be abnormal. Mature red cells are not only larger than normal, that is, they are, macrocytic, but they vary in size and shape. The presence of large numbers of deformed red cells is indicated by the term "poikilocytosis." The term "anisocytosis" refers to the marked variations in size. In conditions in which vitamin B_{12} is deficient, mature red cells are generally larger than normal (macrocytic), a large proportion of them are deformed (poikilocytic), and they vary in size (anisocytic). Their cell membrane is unusually fragile with the result that the cell is destroyed sooner than a normal erythrocyte. Because the erythrocytes are poorly formed in vitamin B_{12} deficiency, vitamin B_{12} is said to be a maturation factor. Without it, the red cells are incapable of maturing normally.

Despite defects in the maturation of red blood cells in vitamin B_{12} deficiency, the formation of hemoglobin is normal and the red cells contain a full complement of hemoglobin. One hundred ml of erythrocytes (not whole blood) contains 34 gm of hemoglobin. Since the cells are macrocytic, the proportion of hemoglobin to whole blood is reduced less than are the number of erythrocytes. The color index is therefore greater than one and the cells appear to be more highly colored than ordinary erythrocytes.

Unlike iron-deficiency anemias, most anemias resulting from a lack of vitamin B_{12} are not due to an inadequate intake, but from failure of absorption. Failure of absorption can be demonstrated by the Schilling or a similar test. This test is based on the discovery that the cobalt in vitamin B_{12} can be labeled, by making it radioactive. The radioactive vitamin B_{12} is administered by mouth and the urine is then collected and tested for radioactivity. Normal individuals excrete from 11 to 26 per cent of the dose within 24 hours. Excretion in patients with anemias due to failure to absorb vitamin

B_{12} is much reduced. There may, in fact, be no excretion of radioactive material.

What are the sources of supply of vitamin B_{12}?

An ample supply is provided by a small intake of animal proteins. Absorption is dependent on a mucoprotein or some substance bound to the mucoproteins in the mucus secreted by the stomach. This factor was named the intrinsic factor by Castle. It combines with vitamin B_{12} and makes it more soluble, thus facilitating its absorption. In the absence of the intrinsic factor, the absorption of vitamin B_{12} is poor. The most common cause of lack of the intrinsic factor is atrophy of the gastric mucosa. It is most frequently associated with pernicious anemia. Until the underlying defect of pernicious anemia was discovered, it led to a disabling illness and death which accounts for the word "pernicious." Despite the inability to cure this form of anemia, it can now be controlled by regular injections of vitamin B_{12}. Though there are individual differences, anemia and other effects of deficiency can be prevented in most persons by monthly intramuscular injections of vitamin B_{12}. Vitamin B_{12} is stored in the liver and released as needed for the maturation of erythrocytes. As stated earlier, vitamin B_{12} is also required by other cells and its deficiency in the young leads to poor growth. One of the most serious consequences of its deficiency is the development of degenerative changes in the nervous system.

The discovery of the therapy of pernicious anemia is one of the classics of American medical science. In 1925 Whipple reported a study made for the purpose of finding a method for creating a constant anemia in dogs. In 1926 Minot and Murphy introduced the treatment of pernicious anemia with liver. For the liver to be effective, the patient was required to ingest at least a pound and a half of raw or lightly seared liver each day. Some patients found this treatment almost as distasteful as the effects of the disease. Efforts were made to disguise the taste by mixing ground raw liver with grape or orange juice. Methods were soon found to dry the liver without destroying the antipernicious anemia factor, as it was called. The role of the stomach in the pathogenesis of pernicious anemia was reported by Castle in 1929.[120] He observed that the lining of the stomach of patients with pernicious anemia was atropic. Subsequently, a preparation of pig stomach was prepared to be taken orally. Not too much time elapsed until an extract was made from liver tissue which could be injected intramuscularly. Since it was made from beef liver, it contained foreign proteins to which some patients became hypersensitive. Unless crude liver extract was injected deep into the muscle, it was also likely to cause a foreign-body reaction with the formation of an abscess. In 1948, vitamin B_{12} was isolated in pure form and identified as a chemical entity. It

[120] W. B. Castle, "Development of Knowledge Concerning the Gastric Intrinsic Factor and Its Relation to Pernicious Anemia," *New England Journal of Medicine,* CCXLIX, 1953, p. 603.

has now supplanted liver extracts in the treatment of pernicious anemia. It prevents not only the macrocytic anemia characteristic of pernicious anemia, but the degenerative changes in the nervous system as well.

Once the diagnosis of pernicious anemia is established in a patient, the manifestations of the disease can be corrected and controlled for the rest of his life by regular intramuscular injections of vitamin B_{12}. In the beginning vitamin B_{12} may be administered at weekly or biweekly intervals. Later the interval can be lengthened to monthly or even bimonthly. The need for the patient to continue these injections for the rest of his life cannot be emphasized too strongly. In the present state of knowledge, no methods for the primary prevention of pernicious anemia are available. Methods for the prevention of the harmful effects are, however, highly successful. It is one of the best examples of a chronic disorder which cannot be cured, but can be well controlled. The patient should be encouraged to continue treatment and medical supervision for the rest of his life. Whether or not patients with macrocytic anemias associated with other disorders such as cirrhosis of the liver will have to continue to take vitamin B_{12} for the remainder of their lives depends on the nature of the condition predisposing to it.

Mrs. Oaks is an excellent example of the patient who has had a long history of pernicious anemia. She is now 89 years of age. Despite her present state of ill health, this stems not from the presence of pernicious anemia for more than 40 years, but from other disorders. She became aware of symptoms of pernicious anemia at about 50 years of age. Manifestations of pernicious anemia are uncommon before 30 years of age. Mrs. Oaks has many of the characteristics of persons developing this disease; she is blue-eyed and has a light skin. Though she is now white-haired, in her youth she was a golden blonde. When asked, she states that she grayed early. Pernicious anemia is more common in blue-eyed blondes who are of Scandinavian descent or from the British Isles or other northern European countries. It is less common in dark-skinned individuals, though it does occur. She is of German descent. Early graying of the hair is also frequently observed. Mrs. Oaks's father died from the effects of pernicious anemia. A family history of this disease is not at all unusual. As in other persons with pernicious anemia, the mucosa of Mrs. Oaks's stomach is atrophied with the result that it does not secrete the intrinsic factor. Neither does it secrete hydrochloric acid. The finding of a macrocytic anemia in a patient with persistent achlorhydria, even after the injection of histamine, is highly suggestive of pernicious anemia. Despite the association of achlorhydria with pernicious anemia, it is not responsible for the anemia, nor does it cause the degenerative changes in the nervous system. Many patients, and Mrs. Oaks is one of them, have indigestion which is corrected by the regular replacement of hydrochloric acid with meals. It has no effect on any other manifestation of the disease, however. With the atrophy of the lining of the stomach, secretion of mucus and hydrochloric acid both fail.

At the onset of illness Mrs. Oaks presented the usual manifestations of pernicious anemia. She complained of weakness and a sore tongue which was beefy red in appearance. She had some numbness and tingling of her fingers. On examination of her blood macrocytic anemia with both anisocytosis and poikilocytosis were found. Her red cell count was 2 million cells per cubic millimeter of blood. Her hemoglobin was about 9 gm per 100 ml of blood. Other characteristic changes in the blood in pernicious anemia, but which were not determined at the time the diagnosis was made for Mrs. Oaks, are granulocytopenia with relative lymphocytosis and thrombocytopenia. The thrombocyte count usually is down to 60,000 to 70,000 cells. About two days following the intramuscular injection of crude liver extract, her reticulocytes had risen sharply. About 15 per cent of the total number of erythrocytes were reticulocytes. Later the percentage of reticulocytes fell as the number of mature erythrocytes increased. Shortly after vitamin B_{12} was demonstrated to be effective in the treatment of pernicious anemia, it was substituted for liver extract in her treatment.

Accompanying the response of Mrs. Oaks's bone marrow to treatment was improvement in her general state of health. Soreness of her tongue was relieved. Since Mrs. Oaks was not acutely ill, she was treated in the office of her physician. Patients with degenerative changes in the nervous system and those who are too ill to be treated at home are usually hospitalized. Particular attention should be paid to position and body alignment of those who are weak or who have changes in the nervous system. Extremities should be put through the normal range of motion exercises and the patient should be encouraged to move his arms and legs. Patients who are unable to turn or who do not should be placed on a regular turning schedule. Although an extreme and unusual example, one patient was admitted to the hospital recently with multiple decubiti associated with neglected pernicious anemia. These sores were thought to be due to the effect of prolonged deficiency of vitamin B_{12} on somatic cells. Since pernicious anemia is also accompanied by sensory deficits, this was probably a contributing factor.

With the exception of changes in the nervous system, most of the manifestations associated with pernicious anemia respond quickly to therapy with vitamin B_{12}. Mrs. Oaks was fortunate inasmuch as no permanent changes had taken place in her nervous system. While therapy with vitamin B_{12} can be expected to prevent further progress and may even result in some improvement in symptoms arising from lesions in the nervous system, it will not reverse the changes that have already taken place. Wintrobe[121] suggests that the patients in whom there are neurological changes eat a half-pound of cooked liver a week. He makes this recommendation because the exact nature of pernicious anemia is not known. Otherwise no special diet is required. The patient should be encouraged to eat a diet planned to maintain a good nutritional status. In the absence of neurological changes no special foods are required. Neither is iron required unless there is evidence of iron deficiency.

[121] Harrison, *Op. cit.*, 4th ed., p. 1285.

Besides pernicious anemia, what are some other disorders in which macrocytic anemia occurs?

Macrocytic anemias may result from a deficiency in the intake of vitamin B_{12} or from failure in its absorption. In the United States where meat is generally available, deficient intake is uncommon. Failure of absorption is much more frequent. There are, of course, other causes of failure of absorption of vitamin B_{12} than pernicious anemia. They include total gastrectomy, in which the source of the intrinsic factor is removed; sprue, in which the absorbing membrane in the small intestine is defective; removal of the small intestine, followed by impaired absorption; and strictures or anastomoses, resulting in a diversion of the contents of the alimentary canal around the absorbing surface of the intestine. The anemia in these conditions is similar to that of pernicious anemia. Achlorhydria and neurological changes are not, however, characteristic features in these conditions.

Certain infestations and therapy with certain drugs are associated with macrocytic anemia. For example, persons who are hosts to the fish tapeworm develop a macrocytic anemia. It is believed that the tapeworm competes with the host for vitamin B_{12}, but it is not known exactly how the interference is accomplished. The tapeworm may merely utilize the vitamin or it may interfere with some step in the process of its utilization. The anemia results not because the intake of vitamin B_{12} is below normal requirements, but because it becomes unavailable to the host. Fish tapeworm infestations occur most commonly among persons who eat raw fish. One of the possible toxic effects of drugs such as diphenylhydantoin sodium U.S.P. (Dilantin Sodium) primidone, barbital derivatives, methotrexate (Amethopterin), and Mercaptopurine (6-mercaptopurine) is macrocytic anemia. With the latter two drugs and probably with the others, the effect is due to a deficiency of folic acid.

An adequate intake of all of the B vitamins is undoubtedly essential to hematopoeisis. These chemicals participate in a wide variety of metabolic reactions in cells either as direct regulators or as coenzymes.

Another substance which has a hematopoietic effect is folic acid. In many patients with pernicious anemia, blood cell formation is stimulated by the administration of folic acid. It does not, however, prevent the development of lesions in the nervous system. Wintrobe[122] states that the functions of vitamin B_{12} and folic acid are interrelated. A deficiency of one or both is likely to lead to a number of abnormalities.

A serious lack in any one regulatory substance can be associated with a depression in the production of erythrocytes. Moreover, the problem of deficiency in one required element is often accompanied by a deficiency in others. For example, a diet deficient in vitamin B_{12} would almost certainly be lacking in protein and very possibly in iron. Other regulators are also neces-

[122] *Ibid.,* p. 1282.

sary to the formation and maturation of erythrocytes. Anemia develops in hypothyroidism or myxedema. It may also be associated with chronic adrenal insufficiency and disorders associated with deficiencies of function of the antererior hypophysis.

All the factors in the regulation of erythrocyte formation have not been identified, but certain observations have been made. It is known that the production of red cells is stimulated by a general lack of oxygen or by the loss of blood. It is not known how hypoxia acts to stimulate erythropoiesis. One hypothesis is that hypoxia directly stimulates the bone marrow. Guyton[123] states, however, that localized anoxia of the bone marrow does not result in increased red cell production, but generalized anoxia does. An erythropoietic substance has been postulated to account for these observations. With the possible exception of the kidney, no site has been found in which a greater quantity of an erythropoietic-stimulating substance, erythropoietin, has been produced than in any other. Support is given to the belief that the kidney is an important source of erythropoietin as anemia accompanies chronic renal disease. The erythropoietic substance increases the rate of all phases of red cell production, including the formation, maturation, and release of red cells. In contrast, with an excess of red cells, the formation of the erythropoietic substance is depressed and presumably the production of erythrocytes is depressed.

Although the mechanisms for blood production are only partly understood, those for blood destruction are, if anything, less well understood. Healthy erythrocytes live an average of about 120 days. As the cell ages, its surrounding membrane thins and becomes more and more easily ruptured. Cell destruction may, therefore, merely be the result of the inability of the fragile membrane of the aged cell to withstand the pressure exerted against it as the erythrocyte passes through a capillary. Erythrocytes undergo a certain amount of deformity as they pass through capillaries, and this distortion in shape could place a strain on areas of the cell membrane. According to Guyton, much of the destruction of red cells takes place in the spleen, where the erythrocytes pass through the pulp of the spleen to the venous sinusoids by diapedesis. The walls of erythrocytes undergoing this process would need to be strong to survive. The assumption that the aging of the membrane of the red cell predisposes it to mechanical injury is supported by the observation that poorly constructed cells with fragile membranes have a shorter life span than do normal erythrocytes.

What happens to the contents of the cell after it has been ruptured?

Once the wall of the erythrocyte is disrupted, hemoglobin is released. The shell of the former erythrocyte is called a ghost cell, and it is probably quickly

---

[123] *Op. cit.,* p. 148.

removed from the blood by reticuloendothelial cells. The amino acids and lipids are utilized for energy or are reused in the building of new cells including erythrocytes.

The hemoglobin is also phagocytized by reticuloendothelial cells into globin and heme. The heme is the iron-containing fraction. It is further split into iron and a pigment biliverdin. The iron enters the iron pool of the body from whence it may be drawn to form myoglobin in the muscle, or hemoglobin in new erythrocytes, or stored until it is needed in the liver. The biliverdin is reduced to bilirubin, which is gradually released into the blood. Bilirubin is insoluble in water, but it combines with the blood proteins and it is transported in this form to the liver. The liver separates bilirubin from the blood protein and combines about 80 per cent of it with glucuronide. Bilirubin glucuronide is highly soluble in water. The liver cells secrete it along with the other forms of bilirubin into the bile. Bilirubin is responsible for the greenish-yellow color of bile. After the bile reaches the small intestine, some of the bilirubin is converted by bacterial action to uribilinogen, some of which is excreted in the stool.

Most of the uribilinogen is reabsorbed into the portal circulation and excreted in the bile. A small amount escapes into the circulation and is excreted in the urine. An increase in the level of bilirubin in the blood may be caused by obstruction in the bile ducts or by increased blood destruction. Usually the elevation is greater in the presence of obstructive lesions than in increased blood destruction, though there are occasional exceptions. There are also other differences. (See Chapter 10.)

What are some of the consequences of failure to maintain a balance between erythrocyte production and destruction?

As long as blood production keeps up to the demand for red cells and the rate of red·cell destruction or loss does not exceed cell production, the number of red cells found in the blood remains stable. When, however, production fails to keep pace with the destruction or loss of erythrocytes, anemia develops. In the preceding discussion, some of the causes of failure of the production of erythrocytes were presented. In those conditions anemia developed because the production of red cells failed to keep pace with the normal rate of cell destruction. Anemia may also be the result of any disorder in which the rate of cell destruction or the hemolysis of cells is excessive. These anemias are classified as the hemolytic anemias. The common feature of the hemolytic anemias is an excessive rate of hemolysis of erythrocytes. The etiological agents vary widely. Depending on the nature of the cause, hemolysis may take place in the circulating blood or in the reticuloendothelial system. These disorders also differ widely in symptomatology, severity, and course. In some, the rate of onset may be rapid and the manifestations severe. In others, the onset is slow and the manifestations are mild or absent. A determining factor is whether hemolysis occurs in the circulating blood or in the reticuloendo-thelial system. In all instances in which erythrocytes are hemolyzed at an abnormal rate, some degree of jaundice occurs. It may be barely perceptible or it may be of marked degree. It may develop slowly or rapidly, but jaundice is present to some degree. In chronic hemolytic anemias the liver and spleen are frequently enlarged and complications such as cholelithiasis and leg ulcers may develop.

When the onset of hemolysis is rapid and a large number of red cells are hemolyzed as following the transfusion of incompatible blood, the patient may have a severe shaking chill followed by a high fever, headache, and pain in the back, abdomen, and extremities. The abdominal pain may be so severe that abdominal rigidity results. When the hemolysis is great enough, shock may develop. As in shock from other causes, oliguria and anuria may follow. The urine that is voided is dark in color.

What are some of the etiological agents in the hemolytic anemias?

A very large number of etiological agents have been implicated in the hemolytic anemias. Wintrobe[124] classifies them as causes arising outside the erythrocyte, or extracorpuscular causes, and those associated with defects in the structure or construction of erythrocytes, or intracorpuscular defects. Among the extracorpuscular (outside-the-cell) causes are the acute hemolytic anemias due to immune body reactions. Common examples include the trans-fusion of incompatible blood and hemolytic disease of the newborn due to the Rh factor. Excessive hemolysis of red cells is secondary to a number of diseases, particularly those in which there is a disease involving structures forming part of the reticuloendothelial system. Some examples include Hodg-kin's disease, chronic lymphocytic leukemia, metastatic carcinomatosis, and liver disease. A variety of infectious agents are also responsible for increased hemolysis of erythrocytes. Although not common in the United States, malaria on a worldwide basis is probably the most frequent cause of anemia due to increased hemolysis of red cells.[125]

A wide variety of chemicals may also be associated with increased blood destruction. The effect of some such as acetophenetidin (phenacetin) methyl chloride, acetanilid, benzene, and lead depends on the size of the dose to which the individual is exposed. Others such as the sulfonamides, quinine and

[124] Harrison, *Op. cit.,* 4th ed., p. 1289.
[125] Malaria is a protozoan disease in which the parasites reproduce asexually in the erythrocytes. After they undergo several divisions, they fill the cell and it ruptures, releasing parasites to invade more erythrocytes. At the time the parasites are released by the hemolysis of the erythrocytes, the patient experiences a severe shaking chill, followed by a high fever, malaise, headache, and muscle pain. The spleen is frequently enlarged. As in other disorders associated with hemolysis of erythrocytes, jaundice occurs. The attack is terminated by a drenching perspiration. There are some differences in the manifestations, in their severity, and in the frequency of attacks depending on the species of *plasmodium* infecting the individual.

quinidine, Amphetamine sulfate U.S.P. (Benzedrine), methyl-phenyl-ethyl hydantoin (mesantoin), and vitamin K substitutes depend on hypersensitivity to the chemical agent. It may be noted that some of these chemicals may also cause hypoplasia or aplasia of the bone marrow.

Physical agents such as severe thermal burns are also associated with increased hemolysis of erythrocytes. This is one of the factors predisposing to anemia in the severely burned patient.

Besides exposure to a variety of physical and chemical agents, defects in the construction of red cells or in the type of hemoglobin also predispose to an increased rate of blood destruction. A number of these disorders are hereditary. Among them are hereditary spherocytosis (familial or congenital hemolytic jaundice, hereditary leptocytosis also known as thalassemia or Mediterranean anemia) and sickle cell anemia.

To summarize, anemia results when blood production fails to keep up to blood destruction. The balance between the two factors may be upset by a failure in blood production, by the demands for erythrocytes exceeding the capacity of the bone marrow to produce them, or by an increase in the rate of destruction of erythrocytes over the functional capacity of the bone marrow. Anemia is also caused by the loss of blood. When the loss of blood is rapid, the most acute problems are created by a loss of blood volume.

Anemias have a great number of causes. They may be primary, that is, arise from some disturbance in the functioning of the hematopoietic tissues, or they may be secondary to disturbances in other parts of the body. There are few chronically ill patients who, because of the effects of the disease on blood production or destruction or both, as well as on food intake, escape some degree of anemia. It is not unusual for the chronically ill patient with a marked degree of anemia to feel much improved after his anemia is corrected. The characteristic feature of all anemias is a reduction in the normal number of erythrocytes or in the total quantity of hemoglobin or both. Anemias arising from various etiological factors differ from each other in some respects. In the hemolytic anemias, the products of increased blood destruction are responsible for some of their major manifestations. One aspect common to all anemias is that the oxygen-carrying power of the blood is diminished. In slowly developing anemias, the major manifestations are usually due to the decreased oxygen-carrying power of the blood. The severity of the symptoms experienced by the patient depends in part on the rapidity with which the anemia develops and the degree to which the erythrocyte count and hemoglobin fall below normal. The latter will determine the degree to which the oxygen-carrying power of the blood is reduced. Severity also depends on the effectiveness of the adaptive mechanisms of the patient. The status of the circulatory system is a significant factor in adaptation to anemia.

When the loss of blood is slow, a patient may have a marked decrease in oxygen-carrying power and yet have few symptoms. Allen Maple illustrates this point very well. Allen, a 14-year-old boy, was admitted to the hospital for the purpose of determining why he was subject to fainting spells. Neither his mother nor his teachers had noted any other change in his behavior. To everyone's amazement, his hemoglobin was found to be 2.5 gm per 100 ml of blood. Apparently his cells had adapted quite successfully to a very slow loss of blood. Needless to say, Allen was somewhat less active than a healthy boy.

The functions of the organs of most systems of the body are affected by the decreased oxygen-carrying power of the blood. In some individuals, anemia is associated with pallor of the skin. Despite the widespread belief that pallor indicates anemia, it is not a very reliable sign. Many factors affect the color of the skin, such as the thickness of the epidermis, the quantity and color of the skin pigment, the number of blood vessels in the skin, as well as the nature and quantity of hemoglobin carried in the blood. Some persons have naturally sallow complexions and are not anemic. Certain diseases are accompanied by a pallor, though anemia is absent. Pallor of certain parts of the body such as the finger- and toenails or of the mucous membranes does indicate anemia.

Inasmuch as the respiratory system, the circulatory system, and the blood function together to deliver oxygen to the cells, many of the effects on respiratory and circulatory systems have been previously described as symptoms of circulatory distress. In moderate degrees of anemia, they are initiated by exertion or by excitement. When anemia is severe, they may even occur at rest. Among the signs and symptoms referrable to the respiratory system are dyspnea and rapid breathing. Both are adaptive inasmuch as dyspnea discourages exertion, and the increase in the rate of breathing if not excessive increases ventilation.

The most frequent cardiac manifestation is palpitation, or awareness of the heart pounding. The heart also adjusts to anemia by increasing its rate and stroke volume. Arterial pulsation and pulse pressure increase. Sometimes the capillaries in the fingertips can be seen to be pulsating. Under some circumstances the patient may have angina or present evidence of developing congestive heart failure. Cardiac failure occurs when adaptation is inadequate or fails.

Any person reporting symptoms of circulatory distress should be encouraged by the nurse to seek medical attention. Relief of these and other symptoms depends on the identification and correction of the cause. In patients with marked symptoms, the nursing requirements of the patient are similar to those of the patient in congestive heart failure. As the anemia is relieved, symptoms lessen and the patient will be able to assume more responsibility for his own care.

The neuromuscular system is also affected in anemia. Among the signs and symptoms referable to this system are headache, dizziness or vertigo, fainting, sensitivity to cold, tinnitus (ringing in the ears), muscular weakness, easy fatigability, and irritability. Parasthesias, or abnormal sensations, are common. The headache may be very severe. The patient who is dizzy or faint should be protected from falling. These symptoms may be less troublesome if he learns to change position slowly. The patient requires a warm room, extra blankets and clothing, and protection from drafts. Although the patient should also be protected from overexertion, he should not be allowed to be in one position for endless periods of time. If he is unable to move himself, he should be moved and turned, and his extremities should be put through the normal range of motion exercises. As the patient improves, he can be expected to be more energetic.

In anemia, a number of signs and symptoms indicative of disturbances in the function of the alimentary canal are frequent. Most patients have a loss of appetite. They may need to be encouraged to eat and may require some assistance. Nausea, vomiting, flatulence, abdominal discomfort, and diarrhea or constipation may also occur. When one or more of these are present, they may also discourage the patient from eating. In pernicious anemia, glossitis with a sore tongue is a common event. In aplastic anemia, leukemia, and agranulocytosis, necrotic lesions develop in the mouth and pharynx. In these latter conditions gums tend to bleed either spontaneously or on slight trauma. These patients not only have problems in eating, but their mouths are difficult to keep clean and relatively free from crusts.

In the patient with a painful tongue or who has sores in his mouth, the diet should be low in roughage and bland. To spare the patient unnecessary discomfort and to encourage eating, hot, spicy, or highly acid foods should be avoided. If a toothbrush is used to cleanse the teeth, it should be soft and brushing should be gentle. Application of toothpaste with large cotton balls or well-moistened pieces of cotton is less likely than toothbrushes to traumatize fragile tissues and thus cause bleeding. In some patients the cleansing of the mouth should be limited to the use of a mouthwash. Solutions such as 1 per cent hydrogen peroxide or of sodium perborate, Dobell's solution, or flavored mouthwashes may be tried. The mucous membranes can be kept moist by rinsing the mouth with milk of magnesia. It forms a coat over the mucosa, which can be removed later by rinsing the mouth with water. Carbonated beverages may be used to break up the crusts collecting in the mouth without causing bleeding. Potentially toxic agents should not be used unless they are prescribed by a physician and the patient should be able to cooperate. In patients in whom the lips have a tendency to crack, liquid petrolatum or some other substance should be applied to keep the skin soft. Whenever mouth care is given, an outstanding feature should be great gentleness.

In severe anemia, menstrual disturbances in the female and loss of libido in the male are not infrequent. The most frequent menstrual disturbance is amenorrhea, although menorrhagia, excessive menstruation, also occurs.

Among the other signs and symptoms frequently associated with severe anemia are increased metabolic rate, a slight degree of fever, and enlargement of the spleen.

In longstanding anemia changes take place in the skin and its appendages. The skin loses its elasticity and tone, the hair thins, and, in iron-deficiency anemias, the nails lose their luster, become brittle, and break easily. They may also become concave instead of being convex. Bruised spots, ecchymoses, and purpura may also be observed in the skin.

From this review of the effects of anemia on the various systems of the body, it should be clear that anemia has widespread effects. Some, such as those in the respiratory and circulatory system, represent adjustments to lessen the effects of the lowered oxygen-carrying capacity of the blood. Others, such as those arising in the gastrointestinal and nervous systems, warn the individual that something is wrong, but do not add to his capacity to adapt. Some, such as loss of appetite, may, when continued, aggravate the pre-existing disorder.

How is the presence and nature of the anemia established?

The first step in the treatment of anemia is the identification of its presence and the nature of the cause. The appearance and general behavior of the patient provide clues leading the physician to suspect the presence of anemia. With experience and careful examination of the patient, he may be able to estimate with some accuracy the degree of anemia. Pallor of the palms of the hands, the nail beds, and the mucosa is present when the anemia is fairly severe. The physician also examines the patient for evidence of circulatory and respiratory adjustments to the anemia as well as for the previously listed effects on other systems of the body. Examination of the blood establishes the presence or absence of anemia. Other evidence may be required to establish its cause.

Besides counting the total number of each type of cell, the blood may be examined in one or more of the following ways:

Blood cells

Erythrocytes. Total count per cubic millimeter of blood; percentage of mature cells; percentage of immature cells and stage of immaturity; presence of abnormal cells; size; variations in size as well as in the shape of cells; fragility test (osmotic and mechanical).

Leukocytes. Total count per cubic millimeter of blood; differential white count (percentage of various types of leukocytes); presence and percentage of immature cells and degree of immaturity; presence and description of abnormal leukocytes.

Thrombocytes. Number.

Hemoglobin. Grams per 100 ml of blood (may be reported in percentage of normal value such as 100 per cent, 50 per cent).

Hematocrit. Volume of packed red cells in proportion to volume of plasma—in some institutions this is used in preference to hemoglobin determination as the result is likely to be more dependable.

Icterus index. Determination of the bilirubin content of the blood.

Sedimentation rate of erythrocytes. Rate at which the red cells settle out of whole blood. The height in mm of the column of plasma which is formed at the top of a tube of blood in one hour. Range 1-3 mm per hour.

Schilling test. Vitamin B_{12} absorption.

Bone marrow. State of activity, percentage composition, morphology.

Urine. Urobilinogen and bilirubin content; evidence of blood in the urine.

Stool. Bilirubin, urobilinogen content; occult (hidden) or obvious blood in the stool.

Gastric juice. Presence or absence of free hydrochloric acid, including response to histamine.

Isotope studies. Red cell survival (Cr^{51}), iron turnover (Fe^{59}).

Bleeding and clotting times.

Capillary fragility test. (Rumpel-Leeds).

As a result of the examination of the blood and the bone marrow the physician learns: (1) the degree of the anemia, (2) something about its cause, (3) the extent to which blood production is normal or abnormal, and (4) the degree to which blood destruction is increased.

Obviously not every patient is subjected to all the above examinations. Moreover, in individual instances other tests may be utilized in the process of making the diagnosis. Most of these tests do not require special or elaborate preparation of the patient. The patient may need some help in understanding why blood must be removed for the purposes of examination. Even when the patient accepts, on an intellectual level, that blood is required, he may not accept it on an emotional level. He expresses this lack of acceptance in a number of ways. He repeatedly asks questions, such as, "Is it really necessary to take all that blood?" "Doesn't the physician know that I am already short of blood?" "How can I get well when they take my blood each morning?" He calls the laboratory technicians, nurses, or doctors who take the blood "blood suckers." Among healthy people the loss of a few milliliters of blood can be frightening or believed to be dangerous. Understanding how the patient feels about the removal of blood for examination should help the nurse to be supportive to the patient. Since the anemic patient is frequently hyperirritable, the taking of blood may be associated with expressions of this irritability. As the patient responds to treatment, he will be better able to tolerate frustration and discomfort.

*What factors are taken into consideration in the treatment
of anemia?*

Therapy in anemia must be directed to the cause and pathogenesis of the disorder in each patient. In anemias caused by blood loss, the condition causing the loss of blood must, if possible, be corrected. In acute blood loss, the first consideration is the maintenance and restoration of the blood volume.

When there is a great loss of blood with a marked decrease in its oxygen-carrying power, the cellular elements must also be replaced. In serious hemorrhage, replacement of blood cells, although not lifesaving, may facilitate the recovery of the patient.

In chronic blood loss such as occurs in hookworm disease or other disorders accompanied by prolonged loss of small amounts of blood, volume is not a problem. The loss of iron from the body is. Therapy is therefore directed toward identifying and eliminating the cause and restoring the level of iron in the body to normal. Iron is administered as ferrous sulfate or as whole blood. Attention is also paid to the state of the nutrition of the patient.

There are few disorders in which knowledge of the underlying disorder is more important to the therapy than in the treatment of the anemias. In iron-deficiency anemia, the patient responds to an increased intake of iron, but does not benefit from an increased intake of vitamin B_{12}, unless it is also lacking. The same is true of patients who have a vitamin B_{12} deficiency. In some instances, such as in the patient with sickle cell anemia or thalassemia, an increase in the intake of iron, particularly in the form of red cells, may actually be harmful, because the body has no mechanism by which it can eliminate iron once it is absorbed into the body. Probably the greatest harm to the largest number of people comes from the waste of money spent on "shotgun" preparations prepared to cure all blood deficiencies. Many of them are expensive and, with the possible exception of one constituent, useless. In the absence of a disease of the blood or a condition causing the loss of blood, money spent for a nutritious diet is a good anemia preventative.

The patient who suffers from a deficiency of vitamin B_{12}, either from lack of absorption or from an actual dietary deficiency, requires this substance in his treatment.

Although not effective in all anemias characterized by periods of increased blood destruction, in some types, removal of the spleen may prevent episodes of massive hemolysis of blood. In certain anemias, such as sickle cell anemia, there is no specific therapy and no way to prevent the progress of the disorder.

What is polycythemia?

As in other homeostatic conditions, homeostasis may fail because too few cells and/or too little hemoglobin is produced or erythrocytes are formed in excess. The latter condition is known as polycythemia. The term itself means a large or excessive number of blood cells. In some instances polycythemia results from a physiological stimulus, that is, generalized hypoxia. In a few persons, there is no ready explanation for the disorder. This form is called polycythemia vera.

What factors are involved in the self-sealing mechanism?

A second function of the blood which may be disordered is the self-sealing mechanism. As the term implies, this mechanism defends the body against the loss of blood. Three elements enter into the self-sealing mechanism. They are (1) the surrounding tissues (extravascular); (2) the blood vessels (vascular); and (3) the coagulation of the blood (intravascular). Were it not for the self-sealing mechanism, even minor tears in a blood vessel would permit enough blood to escape to cause death. In every individual, small blood vessels are disrupted many times a day. When the self-sealing mechanism is effective, little or no loss of blood occurs. When for some reason it is defective, blood loss may threaten or take the life of the individual. Defects in the self-sealing mechanism may be acquired or hereditary. Walter Thomas is an example of an individual with one of the hereditary disorders of the self-sealing mechanism. He lacks one of the factors necessary to the clotting of the blood, the antihemophilic factor. As a result of this hereditary defect, minor trauma or other injuries induce severe bleeding. Despite his youth (he is only 15 years of age), he has been hospitalized 29 times for episodes of bleeding. His weight-bearing joints are ankylosed (rigid) from bleeding into the joint capsule. Were it not for excellent medical and nursing care, Walter would not have been able to survive. An older brother died from hemorrhage at the age of two.

The characteristic tissues in which the ruptured blood vessels are located have a significant influence on the extent of bleeding. Firm or nondistensible tissues tends to limit bleeding because the addition of blood quickly raises the tissue hydrostatic pressure. With the elevation of the pressure in the tissue blood flow is impeded. In contrast, when bleeding occurs in distensible tissues or from an area where the blood escapes from the body, hydrostatic pressure may be slow to rise or not rise at all. Consequently, bleeding into an area involving a break in the skin, mucosa, or serous membrane is likely to be more profuse than bleeding into a solid tissue, because the flow of blood is unopposed by tissue hydrostatic pressure. To illustrate, some months ago, while closing a car door Mary Silver slipped and her thumb was caught between the door and the frame of the car. Many blood vessels were ruptured and the soft tissues appeared bruised. The actual quantity of blood lost into the injured area was minimal as the nail is nondistensible and the skin of the thumb is firm. The hydrostatic pressure rose rapidly in the bruised area and bleeding was stopped promptly.[126]

The use of tissue hydrostatic pressure in controlling bleeding is illustrated by the following instance. A young man was admitted to the emergency service of a well-known hospital. He was bleeding profusely from a gash in his right thigh made by a sharp razor. As far as the physician could determine, large nerves and muscles had escaped injury. The intern who was assigned to care for the wound was busily trying to ligate all the severed blood vessels when an experienced nurse came into the room, evaluated the situation, then leaned over his shoulder, and said in a low tone of voice, "Sew it up, and it will stop itself." What she was saying was that if the wound is closed, pressure

---

[126] Needless to say, the pain was exquisitely severe. Loss of the nail can usually be prevented, if the nail is pierced with a red-hot pin and the blood is allowed to escape.

within the tissues will soon exceed the hydrostatic pressure of the blood and bleeding will stop.

In contrast, in the absence of increasing hydrostatic pressure, disruption of a blood vessel may lead to copious and at times fatal bleeding. Examples such as a ruptured esophageal varix and a bleeding peptic ulcer have been discussed elsewhere.

To recapitulate, one factor in the self-sealing mechanism is the character of the tissues into which bleeding takes place. In tissues relatively resistant to distention, a small amount of bleeding may quickly elevate the intratissue pressure above the hydrostatic pressure of the blood. Blood flow is thereby impeded and other factors in the self-sealing mechanism can come into play and plug the rent in the blood vessels. Where bleeding is into distensible tissue or cavities and the blood escapes from the body, bleeding is likely to be more profuse because the opposing hydrostatic pressure is not developed rapidly or does not develop at all.

Another factor in the self-sealing mechanism is the blood vessel. Following disruption the cut end of the blood vessel constricts. An interesting point about this is that the more the tissue is traumatized, the greater the degree of constriction. Thus instances have been known in which amputation of an extremity by crushing were associated with little bleeding. Vasoconstriction is least with the type of injury in which the blood vessel is subject to minimum trauma. Three factors contribute to vasoconstriction, the spasm of the muscle in the wall of the blood vessel, reflex nervous stimulation, and the release of serotonin by the injured tissues. One other factor enters into the decrease in the diameter of the cut end of the vessel; as the clot retracts, it pulls the blood vessel together. This will be discussed in more detail later.

The third factor in the self-sealing mechanism is the clotting of the blood. Healthy blood is capable of clotting in response to a break in the wall of a blood vessel and surrounding tissue. If, however, blood is to accomplish its function as a transporting media, it must be in a fluid state. Two general elements protect the blood against clotting. One is the structure of the blood vessel and the nature of blood flow; the other the presence in the blood of anticoagulant chemicals.

Healthy blood vessels have a smooth endothelial lining, which lessens trauma to blood cells as they pass through. A second source of protection is a layer of negatively charged protein absorbed on the lining surface of the intima. It repels the negatively charged platelets and thereby prevents them from sticking.

Furthermore, the flow of blood in the blood vessels is laminar, that is, in layers. The fluid elements are to the outside and the cellular elements are in the inner core. This enables blood cells in larger vessels to slip along with little or no contact with the lining. When blood flow is slow due to lack of exercise of the extremities or obstruction of a vessel, cellular elements tend to settle to the wall of the vessel. The possibility of intravascular clotting is therefore increased. Patients confined to bed can be protected from venous stasis by exercising the extremities and avoiding pressure at points where blood flow is likely to be impeded. The blood contains two types of substances, the anticoagulants and the procoagulants. The function of the anticoagulants is to keep the blood in its circulating or fluid state. Among the substances postulated are those with antithromboplastin and antithrombin activity. A chemical known to act as an anticoagulant is heparin. Heparin is believed to be secreted by basophilic mast cells located around capillaries throughout the body. These cells are most abundant in the liver and lungs.[127] Heparin is thought to act by preventing the conversion of prothrombin to thrombin. It may also destroy thrombin. Healthy blood is capable of clotting in response to a break in the wall of a blood vessel. The proclotting factors are normally kept in check by anticoagulant factors in the blood. This is necessary if the blood is to carry out its defensive and transporting functions.

Important as the fluid state of the blood is to its functions, its capacity to clot is an essential defense against the loss of blood. Normal blood contains a number of substances capable of acting together to cause the blood to clot. Some of these substances are normally held in check and do not act unless they are activated by some other substance. Once blood clotting is initiated, however, the process tends to keep itself going. Blood clotting acts as a positive feedback system; that is, it is a process which is self-perpetuating or creates more of the same. This is different from many homeostatic mechanisms in which a change in one direction is counteracted by a change in the opposite direction.

One disorder in which the positive feedback effect in blood clotting can be seen is thrombophlebitis or phlebothrombosis. In these disorders, a blood clot is formed on the wall of a vein. When such a vein is opened, the clot is frequently seen to be in all stages of development from the well-organized clot adherent to the wall of the vessel to the amorphous newly forming clot in its tail. The stimulus to clot formation is usually some type of injury to the wall of the blood vessel. Occasionally, however, the clots are formed in the blood vessels in the absence of apparent damage. This situation is maladaptive.

Knowledge of the final stages of blood clotting is fairly complete, but less is known about the initial stages. A deficiency or absence in any one of the essential factors results in defective coagulation of the blood. Traditionally four factors have been identified as being necessary. They are: thromboplastin, prothrombin, calcium, and fibrinogen. Wintrobe[128] lists 12 different factors. In some instances three or more substances are included under one of these factors. All of these, and possibly others, are believed to play a role in blood coagulation. Although a deficiency of calcium was once believed to be a cause of failure of the blood to clot, this is no longer thought to be true. Calcium must be present in the ionized form, but the quantity required is

---

[127] Guyton, *Op. cit.,* p. 207.
[128] Harrison, *Op. cit.,* 4th ed., p. 219.

small. Because calcium is also required to regulate the irritability of nerve tissue, a significant fall in the level of calcium causes disturbances in neuro-muscular functioning before it affects blood coagulability. Before the quantity of calcium could drop enough to affect the clotting of the blood, death would have occurred from respiratory failure.

What are the steps in blood clotting?

The first step in the clotting of the blood is the activation of thromboplastin which is released by the injured tissues or platelets. Pure platelet thrombo-plastin cannot by itself initiate blood clotting. Three plasma cofactors are especially important in the activation of platelet thromboplastin. A deficiency of any one of them will prevent the clotting as a consequence of a lack of degeneration of platelets. The three factors include: (1) antihemophilic fac-tor, (2) plasma thromboplastin component, and (3) plasma thromboplastin antecedent. Walter Thomas, who was described earlier, had difficulty in the coagulation of his blood because he had a hereditary lack of the antihemo-philia factor.

After thromboplastin is activated, it combines with ionized calcium in the blood and acts as an enzyme to catalyze the conversion of prothrombin to thrombin. As stated previously, sufficient ionized calcium is always available for this reaction to occur. The same cannot be said for prothrombin. One of the precursors of prothrombin is vitamin K. In diseases in which bile fails to reach the small intestine, vitamin K is not absorbed. As a fat-soluble sub-stance, its absorption depends on the presence of bile. Formerly, patients with obstructive jaundice often continued to bleed for hours from minor breaks in the skin, such as those caused by the introduction of an intravenous needle into a vein. Needless to say in these patients surgical procedure was fraught with great danger. Vitamin K can now be administered by intramuscular injection. Within about four hours, provided the patient has sufficient liver tissue, enough prothrombin will be synthesized to make a surgical procedure safe. Occasionally a baby is born who experiences serious bleeding because the store of vitamin K in his liver is inadequate. Like the patient with obstruc-tive jaundice, he bleeds because he lacks a sufficient quantity of prothrombin.

Since prothrombin is manufactured by the liver, in disease involving the parenchyma of the liver, prothrombin levels may be low. The production of prothrombin may also be depressed by certain anticoagulant preparations of coumarin. These substances are employed in disorders in which there is a tendency for the blood to clot in the blood vessels. Though the danger of spontaneous hemorrhage is less with some of the newer anticoagulant prepa-rations, it is always a possibility. Any bleeding should be brought to the attention of the physician immediately, and the patient receiving an anticoagu-lant on an outpatient basis should be under regular medical care. The patient may bleed spontaneously from the gastrointestinal or genitourinary tract or into serous cavities. Areas of purplish discoloration of the skin or mucous membrane may indicate bleeding into these tissues. When these areas occur in the skin, they are called ecchymoses. The term "purpura" is also used to describe spontaneous bleeding into the skin and mucous membrane. For reasons not completely understood, large doses of salicylates also decrease the prothrombin content of the blood plasma.

In the third step in the process of blood clotting, thrombin catalyzes the conversion of fibrinogen, a blood protein synthesized in the liver, to fibrin. In the process the fibrinogen molecule is split and the resulting fragments are polymerized[129] and form a threadlike structure. The fibrin strands run in all directions and form a mesh that catches plasma, blood platelets, erythrocytes, and leukocytes. As the fibrin strands contract, they squeeze out fluid or serum, and the size of the clot is reduced. This process is called clot retraction. Large numbers of platelets are required for the formation and satisfactory retraction of the clot. Since the fibrin threads are sticky, they adhere to the wall of the damaged blood vessel. As they shorten they pull the blood vessel wall together, thus diminishing its diameter and acting as a plug or cork.

Sometimes in surgical procedures involving the surface of a mucous membrane, a large, loose clot forms over the surface. It acts like a curtain with the vessels behind it continuing to bleed. For bleeding to be controlled, the sheltering clot must be prevented from forming, or, if it does, it must be removed, so that the blood clots in the end of the exposed blood vessels. Two common sites of hemorrhage of this type are the pharynx following tonsillectomy and surgery on the prostate or urinary bladder. Following the latter type of surgery, the physician often prescribes bladder irrigations frequently enough to prevent the formation of blood clots. If one or more clots form, they can also be removed by irrigation. Unless the bladder irrigations are performed thoroughly, the patient may lose an unnecessary quantity of blood.

Although primary fibrinogenemia or fibrinogenopenia can cause bleeding, this is a rare event. As a rule, a low level of fibrinogen in the blood is associated with diminished quantities of other procoagulation factors such as prothrombin and the blood platelets and is secondary to a serious injury or illness. Massive and spontaneous hemorrhage may occur. The events leading to spontaneous bleeding are complex and are not well understood One hypothesis suggested to explain the changes is that the elements required for clotting are used more rapidly than they can be replaced by the body. In other words, demand exceeds supply. This is followed by an increase in the destruction of fibrin or fibrinolysis. The presence of this condition is heralded by large ecchymoses in the skin and spontaneous bleeding from mucous membranes. Wintrobe[130] lists five different types of pathological disorders in which fibrinolysis is observed. They are: (1) following severe traumatic in-

---

[129] The joining of like molecules so that the resulting compound is a multiple of each unit.
[130] Harrison, *Op. cit.*, 4th ed., p. 226.

juries or burns, (2) following surgical procedures such as those involving the lung, (3) obstetrical complications such as abruptio placentae, (4) neoplastic disease, and (5) a variety of disorders such as leukemia, polycythemia vera, and cirrhosis of the liver.

The bleeding resulting from acquired fibrinolysis is often massive. The nurse should observe the patient for indications of an increased tendency to bleed, such as ecchymosis in the skin. Bleeding from any area should be brought to the attention of the physician immediately. The life of the patient depends on the prompt administration of fresh whole blood and fibrinogen.

Summary

The self-sealing mechanism consists of the tissue of the body, the blood vessels, and the blood-clotting mechanism. The importance and effectiveness of any one of these elements in health depends on the nature, location, and extent of injury to blood vessels. Through the efficient operation of the self-sealing mechanism, breaks in blood vessels are repaired before appreciable amounts of blood escape from them. For the blood to perform its function as a vehicle in the transportation of materials throughout the body, however, its fluid state must be preserved. The blood-clotting process must be held in check so blood does not clot in the blood vessels thereby obstructing the flow of blood to or from the tissues. Whether or not blood clots depends on the balance between the anticlotting and the proclotting factors. Because the factors favoring intravascular clotting have been discussed elsewhere, they have not been presented in detail here.

The process of blood clotting is very complex. Despite significant advances in knowledge of the process, it still is not completely understood. Certain substances such as thromboplastin must be present and activated to initiate blood clotting. Thromboplastin is released by injured tissues and thrombocytes. Platelet thromboplastin further requires a number of plasma factors for its release and activation. A lack in any one of these factors is accompanied by an increase in the tendency to bleed. The platelets release serotonin, a vasoconstrictor substance, and they are required in large numbers to fill in the spaces in the fibrin network of the clot. Any considerable decrease in the platelet count is a potential source of bleeding. Abnormalities in the structure of the platelets increase the difficulty with which they disintegrate and thereby increase the tendency to bleeding.

Activated thromboplastin acts on prothrombin to produce thrombin. For the liver to synthesize prothrombin, vitamin K must be available in adequate quantities. Prothrombin deficiency accompanies diseases of the liver in which large numbers of parenchymal cells are destroyed or in which there is failure to absorb vitamin K from the gastrointestinal tract. As a fat-soluble substance, vitamin K requires bile for its absorption. Any disorder preventing bile from reaching the gastrointestinal tract will therefore result in inadequate absorption of vitamin K and a deficiency in prothrombin. A not uncommon cause of insufficient prothrombin is iatrogenic; that is, it results from treatment. Therapy with anticoagulants such as preparations of coumarin is most likely to be responsible.

Fibrinogen, also synthesized by the liver, is acted upon to form fibrin. Strands of fibrin form the structural framework for the clot. Being sticky, fibrin adheres to the lining of the blood vessel and catches the constituents of the blood in its mesh to fill in the spaces. As the fibrin contracts, the wall to which it adheres follows and diameter of the vessel diminishes. Contraction, or retraction, of the clot, as it is called, makes a strong, firm clot.

The principal anticoagulant agents used in therapy interfere with blood clotting by preventing the formation of prothrombin or by inhibiting a step in the clotting process.

In the therapy of disorders characterized by bleeding, the most frequently used agent is fresh whole blood. It is employed because it provides not only for the replacement of blood volume and blood cells, but for the replacement or addition of the substances required in blood clotting. There are a number of hemostatic agents, that is, substances causing the blood to clot rapidly, used to accelerate coagulation of the blood. These include thrombin and purified fibrinogen. Gel foams containing procoagulant substances are sometimes applied to bleeding surfaces to hasten coagulation.

Nursing the patient with a disorder characterized by a tendency to bleed can challenge the most competent nurse. As emphasized earlier, the loss of even small quantities of blood provokes fear in almost everyone. A large hemorrhage with a sudden onset may frighten the nurse as well. Some of the disorders characterized by a tendency to spontaneous hemorrhage, such as leukemia, have a poor prognosis. Patient, family, and nurse live day by day in the presence of death. Especially when the sick person is a child or a young adult, family members may suffer from a variety of negative emotional states including grief, disappointment, depression, panic, and guilt. Their demands on the nurse and physician for emotional support may be greater than those of the patient. Parents and families can be referred to local branches of the Leukemia Foundation for help and emotional support. This does not mean that the nurse is thereby relieved of all further responsibility in this area. What it means is that she shares it with others. In working with the patient with a poor prognosis, the situation for both the patient and his family can often be improved by concentrating attention on what can be done rather than on the hopelessness of the situation. Attention to the comfort of the patient when he is ill, acceptance of his behavior as part of his illness, as well as gentleness and kindness, may not lengthen his life, but they should ease his suffering. The trend toward care of the patient at home, when this is feasible, often makes individualized care easier to attain.

Team conferences, in which nurses, doctors, social workers, occupational and physical therapists, and dietitians meet to discuss the problems involved and possible solutions to them, can do much to improve the quality of care of a patient. When appropriate, the patient and/or a member of his family may also be invited to participate. If this is done, they should be treated as a contributing member of the group. These conferences can also be used to provide support to the various members of the team. A planning conference in which goals and problems are identified, difficulties recognized, and plans made to utilize available resources often helps the personnel to gain a positive perspective in a difficult situation.

For persons such as Walter Thomas, medical and nursing care may save the life of the patient for extended periods of time. However, progressive disability is more difficult to prevent. This leads to a variety of social, economic, psychological, and educational problems. At the last admission of Walter to the hospital, he was bedfast and had been for some time. After the age of nine, he no longer attended school. Although he was assigned a visiting teacher, his progress was slow. His one interest was to be a "ham" radio operator. Since this seemed possible, his nurse encouraged him in his ambition. After discussing possible activities with him and his physician, the help of the occupational therapist was enlisted. Walter illustrates some of the problems involved in the life of an individual who has a severe bleeding tendency from early life. Economic problems were not as great as they are in many instances, since his father had a high income.

In addition to emotional support, another goal in the nursing of the patient with a tendency to bleeding is to prevent incidents predisposing to tissue trauma. Care of the mouth was discussed earlier in the chapter. Bleeding from the nose, or epistaxis, is a common problem. Crusting of the mucosa of the nose predisposes to and follows episodes of bleeding. The crusting may be lessened by inserting a wick of cotton soaked with mineral oil. Only one nostril should be treated, and all excess of oil should be removed from the wick before it is inserted to prevent the possibility of its aspiration.

Another problem arises when subcutaneous or intramuscular injections are administered. To minimize the danger of bleeding, a sharp needle of as small diameter as is compatible with the solution to be injected should be selected. The selection of the sites to be used for injection should be discussed with the physician. When repeated injections are required, the sites should be rotated according to a plan and recorded each time. Steady pressure over the injection site for a period of three to five minutes lessens the likelihood of bleeding into the tissue with the formation of a hematoma.

Patients who are ambulatory should be instructed to avoid bumping themselves against furniture or other hard objects. Care should be taken to perform nursing procedures with extra gentleness. The patient should be protected from sources of infection, not only to protect him from unnecessary discomfort, but because infection increases his tendency to bleed.

Despite every effort to prevent hemorrhage, bleeding does occur, and the nurse should be alert to evidences of it. Petechiae, small capillary hemorrhages, occurring about the ankle or in the antecubital space after a blood pressure determination is made may be the first warning that bleeding is threatened. Purpura and ecchymosis of the skin should be watched for. Bleeding or serous drainage from the nose, gums, or vagina or the vomiting or expectoration of blood should be noted and the quantity of blood lost estimated. The first evidence of bleeding may be as bright-red blood in the stool or in the form of tarry stools. Bright-red blood in the urine is easily recognized, but lesser amounts causing urine to be smoky may be missed.

To summarize briefly, the maintenance of the conditions required for the healthy functioning of cells depends upon a system to supply the needed substances and to remove the products of cell activity. In large multicellular organisms such as man, conduits deliver and remove materials from the capillaries where exchange takes place between the blood and the interstitial fluid. A variety of mechanisms are required to regulate the diameter of the blood vessels and the pressure of the blood within the system. A source of power is necessary to keep the fluid circulating through the system. Through regulation blood supply to vital organs is maintained and the localized needs of tissues are met. Since the transporting medium is in a fluid state, it must be kept fluid and at the same time be capable of being converted into a solid state when blood vessels are disrupted. In health, tissues are protected from a failure of supply by the capacity to adapt function to needs and by a reserve that can be called upon. In disease, cell function or even survival are threatened by failure of supply and/or removal of cell products. Care is directed toward reducing the requirements of affected tissues and/or improving the functioning of diseased organs.

REFERENCES

Books

Allen, Edgar, Nelson Barker, and Edgar Hines, Peripheral Vascular Diseases, 3rd ed., W. B. Saunders Company, Philadelphia, 1962.

Bailey, Charles P. (edited by), *Cardiac Surgery,* F. A. Davis Company, Philadelphia, 1960-61.

Bailey, Charles P., *Surgery of the Heart,* Lea and Febiger, Philadelphia, 1955.

Baker, Wiley F. (edited by), *Surgical Treatment of Peripheral Vascular Disease,* McGraw-Hill Book Company, Inc., New York, 1962.

de Gruchy, G. C., *Clinical Haematology in Medical Practice,* Charles C Thomas, Springfield, Illinois, 1958.

Eick, Ronald E. (ed.), *Can Cardiacs Work? A Conference on the Heart in Industry,* Michigan Heart Association, Detroit, 1960.

Foote, R. Rowden, *Varicose Veins,* 3rd ed., John Wright and Sons Ltd., Bristol, Great Britain, 1960.

Fordham, Mary E., *Cardiovascular Surgical Nursing,* The Macmillan Company, New York, 1962.

Hoebler, Sibley, *Hypertensive Disease,* Hoeber-Harper, New York, 1959.

Hurst, Willis J. (edited by), *Cardiac Resuscitation,* Charles C Thomas, Springfield, Illinois, 1960.

Levine, Samuel A., *Clinical Heart Diseases,* 5th ed., W. B. Saunders Co., Philadelphia, 1958.

Luisada, Aldo A. (ed.), *Cardiology: An Encyclopedia of the Cardio-Vascular System. Vol. I. Normal Heart and Vessels. Vol. II. Methods. Vol. III. Clinical Cardiology. Vol. IV. Clinical Cardiology-Therapy. Vol. V. Related Specialty Fields,* The Blakiston Division, McGraw-Hill Book Co., Inc., New York, Vol. V, 1961.

Modell, Walter, Doris Schwartz, Louis Hazeltine, and Frederic T. Kirkham, *Handbook of Cardiology for Nurses,* 4th ed., Springer Publishing Co., New York, 1962.

Nite, Gladys, and Frank N. Willis, *The Coronary Patient,* The Macmillan Company, New York, 1964.

Prankerd, T. A. J., *The Red Cell,* Charles C Thomas, Springfield, Illinois, 1961.

Peddie, George H., and Frances E. Brush, *Cardio-Vascular Surgery—A Manual for Nurses,* G. P. Putnam's Sons, New York, 1961.

White, Paul, *et al.,* eds., *Cardiovascular Rehabilitation,* McGraw-Hill Book Co., Inc., New York, 1957.

Whitby, Sir Lionel E. H., and C. T. C. Britton, *Disorders of the Blood,* 8th ed., Grune & Stratton, New York, 1957.

Wintrobe, Maxwell M., *Clinical Hematology,* 5th ed., Lea & Febiger, Philadelphia, 1961.

Articles

American Journal of Cardiology, VII, March, 1961, pp. 317-19, Williams, Bryan, and Paul D. White, "Rehabilitation of the Cardiac Patient"; pp. 320-29, Jokl, Ernst, "Cardiovascular Responses to Exercise in Rehabilitation of Cardiac Patients—Physiologic Considerations"; pp. 330-34, Levinson, Robert M., and Donald R. Sparkman, "Exercise Testing of Cardiac Patients in Evaluating Work Potential"; pp. 340-49, Master, Arthur, M., "Survival and Rehabilitation in Coronary Occlusion."

Anderson, Milton W., "The Management of Acute Myocardial Infarction," *Medical Clinics of North America,* XLII, No. 4, July, 1958, pp. 849-58.

Aviado, Domingo, and Carl F. Schmidt, "Physiologic Bases for the Treatment of Pulmonary Edema," *Journal of Chronic Diseases,* IX, No. 5, May, 1959, pp. 495-507.

Bellet, Samuel, "Treatment of Cardiac Arrhythmias," *Geriatrics,* XVI, No. 1, January, 1961, pp. 1-12.

Berge, Kenneth G., "Usefulness and Limitations of Determinations of Serum Transaminase in the Diagnosis of Acute Myocardial Infarction," *Medical Clinics of North America,* XLII, No. 4, July, 1958, pp. 859-60.

Bing, Richard J., William H. Danforth, and Fred B. Ballard, "Physiology of the Myocardium," *The Journal of the American Medical Association,* CLXXII, January 30, 1960, pp. 438-44.

Bing, Richard (ed.), "Heart Disease—Selected Aspects of Pathophysiology, Evaluation and Treatment," *Medical Clinics of North America,* XLVI, No. 6, November, 1962, whole issue.

Blalock, Alfred, "External Cardiac Massage," *Journal of the American Medical Association,* CLXXVI, No. 7, May 20, 1961, p. 609.

Borg, Joseph F., "Long-term Anticoagulant Therapy in Coronary Artery Disease," *Geriatrics,* XVII, June, 1962, pp. 372-78.

Briller, S. A., "Important Uses of Electrocardiography," *American Journal of Nursing,* LV, No. 11, November, 1955, pp. 1378-80.

Brinkhous, K. M., and H. R. Roberts, "Thrombolysis and Thrombolytic Agents," *Journal of the American Medical Association,* CLXXV, No. 4, January 28, 1961, pp. 284-89.

Brown, Amy Frances, "Coronary Occlusion," *American Journal of Nursing,* XLII, No. 3, March, 1942, pp. 248-51.

Burch, George E., and John H. Phillips, "Hypertension and Arteriosclerosis," *American Heart Journal,* LX, August, 1960, pp. 163-67.

Byrne, John J., "Phlebitis," *Journal of the American Medical Association,* CLXXIV, No. 2, September 10, 1960, pp. 113-18.

Cady, Lee D., *et al.,* "Clues to the Development of Coronary Heart Disease," *Geriatrics,* XVI, No. 2, February, 1960, pp. 69-73.

"Cardiacs at Work," *Industrial Medicine and Surgery,* XXX, No. 5, May, 1961, entire issue.

Coe, Myrtle, "Some Roles of Nursing in Cardiac Disease," *Nursing World*, CXXX, No. 2, February, 1956, pp. 7-9.

Cohen, S. I., and Richard Warren, "Fibrinolysis," *The New England Journal of Medicine*, CCLXIV, No. 2, January 12, 1961, pp. 79-83, and CCLXIV, No. 3, January 19, 1961, pp. 128-33.

Crawley, Mildred, "Care of the Patient with a Myocardial Infarction," *American Journal of Nursing*, LXI, February, 1961, pp. 68-70.

Creighton, Helen, "The Nurse's Role in Cardiac Catheterization," *Nursing World*, CXXXIII, No. 2, February, 1959, pp. 25-28.

Cross, Joseph, "Back to Work After Myocardial Infarction," *American Journal of Nursing*, XLII, February, 1962, pp. 58-61.

DeBakey, Michael, and Leonard Engel, "Blood-Vessel Surgery," *Scientific American*, CCIV, April, 1961, pp. 88-101.

Delit, Clement, *et al.*, "Thyrocardiac Disease and Its Management with Radioactive Iodine I^{131}," *Journal of the American Medical Association*, CLXXVI, No. 4, April, 1961, pp. 263-67.

Dickson, Laurie C., Jr., "A Philosophy of the Management of Coronary Occlusion," *Postgraduate Medicine*, XXIV, July, 1958, pp. 3-6.

Donald, Kenneth W., "Hemodynamics in Chronic Congestive Heart Failure," *Journal of Chronic Diseases*, IX, No. 5, May, 1959, pp. 476-92.

Dustan, Harriet P., "Diet and Diuretics in the Treatment of Hypertensive Cardiovascular Diseases," *Journal of the American Medical Association*, CXXVII, No. 18, April 30, 1960, pp. 2052-56.

Elliott, Florence C., and Paul Winchell, "Heart Catheterization and Angio Cardiography," *American Journal of Nursing*, LX, October, 1960, pp. 1418-22.

Elliott, Florence, "Emotional Needs of the Cardiac Patient," *Nursing World*, CXXXIII, No. 2, February, 1959, pp. 14-17.

Estes, J. Earle, "Hypertension in 1958: A Tale of Pills, Philosophy, and Perplexity," *Medical Clinics of North America*, XLII, No. 4, July, 1958, pp. 899-915.

Freis, Edward, "Hypertensive Emergencies," *Medical Clinics of North America*, LXIV, March, 1962, pp. 353-58.

Freis, Edward D., "Treatment of Hypertension with Chlorothiazide," *Journal of the American Medical Association*, CLXIX, No. 2, January, 1959, pp. 105-8.

Ford, Ralph, "The Newer Diuretics," *Medical Clinics of North America*, XLV, July, 1961, pp. 961-72.

Friedburg, C. K., "Evaluation of Cardiac Function in Clinical Practice," *Postgraduate Medicine*, XXIII, No. 3, March, 1958, pp. 213-20.

Frohman, I. Phillips, "Digitalis and Its Derivatives," *American Journal of Nursing*, LVII, February, 1957, pp. 172-75.

Gallagher, J. C., and David Seligson, "Significance of Abnormally Low Blood Urea Levels," *New England Journal of Medicine*, CCLXVI, March 8, 1962, pp. 492-95.

Gauder, Peter J., F. William Blaisdell, and Doris Vonmorpurgo, "Cardiac Resuscitation From Theory to Practice," *Postgraduate Medicine*, XXX, No. 3, March, 1963, pp. 228-32.

Glenn, Frank (ed.), "The Circulatory System in Surgery," *The Surgical Clinics of North America*, XLI, No. 2, April, 1961, entire issue.

Glover, Robert P., and Howard L. Gadboys, "Practical Management of Aortic Stenosis," *Journal of the American Medical Association*, CLXVIII, No. 3, September 20, 1958, pp. 229-36.

Goldsmith, Grace A., "Highlights on the Cholesterol—Fats, Diets and Atherosclerosis Problem," *Journal of the American Medical Association*, CLXXVI, No. 9, June 3, 1961, pp. 783-89.

Greer, William E. R., "Rehabilitation and Employment of Industrial Workers with Cardiovascular Disease," *The American Journal of Cardiology*, VII, March, 1961, pp. 350-53.

Groch, Sigmund N., and Irving S. Wright, "Recent Trends in Therapy of Cerebral Vascular Disease," *Circulation*, XXIII, March, 1961, pp. 458-65.

Hartman, John R., and Rose A. Bolduc, "Hemophilia," *American Journal of Nursing,* LVI, February, 1956, pp. 169-74.

Hashim, Sami A., "The Relation of Diet to Atherosclerosis and Infarction," *American Journal of Nursing,* LX, March, 1960, pp. 348-52.

Hayter, Jean, "Acute Myocardial Infarction," *American Journal of Nursing,* LIX, November, 1959, pp. 1602-4.

Heap, Beth, "Sodium Restricted Diets," *American Journal of Nursing,* LX, February, 1960, pp. 206-9.

Heller, Anne F., "Nursing the Patient With an Artificial Pacemaker," *American Journal of Nursing,* LXIV, No. 4, April, 1964, pp. 87-92.

Henrie, John N., and John C. Ivins, "Surgical Treatment of Peripheral Arterial Occlusions," *Medical Clinics of North America,* XLII, No. 4, July, 1958, pp. 997-1006.

Herrmann, Louis, "Peripheral Venous Diseases: Value of Signs and Symptoms in Clinical Practice," *Medical Clinics of North America,* XLVI, May, 1962, pp. 659-68.

Hosler, Robert M., "Cardiac Resuscitation," *American Journal of Nursing,* LVI, April, 1956, pp. 424-28.

Hufnagel, Charles, and Peter Conrad, "Calcific Aortic Stenosis," *New England Journal of Medicine,* CCLXVI, January 11, 1962, pp. 72-75.

James, George, "A Stop Smoking Program," *American Journal of Nursing,* LXIV, No. 6, June, 1964, 122-25.

Juergens, John L., "Intermittent Claudication," *Medical Clinics of North America,* XLII, July, 1958, pp. 981-88.

Kannel, William B., *et al.,* "Epidemiology of Coronary Heart Disease," *Geriatrics,* XVII, October, 1952.

Karpman, Harold, *et al.,* "A Practical Systematic Laboratory Approach to the Study of the Peripheral Circulation," *Annals of Internal Medicine,* LIII, No. 2, August, 1960, pp. 306-18.

Kayden, Herbert, "Some Clinical Aspects of Complete Heart Block," *Postgraduate Medicine,* XXVI, November, 1959, pp. 588-98.

Kelly, Ann, and Goffredo Gensini, "Coronary Arteriography," *American Journal of Nursing,* LXII, February, 1962, pp. 86-90.

Keyes, John W., and Franz J. Berlacher, "Chlorothiazide (Diuril)—A New Nonmercurial Orally Given Diuretic," *Journal of the American Medical Association,* CLXIX, No. 2, January 10, 1959, pp. 109-22.

Kilgour, Frederick G., "William Harvey and His Contributions," *Circulation,* XXIII, February, 1961, pp. 286-96.

King, Harold E., and Talbert Cooper, "Thrombocytopenia," *Postgraduate Medicine,* XXXI, June, 1962, pp. 532-38.

Kroeker, Edwin, "Diagnosis and Management of Chronic Cor Pulmonale," *Postgraduate Medicine,* XXXIII, January, 1963, pp. 48-58.

Kurtz, Chester, "The Management of the Patient with Acute Myocardial Infarction," *Medical Clinics of North America,* XLVI, March, 1962, pp. 317-29.

Laki, Kolman, "The Clotting of Fibrinogen," *Scientific American,* CCVI, March, 1962, pp. 60-65.

Lillehei, Walton, and L. Engel, "Open-Heart Surgery," *Scientific American,* CCII, February, 1960, pp. 76-90.

Marcus, Emanuel, and Earl N. Silber, "Preparation of the Cardiac Patient for Surgery," *Surgical Clinics of North America,* XXXIX, No. 1, February, 1959, pp. 171-76.

Marple, Charles D., and Marie J. McIntyre, "Anticoagulant Therapy," *American Journal of Nursing,* LVI, July, 1956, pp. 875-79.

McCabe, Edward S., "Long-Term Anticoagulant Therapy," *Geriatrics,* XVII, April, 1962, pp. 200-4.

McKusick, Victor A., *et al.,* "Buerger's Disease: A Distinct Clinical and Pathological Entity," *The Journal of the American Medical Association,* CLXXXI, July 7, 1962, pp. 5-12.

Morris, Alton J., "Antibacterial Drugs in the Prevention of Rheumatic Fever," *Postgraduate Medicine,* XXIII, No. 2, February, 1958, pp. 121-26.

Morse, William, and Richard Bing, "Congestive Heart Failure," *Postgraduate Medicine,* XXX, October, 1961, pp. 293-99.

Morson, Betty J., and David M. Sensening, "Buerger's Disease," *American Journal of Nursing,* LVII, March, 1957, pp. 337-40.

Newman, Elliot V., "Regulation of Electrolytes in the Management of Heart Disease," *Journal of the American Medical Association,* CLXXII, No. 18, April 30, 1960, pp. 2046-52.

Ochsner, Alton, "Venous Thrombosis," *Postgraduate Medicine,* XXXI, June, 1962, pp. 539-45.

Olwin, John H., and J. L. Koppel, "Anticoagulant Therapy," *American Journal of Nursing,* LXIV, No. 5, May, 1964, pp. 107-10.

Osmundson, Philip J., "Preoperative and Postoperative Management of Patients with Hypertension," *The Medical Clinics of North America,* XLVI, No. 4, July, 1962, p. 963.

Pack, Sarah, and E. S. Craig, "Nursing Care of the Child After Open-Heart Surgery," *American Journal of Nursing,* LXI, February, 1961, pp. 78-80.

Page, Irving H. (ed.), "Hypertension and Its Treatment," *The Medical Clinics of North America,* XLV, No. 2, March, 1961, entire issue.

Page, Irving H., "The Changing Outlook for the Hypertensive Patient," *Annals of Internal Medicine,* LVII, July, 1962, p. 96.

Pollack, Byron E., "The Early Management of Myocardial Infarction," *Journal of the American Medical Association,* CLXI, No. 5, June 2, 1956, pp. 404-9.

Rabwin, Marcus H., and Arthur Hoffman, "Present Status of Surgery in Hypertension," *Medical Clinics of North America,* XLIII, No. 4, July, 1959, pp. 1049-53.

Rath, Charles E., "The Prevention and Management of Blood Transfusion Hazards," *American Journal of Nursing,* LV, March, 1955, pp. 323-26.

Rosenman, Leonard, "Diseases of Vasoconstriction," *Postgraduate Medicine,* XXVII, April, 1960, pp. 455-60.

Russek, Henry I., "Role of Heredity, Diet and Emotional Stress in Coronary Heart Disease," *Journal of the American Medical Association,* CLXXI, No. 5, October 3, 1959, pp. 503-8.

Scher, Allen, "The Electrocardiogram," *Scientific American,* CCV, November, 1961, pp. 132-41.

Schwartz, M., and R. C. Little, "Physiologic Basis for the Heart Sounds and Their Clinical Significance," *The New England Journal of Medicine,* CCLXIV, No. 6, February, 1961, pp. 280-85.

Shapiro, Alvin, "Psychophysiologic Mechanisms in Hypertensive Vascular Disease," *Annals of Internal Medicine,* LIII, No. 1, July, 1960, pp. 64-84.

Smirk, F. H., "Recent Developments in Hypertensive Therapy," *American Heart Journal,* LXI, February, 1961, pp. 272-81.

Smith, Genevieve Waples, "A Stroke Is Not the End of the World," *American Journal of Nursing,* LVII, March, 1957, pp. 303-5.

Sparkman, Donald, "Useful Life After Development of Congestive Heart Failure," *Postgraduate Medicine,* XXXI, April, 1962, pp. 371-80.

Sprague, Howard B., "Emotional Factors in Coronary Heart Disease," *Circulation,* XXIII, May, 1961, pp. 648-54.

Spurr, Charles L., and Donald Hayes, "Treatment of Various Hematologic Disorders," *American Practitioner and Digest of Treatment,* December, 1959, pp. 2113-21.

Stare, Fredrick, Nutrition in Relation to Arteriosclerosis," *Postgraduate Medicine,* XXIX, February, 1961, pp. 133-37.

Steiner, Alfred, Elliot J. Howard, and Suat Akgun, "Importance of Dietary Cholesterol in Man," *The Journal of the American Medical Association,* CLXXXI, July 21, 1962, pp. 186-90.

Strauss, Maurice, and Solom Papper, "Sodium and Water Retention in Chronic Congestive Heart Failure," *Journal of Chronic Diseases,* IX, No. 5, May, 1959, pp. 536-53.

Stirling, George, *et al.,* "Open Heart Surgery Using Total Body Perfusion," *Postgraduate Medicine,* XXV, No. 2, February, 1959, pp. 156-63.

Surgical Clinics of North America, XL, No. 1, February, 1960, entire issue devoted to peripheral vascular diseases.

"Symposium: Hematologic Disorders," *Medical Clinics of North America,* XL, July, 1956.

Swan, Henry, "The Current Status of Open Heart Surgery," *Postgraduate Medicine,* XXIII, No. 2, February, 1958, pp. 127-31.

Takats, Geza, "Symptoms and Signs of Peripheral Arterial Disease," *Medical Clinics of North America,* XLVI, May, 1962, pp. 647-57.

"The National Diet-Heart Study," *New England Journal of Medicine,* CCLXVIII, April 25, 1963, pp. 956-57.

Turner, Gwendolyn E., "The Cerebral Vascular Accident Patient," *Nursing Outlook,* VIII, June, 1960, pp. 326-30.

Unglaub, Walter, Amos Prevatt, and Grace Goldsmith, "Recent Experiences in Diagnosing and Treating Pernicious Anemia," *Postgraduate Medicine,* XXIX, April, 1961, pp. 399-407.

Vernon, Charles R., Dan A. Martin, and Kerr L. White, "Psychophysiological Approach to Management of Patients with Congestive Heart Failure," *The Journal of the American Medical Association,* CLXXI, December 5, 1956, pp. 1947-54.

Wilson, Henry E., and Geraldine Price, "Leukemia," *American Journal of Nursing,* LVI, May, 1956, pp. 601-5.

Wilson, William R., and James W. Culbertson, "Drug Therapy of Cardiac Arryhthmias," *Postgraduate Medicine,* XXIII, No. 4, April, 1958, pp. 360-71.

Wintrobe, Maxwell M., "Blood Dyscrasias," *American Journal of Nursing,* LX, April, 1960, pp. 496-500.

Wolfman, Earl, and C. Thomas Flotte, "Surgical Management of Arterial Peripheral Vascular Disease," *Postgraduate Medicine,* XXVII, January, 1960, pp. 40-45.

Zucker, Marjorie, "Blood Platelets," *Scientific American,* CCIV, February, 1961, pp. 58-64.

10 : Nursing the Patient Having a Problem with Some Aspects of Nutrition

> Spurred by hunger from his remote past, man suffered, starved, struggled for food, survived, and is there to tell the tale. But only just.[1]

A continuous supply of nutrients and oxygen are required by cells if they are to survive and carry out their functions. Because most nutrients are stored in the body and cells are able, within limits, to sacrifice some of their substance for use as energy and to adapt energy output to energy intake, the need for a continuous supply of food is less acute than is the need for oxygen. Despite some degree of protection against a lack of food intake, continued deprivation threatens survival. Moreover, unless the supply of food more than meets minimum requirements, growth, health and productivity are threatened.

The earliest written record describing the effects hunger due to famine might have been written today in many parts of the world. The following record was found on a stone in the tomb of an Egyptian Pharaoh:

> Pharaoh: From my throne 1 grieve over this calamity. During my reign, the Nile has failed to flood for seven years. Corn is scarce and there is no other food. My people thieve and pillage their neighbors. Those who would run cannot even walk. Children weep and the young falter and totter like old people. Their legs drag or give way under them. Their spirits are broken. My council chamber is deserted, my food stores have been pillaged and emptied. It is the end of everything.[2]

Before discussing the role of the nurse in meeting the nutritional needs of people and some of the knowledge required to function with understanding, the terms "nutrition" and "diet" will be clarified. All too often nutrition and diet are used synonymously. Nutrition is the broader term as it includes all the bodily processes involved in the use of food. It depends not only on a supply of food, but on the requirememts of cells. Good nutrition implies, therefore, that the supply of food is adequate in quantity and quality to the needs of the cells, and that the cells are able to utilize nutrients in a physiological manner.

---

[1] Morris Sinclair, "Another Man's Hunger," *World Health,* XV, September-October, 1962, p. 8.
[2] *World Health,* March, 1963, p. 30.

Whereas nutrition covers all aspects of nutrition, diet is limited to the regime of food required to support nutrition.[3]

A good or nutritious diet is one providing the quantity and quality of food required to sustain good nutrition. Whether or not good nutrition follows depends on many other factors. The food must be eaten, digested, absorbed, transported, and finally utilized by the cells.

Knowledge of the science of nutrition, coupled with the ability to apply it, is important not only to members of the health professions, but to all persons. Health, well-being, strength, and the ability to resist and to recover from disease are all influenced for good or for ill by the nutritional state. Not only is nutrition a significant factor in the capacity to survive, but adequate nutrition is known to be essential to productive and zestful living. Moreover, nutrition is a factor in the etiology of or recovery from most diseases. Some diseases such as anemia, scurvy, kwashiorkor, pellagra, beriberi, and goiter result from the lack of specific food elements. Resistance to others, such as tuberculosis and pneumonia, is diminished among the undernourished. According to *World Health*,[4] the mortality rate for children of ages one to five who do not get proper food may be as much as 15 times that of children who do. Despite a considerable body of knowledge of nutrition, comparatively few people in the world are well fed. In fact, malnutrition is one of the major health problems in the world. Even in the United States and Europe, where food is in overabundant supply, undernutrition is not unknown. Overeating with its attendant problems is, however, more common. Health is threatened by either an excess or a deficiency in the supply of food. As with other homeostatic mechanisms, within limits the individual is able to adapt to variation in supply. Although the nature of the effects differ, either a deficiency or an excess supply of food may impair structure and function.

In addition to problems of supply of food per se, selection of food is also a factor. The American public is constantly exposed to unjustified claims about foods and diets, as well as vitamin and mineral supplements. All communications media present information in the form of scientific or pseudoscientific articles or reports of research and in advertisements. The accuracy and validity of some of the above are open to question and some of it is actually misleading or false. For example, one evening a local newspaper quoted two different "nutrition experts." The first is purported to have said that the average person who eats a variety of foods is supplied with all the nutrients that he needs. He does not require extra vitamins or mineral supplements, and money spent for unnecessary food supplements is wasted. The second was cited as saying that few, if any, diets contain an adequate quantity of vitamins and minerals. To be well nourished, supplementation is necessary. What is the average lay person to believe? What, if any, function does the nurse have in interpreting present-day knowledge to the public?

---

[3] H. D. Kruse, "The Interplay of Noxious Agents, Stress, and Deprivation in the Engenderment of Disease," *The Milbank Memorial Quarterly*, XXXI, April, 1953, p. 112.
[4] *Op. cit.*, March, 1963, p. 5.

What is the role of the nurse in meeting the need of the patient for food?

In general, the physician prescribes a diet designed to meet the special as well as the usual or normal requirements for food. The dietary prescription is based on knowledge of the nutritional state of the individual as well as the modifications imposed by the nature of his illness. To illustrate, Mrs. Smith, aged 65, has a diagnosis of diabetes mellitus and obesity. The dietary prescription written by her physician is based on the following knowledge of Mrs. Smith. She is a 65-year-old woman who leads a sedentary life. She is 25 lb overweight and has diabetes mellitus. A loss of excess weight will probably be accompanied by a lessening in the severity of her diabetes mellitus. The physician prescribes sufficient calories to meet her basal needs and adds 15 per cent to cover her activity. Both carbohydrate and fat are restricted. The prescription allows for an adequate quantity of protein and protective nutrients. By restricting calorie and carbohydrate intake, the physician hopes to lessen the quantity of insulin required by Mrs. Smith. The restriction in fat and carbohydrate lessens her intake of calories and should result in a gradual loss of weight and some reduction in the severity of her diabetes.

In many hospitals, dietitians translate the dietary prescription into food. They plan the menus and supervise the preparation of food. Like the physician, they depend to a considerable extent on the nursing staff to relay problems encountered by the patient which interfere with his ability to eat or to enjoy his food. Dietitians also give diet instructions to the patient who will continue to modify his food intake after he leaves the hospital. In public health agencies dietitians may act as consultants to nurses, as well as instruct patients and their families.

The responsibilities of the nurse in meeting the nutritional needs of patients are many and varied. The extent of these responsibilities differs somewhat in different hospitals and health agencies. In the small community hospitals nurses frequently perform many of the functions of dietitians. No matter how highly organized the food service is, however, the nurse has a significant contribution to make in meeting the nutritional needs of patients. She has as her objectives to help the patient to understand why food is essential to his health, and to help him accept and follow the diet as prescribed by his physician. To achieve these objectives, the nurse has the following responsibilities: (1) to obtain the diet prescription, if one has not been provided; (2) to plan with food service so that the patient receives food suited to his needs and, inasmuch as is possible, his desires; (3) to prepare the environment of the patient so that it is conducive to eating; (4) to prepare the patient so that he is in a comfortable position and in condition to eat; (5) to prepare the patient for what to expect, if his diet is different from his usual food pattern and to explain the reasons for modification in his diet; (6) to observe and report the appetite and food preferences of each patient; (7) to observe and report the adequacy of the food intake of the patient; (8) to observe his attitude toward food; (9) to feed or supervise the feeding of patients who are unable to feed themselves; (10) to give appropriate emotional support to those who must be fed or must learn to feed themselves or whose food habits require modification; (11) to give appropriate assistance to those who need some help; (12) to instruct the patient and his family and to answer his questions about his diet;[5] (13) to assist in the collection of data about the food pattern of the patient, his likes and dislikes, and the methods of and facilities available to him for food preparation or for the securing of food after he leaves the hospital; (14) to identify those patients who will require some assistance in obtaining or preparing a suitable diet after dismissal from the hospital; (15) to communicate with the patient, his family, the physician, and the dietitian in such a way that the needs of the patient are met and the lines of communication are kept open; (16) to assist the patient and/or members of his family in meal planning, budgeting, buying, and preparing a nutritious diet; (17) to provide assistance to patients and/or members of the family in the home to: (a) make required adjustments at home after he is discharged from the hospital; (b) provide assistance to the patient who requires a therapeutic diet, but does not require hospitalization; (c) assist the patient to modify his usual food pattern so that his basic and special needs are met; and (18) to feed the patient by an abnormal route and to aid the patient and/or members of his family in learning how to perform the necessary procedures.

What kinds of information does the nurse require if she is to assist the patient to meet his nutritional needs?

The maintenance of the nutrition of cells involves the same general processes and structures as do other homeostatic conditions. Food must be available in adequate quantity and quality and of the type accepted as being suitable to eat. Food requires a special service facility, the digestive system, to receive and to transfer nutrients from the external to the internal environment. Since the nutrients contained in food are not usually in an absorbable form at the time they are eaten, foods must undergo digestion, which consists of a series of physical and chemical changes by which nutrients are prepared for absorption. The residue remaining after digestion and absorption is then ejected from the alimentary canal. Like oxygen, nutrients must be transported to the cells where they are utilized. The various nutrients provide cells with materials required for energy, for building or replacement of cell structure, and for the regulation of cellular processes. Excesses of supply are stored for future use or are excreted. As with other homeostatic conditions, processes are subject to regulation. Cells are, within limits, capable of adapting to differences in supply. Like other physiological needs, the need for food must be met before higher needs can be manifested. Ill health can result from an

---

[5] These functions may be referred to others.

imbalance between food intake and cell requirements. The causes for this imbalance are many and varied. There are few, if any, illnesses, of any length or severity, in which nutrition is not of significance.

What are some of the factors in the supply of food?

Despite a plethora of food in a few areas of the world, such as in the United States, a lack of sufficient food to meet minimum nutritional requirements is one of the most critical public health problems in the world. In many countries, the vast majority of the population is adapted to a chronic state of undernutrition. In fact, the effects of nutritional deficiency may be accepted as a normal condition. For example, in the Andean Altiplano, where goiter due to a deficiency in iodine has been present for generations, dolls are made with the characteristic neck deformity of goiter, indicating that it is accepted as usual or normal. Insufficient food is not a new problem, nor is it one subject to easy solution. For thousands of years man in most parts of the world has led a hand-to-mouth existence. Most, if not all, of his energy is expended in obtaining just enough food to sustain life. Food supply, and with it survival, are continuously threatened by drought, floods, windstorms, and pestilence. Lack of facilities for preserving and transporting food may result in relative abundance during the warm months of the year and scarcity during the cold winter months. In other areas, hunger is continuously present. Food supplies are limited to plants and animals indigenous or native to the region. As is true in the United States, not all plants and animals suitable for food are utilized.

In the early history of mankind and among some present-day primitive societies, the principal methods for obtaining food were hunting and fishing or gathering berries, nuts, and roots. One of the most significant steps in the progress of man occurred when he began to cultivate plants and animals as sources of food. The cultivation of plants and of animals is known as agriculture. Not until agriculture became a reality did the prevention of periodic or continuous hunger become a real possibility. In addition to increasing the supply of food, the development of agriculture has other far-reaching effects. Successful cultivation of sources of food made it necessary for man to give up being a nomad and to settle in one place. Once man was able to produce more than enough food to feed himself and the members of his immediate family, some members of the group were released for other activities. Thus specialization was born. In addition to the food producers or farmers, other men became butchers, bakers, carpenters, and teachers. As the food supply became relatively secure, man had time and energy to think of ways by which his external environment might be changed or improved. Without the development of agriculture, the industrialized societies of today would be impossible.

Despite the importance of the development of the tools and techniques essential to modern agriculture, food supply also depends on suitable means for its preservation and distribution. Without suitable means of preserving food, it is likely to deteriorate in quality or actually spoil before it reaches the consumer, who may live far from where food is produced. Food preservation also makes it possible to save perishable foods for use throughout the year. Modern methods of food preservation combined with efficient and economical methods of transportation make possible the distribution of food far from its site of production. The accomplishment of all of the above requires highly trained and skilled manpower. Thus, in Big City one Sunday in January, the menu consisted of fresh chicken from Alabama, lettuce from Arizona, potatoes from Idaho, peas from Minnesota, and ice cream and butter from Wisconsin. This was not only possible, but was in no way unusual.

Although remarkable progress has been made in developing methods of food production, preservation, and transportation, too little available food remains a problem in much of the world. Sinclair[6] states that, according to one estimate, one third of the population eats three quarters of the food of the world. This means that about two thirds of the people subsist on one quarter of the available food. Many factors contribute to the unequal availability of food. In some parts of the world food supplies are limited by either a lack of or a failure to exploit natural resources. An increase in food supplies in these areas depends on the modernization of agricultural methods, the introduction of suitable methods of food preservation, and the development of transportation facilities. The introduction of suitable methods of home preservation of foods by drying, smoking, and pickling, and in some instances by home canning, may do much to bring about immediate improvement in the supply of food. The United States has a long history of working for the improvement of the health of people living in other lands. The U.S. Interdepartmental Committee for National Defense (ICND) illustrates the scope of the interest of the United States in the nutritional problems of other peoples. Since 1955 ICND has been assisting the less-developed countries "in assessing their nutritional status, pinpointing existing problems of malnutrition and identifying means for solving their problems." [7]

The United Nations has also expended time, money, and effort to assist the people of many countries to help themselves improve their nutritional status. In February, 1963, The United Nations Conference on the Application of Science and Technology for the Benefit of Less Developed Areas was held to consider a wide range of subjects related to nutrition. They included "agricultural practices, development of natural resources, industrial development, transportation and communications, public health, social problems of urbanization, organization and planning, and training of scientific and technical personnel."[8, 9]

[6] Sinclair, *Op. cit.*, p. 8.
[7] "U.S. Activities Supporting International Nutrition Research," *Public Health Reports*, LXXVIII, April, 1963, p. 338.
[8] "U.S. Science and Technology Conference," *Public Health Reports*, LXXVIII, April, 1963, p. 336.
[9] Summaries of papers on problems relating to nutrition are published in *Public Health Reports*, LXXVIII, April, 1963, pp. 336-44.

In the 22 countries that have been surveyed so far, the principal nutrition problems encountered are deficiency of proteins (kwashiorkor), insufficient calories, endemic goiter due to a lack of iodine, nutritional anemias, inadequate supplies of vitamins—A, thiamine (beriberi), riboflavin (ariboflavinosis), vitamin C deficiency (scurvy), and deficiency of niacin (pellagra). With the exception of goiter and scurvy, most of the nutritional deficiencies could be corrected by the addition of meat and milk to the dietary.

Why does malnutrition continue to be a problem in the United States?

In the United States, despite the production of an abundant supply of food and adequate means for its distribution, malnutrition has not been eliminated. Factors responsible include poverty, ignorance, ill-planned dieting, and food fads. Malnutrition may also be secondary to conditions such as alcoholism and chronic illness.[10] Almost all sick people have some disturbance in their capacity to ingest, digest, absorb, or utilize food. When an illness is mild and of short duration, the deleterious effects on the nutritional state of the individual may be minimal. However, serious illnesses and those of long duration are likely to be accompanied by some degree of malnutrition.

The maintenance of health as well as the successful control of certain diseases sometimes necessitates a change in food habits. In order to be most helpful to persons, well and sick, who must make some change in their food habits, the nurse must have some knowledge of the elements contributing to the acceptance or rejection of food.

What are some of the factors influencing the acceptance of food?

As stated by Eppright,[11] "Acceptance of food is a complex reaction determined by the biochemical conditions in the body, the response of the sense organs, and the mental state of the individual." The latter, in turn, is influenced by social, economic, and environmental conditions as well as the past experience of the individual. In the following pages some of the biochemical, physiological, psychological, social, economic, and educational factors affecting the acceptance of food will be discussed. For those who would like to explore one or more of the above in detail, references have been included at the end of the chapter.

Four terms used to indicate some aspect of desire for food are appetite, hunger, satiety, and anorexia. Although appetite and hunger are sometimes used synonymously, they are not the same physiological state. Some of the confusion in the use of these terms may result from the fact that neither term has been precisely defined. Though one may exist in the absence of the other,

[10] James M. Hundley, "Diet in Health," *Public Health Reports,* LXXVII, April, 1962, p. 277.
[11] Ercel D. Eppright, "Factors Influencing Food Acceptance," *Journal of the American Dietetic Association,* XXIII, July, 1947, p. 579.

appetite and hunger are closely related. In general, appetite implies a psychic desire for food and is a pleasant sensation. Unlike hunger, it may persist after sufficient food has been ingested to appease hunger. It is conditioned by previous experiences and habit as well as by the sight, smell, and taste of food. For example, Mr. Francis arrives at home in the evening. As he enters the house, he smells the aroma of his favorite stew. His mouth waters as he anticipates eating his dinner. He had eaten a big lunch and is not particularly hungry.

In contrast, hunger is the most basic drive for food. There is an awareness of the need to ingest food which is accompanied by increased salivation and food-searching behavior. It is associated with unpleasant or even painful contractions of an empty stomach or intestine. As hunger increases, it occupies more and more of the attention of the individual. For example, Mr. Francis arrived at his hotel late last night. He had not stopped for dinner as he expected to eat after arriving at his destination. The dining room was closed, as were all the nearby restaurants. After retiring, Mr. Francis tried to sleep, but he could not. He finally arose and drove 20 miles to find an all-night restaurant where he ate a large meal. Despite the consumption of a high-calorie meal, Mr. Francis continued to experience hunger pangs for an hour or so after eating.

Appetite and hunger are terms indicating desire for food. Most persons do not distinguish sharply between appetite and hunger. Both may be accompanied by physiological changes. For example, thoughts of a lemon pie or a thick steak can stimulate the flow of saliva almost as effectively as the sight or smell of either. The extent to which the physiological changes characteristic of hunger are initiated by biochemical changes in the body is not completely understood. Hunger, however, is one of the frequent manifestations in certain hormonal imbalances such as in hyperthyroidism, as well as in both hyper- and hypoinsulinism. In the preceding examples the individual did not experience a desire for any particular food; the need was for food. In certain disorders, the individual is aware of a craving for a special food. For example, in adrenal insufficiency, the patient is often aware of an increased consumption of sodium chloride. Although much remains to be learned about the biochemical and physiological aspects of the acceptance of food, it appears that they are of some importance.

Appetite and hunger also appear to be affected by the hormonal responses to a severe injury or to a major surgical procedure. During the adrenergic and glucocorticoid response to injury, appetite and hunger are suppressed and anorexia is the rule. In fact, the sight or smell of food may induce nausea and other unpleasant sensations. During the glucocorticoid withdrawal phase, appetite begins to return. During convalescence, appetite may, unless curbed in time, be so great as to lead to an excessive gain in weight. The hormonal responses to illness are discussed in more detail in Chapter 13, Part A.

The third term "satiety" is defined as a state of satisfaction or lack of desire for food following the ingestion of food. Unless an unusual quantity of food is ingested, it is a pleasant state. For example, after eating a big dish of stew, Mr. Francis leaned back from the table, relaxed and comfortable. The fourth term, "anorexia" is descriptive of an abnormal state, since it implies an absence of hunger under circumstances in which it should be expected. At lunchtime John, aged 14, refuses to eat, saying, "I'm not hungry." Because he has not eaten since breakfast, and then only lightly, his mother asks him, "Are you ill?" John has anorexia. He is not hungry under circumstances in which he could be expected to be. When his mother investigates further, she finds that he has a fever and a rash.

The sensations of taste and smell also affect appetite and the acceptability of food. Everyone has experienced the lack of enjoyment of food which accompanies a common cold. Inasmuch as taste and smell enable the individual to identify poisonous substances, these senses are protective. Since both senses are subject to conditioning, they are not completely reliable guides to the selection of foods that are safe. Familiar foods prepared in accustomed ways taste and smell "good." Unaccustomed foods, most particularly those with strong odors, are rejected because they taste and smell "bad." Thus Limburger cheese is a delicacy to one person and spoiled cheese to another.

Because taste buds disappear gradually throughout life, taste becomes less acute as the individual grows older. Since children have more taste buds, they may well have different taste sensations than adults. Although conditioning is probably a factor, greater sensitivity to taste may account for the tendency of young children to reject strongly flavored foods. With advancing years the preference for sweet foods tends to lessen and tart fruity flavors are preferred. As in many other aspects of life, the ability to taste varies among individuals as well as in the same individual from time to time.

Most sick people have some defect in their ability to taste food, with the result that they complain of its being tasteless or flat. Although illness is responsible for the inability to taste food, something can be done to improve the acceptability of food to the patient. First, since a clean, moist mouth minimizes the loss of taste, the patient should be provided with the opportunity to brush his teeth or have them brushed before food is offered, and the mouth should also be cleansed after meals to remove food particles. The nurse can also relate the tastelessness of the food to the illness. Loss of taste is usually temporary and taste will return as the patient recovers. When the consumption of food is important to the recovery of the patient, he should be encouraged to eat. Eating is a way he can help himself to recover. Recognition by the nurse that eating is difficult when food is without taste may also strengthen the efforts of the patient.

Although few people distinguish between the sensations of taste and smell, much of what is loosely called taste results from the odor of food. Odors may also be responsible for unpleasant sensations associated with food. Most persons are aware that when they have a cold, food becomes flat or tasteless. In healthy persons the fragrance of baking bread or broiling steak arouses pleasant sensations. In the sick person, these same odors may be highly unpleasant. Odor is often accepted as an indication of the safety of a food; for example, meat smells fresh or spoiled. A procedure now being advocated is to smell all canned food before tasting it. If it has a peculiar smell, canned foods should be discarded without tasting. Appetite may be depressed by disagreeable odors and stimulated by pleasant ones. Patients with foul-smelling wounds may find eating difficult. Keeping dressings clean and minimizing the odor may do much to promote appetite.

In addition to taste and smell, the texture of food affects its palatability. According to Eppright,[12] people have, since early times, preferred smooth food. Smooth food has the disadvantage of increasing the tendency of the food to adhere to the teeth. Some foods, such as peanut butter, tend to cling to the teeth more than others. Nurses should recognize this possibility and provide an opportunity for patients to have their teeth cleaned after eating.

The temperature at which food is served also influences its acceptability. Despite provisions made in hospitals to ensure the correct temperature of the food served, foods do not always arrive at the bedside of the patient at either the proper temperature or consistency. For example, hot foods such as coffee, soups, and entrees are all too frequently tepid by the time they reach the patient. Cold foods, such as gelatin salads and ice cream, may have melted before they are served to the patient and are therefore unacceptable. When a tray must be delayed, hot food should be kept hot or heated and cold food should be refrigerated during the delay. Attention to the condition of the food at the time it is presented to the patient not only increases the likelihood of its being eaten, but affords an opportunity to reinforce the feeling of the patient that what happens to him is important to those responsible for his care.

How do psychological and social factors influence the acceptability of food?

Despite the significance of biochemical and physiological factors in influencing the acceptability of food, psychological factors are probably even more important. Though knowledge of the psychological and social factors in eating is incomplete, there is an increasing literature emphasizing that eating is motivated, not by logic, but by feelings. Mead[13] summarizes the psychological, social, and cultural aspects of food as follows: "In most societies, food is the focus of emotional associations, a channel for interpersonal relations, for the communication of love or discrimination or disapproval; it usually has a symbolic reference." Galdston[14] emphasizes the importance of psychological factors by saying: "Few functions in life are more freighted with emotions, prejudices, taboos, and prestige symbols than is eating." He further states that

---

[12] *Ibid.*

[13] Margaret Mead, *Cultural Patterns and Technical Change,* UNESCO, 1953, p. 213.

[14] Iago Galdston, "Nutrition from the Psychiatric Viewpoint," *Journal of the American Dietetic Association,* XXVIII, May, 1952, p. 40.

a person does not eat for health, but because he is hungry, jealous, or frustrated.

The hypothesis that likes and dislikes are more important factors in the selection of food than health is supported by a study reported by Shapiro, *et al*.[15] Food selection was studied in families from different income groups. All families had sufficient income to purchase an adequate diet. Little difference was found in the food selected by the families of the various economic levels. In all groups, likes and dislikes far outweighed health as a consideration in food selection.

If the nurse is to be effective in assisting people to establish sound habits of eating or to change their present ones, she requires some understanding of the influence of the established food habits on the people with whom she is working and of how food and eating fit into their value system.

To be really effective in helping people to meet their nutritional needs, the nurse must know not only what people should and do eat but what food and eating means to them, as well as what some of the possible consequences of suggested changes may be. Clear distinctions among the cultural, psychological, and social aspects of food and eating are not easy to make. In the discussion of these factors, the following points will be made and illustrated: a cultural definition of food; the influence of conditioning or habit on food selection; factors modifying selection of food and food intake; and general principles basic to changing food habits.

Earlier in the chapter, diet was defined as a regime of food to support nutrition. By implication, food was defined as a substance, generally a plant or animal, containing one or more substances required to support cell activity. To be safe, a foodstuff must not contain anything harmful to the organism ingesting it. Among many potentially nutritious plants and animals available as food, only a few are used by any group of people. An explanation offered to account for this failure to use all suitable and nonpoisonous plants and animals as food is that the definition of food is of cultural origin. Some plants and animals are designated as being fit for human consumption without regard for their nutritional value. In some cultures, there are religious prohibitions against certain foods. In Moslem countries pork is forbidden. Hindus do not eat beef. Even in the absence of religious proscription, nutritious foods may be rejected. To most Americans, horse meat is not fit for human consumption. In America sweet corn is a treat; in France it is considered fit only for animals. In the southeastern United States grits are served with every meal. In the North they are seldom, if ever, eaten. Children learn very early which plants and animals are not acceptable to eat. Not quite five-year-old Mary supported the above by commenting during a conversation about the use of horse meat as food, "I like horses, but not to eat."

In addition to defining the types of plants and animals suitable for use as

[15] Leona R. Shapiro, Ruth L. Huenemann, and Mary C. Hampton, "Dietary Survey for Planning a Local Nutrition Program," *Public Health Reports*, LXXVII, March, 1962, pp. 257-66.

food, the culture and the family also designate those to be eaten during illness and how they are to be prepared. The old saying "Feed a fever and starve a cold" is well known. Milk may be eliminated from the dietary of the sick person because it is believed to be constipating or it may be boiled to make it constipating in the treatment of diarrhea. Tea and toast are frequently believed to be suitable foods for sick people. Other foods such as rich desserts and cucumbers are designated as unsuitable.

A study of the symbolic reference of different foods in various cultures could easily take a lifetime. Only a few examples will, however, be cited. At the Seder feast which is celebrated at the beginning of the Passover, food is used to symbolize certain events in Jewish history. Three matzo crackers, or pieces of unleavened bread, are placed in a linen napkin on the table to represent the unity of Israel and to recall the departure from Egypt, so rapid that there was no time to take leaven. A roasted egg symbolizes life and its continuity, and bitter herbs symbolize the bitterness of slavery in the land of bondage.

In the Christian religions the egg is the symbol of the rebirth of the spiritual life of man through the death and resurrection of Christ. Eggs are colored and, in some cultures, highly intricate designs convert the egg into a thing of beauty.

Outside the realm of religion, certain foods are symbolic of certain events, status, wealth, or hospitality. Although turkey is available in the United States throughout the year, it remains the symbol of Thanksgiving. In terms of status, hamburger may be eaten by family members, but except for a cookout, it is not served to guests, as it is equated with a limited income.

Evidence of a high or low food intake can also be a status symbol. In some groups, plump children and a wife of ample proportions are accepted as evidence that "mama" is a good cook and "papa" is a good provider. In contrast, to be employed as a high fashion model, a young woman is required to restrict her food intake sufficiently to maintain a lean look.

Though the culture into which the individual is born defines what is fit to eat and how and under what circumstances foods are to be eaten, conditioning or habit influences what he will eat throughout his lifetime. Although some foods are accepted more readily than others and some infants accept new foods more easily than others, babies learn to eat the foods offered to them. Food habits are established quite early in life. Most individuals prefer foods to which they became accustomed as young children, and they may be quite resistant to changing their food habits. Some may even prefer ill health or starvation to eating unaccustomed or unfamiliar foods or known foods prepared in unfamiliar ways. One of the difficult adjustments international students in the United States frequently have to make is the adjustment to American food. Nor is the problem of adjusting to strange food limited to persons from other lands, as some Americans insist on familiar foods when they visit other countries. For example, to attract American tourists, signs on restaurants in Quebec advertise hamburger, hot dogs, and steak. In Santiago, Chile, a waitress eagerly approached the writer with "Ham and eggs for breakfast?" The usual Chilean breakfast consisted of a hard roll and coffee with milk. Americans working in Chile had taken their food habits with them and Chilean hotels had adapted to their demands.

Although the foods eaten by an individual are those to which he is conditioned early in life, most individuals eat more food if there is a variety of foods from which to select and a variety in methods of preparation. Variety is as important to the sick as to the healthy. The effects of the repeated serving of one food to hospitalized patients were well illustrated when a general hospital was given several hundred bushels of apples. Storage space was limited and the apples were served several times a week. Since most patients remained in the hospital only a short time, no problem was anticipated. However, a near rebellion occurred among patients undergoing rehabilitation following poliomyelitis. After several weeks, the monotony of almost daily servings of apples in some form resulted in these patients organizing a mass protest. Particular attention should be given to planning for variety for the patient who is chronically ill or who is faced with numerous adjustments and frustrations.

Something can be learned about the food habits of different groups by visiting supermarkets in various areas in a city or the country. For example, beef or pork is preferred to lamb in Iowa, with the result that lamb is seldom available in a market. In a community in which Jewish people are concentrated, kosher corned beef and bagels are easily obtained. In non-Jewish communities, these foods are frequently unknown. In Minneapolis during the Christmas season, lutefisk is found in every grocery store. In one section of Detroit, signs on store windows advertise mustard greens and possums. In northern Michigan, pasties—beef, potatoes, and onions, enclosed in pastry and baked—remind one of the Welsh miners who brought their food habits with them when they migrated to America. To any one person reading this, depending on conditioning, some of the above foods are delicacies, others are unknown, and still others are rejected as being unfit to be used as food. In the true sense, all are nutritious.

As previously stated, food habits are culturally based. Within the framework of a culture, the family translates and modifies the cultural attitudes toward food and eating for its members. In the family, food is an important and continuing aspect of the mother-child relationship. From the beginning, the mother not only provides or makes available nutrients for the child, but, by the manner in which she feeds him, shows her love and affection.

In the family, mealtime provides more than food. In a modern industrial society, the evening meal may be the only time the entire family regularly meets together as a group. This coming together of the family contributes to morale and a sense of unity among the members. Experiences of the day can be shared, plans made, events reviewed. For a little while each day, each person can feel a part of a group in which he is accepted and respected. In some families eating food is looked upon as a pleasure, and much time and effort are spent in its preparation. Foods may be prepared to please one or more of the family members. Mother communicates her love and affection by preparing the foods they enjoy. Significant events are celebrated with food, and individual members are made to feel important by being served a dish they particularly enjoy.

In other families eating may be merely a necessary activity; food is prepared and eaten and the dishes are washed promptly. Little or no sociability accompanies eating; for members of the family, eating is necessary to sustain life but has few other tangible values. In still others, mealtime is utilized to discipline the children and settle the problems of the day. Instead of a relaxed atmosphere, meals are accompanied by strife and tension.

Whatever the attitude of the adults in the families, children develop values associated with food and eating. They learn what is and is not fit to eat and how it should be prepared. From their parents they learn not only what foods are good for them, but what foods are not good to eat. They learn to enjoy, tolerate, or reject food and eating.

One of the problems that nurses and other health workers have stems from a failure to identify and utilize knowledge of the psychosocial aspects of eating. As a subcultural group, health workers expect the recipients of their services to accept their direction and advice without question. Moreover, they themselves may not follow the advice they give to others. Further, nurses may not recognize that patients do have at least two alternatives, to reject or to accept advice. The point of view of patients may be quite different from that of nurses who are trying to be helpful. Unless these differences in points of view are clarified by the nurse, she may never know why the patient fails to "cooperate." After the point of view of the patient has been identified, his alternatives can also be clarified.

One of the problems in feeding the sick and the aged without families is the lack of a social group with whom to eat. In some hospitals, particularly those for the chronically ill, group dining rooms are provided in order to provide a social atmosphere at mealtime. For patients who are confined to their rooms, attention to the environment before food is served may help to improve the appetite. The presence of a family member or a good friend at mealtime, or a flower on the tray, may aid in creating a more homelike atmosphere and encourage eating. When failure of a patient to eat is a problem, attention to the social aspects of eating sometimes contributes to its solution.

Food may provide the group or the individual with an emotional outlet. The individual eats to satisfy not just a physiological hunger, but a psychological hunger. He may also eat or refuse to eat to gain some measure of control over others. Mary Ellen feels comforted by eating when she feels depressed, lonely, or sad. She knows she eats too much and is too fat, and she envies her slender classmates, but she continues to seek solace in food. She also knows that she gets more attention from her mother when she is fat than when she is thin. Despite the negative character of the remarks made by her mother and the fact that they increase her depression, Mary Ellen has the attention of her mother.

Some of the psychological implications of food stem from the value placed on certain foods as rewards. In the American culture desserts such as cake, pie, ice cream, cookies, and candies have a reward value. They are served at the end of the meal after "wholesome" foods such as meat, bread, potatoes, and vegetables have been eaten. Whether or not desserts are included with the meal depends on specific conditions. They may be withheld if the individual fails to eat the foods that are "good for him" or as a punishment for some transgression. They are also used as a treat or as a reward for good behavior. They play a significant role in special events such as birthday parties, teas, and weddings. Although using specific foods as rewards may accomplish a desired result at the time, this practice may also be responsible for engendering negative attitudes toward food.

Increasing recognition is being given to the knowledge that certain foods have a reward value in the planning of special diets. For example, ice cream is included in the diabetic diet. The food industry has recognized the psychological value of candy and other reward foods and makes them available as diabetic candy and cookies for purchase. Education is needed to acquaint parents and teachers with the undesirable effects of using food as a threat or reward. The reward-and-punishment aspect of food should also be taken into account in planning to meet the food requirements of any patient. In the past, this has often been neglected.

The basis for the use of food as a reward or punishment is to control the behavior of another. Thus a parent seeks to control his child by rewarding him with food or withholding it. The child or other individual, however, can gain some measure of control in the situation by eating or refusing to eat. By eating, he may win the approval of his mother and other members of the family. By refusing to eat, he may be able to arouse the concern and attention of his mother and gain some measure of control over her.

Recognition that food has psychological as well as nutritional values is important to meeting the nutritional needs of patients. Unless the psychological values of food are identified, understood, and translated into the diet plan for the patient, the diet may fail to be eaten. To nourish, food must be ingested.

Both physiological and psychological factors influence the acceptance or rejection of food. For example, a healthy person who has been exercising out of doors is likely to be hungry at mealtime. This same person may develop anorexia on being frightened or angry. Neither is he likely to feel like eating or to be hungry if he is in the acute phase of an illness or in pain. When at all possible, painful procedures should be performed between meals and not just before or during meals. One reason for encouraging activity in the chronically undernourished is to increase appetite and hunger.

Not only do many factors influence what man eats, but his behavior is affected by whether he is hungry or well fed. He may be irritable, withdrawn, or restless when hungry, and happy and relaxed when he is well fed. Shakespeare relates the behavior of men to food when he has Caesar say, "Let me have men about me who are fat; sleek-headed men and such as sleep o'nights. Yon Cassius has a lean and hungry look; he thinks too much; such men are dangerous."

In the preceding discussion, some of the psychological, cultural, and social aspects of eating have been presented. From this content it should be clear that food serves many functions beyond providing the materials required by cells to carry out their functions. As a matter of fact, food is associated with most aspects of life. Very early in life one is conditioned to select certain plants and animals as being fit to eat and to reject others as being unfit. Throughout the lifetime of an individual, food is used to express feelings or emotions not only toward one's neighbors, but toward oneself. Unless the nurse understands the social and psychological implications of food, she will at times be unable to assist a patient in meeting his nutritional needs, which is to say, the food will remain on the plate, rather than be ingested by the patient.

What are some of the factors that should be taken into consideration when a person is required to change his food habits?

Probably the most frequent reason for a change in food habits is illness. Travelers to parts of the world where food differs from that to which they are accustomed are likely to have to make some alterations in their pattern of eating. In the past, health workers acted on the premise that if the person was properly instructed about what he should eat, and he had enough money to buy food, he would eat a nutritious diet. Although knowledge is of significance, it by itself is not sufficient.

Studies of efforts to change food habits demonstrate that once food habits are established, they are very difficult to change and they cannot be changed overnight. Immigrants change their language before they change their pattern of eating. During a period of famine in the rice-eating part of India, wheat was sent in to relieve starvation, but the population preferred death by starvation to eating wheat. Not only was wheat a strange food, but the familiar methods of food preparation were suited to rice and not to wheat. Before wheat could be expected to be used as food, it would have had to be accepted as being suitable to eat and new methods of food preparation learned. At best, changing food habits is a slow process. It took 250 years to establish the potato as food in Europe. Two procedures, giving the potato prestige by planting it in royal gardens and feeding it to soldiers during the wars in the sixteenth century, finally accomplished acceptance of the potato as food in Europe. After the potato was planted in the royal gardens, guards were stationed about but were instructed to look the other way when the potatoes were stolen. The process was completed by feeding soldiers potatoes so that they developed a taste for them. In our present state of knowledge and with the variety of communications media available, it should not take 250 years to make a change in the eating habits of a people. Nevertheless, food habits, once developed, continue to be difficult to alter.

What are some of the general principles which should guide those who wish to help others change their food habits?

There are several general principles which should be observed by those who desire to assist others to change their food habits. The first is, study existing beliefs, values, and practices before attempting to make a change. The cause of or reason for food practices should also be identified if possible. For example, in the United States frequent causes of inadequate diets are lack of money, poor money management, lack of interest in food, insufficient knowledge, food fads, and misguided dieting. As in other parts of the world, food intake is sometimes limited by misconceptions about food or by values ascribed to it. Beliefs about certain foods may bear little relation to their actual characteristics. For example, Mrs. Thoms never serves milk with acid foods as she believes acids curdle milk. The following illustration which was observed in a primitive culture, illustrates the relation of beliefs to practice. Despite the continued efforts of health workers and an adequate supply of eggs, the women refused to eat eggs. Eggs were not taboo as the men and children ate eggs. When the underlying reason for the women rejecting eggs was finally uncovered, it was learned that the women believed that eggs made them aggressive and therefore were undesirable. Attention was given to changing this belief, and as the belief was changed, eggs were eaten by the women.

In the United States values motivating people to eat or not to eat include: staying slim, looking well, and keeping up with the neighbors next door. Studies indicate that the majority of people do not eat to be healthy per se. Motivation is through feelings, not logic. Unless the feelings of people about food are understood, information may fall on sterile soil. To date, relatively little attention has been paid by health workers to the factors motivating eating and to the utilization of what is known in practice.

Another general principle that must be observed if change is to be effected is to avoid direct or implied criticism of what is done or believed. The principal effect of criticism is to arouse stubborn resistance to change. An instance is related in which a public health nurse who was trying to encourage a group of mothers to feed their babies milk instead of beans was unsuccessful. Finally she suggested the babies be given the water in which the beans were cooked. Later, when visiting the mothers, she found that they were feeding milk to their babies. When the nurse expressed surprise, one of the mothers said, "You accepted our way. We do your way."

In the American culture the nutritional problems of adolescents and the aged have received considerable attention. Numerous studies of the dietary of teen-age girls indicate that their intake of nutrients is deficient in some respects. The dietary of boys is less likely to be inadequate. Some authorities are, however, quoted in the public press as saying that the large quantity of food ingested by teen-age boys may be a factor in the earlier development of coronary artery disease in men than in women. Like the adult, the adolescent has little interest in nutrition and diet as such. A number of characteristic features of adolescence influence how and what he eats. The adolescent wants to be liked and do what his peers do. Since adolescence occurs at different ages with different individuals, they differ in rate of growth, size, and general appearance. The adolescent is concerned about the changes he is undergoing and his relationships with members of the opposite sex and with his peers. He worries about pimples and being attractive. Girls are terrified lest they become fat. They skip breakfast, try fad diets, and take other short cuts to a slender figure. The adolescent is in a period in which he has an exaggerated concern about himself. He wants others to be interested in him and to make their interest known. He requires respect. At the same time, adolescence is a period when the individual is developing an independent life. He may be torn between his wish to remain a child and his desire to be an adult. During adolescence he is developing his own ideas and making plans for his future. Physiologically, adolescence is a period of rapid growth. Especially in boys, food is required to build muscles. Girls are preparing themselves for pregnancy and lactation. Boys and girls require the quantity and quality of food required for growth and development into healthy adults, as well as for their current activities.

Gallagher[16] summarizes the qualities required to work with the adolescent and his nutritional problems. Many of these qualities are necessary to work with adolescents whatever their problems. Knowledge of the nutritional needs of this age group, although necessary, is not enough. Knowledge of the changes the adolescent is undergoing and their meaning to him is indispensable. Without an understanding of the characteristics of this age group, nothing can be accomplished. The problems with which the adolescent is concerned are those of popularity in school, sex, growth, relationships with his parent and siblings, and his future. Adolescence is the period during which the boy or girl works through the processes of becoming an independent adult with mature conscience and mature attitudes toward his parents. During this period he forms his own ideas about life and his future. According to Gallagher,[17] the adolescent also has a great capacity for change. The adolescent wants respect and understanding as an individual. He wants those who work with him to believe in him and in his potential for becoming a mature adult.

Another period of life when nutritional problems may be exaggerated is old age. An individual brings to old age the food habits of a lifetime. Appetite

16 J. Rosswell Gallagher, "Some Aspects of Adolescents' Medical Care," *Postgraduate Medicine,* XXXI, February, 1962, pp. 190-94.
17 *Ibid.,* p. 192.

may, however, be impaired by gradually diminishing activity, loss of the sense of taste, and loss of teeth. Ability to masticate food may be lessened by failure to replace teeth or by poorly fitting dentures. For some old people, money may be a real or perceived problem. Persons living on pensions, welfare, or social security may have barely enough to take care of their needs. Others may have sufficient funds, but fear their money will be exhausted before they die. The cost of illness or other emergencies may strain the budget to the point where the amount left for food is inadequate. Pride or lack of knowledge of the means available to supplement the income may be responsible. Sometimes the food money is spent for food for a dog or cat. To a lonely aged man or woman, a pet may have more value than an adequate or nearly adequate diet. In order to feed her dog, Mrs. Frisk eats meat only twice a week. She speaks with pride when she says that Skippy has a nice, juicy hamburger every day. A deficient food intake may result from a lack of incentive or energy to secure or prepare food. People who live alone, such as the elderly or the chronically ill, are especially prone to neglect their food intake. In some cities *Meals on Wheels* have been developed to make meals available to the homebound at a reasonable cost.[18]

As implied earlier, poverty among the elderly is not limited to money. With the passage of time, the elderly man or woman often becomes increasingly isolated. As relatives and friends die or move away, the opportunity to share meals with others diminishes. With the decrease in or loss of the social aspect of eating, incentive for eating diminishes. The positive effects on the appetite of eating with others can be observed when company comes for dinner or the elderly person is invited out to eat. Mrs. Marshall illustrates this point very well. She lives alone in a small apartment. When she prepares her own meals and eats alone, she, in her own words, "eats like a bird." On Sundays, when she is invited to the home of her granddaughter, she eats about as well as the other members of the family. Her explanation is, "The food tastes better." The combination of well-prepared food, friendly conversation, and the example of others eating with pleasure has a favorable effect on Mrs. Marshall's appetite.

In addition to the physiological, psychological, and social aspects of nutrition and the influence of age on food selection, at least a minimum amount of money must be available to purchase the food required for an optimal nutritional state. If the study of Shapiro, *et al.*,[19] is generally applicable, an increase in income above that required to purchase an adequate diet does not result in improved food selection. A certain amount of money is, however, required to purchase food. Persons whose incomes fall below the minimum required to purchase an adequate diet are likely to have difficulty securing enough food of good quality and variety.

Any plan made to assist a person to change his food habits should also

[18] M. D. Keller and C. E. Smith, "Meals on Wheels; 1960," *Geriatrics*, XVI, May, 1961, pp. 237-47.
[19] *Op. cit.*

include an exploration of the wants of the individual that are competing for his income. For example, a young woman with a baby had just enough money to buy a small can of peaches or a box of oatmeal. After much thought and indecision, she bought the peaches. Other individuals may want items other than food. When a person has an increase in salary, he may be faced with a number of alternatives. Should the new money be spent on powdered skim milk, candy, carbonated beverages, cigarettes, liquor, or a television set? Objectively the answer seems clear. To the individual who makes the choice, other answers may well take priority.

Although knowledge by itself is insufficient to ensure or change food habits, it is one necessary requirement. During the twentieth century, communications have improved and more people are exposed to more information than in the past. Educated people tend to be more flexible in their selection of food than the uneducated. Though the problem of changing food habits is poorly understood, they do change. For example, fewer potatoes and more citrus fruit and milk products are eaten today than at the beginning of the century. The extent to which education has played a part in these and other changes is not known.

Summary

Survival, growth, productivity, and health all depend on a continuous supply of food. In some areas of the world the amount of food available is insufficient to support the population at much more than a survival level. The reasons for the inadequate food supply include poor soil or unfavorable climate and lack of transportation or food preservation facilities. As the result of experiences during and following World War II, there has been growing appreciation of the fact that a supply of food is only one aspect of eating. Eating is a voluntary act. Before a plant or animal is utilized as food, it must be accepted as being fit or suitable to eat. This acceptance involves a variety of psychological and social factors having little or nothing to do with the nutritional value of a substance. A man as well as a hen may starve to death while sitting beside a sack of wheat. There are few events in the life of the individual where food does not play a part. Often the improvement of the nutrition of an individual or of a nation depends on a change in food habits. Though knowledge of how to effect change is limited, a few guides to action have been suggested. They include: (1) Take time to discover the what and why of the pattern of the group. (2) Do not criticize as criticism only arouses stubborn resistance. (3) Remember that changing food habits is a slow process. (4) Motivation for eating is more psychological and social than it is intellectual. (5) Although knowledge of what constitutes good nutrition is usually insufficient to effect change, it is one factor in change.

As stated earlier, nutrition plays a role in the etiology of or recovery from almost all diseases. It may, of course, be an element throughout the course of an illness. The biochemical, physiological, and psychological changes taking place during illness frequently affect the desire for food. Not uncommonly the sick person is faced with a change—temporary or permanent—in his pattern of eating. Sometimes the problem is easily solved, as it was for Mrs. Brown who was wondering how she could ever adjust to a diabetic diet. She thought that she would be denied greens, corn bread, and ice cream. The greens presented no problem. Within limits, neither did the corn bread nor the ice cream.

When significant changes are required, the patient may appear to accept the change but may actually continue his usual food pattern. Mrs. Smith, also a diabetic, was such a person. At one time she was under the supervision of a physician who believed in a strict control of the diet. Later she was cared for by a physician who believed a diabetic person could and should eat the same food as a nondiabetic. When asked by a nurse about how confusing the change must have been, she said, "Not at all, I've followed about the same regime all the time. Both physicians were so enthusiastic that I couldn't bear to disappoint them."

Some patients react with what appears to be unreasonable resistance to change. If the professional staff reacts with hostility or indifference, the resistance of the patient is likely to increase. If the cause of the reaction of the patient can be determined, then the patient may be more willing to modify his behavior. Not infrequently the reasons for the rejection of the diet plan are reasonable, not only to the person, but, when the trouble is taken to identify them, to the nurse. What appears to be irrational behavior to the observer may be rational to the behaver. Often the diet plan can be altered in such a way as to make it more acceptable to the individual. Success is, at least in part, dependent on learning what the change means to the individual and working with him in making an acceptable plan.

Why is a service facility required and what purposes does it serve in nutrition?

As with oxygen, a service facility is required for receiving foodstuffs from the external environment and absorbing nutrients into the internal environment. Because nutrients are usually ingested in a complex state, foods—plants or animals—must be subjected to a series of chemical and physical changes by which they are converted to a state in which they can be absorbed. Large multicellular organisms, such as man, have specialized structures which receive, temporarily store, and convert, by mechanical and chemical means, crude materials to utilizable forms, following which they are transferred from the external to the internal environment. The remaining residue is temporarily stored, water is absorbed, and the remainder is ejected at regular intervals.

Before discussion of individual organs, some of the common features of the digestive system and the effects of disturbances in function on the body economy as well as on the general nutritional state will be presented. The alimentary canal, along with the accessory organs of digestion, functions as a unit. Under nervous and hormonal control, the activity of each organ of the digestive system is coordinated and integrated so that its functions are accomplished and the nutritional needs of the entire organism are met.

The alimentary canal is a hollow muscular tube passing through the center of the body and extending from the mouth to the anus. The two primary functions are the digestion and the absorption of nutrients. Despite the impor-

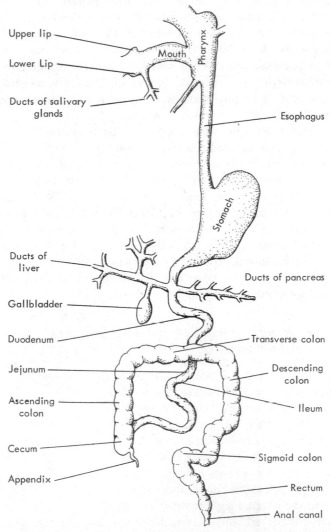

F I G U R E   10 — 1.   Schematic diagram of the digestive tract of the human being, and accessory organs. (Adapted with permission of The Macmillan Company from *Anatomy and Physiology*, 14th ed., Fig. 41, p. 54 by Diana Clifford Kimber, Carolyn E. Gray, Caroline E. Stackpole and Lutie C. Leavell. Copyright © The Macmillan Company, 1961.)

tance of the regular evacuation of the residue remaining after digestion is completed, in health the alimentary canal does not play a significant role in the elimination of substances from the internal environment.

In relation to the functions performed by the alimentary canal, it can be divided into three general regions: upper, middle, and lower. The upper alimentary canal includes the esophagus, stomach, upper duodenum, liver, and pancreas. Similar to other regions, the upper alimentary canal conveys food from upper to lower parts. Its other principal functions are the secretion of digestive juices; the breaking up and mixing of food particles with them, and the beginning of chemical digestion. The importance of the various structures comprising the upper alimentary canal to life and health varies. Persons with strictures of the esophagus can and do live for many years. Removal of the stomach is compatible with life, but is frequently associated with some loss of health.

The middle alimentary canal extends from the duodenal papilla to the mid-transverse colon. From the viewpoint of function, this is the most important region of the alimentary canal, for it is here that digestion is completed and absorption of nutrients takes place. In our present state of knowledge, adequate nutrition cannot be maintained without the absorbing surface of the mid-alimentary canal. The available surface for absorption in a healthy person is greater than is required, and although the small intestine cannot be removed in its entirety, some of it can be removed without threatening the nutritional status of the individual. Many nutrients can be supplied parenterally, but neither calories nor amino acids can be infused in sufficient quantities to meet tissue requirements. The middle portion of the alimentary canal is therefore a vital organ.

The lower portion of the alimentary canal extends from the mid-portion of the transverse colon to the anus. Its primary function is to store refuse until it can be conveniently evacuated. The lower alimentary canal is not necessary to either life or health. An artificial opening in any portion from the lower ileum downward can be made to function satisfactorily in the elimination of wastes. Since the ascending and transverse colon absorb water from the fluid content of the alimentary canal, the lower the opening, the less physiological adjustments have to be made. For example, the drainage from an ileostomy is watery, but the feces in the sigmoid colon are semisolid. Following an ileostomy, the lower ileum adapts by increasing water absorption, but the process of adaptation takes time and the patient needs to be protected from the loss of water and electrolytes. The skin around the ileostomy requires protection from the fluid feces. Following a sigmoidostomy, the feces may be fluid or semifluid for a few days, primarily as a result of hypermotility, but within a short time the feces assume their normal semisolid consistency.

Most of the regions of the alimentary canal have a rich blood and lymphatic supply. The exceptions include a portion of the esophagus and of the colon. The parts richly supplied with blood have the advantages of healing rapidly after planned or accidental injury. The abundant blood supply also makes hemorrhage a greater possibility when blood vessels are ruptured. Venous drainage from the alimentary canal is through the portal system which supplies the liver. In diseases of the liver in which there is obstruction of the portal venous system, varicosities of the esophageal and hemorrhoidal veins occur. Rupture of esophageal varicies is attended by massive hemorrhage.

The function of the alimentary canal is regulated by the nervous and hormonal systems. As a service facility in which all nutrients required by cells are prepared for and absorbed into the internal environment, its functioning is regulated in relation to the needs of the entire organism. As emphasized elsewhere, the alimentary canal is exceedingly sensitive to conditions in the body as a whole. The various organs of the alimentary canal are also regulated in relation to each other. Food in one organ acts as a stimulus to alert the next organ to prepare for it or to delay the rate at which the preceding organ empties. For example, a factor in the rate at which the stomach empties into the duodenum is the degree of fullness of the small intestine. When the intestine is distended, inhibitory messages are sent to the stomach in the form of an inhibitory hormone, enterogastrone, secreted by the intestinal mucosa.

Two groups of hormones participate in the regulation of the alimentary canal. The first are the hormones participating in the regulation of activities throughout the body. The second group are classified as local hormones as they are secreted by some part of the alimentary canal and alter action by stimulating or inhibiting another part. Examples of hormones of the first group are insulin and the adrenal glucocorticoids. Insulin increases the secretion of acid gastric juice. The adrenal glucocorticoids probably reduce the resistance of the mucosa to the digesting action of gastric juice. In some individuals, the administration of the adrenal glucocorticoids predisposes to peptic ulcer formation. A history of peptic ulcer is therefore a relative contraindication to the employment of adrenal glucocorticoids in treatment. When they are prescribed, the patient should be observed for symptoms associated with ulcer formation.

The alimentary canal is richly supplied with nerves from the autonomic nervous system and from an intramural (within the wall) nerve plexus. This plexus extends all the way from the esophagus to the anus. It consists of two layers of neurons. The outer layer lies between the longitudinal and circular muscles of the digestive tube and is known as the myenteric (or Auerbach's) plexus. The inner layer of neurons lies in the submucosa and is known as the submucous (or Meissner's) plexus. These plexuses, often referred to, collectively, as the myenteric plexus, regulate many of the local actions of the digestive tube. According to Guyton,[20] the plexuses increase the muscle tone.

[20] Arthur C. Guyton, *Textbook of Medical Physiology,* 2nd ed., W. B. Saunders Co., Philadelphia, 1961, p. 82.

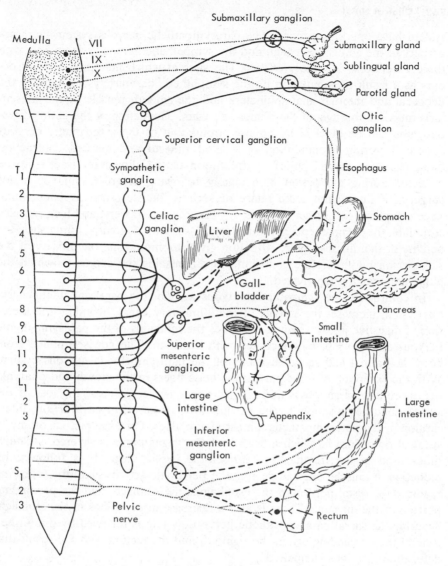

FIGURE 10-2. Innervation of the digestive pathway. Parasympathetic fibers are dotted. The ganglia of the vagus and the pelvic nerves lie in or near the organs. (Reprinted with permission of The Macmillan Company from *Textbook of Physiology*, Fig. 101, p. 279, by Caroline E. Stackpole and Lutie C. Leavell. Copyright 1953 by The Macmillan Company.)

the intensity and rate of rhythmical contraction, and the speed with which excitatory waves spread along the wall of the gastrointestinal tract.

The alimentary canal receives nerves from both the parasympathetic and the sympathetic divisions of the autonomic nervous system. (See Figure 10-2.) Centers in the central nervous system act through the parasympathetic and sympathetic nervous systems to increase or decrease the activity of the gastrointestinal tract. In general, these two divisions of the autonomic nervous

761

system have opposing actions. The parasympathetic nervous system increases activity of the alimentary canal, and the sympathetic nervous system has, with three exceptions, inhibitory effects. The sites at which increased activity occurs as a result of stimulation by the sympathetic nervous system include the ileocecal and internal anal sphincters and the smooth muscle of the muscularis mucosae throughout the alimentary tract. The action of the entire digestive tube can be blocked by intense stimulation of the sympathetic nervous system. It results in inhibition of wall of the gut and marked contraction of at least two major sphincters. Inhibition of the alimentary tract is to be expected during the period immediately following severe trauma or major surgery, or during the acute phase of serious illnesses such as pneumonia. (See Chapter 5 for further discussion.) Excitement, anxiety, and fear can also stimulate the sympathetic nervous system so that it greatly diminishes the activity of the digestive tube. Attention given to minimizing the anxiety of the sick person may therefore contribute to diminishing the degree to which the alimentary canal is inactivated.

In contrast to the sympathetic nervous system, the parasympathetic nervous system increases the activity of the alimentary canal, including the secretion of digestive juices. Cannon describes the functions of the parasympathetic nervous system as being concerned with nutrition. The gut is supplied from both the cranial and sacral divisions of the parasympathetic nervous system. With the exception of some parasympathetic fibers in the mouth and pharynx, the entire cranial supply is through the vagus nerve. Whereas the loss of the sympathetic nerve supply to the gut has little or no effect on function, interruption of the parasympathetic almost always does. For example, vagotomy, a surgical procedure in which a branch of the vagus nerve is severed, is sometimes used in the treatment of intractable peptic ulcer. It is followed by reduction in muscle tone and decrease of peristaltic activity in all the following regions: the distal portion of the esophagus, the stomach, and the proximinal portion of the intestine. There is also a decrease in secretions in the stomach. Severing the sacral parasympathetic nervous system is followed by diminished tone of the descending colon, the sigmoid, and the rectum with the result that defecation is seriously impaired.

What are some of the factors in and characteristics of the movement of food through the alimentary canal?

The rate at which the contents are moved diminishes progressively from the mouth to the anus. Motion is accomplished by smooth muscle arranged in longitudinal and circular layers. The muscle fibers lie so close together that contraction initiated at one point tends to spread to adjacent areas. The muscles of the alimentary canal exhibit the two types of contraction characteristic of smooth muscle in any part of the body—tonus contraction and rhythmical contraction. Tonus contraction determines the degree of pressure in any organ and the resistance to movement by the sphincters. Rhythmical contraction, or peristalsis, moves the contents toward the anus. Excessive tonic contractions of a segment or of a sphincter may interfere with the forward movement of the contents of the digestive tube. It may also be a source of pain.

Each major segment of the alimentary canal is separated from other segments by sphincter muscles. The sphincter muscles control the rate at which the contents of the gastrointestinal tract are moved from one organ to another, and they prevent backflow. The sphincters at the inlet and at the outlet of the stomach also regulate the size of particles allowed to move forward. Food is retained in the stomach until particles are finely divided and converted into a fluid state and acidified. The resulting mixture is known as chyme.

The rhythmical contraction of the smooth muscle is known as peristalsis. Peristalsis mixes the contents of the alimentary canal and propels them forward. Peristalsis is characterized by contraction of the muscle behind the bolus and simultaneous relaxation of the muscle ahead of it. Any increase or decrease in the activity of smooth muscle will disturb in some manner the capacity of the alimentary canal to receive, retain, digest, or absorb food.

Both the tone and the rhythmical contractions of the alimentary tract are regulated by the nervous system. As a consequence of the action of the nervous system, the rhythmical contractions of the alimentary canal can be increased or decreased in intensity or rate. In addition, peristalsis (the major propulsive movements of the gastrointestinal tract) is coordinated and the secretion of digestive juices is regulated so that each ferment is provided at the time and place it is needed.

Another anatomical characteristic of the alimentary canal, of importance in understanding possible effects of disease, is that the lumen of the gut lies outside the body proper. The entire lumen from the mouth to the anus is surrounded by the body, but it is not part of it. (See Figure 10-1.) The wall surrounding the lumen of the alimentary canal either is impermeable to its contents or is permeable only to water, alcohol, small molecules, and ions. In fact, many molecules and ions require a transport or carrier system to move across semipermeable membranes in appreciable quantities.[21] Any break in the integrity of the wall therefore carries with it the possibility of the escape of the contents of the alimentary canal into the internal environment. Superficial disruption of the mucous membrane is not usually serious. If, however, the break penetrates through all the layers and extends through the entire wall, the contents of the organ can and do escape into a body cavity.

How is the individual protected against the invasion of the internal environment by foreign materials by way of the alimentary canal?

Similar to other structural facilities serving as points of exchange between the internal and external environment, some system of defense or protection

---

[21] Fat solvent liquids such as carbon tetrachloride are readily absorbed.

against the ingestion of harmful substances is required. The senses of sight, taste, and smell all function in protection. Foods are accepted or rejected on the basis of general appearance, odor, taste, and feel. Meat may be accepted because it is bright in color and rejected because it is dull red or black. If the meat smells fresh, it is more likely to be eaten than if it has a peculiar odor or is putrid. The same is true of taste. Inasmuch as these senses enable the individual to correctly evaluate the safety of a food, they are protective. Because they are subject to conditioning and are not very accurate, wholesome food may be rejected and harmful foods accepted. When there is any doubt about the safety of food, it should be rejected.

The mucous membrane which extends from the mouth to the anus acts as a barrier to the entrance of excessively large molecules and of some microorganisms into the body proper. As in other areas of the body, the mucous membrane must be unbroken or intact. Glands in the mucous membrane secrete mucus which tends to coat the mucous membrane lining the alimentary canal and to lessen the extent of direct contact with its contents. The mucous membrane is thereby protected from mechanical injury by rough or harsh foods and from the digesting action of enzymes contained in the digestive juices. As in the respiratory tract, the mucous glands in the membrane lining the alimentary canal respond to irritation by increased secretion. After a harsh laxative has been taken or hard feces are defecated, mucus can sometimes be seen in or around the stool. In a disorder known as mucus colitis, hyperactivity of the colon may be sufficient to be accompanied by the discharge of large quantities of mucus. Sometimes the sheets of mucus are in the form of a cast of the bowel. In disorders in which there is a disruption of the mucous membrane lining of the large intestine, such as in chronic ulcerative colitis, mucus secretion is also increased over the normal. Any break in the integrity of the mucous membrane predisposes to the entrance of microorganisms and/or other foreign particles into the internal environment.

A third barrier to the entrance of microorganisms from the alimentary canal into the internal environment is the character of its secretions. The acid gastric juice is of particular importance. Under conditions of health, few microorganisms are found in the gastric secretions.

Three closely related mechanisms serve to protect the individual against the ingestion of harmful material or remove it from the gastrointestinal tract after it has been ingested. They are anorexia, nausea, and vomiting. Anorexia, as defined earlier, is the absence of the desire for food when this desire should be present. The person suffering from anorexia says, "I have no appetite," or "I don't feel like eating," or "Nothing tastes good." He may dawdle with his food or force himself to try to eat. Whereas anorexia is characterized by loss of appetite, nausea is an unpleasant or disagreeable sensation characterized as a revulsion for food. When food is offered to the nauseated patient, he says "Take it away." "I can't stand the sight or smell of it." "It makes me feel sick to even think of it." He looks and feels miserable. Usually the nauseated person cannot force himself to eat. There are exceptions, of course. As a rule, the patient who is nauseated has other symptoms arising from imbalance in the autonomic nervous system, such as increased salivation and secretion of mucus, sweating, and tachycardia. Evidence of increased activity of the vagus nerve may result in bradycardia and hypotension. In nausea, the tone and activity of the stomach and small intestine are probably diminished.

Although nausea and vomiting are frequently associated, they may appear independently of each other. Because of the close relationship of nausea to vomiting, factors in its cause and treatment will be discussed with vomiting. Vomiting is defined as the sudden forceful ejection of the contents of the stomach, duodenum, and proximal jejunum through the mouth. It is frequently, but not invariably, preceded by nausea. A projectile type of vomiting, occurring without warning nausea, accompanies rapidly increasing intracranial pressure, such as follows head injuries.

In the past, vomiting has been classified as reflex and central. Because of new knowledge, this classification is being discarded. Although all vomiting results from reflex activity, the point at which the reflex is initiated varies. The basic pattern for the vomiting reflex is similar to that of any reflex. It involves a receptor connected by way of nerve fibers and cells to an effector. As in other reflexes, a group of nerve cells located within the brain, the vomiting center, regulates and coordinates the act of vomiting. Sensory receptors capable of initiating the vomiting reflex are located outside as well as within the wall of the alimentary canal. Within the alimentary canal, receptors are located in the fauces and pharynx, the stomach, and the intestine. The most acutely sensitive area is the first portion of the duodenum. Outside the alimentary canal, sensory receptors for vomiting are located in the uterus, kidneys, heart, and semicircular canals. Receptors may be stimulated by excessively irritating substances or by overdistention of an organ supplied with sensory receptors. The degree of excitability of the receptors is an element in the intensity of stimulation required to trigger the vomiting reflex. The more irritable the receptor, the easier it is to stimulate it.

Even a cursory glance at the variety of sites containing sensory receptors for vomiting and the types of conditions likely to stimulate them suggests that vomiting is a frequent event in disease. Moreover, it occurs not only in disorders involving the gastrointestinal system, but in those of the heart, kidney, uterus, and semicircular canals. Inflammatory conditions of the alimentary canal, such as acute appendicitis and gastroenteritis, frequently cause vomiting. The vomiting associated with motion sickness results from the effects of motion on the semicircular canals in sensitive persons. Motion sickness is caused by any form of transportation in the air or on water or land. As in many other situations, fear and anxiety increase the tendency to motion sickness.

Since the fauces and pharynx are areas where the vomiting reflex may be triggered, care should be taken during mouth hygiene to avoid initiating the vomiting reflex by mechanical stimulation of these areas. Particular attention should be paid to this in patients who have been vomiting. Mechanical stimulation of the pharynx or fauces during the passage of a nasogastric tube or the introduction of a nasopharyngeal catheter initiates the gag reflex in many people. Procedures such as asking the patient to breathe deeply or to swallow are often beneficial as they distract the attention of the patient and help him to relax. The most useful effect of the voluntary initiation of swallowing is that swallowing suppresses the vomiting reflex.

Easy access to receptors initiating the vomiting reflex can be lifesaving in some instances. After a toxic substance has been ingested, vomiting can sometimes be induced by stimulating the fauces with a finger or a blunt instrument. This is probably the most commonly used technique for self-induction of vomiting. Emotionally disturbed persons sometimes induce vomiting by this method. Should a person who is vomiting be observed to be inducing the vomiting reflex, this fact should be recorded and brought to the attention of the physician.

Receptors in the stomach can be stimulated by drinking water containing an irritating substance or by the rapid distention of the stomach. A common, though not always effective, method is to drink a glass of tepid water to which a teaspoonful of dry mustard has been added. Mustard has the undesired effect of increasing any previous irritation. Distention of the stomach is accomplished by drinking ordinary tap water, or starch water, as rapidly as possible until vomiting occurs. Water or a mixture of starch and water will always induce vomiting, if ingested in sufficient quantities. Water has the advantage of diluting the contents of the stomach and it facilitates the removal of toxic substances.

Vomiting may also be initiated by impulses at the vomiting center by the way of the cerebral cortex. Unpleasant sights, sounds, odors, tastes, and thoughts as well as sensations, such as severe pain, can initiate the vomiting reflex. In some persons, the sight of blood induces vomiting. It is not unusual for a person arriving at the scene of an accident where blood has been spilled to complain of nausea or to actually vomit. Fetid odors or the odor of vomitus can have a similar effect.

A third general site where vomiting may be initiated is the chemoreceptor zone. It is located in the medulla, but outside the vomiting center. At one time it was thought that circulating toxic agents caused vomiting by acting on the vomiting center. Emetic drugs such as apomorphine, toxic dosages of digitalis, and the "toxins" of acute infectious disease, as well as the retention of products normally excreted by the kidneys, are believed to induce vomiting by stimulating the chemoreceptor center. Vomiting is a problem in disorders accompanied by disturbances in metabolism such as pernicious vomiting of pregnancy, diabetic acidosis, and Addisonian and hyperthyroid crises. As indicated earlier, vomiting also occurs in patients with traumatic head injuries,

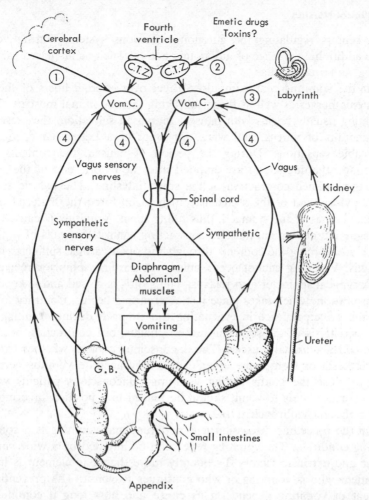

FIGURE 10−3. Mechanisms in the initiation of vomiting. C.T.Z., Chemoreceptor trigger zone; Vom. C., vomiting center; G.B., gall bladder; 1, cerebral stimulation of vomiting center; 2, drug stimulation of chemoreceptor trigger zone; 3, labyrinthine (motion, etc.) stimulation of vomiting center; 4, visceral afferent stimulation of vomiting center. (Adapted. Courtesy of Ruth D. Musser and Joseph G. Bird, *Modern Pharmacology and Therapeutics*, 2nd ed., The Macmillan Company, New York, 1961, Fig. 14, p. 390.)

with infections involving the brain and meninges, and with increasing intracranial pressure.

In Figure 10-3[22] the location of common receptors which, when stimulated, initiate the vomiting reflex can be seen. Impulses are carried from these receptors to the vomiting center by way of peripheral, cranial, and autonomic sensory fibers. The vomiting center is located in the lateral reticular formation of the medulla oblongata. It is one of a number of visceral centers such as the vasomotor, the defecation, the respiratory, and the salivation centers. These

[22] Ruth D. Musser and Joseph G. Bird, *Modern Pharmacology and Therapeutics*, 2nd ed., The Macmillan Company, New York, 1961, p. 390.

are all centers regulating the autonomic nervous system. During vomiting there is additional evidence of autonomic activity such as increased salivation, sweating, and bradycardia.

From the vomiting center impulses travel over efferent fibers of the vagus and phrenic nerves as well as those supplying the abdominal muscles. The act of vomiting usually begins with nausea, increased salivation, the secretion of large amounts of mucus, and what, for want of a better name, are called disagreeable sensations. During the period of nausea, the contents of the jejunum and the duodenum are emptied into the pyloric end of the stomach by strong sustained contraction of the small intestine. The pyloric sphincter and the pyloric end of the stomach contract and force the material into the body and fundus of the stomach, thus filling them. Vomiting is caused by the diaphragm and abdominal muscles contracting against the walls of the dilated stomach and forcing the contents through the open cardiac sphincter into the esophagus. Vomiting cannot occur unless the cardiac sphincter relaxes. The hypopharyngeal sphincter also relaxes. The glottis is closed and is kept closed after inspiration, which takes place just as vomiting begins. Contrary to an old belief, the principal force in evacuating the stomach during vomiting is not reverse peristalsis of the stomach and esophagus, but contraction of the diaphragm and abdominal muscles. The unconscious patient, whether from general anesthesia or from some other cause, may aspirate vomitus because of failure to close the glottis during vomiting. Unconscious patients who are vomiting or are likely to vomit should be placed in a position favoring drainage from the tracheobronchial tree.

From the preceding discussion it is apparent that vomiting is a commonly occurring condition. The vomiting reflex can be initiated by a wide variety of intrinsic and extrinsic factors. Frequently more than one element is involved in a patient who is vomiting or who continues to vomit. The prevention and treatment of vomiting depend on its cause and how long it continues. Although vomiting removes irritating materials from the gastrointestinal tract, it also removes water and electrolytes as well and it interferes with the ingestion of food. In a well-nourished person who vomits for a brief period of time, the latter effects are of little moment. Some emotionally disturbed persons who vomit do not lose weight because they actually vomit very little food. In the patient who is debilitated or who continues to vomit not for a few hours, but for days, vomiting may result in dehydration, metabolic alkalosis, and serious loss of weight. It may also contribute to the problem of maintaining or improving the nutritional state of the individual. In patients who have had surgery, vomiting may place strain on the site of the incision by increasing pressure within the abdominal, ocular, and cranial cavities. Vomiting after surgery on the eye predisposes to intraocular bleeding. If vomiting occurs in a patient who has undergone surgery on the eyes, it should be brought to the attention of the physician immediately. Orders for antiemetic drugs should be carried out faithfully.

Treatment of the patient who is vomiting is based on its cause and effects. If vomiting is associated with acute appendicitis or diabetic acidosis, the obvious treatment is to remove the inflamed appendix or restore glucose metabolism and correct the disturbances in water and electrolyte balance. When treatment is directed toward the control of vomiting, procedures are selected which relieve vomiting by: (1) removing irritating substances from the stomach; (2) relieving or preventing distention of the stomach; (3) diminishing the sensitivity of the chemotherapeutic trigger zone; (4) discontinuing the administration of drugs stimulating the chemoreceptor trigger zone; (5) correcting metabolic disorders in which circulating "toxins" activate the chemoreceptor trigger zone; and (6) correcting imbalances and deficits in water and electrolytes.

As stated earlier, irritating materials may be removed from the stomach by drinking water and vomiting it or by suction through a nasogastric tube. When the stomach is distended because of failure to empty, nasogastric suction is usually prescribed. The advantages of this method of emptying the stomach are that distention can be prevented and repeated and prolonged vomiting can be controlled.

A number of antiemetic drugs act by raising the threshold of the chemoreceptor trigger zone to stimulation. The first drug found to be effective was chlorpromazine. Other drugs include dimenhydrinate (Dramamine[23]), other phenorthiazines, trimethobenzamide hydrochloride (Tigan[23]), and the barbiturates. These drugs are useful, not only in the treatment of vomiting, but in its prevention in motion sickness.

Physical and chemical agents used in the treatment of disease may induce vomiting. Therapy with X ray or radioactive isotopes, particularly when applied over the upper abdomen, frequently causes some degree of nausea and vomiting. Usually treatment with radioactive substances is continued, despite the presence of vomiting. Some drugs such as digitalis cause nausea and vomiting when toxic dosages have been reached. When it has been established that vomiting is due to the toxic effects of a drug, it may be discontinued temporarily or permanently or its dosage reduced. Other drugs such as morphine and meperidine hydrochloride (Demerol[24]) induce vomiting in susceptible persons. When nausea and vomiting regularly follow the administration of a drug and diminish in severity as time elapses after it is given, idiosyncrasy to the drug should be suspected. The discontinuance of the drug is usually all that is required to correct the nausea and vomiting.

In addition to the treatment prescribed by the physician, the nurse can do much to lessen the discomfort of the patient who is vomiting. There are few more disagreeable or unpleasant symptoms than nausea and vomiting. For many persons, the presence of a kindly and solicitous person makes vomiting more bearable. The nurse herself may experience nausea as she assists the

[23] Trade name.
[24] Trade name.

patient, with the result that she finds it difficult to stay with him. The nurse can suppress the vomiting reflex by swallowing and by concentrating on what she can and should do to assist the patient. Should simple measures be ineffective, the nurse should discuss her problem with her instructor or supervisor or her physician.

During vomiting, nursing care of the patient should be based on two objectives: (1) to prevent the aspiration of vomitus and (2) to increase the comfort of the patient. To lessen the possibility of the aspiration during emesis, if at all possible, the patient should be turned to one side and the head should be flexed at the neck. Factors predisposing to nausea and vomiting in susceptible patients should be identified and controlled. In so far as possible, pain should be prevented or kept under control. The room should be well ventilated. Strong odors—dressings, emesis, perfumes—should be eliminated from the environment. The emesis basin should be emptied and washed immediately after use. On the basis that there is a psychic element in vomiting, the suggestion is usually made to keep the basin within easy reach, but out of sight. If, however, the patient is more relaxed when the basin is where he can see it, this factor should be taken into consideration before deciding on its placement. After vomiting, the patient should have an opportunity to rinse out his mouth. Soiled bed linen should be changed. Since moving predisposes to an attack of nausea and vomiting, necessary changes in position should be made slowly. Sometimes the vomiting reflex can be suppressed by deep breathing and by initiation of the swallowing reflex. If the condition of the patient allows, carbonated beverages such as ginger ale or soda may be tolerated when other fluids are not. Either cold or hot fluids are generally better tolerated than tepid ones. A combination of measures is sometimes necessary to control vomiting. The patient should be encouraged in the belief that something can be and is being done to control the vomiting.

The following case illustrates the value of simple measures in the control of vomiting triggered by anesthesia and prolonged by metabolic and emotional factors. Alexandra Berry, who was attending college far from home, fell and fractured the radius of her left arm. The fracture site was placed in a splint immediately, but several hours elapsed before Miss Berry was admitted to the hospital and the fracture was reduced under Pentothal Sodium[25] anesthesia. As soon as Miss Berry regained consciousness, she was discharged to the college dormitory. For the next 24 hours, she continued to vomit. Since psychic factors were undoubtedly important, the dormitory nurse cleared the room of anxious friends. She also removed the bucket being used as an emesis basin. She obtained a large bottle of chilled ginger ale and encouraged Alexandra to sip it slowly. Each time Alexandra retched, the nurse encouraged her to swallow and breathe deeply. After an hour or so Alexandra was able to rest comfortably without vomiting. The nurse bathed Alexandra, changed her bed,

[25] Trade name for thiopental sodium.

aired the room, and suggested firmly that the measures that she had instituted would cure her. They did.

Although vomiting was probably induced by the effect of the anesthetic on the chemoreceptor trigger zone, psychic factors were undoubtedly important in its continuance. Miss Berry had a frightening experience, she was far from the comforting presence of her family, and she was treated by a strange physician. Futhermore, with the loss of fluid and failure to ingest food, some degree of electrolyte imbalance presumably increased the activity of the chemoreceptor trigger zone. Factors contributing to the control of vomiting included deep breathing, swallowing, and the drinking of ginger ale. The ginger ale provided fluid required to correct dehydration, and it provided a ready supply of glucose. With the correction of glucose starvation, the rate of mobilization of fat is depressed and the degree of metabolic acidosis is lessened. The probability also exists that Miss Berry responded in a positive way to the presence of an individual who was in control of the situation and who appeared to be convinced that the vomiting could and would disappear. Of course, not all patients are as easily helped as Alexandra. The specific measures utilized in the therapy of vomiting depend on its cause and its effects.

Although implied, the importance of observation in the care of the patient who is vomiting has not been explored. Observation is of great significance in any disturbance in which vomiting occurs. Among the pertinent observations are the nature of the onset and the circumstances surrounding it. Had the patient been apparently well and then become suddenly ill or had he been unwell for a period of time? How long has the patient been vomiting? Is vomiting preceded by nausea? What other signs and symptoms does the patient have? When does the patient vomit in relation to food intake or to the ingestion or injection of drugs? The emesis should be observed for amount, odor, general appearance, and presence of blood. Fresh blood is bright red, while flecks of partly digested blood give the vomitus a coffee ground appearance. In addition to the making of pertinent observations, they should be accurately recorded. Whether or not they are immediately drawn to the attention of the physician will depend on the extent to which prompt action is required. When in doubt, the nurse should notify the physician.

Like vomiting, diarrhea results in the removal of irritating substances from the alimentary canal. It is, however, almost always associated with a disease process or with an emotional disturbance. It will be discussed with disorders of motility.

Despite the effectiveness of primary defense mechanisms in preventing harmful agents from getting beyond the first lines of defense, they sometimes do. The internal environment is protected from general dissemination of injurious agents from the alimentary canal by lymph nodes and phagocytes. They function in protection just as they do in other parts of the body. The internal environment is further protected from the general dissemination of microorganisms and some potentially toxic agents by the liver. Bacteria in the blood circulating through the liver are destroyed by reticuloendothelial or Küpffer cells. Chemicals of extrinsic or intrinsic origin are detoxified or inactivated in the liver. To illustrate, the liver is the chief site of degradation of most barbiturates. Barbital and phenobarbital are exceptions, as they are mainly excreted by the kidney.[26] Barbiturates excreted by the kidney have a more prolonged effect than those that are inactivated by the liver. Since persons who have severe liver damage are dependent on the kidney for the excretion of barbiturates, they are likely to experience toxicity when receiving barbiturates other than phenobarbital or barbital. Steroid hormones such as estrogen are degraded by the liver. Thus the liver plays a role in the regulation of the level of estrogen in the blood. An explanation frequently offered to account for evidence of feminization in some men with cirrhosis or other diseases of the liver is that the balance between the synthesis and degradation of estrogen is upset. Because it implies a loss of control through the negative feedback system, many authorities seriously question its validity.

As in other structures in the body, tissues of the alimentary canal are capable of responding to injury by inflammation and by the formation of scar tissue. Inasmuch as these responses help to limit the extent of injury and to protect the organism from further injury, they are beneficial. Scar tissue may be required to restore the continuity of injured tissue. Scar tissue located near or at the orifice of an organ or duct or encircling a part can cause obstruction as it contracts with maturity.

To recapitulate, in a structural facility where materials are transferred from the external into the internal environment, provisions for the protection of the internal environment from harmful agents are required. The internal environment is protected from the ingestion, absorption, and dissemination of potentially injurious substances by a variety of structures and mechanisms. The senses of sight, taste, smell, and touch serve to warn the individual of the possible unsuitability of food or water for ingestion. Since they are not very accurate and are subject to conditioning, wholesome substances are sometimes rejected and harmful ones ingested. A continuous sheet of mucous membrane extending from the mouth to the anus acts as a mechanical barrier to the transfer of substances from the external to the internal environment. Mucus, secreted by the glands of the mucous membrane, provides a protective layer of material between the contents of the alimentary canal and the mucosa. Vomiting and diarrhea provide means for the removal of irritating materials. Semipermeability of the gastrointestinal mucosa as well as specific transfer mechanisms determines the size and type of materials absorbed into the internal environment. All of the above are only partly effective in preventing the absorption of injurious substances. The individual is protected from absorbed substances by phagocytic cells in the blood, lymph nodes, and liver. In addition to phagocytizing bacteria and other foreign substances, the liver decreases the activity of a variety of chemicals by altering their structure.

[26] Louis S. Goodman and Alfred Gilman, *The Pharmacological Basis of Therapeutics*, 2nd ed., The Macmillan Company, New York, 1956, p. 136.

The mucous membrane lining the alimentary canal also requires protection from mechanical, chemical, and living agents and from the digesting action of enzymes. It is really quite remarkable that the protective mechanisms are successful in preventing self-digestion as the protein-digesting enzymes of the alimentary canal do digest living tissue. The capacity of protein-digesting enzymes to act on living tissue can be observed when unprotected tissue is exposed to intestinal and pancreatic secretions or when the balance between the mechanisms protecting the lining of the alimentary canal from the proteolytic actions of digesting secretion is upset as in peptic ulcer.

What determines the effects of disease or injury of the alimentary canal?

Any disorder interfering with the capacity to ingest, digest, or absorb one or more nutrients will interfere with the nutritional status of the affected individual. Other effects will depend on the nature of the disorder and the organ or organs affected. As repeatedly emphasized, the gastrointestinal tract is sensitive to the general condition or status of the body as a whole. Disorders in other parts of the body are frequently accompanied by one or more disturbances in the gastrointestinal function.

The structures forming the gastrointestinal system are also subject to the same general types of disorders as other portions of the body. Disturbances in gastrointestinal functioning may result from messages sent by the mental apparatus, from direct injury to cells, or from a response to injury or threat of injury. As a muscular structure, under control of the autonomic nervous system, disorders of motility and secretion are not infrequent. As is true of all cells, blood supply is necessary to survival. Because of the rich blood supply of the mucosa, the relationship of the veins draining the alimentary canal and the portal circulation to the liver, and the fact that when bleeding into the lumen of the gut occurs, it is not opposed by a rapid rise in tissue fluid pressure, life-threatening hemorrhages are not an infrequent problem.[27] Massive bleeding into the lumen of the alimentary canal usually initiates the vomiting or defecation reflex and blood is evacuated in vomitus or from the rectum. Bleeding into the lumen of the alimentary canal is not always massive. Small quantities may be lost at one time or continue to be lost over an extended period of time causing a microcytic anemia.

Blood supply to a portion of the alimentary canal may be cut off by arterial or venous thrombosis or by twisting of the small intestine or by incarceration of a viscus or the mesentery by a ring through which one or more body structures normally pass. For example, mesentery of intestine may slip through the inguinal or femoral ring. Neither the mesentery nor the intestine normally passes through either of these rings, and protrusion into one of them

[27] In solid tissues, bleeding raises the intertissue pressure, which opposes further bleeding.

is known as an inguinal or femoral hernia.[28] Should the contents be trapped, the venous return is impeded and swelling occurs. Unless the incarcerated tissue or organ is removed from the hernial sac, the intertissue pressure will be raised sufficiently to prevent blood from entering the area and tissue necrosis will occur.[29]

Epithelial and other types of cells in the mucosa of glands along the alimentary canal can and do undergo neoplastic change. Neoplasms can be either benign or malignant. For some unexplained reason, neoplasms rarely are found in the small intestine. Neoplasms in the alimentary canal cause harmful effects by obstructing the lumen of the gut and thereby preventing the normal passage of food. Pedunculated neoplasms may twist on their pedicles and cause symptoms associated with the necrosis of tissue. In the small intestine they may act as a focus predisposing to the twisting or volvulus of the intestine. The neoplasm may undergo necrosis and predispose to bleeding from ulcerations formed at its surface. Specific effects of any neoplasm will depend on its nature and location in the alimentary canal. Neoplasms are discussed in detail in Chapter 12.

The lining mucosa is exposed to a variety of mechanical, chemical, and living agents of extrinsic origin as well as to the digestive juices. Cells may be sensitive to ordinarily harmless substances; that is, they are or become allergic. Depending on the nature of the etiology and the extent of the injury, the mucosa may be acutely or chronically inflamed, infected, or ulcerated. If there is sufficient tissue destruction, scar tissue may be formed in the process of healing. Depending on its location and extent, the scar tissue, as it matures and contracts, can reduce the size of the lumen of the gut or block a duct opening into it.

To illustrate the above, Mr. Brave has a peptic ulcer in the proximal portion of his duodenum. Ulceration is due to an imbalance between the capacity of the mucous membrane lining his duodenum to resist digestion and the action of the digestive ferments. In the healing of the ulcer, scar tissue was formed, and as it matured, it shrank or contracted. Since the area of ulceration was small and not close to the opening of the ampulla of Vater,[30] healing took place without causing obstruction.

As mentioned previously, the wall forming the alimentary canal acts as a barrier protecting the internal from the external environment. In health, the internal environment is protected not only from unusable or partly digested nutrients, but from the entrance of digestive enzymes and large numbers of microorganisms. When, as a result of surgery, trauma, or disease, the wall of

---

[28] A hernia is the protrusion of the contents of a body cavity through a defect in the wall of the cavity. When the protrusion occurs near the surface of the body, it can be felt as a bulge.

[29] When herniated tissue can be returned to its proper cavity, the hernia is said to be reducible. When it cannot be removed, it is irreducible or incarcerated, and when the venous return is obstructed and swelling takes place, it is said to be strangulated.

[30] The duct formed by the union of the common bile duct from the liver and the duct of Wirsung from the pancreas.

the alimentary canal is penetrated, its contents escape into the surrounding cavity. When the esophagus is perforated, secretions and food can enter the trachea or mediastinum depending on the level of the lesion. Either is serious. The effects of food and fluids entering the trachea have been discussed in Chapter 7. In the mediastinum, the esophagus is near the heart, aorta, lungs, vagus nerves, thoracic duct, vertebral column, and diaphragm. Food escaping into the mediastinum carries bacteria with it. Either food or bacteria can be responsible for abscess formation. Because of its location and poor blood supply, lesions of the esophagus are difficult to treat. For example, Mrs. Bird swallowed a large fish bone. It became lodged in and perforated her esophagus, resulting in secretions and microorganisms gaining access to the mediastinum. A mediastinal abscess was formed as a result. Because of the possibility of perforating the wall of the esophagus, a person should neither manipulate nor allow anyone except a physician attempt to remove an object caught in his esophagus. In the event that a chicken or fish bone or other object becomes lodged in the esophagus, no time should be lost in seeking assistance from a physician. No other person should be allowed to try to remove it.

Penetration of structures below the diaphragm allow the contents of the stomach or intestine to escape into the peritoneal cavity. According to Gius,[31] the peritoneum has remarkable protective and reparative powers. The capacity of the peritoneum to defend and heal itself is one of the factors making abdominal surgery possible and successful. When leakage is small, the body may be able to wall off the area and prevent the dissemination of the contents of the alimentary canal throughout the peritoneal cavity. At the time Mr. Brave had a recurrence of his ulcer, it penetrated through the wall of the duodenum and into the peritoneum. He did not have generalized peritonitis, however, because his body was able to wall off the area. Mary Alice Todd had acute appendicitis with the formation of an appendiceal abscess. The inflammatory process around the diseased appendix was sufficient to wall off the leakage from it and to prevent generalized peritonitis.

When, however, a viscus is suddenly perforated and a large quantity of stomach or intestinal content enters or continues to gain entrance to the peritoneal cavity, the protective and reparative powers of the peritoneum may be overcome and generalized peritonitis may result. Even with a fairly large opening, the peritoneum is able to defend itself against most bacteria for 24 hours.[32] Thereafter, its defensive capacity fails rapidly. Prompt closure of an opening between the digestive tube and the peritoneal cavity is therefore of the greatest importance.

Peritonitis is frequently secondary to perforation of the alimentary tract, or leakage from the liver, biliary tract, or pancreas. Disease or injury of the alimentary tract, in which perforation of viscus occurs, includes stab and

[31] John Armes Gius, *Fundamentals of General Surgery,* 2nd ed., Yearbook Medical Publishers, Chicago, Illinois, 1962, p. 336.
[32] *Ibid.,* p. 341.

gunshot wounds in the abdomen, perforated peptic ulcers, ruptured appendices or diverticuli, postoperative leakage, and strangulating obstruction of the intestine. One of the hazards in cholelithiasis (gall stones) is that a stone can act as a ball valve, allowing bile to enter the gall bladder, but not to escape. As the wall of the gall bladder distends, its blood supply lessens and predisposes the wall to necrosis and gangrene. With necrosis of its wall, bile escapes into the peritoneal cavity and causes peritonitis.

When contents of the alimentary canal escape into the peritoneal cavity, the patient usually experiences abdominal pain. This pain is usually severe, but it may be either localized or generalized. The patient also presents signs and symptoms of shock, that is, pallor, sweating, an anxious expression, and rapid pulse and respiration. He will eventually have signs and symptoms of sepsis; fever and rapid pulse and respirations. The alimentary tract responds first by vomiting, but eventually gastrointestinal activity is depressed and the patient becomes distended. The abdominal wall is tender and rigid, and splinting of the diaphragm results in shallow, grunting respirations. Leukocytosis indicates a general response to the injury. Patients who fail to develop leukocytosis generally have a poor prognosis.

What are the responsibilities of the nurse in the prevention of peritonitis?

The responsibilities of the nurse differ somewhat with the potential causes of peritonitis. Individuals who have an acute gastrointestinal disorder or what is commonly referred to as "stomach flu" should avoid ingesting food or fluid during the attack. They should *not* take either a laxative or an enema. If the attack lasts more than a few hours, they should be advised to call their physician. When a patient who has a peptic ulcer experiences sudden severe pain, his physician should be notified immediately. Time should not be wasted on the hypothesis that given time the pain will disappear. No fluid, food, or drugs should be administered orally. When there is any doubt about the cause of abdominal pain, or pain continues for more than a few hours, a physician should be consulted.

Should the pain be caused by perforation of the alimentary tract and the physician decide that the opening is to be closed surgically, the operation is usually performed as soon as possible. The care of the patient following closure is similar to that of any patient having abdominal surgery. Whether or not surgical closure is effected, the prevention of gastrointestinal distention is important. To prevent distention, a long tube is introduced by way of the nose, pharynx, esophagus, and stomach into the small intestine. Suction is applied to establish and maintain decompression, Since the patient is unable to take fluids and foods orally, fluids must be administered parenterally as prescribed by the physician. Antibiotics are usually prescribed to combat bacterial infection.

Pain should be prevented, without depressing the patient unduly. Small doses of morphine or one of the morphine substitutes may be used for this purpose. Morphine has the particular advantage of splinting the intestine.

Care directed toward making and keeping the patient comfortable is very important. Since the patient with peritonitis is very ill, he should be allowed to be sick. His needs should be anticipated and the responsibility for his care assumed by his attendants. He should be placed in a comfortable position. He should be moved and turned as necessary to prevent respiratory and circulatory complications. He should have a quiet, nonstimulating environment. Talking should be limited to that required for his care. Personal care, such as mouth hygiene and bathing, should be performed by the nurse. The patient should be protected from unnecessary exertion. As the patient recovers, his activity should, of course, be increased.

With the preceding general background discussion, it should be clear that no serious disorder in the structure or function of any part of the digestive system is without its effects on the functioning of the entire system or on the body as a whole. It is easier, however, and the presentation is likely to be clearer, if the function or functions of each organ and the effects of alterations in function are presented separately. Discussions will be related primarily to the effects of disturbances in functions of the various organs and the implications of these to nursing. Specific diseases are outlined at the end of the chapter.

What are the functions of the mouth and how are these functions accomplished?

The normal entrance to the alimentary canal is the mouth, which also serves as a second entrance and exit for air. The function of the mouth in nutrition is to prepare food for digestion and swallowing. Enzymes act only on the surface of particles. Therefore, if enzymes are to be effective, large particles must be broken up into small ones so that the surface area exposed to the action of enzymes is increased. Reduction in the size of food particles also facilitates swallowing. In the mouth, food is mixed with saliva and converted to a semifluid state. Although the changes in the food are almost entirely physical, they are indipensable to digestion. When, for any reason, an individual is unable to chew food, it must be liquefied before it is introduced into the alimentary canal. Either liquid or semiliquid foods such as milk, cream, oils, eggs, and fruit and vegetable juices may be used, or solid foods may be liquefied in a blender. The latter has the advantage of making it possible to utilize a wider variety of foods in the diet.

Lack of teeth is probably the most common factor in the inability to properly masticate food, but teeth that are painful and carious (decayed) can and do interfere with chewing. Painful lesions of the gums, tongue, or buccal mucosa may interfere with the chewing and mixing of food. Inability to open or close the jaws will obviously make chewing difficult, if not impossible. As the result of rheumatoid arthritis, Mr. Gerald has an ankylosis (stiffness or fixation) of the mandibular joints. He can separate his teeth only about 2 cm, which makes it difficult to introduce food into his mouth and for him to grind it. He is given soft and liquid foods. Mr. Elmer fractured his mandible in an automobile accident and his jaw has been wired. All food and fluids have to be introduced into his mouth through a tube.

Patients who cannot properly masticate their food should be served food in a state that does not require chewing; that is, the food should be in a liquid or semisolid form. The nurse has a responsibility for determining whether or not the patient needs to have some or all of his food altered in order to eat it. For example, some people with poor natural teeth or dentures can eat most foods, but cannot eat meat unless it is tenderized or ground.

Because the teeth are essential to proper mastication of food, their care is important. According to some dentists, the baby should be taught to brush his teeth with his first tooth. Regular dental care, as well as good nutrition, is also important in the care of teeth.

In addition to the grinding surface provided by the teeth, the act of chewing requires the power or energy to open the jaws and to close them with force on the food. Power is provided by the muscles of mastication. In disorders such as myasthenia gravis—great muscle weakness—the patient may quickly tire if he is required to masticate an ordinary diet. In order to conserve his energy and maintain his food intake, his food may have to be ground or be soft in character.[33]

In addition to the breaking of food into small particles in the mouth, food is mixed with saliva and converted to a semisolid state. Saliva contains an enzyme, ptyalin, which starts the digestion of starch. Saliva is secreted by three pairs of glands. These glands are the site of the common infectious disease mumps. Debilitated patients, in whom oral intake is restricted, are susceptible to an infection called surgical parotitis. Prevention of surgical parotitis is based on an adequate fluid intake, cleanliness of the mouth, and stimulation of the flow of saliva. An adequate intake of fluid makes an important contribution to keeping the mouth clean and moist. The maintenance of oral fluid intake in sick and debilitated patients requires time, planning and attention of nursing personnel. It should not be left to chance. Mouth care, including the brushing of the teeth, should be performed at least every four hours. Stimulation of the flow of saliva is essential. Measures such as chewing gum and sucking on lemon or orange slices or lemon sour balls are all useful in encouraging salivation. Care taken to prevent parotitis is important, as it is a serious complication. After the introduction of antibiotics, its incidence decreased. However, recent statements about parotitis indicate that it is in-

---

[33] Myasthenia gravis is a disorder in which there is a defect in transmission of impulses at the myoneural junction. The patient experiences weakness. For some reason, many patients with this disorder have difficulty breathing and swallowing before other muscle function is seriously impaired.

creasing in incidence. The nurse is responsible for keeping the mouth clean and, if necessary and appropriate, for introducing measures to stimulate the flow of saliva. Although the physician prescribes the route by which fluids are administered, it is the nurse who carries the responsibility for their administration.

Not only does the taste and aroma of food stimulate the flow of saliva, but they initiate reflexes which increase secretion in the stomach. In persons who are unable to taste or smell food, not only is the enjoyment of food diminished, but there may be some impairment in digestion. As will be discussed later, the capacity to secrete gastric juice in response to external stimulation may be a factor in peptic ulcer

After food has been masticated, it passes from the mouth by way of the pharynx and esophagus to the stomach by the act of swallowing. Swallowing takes place in three stages. The first, or oral, phase is voluntary. The second, or pharyngeal, stage and the third, or esophageal, stages are involuntary. In the act of swallowing, food passes through the pharynx, which also serves as a passageway for air, and therefore food must be transferred without entering either the nares or the glottis. Furthermore, particles too big to pass easily through the esophagus must be prevented from entering the pharynx.

What are some of the causes and results of failure of the swallowing reflex?

The first stage of swallowing is initiated after the food has been masticated and mixed with sufficient saliva to form a soft mass. It is then squeezed and rolled toward the posterior portion of the mouth by the pressure of the tongue moving upward and backward toward the palate. The tongue forces the bolus of food into the pharynx. At any time before the bolus reaches the pharynx, the act of swallowing can be stopped.

As the food is pushed back, it stimulates sensory receptors located in and around the pharynx. Impulses are carried to the swallowing center located in the brain stem. Messages are sent from the brain to the pharyngeal area and a number of automatic actions are initiated. These begin with the closure of the posterior nares by the upward movement of the soft palate. This action prevents food from entering the nares. One of the characteristics of disorders in which the soft palate is paralyzed or defective is the escape of food or fluid into the nose. In the patient who has a lesion in the nervous system, including the peripheral nerves, the escape of fluid or food through the nares should be regarded as prima facie evidence of paralysis of the soft palate. Food and fluid should be discontinued until the patient has been examined by his physician.

Even more important than preventing food from entering the nares is the protection of the airway below the glottis from the introduction of food. The swallowing, or deglutition, center in the brain acts to inhibit respiration as well as to facilitate the passage of food through the pharynx and into the esophagus. The glottis is closed by the approximation of the vocal cords, and the epiglottis moves backward to shield the superior opening into the larynx. The larynx is raised and moved out of the way and the esophagus is opened. All of this happens very quickly, and the bolus of food is moved rapidly through the pharynx into the esophagus. The pharyngeal stage of swallowing takes only about two seconds. Failure to closely approximate the vocal cords during swallowing always results in the introduction of food or fluid into the trachea. (See Chapter 7.) When food or fluids enter the larynx and trachea, a paroxysm of coughing or choking is initiated. Particularly in patients who have lesions in the nervous system, choking should be regarded as an indication that food and fluids should be discontinued until the patient has been examined by his physician.

The third stage of swallowing takes place in the esophagus. After the bolus of food enters the esophagus, it is conveyed by peristalsis to the stomach. If the primary peristaltic wave, which begins when food enters the pharynx and continues over the length of the esophagus, is insufficient, secondary waves are initiated at the sites where the esophagus is distended. Under normal conditions, the average length of time it takes food to pass through the esophagus is about five seconds.

Although the most immediate and serious danger attending failure of the swallowing reflex is aspiration of food or fluid into the airway, other problems are also created. One troublesome problem is the handling or disposal of saliva and other secretions in the mouth and upper respiratory tract. According to Guyton,[34] about 1200 ml of saliva is secreted per day, or about 100 ml is secreted each waking hour. When swallowing fails, saliva must be removed from the mouth by suction or by expectoration. Drooling is not only unpleasant and unesthetic, but saliva is injurious to the skin around the mouth as a continuous state of wetness predisposes to maceration of the skin. When drooling cannot be prevented, the skin should be protected by the application of some water-repelling agent, such as aluminum paste or zinc oxide.

Another problem created by the inability to swallow is the maintenance of the fluid intake and the nutritional status of the patient. Although fluids can be administered by intravenous infusion, at the present time nutrients are not available on a practical basis for the maintenance of even minimal nutrition. If the individual is unable to swallow, but a tube can be passed through the esophagus, a nasogastric tube may be introduced into the stomach. Food or fluids may be introduced into the tube at regular intervals or continuously. The latter method requires some means of keeping the food cold to prevent the multiplication of bacteria which cause food poisoning. When a tube cannot be passed through the esophagus, a tube may be placed directly into the stomach by way of an incision in the abdominal wall and stomach. The procedure by which this opening is made is called a gastrostomy. In some

[34] *Op. cit.*, p. 838.

instances, the tube is inserted into the jejunum; that is, a jejunostomy is performed. Following either a gastrostomy or a jejunostomy, food and fluid can be introduced into the stomach or jejunum.

For food to be introduced through a tube, it must be in a liquid state. For reasons previously stated, satisfactory digestion also depends on food being liquefied either in the mouth or in a blender. Some patients prechew food before placing it in the tube. Though the spitting of food into a funnel after it is chewed may appear unesthetic or even revolting to the onlooker, an effort should be made to concentrate on the benefit the patient receives from this practice. The patient should be protected from onlookers and embarrassment by adequate screening. Unless the patient plans to chew his food before it is placed in the tube, it should be liquefied. When the patient is physically able and emotionally ready to feed himself, he should be taught to perform the procedure. The nurse should be certain that the food served to the patient has been properly liquefied. For weeks Mr. Good, who had developed an esophageal fistula following a laryngectomy and radical neck resection, was repeatedly served lumpy wheat cereal for breakfast. The lumps were large enough to obstruct the feeding tube and they could have been removed easily by straining the cereal. Because of the nature of his surgery, Mr. Good was not able to chew the cereal before introducing it into the tube. Quite understandably Mr. Good interpreted the lumps to mean that the hospital personnel were persecuting him.

What is dysphagia and how is it manifested?

Difficulty in swallowing is known as dysphagia. How dysphagia is manifested depends on its cause and the degree to which the passageway is obstructed. The person with dysphagia may be unable to swallow either food or fluids, or he may be able to swallow foods of one consistency, for example solids, and not be able to swallow those of another, possibly liquids. The patient may also have periods of dysphagia with little or no difficulty in between. Accurate descriptions of the type and timing of the difficulty in swallowing experienced by the patient are very important in establishing the cause of dysphagia. When an individual is unable to swallow any food or fluids, evidence of dehydration and starvation appear very quickly.

Dysphagia may be of reflex origin or due to an obstruction in the pharynx or esophagus. Reflex disturbances are usually responsible for interference with the second stage of swallowing, while obstructing lesions are more likely to be responsible for dysphagia in the third stage.

The factors in dysphagia due to a disturbance in reflex activity are similar to those causing disorders in reflexes in any part of the body. Dysphagia can conceivably arise from disordered function in any part of the reflex arc—receptors, centers in the central nervous system, or effector nerves or cells.

The swallowing centers in the brain can be stimulated or inhibited, with the result that swallowing or the coordination of the various activities involved in swallowing fails. Inhibition of or failure of transmission of impulses over some part of the reflex arc may also be responsible for failure in swallowing.

Similar to other centers regulating bodily functions, the swallowing center receives messages from the higher centers in the brain, including the cerebral cortex. Dysphagia may therefore be a manifestation of emotional disturbance. Frequently the patient says that he cannot swallow because he has a lump in his throat which he believes to be caused by a neoplasm. Despite a thorough examination of the esophagus and the information that his esophagus is healthy, the patient states that he knows there is a tumor but it cannot be seen.

Although it is sometimes difficult to demonstrate, the interference with swallowing may be due to a spasm at some point of the esophagus.[35] In the absence of a demonstrable lesion, the disturbance is said to be functional. Mrs. Clifford is a good example of the patient who is starving because she believes that she has an invisible tumor. She is a lonely widow whose husband died after a long and trying illness. Her children are married and live at a distance. For Mrs. Clifford, life holds little promise. She suffers from marked dysphagia. As far as can be demonstrated by fluoroscopy, esophagoscopy, and studies of cells taken from the mucosa, her esophagus is free from any evidence of neoplasia or other structural disease. Despite evidence to the contrary, Mrs. Clifford believes that she has cancer. When she tries to swallow, she says there is a lump in her throat that prevents swallowing. Her food intake is limited almost entirely to small quantities of milk. She has lost so much weight that her skin hangs loosely. As is characteristic in starvation, she lacks energy. The preparation of adequate meals requires more effort than she can muster. Despite the fact that Mrs. Clifford's illness was precipitated by the loss of her husband, she is now physically ill from a lack of food. Unless her food intake is increased in quantity and quality very soon, irreversible changes will have taken place in her cells and she will die from the direct effects of starvation. Attention must therefore be given to improving the nutritional status of Mrs. Clifford, if she is to survive. There are no easy answers to the problem of how to bring about an increase in food intake in patients such as Mrs. Clifford. In the instance of Mrs. Clifford, a close relative spent some weeks with her. The relative planned the meals around what Mrs. Clifford could and would eat. Progress in the beginning was slow, but as Mrs. Clifford made an effort to eat, she gained strength and her general outlook improved. More food did not cure Mrs. Clifford's basic problems, but it did contribute to her capacity to cope with them. The maintenance of food intake is of no less importance in the patient whose dysphagia is due to an emotional problem than it is in the patient who has an organic lesion.

In addition to dysphagia due to disturbances in function, lesions within the cranial cavity interfere with the function of the swallowing centers in the brain

[35] Joseph B. Kirsner and Walter L. Palmer, "The Esophagus," in William A. Sodeman, *Pathologic Physiology*, 3rd ed., W. B. Saunders Co., Philadelphia, 1961, p. 662.

stem. Lesions are of two general types, those that lessen the blood supply to the area and those resulting in inflammation. Inflammation, by causing swelling, also diminishes the blood supply. The blood supply to the swallowing center may be lessened due to the obstruction of a blood vessel by a thrombus or an embolus. Intracranial pressure may be raised by neoplasms, particularly those obstructing the free flow of cerebrospinal fluid, and by edema of the brain resulting from the response of the brain tissue to injury. Infections such as bulbar poliomyelitis are accompanied by difficulty in swallowing. Usually the difficulty with swallowing is manifested as a failure to coordinate swallowing with breathing, so that the patient is in danger of aspirating saliva and secretions from the nasal and pharyngeal cavities as well as food and fluids. Disturbances in the regulation of swallowing can originate from injury to peripheral nerves supplying the muscles involved in swallowing. Finally, failure of transmission of nerve impulses from the nerve to the muscle will cause dysphagia.

Since the patient cannot manage his own secretions, they must be removed by gravity and by suctioning. Oral fluids, food, and drugs must be withheld until such time as the patient is able to swallow. The objective is to protect the patient from aspiration of foreign material into his airway. The patient with myasthenia gravis can swallow normally until he becomes fatigued. Measures should be taken to limit fatigue.

In the esophagus itself, dysphagia can be caused by a variety of disorders which obstruct the lumen and block the passage of food and/or fluid. Among the causes of obstruction of the esophagus are neoplasms, malignant and benign, inflammatory strictures, congenital defect, hiatus hernia,[36] foreign bodies, achalasia, and extrinsic pressure. The most frequent causes of mechanical obstruction of the esophagus are neoplasms and strictures due to the formation of scar tissue. All obstructing lesions have a common effect. They interfere to a lesser or greater extent with the ability of the individual to ingest enough food to meet his nutritional needs. Patients with one of the above disorders are often in a poor nutritional condition when admitted to the hospital. As a matter of fact, they are all too often in a state of near-starvation. They are usually treated surgically after the diagnosis is made and the gross nutritional, water, and electrolyte deficiencies and anemia are corrected. Since the route of approach to the esophagus is through the thorax, attention must be paid to re-establishing and maintaining the expansion of the lungs during the immediate postoperative period.

Careful and accurate observation of the patient who is dysphagic is important. What, if anything, is the patient able to swallow? Are there any circumstances that affect the ability of the patient to swallow? If the patient regurgitates, what are the characteristics of the emesis? For example, does the

---

[36] A hiatus is a gap or opening in the diaphragm. In hiatus hernia contents of the abdominal cavity escape through the hiatus into the thoracic cavity. A lay term for hiatus hernia is "upside-down stomach."

regurgitated material contain digested or undigested food particles? Does it contain blood? Does the patient complain of pain or other sensations before, during, or after swallowing? When are the symptoms intensified or relieved? The patient may be aware of the point where food is delayed as it passes through the esophagus. When the patient complains of pain or discomfort, where is it located and what is its general character?

Other symptoms associated with alterations in the function or structure of the esophagus include pain and heartburn. Painful sensations accompany the ingestion of irritating substances such as dilute hydrochloric acid. Regurgitation of the acid chyme from the stomach into the esophagus also causes pain. Spasm or distention of the esophagus, particularly when associated with ulceration of the esophagus, is a cause of pain. When the pain-evoking stimulus is continuously present, the pain is burning in character. When the stimulus is applied intermittently, it is likely to be griping and intense.

What is heartburn?

Heartburn, or pyrosis, is a condition experienced by most persons at some time in their lives. Despite its name, heartburn has no relation to the heart or to its function. It is characterized by a burning sensation over the precordium or beneath the sternum and is accompanied by the regurgitation into the esophagus or mouth of the acid gastric juice. Heartburn is one of the discomforts of pregnancy. In persons with hiatus hernia or cardioesophageal hernia, foods such as cake, sweet rolls, and orange juice induce heartburn. The mechanism for this disorder is not known, though the associated sensations may be due to the lowering of the pH in the esophagus by the regurgitation of the contents from the stomach.

What are the functions of the stomach and adjacent portions of the duodenum?

Because the stomach and the adjacent portion of the duodenum perform common functions and are the site of several serious diseases, they will be discussed as a unit. The diseases are peptic ulcer, gastric carcinoma, and hypertrophic pyloric stenosis. Inflammation of the stomach, or gastritis, is not uncommon. Knowledge of the physiology of the stomach and duodenum is essential to understanding the disorders of this region.

The lower end of the esophagus is guarded by the cardiac sphincter, which prevents the reflux of acid chyme from the stomach into the esophagus. The esophageal mucosa is not protected against the digesting action of gastric juice, and repeated reflux of the acid gastric juice predisposes the esophagus to acid ulceration. The pyloric sphincter regulates the movement of gastric contents into the duodenum.

The functions of the stomach to be discussed are those relating to the preparation of food for absorption. The secretion of the intrinsic factor which facilitates the absorption of vitamin B_{12} is no less important in nutrition; however, since vitamin B_{12} is essential to the maturation of red blood cells, its functions are discussed in the chapter on blood formation.

The stomach is divided into three parts, the fundus, the corpus, or body, and the antrum. Tha antrum is frequently, though incorrectly, called the pyloric or prepyloric region. Because the wall of the stomach has relatively little tone and the mucous and submucous coats form folds or rugae as the stomach empties, the size of the stomach is determined by the quantity of its contents. As food enters the stomach, it forms concentric rings with the most recently ingested food lying nearest to the cardiac sphincter, that which had been in the stomach the longest being nearest the pyloric sphincter.

During the time food remains in the stomach, it is mixed with the gastric secretions until a semifluid mixture called chyme is formed. When the stomach is empty and the pyloric sphincter is relaxed, liquids may not remain in the stomach, but may pass immediately from the esophagus to the duodenum. When, however, a mixed diet is ingested, food remains in the stomach for varying periods of time and is slowly emptied into the duodenum. The rate of emptying depends on two factors, the fluidity of the gastric chyme and the receptivity of the duodenum to receiving more chyme. The fluidity of the gastric chyme is determined by the type of food ingested, the completeness of mastication, the length of time food has been in the stomach, and the intensity of peristaltic waves. For reasons to be explained later, fat remains in the stomach longer than carbohydrates. Relatively large particles of food must be reduced in size before they can be emptied into the duodenum. Obviously food remaining in the stomach for some time is nearer the outlet of the stomach and has had a longer period in which to be mixed with gastric juice than food entering more recently. The more intense peristaltic waves are, the less time chyme is likely to remain in the stomach.

How is the duodenum protected from overloading?

The duodenum is protected from overloading by the factors regulating the receptivity of the small intestine to chyme. Receptivity of the duodenum is determined by the quantity of chyme already present in the upper intestine, the acidity of the chyme, and the type of food in the chyme. As the duodenum fills, receptors initiate impulses which depress gastric peristalsis and at the same time increase contraction of the pyloric sphincter. A high concentration of fats in the chyme also diminishes gastric secretion. As fat or fatty acids enter the duodenum, glands in the mucosa secrete a hormone called enterogastrone which is carried by way of the blood to the musculature of the stomach. Enterogastrone has an inhibitory effect not only on gastric muscle, but on secretion of the gastric glands as well. With powerful inhibitors of the activity of the stomach, such as fat, peristalsis may be reversed and intestinal secretions regurgitated into the stomach. In general, products of protein digestion, acid, and nonspecific irritants in the duodenum act reflexly to diminish gastric activity and secretion. The effect of fats and fatty acids is mainly through the hormone enterogastrone. The coordinated functioning of the stomach and duodenum enables the stomach to be a storehouse for food and to prepare it for digestion. The duodenum is protected from overdistention and is provided with a more or less continuous stream of chyme. The importance of the regulation of the rate at which chyme enters the intestine is illustrated by the dumping syndrome.

What causes the dumping syndrome and what are some of its effects?

After gastroenterostomy or gastric resection some patients develop the dumping syndrome. According to Hardy,[37] 15 to 25 per cent of patients who undergo gastric resections in which more than 70 per cent of the stomach is removed develop the dumping syndrome. Various explanations are offered to account for the signs and symptoms that are observed in the dumping syndrome. Authorities are agreed, however, that the manifestations are due to the rapid entry of the contents of the stomach into the jejunum, thus the term "dumping." Shortly after a meal, particularly one containing large amounts of carbohydrate, the patient experiences weakness, profuse perspiration, nausea, dizziness, flushing, epigastric fullness, and palpitation. His symptoms may be so severe that he is forced to lie down. Ricketts and Krahl[38] state that the symptoms are due to hypoglycemia.

The sequence of events leading to hypoglycemia is as follows. The rapid entry of a large amount of carbohydrate causes a marked, but transient, hyperglycemia. Insulin is secreted in excess of the quantity required to restore the level of glucose in the blood to physiological limits, resulting in hypoglycemia. Therefore, according to this theory, the symptoms are due to hypoglycemia.

Hardy[39] states that the cause of the symptoms occurring in the dumping syndrome is unknown, but he favors the theory that they are due to hypovolemic shock. According to this explanation, as food is moved rapidly through the stomach and into the intestine, large volumes of fluid are drawn from the blood into the intestine. Since the rate at which fluid is transferred from the blood is more rapid than replacement from the interstitial fluid, the blood volume drops sufficiently to induce a state of shock.

Despite uncertainty about the etiology of the overt manifestations of the dumping syndrome, they are physiological phenomena occurring as a consequence of alterations in anatomical relationships. After gastroenterostomy

[37] James D. Hardy, *Pathophysiology in Surgery,* The Williams and Wilkins Company, Baltimore, 1958, p. 317.

[38] Henry T. Ricketts and Maurice E. Krahl, "Carbohydrate Metabolism," in Sodeman, *Op. cit.,* p. 83.

[39] *Op. cit.,* p. 319.

or gastrectomy, the individual is no longer able to regulate the rate at which chyme enters the intestine with the result that the intestine is dilated by a large volume of concentrated material. Most patients adapt to the altered anatomy within a year, though a few continue to have symptoms.

The treatment of the dumping syndrome is usually medical. Some patients can control their symptoms by eating frequent small meals and then lying down after they have eaten. The secondary hypoglycemic phase, which follows initial hyperglycemia, can be prevented or minimized by a diet high in protein and low in carbohydrate. Meals should be started with dry foods such as toast and high-protein foods such as poached or boiled eggs. Liquids should be taken at the end of the meal or between meals. Sweetened liquids such as milk shakes and other sweet foods should not be eaten when the stomach is empty.

Although the manifestations accompanying the dumping syndrome are frightening and highly unpleasant, they usually disappear with time. The patient should therefore be reassured that the disorder, though highly unpleasant, is not dangerous and given time he will recover. He can minimize his symptoms by following suggestions about his diet. In the words of Barborka,[40] "Reassurance seems the best treatment and time the best cure." For the American who judges the success of therapy by the immediacy of results, the waiting period may well be a trying one.

Secretion into the stomach and duodenum is important in both health and disease. In the stomach and small intestine, foods undergo chemical as well as physical alterations in preparation for absorption. Chemical reactions are catalyzed by enzymes capable of digesting not only food but living cells. One of the factors in the activity of each enzyme is the pH of the fluid in which it works. Pepsin, an enzyme secreted into the stomach, is most active in an acid medium. In the absence of hydrochloric acid, pepsin is inactive. Chemical digestion in the stomach therefore depends on the presence of both hydrochloric acid and pepsin. Direct contact with the cells lining the stomach is prevented by the secretion of mucin. Other factors, such as the blood supply to the mucosa, are also important to the defense of the gastroduodenal mucosa. Any condition upsetting the balance between digestion and protection predisposes to ulceration.

Regulation of the secretion of hydrochloric acid into the stomach is complicated. It involves the autonomic nervous system as well as systemically and locally acting hormones. As a result of the interaction of the various regulators, a balance between stimulation and inhibition is maintained. Digestion is accomplished, and at the same time the mucosa protected.

Hydrochloric acid is secreted by the parietal cells in the corpus of the stomach. Three phases, cephalic, antral, and intestinal, are involved in secretion. The cephalic phase of secretion is under nervous control. Stimulation of

---

[40] Clifford J. Barborka, "The Stomach," in Christopher's *Textbook of Surgery*, 7th ed., W. B. Saunders Company, Philadelphia, 1960, p. 661.

the vagus nerve increases the production of hydrochloric acid, while stimulation of the sympathetics, either by their direct effect on the acid-secreting glands in the stomach or by inhibition of the action of the vagi, lessens it. Usual stimuli initiating the cephalic phase of gastric secretion include sight, smell, and taste of food. Even thoughts of good food, such as a thick steak or luscious lemon pie, may be sufficient to initiate the cephalic phase of gastric secretion. Impulses from distance receptors, such as the retina of the eye, travel to the cerebral cortex, where they are relayed to the hypothalamus. From the hypothalamus, secretory impulses are relayed to the glands in the stomach by way of the vagi. The cephalic phase of gastric secretion can be prevented by the sectioning of the vagus nerves. The procedure is known as vagotomy.

According to Harkins,[41] hypoglycemia of less then 50 mg per 100 ml of blood plasma stimulates gastric secretion by way of the hypothalamus and vagi. After vagotomy, insulin-induced hypoglycemia is utilized to test the completeness of the division of the vagus nerve. After the injection of sufficient insulin to lower the blood sugar to 50 mg or less, no hydrochloric acid should be secreted by the stomach if the vagus nerve supply to the stomach has been completely interrupted. Hypersecretion of insulin with associated hypoglycemia may be a factor in the development and persistence of peptic ulcers in some patients.

The second phase in gastric secretion is the antral phase. Whereas the cephalic phase prepared the stomach for food, the antral phase regulates the amount of acid secreted after food enters the stomach. The antrum does not secrete hydrochloric acid, but it secretes a hormone, gastrin, that stimulates the acid-secreting glands in the corpus of the stomach. When the acidity of the chyme is high, gastrin secretion lessens. When partial gastrectomy is performed in the therapy of peptic ulcers, the antrum is often removed, not because it secretes hydrochloric acid, but because it regulates the production of hydrochloric acid. Marginal ulcers[42] are more frequent in patients in whom the antrum has not been removed.

The third phase in the secretion of hydrochloric acid is the intestinal phase. A hormone similar to, but not as powerful as, gastrin is believed to be secreted by the intestinal mucosa, but it has not been identified. The basis for the hypothesis that the intestinal mucosa produces a hormone is that gastric juice continues to be secreted when the stomach is empty. As indicated earlier, a high concentration of fat in the chyme entering the duodenum stimulates the production of enterogastrone and thereby decreases both gastric secretion and motility. Thus, secretion into the stomach is regulated by nervous and hormonal factors. In health, secretion in the stomach illustrates one of the characteristics of a homeostatic mechanism; that is, a change in one direction

[41] Henry N. Harkins, *et al.*, Principles and Practice, 2nd ed., J. B. Lippincott Company, Philadelphia, 1961, p. 662.
[42] Ulcers formed at the site of junction or anastomoses of the stomach and jejunum.

is counteracted by increasing activity of processes acting in the opposite direction.

How is the mucosa of the stomach and adjacent structures protected from the digesting action of the gastric juice?

The mucosa lining the stomach is protected from digestion by a covering sheet of mucus. Mucous glands are located in the mucous membrane throughout the stomach. The mucosa of the duodenum is protected by alkaline mucus secreted by Brunner's glands. Secretion of mucus is constant, though the volume can be increased by the ingestion of irritating agents. Any failure to secrete mucus in adequate quantities reduces the protection of the underlying mucosa and increases its susceptibility to digestion.

In health, the mucosa of the stomach and adjacent duodenum is protected from digestion by the gastric juice, but other parts of the alimentary canal, such as the esophagus, lower duodenum, jejunum, and ileum, do not have the same degree of resistance. However, since bile and pancreatic juices are alkaline in reaction, they neutralize the acid chyme with the result that the lower duodenum, jejunum, and ileum are protected from injury by the acid gastric juice. When the mucosa of organs lacking protection is exposed to acid chyme over a period of time, ulceration is likely. Ulceration of the area normally exposed to acid chyme, that is, the stomach and proximal duodenum, also occurs and is called peptic ulcer. The word "peptic" is derived from the Greek and pertains to digestion or to pepsin. A peptic ulcer is an ulcer caused by the digesting action of gastric juice. More exactly, ulceration results from an imbalance between the digesting action of gastric juice and the capacity of the gastric and duodenal mucosa to resist digestion. In effect, the digesting action of the gastric juice may be increased or the resistance of the mucosa lining the stomach and duodenum decreased or both. Continuous or intermittent hypersecretion of hydrochloric acid is believed to be responsible for the increase in the digesting action of the gastric juice. Hypersecretion can be the result of overstimulation of the secretory mechanisms or failure of the mechanisms inhibiting secretion, or it can be the effect of failure of the mechanisms inhibiting secretion, or it can be the effect of failure of the mechanisms for neutralizing hydrochloric acid. Rough and highly spiced foods, failure to secrete an adequate quantity of mucus, and a poor blood supply can all predispose to ulceration. Although peptic ulcers in the duodenum are always benign, ulcers in the stomach can be either benign or malignant. Malignant neoplasms in the stomach may eventually ulcerate. Although peptic ulcers are usually chronic, they may also be acute.

Acute ulcers are of two types: Cushing's and Curling's. The acute ulcer of Cushing is found in disorders involving the nervous system, particularly in disorders involving the anterior hypothalamus. It sometimes occurs in bulbar poliomyelitis.

Curling's ulcer was first described by Curling, who noted the formation of ulcer of the stomach and duodenum in patients who had been burned. More recently, the formation of acute gastric and duodenal ulcers has been reported in patients who have experienced various types of trauma. Because some degree of stress is involved, one explanation for the formation of Curling's ulcer is that it results from the effect of the adrenal cortical hormones on the secretion of gastric juice. According to Harkins,[43] experimental evidence indicates that increased gastric secretion occurs even after sectioning of the vagi. The increase in adrenal corticoids results from stimulation of the adrenal cortex by corticotrophin (ACTH). Corticotrophin is secreted by the anterior hypophysis. Its secretion is thought to be increased by a humoral substance secreted by the anterior hypothalamus. In patients who have had a history of gastric hypersecretion or peptic ulcer, symptoms are often aggravated by treatment with corticotrophin or adrenal corticoid hormones. It is not known whether activation of the ulcer is due to increased gastric secretion or to the nitrogen-depleting effect of the adrenal corticoids. If the first is true, increased gastric secretion heightens the digesting action of gastric juice. If the latter is the main effect of the adrenal steroids, the loss of nitrogen from cells presumably decreases the resistance of the gastric and duodenal mucosa to digestion. To reduce the likelihood of ulcer formation in susceptible patients, that is, those who have been seriously injured or are under corticotrophin or adrenal steroid therapy, antacids and an ulcer diet may be prescribed by the physician. To lessen the likelihood of peptic ulcer formation, as well as for other reasons, seriously injured patients should be protected from preventable physical and emotional stress.

Patients who are predisposed by disease or injury to acute ulcer formation should be observed for symptoms and signs indicating ulcer development. Any type of pain or discomfort in the upper abdomen should be brought to the attention of the physician. Onset may be ushered in with hemorrhage or perforation. Either is an emergency and should be treated as such; that is, the physician should be notified immediately. Fluids and food should be withheld until the physician indicates that they can be safely given. The patient should be kept quiet and as comfortable as his situation permits.

What are the characteristics of the common type of ulcer?

The common type of ulcer is the chronic peptic ulcer located in either the stomach or duodenum, usually in the part of the stomach or duodenum exposed to the highest concentration of acid chyme. Peptic ulcer is an important cause of morbidity and, because of the serious nature of its complications, of mortality. The exact incidence is not known, although Sleisenger,[44] from observations derived at postmortem examinations, indicates the incidence is

---

[43] *Op. cit.,* p. 674.
[44] Marvin H. Sleisenger, "Duodenal Ulcer," in Harrison *Principles of Internal Medicine,* 4th ed., The Blakiston Division, McGraw-Hill Book Company, Inc., New York, 1962, p. 1592.

from 7 to 10 per cent. The ratio of men to women is about 3.4 to 1. Early in the century, the ratio was reversed as the incidence was higher among women than men. The disorder is found in all parts of the world and in all groups of people. The incidence varies from one group to another and in the same group from one time to another. Sleisenger states that despite efforts to establish peptic ulcer as a disease of the white-collar class or as associated with a particular personality, this has not been accomplished.[45] Certainly the diagnosis of peptic ulcer is made with some degree of frequency in hospitals and clinics where indigent patients are treated. Since peptic ulcer results from an imbalance between secretions of hydrochloric acid and the resistance of the gastric mucosa to secretion, a single cause or factor should not be expected to be responsible. Various forms of stress, including emotional stress, undoubtedly are associated with changes that upset the balance between digestion and resistance to digestion and thus predispose to ulcer formation.

Mrs. Carrie Maple, a 43-year-old charwoman, illustrates some of the problems of the patient with peptic ulcer as well as the methods employed in the treatment of peptic ulcer. Five years previous to her present admission to the hospital, Mrs. Maple had undergone a subtotal thyroidectomy for the treatment of hyperthyroidism. Shortly thereafter, she experienced pain in the epigastric region about one and one-half to two hours after eating. X ray examination of the stomach and duodenum revealed an ulcer in her duodenum. She was treated by diet and an aluminum hydroxide antacid. She responded well and treatment was discontinued after three months. Mrs. Maple continued to be well until two days prior to her admission to the hospital, when she noted that her stools were tarry. The following day she had lower abdominal pain radiating to her upper abdomen and she had several loose, tarry stools.

At the time of her admission she was feeling weak and dizzy. Her hemoglobin was 7.8 gm per 100 ml of blood and her erythrocyte count was 2,370,000 cells per cubic millimeter of blood. Both the hemoglobin level and the erythrocyte count were reduced to approximately half of normal, indicating serious blood loss. Although her hematocrit was 28 per cent (the normal is about 48 per cent), her blood pressure was 142/88, indicating the blood volume had been maintained despite the loss of blood. See Chapter 9. She required 2,000 ml of blood to raise her hemoglobin to 13.4 gm.

In many respects, the history presented by Mrs. Maple is characteristic of the patient with peptic ulcer. As is most frequently true among residents of the United States, Mrs. Maple's ulcer was located in her duodenum. Although peptic ulcer occurs in women, its incidence is higher among men.

Which of the factors believed to predispose to peptic ulcer did Mrs. Maple demonstrate?

As stated earlier, peptic ulcer occurs where there is an imbalance between the digesting action of gastric juice and the capacity of the mucosa in the

[45] *Ibid.*, p. 1953.

stomach and duodenum to resist digestion. Exactly why ulceration occurs is not known. Authorities agree that certain factors are predisposing. One is that too much acid secretion must have a role in ulcer formation. Not all patients, however, can be shown to have hyperchlorhydria, as there is some overlapping between the level of secretion in patients with ulcer and the upper limits of normal secretion. No information was available about acid secretion by Mrs. Maple's stomach. She had been in another hospital at the time of her first illness and was in no condition at this time to have her gastric acidity evaluated. It can be assumed that she did have either absolute or relative hyperchlorhydria as there is general consensus among authorities which supports the maxim: no acid, no ulcer.

There is less agreement about why acid secretion is increased. In the earlier review of the regulation of the secretion of hydrochloric acid, the fact that gastric secretion occurs in three phases—cephalic, gastric, and intestinal—indicates the complexity of its regulation. Of the three phases of stimulation, the first two are probably the most important. There are at least two views about the immediate cause of hyperchlorhydria. One is that the acid-secreting, or parietal, cells in the stomach are hyperactive. The other is that the number of parietal cells is increased. That factors other than hyperacidity are involved in peptic ulcer formation is demonstrated by the observation that hypersecretion of hydrochloric acid and healing of the ulcer can and do occur simultaneously.

What are some other factors in peptic ulcer formation?

One factor is the relatively recent observation that duodenal ulcer occurs more frequently among persons of blood group O than among other groups. It is also associated with the nonsecretion by the stomach of ABH substances. Both of these are hereditary traits which are inherited independently of each other, but their effect is additive. The person who belongs to blood group O and who secretes the ABH substances is less likely to develop duodenal ulcer than the person who inherits both traits. Although these observations have been made, proof is lacking that there is an hereditary factor predisposing to duodenal ulcer. Mrs. Maple had type A blood and was Rh-positive. No determination was made of the secretion of ABH substances in her gastric juice or saliva. As far as she knew, no one in her family had ever had an ulcer, nor had they had bleeding into the alimentary canal. There was no evidence suggesting that heredity contributed to the development of a duodenal ulcer by Mrs. Maple.

A second factor long known to predispose to hypersecretion is that the stomach responds to many different stimuli by hypersecretion. The first to report this effect was Beaumont. He made his studies by directly observing the lining of the stomach of Alexis St. Martin, who had a gastric fistula. The later work of Wolf and Wolff[46] further supported and extended the concept that

[46] Stewart Wolf and H. G. Wolff, *Human Gastric Function,* 2nd ed., Oxford University Press, New York, 1947.

the stomach responds to many forms of stimuli by secretion. Prolonged emotional disturbance associated with anxiety, guilt, resentment, anger, or hostility has been demonstrated to evoke vascular engorgement accompanied by increased secretion and motility of the stomach.

It will be remembered that the onset of ulcer symptoms in Mrs. Maple followed thyroidectomy to correct hyperthyroidism. Similar to peptic ulcer, the onset of hyperthyroidism may be coincident with a period of emotional stress. As a shy, retiring person, Mrs. Maple did not conform to the stereotype of the "ulcer personality" of the hard-driving, anxious-to-succeed, "wants what he wants when he wants it" person. She gave some evidence of being depressed, as she was found crying on several occasions. Despite her outward appearance, she may have felt angry but turned her anger against herself. Despite the absence of any positive evidence of emotional stress, she may well have been experiencing it.

In the previous discussion of the factors in the development of peptic ulcer, the roles of the nervous and endocrine systems were presented. The effect of stress on the capacity of the stomach to resist digestion and on the secretion and motility of the stomach is mediated by the nervous and the hormonal systems. In terms of the above, duodenal ulcer is a localized manifestation of a constitutional disease.

The clinical history of Mrs. Maple's ulcer illustrated an almost textbook picture of the behavior and manifestations of duodenal ulcer. Five years prior to her present attack, she had had pain and nausea, appearing one and one-half to two hours after eating. The pain responded to treatment with hourly feedings on the hour alternating with hourly doses of an aluminum hydroxide antacid taken on the half-hour. As a result of this schedule, she ingested either food or medication each half-hour.

Pain is the most frequent symptom associated with peptic ulcer. Opinion as to why pain occurs differs among authorities. One hypothesis is that the hydrochloric acid irritates the exposed sensory nerve endings in the edges and base of the ulcer. According to this view, the hydrochloric acid causes a chemical inflammation and lowers the pain threshold of the nerve endings in the ulcer. As a result, pain is present when the concentration of acid is elevated in the stomach and disappears when it is low. Evidence casting doubt on this hypothesis is that pain occurs when the concentration of hydrochloric acid is within normal limits.

Another hypothesis is that the pain associated with duodenal ulcer results from increased motility or spasm of the muscle at the ulcer site. Hardy[47] is of the opinion that both factors are involved in causing pain.

Although Mrs. Maple did not remember the exact nature or location of the pain associated with her first ulcer, the pain of uncomplicated ulcer is almost always located in the epigastrium and is limited to a small, localized area. When an ulcer is located on the posterior wall of the duodenum, the pain

[47] *Op. cit.,* p. 306.

sometimes is referred to the back. Pain is steady, and it may be described as gnawing, or it may be dull, aching, or ourning.

Three characteristic features of the pain, its chronicity, periodicity, and relationship to the ingestion of food, are considered to be pathognomonic of the disease. Although not true of Mrs. Maple, patients not infrequently have periodic attacks of pain for five or six years before seeking medical attention, and ulcers may have been present for as many as 40 or 50 years. Recurrences are common, even among patients who continue under medical supervision, and are often triggered by a situation associated with an increase in stress. Sources of stress may include a traumatic injury or a frustrating situation at the office.

During her first attack, the pain experienced by Mrs. Maple demonstrated the characteristic relationship to the ingestion of food inasmuch as it occurred from one and a half to two hours after meals. Most patients have pain from one to three hours after eating and secure relief by the ingestion of food or antacids.

At the time of Mrs. Maple's current admission to the hospital, she had one of the complications associated with peptic ulcer, hemorrhage. At the time of her admission, the priority objective in her care was to stop the bleeding and to restore the elements lost as a result of hemorrhage. (See Chapter 15 for details.)

The most common complication of the ulcer is intractability, or the failure to heal with treatment. Jim Snow was a 19-year-old premedical student who had an intractable duodenal ulcer. Despite intensive medical therapy, his ulcer did not heal and so about four fifths of his stomach was removed. A few months later, he returned to his physician with a marginal ulcer. Possibly Jim was born 15 years too soon, inasmuch as neither vagotomy nor anticholinergic drugs were available to him. He does illustrate, however, the persistence of ulcer formation in some individuals.

The dangers and problems of the two other relatively frequent complications, penetration of the duodenal wall (perforation) and obstruction of the pylorus, have been discussed earlier. Obstruction may be due to edema, inflammation, muscle spasm, or the contraction of scar tissue. Unless there are frequent recurrences of the ulcer with the formation of scar tissue in healing, obstruction is likely to be temporary.

In addition to the care and observation which Mrs. Maple required because she was having a hemorrhage, therapy was initiated to heal the ulcer. The basic objective of treatment is to suppress the secretion and activity of the pepsin and hydrochloric acid in the gastric juice. Four different types of measures are employed—diet, antacids, antisecretory compounds, and attention to psychic or emotional factors. Surgical therapy may also be utilized to bring about a similar effect. Gastric resection with the removal of the part of the stomach containing the parietal cells and vagotomy, either one alone or the two in combination with each other, may also be performed to decrease gastric secretion. Mrs. Maple was successfully treated by medical means.

Diet and antacids are usually prescribed in relation to each other in order to secure and maintain the continual neutralization of the gastric juice. Physicians vary in the emphasis they place on the traditional ulcer diet. Some physicians prescribe half-hourly feedings of milk and antacid during the phase of acute ulcer activity. Mrs. Maple was allowed clear liquids and milk for the first two days of her hospitalization. She was given 3 oz of milk every two hours and an ounce of Maalox[48]—a creamy-white, colloidal suspension of magnesium and aluminum hydroxides.[49] By the third day of her hospitalization there was no longer any evidence that Mrs. Maple was bleeding, and the physician prescribed a modified ulcer diet for her. The modified ulcer diet is a transitional diet between a restricted ulcer diet and an ordinary house diet. Food is distributed in six meals with the sixth meal served at nine in the evening or before the patient retires. Since one of the major objectives of the diet is to neutralize gastric acidity, all meals are important and none should be omitted. Food is selected from a variety of sources, but is subjected to the test, is it bland? Fruit juices are strained and may be diluted. Foods with a high content of roughage are eliminated. Cabbage, kale, and cereals containing bran are not included. Vegetables such as peas and string beans are strained to remove the fiber. When Mrs. Maple's ulcer was shown to have healed, she returned to a regular diet.

In addition to minimization of possible trauma to the stomach and duodenum by control of the fiber content of food, nothing should be ingested that stimulates the secretion of acid without neutralizing it or that directly irritates the gastric mucosa. For example, alcohol is a potent stimulator of gastric secretion, but it does not neutralize the acid after it is secreted. Neither should the patient be given, or take, a drug that directly irritates the gastric mucosa, such as the salicylates. They appear to exert a direct irritating effect without increasing acid secretion. The most frequently used form of this drug is acetylsalicylic acid, or aspirin. The daily or very frequent ingestion of aspirin appears to predispose to hemorrhage from the stomach. Mrs. Maple was given codeine, 32 mg, when she complained of headache. Patients with a diagnosis of peptic ulcer should be instructed *not* to take either aspirin or drugs containing it or other salicylates without a specific prescription from a physician who knows that they have an ulcer.

Because there is evidence that smoking increases the secretion of acid by the stomach, some physicians discourage their patients from smoking. In fact, some physicians feel so strongly about smoking, they refuse to treat patients who do not cooperate. (See Chapter 9 for a discussion of some of the aspects of discontinuing smoking.)

Since hydrochloric acid is one of the essential factors in ulcer formation, an ideal drug would appear to be one that depresses its secretion. These drugs would, in effect, produce a chemical vagotomy. There are a number of drugs

[48] Trade name.
[49] See Elsie E. Krug, *Pharmacology in Nursing,* 9th ed., The C. V. Mosby Company, St. Louis, 1963, pp. 376-83, for a discussion of antacids.

available that do block the action of acetylcholine on smooth-muscle and gland cells. Since stimulation of the vagus nerve results in the release of acetycholine and increases gastric secretion and motility, the effects of the anticholinergics or cholinergic-blocking agents are to decrease secretion and motility. Among the most widely used anticholinergics or cholinergic-blocking agents are the alkaloids of belladonna. Authorities differ as to the effectiveness of the alkaloids of belladonna in decreasing gastric secretion and motility in human beings. They do decrease both in experimental animals.

Among the synthetic anticholinergic agents are Methantheline Bromide (Banthine Bromide[50]) and Propantheline Bromide (Pro-Banthine Bromide[50]). At the time Banthine Bromide was introduced, it was believed that an effective chemical agent had been found to control gastric secretion and motility. It has been largely replaced by Pro-Banthine Bromide, which is said to be more effective in reducing gastric secretion and motility and to have fewer toxic effects. Readers who wish a more detailed description of the above drugs should refer to a textbook on pharmacology.

One of the most important aspects in the care of the patient with a peptic ulcer is attention to the psychic factors in his illness. As indicated earlier, gastric secretion, motility, and blood supply to the gastric mucosa are all responsive to a wide variety of stimuli in the environment. Some patients respond positively, that is, by healing their ulcers, when they are removed from a stressful environment. For example, Mr. George fits the stereotype of the patient with a peptic ulcer. He was a tense, hard-driving executive. He smoked cigarettes excessively, and, although he never became intoxicated, he consumed several cocktails in the course of most days. He often took work home at night, and his weekends were spent playing golf with business associates. When his ulcer symptoms finally became so severe that he could no longer ignore them, he consulted a physician and the diagnosis of peptic ulcer was confirmed. Instead of being admitted to a hospital, Mr. George and his physician decided that he should take a long-planned hunting trip with his wife. Plans were made for the trip. Mr. George agreed to eliminate smoking and the drinking of alcoholic beverages. He also took a bottle of an aluminum hydroxide antacid with him. Most of all, he planned to relax and enjoy himself. Within a few days of his arrival at the hunting lodge his symptoms had disappeared. At the time of his return to his physician one month later, his ulcer was found to be healed and he was free from symptoms.

For some patients, hospitalization is therapeutic because it provides a setting in which the patient can be dependent without feeling guilty about wanting to be dependent. A hospital is a place where he can be looked after. He can feel comfortable in allowing others to assume responsibility for his care. For this patient, the healing of his ulcer is favored by an atmosphere in which he is allowed and encouraged to be dependent. He not only wants, but needs,

[50] Trade name.

to have his needs anticipated and met. He wants and needs to be freed from responsibility for a time. If he is a patient who is undemanding, his need for dependence may be overlooked. Mrs. Maple, who was shy and quiet, was such a patient. One statement that she made to the nurse indicated that she had the desire to be dependent. She said, "I'm so glad to have a nurse who does things for you." "At home, Joe always makes me make the decisions about how the money is to be spent and when to discipline the children. I wish that he would take more responsibility."

At the other extreme is the patient who is unable to allow others to assume responsibility for his care and overtly overreacts at the slightest frustration. For example, Mr. Johns watches a clock, to be sure that he gets his medication at the exact time it is scheduled. As the hour approaches, his muscles become tense and he becomes more and more angry. Should the nurse be two minutes late, he becomes highly distraught. The nurse knows that she cannot possibly distribute medications to all 30 patients at the same time and that a reasonable interval before or after the hour is acceptable. Because the patient attacks an approved practice and the nurse herself feels attacked, she too may feel angry. If she can recognize that the behavior of the patient is his usual way of reacting in frustrating situations and that she just happens to be the person who is present, then she may be able to avoid personalizing his remarks and to remain objective. She will be better able to develop a plan to increase the confidence of the patient that he will, in fact, receive the care he requires. Instead of responding with anger, she may try to administer Mr. Johns's medication at the scheduled hour. When the medication is one that can be safely left at the bedside of the patient, this possibility may be discussed with the physician and, with his approval, the drug may be left with the patient. Once the nurse has established a trusting relationship with the patient, problems such as the above tend to be less acute.

Because of the importance of psychic stimuli in promoting gastric secretion and motility, drugs are also prescribed to decrease the responsiveness of the individual. The physician prescribed phenobarbital, secobarbital (Seconal[51]) and prochlorperazine maleate (Compazine[51]) for Mrs. Maple. Phenobarbital, 30 mg, was administered every four hours during the daytime. Because of its relatively prolonged sedative action, phenobarbital maintained Mrs. Maple in a continuous state of relaxation. Secobarbital 0.1 gm, a relatively short-acting barbiturate, was prescribed for the hour of sleep, should Mrs. Maple require it for restful sleep. After the first evening, Mrs. Maple did not require it. Mrs. Maple, as well as other patients who are receiving relatively large doses of barbiturates, should be observed for indications of excessive depression of the nervous system. Furthermore, the patient who sleeps most of the time should be moved and turned regularly as well as be offered fluids.

In place of, or in combination with, phenobarbital, any one of a number of

[51] Trade name.

tranquilizing agents may be prescribed for the patient. The desired effect is to lessen the response of the individual to stimuli. These drugs modify the cephalic phase of gastric secretion; that is, they lessen secretion in response to sight, smell, or taste of food. With a decrease in the cephalic phase, the gastric phase of secretion may also be less intense.

The indications for and the effects of surgical therapy in the treatment of peptic ulcer have been discussed elsewhere. Should bleeding recur or her ulcer fail to heal, surgery may be considered in the treatment of Mrs. Maple.

To summarize briefly, at the time of the admission of Mrs. Maple to the hospital, she was suffering from the effects of blood loss. Because an adequate volume of blood is essential to maintaining tissue nutrition, the restoration of the lost blood was the objective receiving priority. As soon as bleeding stopped and the blood which had been lost was replaced, attention was then directed toward treating her ulcer. Because an ulcer is a local manifestation of a constitutional disease, attention to Mrs. Maple as a person was as important as treating her ulcer. The fundamental objective of care was to reduce the effect of acid-pepsin in gastric juice on the lining of the duodenum. Since the stomach responds to a wide variety of stimuli by increased secretion and motility, treatment was planned to decrease Mrs. Maple's responsiveness to environmental stimuli as well as to neutralize gastric acidity.

Since peptic ulcer is a chronic disease characterized by periodic recurrences, Mrs. Maple should know that the ulcer may be reactivated at a later time. She should be advised to see her physician immediately should she develop pain or nausea. Delay not only increases the difficulty in healing the ulcer, but predisposes to complications. Inasmuch as she is able, Mrs. Maple should try to avoid situations that are upsetting to her. Possibly, Mr. Maple could be encouraged to assume more responsibility for family matters. Before approaching this problem with either Mr. or Mrs. Maple, the nurse should discuss the problem with the physician, who may decide to refer Mr. and Mrs. Maple to social service or to some other agency, such as the Family Service Society. As with other chronic illnesses, one of the important factors in the control of peptic ulcers is the strengths and resources of the patient and his family.

What are the functions of the middle portion of the alimentary canal and how does disease of the structures affect the individual?

The middle portion of the alimentary canal extends from the duodenal papilla to the mid-transverse colon. It consists, therefore, of the lower duodenum, the jejunum, the ileum, the cecum, the ascending colon, and the first portion of the transverse colon. This portion of the digestive tube functions as do other parts of the alimentary canal to move its contents analward (toward the anus). Its specific functions are to dilute, digest, and absorb nutrients. Because the mid-portion of the alimentary canal is where nutrients are transported from the external to the internal environment, the most critical function of the alimentary canal as a service facility is accomplished here. With the exception of water, absorption of nutrients is largely completed before the intestinal contents reach the ileocecal valve. The ileocecal valve acts to regulate the movement of material into the cecum and normally prevents the reflux of the contents of the colon into the small intestine. Acute obstruction of the colon distal to the ileocecal valve induces reverse peristalsis and relaxation of the ileocecal valve. Reverse peristalsis may be sufficiently active to carry fecal material to the stomach after which it is vomited. The emesis which results has a fecal odor. Needless to say, observation of the odor of vomitus is important. In terms of survival, the mid-alimentary tract is the most important region of the alimentary canal. Although a portion can be sacrificed, enough of the ileum must remain for the absorption of nutrients. Large quantities of fluid enter the jejunum from the duodenum and stomach, and secretions are added by the jejunum. Disturbances in the motility, secretion, or absorption in the mid-portion of the alimentary canal impair nutrition and hydration by decreasing the length of time nutrients and water remain in the intestine or by interfering with their absorption. Important disorders are summarized at the end of the chapter.

What are the functions of the lower portion of the alimentary canal and how does disease of the structures affect its function?

The lower portion of the alimentary canal extends from the mid-portion of the transverse colon to and including the anal sphincters. Because the portion distal to the ileocecal valve forms the large intestine and many of the disorders involving these structures are similar or involve the whole area, the entire large-intestine wall will be discussed here.

Although the surgical removal of the entire large intestine is possible, it is attended by considerable risk. A part or all of the large intestine can be bypassed by anastomosing two sections of the intestine or by bringing a portion of the intestine to the outside, usually through the abdominal wall. Complete or partial resection or bypassing of the large intestine with or without the formation of an artificial anus is not only compatible with life, but, once the individual has adjusted to the change, is compatible with a full and active life. Although the large intestine completes the absorption of water and stores and evacuates the residue left from the digestion of food, these functions can be accomplished by the remaining portion or by the distal end of the ileum.

The large intestine is the site of a number of important diseases. They include cancer, chronic ulcerative colitis, diverticultiis, and hemorrhoids. Abscesses and fissures in the region of the external anal region are not uncommon. Since the above disorders are summarized at the end of the chapter or discussed elsewhere, they will not be presented here. Two common effects of disease or disturbances on the function of the large intestine include diarrhea and constipation. Lesions, such as benign and malignant neoplasms or strictures formed in the process of healing, that narrow the lumen of the intestine will in time prevent the passage of the contents through the large intestine, that is, block or obstruct it.

Diarrhea and constipation are terms used to indicate alterations in the normal pattern of defecation. Because of the wide range in bowel habits among healthy individuals, these terms are difficult to define precisely. For the purpose of this discussion, diarrhea is defined as the passage of several unformed stools as a result of the rapid movement of the fecal contents through the large intestine. By way of contrast, constipation is associated with undue delay in the passage of feces. Because the feces remain in the intestine for an unduly long period of time, water is absorbed, and they are hard and dry. Defecation may be accompanied by discomfort. Both diarrhea and constipation are relatively common, and either can be due to a disturbance in the regulatory mechanisms controlling the functioning of the large bowel or to mechanical interference with the progress of its contents. Inflammatory disorders of the large intestine are more likely to cause diarrhea than constipation. Hyperactivity of the stomach and small intestine predispose to diarrhea for reasons to be explained later.

Acute disturbances in the function of the digestive system are second only to acute respiratory disease as a cause of morbidity. Any acute disorder increasing the activity of one part of the alimentary canal is likely to affect the function of other parts. An affected individual is likely to experience both vomiting and diarrhea. Similar to vomiting, diarrhea is one of the defense mechanisms utilized by the gastrointestinal tract to rid itself of harmful agents. In diarrhea, the intestine is hyperactive.

The intestine, like other areas in the alimentary canal, is under control of the autonomic nervous system. Although defecation is largely a reflex action, it is subject to some voluntary control. Unless the contractions of the bowel are very powerful, defecation can be delayed for a time. The defecation reflex is similar to other reflexes in the body. Receptor cells in the rectum, which is normally empty, are stimulated by material entering the rectum. Impulses are carried to the defecation centers in the hypothalamus, where they are relayed to the intestinal muscles. Interconnections between the hypothalamus and the cerebral cortex make it possible for messages to be sent from the cerebral cortex to the hypothalamus which modify the activity of the defecation center. As indicated above, feces are not normally stored in the rectum, but they are stored in the sigmoid and adjacent portions of the colon. The fecal content is moved to the storage areas by the same type of peristaltic action found in other parts of the alimentary canal.

A mass type of movement, known as the gastrocolic reflex, also occurs. It usually follows a meal or the ingestion of a glass or two of cold water or fruit juice on arising in the morning. Some persons make a practice of drinking a glass or two of fluid shortly after arising in the morning to prevent constipation. The cold fluid moves rapidly through the stomach and into the duodenum and acts as a stimulus to activate the gastrocolic reflex. The entire small intestine is excited and the wave of contraction passes rapidly along the colon with the result that feces enter the rectum. Whether or not the anal sphincters are relaxed at this time will depend on the propulsive power of intestinal contractions and the cooperation of the individual with the reflex. For this treatment to be successful, the person should pay attention to the call to defecate. If he successfully inhibits defecation, future efforts will be increasingly unsuccessful.

As defined earlier, diarrhea is a condition in which a number of unformed stools are defecated. From the above description of the defecation reflex, it is evident that diarrhea can result from any condition in which peristalsis becomes hyperactive. As in other reflex activity, stimuli may act on receptors in the lining of the alimentary canal or be of central origin. Simply, diarrhea can result from irritation of the lining of the intestine resulting in hyperactivity of the intestine or it may be of nervous origin.

Two examples of diarrhea of neurogenic origin follow. One is Joan Book, who usually has diarrhea just preceding an examination. She calls her condition "nervous diarrhea." Jean Servus is the second example. When Jean consulted her physician because she had had repeated attacks of diarrhea over the past few months, no evidence of an organic lesion was found to account for her difficulty. After some discussion, Jean remembered that her episodes of diarrhea began following a violent quarrel with her father. The problem had not been resolved and she felt that her father was continuing to harass her. Each time Jean and her father had an argument or he was sarcastic, Jean had an episode of diarrhea. Once she understood the relationship of her feelings to diarrhea, it became less troublesome.

Although diarrhea of neurogenic origin is not uncommon, the usual cause is some agent irritating the intestinal mucosa. Irritants can be of endogenous or exogenous origin. Microorganisms are among the more frequent causative agents of acute diarrhea. In the United States infection is most frequently caused by a virus, a *Salmonella* or the *Endamoeba histolytica*. The nature of each of these is summarized at the end of the chapter. Diarrhea, as well as nausea and vomiting, is frequently associated with the onset of acute diseases of the gastrointestinal tract.

Whenever a person experiences repeated attacks of diarrhea, he should be examined by his physician because it may be associated with a serious disorder, which may respond to treatment if treated early. Furthermore, when diarrhea continues, important nutrients and fluids are lost from the body. In severe diarrhea there is probably always some impairment in absorption. In disorders in which absorption is markedly reduced, large quantities of fat and protein may be lost. For example, in sprue, failure to absorb fat and protein results in large, bulky, foamy feces with a foul odor. Maintenance of even a minimal nutritional status may be difficult.

In obstructive lesions of the large intestine, diarrhea alternates with constipation. As the lumen of the bowel is reduced in size, liquid feces are moved past the site of the obstruction and evacuated. During periods when the feces accumulate behind the obstruction, constipation occurs. The most serious cause of this type of diarrhea is cancer. Fecal impactions can, however, be responsible for the same combination of symptoms. Diarrhea is a manifestation in a number of generalized disorders, such as hyperthyroidism, lymphosarcoma, and tuberculosis. It, too, can be of allergic origin. Radiation therapy of pelvic and abdominal organs predisposes to diarrhea.

From the above, the conclusion that diarrhea occurs frequently and is associated with a variety of disorders is obvious. The effects of diarrhea will depend on its cause and severity as well as how long it persists and the age and state of health of the individual who has diarrhea. Age is a significant factor, as diarrhea in a young infant can soon cause a serious depletion of electrolytes, water, and nutrients. Unless the disorder is promptly corrected, the life of the child can be threatened. A bout of diarrhea in a youth or adult is likely to cause some feeling of unfitness, but need not be the source of alarm unless it is very severe or continues for more than a few hours.

Although few persons escape or fail to recover from an occasional episode of diarrhea, excessive or prolonged diarrhea leads to the loss of water and nutrients from the body and predisposes to malnutrition. Undernutrition may be worsened by the fact that anorexia, nausea, and vomiting discourage the intake of food. When cramping accompanies diarrhea, the individual may be afraid to eat. Loss of nutrients may be exaggerated when diarrhea is due to failure to digest or absorb food, or when there is a large outpouring of mucus into the alimentary canal. Erosion of blood vessels accompanied by bleeding is a frequent observation in patients whose diarrhea is due to an ulcerating lesion or lesions. In chronic or severe diarrhea, nutrition is always affected to some extent by failure to ingest food and by losses of nutrients, mucus, and blood.

Whenever diarrhea fails to clear up in a few hours and the person does not recover completely in a day or two, medical attention should be sought. The physician will try to determine the nature of the cause of the diarrhea and what effect, if any, this has had on the nutritional status of the individual. The medical plan of therapy will then be dependent on the cause of diarrhea and the general status of the individual. The nurse contributes to diagnosis through observations of the patient and by assisting with medical examinations. The nurse usually participates in the therapy by administering medications and other forms of treatment. In addition to the above, the nurse carries the responsibility for the comfort of the patient and for improving his nutritional status. When the patient is known to harbor or is suspected to harbor agents that are transmissible to others, the nurse has the responsibility for planning and enforcing suitable procedures to protect herself and others.

One important way in which information is collected is by observation of the feces. Pertinent observations include color, odor, consistency—formed, liquid, frothy—number and frequency, and the presence of foreign matter such as blood, mucus, pus, and worms. What symptoms accompany defecation; that is, does the patient have cramping, urgency, pain, or tenesmus on defecation? Tenesmus is the term for the sharp, unpleasant contractions in the lower-left quadrant associated with straining during defecation. Following defecation, the patient feels only partly relieved. The nurse is more helpful when she describes the sensations as they are related by the patient in his own words than when she names them. Does he have abdominal or other pain? Where is it located? Under what conditions are the symptoms of the patient worsened? Improved? For example, is defecation initiated by eating or activity? Is the patient relieved following defecation, or does he feel as if he had only partly evacuated his bowels? Observations of vital signs are of particular significance when diarrhea is associated with infection or hemorrhage. Some of the causes of diarrhea are listed in Figure 10-4. The nursing of the patient who suffers from a disorder accompanied by chronic diarrhea taxes the patience and ingenuity of any nurse. Mrs. John Reddy, who is 24 years of age, has a diagnosis of chronic ulcerative colitis. A year ago, shortly after her marriage to a promising young businessman, she suffered an attack of diarrhea with pus, blood, and fibrin in the stool. At the time of her admission to Special Hospital, she looked and felt sick. She presented evidence of a poor nutritional state as she had lost 20 lb in weight, her hemoglobin was reduced to 6 gm, and her blood proteins were 5.2 gm per 100 ml. Each day she passed from 10 to 20 rectal discharges of blood, mucus, and pus. With each defecation, she experienced intestinal cramping and straining. Despite frequent defecations, she was not relieved by defecation. The area around the anus was inflamed and sore. When she tried to eat, cramping was intensified. She was aware of the disagreeable odor of her stools. Because of the urgency associated with defecation, Mrs. Reddy was not always able to get on the bedpan in time, and the bed was soiled. Since she was chronically ill and many aspects of her illness were unpleasant, if not repugnant, to others, Mrs. Reddy worried about her marriage and the reaction of her husband to her illness. Quite understandably, she was anxious and depressed.

In making a nursing care plan for Mrs. Reddy, her nurse established two objectives. The *first* was to increase her comfort and the *second* to try to improve her nutritional status. To accomplish the first objective, the nurse planned to wash, dry, and powder the anal region after each defecation. To protect the bed from soiling, an absorbent pad of the type used in disposable diapers was placed under Mrs. Reddy's buttocks. It was changed each time it was soiled. The bedpan was washed after every use. To help minimize odor, the room was aired after each defecation. Since the outside temperature was cold, a screen was placed in front of the window and an extra blanket was spread over Mrs. Reddy to prevent chilling. After each defecation, Mrs.

FIGURE 10–4
Causes of Diarrhea

Psychogenic and/or neurogenic innervation
1. Vagal (generalized hypermotility of entire alimentary tract)
   - a. Stomach
   - b. Small intestine   } Treatment: surgical { a. Vagotomy
   - c. Ascending colon   b. Gastrectomy
   - d. Transverse colon
2. Sacral (diarrhea alternates with constipation; irritable colon, mucous colitis)
   - a. Descending colon

Classification of diarrhea
1. Inflammatory
   - a. Regional enteritis: distal portion of small intestine
   - b. Ulcerative colitis: distal portion of descending colon
2. Irritative
   - a. Mechanical: small intestine, transverse and descending colon
     1. Fecal impaction
     2. Foreign body
     3. Neoplasm
     4. Intussusception
     5. Extraluminal compression
     6. Angulation
   - b. Chemical: descending colon
     1. Poisons
     2. Cathartics
   - c. Bacterial: small intestine, descending colon
     1. Salmonellae
     2. Shigellae
     3. Staphylococci
     4. Streptococci
     5. B. coli
     6. Clostridia, et al.
   - d. Parasitic: descending colon
     1. Amebiasis
     2. Trichinosis
     3. Ascariasis
3. Malabsorption: small intestine
   - a. Tropical sprue
   - b. Symptomatic sprue
   - c. Celiac disease (adult celiac disease)
   - d. Nontropical sprue
   - e. Whipple's disease
4. Osmotic: small intestine and descending colon
   - a. Saline cathartics
5. Endocrine
   - a. Thyroid
     1. Hyperthyroidism
   - b. Adrenals
     1. Adrenal cortical insufficiency
   - c. Liver
     1. Secreting carcinoid tumors (serotonin)
6. Dietary: descending colon
   - a. Food intolerance
   - b. Coarse food
   - c. Vitamin deficiencies
7. Allergic: descending colon
   - a. Drug sensitivity, or
   - b. Food sensitivity

Reddy was provided with an opportunity to wash her hands. For the first few days, the nurse gave care to Mrs. Reddy; that is, she allowed her to be sick and dependent. She made few demands on her, accepting her as a very sick woman whose behavior could be explained by her illness and who needed a high quality of nursing care.

For the first three days Mrs. Reddy was in the hospital, fluids containing multivitamins were administered by intravenous infusion and she was given 1,000 ml of whole blood. To decrease intestinal peristalsis, her physician prescribed tincture of opium (Laudanum), 0.6 ml (10 minims), every four hours during the daytime. If required, a fifth dose could be administered during the night. For two weeks, she was given 100 ml of water containing 20 mg of prednisolone rectally, morning and evening. Because of her improved condition, a soft diet was prescribed to be started on her fourth day in the hospital. Before Mrs. Reddy's food arrived, she was prepared for the meal by having an opportunity to brush her teeth and wash her face and hands and was assisted to a comfortable position. The room was aired and a clean bedpan was conveniently placed, but covered. Mrs. Reddy had been encouraged to choose what she wanted for breakfast. She asked for a white wheat cereal and toast. The suggestion was made that she eat slowly and drink only a minimum of fluid during her meal. Fluids were encouraged between meals. Iced fluids are generally avoided because they tend to stimulate peristalsis. When Mrs. Reddy complained of a cramping sensation, the suggestion was made that she contract her buttocks and pull them together and try to contract the anus. By practicing this maneuver, she was sometimes able to prevent defecation.

As her nutritional and general status improved, Mrs. Reddy widened her selection of foods. To occupy her time and attention, and to promote relaxation, her physician prescribed occupational therapy. The occupatioal therapist suggested she make pot holders on a "Weave It" frame. By using different colored strands, she could design varying patterns. The motions are, however, repetitive and relaxing. The product is useful and could be sold or given to relatives and friends. To encourage relaxation, her nurse planned regular rest periods for her. She tried to control conditions in her external environment, so that Mrs. Reddy was protected from unnecessary stimulation or irritation. Since any kind of stress, including infection, aggravates the disorder, people with colds were banned from her environment.

In addition to medical therapy, surgical procedures are sometimes indicated. To provide rest and allow the diseased portion of the bowel to heal, an ileostomy may be performed. Since there is a tendency for islands of healthy tissue that are surrounded by areas of disease and cicatrization (scarring) to undergo polyp formation and malignant degeneration, resection of the diseased bowel may be required.

Whatever form of therapy is instituted, the patient with chronic ulcerative colitis is sick. Minimizing the disagreeable effects of the disease includes the control of odors, protection of the skin, and control of conditions in the environment tending to stimulate peristalsis. Owing to the nature of the disease, nutrition is a problem. One of the major problems in nursing the patient is to improve his intake of food. Unless his food intake is improved, however, recovery is doubtful.

In constipation, in contrast to diarrhea, evacuation of feces is delayed, and when they are finally evacuated, feces are frequently hard and dry. Because of the great variability among people, constipation is difficult to define exactly. Many people, though by no means all, defecate once daily. Probably the most frequent cause of constipation is neglect to respond to the normal defecation reflex. With failure to respond, the reflex itself becomes less powerful and constipation results. Constipation can also be the result of a disease process or of agents used in the treatment of disease. Constipation occurs in degenerative diseases of the central nervous system, in severe psychoses, and with the use of drugs such as the ganglionic blocking agents and morphine.

The treatment of simple constipation is primarily education. A regular and convenient time should be selected for defecation. For most people, the defecation reflex is most active after meals, particularly after breakfast. In a family of six or eight with only one bathroom, obviously it will not be available to all members of the family immediately after breakfast. The time selected should be one when the individual can be comfortably relaxed. The individual should be encouraged to "obey" the urge to defecate when it does occur. A diet containing a reasonable amount of bulk and regular exercise, especially before breakfast, are other useful measures in the prevention and treatment of constipation.

For the elderly patient who is poorly motivated or who has a disease which makes change difficult or impossible, the correction of constipation by changing habits of living may not be possible or practical. Measures such as bulky laxatives and oil-retention or other types of enemas may be the most reasonable solution to the problem. In elderly patients and in those who have neurological disorders affecting bowel function, observation of the regularity of defecation as well as the size and consistency of feces is important to the prevention and early detection of fecal impactions. Sick and debilitated individuals, especially if elderly, and persons with lesions in the nervous system that interfere with the regulation of bowel function are especially predisposed to impaction. Size of the stool is significant as the patient may pass a small amount of feces while retaining and accumulating feces in the lower bowel. Water is absorbed from the fecal material remaining in the bowel, increasing the difficulty with which it is evacuated. In patients who are predisposed to fecal impactions measures such as bulk-producing cathartics and oil-retention enemas may be successful in the prevention of their formation. Once an impaction is formed, it usually has to be broken up manually and removed. Impactions should not occur if the patient is observed and appropriate actions are taken when there is evidence that feces are being retained. Prevention is to be preferred to cure.

What are the causes and effects of obstruction of the lumen in the alimentary canal?

Any disorder interfering with the forward movement of the contents of the alimentary canal is called an obstruction. As indicated earlier, an obstruction in the esophagus interferes with the ability to ingest food. An obstruction of the outlet of the stomach delays or prevents chyme from entering the duodenum. Either the small or large intestine may be the site of an obstruction. For the most part, the discussion of obstruction that follows will be related to blocking of the intestine, large or small. Whatever the nature of obstruction or its site or location, however, it interferes with the accomplishment of the function of the alimentary canal. Three primary types of disturbances predispose to obstruction. They are mechanical blocking of the lumen, reduced or absent peristalsis, and impaired circulation due to the occlusion of the blood supply.[52] Mechanical blocking may have its origin in abnormalities within the wall of the alimentary canal or outside it. Neoplasms, unreduced volvulus, and incarcerated hernias are a few of many causes of mechanical obstruction.

Absent peristalsis is usually due to some disturbance in the function of the autonomic nervous system associated with surgical or other trauma. As a result of reflex inhibition of the gastrointestinal tract, the stomach may be acutely dilated by retained secretions and swallowed air. Complete cessation of motor activity of the small intestine produces a functional obstruction and is referred to as paralytic ileus. Impairment of the circulation may be caused by a thrombosis of the mesenteric artery. In both the neurogenic and the vascular types of obstruction, the lumen of the bowel is open. The effect is that of obstruction, however, because the affected parts of the bowel do not propel its contents forward. Decompression is necessary to restore normal blood flow to the bowel wall and to relieve shock. As a result of the obstruction the intestine and stomach are distended by gas and fluids. The gas is presumed to have its origin in the air that is swallowed. As the pressure within the bowel increases, absorption decreases. When the pressure within the intestine equals the diastolic blood pressure, absorption ceases. The effect of distention on the circulation of blood to the wall of the intestine is similar to that of pressure on any tissue. First the venous outflow from the tissue is impaired. This leads to a slowing of the blood flow through the tissue and the development of edema. If the condition is allowed to continue, arterial blood flow is impaired and finally ceases. With the failure in the flow of blood to the tissue, tissue necrosis occurs. Death of a portion of the alimentary tract may lead to perforation of the viscus and to the death of the individual.

Obstruction in the gastrointestinal tract also leads to shock. One of the factors in the development of shock is that distention of the stomach and intestine is a powerful stimulus to secretion.[53] Secretion combined with a failure of absorption leads to the trapping of a large volume of fluid within the

[52] Gius, *Op. cit.*, p. 376.
[53] *Ibid.*, p. 377.

gastrointestinal tract and to a reduction in the blood volume. Therefore, when obstruction is allowed to progress, shock eventually develops. As the stomach and/or bowel distends, the increase in their volume has an adverse effect on respiratory and circulatory function. Increased intra-abdominal pressure reduces vital capacity by interfering with the depression of the diaphragm. It also interferes with the return flow of blood from the lower extremities by direct pressure on the veins.

Before definitive treatment can be instituted, the stomach and/or intestine must be deflated by the removal of gas and fluid. Decompression is accomplished by the introduction into the stomach or intestine of a tube to which suction is applied. The principles on which decompression therapy is based are described in Chapter 15. As the bowel is decompressed, the blood supply to the wall improves. With the improvement of the nutrition of the wall, functional disorders such as paralytic ileus tend to correct themselves. Structural lesions usually require some form of surgical therapy to remove or relieve the effects of obstruction. One of the important responsibilities of the nurse in the care of the patient who has a gastric or intestinal obstruction is to maintain the suctioning apparatus in good working order. Since respiratory and circulatory function is impaired, attention must be given to nursing measures that support these functions.

Summary

Understanding of the effects of disease on some portion of the alimentary canal requires knowledge of the following:

1. The structure and function of each part.
2. The mechanisms regulating each part, so that it performs its function and its activity is coordinated with that of other parts of the alimentary canal.
3. The mechanisms for regulating the function of the alimentary canal so that the nutritional needs of the individual are met.

Disease may be due to disorders in the regulation of function or to alteration in the structure of the alimentary canal. The manifestations of disease of the alimentary canal result from the effect of injuring agents (in a broad sense) on the structure and function, from failure of the canal to defend the integrity of its lining, and from interference with the intake of food and water. Furthermore, most of the wall of the alimentary canal is richly supplied with blood. Disorders in which the lining membrane is damaged predispose to bleeding. Thrombosis of arteries or veins supplying any part of the alimentary canal predisposes to tissue necrosis. Esophageal and hemorrhoidal veins have the tendency under certain circumstances to dilate and become tortuous, that is, to form varicosities. Although rupture of varices may occur in either location, those in the esophagus are more likely to be the site of serious hemorrhage. Varicosities of hemorrhoidal veins (hemorrhoids) may become thrombosed and painfully inflamed.

To what types of herniation is the alimentary canal predisposed and how do the effects differ?

The alimentary canal is subject to two general types of herniation. In the first type the mucosa prolapses through the muscle wall forming a sac or pouch known as a diverticulum. The two most common sites for the formation of diverticuli are the colon and the esophagus. Similar to the appendix, the diverticuli may become filled with food or feces and become inflamed or perforated. Inflammation of a diverticulum is known as diverticulitis.

In the other types of herniation, the mesentery or one or more of the organs escape through a ring through which body structures pass. Common types of hernias involving the alimentary canal include esophageal hiatus hernia and inguinal, femoral, umbilical, and postoperative ventral hernia. The name indicates the ring through which the organ prolapses. Thus in an esophageal hiatus hernia, contents of the abdominal cavity protrude through the gap in the diaphragm into the thoracic cavity. Most types of hernia predispose the patient to two dangers, obstruction of the alimentary canal and necrosis of the trapped tissues.

What are the nurse's contributions to making the medical diagnosis?

Although the making of the medical diagnosis is a primary function of the physician, the nurse assists in a number of ways. One of the most valuable contributions a nurse can make to medical diagnosis is to accurately observe and report and record her observations. The nurse uses her senses, hearing, touch, sight, and smell to gain information about the patient and the effects of his disease and therapy. One of the significant aspects of observation is an alertness to changes in the behavior of the patient and any conditions in his environment that appear to be related. For example, each time Mrs. Smathers receives morphine sulfate, 15 to 20 minutes later she vomits. Mrs. Cletus, who has had a gastric resection, suffers an attack of severe pain on each of her husband's infrequent visits. After Mr. Brave returned to his room following a gastric resection, he vomited bright red blood. Each of the above has implications for the diagnosis and treatment of the respective individuals. Mrs. Smathers probably has an intolerance to morphine and another drug should be substituted for it. Unless the nurse makes the connection between the time the drug is administered and the time vomiting occurs, Mrs. Smathers may continue to be made uncomfortable. Unless the observation is made about the time Mrs. Cletus' pain occurs, the emotional factors in her illness may be missed. Finally, unless the nurse knows how much blood Mr. Brave has vomited and knows whether it is within the amount to be expected, the survival of the patient may be threatened.

In addition to collecting information through observation of the patient, the nurse assists in diagnosis by preparing the patient for examination, by performing certain parts of some diagnostic tests, and by collecting secretions or excretions from the alimentary canal. Examinations for disease of the alimentary canal are of three different types. The canal or some part of it is directly or indirectly visualized, the contents are collected for examination, or determinations are made to assess the effects of the disorder on the nutritional status of the individual.

The details for the preparation of patients for different diagnostic tests vary from one institution or physician to another. A few generalizations will, however, be made that should be helpful. The different types of tests will be defined or described and the conditions necessary to their performance suggested.

Earlier, it was stated that the direct observation of the lining mucosa of an organ is known as endoscopy. The term for a particular endoscopic examination is formed by joining the combining form for the organ with the suffixscope: thus, esophagoscope, laryngoscope, gastroscope, or proctoscope. Obviously, direct visualization of the mucosa is limited to the organs that are accessible from the natural orifices, the mouth and the anus. An exception is a peritoneoscopic examination. A small incision is made in the abdominal wall to gain entrance into the peritoneal cavity. In addition to providing a means for the examination of the appearance of the mucosa or peritoneum, tissue and secretions can be removed for purposes of examination.

X ray is utilized in fluoroscopy and in making shadow photographs of all organs of the alimentary canal from the esophagus to the anus. In both procedures a contrast medium is introduced into the organ to be studied. In fluoroscopy the progress or movement of the contrast medium through the canal can be followed. As the roentgen rays pass through the body, they are projected onto a fluorescent screen. X rays are shadow photographs that provide a permanent record.

Secretions from the upper and mid-portions of the alimentary canal can be removed for examination. Secretions are examined for the concentration of normal constituents and for substances not normally present in the secretion. The capacity of the glands of the stomach to respond to food or other secretory agents can also be determined. Both secretions and excretions are examined for blood, pus, and microorganisms. Feces are also examined for parasites and ova.

Examination for the effect of disease on the nutritional status of the individual includes weighing the patient and observing for signs of rapid loss of weight and for evidence of dehydration. Hemoglobin, erythrocyte determinations, and hematocrit all provide evidence for or against nutritional anemia. In the seriously dehydrated patient, hemoglobin level and erythrocyte count may be within normal levels despite the presence of anemia. With the restoration of a normal state of hydration, hemoglobin and erythrocyte levels fall.

The preparation of the patient for examination of the alimentary canal will, of course, depend on the nature of the test to be performed. In general, food and fluid are withheld in preparation for examinations of the upper and middle alimentary canal and previous to roentgen examination of the large bowel. Obviously food or fluids in the stomach or intestine will interfere with the performance of the examination by getting in the way of the instrument or by occupying space. In studies made on gastric juice, the physician is interested in determining the concentration of hydrochloric acid before and sometimes after the acid-secreting glands are stimulated. Therefore, gastric juice is tested for acid while the patient is in the fasting state. The patient may then be given a test meal consisting of dry toast or arrowroot cookies and weak tea or water and the test repeated. Secretion of gastric juice can be further increased by the ingestion of ethyl alcohol or the subcutaneous injection of histamine phosphate U. S. P. Since histamine dilates arterioles and capillaries, susceptible patients may experience a marked drop in blood pressure. It is probably well for the patient who is to receive histamine to be in bed. If the fall in blood pressure is marked, it may be necessary to place the patient in a Trendelenburg position. Other effects of histamine include intense headache, shortness of breath, vomiting, and diarrhea. According to Resnik,[54] gastric analysis no longer occupies the position of importance that it once did in the diagnosis of disease of the stomach and intestine.

In endoscopic examinations of the upper alimentary canal, food and fluid should be withheld because the swallowing reflex is depressed when the pharynx is anesthetized before the tube is passed. Should the patient vomit, he is in danger of aspirating food or fluid into the airway. Care of the patient during and following endoscopic examination of the esophagus is similar to that following bronchoscopic examination and will not be further described.

Preparation of the large intestine for examination by X ray or endoscopy requires a number of procedures to cleanse the bowel. The procedures should be conscientiously performed, as either feces or gas interferes with the filling of the bowel with the contrast medium and thereby distorts the resulting shadow.

Following roentgen examination of the gastrointestinal tract, particularly after colon X rays, the barium sulfate introduced into the bowel as a contrast medium should be evacuated. The patient may be instructed to take or be given an enema to wash out the barium remaining at the end of the procedure. Unless it is removed, it may form a hard mass in the bowel because the water is absorbed.

During the period when the patient is undergoing diagnosis, the nurse makes a number of valuable contributions. Through conscientious and in-

[54] William H. Resnik, "Indigestion, Dysphagia, Nausea and Vomiting," in Harrison, *Op. cit.,* p. 131.

formed observations, she collects information about the patient and his reactions to his disease, to diagnostic procedures, and to therapy. She helps to prepare the patient both physically and psychologically for the different diagnostic procedures. She cares for the patient during and after the examinations are performed. One point that has not been made that bears emphasis is that many of the methods utilized in the examination of the alimentary canal are unpleasant. They require that meals be withheld and the contents of the canal be removed by catharsis, enema, and stomach tube. In the performance of some examinations a tube may be introduced into the mouth or the anus. Neither is accompanied by pleasant sensations. Although the patient knows that the various procedures are necessary, he still feels miserable. In all probability he is anxious about the outcome of the various examinations. He may, with or without reason, fear that he has cancer. Insofar as is possible, the patient should be protected from preventable sources of distress. He should be prepared for what to expect and what he can do to help himself. Attention to his personal hygiene and to serving his meals promptly after a test is completed may not seem to be crucial to the onlooker, but can do much to remove controllable sources of irritation.

In the preceding discussion, the functions of the alimentary canal, as well as something about the nature of disorders in function, have been discussed. In addition to the secretions from glands in the mucosa of the alimentary canal, secretions from two glands external to but emptying into the duodenum have a significant role in digestion. These glands are the liver and the pancreas.

What are the functions of the liver?

The liver is not only the largest, but it is the most complex, organ in the body. Ingelfinger[55] states that the liver has four main systems—blood vessels, reticuloendothelial Küppfer cells, parenchymal cells, and the biliary channels. All these systems are so intimately related that any considerable or continuing pathology in one inevitably leads to disturbances in others. Injury can be the result of direct extension of a pathological process or the response of the tissues to injury. In the adult, the vascular system of the liver stores and filters blood. The Küppfer cells—a specialized type of reticuloendothelial cells—in the lining of the venous channels of the liver play an important role in defense as they phagocytize potentially harmful agents circulating through the liver. Parenchymal cells secrete bile and play an essential role in the intermediary metabolism of most nutrients. The biliary channels store, concentrate, and conduct bile from the liver to the alimentary canal.

In the study of the liver, one is impressed with the interrelatedness of bodily functions and structure. For example, the most frequent cause of vascular congestion in the liver is congestive heart failure due to the failure of

---

[55] Franz J. Ingelfinger, "The Liver," in Sodeman, *Op. cit.,* p. 750.

the right side of the heart as a pump. In health, the heart is able to eject as much blood into the circulation as is delivered to it and to accommodate its output to the quantity of blood returning by way of the venous system. (See Chapter 9.) In right-sided heart failure, stasis of blood in the right atria impedes the flow of blood from the inferior vena cava with the result that the blood pressure rises in the inferior vena cava. As the blood pressure rises in the inferior vena cava, pressure is transmitted to the hepatic veins and blood accumulates in the liver, causing the liver to swell. As the liver swells, it enlarges. Because the capsule surrounding the liver offers resistance to swelling, pressure within the liver rises. As in any other tissue in which venous congestion occurs, blood supply to the tissue is impeded by failure to remove blood at about the same rate as it enters.

Approximately three fourths of the blood delivered to the liver is venous blood and is carried by the portal system. The other one quarter is arterial blood conveyed by the hepatic artery. Because such a high proportion of the blood circulated to the liver is venous blood, oxygen supply, under the most favorable circumstances, tends to be marginal. Any condition decreasing the blood supply through the liver, therefore, predisposes to some degree of hypoxia. In addition to causing a deficient supply of oxygen to liver cells, congestion in the liver elevates the blood pressure in the veins forming the portal system. Since fluids move in the direction of least resistance, the elevation of blood pressure within the portal system is reflected by congestion of the wall of the stomach, esophagus, and duodeum. In the esophagus, elevated venous pressure predisposes to esophageal varices. In the stomach and duodenum, elevated portal pressure predisposes to peptic ulcer.

In the liver itself, swelling interferes with parenchymal cell function and may, when severe, obstruct ducts of the biliary canal. Jaundice due to a failure to remove bile pigments is a frequent sign in severe right-sided heart failure.

What is the function of the liver in digestion?

At this point, the function of the liver in digestion and absorption will be presented. Metabolic functions will be discussed later in the chapter. The liver functions in digestion by the secretion of bile. Since bile contains substances which are discharged into the internal environment, it is an excretion as well. From 600 to 800 ml of bile is formed each day. Drainage of all of the bile secreted each day results in the loss of fluid and requires replacement. In addition to water, the important constituents of bile are cholesterol, bile salts, bile pigments, and lecithin. Since the biliary tract is lined with mucous membrane, bile contains some mucus.

Bile formed in the liver is conveyed by way of a series of channels or ducts to the duodenum. Liver cells are arranged around ducts which join together to form larger ducts and finally leave the liver as the common hepatic duct. The common hepatic duct branches to form the cystic duct leading to the gall bladder where bile is stored and concentrated. The duct formed by the common hepatic and cystic ducts is the common bile duct. It opens, usually in common with the duct of Wirsung from the pancreas, into the duodenum. The terminal portion of the common bile duct and the duct of Wirsung are known

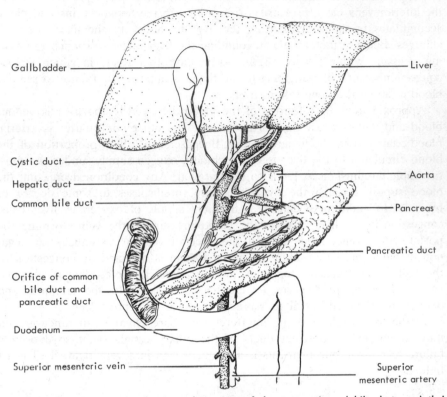

Gallbladder — Liver

Cystic duct —

Hepatic duct — Aorta

Common bile duct — Pancreas

Pancreatic duct

Orifice of common bile duct and pancreatic duct

Duodenum —

Superior mesenteric vein — Superior mesenteric artery

F I G U R E   10 – 5.   Diagram showing relationships of the pancreatic and bile ducts and their entrance into the duodenum. Where might obstructions be located to produce jaundice? (Adapted with permission of The Macmillan Company from *Textbook of Physiology,* Fig. 100, p. 278, by Caroline E. Stackpole and Lutie C. Leavell. Copyright 1953 by The Macmillan Company.)

as the ampulla of Vater. The opening into the duodenum is guarded by a muscle called the sphincter of Oddi. For the structural relationships of these organs see Figure 10-5.

Between meals, bile, which is secreted more or less continuously, is stored in the gall bladder, where it is concentrated. When fat enters the intestine, a hormone, cholecystokinin, is secreted by the intestinal mucosa and carried to the gall bladder by way of the blood. It stimulates the muscle in the gall bladder to contract thus forcing the bile out into the bile ducts. At the same time the sphincter of Oddi relaxes and bile enters the duodenum along with the pancreatic juice.

The patency of the bile ducts and the capacity of the gall bladder to store and concentrate bile are evaluated by the administration of an iodinated organic compound which is opaque to X ray. The usual method for the administration of the dye is by mouth, but it may be given by intravenous injection. Dye may also be injected directly into biliary canals in patients having a T tube or at the time of surgery involving the biliary tract. After absorption of the dye into the blood, it is removed by the liver and secreted into the bile. When the substance is administered orally to a healthy person, sufficient dye will have been excreted into the biliary canals to render them opaque to X ray in about 12 hours. The success of the examination depends on normal motility and absorbing powers of the alimentary canal, normal liver function, patent biliary channels, an empty gall bladder at the time the test is initiated, and a gall bladder capable of concentrating and storing bile. To make sure the gall bladder has been emptied before the dye is administered, the patient may be given a fatty meal the morning and noon before the tablets are administered. The evening that the dye is given the patient has a liquid low-fat meal. Following the initial X rays, the capacity of the gall bladder to empty can be checked by the ingestion of a fatty meal. Throughout the period of the examination, food and fluid are limited to those indicated in the directions for the examination. Stimulation of gastric motility and foods stimulating the flow of bile into the alimentary canal are to be avoided after the dye is administered and until the first X rays have been taken, as they will prevent the dye from being concentrated in the gall bladder.

How do the bile salts function in digestion and absorption?

Of the constituents of bile, the only ones functioning in digestion and absorption are the bile salts. Bile salts are formed by the neutralization of cholic acid in the liver and secreted as sodium and potassium salts. Cholic acid is probably formed from cholesterol. The action of bile salts is similar to that of a detergent. They lower the surface tension of fat. In the presence of the bile salts, the fat globules suspended in the watery chyme can be broken up and prevented from merging again. Many small droplets offer a larger surface on which enzymes can act.

Even more important than their action in facilitating the digestion of fat, bile salts are required for the absorption of fatty acids, monoglycerides, and fat-soluble vitamins. In the process of the absorption of fats, bile salts are reabsorbed and returned to the liver to be resecreted. One of the earliest effects of injury of liver cells is a decrease in the secretion of bile salts. Obstruction of the common hepatic or the common bile duct can prevent bile salts from reaching the intestine. One of the most distressing effects observed in patients with lesions associated with obstruction of the biliary tract is pruritus. It is believed to be due to excessive amounts of bile salts in the blood. Mr. Pine, who was admitted with a diagnosis of cancer of the head of the pancreas obstructing the common bile duct, had deep scratches over every part of his body that he could reach. To minimize itching he was given tepid baths to which starch was added and calamine lotion was applied to his skin. Room temperature was regulated not to exceed 68° F. as heat increases the intensity of itching. To lessen the damage to his skin from scratching, his nails were cut short.

In the absence of bile salts, a large part of the ingested fat is lost in the stool in the form of soaps. The stool is pale and frothy in appearance. Fat-soluble vitamins A, D, K, and E are also lost in the stool. Since vitamins A and D are stored in sufficient quantities to last for some time, evidence of vitamin A or D deficiency does not usually occur unless the deficiency continues for months. In contrast, absence of bile salts for more than a few days leads to deficiency in vitamin K. Vitamin K acts as a catalyst in the formation of prothrombin. In the absence of prothrombin, whether due to a vitamin K deficiency or to the administration of one of its antagonists such as bishy-droxycoumarin, the blood fails to clot in the usual period of time. Before the discovery of vitamin K, the surgical treatment of the patient with a common bile duct obstruction was difficult because of the tendency of the patient to bleed. Even small breaks in a blood vessel resulted in bleeding that was difficult to control.

Since bile is alkaline in reaction—its pH is between 8.0 and 8.6—it helps to neutralize the acid chyme entering the duodenum. Under some circumstances bile is regurgitated into the stomach, where it has a similar effect. Enzymes in pancreatic and intestinal juice require a pH of about 7 for optimum function.

In addition to the secretion of bile salts, bile contains substances that are excreted from the body, such as cholesterol and bilirubin. Cholesterol is synthesized in the body and ingested in food. The liver is the chief organ in which cholesterol is synthesized but it is formed in lesser quantities in other tissues, such as the adrenal cortex and skin. Cholesterol is found in fats of animal origin and is readily absorbed from the intestine. Food sources include egg yolk and the fats of meat, liver, liver oils, and brain. Although the level of cholesterol in the blood can be lowered by decreasing the quantity ingested in the diet, synthesis by the liver and other tissues prevents it from being eliminated from the blood. Cholesterol continues to appear in the bile despite its elimination from the diet. The quantity of cholesterol in the bile is not affected by its concentration in the blood.

From what are gall stones formed and what factors contribute to their formation?

Although cholesterol is nearly insoluble in water, it is kept in solution in the bile by bile salts, fatty acids, and lecithin. In some persons, cholesterol and/or bilirubin and calcium carbonate precipitate and form stones (cholelithiasis). Almost all gall stones contain in varying proportions some of each of the above constituents. Even so-called pure stones contains other bile constituents. For example, a "pure" cholesterol stone is about 98 per cent cholesterol. The other 2 per cent is bile pigment and calcium carbonate. Cholesterol, mixed, and pigment stones are relatively common in man. Calcium carbonate stones are uncommon in man but are common in cattle. About 50 per cent of gall stones contain sufficient calcium carbonate to be opaque to X ray. Stones with little or no calcium cannot be detected by X ray without use of contrast media. Cholesterol stones are cream-colored. Pigment stones are dark-colored.

Despite knowledge of the incidence of cholelithiasis as well as of some of the conditions seeming to predispose to the formation of stones, the mechanisms by which stones are formed in bile are not known. Cholelithiasis is presumed to result from some condition upsetting the balance between the factors keeping cholesterol, bile pigments, and calcium carbonate in solution and those favoring their precipitation. Best and Taylor list four general factors favoring precipitation.[56] They are: (1) injury to the lining of the gall bladder, usually by infection, (2) a disturbance in the metabolism of cholesterol, (3) stasis of bile, and (4) a change in the reaction of pH of bile. Each of these conditions acts in some way to decrease the solubility of the constituents of bile or to lessen the effectiveness of the substances or conditions keeping them in solution.

The incidence of cholelithasis is higher among women than among men. According to Ingelfinger,[57] at the time of death, 25 per cent of women and 10 per cent of men have gall stones. Women having had several children are believed to be more susceptible to cholelithiasis than nonparous women. The incidence of cholelithiasis is high among persons having hemolytic jaundice, a condition in which red blood cells are destroyed at an excessive rate. Stones are believed to form because the concentration of bile pigments in the bile is so high that they cannot be kept in solution. They precipitate out and form stones. Infections of the gall bladder, one notable example being typhoid fever, predispose to the precipitation of cholesterol. Changes in the secretion of lipids in the bile may account for the association of gall stones with diabetes mellitus and obesity.

The number of stones found in the gall bladder of any one person varies from 1 to more than 200. They vary in shape and size. Single stones are likely to be smooth and round or oval in shape, while multiple stones are likely to be small and faceted and vary in size and shape.

Signs and symptoms accompanying cholelithiasis are highly variable. About half of the patients have no signs or symptoms referable to the biliary tract, but have so-called silent cholelithiasis. In those who have stones containing

[56] Charles H. Best and Norman B. Taylor, *Physiological Basis of Medical Practice,* 7th ed., The Williams and Wilkins Company, Baltimore, p. 650.
[57] Franz J. Ingelfinger, "Diseases of the Gall Bladder and Bile Ducts," in Harrison, *Op. cit.,* p. 1710.

sufficient calcium carbonate, their presence may be demonstrated by an X ray over the area. Stones may be identified during abdominal surgery or after death during postmortem examination. Signs and symptoms vary from belching and bloating to periodic attacks of biliary colic. Biliary colic is characterized by attacks of pain in the right upper abdomen accompanied by nausea, vomiting, and difficulty in taking a deep breath. The attacks are believed to be due to muscle spasm initiated by a stone passing through the common duct. Attacks may be precipitated by a fatty meal, but they may also occur during the night when the stomach is presumably empty.

Mrs. Helmer is illustrative of the patient who is assumed to be predisposed to cholelithiasis. She is 40 years of age, about 20 lb overweight, and has four daughters. Although gall stones do develop at any age, they are uncommon before the age of 30. Mrs. Helmer was among the 50 per cent of the persons who have cholelithiasis with symptoms. About two o'clock one night, she awakened with excruciating pain in her right upper abdomen. It extended through to the region just under the central side of the right scapula. Her pain was so severe that she arose and walked the floor, bending forward with her arms folded firmly across her chest. Though the room was cool, beads of perspiration stood out on her forehead. She complained of nausea, and her breathing was shallow. Because of the severity of her pain, Mr. Helmer called the family physician, who came and gave Mrs. Helmer 15 mg (gr ¼) of morphine sulfate and suggested that she come into his office as soon as possible for diagnostic tests and probably surgery. In the meantime, Mrs. Helmer was to avoid greasy, fatty, or fried foods and those having strong odor when cooked such as cabbage, turnips, and kale.

The pain was relieved by the morphine and Mrs. Helmer went to sleep. When she awakened in the morning, she had some residual soreness in the affected area, but she felt much better. Although some patients have frequent attacks, Mrs. Helmer continued to feel well for several months. She found that if she avoided fatty foods and cabbage, she was free from symptoms. Being comfortable, busy, and human, she did not make an appointment to see her physician.

Because Mrs. Helmer's gall bladder contained many small stones—over 100 were found in her gall bladder at the time of cholecystectomy—she might have had biliary colic at any time. By delaying treatment Mrs. Helmer was exposing herself to the danger of several serious complications. They include acute and chronic cholecystitis, choledocholithiasis, cholangitis, fistula from the biliary tract to surrounding organs, biliary cirrhosis, carcinoma of the gall bladder, and gall stone ileus. She did develop choledocholithiasis—a stone was lodged in the common duct causing obstruction. On examination in the laboratory her gall bladder was found to be acutely inflamed.

About a year after the attack described above Mrs. Helmer experienced several acute bouts of pain. None were as severe as the first and she could usually relate an attack to a dietary indiscretion. Her final attack was not quite as severe as the first, but instead of disappearing, her symptoms persisted. She could no longer avoid facing the fact that she was ill and she sought admission to the hospital for diagnosis and treatment. At the time of admission, she had pain in the right upper quadrant, nausea and vomiting, a temperature of 101° F., and leukocytosis. She looked and felt sick. Although chills may precede a rise in temperature, she had none. Careful inspection of the sclera of her eyes revealed some icterus. The level of bilirubin in her blood was 2 mg per 100 ml of blood plasma. The normal range is 0.1 to 1.2 mg per 100 ml. Even in the absence of stones in the common duct a transient icterus can occur. Jaundice is probably due to edema, spasm, or inflammation of ducts draining the liver.

Although the history and clinical picture pointed toward choledocholithiasis, a few days were required before Mrs. Helmer was ready for surgery. In addition to the diagnostic procedures cited above, she had an X ray of the abdomen. No preparation was required for it. Her urine was examined for, and, as expected, contained, bilirubin. Urine containing bilirubin is dark in color and forms large bubbles when shaken. Feces were pale or clay-colored.

Because Mrs. Helmer had fever and had been vomiting, she was somewhat dehydrated. She was given fluids containing glucose in physiological saline solution to correct the loss of water, chlorides, and calories. Because her biliary tract was obstructed and she had not been eating for several days, she was given multivitamins plus vitamin K in the intravenous infusion each day. Nursing of Mrs. Helmer during the period of diagnosis and preparation for surgery was directed toward providing comfort and emotional support and preventing complications as well as carrying out the aspects of diagnosis and treatment usually delegated to the nurse. Mrs. Helmer was a very sick woman who was fighting for survival and she behaved as sick people are likely to do. She regressed to a childlike state. Her tone of voice was whining. She complained repeatedly about how miserable she felt when she had to wait for care even briefly. She was petulant and irritable. She required and was provided with the same kind of care any acutely ill person needs. She was given mouth care, was bathed, and had her back rubbed. The external environment was regulated to her need for quiet and comfort. Since she was a member of a large family and had many friends, she required protection from too many visitors and from those who stayed too long. To prevent respiratory and circulatory complications, she was moved and turned and her extremities were passively exercised. Instructions were limited to preparing her for what was to be done at the time and to answering her questions. The nurse assumed full responsibility for the nursing care of Mrs. Helmer. The nurse anticipated her needs and she limited the demands made on Mrs. Helmer for adapting to her environment, including other people.

Although any change in the condition of a patient should be noted and recorded, observations of particular significance, in the instance of Mrs.

Helmer, included increasing jaundice, color of stools and urine, and abdominal pain.

What are other causes of obstruction in the biliary tract?

The second substance excreted by the liver, bilirubin, has been referred to in the discussion of cholelithiasis. Bilirubin is a product of the degradation of heme, the pigmented portion of hemoglobin. It is discussed in greater detail in Chapter 9.

The level and type of bilirubin or its products found in the blood, feces, or urine have several uses in diagnosis. As a product of the breakdown of hemoglobin, they can be used as a measure of the rate of blood destruction. As an excretion product, they can be used as a measure of liver function or of the patency of the biliary tract. In some instances, the site of failure may be indicated by the form in which the substance occurs. For example, bilirubin levels in the blood rise when the rate of blood destruction is excessive, in certain types of injury to liver cells, and in biliary-tract obstruction. In the first instance bilirubin is formed more rapidly than the liver can excrete it. In the second, the liver forms bilirubin, but cannot excrete it. In the third, the flow of bile from the liver to the intestine is blocked. As bilirubin passes through the liver, glucuronic acid combines with the bilirubin molecule to form bilirubin glucoronide,[58] which is soluble in water. Bilirubin is not. Variations in solubility explain the direct and indirect van den Bergh reactions in different types of jaundice. In obstructive jaundice, the reaction is likely to be positive because some of the bilirubin is converted to bilirubin glucuronide by the liver cells. In hemolytic jaundice, the van den Bergh reaction is indirect; that is, the plasma must be treated with alcohol before the color change occurs.

Bilirubin can be measured and expressed in terms of milligrams per 100 ml of blood plasma, or the color of the blood plasma may be compared with a standard. The latter is known as the icterus index. When the level of bilirubin glucuronide in blood plasma increases, it is eliminated in the urine. The amount and type can be measured by the same tests used on blood plasma.

Since bilirubin is responsible for the color of the stool, failure of bilirubin to reach the intestine is indicated when the stool is clay-colored. The stools and urine can be examined for urobilinogen and urobilin, breakdown products of bilirubin. Urobilinogen is increased in hemolytic jaundice and decreased or absent in jaundice due to obstruction.

In another type of excretion test of liver function, a dye is administered by intravenous injection and the rate at which the dye is removed from the blood is measured. Although a number of dyes are available for use, the bromsulfalein (BSP) excretion test is most widely used. In normal persons, 10 to 15

---

[58] Harold A. Harper, *Review of Physiological Chemistry*, 8th ed., Lange Medical Publications, Los Altos, California, 1961, p. 274.

per cent of the dye is removed per minute. Forty-five minutes after the dye is injected less than 5 per cent should remain. The greater the retention of bromsulfalein, the greater is the liver injury.

What are the causes and effects of failure of the liver parenchyma?

In addition to disorders involving the vascular system of the liver and the biliary canals, the liver parenchyma may fail. Because of the large reserve of liver parenchyma, evidence of failure of the metabolic and excretory functions is a relatively late manifestation in liver disease. Approximately 80 per cent of the liver can be destroyed before signs of liver failure appear. The liver is further protected by the great regenerative power of its cells. For example, in acute infectious hepatitis, areas of necrosis regenerate leaving no evidence of previous disease.

As stated earlier, the most frequent cause of vascular congestion is failure of the right side of the heart as a pump. Parenchymatous cells can be injured by a wide variety of agents. They include viruses, bacteria, and animal parasites, chemical poisons, hypersensitivity reactions, metabolic disturbances, nutritional deficiencies, and hypoxia. Parenchymal injury can also result from the disease or obstruction of the biliary tract.

According to Ingelfinger,[59] the effects of the various etiological agents on parenchymous cells of the liver are similar. Three principal factors probably account for similar morphological effects of different etiological agents. With the exception of hypoxia and certain specific poisons such as carbon tetrachloride and carbon trichloride (chloroform), etiological agents are poorly defined. In some patients a number of factors may be interacting to cause injury. Second, the number of ways in which liver cells can respond to injury are limited. Third, by the time the effects of disease of the liver are manifested, the defensive reactions of the liver tend to obscure the original injury.

To illustrate, Mrs. Clarence, aged 42, had a diagnosis of advanced portal cirrhosis of the liver. For the last ten years she had consumed increasing quantities of alcohol. For three or four months preceding her admission to the hospital, she had been drinking heavily and eating very little food. The only food that she ingested consistently was an 8-oz glass of orange juice on arising. Biopsy of her liver demonstrated necrosis of the parenchyma of her liver and extensive fibrosis. What factor or factors were responsible for the injury of Mrs. Clarence's liver? Was it due to the alcohol or poisons contained in it or was it due to lack of important nutrients such as protein and the B vitamins? Probably all these factors played a part.

Manifestations in diseases of the liver depend on a number of factors such as the acuteness or chronicity of the disorder, the extent to which liver function is impaired, and the nature of the response of the liver to injury. Unless

[59] Sodeman, *Op. cit.*, p. 751.

cirrhosis of the liver develops, the patient is not likely to develop ascites. Serious disease of the liver affects to a greater or lesser degree the functioning of all parts of the body.

As might well be expected, disorders of gastrointestinal function frequently accompany liver disease. Many of the gastrointestinal manifestations are due to disorders in motility and are nonspecific, inasmuch as they are commonly seen in illness. They include anorexia, nausea, vomiting, flatulence, diarrhea, constipation, and cramping.

One of the manifestations frequently observed in patients with a diagnosis of disease of the liver is anorexia. Anorexia is of especial significance in the nursing of the patient because one of the keystones in the therapy is a nutritious diet. As indicated above, malnutrition, particularly of protein and the B vitamins, predisposes to injury of liver parenchyma. Despite disagreement among authorities about whether or not protein should be forced in the treatment of acute hepatitis or in cirrhosis of the liver, there is general agreement that a nutritious diet with at least an average intake of protein is a fundamental aspect of treatment. To be of value, food must be eaten. When a patient is severely anorexic, he will usually require considerable attention and support to overcome his disinclination to eat. For example, Mr. Clarence, who has acute infectious hepatitis, in anorexic to the point that the thought of food causes a feeling of revulsion. His doctor has explained to him that anorexia is a cardinal manifestation in acute hepatitis, but that he will recover more rapidly if he will force himself to eat. Kark[60] emphasizes the importance of the patient eating the prescribed diet by saying that food is more than food, it is medicine. By eating, the patient is helping himself to get well. The patient should know why eating is important and he should be given whatever encouragement and assistance he requires. Within the limitations of the dietary requirements, his food preferences should be taken into account in the selection of his food. The patient should be expected to be a "fussy" or "finicky" eater, even if he eats everything when he is well. Food should be served in its most appetizing forms. As long as the patient is acutely ill or becomes exhausted before he has completed eating, he should be fed. If his relationship with family members or friends is such that he will eat when they feed him, they may be enlisted to assist. Emphasis should be on the patient eating. If he does not eat all the food on his tray, the quantity of food remaining should be recorded. If he will eat it or an acceptable substitute at a later time, food should be obtained for him. The nurse often performs a service to the patient by keeping the lines of communication open between the dietitian and the physician. Only by all persons working together in the interest of the patient can his nutritional needs be met.

In disorders of the liver and the biliary tract, digestion of food usually

60 Robert M. Kark, "Nutritional Aspects of Liver Disease in Man," in Michael G. Wohl and Robert S. Goodhard, *Modern Nutrition in Health and Disease,* 2nd ed., Lea and Febiger, Philadelphia, 1960, p. 651.

proceeds normally unless bile is prevented from reaching the alimentary canal. When bile does not reach the duodenum, the usual cause is an obstruction of the biliary tract.

In addition to the manifestations due to effects of illness on gastrointestinal motility and to the absence of bile, changes in gastrointestinal function can also be due to organic changes associated with liver disease. In portal cirrhosis, the alimentary canal may be congested as a consequence of portal hypertension. Not only do the previously listed manifestations of disturbed gastrointestinal function add to the discomfort of the patient, but they interfere with his intake of food, one of the most necessary aspects of his therapy.

What changes in the blood are observed in disease of the liver?

Disease of the liver is frequently accompanied by changes in the blood. These changes can be due to the response of the organism to infectious agents or to cellular necrosis. In infectious hepatitis, neutrophils are frequently decreased and monocytes increased. As indicated above, these changes are probably due to a response of mesenchymal tissues to the infectious agent and are not due to the involvement of the liver per se.

Anemia is a second change not infrequently associated with disease of the liver. The type of anemia found in a particular patient will depend on the factors contributing to its cause. For example, Mrs. Helmer, whose biliary tract was obstructed, developed hypoprothrombinemia from failure to absorb vitamin K. She had a microcytic anemia; that is, her red cells were small in size and pale in color. Patients who have repeated bleeding from esophageal and hemorrhoidal varices may also have a microcytic anemia. Mrs. Clarence had a macrocytic anemia. Her red cells, though decreased in number, were larger than normal size. Normocytic and macrocytic anemias are common in the patient with cirrhosis of the liver. It is not known whether this anemia is due to an increase in blood destruction or to a nutritional deficiency, such as a lack of sufficient folic acid.

A third change in the blood in disorders of the liver is an increase in the tendency to bleed. A common cause is hypoprothrombinemia due to failure to absorb vitamin K. In the patient who has an increased tendency to bleed, despite a normal blood prothrombin, other factors, such as increased capillary permeability or the lack of some other element essential to clotting, are usually at fault. Patients who have a disorder of the liver or biliary tract should be observed for evidences of bleeding. Should they occur, the physician should be apprised of the fact.

Synthesis of blood proteins takes place in the liver. In serious liver disease, synthesis may be deficient and the level of protein in the blood falls.

A phenomenon associated with cirrhosis of the liver is spider telangiectases. These are small, dilated blood vessels resembling a spider in form. They may be observed in the skin in various parts of the body.

What are some of the disturbances in water and electrolyte balance in liver disease?

In the disease of the liver, the patient retains sodium and water. Retained water may be generally distributed over the body as generalized edema or be concentrated to some extent in body cavities, particularly in the abdominal cavity as ascites and in the pleural cavity as hydrothorax. In the development of edema in liver disease a number of mechanisms are usually implicated. Not all are involved in every patient. In all instances sodium and water are retained. Some authorities state that failure to inactivate aldosterone is a factor in the retention of water and electrolytes in cirrhosis of the liver. Others state that it is doubtful if failure to inactivate aldosterone plays a significant role in fluid retention in cirrhosis. A more important factor is fluid sequestration (ascites) and cutaneous vasodilation with a relative hypovolemia.

Another factor predisposing to edema formation is a decrease in synthesis of albumin. Albumin is the most important of the blood proteins in determining the colloid osmotic pressure of the blood. A significant fall in the concentration of albumin in the blood, therefore, decreases the water-holding power of the blood. All of the above factors contribute to generalized edema as well as to development of ascites and hydrothorax.

In the liver itself, two changes may occur which increase the likelihood of the development of ascites. In cirrhosis of the liver, contraction of the liver by scar tissue leads to portal hypertension and to an elevation of the hydrostatic pressure of the blood in the portal capillaries. With increased capillary permeability, albumin and fluid escape into tissues and serous cavities and increase the water-holding power of the tissue and serous fluids. All of the following may contribute to a greater or lesser extent to the development of edema: (1) possibly an increase in the retention of sodium and water by the kidney as a result of increased activity of aldosterone and possible increased release of the antidiuretic hormone; (2) a loss of water-holding power of the blood as a result of a decrease in serum albumin; (3) an increase in the force driving the fluid out of the capillaries; (4) an increase in the permeability of the capillaries; and (5) heightened water-holding power of fluids in tissue spaces and body cavities.

What types of therapy are used in the treatment of edema?

The treatment of edema in the patient with disease of the liver is similar to that in the patient with an apparently healthy liver. Because of the importance of the sodium ion in the formation of edema, intake must be restricted. Sodium restriction adds to the problem of getting the patient to eat. The use of lemon juice, onion, garlic, and other nonspicy flavorings may be tried to improve the flavor of vegetables, fish, and meats.

When ascites or hydrothorax becomes so great that either interferes with the function of the alimentary canal or with breathing, fluid may be with-drawn from the peritoneal or thoracic cavity. Removal of fluid from either cavity involves intrusion in the internal environment, and both procedures should therefore be performed under sterile conditions. The general precautions to be taken when the pleural cavity is entered are discussed in Chapter 7.

Paracentesis is usually performed in the room of the patient or in the treatment room. The nurse has two general responsibilities. One is to prepare the patient and to support and comfort him during the procedure and the other is to assist the physician. The latter is also a service to the patient, inasmuch as assistance given by the nurse to the physician facilitates the care provided for the patient. The patient should be so prepared that he knows what to expect. Emphasis should be placed on the fact that as the result of the removal of fluid, he will be able to breathe more easily, move about more freely, and eat better. To prevent puncturing of the bladder during the procedure, the urinary bladder should be emptied by the patient or by catheterization before the procedure is attempted. If the paracentesis is performed on the patient in bed, he should be brought to the side of the bed and supported in a sitting position. If he is able, he may sit in a chair or with his feet over the edge of the bed. In whatever position he is placed, his back should be adequately supported. The skin should be shaved if necessary and thoroughly cleansed.

To lessen the danger of puncturing the colon, the cannula is introduced at the mid-line and below the umbilicus. After the cannula has been introduced into the peritoneal cavity, tubing is attached to it and the ascitic fluid is drained into a pail or a bottle. Although either is a satisfactory receptacle, the physician may wish to collect the fluid under sterile conditions for purposes of examination or to infuse it into the patient.

After the procedure is completed, the skin at the site of puncture may require a stitch or two to close the incision. A small dressing may be all that is required. When it becomes wet, it should be replaced. The clothing of the patient and bedding should also be checked at the same time and changed as often as necessary. When ascites develops rapidly and the patient requires repeated paracenteses, the problem of keeping him dry may be considerable.

During the performance of paracentesis, fluid is withdrawn slowly to prevent syncope resulting from a too rapid reduction in intra-abdominal pressure. At the completion of the procedure a scultetus binder may be applied until the patient has adjusted to the decrease in intra-abdominal pressure.

Throughout the procedure the patient should be apprised of what is expected of him, of what is being done, and of his general progress. For example, when the nurse cleanses the skin, she should tell the patient what she is doing. When a solution that evaporates rapidly is placed on the skin, the patient should be prepared for the fact that it will be cold. As the physician injects the anesthetic into skin, or introduces the cannula into the peritoneal cavity, the patient should be informed of what is happening. After the peritoneal cavity has been entered and the fluid has started to flow, the patient should be informed. Whether the patient is undergoing paracentesis for the first or the hundredth time, he should be included as a participating member of the team. Attention should be given to the physical status of the patient. His pulse, respiration, and color should be noted and any undue change reported to the physician.

In patients with serious disease of the liver, changes in the mental status from mild confusion, disorientation, and irrational behavior to stupor and deep coma may appear. Hyperventilation and flapping tremor may also occur. In hyperventilation the depth of respiration is increased, but not the rate. In fact, the rate of respiration may be slower than normal. Not all patients with severe liver disease develop coma, nor do those who become comatose necessarily present the milder signs before developing coma.[61]

Although the reasons for the development of mental changes have not been completely identified, two mechanisms appear to be involved. They are the accumulation of metabolites, probably of a nitrogenous nature, in the internal environment of cells and an abnormal sensitivity of cerebral cells to changes in their fluid environment.[62] Among the nitrogenous substances, ammonia and ammonia-bearing compounds are implicated. Hepatic coma can be precipitated in susceptible patients by orally administered ammonia compounds as well as by certain bacterial metabolites containing methionine. In the healthy liver, substances absorbed from the intestine, such as ammonia, are detoxified before they reach the general circulation. Ammonia is converted to urea. In severe liver disease, the liver cells are assumed to be unable to convert ammonia and other potentially harmful nitrogenous materials to harmless ones. Another possibility is that blood containing these substances does not pass through the liver before it enters the general circulation. Blood flow may be detoured around the liver by naturally occurring or surgical shunts.

Coma can be precipitated in susceptible patients by agents increasing the load of nitrogenous substances or by sodium-excreting diuretics. Thus a high-protein diet or ammonium drugs, such as ammonium chloride, predispose to coma by increasing the load of nitrogenous substances to be excreted. Carbonic anhydrase inhibitors such as acetazolamide (Diamox[63]) also predispose to coma by increasing the excretion of the sodium ion.

Since these agents are also of value in the therapy of the patient with liver disease, the physician may prescribe one or more for a given patient. In any patient who has disease of the liver, the nurse should be alert to and promptly report changes in his mental alertness and status. Nursing of the comatose patient is discussed in Chapter 7.

In addition to a nutritious diet, the other form of treatment used in the therapy of patients with disease of the liver is rest. Currently the subject of the

[61] In stupor, the patient can be, but is not easily, aroused. In coma he cannot be aroused.
[62] Ingelfinger, *Loc. cit.,* Sodeman, p. 791.
[63] Trade name.

extent to which rest should be prescribed is highly controversial. Some, but not all, physicians advocate complete bed rest until the serum bilirubin is reduced to 3 mg or less per 100 ml. Bed rest is thought to shorten the length of illness. Everything should be done to promote relaxation of the patient. All activities that can be done by someone else should be performed for the patient, and the physical, emotional, and social climate should be regulated so that rest is encouraged.

Although the physician prescribes the therapeutic regime for the patient with a disease of the liver, much of the responsibility for carrying it out is borne by the nurse. Whether the food served to the patient is eaten frequently depends on the patience and the persistence of a nurse who appreciates the importance of a nutritious diet to the recovery of the patient. Whether the patient is provided with an environment in which rest is possible also depends on a nurse who understands the importance of rest to recovery and who acts in accordance with her understanding.

What factors other than a supply of food are of significance in nutrition?

To this point all of the processes involved in supplying the cell with the materials it requires for its activities have been discussed. Nutrition, however, depends not only on the supply of food, but on the requirements of cells and on the capacity of cells to utilize nutrients. A specific quantity of food may at one time be adequate, at another time inadequate, and at still another time excessive. In the following section attention will be devoted to the factors influencing the requirements of cells for nutrients and processes whereby cells utilize food stuffs.

Intermediary metabolism includes all the changes taking place in a nutrient from the moment it enters the internal environment.[64] To illustrate, the intermediary metabolism of glucose includes all the chemical processes it undergoes after it is absorbed from the gastrointestinal tract until its potential energy is released and carbon dioxide and water are eliminated into the external environment or the excess of glucose is stored as glycogen or as fat. Since intermediary metabolism includes only those changes occurring after glucose enters the internal environment, digestion is not a part of intermediary metabolism.[65] Intermediary metabolism has two aspects, anabolism and catabolism. Because of increasing knowledge in the field of biochemistry, older definitions of anabolism and catabolism are somewhat misleading. In general, however, the term "anabolism" covers those processes in which there is a synthesis or combination of molecules, with the formation of larger ones. The reactions involved in anabolism are usually energy-saving. Catabolism includes those processes in which larger molecules are broken down with the

[64] Abraham White, Philip Handler, Emil L. Smith, and DeWitt Stellen, Jr., *Principles of Biochemistry*, 2nd ed., The Blakiston Division, McGraw-Hill Book Company, Inc., New York, 1959, p. 275.
[65] Some authorities include digestion with intermediary metabolism.

release of energy. However, energy is sometimes released without an obvious change in the size of molecules.

With an increase in knowledge of the nature of intermediary metabolism has come greater understanding of the chemical processes occurring in the cells in health, as well as of their response to injury and disease. The work of Moore, Selye, as well as other scientists, is beginning to provide knowledge of the nature of the metabolic responses of individuals following surgery and injury. These are discussed in Chapters 5 and 15

At the beginning of the chapter, nutrition of tissues was defined as depending on the capacity of the organism to supply the substances required to support the chemical processes within its cells. Nutrition depends not only on food supply, but on the degree to which tissue requirements are met. The effects of failure or excesses of supply will be discussed with the varying types of nutrients.

What nutrients are required by cells?

Nutrients known to be required by cells include calories, protein, minerals, and vitamins. Recently the roles of minerals such as magnesium and molybdenum have been identified. The possibility exists that other elements will be found to have a significant role in some aspect of metabolism. This discussion, however, will be limited to the needs of the cells for calories, proteins, vitamins, and the minerals iodine, fluorine, iron, and phosphorus. The electrolytes sodium, potassium, calcium, and chlorides are discussed in Chapter 8.

Despite the general belief to the contrary, the basic nutritional requirement is for energy-producing materials or calories. Before protein can be used for growth, sufficient calories must be available to provide energy for metabolic processes. Because of the ease with which food is obtained in the United States, an abundance of calorie-containing foods is available, and there is a tendency to look upon calories as harmful. When food is plentiful, overeating is a common problem. Unless care is taken to balance caloric intake and output, more food is ingested than is required to meet the need for calories and possibly for other nutrients. Unlike many other homeostatic mechanisms, the regulation of food intake in relation to the expenditure of energy is far from perfect. A low expenditure of energy is not followed automatically by a proportionate decrease in the intake of food. For many people, habit rather than energy expenditure determines food intake. For a not inconsiderable number, psychological factors contribute to an actual increase in food intake during periods of inactivity or limited activity.

Release of energy is essential to all bodily processes. The release of energy is fundamental to the constancy of the composition and structure of the cell itself. For example, the sodium ion constantly leaks into the cell, yet in health it does not accumulate in it. Energy is required to eject the sodium ion from the cell and to maintain the normal concentration of intracellular sodium.

Among other bodily processes requiring an expenditure of energy are the maintenance of the semipermeability of cell and capillary membranes; the maintenance of the composition of the extracellular fluid environment of cells; secretion by glands; the transmission of nerve impulses; and the conctraction of muscles. An insufficient intake of calories in relation to cellular requirements has an adverse effect on all of the above.

In acute starvation of short duration, calories are obtained from depots of fat stored in the body. When starvation continues, some cellular substance is sacrificed to supply calories. With the loss of fat and other tissue substance, weight declines. Eventually, strength is also adversely affected. Loss of weight and strength serves to protect the individual against the effects of starvation. Loss of weight decreases the quantity of tissue requiring support; and with a loss of strength, less energy is utilized for nonsurvival purposes than when more calories are available. The starving person may appear to be better nourished than he really is because he becomes edematous. Although the emphasis here has been on the inadequate ingestion of calories, any increase in energy expenditure without a comparable increase in caloric intake has a similar effect. Some illnesses increase caloric requirement and at the same time interfere with the ingestion of food. Unless the disorder is corrected, life is soon threatened. For example, in hyperthyroid crises, the metabolic rate increases greatly and vomiting and diarrhea limit or prevent the ingestion and absorption of food. Because the caloric requirements of cells are greatly in excess of the calories provided, life is soon threatened. All functions involved in supplying cells with nutrients are increased. Heat production is increased, and the mechanisms for eliminating heat as rapidly as it is produced may fail and the body temperature continue to rise until death.

What are some of the factors affecting caloric requirements?

Requirements for calories are modified by age, body size, climate, body temperature, pregnancy, lactation, exercise, and certain internal secretions. The need for calories diminishes with age. It is interesting to note that calories are the only element for which there is a decreasing requirement with advancing years.[66] Two changes, diminishing activity and some decrease in metabolic rate, are believed to be mainly responsible. There is no decrease in the number of calories required by the older person to perform any activity. Mrs. Bird requires as many calories to walk a mile as her nine-year-old grandchild, but she walks fewer miles in a day.

For centuries farmers have known that active animals are difficult to fatten and inactive ones gain weight. Consequently, they limit the exercise of the animals that they wish to fatten by placing them in a cage or small pen.[67]

[66] The Food and Nutrition Board of the National Research Council in *Recommended Allowances* recommends decreased intake of calories as age increases.

[67] Jean Moyer, "Genetic Factors in Obesity," *Bulletin New York Academy of Medicine,* XXXVI, May, 1960, pp. 323-41.

Some, but not all, studies made on obese adolescents indicate that they are less active than their thinner peers. In the recent past, exercise has not been emphasized as an aspect in the control of weight. There are two principal reasons for this. One is that a person must walk 36 miles to utilize the calories in a pound of fat and the other is that strenuous exercise increases the appetite. Recent literature indicates that regular exercise should be encouraged to aid in the control of body weight. Over the period of a year, a daily walk of 1 mile will result in the loss of or in the prevention of the gain of 10 lb, and this moderate exercise is not accompanied by a comparable gain in appetite. On a day-to-day basis, the effect of the walk of a mile is negligible. Over time, however, it is significant.

In the American culture, machines have largely replaced human beings in the performance of manual labor. In fact, the machine has greatly reduced physical activity in all aspects of the life of man. The farmer not only uses a tractor to cultivate his fields, but both he and his city cousin use a machine to mow their lawns. When a man plays golf, he rides a motorized cart because it speeds his game and is easier. When he needs something from the corner store, he rides in a car. Even children ride to school or to the park. Elevators make it unnecessary to walk from one floor to another. The home is equipped with labor-saving devices from vacuum cleaners to electric beaters and dishwashers. Many recreational activities are for the spectator rather than the participant. Because machines have reduced the need for physical exercise, control of caloric intake combined with regular exercise is necessary for control of weight.

Body size also influences caloric requirements. In general, the larger individual needs more calories than a smaller one. Small animals, however, have a higher metabolic rate than larger ones with the result that they require more food per unit of mass. A bird or a mouse requires more food per gram of weight than an elephant. Sex also influences metabolic rate as males have a higher rate than females. Metabolic rate is higher in the young than in the old. Baby Martin has a higher metabolic rate, and therefore requires more calories per kilogram of weight, than his grandmother, Mrs. Bird. During childhood and adolescence, proportionally more calories are required than later in life. For example, the recommended allowance of calories for a 10- or 12-year-old child weighing 36 kg (79 lb) and 57 in. tall is 2,500. For his 65-year-old grandmother who weighs 58 kg (128 lb) and is 64 in. tall, 1,800 calories is recommended.[68] These allowance levels are for persons living in the United States.

Persons exposed to cold climates, such as those living in Arctic regions, require a high intake of calories to survive. In America the effects of climate on the need for calories have been minimized by air-conditioned buildings, central heating and heated automobiles.

[68] Food and Nutrition Board, National Research Council, *Recommended Dietary Allowances,* 1958.

During the latter half of pregnancy and during lactation, women require some increase in calories, but attention should be given to preventing the addition of undesired adipose tissue. The effect of internal secretions on caloric requirements is discussed elsewhere. However, there is a direct relationship between caloric requirement and the secretion of thyroid hormones as an increase in the secretion of thyroid hormones increases the caloric requirement. Likewise, a decrease in thyroid secretion lessens the need for calories. Although thyroid hormones affect caloric requirements, hypothyroidism is not usually responsible for true obesity. A variety of internal and external factors affect the caloric requirements of cells. As long as food intake and caloric requirements are in balance, weight and strength can be expected to remain stationary. When intake of calories exceeds energy output, weight is gained in the form of adipose tissue.

From what sources are calories obtained?

Calories are obtained from carbohydrates, proteins, and fats. From 85 to 90 per cent of the calories in the diet of persons living in the United States are from carbohydrates and fats.[69] Authorities recommend that no weight be gained after 25 years of age. Even when weight remains stationary, the proportion of adipose to other tissues increases. At one time, a moderate amount of overweight was an advantage to those under 25 years of age because these individuals had a greater resistance to tuberculosis and pneumonia. As these diseases are being brought under control, overweight no longer increases chances of survival.

Besides a variety of physiological conditions affecting the caloric requirements of tissues, there are many pathological states in which tissue requirements are increased or diminished. In some disorders the imbalance between intake and expenditure of energy is aggravated by a diminished desire for food or by the inability of the alimentary canal to tolerate it. Conditions increasing tissue requirements include hyperthyroidism, surgical operation, fractures, burns, fever, leukemia, severe anemia, and advanced neoplastic disease. Effects of illness, such as restlessness, dyspnea, or orthopnea, intensify the need of the patient for food.

The degree to which the basal metabolic rate is elevated in the orthopneic patient is illustrated by Mrs. Thims. She had a basal metabolic rate of $+100$ per cent. Unless there is a corresponding increase in food ingested, weight loss accompanies any condition in which tissue requirements are increased. In some disorders such as congestive heart failure, retention of salt and water may mask the loss of body substance. With the removal of the edema fluid the patient is found to be emaciated. Sometimes the state of nutrition of the edematous patient is so poor that he does not respond to the usual measures to eliminate the edema until his nutrition is improved.

[69] *Ibid.*

In some disorders, the total quantity of food required by the patient may be increased, not by an increase in the requirement of cells, but by excessive losses of nutrients from the body. For example, some disorders of the alimentary tract are accompanied by loss of nutrients. Patients who have large burns or draining wounds or abscesses may lose enormous quantities of nutrients. Large quantities of protein may be lost through abnormally permeable glomeruli in the kidney. In uncontrolled diabetes mellitus, weight loss results from the loss of glucose in the urine. Inasmuch as protein and fats are mobilized for energy and to form glucose, they are also lost. Whatever the cause of the loss, the extent and type of nutrient lost must be estimated and every effort made to restore the balance between supply and demand. The nurse contributes to the estimation of the extent of tissue requirements by making pertinent observations. Methods which the nurse can use to improve the food intake of the patient have been presented.

Not only may tissue requirements be increased, but they may be decreased. As might be predicted, the factors that decrease the metabolic requirements of tissues are the opposite of those increasing it. Hence, metabolism is decreased by inactivity, starvation, and lower tissue temperature due to hypothermia. The reduction of the metabolic rate combined with a voluntary reduction in activity is an important mechanism in the protection of tissues during starvation. Pathological conditions in which there is a decrease in tissue requirements include hypothyroidism, Addison's disease, starvation, malnutrition, shock, and hypothermia. Hypothermia is utilized in cardiac and brain surgery, as well as in the treatment of patients with brain injuries, to reduce the rate of cell metabolism. As a consequence the length of time that cells in the nervous system can tolerate a reduction in the supply of oxygen and nutrients is extended.

Since the mechanisms for the regulation of caloric intake and output are not very accurate, caloric under- or oversupply is always possible. In the United States the latter is perhaps more common. In the world as a whole, however, undernutrition is the more frequent problem. Approximately 75 per cent of the people in the world have a diet that is deficient in calories and protein.[70] Among the multiple causative factors are: (1) a lack of facilities for the transportation and preparation of food, (3) poorly developed natural resources, (4) illiteracy, (5) poverty, (6) alcoholism, and (7) chronic illness.

In the United States, despite continued overproduction of food, undernutrition has not been eliminated. In some parts of the country undernutrition is endemic. This is especially true in regions where poverty and low educational standards are the rule and food habits and customs limit food intake to a few foods. Undernutrition is not limited to those who are poor and uneducated, however. Concern is frequently expressed in popular as well as in scientific

[70] Francisco Gomez Mont, "Undernutrition," in Wohl and Goodhart, *Op. cit.,* p. 873.

literature about the inadequacy of the food intake of teen-aged girls. Fad diets, particularly when prolonged, may lead to undernutrition. Chronic illness, aging, and alcoholism are other conditions that predispose to an inadequate intake of food.

Loss of appetite is a common cause of undernutrition. Anorexia is frequently associated with organic disease as well as with psychological disturbances. In the latter, it occasionally leads to extreme emaciation. Acute illness in the well nourished and the temporary loss of appetite are not likely to be serious. In the chronically ill or in those who are undernourished at the onset of illness, anorexia is of more serious import. Undernutrition may also result when tissue requirements exceed food intake. Conditions which are likely to increase tissue requirements include strenuous exercise, fever, hyperthyroidism, and diabetes mellitus.

To recapitulate, in the United States undernutrition is most frequent among: (1) people whose incomes are insufficient and/or whose habits and customs limit the quantity and variety of foods in their dietary, (2) people who lack appetite for food, and (3) persons whose tissue requirements exceed their intake of food.

Correction of the undernutrition is effected through an increase in the intake of calories and protein. Easy as this may appear to be to those who have a problem with overweight, the correction of caloric and protein undernutrition may take weeks and months of effort. It often requires: (1) a fundamental change in attitudes of the individual and/or his family, (2) a building up of the tolerance of the gastrointestinal tract for food, (3) more money to buy food as well as (4) the patience, understanding, and cooperation of the various members of the health team to achieve success. The reasons for undernutrition vary from one person to another. Therefore, inasmuch as is possible, each person must be treated as an individual.

The following individuals illustrate some of the problems that contribute to caloric undernutrition. When caloric intake is inadequate, other nutrients are almost certain to be deficient as well.

Sharon, aged 15, had been a plump baby and child and had always eaten well. At the close of the school year she decided to lose weight so that she would be more nearly like her friends in appearance. Since her previous attempts had been unsatisfactory, she felt that her situation was desperate. With the exception of a glass of skim milk and a piece of fruit, three times a day, she refused to eat. Her parents became frantic. The less she ate, the more they scolded and the greater was Sharon's determination to stick to her diet and to lose weight rapidly.

Mrs. Ross, aged 75, lives across town from Sharon. She lives alone in a one-room apartment. Though she has a modest income, her meals consist of health bread and tea. She says other foods disagree with her and that her food intake is adequate. She supports her position by stating that printed on the wrapper covering of the bread is a statement that this bread contains all of the elements required for health. Mrs. Ross has never been fat. She is weak and tired, but after all, as she says, she is an old woman. Her family and friends are gone. She lived during the period when family life was the most intense at any time in American history. When she was a child and until her children left home and her husband died, meals were a social event. The entire family gathered round an abundantly supplied table to eat and enjoy each other's company. Now all that is gone and Mrs. Ross has little incentive to eat.

Mary Alice, aged 17, has arthritis. She was hospitalized for rehabilitation, during which time she made considerable progress. After her return home, she soon returned to almost full-time bed rest. She says that she is too weak and tired to get out of bed. A three-day food-intake study revealed that her caloric intake was only about 800 calories. Among a number of possible factors contributing to the situation, the easiest to identify and correct is the fact that Mary Alice's mother is a poor cook.

Many of the elements that contribute to problems that arise in he chronically malnourished patient are well illustrated by Mrs. Muncie. As is often true, Mrs. Muncie's malnourished state did not arise suddenly nor was it the result of a single cause. At the time of her admission to the hospital Mrs. Muncie presented an emaciated appearance. Her skin was tightly drawn over her slight frame. She had a large infected decubitus ulcer over her sacrum. Although she had not felt well for some years, she had been able to care for a five-room flat, prepare meals for herself and her husband, and be active in church work. Her present illness had its onset about a week previous to her admission for an episode of diarrhea. Her husband had cared for her at home, because he wanted her to die in peace. A neighbor finally persuaded him to have her admitted to the hospital.

Some of the factors contributing to Mrs. Muncie's chronically malnourished state were revealed by her personal history. She was the thirteenth child born to sharecropper parents in Mississippi. She had completed about the fourth grade in school. Her diet throughout her lifetime was that which she ate as a child. She and her husband had moved to Big City 25 years ago. Insufficient income to cover expenses had been a constant problem. At the time of her admission to the hospital, her husband's wages as a janitor were only $270 a month, but he did have sufficient hospital insurance to cover Mrs. Muncie's hospital expenses. Only by the most careful management were they able to meet all of their obligations. Because her appetite was poor and her husband left early in the morning, she usually ate only two meals a day. The first consisted of either tea or coffee and toast and soup or orange juice. The second meal, which she shared with her husband, usually consisted of a vegetable, preferably greens cooked with fat pork, and cornbread or hot biscuits. Mrs. Muncie had worn dentures since she was 25 years of age. When she was between the ages of 13 and 25, her father pulled her teeth, one by one, because they were painful. When asked about her weight, she said that she had always been "skinny." From her dietary, Mrs. Muncie's nutritional status was probably always marginal. Significant factors in her background include poverty, a low educational level, loss of her teeth at an early age, and customs in food selection and preparation that tended to restrict her intake of protein and calories as well as other important nutrients.

An appropriate question at this point is, "How is it that Mrs. Muncie managed to live for more than 60 years on a diet of cooked vegetables, corn bread, and fat pork?" Adults show considerable resistance to food deprivation. In the presence of an inadequate supply of nutrients, cells adapt by decreasing their rate of metabolism. Stores of fat and protein are mobilized and utilized for energy. The only evidence that food intake is less than that required may be loss of weight or a weight that is less than normal. Although the individual is able to do heavy work, he rests at every opportunity. During the period in which the individual is able to adapt the metabolic rate of his cells to his limited food intake, his malnourished state is said to be compensated. He may survive in this state for a long period of time. When some condition develops, such as an infection, that places added stress on the individual, adaptation fails and evidence of uncompensated undernutrition appears.

Mrs. Muncie indicated that she had been underweight most of her life when she said, "I've always been skinny." Until she had a nephrectomy six years ago, she had always been reasonably well. Since that time she had been in her words "poorly." Her present illness was ushered in by an episode of diarrhea. Though she attributed this to some cabbage that she had eaten, diarrhea is frequently the first evidence that chronic undernutrition has entered the uncompensated phase. When she entered the hospital a week later, she was also found to have pyelonephritis in her remaining kidney. As stated earlier, an infection is frequently the stress that upsets the unstable balance in chronic undernutrition. Soon after the onset of her illness a decubitus ulcer formed at the base of her spine. It was infected. Once compensation failed, Mrs. Muncie was no longer able to protect her tissues from the effects of pressure. Resistance to infection was also impaired.

On physical examination, Mrs. Muncie presented many signs and symptoms of chronic undernutrition. Despite the fact that she was 5 ft 5 in. tall, she weighed only 88 lb. The desirable weight for a woman of small frame and 65 in. tall is from 119 to 128 lb.[71] She did not give the appearance of having lost weight recently. In older individuals, rapid losses of weight are usually accompanied by wrinkling of the skin and loose folds of skin over areas where subcutaneous fat is stored. As the skin ages, it loses its elasticity, and with the loss of elasticity, the ability to adapt the skin to the size of the underlying tissue is diminished. After 50 years of age or so, the skin of the person who loses weight rapidly is likely to be too large for him. The severely undernourished person tends to retain water. Although this is more likely to occur in

[71] Metropolitan Life Insurance Company, *Ideal Weights for Women*, Metropolitan Life Insurance Bulletin, XL, 1959, p. 1.

children than in adults, the absence of wrinkling of Mrs. Muncie's skin may have been due in part to water retention.

Among the other signs and symptoms of chronic undernutrition presented by Mrs. Muncie were: wasting of tissues including her muscles, edema, dry, scaling skin, numbness and tingling of her toes, hyperesthesia of feet and legs, weakness and pallor, glossitis (sore tongue), diarrhea, poor wound healing, and anorexia.

Her laboratory findings, which are summarized below, were consistent with a state of chronic undernutrition.

Laboratory Test	Finding—Mrs. Muncie		Normal Range	
Blood protein—total	6.6	gm/100 ml	6.5 —	8.3
Serum albumin	1.82		3.5 —	5.5
Beta globulin	2.51		0.52–	1.01
Gamma globulin	2.25		0.61–	1.39
Blood urea nitrogen	35	mg/100 ml	10 —	20
Electrolytes				
Sodium	120	mEq/l	125	–147
Potassium	4.8	mEq/l	3.5 —	5.5
Carbon dioxide	26.1	volumes per cent	50 —	70
Hemoglobin	8.1	gm 100 ml	12 —	16
Hematocrit	31	per cent	36 —	47
Urine				
Albumin		Negative		Negative

It will be noted that her total blood proteins are within the lower limits of normal, but that the albumin-globulin ratio is reversed. This indicates that albumin is being broken down or lost from the body more rapidly than it can be replaced. Multiple factors probably account for the deficit of albumin. Lack of sufficient intake of protein to provide the amino acids required to replace albumin lost from the body, loss of albumin in the exudate from the decubitus ulcer, and possibly in the diarrheal fluid, utilization of serum albumin to provide energy, and possibly inability of the liver to synthesize albumin—all probably contribute to the reversal of the albumin-globulin ratio. This condition also occurs when large quantities of albumin are lost in the urine. Loss of albumin by this route was not a factor in the instance of Mrs. Muncie. Some degree of dehydration may have also contributed to maintaining the level of protein within normal limits. The blood urea nitrogen elevation may be due to some degree of dehydration. The lowering of her carbon dioxide-combining power is consistent with acidosis. It will be noted that her serum sodium is slightly decreased; this indicates some loss of cations. Acid-base balance is discussed fully in Chapter 8. Acidosis is common in starvation. As might be expected, Mrs. Muncie's hemoglobin is low. Associated with this is a low hematocrit. Anemia is a common occurrence in menstruating women who are undernourished. Although Mrs. Muncie is well past the menopause, she has been undernourished for much, if not all, her life.

After Mrs. Muncie was admitted to the hospital, three interrelated problems required immediate attention. The first and central problem was to improve her nutritional status. The second and third were to heal the decubitus and to eliminate the infection in her kidney—the pyelonephritis. In the early part of her hospitalization, these problems required urgent attention. Others were secondary. To correct her undernutrition, a plioform nasogastric tube was introduced into her stomach. The formula was made by liquefying natural foods in a blender. It contained 1,500 calories per liter. In the beginning the formula was administered over a 24-hour period with the pump adjusted at the slowest rate of speed. In addition, she was served an 1,800-calorie low-salt diet and a multivitamin capsule which contained the recommended daily allowance for minerals and vitamins. Nutrients were not administered parenterally.

To prevent the loss of nutrients and fluid by diarrhea, she was given 1 dram of paregoric (camphorated tincture of opium) in each liter of formula. Paregoric was discontinued when the diarrhea ceased. The tolerance of the digestive tube for food is diminished in undernutrition. Therefore, the ingestion of more than the usual amounts of food is likely to aggravate or induce diarrhea. Paregoric acts by increasing the tone of the stomach and intestine and by decreasing propulsive peristalsis. The latter action is important in the control of diarrhea.

In addition to efforts to improve her nutritive state, measures were instituted to hasten the healing of her decubitus ulcer. She was placed on a Stryker frame, which was turned every two hours day and night. Attention was paid to all sites of pressure in order to prevent further tissue breakdown. Warm saline compresses were applied to the decubitus twice daily for an hour, followed by exposure of the area to a heat lamp for one-half hour. When she was first admitted to the hospital she was incontinent of urine. A retention catheter was inserted. Every effort was made to keep the area clean and dry. Plastic surgery was considered, but not performed because of her poor nutritive state.

Mrs. Muncie's progress was slow. During the first three weeks of therapy she gained only 2 lb in weight but she had gained enough strength that she was able to walk with assistance. She was encouraged to walk because ambulation improves morale and appetite as well as the normal functioning of the alimentary canal. In order to increase her food intake, her request for a soft diet was granted. As she tired when eating, she was given assistance at mealtime.

Mrs. Muncie had some assets not available to all patients. She had a devoted husband. She had a strong religious faith. Her husband, who had an excellent work record, was assisted by his employer in establishing that he was 65 years of age and therefore eligible for social security. He planned to retire so that he could care for his wife at home. As soon as the decubitus ulcer was healed, Mrs. Muncie was to be discharged home under the supervision of the outpatient clinic and a visiting nurse. Efforts were made to instruct the husband and wife in selection of food that would meet at least minimal nutritional requirements. Because of their age, limited education and money, and a lifetime of habits, the outlook for marked improvement was poor.

There were also other problems in the care of Mrs. Muncie. The purpose however, of introducing her case here was to present some of the problems that cause and result from chronic undernutrition. Mrs. Muncie was not from a far-off land, but lived in a large city in the United States. The factors in her condition are those that underlie undernutrition over the world—poverty and illiteracy perhaps being the most fundamental. She did not have a so-called deficiency disease, such as arises when one nutrient is lacking in the dietary. Rather she suffered to a greater or lesser extent from a lack of all nutrients, calories, proteins, vitamins, and minerals.

Had Mrs. Muncie's state been discovered before decompensation occurred, her illness might have been prevented. This would have taken an increase in the ingestion of all nutrients. For each pound gained, an intake of 3,500 calories in excess of those utilized is required. In persons whose food habits and patterns are set, an increase in food intake is often difficult to achieve. It takes time and patience. The individual needs to understand and accept that increase in the intake of food is necessary to health and well-being and to want to improve his food habits.

Some of the questions to be asked here include: What is the presenting problem or problems in each of the four individuals? What are the possible outcomes? Suggest appropriate ways in which a nurse might contribute to the solution of each. In which of these patients presented above is the prognosis favorable, if appropriate action is taken in time?

The converse of too little food is too much. In the United States with its economy of plenty, the problem for many people is that too many calories are available. When the number of calories ingested is in excess of tissue requirement, they are stored as fat. Continued addition to fat stores eventually leads to obesity. Obesity is commonly defined as a condition in which the weight for a specified height, age, and sex is more than 10 per cent above the ideal weight and the excess weight is due to adipose tissue. Overweight due to large bones and muscles is not obesity, for obesity is not just a matter of weight. In obesity the excess in weight is due to adipose tissue. Moderate stores of fat in adipose tissue are of value as a ready source when calories are needed but are not readily available for outside sources. Adipose tissue also serves to insulate underlying tissues and organs and to prevent the excessive loss of heat.

Although the incidence of obesity is high among Americans, obesity neither is confined to Americans nor is it a new problem. It is found among the wealthy, sedentary individuals in all parts of the world. Art objects uncovered in the ruins of ancient civilizations attest to its antiquity. The Venus of Willendorf is a limestone statuette named for the Austrian village in which it was discovered, and the figure is indistinguishable from the present-day fat woman. The Venus of Willendorf, however, is the figure of a Stone Age woman and antedates the development of agriculture by 10,000 years. The group in which the Venus of Willendorf lived were hunters. They probably gorged themselves when food was plentiful, as after a successful hunt, and fasted or starved when food was scarce. Statues and portraits of people living in various periods of time and in different civilizations support the assumption that obesity is not a new problem.

What are some of the factors involved in obesity?

An understanding of obesity depends on understanding the function and behavior of fat tissue in the body. In the healthy young adult, body fat accounts for about 15 per cent of total body weight. Even in the adult whose weight remains stationary, the proportion of adipose tissue increases as he advances in age. Adipose tissue cells account for about 2 per cent of the total amount of body fat, and fat substance for about 95 per cent. The other 3 per cent of adipose tissue is made up of blood vessels, nerves, and other types of connective tissue.[72] Because of the relatively small proportion of cells, adipose tissue was long believed to be relatively inert or inactive. Recent tissue studies using radioactive isotopes of carbon and the electron microscope have demonstrated that, contrary to earlier beliefs, fat tissue is not just an inert storage depot for calories, but it participates actively in the metabolism of the body. A considerable amount of the ingested carbohydrates—sugars and starches—is converted to fat before it is utilized in metabolism. Regulated by hormones, fatty acids are released from fat depots to supply the needs of working cells for energy. All the processes in fat tissue are involved in obesity, that is, conversion of carbohydrates to fat, storage, release of fatty acids to be used as energy, and regulation by hormones. From the growing knowledge of fat metabolism, the theory that obesity is simply due to overeating appears to be inadequate.[73] Similar to many other chronic disorders, obesity probably has many etiologies derived from a disturbance in the ratio between synthesis and storage to mobilization and utilization of fat.

The most obvious and most emphasized cause of obesity is the excessive ingestion of food. In the recent past, some authorities have gone so far as to say that overeating, with rare exceptions, is the sole cause of obesity. Obesity due to failure to adapt food intake to decreasing metabolic needs is a common factor in middle-aged and older people. They continue to eat about as much throughout their life span as they did in their youth. Mrs. Simon, aged 45, is a good example. Despite lessening activity, she eats about as much as she did when her children were young and she was very active. She has gained 10 lb over the last eight or ten years and complains of her thickening waist. Her weight gain is probably due to a failure to adjust her food intake to her diminishing energy requirements.

A second factor in food intake is regulation of appetite by the nervous

[72] Vincent P. Dole, "Body Fat," *Scientific American*, CCI, December, 1959, p. 73.
[73] *Ibid.*, p. 71.

system. Feeding or appetite and satiety centers have been identified in the hypothalamus. Electrical stimulation of the feeding centers in animals leads to overeating. In human beings, lesions in these centers are accompanied by extreme degrees of obesity. There are connections between the feeding and satiety centers and the cerebral cortex which allow the cerebral cortex to exert some degree of control over the ingestion of food. As it is a homeostatic mechanism, there must be some sort of feedback relationship between the quantity of food ingested and the regulatory agencies. As food is ingested, the satiety center must receive a message to this effect and initiate impulses interpreted as a feeling of satisfaction. As the stomach and intestine empty, messages arrive at the appetite center signaling that food is required. Exactly how the feedback relationship between the need for food and satisfaction of this need works has not been identified.

Because the nervous sytem participates in the regulation of eating, overeating frequently has a psychological basis. In some persons overeating accomplishes two psychological purposes or gains. The first is a primary gain. Food is used to substitute for gratification in life situations. Eating relieves unpleasant feelings—loneliness, frustration, guilt, depression, insecurity, or anxiety. As an example, everyone is acquainted with someone who eats when bored or who makes additional trips to the refrigerator when preparing for an important examination.

In a more serious vein, some persons who are obese become seriously depressed when they attempt to reduce. Overeating in these individuals is a defense against feelings of depression. Psychiatrists consider obesity in these individuals the lesser of two problems.[74]

Secondary psychological gains involve the use of eating not for its direct effect on relieving unpleasant feelings, but to bring about desired changes in interpersonal relationships. It may be used offensively to control or gain attention of others. For example, a boy or girl overeats because by so doing he pleases his mother. Overeating may be a defensive maneuver utilized by the individual to protect himself from contact with others. For example, Dorothy, aged 15, is 50 lb overweight. She is a shy, anxious girl who fears rejection by her peers. She uses her obesity as a reason for avoiding others. In effect, a thick layer of fat serves to insulate her from people in her environment.

Because of the importance of hormones in the regulation of various aspects of metabolism, attempts have been made to implicate hormones as a factor in the development of obesity. According to Murphy,[75] there is no physiological basis for implicating either the pituitary or thyroid gland. However, some of the experimental work with tissue cultures shows that insulin not only pro-

[74] Robert I. Simon, "Obesity as a Depressive Equivalent," *Journal of the American Medical Association,* CLXXXIII, January 19, 1963, pp. 208-10.
[75] Rosemary Murphy, "The Complexities of the Problem of Obesity," *Medical Clinics of North America,* LXXII, March, 1960, pp. 439-45.

motes the synthesis of fat, but it also favors retention of fat tissue.[76] According to Dole, at least three other hormones affect the behavior of isolated slices of fat tissue. Prolactin, similar to insulin, increases the synthesis of fat in adipose tissue. Two hormones, corticotrophin or a closely related hormone and epinephrine, promote the release of fatty acids from fat tissues. In the intact individual, the distribution of fat is regulated by the sex hormones. After castration, the distribution of fat changes. Despite what is known about the regulation of fat metabolism by hormones, knowledge is still in its infancy.

Another factor frequently used to explain obesity is heredity. Mr. Johns says, "I'm fat. My father and mother were fat as were their fathers and mothers." There has been tendency to blame conditioning and family patterns of eating for obese families. In some instances, a table laden with rich food and everyone eating heartily provides a ready explanation for the family tendency to overweight.

Recent reports of experiments throw some doubt on overeating per se as a universal cause of obesity. Strains of rats have been identified in which obesity develops on a genetic basis. In one strain, obesity is due to the inefficient mobilization of fat from fat tissue. In these animals, the synthesis and storage of fat proceeds normally, but due to a deficiency of an enzyme lipoprotein lipase, fat mobilization does not occur at a normal rate. This disorder has not as yet been identified in human beings.

Other observations made on animals may or may not have implications in understanding obesity in human beings. Some species, such as hogs, store large quantities of fat. Despite extensive research, the development of a lean hog that continues to breed true through successive generations has not been too successful. The rate at which animals can be fattened and the efficiency of weight gain in animals possibly have implications on meal spacing in human beings. Rats are natural nibblers, eating from 20 to 30 times a day. When they are fed through a stomach tube twice a day the same quantity and quality of food that they usually eat, they exhibit a number of changes in their body metabolism. Among these is an increase in total body fat.[77] Other animals, such as the sheep, steer, and pig, deposit less fat and more protein when they are fed the same quality and quantity of food distributed in a number of feedings than when fed a few large meals. An important point here is that the quantity and quality of food are the same in both instances. The extent to which observations made on animals throw light on the problem of obesity among human beings has not been fully explored.

Whether or not an individual becomes obese depends on the relationship of synthesis and storage to mobilization and use of energy. Any disturbance which increases synthesis and storage out of proportion to mobilization and use of energy will cause obesity. Too much food, whatever the reasons, and excessive eating favor synthesis and storage. From tissue culture studies,

[76] Dole, *Op. cit.,* p. 75.
[77] Clarence Cohn, "Meals?" *Nutrition Reviews,* XX, November, 1962, p. 321.

insulin is probably required for synthesis and storage of fat. Too little activity, or making too few demands on the fat stores for energy, also contributes its share to the accumulation of fat. Possibly an imbalance between the hormones favoring synthesis and those favoring mobilization of fatty acids from fat stores may be involved. Enzymes are required for both the synthesis and mobilization of fat. Inadequacy of those required for fat mobilization facilitates the entrance of fat into storage depots, but limits the extent to which it can be removed. When fat is deposited in greater quantity than it is or can be removed, obesity results.

From the above, the treatment of obesity would appear to be a relatively simple matter—balance energy input with energy output. In actual practice, it is often very difficult to treat. Despite the implication that obesity is a problem arising out of the supply of calories exceeding the demand for them, not all the factors involved are known. Certainly in individual instances, the role of a particular element may be difficult, if not impossible, to identify. Food is not only essential to biological functioning, but it is the center of a complex value system. As such the intake of food is influenced by genetic, physiological, and environmental factors.

In the past the obese person has been exhorted to use his will power to reduce his food intake, and has been treated with hormones, appetite-depressing drugs, and psychoanalysis. Whatever form of therapy is planned, the regulation of food intake is an essential part of treatment of obesity. Essentially, food intake should be adequate in all respects except calories. The degree to which caloric intake is reduced below energy expenditure depends on the age and status of health of the individual. In general, a slow, steady loss of weight has been thought to be better than a rapid rate. According to some recent reports, rapid loss of weight may be more effective in some individuals. In older persons the cosmetic effect of a rapid loss of weight is undesirable. The loose, flabby skin, scrawny necks, and sunken cheeks tend to discourage the dieter and to attract adverse comments from relatives and friends.

The objective of the dietary treatment of obesity is not just the loss of excess weight, but the development of a new habit of eating. A newspaper columnist, in writing of his current experience with a reduction diet, stated that he was waiting for the day when he had attained the desired loss of weight. On that day he planned to eat all of the rich foods he desired so greatly. From the tone of his writing, his aim was to lose weight and not to maintain a desirable weight.

Persons who are obese should be advised to seek medical attention before undertaking a reduction diet. Not all persons who think they are obese are. Self-prescription of crash diets should be discouraged. Diets for the purpose of losing and maintaining weight loss should be adequate in all respects except for calories. They should also be planned so that the individual is encouraged to develop habits of eating that can be continued. Any faulty eating habits should be corrected. In a sense, a reduction diet is a regime of controlled starvation. For each pound lost, intake must be 3,500 calories less than the number expended during the same period. Further, once the weight is lost, the person is faced with a lifetime of caloric control. Loss of weight is only the first step in the treatment of obesity. Some limitation of food intake is usually necessary for the remainder of the life of the person. The real test is not whether he can lose weight, difficult as losing it may be, but whether he can maintain his weight at the desired level. For some persons, the restriction of calories is a dreary business.

The diet prescribed in the treatment of obesity should, as emphasized, be adequate in all respects except for calories. A deficiency in calories forces the organism to utilize its store of fat for calories. Unless carefully planned, a diet lacking in calories is also likely to be deficient in other nutrients. To assure an adequate intake of minerals and vitamins, vitamin and mineral supplements may be prescribed. Some people lack the knowledge or judgment to plan an adequate diet when calories are rigidly restricted and require instruction and help in planning. After the decision to undertake weight reduction has been made, the physician prescribes the diet. The actual number of calories may vary from a minimum of 600 to 1,500 or more. Physicians differ in their views as to whether to encourage the patient to lose weight quickly or slowly. Usually after the first few weeks, a weight loss of 1 to 1.5 lb per week is considered satisfactory. One patient may be more successful if he sees the results of his efforts quickly. Another may be able to restrict his food intake moderately but not stringently. A patient with diabetes mellitus tolerates weight reduction, provided the rate of weight loss is not too rapid.

Once the program of diet and exercise is planned, the patient should be instructed in the regime that he is to follow. Similar to the dietary control of diabetes mellitus, the control of weight is a day-by-day affair. The responsibility is carried by the patient and his family. A major objective is for the patient to develop confidence in his ability to control his food intake. It is not accomplished by frantic reduction in food intake alernating with periods of gourmandizing.

In making the day-by-day, meal-to-meal selections of food, the patient and his family should learn which foods are low in calories and which are high. Except for rich desserts, most nutritionists do not recommend the exclusion from the diet of any food, including potatoes and cereals. Since calories are added by certain methods of food preparation, this point should be emphasized. For example, the caloric value of one egg is approximately 77 calories. Boiled or poached, it still contains 77 calories. When an egg is fried, almost 50 calories of fat are added, bringing the caloric value to 125 calories. Scrambled with milk or cream added, one egg yields 175 calories, more than double the caloric value of a single egg. Therefore, the method by which a food is prepared requires consideration as well as the caloric value of the food itself. In the selection and preparation of food, attention should be given to the likes and dislikes of the individual. Palatability of food may be increased by the use of herbs and spices. For some persons, the satiety value of the diet can be enhanced by increasing the quantity of bulk-containing foods.

Reduction of food intake is accompanied by physiological and psychological effects which have some bearing on the capacity of the individual to tolerate and continue the program. With the loss of weight there may be a loss of energy. There is also a drop in the basal metabolic rate and with it a decrease in the rate of weight loss. Failure to lose weight at the anticipated rate can be quite discouraging to a patient who has been faithfully following his diet. Some expression from the nurse indicating that she knows that failure to lose weight despite adherence to a reduction diet can and does happen lends support to the patient. When a patient becomes severely depressed, weight reduction has to be abandoned.

Since prevention of obesity is easier than its cure, there is a developing trend toward emphasizing prevention. Obesity does not develop suddenly. A rapid gain in weight is usually due to the storage of water. Obesity develops over a more or less extended period of time. Particularly among middle-aged and older persons who become obese, the day-to-day excess in calories is small and is due to failure to adjust intake to diminishing activity. Whenever a person has ingested 3,500 calories in excess of his needs, he gains a pound.

By eating only 100 calories more than he expends each day for a year, an individual gains 10 lb. In terms of food, this is less than a glass of milk, a slice of bread and butter, or one fried egg. Since the gain in weight is gradual, a person may not be aware that he is gaining weight until he has gained several pounds. If this situation can be identified before he has gained excessive weight and while his intake of calories over his needs is still low, he can prevent obesity by small changes in his eating habits. For example, he may eat fruit for dessert rather than pie or heavily frosted cake. He may also increase his exercise moderately and on a regular basis. He should also learn to weigh himself weekly or monthly. A gain in weight from one week or month to the next usually indicates a gain in fatty tissue.

As indicated a number of times, exercise, when taken regularly and in moderate amounts, is an essential part of a weight-reduction program. A walk of a mile each day for a year will result in a loss of 10 lb in weight. An individual playing 18 holes of golf uses from 800 to 1,000 calories. The cause of weight reduction will be lost, however, if as many or more calories are consumed at the nineteenth hole.

Appetite depressants, as well as agents purported to suppress the appetite, come and go. Their numbers attest to their danger or ineffectiveness or both. Drugs suppressing the appetite center in the brain usually cause nausea as well as anorexia. Drugs such as amphetamine phosphate and related compounds depress the appetite by inducing a sense of well-being. Since some drugs have dangerous side effects, they should not be taken by persons who are not under medical supervision.

Metabolic stimulants, including hormones, have been tried in weight-reduction regimes. Since the thyroid hormone stimulates metabolism, it has been used to increase weight loss. In the euthyroid individual, the ingestion of exogenous thyroid hormone decreases secretion by the thyroid gland. When excessive dosages of thyroid are ingested, symptoms of thyroid toxicity appear.

Psychotherapy in conjunction with other forms of treatment or as the principal therapeutic measure is an essential part of a weight-reduction regime. Most people require psychological support to undertake and continue weight loss. In addition to the physical and psychological discomfort associated with a reduction in food intake, the individual is faced with comments of friends and relatives. It is not unusual to see a person manfully trying to resist a second helping or a rich dessert and at the same time being pressed to take it. "He looks so badly." "Not even a fly could exist on that rabbit food." "Just break your diet this once, it can't hurt you." Some husbands discourage their wives from losing weight by saying that they like plump women. In addition to external factors tending to discourage weight reduction, the purposes served by overeating must be identified and the patient helped to meet these needs in acceptable ways.

In the therapy of obesity, knowledge of the factor or factors motivating the person to reduce can be utilized in helping a person to initiate and continue with a weight-reduction program. Among the more common reasons are pride in personal appearance, improved health status, avoidance of jibes of family, friends, and business associates, and desire to improve health or to avoid one of the chronic disorders associated with obesity. Sometimes the obese person finds that to obtain a particular job, he must lose weight. The nurse can sometimes assist the patient in expressing why he wishes to reduce and to support his efforts to continue.

As an example, Mrs. Albert, aged 35, was 55 lb overweight. Her mother had diabetes mellitus, and Mrs. Albert's glucose tolerance curve was indicative of prediabetes. On this basis, the physician recommended that she lose her excess weight over the next year. To encourage her, her husband offered to buy her a new wardrobe when she reached the desired weight. Both Mr. Albert and the physician frequently complimented her on her improved appearance.

What is one psychiatrist's view of obesity?

Aldrich, a psychiatrist,[78] indicates that obesity should be viewed as any other addiction. He recommends that it be studied from the point of view of impulses, controls, and consequences. Obesity is a consequence of failure to control the impulse to eat. According to this concept of obesity, the problem

[78] C. Knight Aldrich, "Mechanisms and Management of Obesity," *Medical Clinics of North America*, XLVII, January, 1963, p. 77.

faced by the patient and by those who are working with him is to help him to learn to control the quantity of food he eats. Emphasis is on the patient exercising the control rather than the control being external. For example, Mrs. Leslie, who is chronically obese, sees her physician about every six weeks. For the two weeks preceding her visit to her physician she literally starves herself. After her visit, she exercises little control over what she eats. Her control is from the physician. Mrs. Leslie wishes to please him or to avoid being scolded. She blames her employer and husband for tempting her with food.

As a consequence of her behavior, Mrs. Leslie feels ashamed. "I should lose weight, I'm a sight." She also rationalizes, "How can I lose weight when you make pie and sweet rolls and leave them out where I can see them?" "Ben won't eat broiled, roasted, or boiled meat. It has to be fried." Many obese people react in a similar manner. They need help in identifying their own responsibility in controlling their weight.

As in the treatment of other forms of addiction, some who wish to lose weight ally themselves with a group, such as Fattys Anonymous. By aligning themselves with a group of persons having a problem similar to their own, some individuals can be helped to develop sufficient control to maintain a desirable weight.

Despite continuing preoccupation with the problem of obesity and a variety of therapeutic approaches, it remains a continuing problem. Previous emphasis on overeating as the single important factor in obesity is an oversimplification. With added study, obesity, similar to many other health problems, appears to be caused by multiple factors. Its therapy therefore depends on some knowledge of its cause. Obesity is of concern primarily because it has an adverse effect on health and life expectancy. Adipose tissue places a double burden on the individual. Excess tissue has to be carried as a weight on the individual. In effect, Mrs. Albert carries a 55-lb weight with her everywhere she goes, upstairs and down as well as on the level. Obese tissue also has to be supported, or supplied with nutrients. Each pound of adipose tissue contains 0.7 mile or more of capillaries through which blood circulates. As the individual gains weight, fatty components in the blood rise and apparently predispose to atherosclerosis. Diabetes mellitus is more frequent among the obese than in those who are of normal weight.

Although not all authorities agree that a moderate degree of overweight (10 to 20 per cent) is harmful, statistics indicate that the mortality rate goes up as the weight rises above the ideal. The adverse effects of obesity are demonstrated in the findings of the Build and Blood Pressure Study made in 1959 by the Society of Actuaries. The men who were included in the study ranged in age from 15 to 69 years. The mortality rate among those who were 10 per cent or more overweight for height and age was one fifth higher than for those insured at standard risks. Among men who were 20 per cent or more overweight, mortality was one third higher. The mortality rate rises with increasing weight. The adverse effects of obesity were found to be somewhat greater for men in the 40-to-69 age group than in the 15-to-39 group. Disorders of the cardiovascular-renal systems accounted for a high percentage of the excess mortality among the overweight men.[79] Other studies made in the United States and elsewhere support the above findings.

As emphasized above, all of the activities within cells depend on a supply of calories to provide energy. Too few calories threaten cellular function and structure by limiting the source of energy. Eventually cell substance may have to be sacrificed to provide energy for vital activities. An excessive supply of calories in relation to output or an interference with the release of fat from stores of fat results in a condition known as obesity. For reasons already cited, obesity has an adverse effect on life expectancy.

What processes are involved in the release of energy from cells?

The survival of each individual cell depends on the continuous release by the cell of energy. The process whereby living cells derive energy from foodstuffs and convert nutrients into cellular constituents is known as oxidation. Actually, oxidation always involves reduction. Oxygen may or may not be involved. According to the electron theory, oxidation is a process whereby one or more electrons are given up. As a result, valence may be raised, oxygen added, or hydrogen removed. In reduction, the basic change is a gain in electrons. This may be accomplished through the lowering of valence, the loss of oxygen, or the addition of hydrogen. To have either oxidation or reduction, a substance donating electrons and another accepting them must be present. According to present theory, one of the ways by which enzymes participate in chemical reactions in cells is to act as electron donators and acceptors.

Although the mechanisms whereby the organism derives energy for its activities have been studied for more than 50 years, they are still not completely understood. Even less is known about the processes involved in the synthesis of cellular proteins or of enzymes, antibodies, and hormones. As stated above, the total of the processes by which cells derive energy and synthesize cells and other bodily components is known by the general term "metabolism." The phase of metabolism which is concerned with the production of energy is known as catabolism. In catabolism molecules are generally reduced in size, though this is not always true, and energy is released to be utilized by the tissues. The phase of metabolism concerned with synthesis is known as anabolism. In anabolism larger molecules are built from smaller units. In the healthy adult whose intake of food is in balance with his output of energy, anabolism and catabolism are equal so that there is neither a gain

[79] Metropolitan Life Insurance Company, *Statistical Bulletin*, XLI, February, 1960, pp. 6-9.

nor a loss of body size. During growth and in the period of recovery following illness or a surgical operation, anabolism exceeds catabolism. During serious illness or following a serious trauma, including a surgical operation, catabolism exceeds anabolism for a period of time.

Because of the limitations and complexity of knowledge, the processes whereby the organism synthesizes body elements will not be discussed. References are included at the end of the chapter. Because of limitations of space, the processes whereby cells liberate energy from food and transform it into a usable form will be summarized. Students who are interested in learning more of the details should consult a reference on biochemistry.

How does the organism extract energy from carbohydrates, fat, and proteins?

In the study of the chemical processes whereby the body extracts energy from foodstuffs, two principles of thermodynamics contribute to their understanding. One of these is that energy must run downhill. Lehninger[80] states this very simply when he says "that energy must run 'downhill' as in a flame." He further states "that all systems of atoms and molecules must ultimately assume the most random configurations with the least energy-content." A simple example is that of water or other liquids which seek the lowest levels, that is, run downhill. To prevent water, or any system of atoms or molecules, from running downhill requires the expenditure of energy. Continuous work is necessary to synthesize cellular constituents and to maintain the composition and structure of cells. The ability to extract energy from nutrients and to use it in an orderly and directed manner is one of the characteristics distinguishing animate, or living, from inanimate, or nonliving, material.

The second principle of thermodynamics is based on the law of the conservation of energy. Lehninger states it as, "the same total amount of energy is always liberated upon combustion of a given weight of a substance, no matter what the mechanism or pathway of the process."[81] Restated in terms of heat, Lehninger is saying that the quantity of heat released is the same whether glucose is burned in one step as in a fire or is oxidized by the tissue through many steps. The by-products of the reaction, carbon dioxide and water, are also the same. Despite the tendency in nature to be economical of effort and to perform in simple rather than complex ways, the cell takes a multitude of steps to liberate and convert energy into a form that it can use. Each step, catalyzed by a specific enzyme, is taken in an orderly fashion. Though some heat is liberated in the process, most of the energy is converted to chemical energy. Failure of any step interferes with the progress of the reaction and results in the accumulation of partly oxidized chemicals. Obviously the rapid release of energy as heat would soon destroy the cell.

[80] Albert L. Lehninger, "Energy Transformation in the Cell," *Scientific American,* CCII, No. 5, May, 1960, pp. 102-14.
[81] *Ibid.,* p. 102.

According to Lehninger, oxidation-reduction reactions, in which the degradation of fuels is accomplished, can be divided into three major stages. In the first stage, glucose, fat, and amino acids to be used as fuel are converted, each through a series of steps and catalyzed by individual enzymes, to a molecule serving as a sort of "common denominator" for all. Little energy is released in the first stage. In the last two stages, this unit is converted to energy and carbon dioxide and water. The energy is stored in the energy-rich phosphate bonds of special molecules called ATP (adenosine triphosphate) and is available to be used by the cells in their activities. ATP is the source of energy for muscle contraction. It transmits energy from the phosphate bond to the muscle fibril and causes it to contract. West and Todd[82] list 11 physiological processes deriving energy from ATP. They include the synthesis of such varied substances as acetylcholine, which functions in the transmission of impulses at nerve endings, as well as the synthesis of sugar phosphates, proteins from amino acids, urea by the liver, and ammonia by the kidney. ATP also provides the energy for the absorption of sugars from the intestine and for the reabsorption of glucose by the kidney.

The second stage in the release of energy is known as the citric acid or Krebs cycle, because the molecule to be metabolized is citric acid and Krebs first described it. In Figures 10-6, 10-7, and 10-8, the routes by which carbohydrates, proteins, and fats reach and enter the Krebs cycle, as well as the changes that take place during the cycle, can be seen. The products of the first stage of metabolism enter a common pool and are treated alike once they enter the citric acid cycle. The end products of the second stage are carbon dioxide and water. When food intake is in excess of current energy needs, molecules from the citric acid cycle are converted into fat. In the third and final stage, hydrogen atoms are removed and combined with oxygen to form water. This is known as the respiratory cycle.

The orderly process by which oxidation-reduction reactions occur depends on a myriad of enzymes each of which acts on a specific chemical bond. Each enzyme has available in its structure a prosthetic group or groups that either donate or receive electrons. The rate at which enzymes catalyze chemical reactions is subject to control by hormones and possibly by the nervous system. Further, the maintenance of metabolic activities depends on the capacity of the cell to synthesize enzymes and to synthesize or recover chemicals needed to keep the process going. For example, in the process whereby pyruvic acid is degraded, it is converted to acetyl coenzyme A. The acetyl coenzyme A is combined with oxaloacetic acid to form citric acid. For the cycle to continue, coenzyme A and oxaloacetic acid must either be recovered or be synthesized so that they are available to enter the reaction at the appropriate point.

The activity of enzymes depends on a number of factors, including pH,

[82] Edward S. West and Wilbert R. Todd, *Textbook of Biochemistry*, 3rd ed., The Macmillan Co., New York, June, 1961, pp. 785-814.

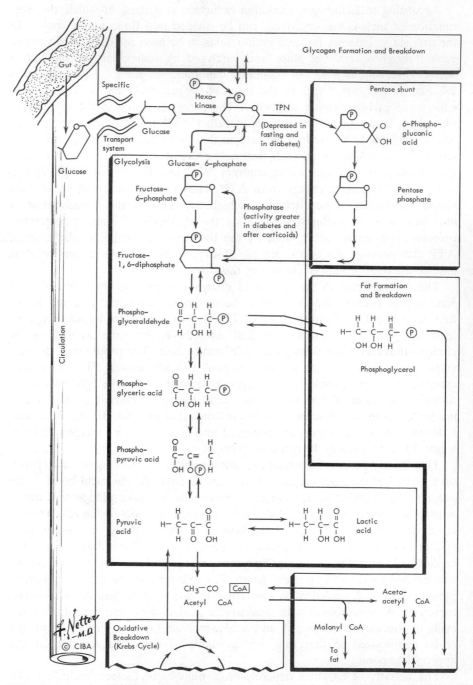

FIGURE 10—6. Glycolysis—the conversion of glucose to pyruvic acid and lactic acid. (Adapted. From Plate IV, *The Ciba Collection of Medical Illustrations* by Frank H. Netter, M.D. Copyright, CIBA.)

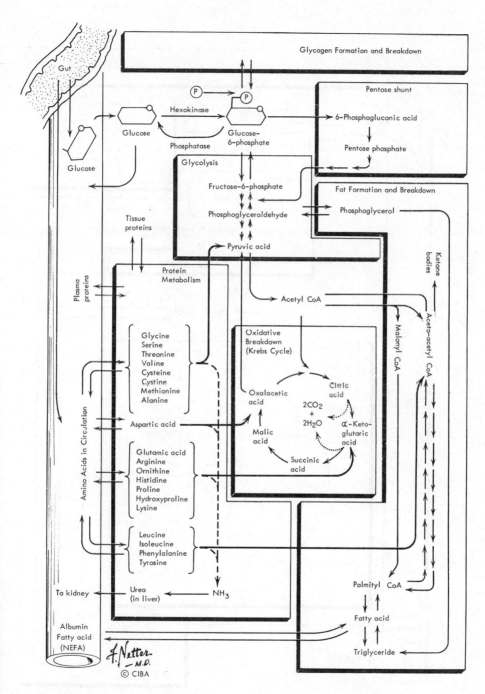

FIGURE 10—7. Oxidative breakdown (the Krebs cycle). (Adapted. From Plate V, *The Ciba Collection of Medical Illustrations* by Frank H. Netter, M.D. Copyright, CIBA.)

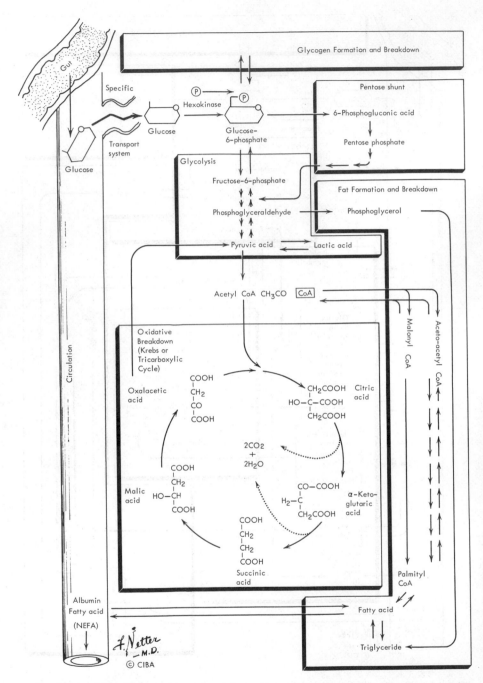

FIGURE 10—8. Protein metabolism. (Adapted From Plate VI, *The Ciba Collection of Medical Illustrations* by Frank H. Netter, M.D. Copyright CIBA.)

temperature, and the presence of coenzymes. For each enzyme there is an optimum pH. Deviations from this pH result in a reduction in activity. Enzymes in the gastric juice function best in an acid medium, while those secreted into the small intestine are most effective in alkaline media. Temperature also influences enzyme activity. Until a temperature of 50° C. is attained, reactions catalyzed by enzymes proceed more rapidly at higher temperatures than they do at lower temperatures. Temperatures of 50° C. or above inactivate enzymes. The use of hypothermia in certain types of surgical procedures is based on the fact that the rate of metabolism in cells is reduced by a lowering of body temperature. As body temperature is lowered, enzyme activity is reduced and the rate of metabolism is diminished.

The action of some enzymes depends on the presence of coenzymes. One such factor is ascorbic acid. Unless ascorbic acid is ingested in the diet, chemical reactions in which it participates do not proceed normally. Since ascorbic acid is not stored, signs of deficiency develop early in its absence from the diet. Although enzymes are protein in nature, some contain a prosthetic group, that is, a non-amino acid group, essential to their function. In some, the prosthetic group is a metal such as iron, magnesium, or copper. In others it is a vitamin such as thiamine, nicotinamide, pyridoxine, pantothenic acid, or vitamin K. Absence of one or more of these substances leads to a breakdown in metabolism and an accumulation of partly metabolized products. For example, thiamine enters into the formation of an enzyme catalyzing the degradation of pyruvic acid, the end product of the first stage of glucose metabolism. In the absence of thiamine, pyruvic acid accumulates in the blood and tissues and is excreted in the urine. The resulting disorder is known as beriberi. (See summary at the end of the chapter.)

The action of enzymes may be inhibited by the action of heavy metals and by certain drugs. Mercury is believed to produce toxicity by inhibiting enzyme reactions. Chemicals such as cyanide are highly toxic because they inhibit enzyme systems catalyzing oxidation-reduction reactions. Death occurs in a matter of minutes following the ingestion or inhalation of cyanide.

The actions of many drugs depend on their ability to depress enzymatic activity. Barbiturates are believed to depress the nervous system by depressing specific enzymes. Acetozoleamide (Diamox) induces diuresis by interfering with the ability of the enzyme carbonic anhydrase to catalyze the reaction enabling the kidney to reabsorb the sodium ion. As a result, the kidney excretes an increased volume of sodium ion in the urine. Sulfonamides are effective in the control of certain bacteria because they depress the enzyme system enabling them to synthesize folic acid from a para-aminobenzoic acid.

In addition to blocking the action of an enzyme by failing to provide something essential to its action or by depressing it with a chemical or physical agent, disorders in metabolism may be due to a deficiency or lack of an essential enzyme. Enzymes are synthesized by the organism in which they act. To synthesize enzymes, the organism must have the capacity for synthesis and be furnished with the necessary materials. The capacity to synthesize enzymes depends on the genetic inheritance of the individual. According to White,[83] a single gene is involved in a single metabolic reaction. A defective gene may be inherited as either a mendelian recessive or dominant. When inherited as a recessive trait, the defect is evident only in individuals inheriting the same trait from both parents. In the absence of a necessary enzyme, a metabolic process is stopped at the point where the missing enzyme acts. The clinical effects depend on the stage of metabolism that is blocked and the need of the organism for the product of the reaction. Diseases such as phenylketonuria (PKU) and alkaptonuria are well-known examples of the type of inborn error of metabolism in which a step in the metabolism of a substance is blocked by the absence of a necessary enzyme. Others will undoubtedly be identified in the future. See Chapter 13A for a discussion of phenylketonuria.

To this point, the discussion has centered around the importance of energy to the activities of the cell. The principal sources of energy are carbohydrates and fats. For neither carbohydrate nor fat has a daily average requirement been established. The small quantity of carbohydrate stored in the body is stored as glycogen in the liver and muscles. The quantity of glycogen deposited in the liver is sufficient to supply the needs of the body for glucose for about five hours. Carbohydrates are hydrolyzed to simple sugars or monosaccharides in the alimentary canal. Before monosaccharides can be absorbed, they must be phosphorylated; that is, a molecule of phosphate must be added. Like other biological chemical reactions phosphorylation requires the presence of an appropriate enzyme. The first step in the metabolism of glucose is its conversion to glucose 6-phosphate. Glucose 6-phosphate may be converted either to glycogen or, by a variety of pathways, to simpler products. The product of the most frequently used pathway is pyruvic acid. The pathway by which glucose is converted to pyruvic acid is known as the Emden-Myerhoff pathway. Enzymes are required for each step in the process of metabolism.

In addition to the production of energy, metabolism of glucose is necessary to prevent the excessive metabolism of fat and protein. At least 100 gm of endogenous or exogenous glucose must be metabolized each 24 hours to prevent the formation of ketoacids at a more rapid rate than they can be utilized. Provided glucose is available, insulin increases the rate at which fat is synthesized and prevents the accumulation of ketoacids in the blood. In severe diabetes mellitus, especially the growth onset type (juvenile or brittle type), failure to utilize glucose is associated with the overproduction of ketoacids by the liver with the development of acidosis. The effects of acidosis are discussed in the chapter on water and electrolyte balance. Severe restriction in the ingestion of carbohydrates to 40 gm or less per day will also result in ketosis. Ketosis is sometimes induced in the therapy of petit mal epilepsy. Patients on very restricted reduction diets usually develop some degree of ketosis, as do those experiencing naturally occurring starvation.

[83] Abraham White, *et al., Principles of Biochemistry,* 2nd ed., The Blakiston Division, McGraw-Hill Book Company, Inc., New York, 1959, p. 609.

The ability of carbohydrate to reduce the degree to which the body utilizes its lean tissue for energy is called its protein-sparing action. An intake of about 100 gm a day is required to produce its maximum effect. Carbohydrate is also essential to protect the liver from the harmful effects of poisons such as chloroform or carbon tetrachloride. It is the preferred fuel of cardiac muscle and appears to be the only fuel metabolized by nerve cells. Although little glucose is stored as glycogen, it makes an important contribution to the reserve supply of calories inasmuch as glucose is converted to fat and stored as such.

Plants and plant products provide the main sources of glucose. In the American culture, the cereals—wheat, corn, and rice—as well as potatoes and sugar are high carbohydrate sources in common use. A variety of vegetables and fruits contribute to the total intake.

In health the level of glucose in the blood is maintained from 70 to 110 mg per 100 ml of blood plasma. As with other homeostatic conditions, constancy depends on the maintenance of supply and the regulation of processes by which glucose is added to or removed from body fluids. The processes are governed in relation to each other with the result that equilibrium is maintained. A change in one direction is counteracted by the activation of mechanisms that correct for the change. The result is change within limits. In terms of glucose, an addition of glucose to the blood results in an increase in the activity of mechanisms for lowering its level in the blood. There appears to be a negative feedback relationship between the factors raising and lowering the concentration of glucose in the blood.

The organism has three general sources of supply of glucose. They are: (1) glucose derived from carbohydrate sources ingested into and absorbed from the alimentary canal, (2) glycogen stored in the liver and muscles and to a lesser extent in other tissues; only liver glycogen is available to raise the level of glucose; (3) protein and fat stores. Glucose is also removed from the blood by three general mechanisms. It is (1) removed by the cells and utilized as energy; (2) removed by the liver and muscles and converted to glycogen and stored; and (3) eliminated by the kidney when the level of glucose in the blood exceeds the renal threshold. In health the renal threshold for glucose is somewhere between 150 and 160 mg per 100 ml of blood. Some authorities cite the upper limit for the renal threshold as 180 mg per 100 ml of blood. In persons in whom prolonged hyperglycemia is present, the renal threshold for glucose may be above 200 mg.[84] As the site in which glucose is stored, the liver serves both to remove glucose from the blood and to restore the level when it falls.

The level of glucose in the blood is regulated by a number of mechanisms. Insulin, which is secreted by the beta cells of the islands of Langerhans in the pancreas, increases the rate at which the liver and muscles store glucose as glycogen and the rate at which glucose enters and is utilized by the cells. Thus

---

[84] The renal threshold is the level at which, when it is exceeded, a substance appears in the urine.

insulin plays an important role in the removal of glucose from the blood. According to Best and Taylor,[85] insulin is also essential for the protein anabolic effect of somatotrophin[86] and for the storage of fat. Regulation of the secretion of insulin appears to be principally by the level of glucose in the blood. The nervous system probably also plays a role, since the islet cells are richly supplied with fibers from the vagus nerve.

Other hormones act to elevate the level of glucose in the blood. Epinephrine acts on the liver to release glycogen as glucose. The adrenal corticoids, cortisone and hydrocortisone, elevate blood glucose by increasing the production of glucose from tissue protein. The production of glucose from noncarbohydrate substances is known as glyconeogenesis. As a result of their action, the adrenal glycocorticoids intensify the severity of diabetes mellitus. According to Best and Taylor,[87] the point at which the adrenal corticoids act in metabolism is not clear. Anterior pituitary hormones also have an anti-insulin effect. Houssay first demonstrated the anti-insulin effect of the pituitary hormones in dogs made diabetic by the removal of the pancreas. The ensuing diabetes could be ameliorated by the removal of the pituitary gland. According to Best and Taylor,[88] the anterior hypophysis influences glucose metabolism through the effect of adrenocorticotrophin and somatotrophin. Adrenocorticotrophin acts by increasing the production of the adrenal corticoids by the adrenal cortex. Somatotrophin acts directly on the cells. In animals the administration of the growth hormones over a period of several weeks results in the development of a permanent state of diabetes mellitus. Examination of the pancreas of these animals reveals severe damage to the islet cells.

Another hormone that has been utilized in experimental studies to elevate the level of glucose in the blood is glucagon. It has been extracted from the pancreas and may possibly be secreted by the alpha cells. To date evidence is not available as to whether or not it has a physiological effect in the control of the blood sugar.

Finally, thyroid hormones affect carbohydrate metabolism in several ways. They increase the utilization of carbohydrate by the tissues and they increase the rate at which glucose is formed from glycogen by the liver. In experimental animals the administration of thyroid hormones results in the destruction of islet tissues.

In addition to the hormonal regulation of the level of glucose in the blood, the nervous system appears to play a role. Evidence of its role in regulation is incomplete, but it has been observed that lesions in certain parts of the hypothalamus are associated with glycosuria.

The liver and certain other tissues have been demonstrated to contain two factors or enzymes, one inactivating insulin (an insulinase) and one inhibiting

[85] Best and Taylor, *Op. cit.*, 7th ed., p. 820.
[86] Growth hormone from the anterior pituitary.
[87] *Op. cit.*, 7th ed., p. 1035.
[88] *Ibid.*, p. 832.

the action of the first or insulinase inhibitor. Though the physiological significance of these substances has not been established, a disturbance in the balance between these two substances may possibly lead to an increase in the rate at which insulin is destroyed.[89]

In the preceding paragraphs, mechanisms for the control of the quantity of glucose in the blood have been discussed. As with other homeostatic conditions, constancy depends on a supply of glucose and the regulation of processes by which glucose is added to and removed from the blood. These processes are regulated in relation to each other so that a change in one direction activates a mechanism or mechanisms to correct the change. In this way constancy within limits is maintained. As far as is known, the principal blood glucose-lowering factor is insulin. At least five internal secretions, as well as the nervous system, and possibly anti-insulin hormones, regulate mechanisms for the elevation of the level of glucose in the blood. Thus the individual appears to be better protected against hypoglycemia than against hyperglycemia. The liver, as the principal site for the storage of glycogen, serves both in the removal of glucose from the blood and as a source of supply. Through the regulation of a number of processes, the organism is able to maintain a continuous supply of glucose to its cells, despite the periodic ingestion of food.

Despite the effectiveness of regulatory mechanisms in keeping the level of glucose in the blood within physiological limits in most people, they sometimes fail. Depending on the nature of the failure, the level of glucose in the blood falls outside physiological limits. When the concentration of glucose in the blood falls below 70 mg per 100 ml, the condition is known as hypoglycemia. Hyperglycemia exists when the concentration of glucose in the blood rises above 110 to 120 mg per 100 ml of blood plasma. In both states, there is a disturbance in the balance between the amount of glucose added to or removed from the blood.

Theoretically, hypoglycemia could result from a failure in the supply of glucose. In diseases of the liver in which its capacity to store glycogen is below physiological limits, hypoglycemia is at times a problem. Hypoglycemia may also result from failure of the mechanisms for adding glucose to the blood. As a consequence, hypoglycemia is associated with adrenal insufficiency. Probably the most frequent cause of hypoglycemia of a severe degree is overactivity of the mechanism for lowering the level of glucose in the blood, that is, an oversupply of insulin. The insulin may be of endogenous or exogenous origin. If the supply of insulin is excessive, the level of glucose in the blood falls below 70 mg per 100 ml of blood. The effects of lowering the level of glucose in the blood will depend on the suddenness and the extent to which it falls below normal limits.

Most of the manifestations of hypoglycemia result from failure to supply

[89] *Ibid.,* p. 822.

sufficient glucose to the cells of the nervous system. Glucose is the only fuel from which it can derive energy. Early symptoms and signs in hypoglycemia result from increased autonomic activity. Hunger, often marked, sweating, increased pulse rate, restlessness, irritability, and headache occur early. The patient who is experiencing hypoglycemia for the first time may say, "I feel funny," or "I feel peculiar." Changes in the usual behavior of a patient who is receiving insulin are frequently the result of hypoglycemia. For example, Steven Anderson, who had been a model patient, suddenly became very amorous. Mary Sema was found sitting upright in bed, her eyes fixed and her arms rigidly extended in front of her. Mild-mannered Mr. Boas became violent when treatment of hypoglycemia was delayed until blood could be drawn for glucose analysis. Mr. Johns was admitted to the hospital in coma. Buddy Reiman, aged 12, developed nocturnal enuresis (bed wetting). Each of the above patients was suffering from the effects of hypoglycemia. In each instance, treatment with a readily available form of glucose restored the patient to his usual mode of behavior. With the exception of Mr. Johns, glucose was administered by mouth in the form of fruit juice. Moments after an intravenous solution of glucose was begun, Mr. Johns regained consciousness and was demanding to know why he was in the hospital.

Because of the possibility of permanent damage to the brain, patients who receive insulin in the treatment of diabetes mellitus should learn to recognize early symptoms and signs of hypoglycemia and how to treat it. Modified insulins create a problem, inasmuch as hypoglycemia may develop without causing warning signs. Persons under insulin therapy should also be taught that exercise improves the utilization of glucose and that hypoglycemia is more likely to develop when unusual amounts of exercise are taken. They should be subject to regular observation when they are hospitalized. Should they develop signs or symptoms indicating hypoglycemia, it should be treated promptly. Usually 100 ml of orange or other fruit juice provides sufficient glucose to correct the condition. Observation of patients receiving long-acting insulin who experience hypoglycemia should be continued. Because of the possibility of recurrence of hypoglycemia in persons receiving long acting insulin, milk and crackers may be used in treatment as they provide for a more sustained source of glucose than do fruit juices or sugar.

Excessive secretion of insulin associated with hyperplasia or an adenoma of islet cells may also be responsible for hypoglycemia. Adenomas are believed to be of infrequent occurrence. Cure is effected by surgical removal. According to Renold and Thorn,[90] functional hypoglycemia is a common occurrence. It is usually associated with anxiety and increased nervous tension. Symptoms such as weakness, faintness, tachycardia, and headache follow a meal. The ingestion of carbohydrate alleviates the symptoms temporarily but because carbohydrates act to stimulate the secretion of insulin, a vicious circle,

[90] In Harrison, *Op. cit.*, p. 663.

or positive feedback, is initiated.[91] Most patients respond well to a high-protein, high-fat, and low-carbohydrate diet. They should be instructed to avoid the ingestion of highly concentrated carbohydrates as they stimulate the secretion of insulin.

In contrast to hypoglycemia, hyperglycemia is a condition in which the level of glucose in the blood exceeds the upper limits of normal. It can result from the excessive ingestion of glucose, from overproduction of glucose within the organism, or from inadequacy or failure of the mechanism for the removal of glucose from the blood. More than one mechanism may be involved. The condition in which hyperglycemia follows the excessive ingestion of concentrated carbohydrates is known as alimentary glycosuria. The term "alimentary" refers to the fact that glucose is absorbed from the alimentary canal. The presence of glucosuria indicates that the renal threshold for glucose has been exceeded with the result that glucose appears in the urine. Therapy is obvious: avoid eating excessive quantities of glucose.

Overactivity of one or more of the mechanisms for the endogenous formation of glucose follows the administration of epinephrine, and this results in an elevated blood glucose. It can also be expected to rise as a part of the reaction of the individual to stressful situations. Many patients have some elevation in blood glucose following a coronary occlusion or major surgery. Because epinephrine stimulates the liver to convert glycogen to glucose, the elevation of the blood sugar depends on glycogen being present in the liver.

Hyperglycemia of sufficient degree to cause glycosuria may also occur in persons with hyperfunctioning adrenal cortices. It is also a finding in acromegaly, a disorder associated with hyperexcretion of the growth hormone by the anterior hypophysis. In these conditions the failure in the homeostasis of glucose is thought to be the result of the overproduction of glucose by the organism. The possibility also exists that some of these hormones also antagonize the action of insulin or interfere with its secretion.

A third source of hyperglycemia derives from a failure of the mechanisms for the removal of glucose from the blood. Although the mechanism that immediately comes to mind relates to the action of insulin, failure of the liver to store glucose is also a cause of hyperglycemia. In serious liver disease, hyperglycemia after a meal, followed by a sharp fall with hypoglycemia, is a common finding.

The second source of failure to remove glucose from the blood at a normal rate is a deficiency in the supply of insulin. Although this is generally believed to be the result of inadequate secretion, it may possibly be caused by an increase in the rate at which insulin is destroyed. Whatever the cause, hyperglycemia occurs when the supply of insulin is insufficient to remove glucose from the blood as rapidly as it is added. All degrees of failure are possible. In some individuals sufficient insulin is secreted to maintain the level of glucose

[91] In a positive feedback, a change in one direction intensifies the tendency to change in the same direction.

within physiological limits provided the ingestion of glucose is moderate or there is no increase in the activity of mechanisms for increasing the production of glucose. In others the deficiency of insulin may be so great that only by restricting the intake of glucose and the administration of exogenous insulin can the blood sugar be maintained within normal limits most of the time. The disease resulting from a failure of the mechanism to remove glucose from the blood at a normal rate is diabetes mellitus.

How can persons who are unable to adapt to a heavy load of glucose be identified?

Individuals who are unable to adapt normally to a heavy load of glucose can be indentified by a glucose tolerance test. The details for performance of this test differ from one physician or agency to another. In all instances the purpose of the test is to determine the adequacy of the mechanism of the patient for removing glucose from the blood, thereby restoring homeostasis. One simple but effective method to determine the adequacy of the mechanisms for lowering the blood glucose is to instruct the patient to eat a breakfast containing 100 gm of glucose. Two hours later a sample of blood is taken. If the concentration of glucose in the blood is within normal limits, the capacity of the person to adapt to glucose is adequate.

To obtain accurate results from a glucose tolerance test, the patient may be placed on a diet containing 300 gm of carbohydrate for two or three days before the test is performed. The nurse has a responsibility to make sure that the patient understands the instructions and, when he is in the hospital, to encourage him to eat the food served to him. On the day of the test fasting specimens of blood and urine to be used as controls are obtained before glucose is administered. The patient is then given 100 gm of glucose dissolved in water and flavored with citric acid or lemon juice. Specimens of blood and urine are obtained one-half, one, two, and three hours later. In one modification, the glucose is divided into two parts. The second 50 gm is given one-half hour after the first. In the person who has a normal adaptive capacity, the level of glucose in the blood does not rise after the second dose of glucose. In the person whose adaptive capacity is impaired, the level of glucose in the blood continues to rise.

The results obtained in individuals with normal and abnormal glucose tolerance curves differ in several respects. The individual who has a normal capacity to respond to an increased supply of glucose has a sharp, but limited, rise in the concentration of glucose in his blood plasma. The maximum elevation should not exceed 150 mg per 100 ml of blood plasma. There is a sharp rise in one-half hour, with little rise thereafter. By the second hour the concentration of glucose in the blood has returned to normal.

The individual with an inadequate capacity to remove glucose from the blood responds to overloading with glucose differently. The fasting blood

sugar is higher than normal. The rise in the blood sugar following the ingestion of glucose is higher, and the return to the pretest level is delayed. This
type of curve is observed in the patient in the early phases of diabetes as well
as in those whose diabetes mellitus is known.

Since the early detection and treatment of diabetes mellitus are believed to
be of advantage to the individual, a modified glucose tolerance test is sometimes used to identify persons who carry the diabetic trait. The individual is
given two glucose tolerance tests. The first test is performed in the usual
manner. Before the second test is performed, 50 mg of cortisone is administered orally twice. The first dose of cortisone is administered eight hours and
the second two hours before the second test is performed. The cortisone
intensifies the strain on the mechanisms for removing glucose from the blood.
In persons with an inadequate insulin reserve, the blood glucose curve obtained during the second test resembles that found in diabetes mellitus. Persons who respond positively to this test are encouraged to follow a regime to
decrease the likelihood of developing diabetes mellitus, that is, to avoid gaining weight.

For example, Mrs. Hale, aged 27, has latent diabetes mellitus. Both her
parents are diabetics. When Mrs. Hale is well and eats moderately and exercises actively and regularly, her fasting blood sugar is within normal limits.
When she overeats, has a cold, or is pregnant, her blood glucose tends to rise.
She sees her physician regularly and eats moderately. She tries to adjust her
food intake so that she maintains her ideal weight. In contrast Mrs. Hale's
sister Clara's response to glucose tolerance tests indicates that her capacity to
adapt to glucose is within normal limits. Present-day knowledge is insufficient
to be sure that Clara will never develop diabetes. Since the ideal weight favors
health and longevity, Clara has been advised to avoid obesity and to exercise
regularly. She has also been assured that she does not have diabetes.

The second important source of calories is fat. It yields 9.3 calories per
gram. Fats found in the body are of three types, triglycerides or neutral fats,
phospholipids, and sterols. Because there appears to be a relationship between
the excessive ingestion of fats and the development of atherosclerosis, considerable publicity has been given to this problem. Emphasis on the danger of
excess fats in the diet, rather than the role of fat in nutrition, is unfortunate. In
animals the unsaturated fatty acids linolinic, linoleic, and arachedonic have
been demonstrated to be essential to nutrition. They are presumed to be
essential in human nutrition. Though the daily requirements of fat are not
known, some fat is probably essential in the diet of everyone.

Fats serve a number of important functions in the organism. They are
sources of calories and are necessary to the absorption and utilization of the
fat-soluble vitamins A, D, E, and K. Choline, which is derived from fat, is
necessary to the health of the liver, and in its absence, fat tends to accumulate
in the liver. Fat also contributes to the palatability and satiety value of the
diet. The basis for the common misconception that fat is difficult to digest is

that it has a high satiety value. Fat enhances the efficiency with which the body utilizes carbohydrates and proteins. Fat deposits serve not only as storage depots for calories, but also to insulate and protect body structures. Studies on the effects of starvation indicate that starving persons are much more sensitive to cold after they lose their fat stores than they were previously.

Sources of fats include meat, fish, poultry, and dairy products as well as vegetables such as corn, peanuts, and other nuts, cotton seed, and coconuts. Fats derived from meats tend to be solid, while those from fish, poultry, and vegetable sources are liquid at room temperatures. Fats from animals indigenous to warm climates tend to be solid, while those from animals from cold climates tend to be liquid. Liquid fats can be made into solid fats by hydrogenation. Despite the implication in some advertisements that artificially hydrogenated fats are more healthful than the naturally occurring ones, this is not true. The type of fatty acids contained in each fat differs with each source. Although the types of fatty acids found in a given animal tend to be characteristic of an animal, they are influenced by feeding. For example, the fat of animals fed corn tends to be solid. When peanuts are used in fattening, the fatty acids are different and the fat is less solid.

The Committee on Fats in Human Nutrition[92] makes a number of pertinent statements about fats. They state that the terms "animal" and "vegetable" fats are meaningless and should be discarded. They emphasize that fats are important in human nutrition, as a source both of energy and of other essential elements. Despite the accumulation of a large body of information about fat, much remains to be learned about its role in nutrition and in the development of disease, including atherosclerosis. The statement has been made that the American diet is as nearly adequate as that of any enjoyed by civilized man. Two characteristics of the diet that should be followed are moderation and reasonableness. If variety in selection of food is added to the above two, adequacy of the diet is likely.

Cholesterol is one of the lipids which is being subjected to extensive and intensive study because of the frequency with which those suffering from atherosclerosis have elevations in blood cholesterol and other blood fats. See Chapter 9.

Though some fat is digested in the stomach, the principal site of digestion is in the small intestine. Bile contributes to the digestion of fat by acting as an emulsifying agent. Absorption of fatty acids from the intestine depends on the presence of bile salts. In the cells of the intestine, the products of fat digestion are resynthesized into fat which passes into the lacteals (lymphatics) and is delivered to the blood via the thoracic duct. Bile salts are absorbed into the

[92] Committee on Fats in Human Nutrition, ed. Willis A. Gortner, *The Role of Dietary Fat in Human Health, A Report of the Food and Nutrition Board.* Publication 575, National Academy of Sciences, National Research Council, Washington, D.C., 1958, pp. 24-25.

blood of the capillaries in the small intestine. They are returned to the liver via the portal system, where they are again secreted into the bile. Any condition which interferes with the secretion of bile or obstructs its flow into the intestine results in the inability to digest and absorb fats. Deficiencies of fat-soluble vitamins, particularly of vitamin K, occur in patients who have long-standing obstructions of the common bile duct.

In the metabolism of fat, fatty acids are oxidized by beta oxidation with the liberation of energy, carbon dioxide, and water. In beta oxidation, which was first postulated by Knoop, the fatty acid chain is dismembered in a stepwise fashion by the removal of two carbon atoms at a time until the chain is reduced to molecules, each containing two carbon atoms. Similar to glucose, activation of the fatty acid requires ATP. The two carbon atom fragments resulting from beta oxidation take one of two possible pathways. They may be converted to acetyl coenzyme A, which combines with oxaloacetate and enters the citric acid pool along with the intermediary products of carbohydrate and protein metabolism, or they may recombine to form acetoacetyl coenzyme A and other ketones. Under normal conditions the quantity converted to ketone is minimal. When, however, too little carbohydrate is ingested or the capacity to utilize it is depressed, the requirements of the body for energy must be met by increased use of fat. With an increase in the metabolism of fat, production of acetoacetic acid is heightened. Glucose, which is necessary to permit the smooth entry of acetoacetic acid into the citric acid cycle, is deficient. This results in the production of ketones at a rate which is more rapid than the body can oxidize them. They accumulate in blood and are excreted in the urine. Since acetoacetic acid and beta hydroxybutyric acid are acids, their continued production results in metabolic acidosis. (See the chapter 8 and 17A.)

The regulation of the level of lipids in the blood is highly complex, and much still remains to be learned. Fats in the blood are all bound to proteins and are therefore lipoproteins. The proportion of fat to protein in the molecule varies. This affects not only the size of the molecule, but the tendency of the molecule to remain suspended in the blood plasma or to settle out. Following the ingestion of a fatty meal, lipemia begins in one to three hours and continues for six to seven hours and then decreases until fasting levels have been reached. A number of chemicals have been identified that appear to increase the rate at which fats are cleared from the blood. They include unsaturated fats containing essential fatty acids, heparin, and lipoprotein lipase. The latter enzyme is also found in high concentrations in certain types of cells. The thyroid hormones have a significant regulatory effect. In hypothyroidism, there is an increase in body fat as well as an elevation of serum cholesterol and other lipids.

As stated earlier, secretions from the gonads also influence the homeostasis of fat. Healthy young women have a relatively greater part of their blood cholesterol in the lipoprotein fraction and less in the β lipoprotein fraction than do normal men of the same age. After the menopause, this difference disappears. Young women rarely have coronary heart disease.

In the homeostasis of fat, excess fats are stored in adipose tissue. All energy-yielding foods, carbohydrates, proteins, and fat, contribute to body fat. Although it is important in the storage of carbohydrate, the liver is not an important organ for the storage of fat. In fact, storage of fat in the liver is an indication of disease. The normal sites for the storage of fat include subcutaneous connective tissue, the abdominal cavity, and muscular tissue. In individuals suffering from extreme obesity, adipose tissue cells may infiltrate the heart and the exocrine pancreas. Fatty degeneration, a disorder in which fat accumulates in abnormal quantities in the parenchyma of organs such as the liver, also occurs. The factors influencing the release and accumulation of depot fat continue to be intriguing and at the same time elusive. As in any highly complicated homeostatic mechanism, there are a number of opportunities for the balance between supply and synthesis and storage and mobilization to go wrong. Despite the poor repute of fats, they are essential in nutrition. Moderate stores are also necessary. Here, as in other areas in life, supply within limits, rather than the all-or-none approach, is probably most appropriate.

What are the requirements for protein and how is it used in the body?

In the preceding discussion, the requirements of the organism for calories and the materials from which they are derived have been presented. The following section will be concerned with the requirements of the body for protein as well as with how it functions in the body. How the organism uses protein depends on the extent to which its need for calories is being met and on the extent to which its protein requirements are met or exceeded. Any condition increasing the total requirements of the body is likely to increase the need for protein. For example, protein requirements are increased during growth, pregnancy, and lactation and during recovery from illness or surgical operation. Protein is necessary for a variety of functions in the body. In addition to growth and repair of tissue, protein is required for the formation of enzymes and antibodies. Blood proteins are responsible for the colloid osmotic pressure of the blood and act as one of the buffer systems in the blood.

Protein differs in chemical composition from carbohydrate and fat, in that, in addition to carbon, hydrogen, and oxygen, it contains nitrogen and sometimes sulfur. A person is said to be in nitrogen balance when his intake of protein equals his output. Nitrogen balance is determined by comparing the amount of nitrogen in the food eaten with the nitrogenous compounds found in the urine. When the quantity of nitrogenous compounds found in the urine is less than in the intake of protein, the individual is said to be in a positive nitrogen balance and he is storing protein. When the intake of protein is less than the output of nitrogenous compounds in the urine, the individual is in negative nitrogen balance and he is catabolizing protein.

The body has the capacity to adapt to differences in protein intake and to maintain nitrogen balance. When the intake of protein is increased, the nitrogen balance is positive for a few days and then the balance is set at a higher level. When intake is decreased, the balance is negative for a short time and then it is established at a lower level. There is, however, a critical level below which the body continues to lose protein despite an inadequate intake. When protein intake and/or caloric intake is insufficient, the body proteins are broken down to provide amino acids and energy.

There is more knowledge of the minimum and optimum requirements for proteins than there is of requirements for carbohydrates and fats. *Recommended Dietary Allowances*[93] suggests that 0.66 gm of protein per kilogram of body weight is the minimum requirement, while 1 gm per kilogram is probably optimum. At the present time there is no evidence that an excessive intake of protein is harmful.

The quality as well as the quantity of protein is of importance. Eight of the twenty-one amino acids must be taken in food as the body cannot synthesize them. However, the so-called nonessential amino acids are important as the body utilizes the essential amino acids more efficiently in their presence. Moreover, the ability of the body to utilize any amino acids depends on the presence at the same time of other required materials.

Proteins are derived from both animal and vegetable sources. Requirements can be met from either source, but since vegetables are less likely to contain all the essential amino acids, a wider variety and larger intake are necessary to meet protein needs. The foods that are good sources of protein also contain considerable amounts of fat. Thus meat, eggs, milk, and cheese are sources of both. Nuts also contain both fat and protein. Cereals and legumes are sources of both protein and carbohydrate as well as of some fat. Dried milk is an inexpensive source of good-quality proteins. In countries where acceptable sources of animal proteins are lacking, dried milk is sometimes added to the dietary. Essential amino acids that can be synthesized without excessive cost can also be utilized to improve the quality of vegetable protein. For example, lysine added to wheat flour raises the usable protein from one half to nearly two thirds.[94]

Protein is digested in the alimentary canal to amino acids which are absorbed into the blood stream. Their fate in the body depends on the needs and conditions within the organism at the time. They may be synthesized into body substance or into antibodies or enzymes. When the quantity taken in is in excess of requirements, they may be stored or deaminized in the liver. The resulting molecules are then utilized as carbohydrate or fat.

[93] *Op. cit.*, p. 18.
[94] UN Technology and Science Conference, "Improving Levels of Nutrition Through Better Health Practices," *Public Health Reports*, LXXVIII, April, 1963, pp. 338.

What are the possible effects of a lack of protein?

Throughout the literature authorities emphasize that deficiences of a single nutrient in the diet rarely occur. Cause-and-effect relationships are thus difficult to establish. In the absence of an inadequate intake of protein, there is likely to be a deficiency in the B vitamins as many of them are found in protein-rich foods. Many of the effects observed in persons whose intake of protein is insufficient could be due in part to a deficiency in vitamins. In patients whose intake of protein is insufficient, loss of weight and strength frequently occur. In young children whose intake of protein is severely restricted a disease known as kwashiorkor, in which severe liver damage occurs, develops. The tendency of the chronic alcoholic to liver disease may be due partly to the fact that diets of alcoholics are deficient in proteins and B vitamins. In starvation the colloid osmotic pressure of the blood is reduced as the level of blood protein falls. Lack of protein may reduce the ability of the organism to react to stress and to resist infections.

What types of disorders predispose to protein deficiency?

Protein deficiency occurs in any condition in which there is an inability to ingest protein, as after a surgical operation, or following trauma, or in a serious illness. The deficit is aggravated by the fact that there is an increase in the rate of tissue breakdown for the first few days after a severe injury or a surgical procedure. Proteins may be lost in excessive amounts into the urine, from draining wounds such as burned surfaces, and in accumulations of serous fluids such as ascites. Chronic abscesses, decubiti, or osteomyelitis may be accompanied by an excessive loss of protein. Continued bed rest, even in the healthy, is accompanied by loss of protein for the first three or four days— then the loss of protein tapers off and the nitrogen balance is restored. Loss of protein from the body is, therefore, one of the undesirable effects of bed rest. Loss of protein-containing fluid represents a loss not only of protein, but of minerals, vitamins, water, and other substances, from the body. The effects on the organism will depend in part on the suddennesss with which the losses occur, the conditions that are responsible, and the length of time that they persist. Sudden large losses of fluid into serous cavities may, by reducing blood volume, lead to shock. Smaller losses over a period of time lead to malnutrition with a loss of weight, strength, and ability to respond to stress. Resistance of tissue to pressure is less in the undernourished than in the well nourished. When decubiti form, they resist treatment unless and until protein and other nutritional deficiences are corrected. Recovery depends on the restoration of nutritive elements.

In addition to calories and proteins, minerals are essential to the economy of the organism. Some minerals, such as sodium, are essential constituents of the environment of cells. Others, such as potassium and calcium, are not only essential components of the extracellular fluid, but are constituents of the cell itself.

In addition to the chemicals discussed in Chapter 8, what others are required for normal function?

Iodine is rapidly absorbed into the blood from the gastrointestinal tract. It is removed from the blood by the thyroid gland, where it is concentrated and utilized in the formation of thyroid hormone. The thyroid hormones stimulate the rate of metabolism. In conditions in which there is a total lack of thyroxin, the basal metabolic rate falls by about 40 per cent. In prolonged deficiency of iodine hypothyroidism associated with hyperplasia of the thyroid gland is a common occurrence. Iodine deficiency is most common in the parts of the world far from the sea. During the history of the world, soil has been leached of iodine and iodine washed into the streams and thence into the seas and oceans. Soil in the great plains, such as the center of the United States, and in mountainous regions, such as the Andean Altiplano or the Swiss Alps, is deficient in iodine. In these areas evidence of iodine deficiency has been common. Conditions increasing the need for thyroxin intensify the deficiency. Pregnancy, adolescence, or infections may be associated with enlargement of the thyroid gland in iodine-deficient areas. Prevention of iodine deficiency is achieved by the use of iodized salt.

When added to water in the amount of 1 part per million of water, fluorine has been demonstrated to reduce the rate of dental caries. Excessive concentrations of fluorine cause mottling of the enamel of the teeth. Despite convincing evidence of the value of fluorides in the prevention of dental caries, there has been organized resistance to the introduction of fluoride into drinking water. Some of the opponents claim the fluorine increases the incidence of heart disease in the areas where it is used. Objective analysis of the statistics indicates the falsity of this belief. Other persons object on the basis that fluorine is of value only to the young and that cities should not use tax funds to support a procedure that benefits only a part of the population. Still others object on religious grounds. Some even object on the ground that it violates the right of the individual to choose what he will or will not ingest. A review of the history of chlorination of water indicates a similar story.

Iron is essential not only to the formation of hemoglobin, but also to enzymes catalyzing reactions in the citric acid cycle. It is obtained from organ meats such as liver, kidney, and heart. Other good sources include whole wheat, egg yolk, oatmeal, fish and clams, nuts, dates, figs, beans, asparagus, spinach, and molasses. The requirements for iron vary. Blood loss, growth, and pregnancy and lactation all increase the need for iron. Only small amounts of iron are absorbed from the intestine, and the quantity of iron in the body is regulated by the rate at which it is absorbed. There is no mechanism for the excretion of excess iron once it is absorbed.[95] In diseases in

[95] Harper, *Op. cit.*, p. 323.

which there is excessive destruction of red blood cells, as in Mediterranean anemia, one of the serious problems is the accumulation of iron in the liver and other tissues. Repeated blood transfusions used in the treatment of non-hemorrhagic diseases also contribute to the excess of iron.

Anemia is the principal manifestation of lack of iron. In longstanding anemias due to a deficient intake of iron or to an excessive loss, the body responds by reducing the size of the red blood cells. These anemias are called microcytic, that is, small-cell anemias. Anemias may, of course, be caused by other conditions than those related to iron deficiency.

As has already been indicated, a number of other elements are essential for prosthetic groups in enzymes. The quantity of each element required is small, but apparently important. Copper, manganese, zinc, cobalt, and molybdenum have been demonstrated to be necessary to enzyme functions in animals. Some of the above elements have been identified in the structures of enzymes found in human cells.

Vitamins are substances that vary widely in chemical structure. Since they are not synthesized in the body, they must be provided from outside sources. Some of them, such as vitamin K, have multiple functions in the body. It is an essential component of an enzyme catalyzing the formation of prothrombin, a substance that is necessary to blood clotting. It is also believed to be a component of enzymes catalyzing reactions in the citric acid cycle. The role of the B vitamins in the formation of enzymes has already been discussed.

For the sake of clarity, each nutritional element was discussed individually. Nutritional deficiencies are, however, usually multiple. Most foods are the source of more than one nutrient. Moreover, chemical reactions require that all elements necessary to the reaction be present simultaneously. Deficiencies of nutrients that are stored develop more slowly than of those that are not. Hence, a deficiency of vitamin A, which is stored in the liver, may take from two to ten years to develop. A deficiency of ascorbic acid, which is not stored, develops quickly. Evidence of deficiences often does not appear until the organism is under stress and requirements are increased. Moreover, the so-called deficiency diseases do not occur unless there is an imbalance among the various nutritional elements.

In this chapter, the role of the nurse in facilitating the maintenance of nutrition in the patient has been presented. Content has been selected to emphasize the importance of nutrition to health and productivity as well as to the susceptibility to disease and the ability to recover therefrom. Emphasis has been placed on the manner in which the body uses nutrients in its processes and the manner in which these processes may be disturbed. Although stress has been placed on the biochemistry of nutrition, the importance of food in the emotional and social life of the individual has been included. Survival depends on the supply to the cells of at least a minimal level of nutrients. Growth, reproduction, and all the higher functions also depend on the nutritional state of the individual.

As with other needs, satisfaction of the need depends on adequate supplies to meet the requirements of the tissues; a facility whereby materials may be taken from the external environment and altered so that they can be transported to the internal environment; transportation from the point of entry to the cell; the capacity of the cell to utilize the nutrients; regulation of the processes so that the needs of the cells are met; and the integration of all activities so that the needs of the whole organism are met. Since some nutrients are stored, provisions for converting them into appropriate substances and storage facilities are necessary.

Facilities are also required to eliminate excesses of intake or end products of metabolism. A disruption or disturbance at any point may interfere with the capacity of the cell to carry on its processes.

Because of the importance of food, physiologically, emotionally, and socially, it provides the nurse with a natural medium through which to convey to the patient her concern for him as a person and as a human being. It is often through her efforts to meet his individual wishes and desires, that the food is "transferred from the plate to his stomach." Though it may be a cliché to say, "It isn't the food that is served to the patient, but what he eats that is important," it is true, nonetheless.

For short periods of time, diets inadequate in one or more nutrients may be ingested without causing serious harm. More or less permanent modifications in the dietary must meet basic nutritional requirements if malnutrition is to be avoided. In general, diets are modified to (1) accommodate to a disturbance in the structure or function of the gastrointestinal tract, (2) correct the effect of an excess or deficit of essential nutrients, and (3) accommodate to a defect in the capacity to utilize one or more nutrients.

The theme of this chapter is summarized in the words of King.

"Nutrition is the science of food, the nutrients and other substances therein, their action, interaction and balance in relation to health and disease, and the processes by which the organism ingests, absorbs, transports, utilizes, and excretes food substances. In addition, nutrition must be concerned with certain social, economic, cultural, and psychological implications of food and eating."[96]

[96] C. Glen King, in Ogden C. Johnson, "A Conference on Nutrition Teaching in Medical Schools," *Nutrition Reviews,* XXI, February, 1963, p. 34.

A Survey of Some Disorders of Nutrition and Conditions Involving the Alimentary Canal and Related Structures

Diagnostic Category	Etiological Factors	Incubation Period and Nature of Onset	Severity of Illness and Course	Part of Gastrointestinal Tract and/or Associated Structures Involved and Response	Effect on Adequacy of Nutrition	Major Medical and/or Surgical Treatment
Psychogenic and/or Neurogenic						
Achalasia (Cardiospasm)	Physiological obstruction. Emotional disturbances may precipitate.	Dysphagia of the kind in which there is a delay of ingested food entering the stomach.	Chronic condition. Progression of dysphagia inconsistent. Regurgitation in recumbent position. Weight loss eventually.	Esophagus: lower end fails to relax with each peristaltic wave. There is esophageal dilation of varying degree except at distal end, which is undilated. Substernal pain, dysphagia, regurgitation.	Nutritional state maintained initially but eventually malnutrition due to insufficient food intake.	Relief of anxiety about organic disease. Deeper psychotherapy if necessary.
Irritable colon	Excessive irritants (laxatives, foods, enemas), or emotional disturbance, or both.	Distention and fullness induced by ingestion of food or liquid to severe cramplike abdominal pain.	Defecation or passage of flatus may afford temporary relief or initiate more cramps and tenesmus. Nausea, belching, rumbling, gurgling in abdomen.	Colon: often palpable and tender. Normal rectum and sigmoid on proctoscopy. Colon irritability noted on barium enema.	Usually well nourished but occasionally varying degrees of malnutrition are seen.	Education of patient in relation to diet and fluids, in obtaining and maintaining satis-

Diagnostic Category	Etiological Factors	Incubation Period and Nature of Onset	Severity of Illness and Course	Part of Gastrointestinal Tract and/or Associated Structures Involved and Response	Effect on Adequacy of Nutrition	Major Medical and/or Surgical Treatment
			Excessive flatus.			factory bowel habits.
			Other physical symptoms related to psychogenesis of disease.			Avoidance of fecal impaction during initial therapy.
			Patient usually wants bowel movement daily and takes laxative or enema to achieve this.			Rest and exercise determined on individual basis.
						Antispasmodics.
Diverticulum (one) Diverticulosis (many) Diverticulitis (Inflammation of) (An outpouching or herniation of the mucosa through a defect in the muscularis.)	In general weakness of the muscular wall of the alimentary canal due to congenital defect or loss of muscle during the process of aging.	Depends on site, size, and presence or absence of inflammation.	May be symptomless, acute, chronic or recurring. Perforation results in mediastinitis or peritonitis depending on location.	Common sites esophagus, duodenum, and colon. May occur anywhere along the alimentary canal. In the presence of diverticulitis signs and symptoms of acute inflammation. Effects intensified by peritonitis or mediastinitis.	Depends on site and effects.	None, a diet avoiding nuts, seeds and fibrous foods, to surgical removal and closure of the defect.

A Survey of Some Disorders of Nutrition and Conditions Involving the Alimentary Canal and Related Structures—Continued

Diagnostic Category	Etiological Factors	Incubation Period and Nature of Onset	Severity of Illness and Course	Part of Gastrointestinal Tract and/or Associated Structures Involved and Response	Effect on Adequacy of Nutrition	Major Medical and/or Surgical Treatment
	Force within the digestive tract pushes outward.	May be few if any symptoms or minor difficulty in swallowing. Prominent complaint is regurgitation of undigested food particles on assuming the horizontal position.	See above.	Esophagus.	Malnutrition in later stages due to failure of food to enter the digestive tract.	Surgical treatment when symptoms occur.
	See above.	Two thirds of persons living to 85 years of age have them. See general comments.	See above.	Colon. See general comments.	None usually.	See Meckel's diverticulum.
Meckel's	Persistence of omphalomesenteric duct. Outpouching of	Lower abdominal	May parallel signs and symptoms of acute appendicitis when inflamed.	Large intestine. Ileum.	Malabsorption syndrome.	Surgical removal if necessary. Bed rest.

Diagnostic Category	Etiological Factors	Incubation Period and Nature of Onset	Severity of Illness and Course	Part of Gastrointestinal Tract and/or Associated Structures Involved and Response	Effect on Adequacy of Nutrition	Major Medical and/or Surgical Treatment
	serosa and mucosa at point where nutrient artery perforates muscularis layer.	pain worsened by defecation.	May cause volvulus, intussusception, or strangulation. Signs of peritoneal irritation. Muscle spasm. Fever. Guarding.			Heat to tender abdominal area. Antibiotic therapy. Very soft diet during acute phase; then diet avoiding nuts, seeds, and fibrous foods. Oil enemas. Surgical resection may be necessary.
Ulcerations						
Chronic nonspecific ulcerative colitis	No known single cause. Relationship between emotional stress and onset and exacerbations.	Diarrhea, abdominal pain, blood in stools.	Anemia, weight loss, anorexia.	Rectum and/or colon: inflammatory reaction involving mucosa and submucosa.	Malnutrition. Avitaminosis. Hypoproteinemia.	Correction of nutrition and electrolyte loss. Discourage bacterial invasion: antimicrobial therapy. Bed rest.
Acute ulcerative colitis		Diarrhea, toxicity, fever, abdominal	Exacerbations and remissions. Little	Rectum and rectosigmoid: intensely		Control diarrhea by

A Survey of Some Disorders of Nutrition and Conditions Involving the Alimentary Canal and Related Structures—Continued

Diagnostic Category	Etiological Factors	Incubation Period and Nature of Onset	Severity of Illness and Course	Part of Gastrointestinal Tract and/or Associated Structures Involved and Response	Effect on Adequacy of Nutrition	Major Medical and/or Surgical Treatment
		pain, distention, tenesmus, spasm, contraction.	systemic sign of active inflammation. Course varies with patient. May have local reaction and involvement. May develop carcinoma (3% to 5% do). May have hyper-immune response.	red, edematous, mucous membrane; tissue friable.		opiates initially and later by sedation and antispasmodics.
				Ileocecal valve to anus: as above.		Psychological support.
				Colon: engorged, hyperactive. Covered with thick, opalescent, tenacious mucus, high in lysozyme concentration; increased friability of mucous membrane; eventual ulceration and submucosal bleeding.		Parenteral feedings. Adrenal cortical steroids. Surgery may be necessary. All the above apply to both forms of the disease.
				Rectum: see above.		
Acute ulcerative proctitis			Bloody exudate on stool with no systemic manifestation.			

Diagnostic Category	Etiological Factors	Incubation Period and Nature of Onset	Severity of Illness and Course	Part of Gastro-intestinal Tract and/or Associated Structures Involved and Response	Effect on Adequacy of Nutrition	Major Medical and/or Surgical Treatment
Peptic ulcer						
Duodenal	Unknown—imbalance between digesting action of contents of the stomach and resistance of stomach and duodenum to digestion—see discussion.	Right epigastric pain. Pain usually 1 to 3 hours after eating. Nocturnal pain between 12 midnight and 2:00 A.M.	Characterized by exacerbations and remissions. Exacerbations occur most frequently in autumn and spring in temperate climates. Increased muscular activity initiates pain. May perforate.	First portion of duodenum: progressively a crater develops in which there is coagulation necrosis at base with infiltration and accumulation of acute and chronic inflammatory cells.		Hospitalization for therapy if possible. Reduction of volume, acidity, and peptic content of gastric juices. Modification of diet: soft, well cooked, non-fibrous, with liberal amounts of dairy products; frequent feedings; initially every two hours milk and cream with additions gradually made.
Gastric	Unknown. May be induced by adrenal steroid therapy; adrenergic blocking drugs (tolazine hydro-	Left epigastric pain. Pain usually one to several hours after eating, relieved by ingestion of food. History of	Vomiting when obstruction occurs. Anemia. Constipation. Chronic disease may lead to perforation.	Stomach: usually in prepyloric area of lesser curvature. Crater develops and area around becomes hyperemic, edema-	Caloric intake may exceed metabolic needs, and overnourishment leading to obesity may occur.	Antacids. Parasympatholytics. Sedatives and tranquilizers. Therapy individualized because of

A Survey of Some Disorders of Nutrition and Conditions Involving the Alimentary Canal and Related Structures—Continued

Diagnostic Category	Etiological Factors	Incubation Period and Nature of Onset	Severity of Illness and Course	Part of Gastro-intestinal Tract and/or Associated Structures Involved and Response	Effect on Adequacy of Nutrition	Major Medical and/or Surgical Treatment
	chloride, hydralazine, and hexamethonium) May develop in connection with practically all diseases.	six to seven years of attacks. Exacerbations occur frequently in spring and fall.		tous, and infiltrated.	Malnutrition may occur if fear of eating is present or prolonged vomiting.	role of stress (emotional and physical) in exacerbations. Surgery (subtotal gastrectomy) may be indicated.
Curling's	Following extensive burns of the skin.	Pain. Hemorrhage.	Nausea and vomiting.	Stomach-duodenum.		
Vascular						
Varices Esophageal	1. Increased pressure in veins of portal system—cirrhosis. 2. Thrombosis of portal and/or splenic vein (uncommon).	Hematemesis.	Chronic illness. Blood loss. Weight loss.	Esophagus: veins are distended and tortuous.	If etiology is cirrhosis, there is generalized malnutrition caused usually by pure carbohydrate intake.	Symptomatic therapy of clinical picture presented. Possible surgery—various shunts.
Mechanical Obstruction Neoplasia—be-						

Diagnostic Category	Etiological Factors	Incubation Period and Nature of Onset	Severity of Illness and Course	Part of Gastrointestinal Tract and/or Associated Structures Involved and Response	Effect on Adequacy of Nutrition	Major Medical and/or Surgical Treatment
nign or malignant neoplasms may occur at any level of the alimentary canal. Occurrence in the small intestine is rare. See Chapter 12.						
Hemorrhoids (dilation of either the internal or external hemorrhoidal plexus or both).	Predisposing factors—constipation, motionless standing, pregnancy, hereditary weakness of the wall of the hemorrhoidal vein. May be found in patients with cancer in the rectum or sigmoid colon.	May be present with few symptoms, or may be highly acute.	When infected, thrombosed, and prolapsed through the anus, symptoms may be exceedingly acute. Severe pain is common. Though bleeding is usually minimal, the loss of large quantities of blood does occur.	Hemorrhoidal veins in anal canal.	None unless continued or excessive loss of blood.	Surgical removal—After-care is very important. Operated area must be kept clean and strictures prevented from forming. Immediately after operation an ice bag may be placed over the dressing to lessen pain. Sitz baths are started about 24 hours after surgery. Mineral oil to keep stool

A Survey of Some Disorders of Nutrition and Conditions Involving the Alimentary Canal and Related Structures—Continued

Diagnostic Category	Etiological Factors	Incubation Period and Nature of Onset	Severity of Illness and Course	Part of Gastrointestinal Tract and/or Associated Structures Involved and Response	Effect on Adequacy of Nutrition	Major Medical and/or Surgical Treatment
						soft. In the treatment of acutely infected and thrombosed hemorrhoids, Sitz baths, stool softeners, keep area clean.
Choledocho-lithiasis	Calculi in common duct.	Biliary colic, fever, and chills.	Jaundice—severity dependent on extent of obstruction. If persistent may lead to distention of the gall bladder.	Extra- and intrahepatic biliary passages may become dilated and edematous.		Vitamin K when jaundice present.
Hernia (protrusion of the contents of the peritoneal cavity through a defect in the wall).	Developmental defects—trauma aging.	Depends on location. Some hernias can be seen and felt as a bulge in the affected area.	May be few symptoms or signs until hernia becomes incarcerated (irreducible), and intestinal obstruction and strangulation occur. If allowed to continue, bowel becomes gangren-	Depends on location and whether or not strangulation occurs. With gangrene of the intestine, peritonitis occurs. Locations include: Inguinal Direct Indirect	Depends on location.	Surgical repair, preferably before complications develop.

Diagnostic Category	Etiological Factors	Incubation Period and Nature of Onset	Severity of Illness and Course	Part of Gastro-intestinal Tract and/or Associated Structures Involved and Response	Effect on Adequacy of Nutrition	Major Medical and/or Surgical Treatment
			ous and peritonitis occurs.	Femoral Umbilical Ventral Post operative incisions Hiatus or diaphragmatic hernia.		
Hiatus Hernia		Gradual onset resulting in substernal or epigastric pressure precipitated by eating. Belching.	Chronic illness which may be quiescent or lead to development of respiratory embarrassment, cardiac irregularities. Bleeding, slow but persistent.	Stomach and esophagus. Stomach herniates into thorax, leads to esophagitis after regurgitation of gastric contents, continues for a long time. Hyperemia of gastric mucosa, due to compression of venous drainage, renders it easily susceptible to trauma.	When acute episode of esophagitis interferes with food ingestion, there is an inadequate quality of nutrition. Anemia, microcytic type.	Avoid excessive filling of herniated pouch: diet is based on small meals, avoidance of spices, high-roughage vegetables, and carbonated beverages. No food for three hours prior to retiring. Sleep with head of bed elevated.

A Survey of Some Disorders of Nutrition and Conditions Involving the Alimentary Canal and Related Structures—Continued

Diagnostic Category	Etiological Factors	Incubation Period and Nature of Onset	Severity of Illness and Course	Part of Gastro-intestinal Tract and/or Associated Structures Involved and Response	Effect on Adequacy of Nutrition	Major Medical and/or Surgical Treatment
Parasites						
Cestodes (tapeworms)	Diphyllobothrium latum. Taenia solium. Taenia saginata.	Asymptomatic.	Transient abdominal discomfort; anemia. Infrequently: severe cramping, vomiting, weakness, loss of weight. Usually seeks medical attention because part of parasite is passed per anus.		Malnutrition. Avitaminosis.	Anthelmintics. High-protein diet. Iron therapy.
Hookworm disease	Necator americanus. Ancylostoma duodenale (Old World).	Have been known to survive 5 years in intestine. "Ground itch" or lesions on feet at point of entry. Later cough is sign of lung infiltration.	Epigastric pain. Abdominal tenderness. Sometimes nausea and vomiting as intestine is attacked. Anemia, dyspnea, palpitation, lassitude, tachycardia, constipation may be manifested as infestation progresses.	Larvae penetrate skin, enter circulation, go to lungs, enter alveoli, ascend respiratory tree, enter pharynx, and are swallowed. In intestine they mature and adults attach themselves to intestine, sucking about 0.5 ml		

Diagnostic Category	Etiological Factors	Incubation Period and Nature of Onset	Severity of Illness and Course	Part of Gastro-intestinal Tract and/or Associated Structures Involved and Response	Effect on Adequacy of Nutrition	Major Medical and/or Surgical Treatment
Ascariasis	Ascaris lumbricoides.			blood daily. Primarily in jejunum. Early transient pulmonary stage followed by larval migration and intestinal infestation. Ingested.		Symptomatic during pulmonary stage, then use chemotherapy.
Amebiasis	Endamoeba histolytica as motile trophozoite and nonmotile cyst.	Chronic: intermittent diarrhea, foul-smelling. Acute: high fever, severe abdominal cramps, bloody diarrhea, tenesmus.	Vague intestinal symptoms; symptoms of appendicitis, gall bladder disease, peptic ulcer. Dysentery or diarrhea. May eventually enter circulation and infest liver. May infest lung from site in liver. May cause granuloma which encroaches on lumen.	Ileum: cyst wall disintegrates and 8 trophozoites result; these pass to cecum, attack mucosa, and divide by binary fission; amebic ulceration: cecum, ascending colon, rectum, sigmoid, appendix, terminal ileum.	Dehydration. Electrolyte imbalance.	Acute: replace fluid, electrolyte, and blood losses; bed rest; relief of pain and tenesmus; specific chemotherapy and terramycin. Chronic: specific drug therapy and terramycin. Hepatic or pulmonary: Chloroquine and terramycin.

A Survey of Some Disorders of Nutrition and Conditions Involving the Alimentary Canal and Related Structures—Continued

Diagnostic Category	Etiological Factors	Incubation Period and Nature of Onset	Severity of Illness and Course	Part of Gastro-intestinal Tract and/or Associated Structures Involved and Response	Effect on Adequacy of Nutrition	Major Medical and/or Surgical Treatment
Enterobiasis	Enterobius vermicularis.	Perianal pruritus most trouble-some at night.		Cecum and colon: adults attach themselves to mucosa. Ingested.		Communal treat-ment.
Trichinosis	Trichinella spiralis.	Diarrhea during intestinal infestation.	Myositis and sys-temic reaction when larvae mi-grate and infest skeletal muscle. Edema, usually periorbital.	Encysted larvae are ingested and parasites are lib-erated in duo-denum and jejunum. There the parasites anchor themselves to mucosa and ex-tract oxygen and liquid food.	Hypoproteinemia. Dehydration.	Symptomatic ther-apy. Relief of pain. Maintain adequate fluid and caloric in-take. Rest; if nec-essary, sedation. ACTH.
Bacillary dysentery	Shigella.	1–6 days; median 48 hours. Colicky ab-dominal pain followed by pro-fuse diarrhea.	Passage of pus and mucus. Fever. Nausea. Vomiting. Headache. Spon-taneous recovery in 2–7 days.	Sigmoid and rectum: acute inflammation leading to coagu-lation necrosis and ulceration. Mild case: mucosa is strawberry-red tint with diffuse inflammation and hyperemia, bleed-ing when traumatized.	Dehydration. Depletion of electrolytes.	Symptomatic plus above. Isolation.

Deficiencies

Diagnostic Category	Etiological Factors	Incubation Period and Nature of Onset	Severity of Illness and Course	Part of Gastro-intestinal Tract and/or Associated Structures Involved and Response	Effect on Adequacy of Nutrition	Major Medical and/or Surgical Treatment
Scurvy	Vitamin C deficiency.		Weakness, fatigue, aching in muscles, joints, and bones. Hair follicles hyperkeratotic, then perifollicular hemorrhages.			Supply. Ascorbic acid.
Pellagra	Nicotinic acid deficiency coupled with protein deficiency and exposure to sunlight. Secondary to diseases of gastrointestinal tract and liver, neoplasia, surgery, infections, pregnancy, and lactation. Chronic alcoholism.		Dermatitis, anorexia, glossitis, lassitude, stomatitis, diarrhea. Later leads to dementia.			Nicotinic acid, adequate diet; high-protein and high vitamin content. Bed rest. Symptomatic therapy.
Beriberi	Thiamine deficiency (Louisiana rice area). Preg-					

A Survey of Some Disorders of Nutrition and Conditions Involving the Alimentary Canal and Related Structures—Continued

Diagnostic Category	Etiological Factors	Incubation Period and Nature of Onset	Severity of Illness and Course	Part of Gastrointestinal Tract and/or Associated Structures Involved and Response	Effect on Adequacy of Nutrition	Major Medical and/or Surgical Treatment
	nancy. Prisons and asylums. Far East. Chronic alcoholism.					
Inflammatory						
Glossitis	Secondary to chronic malabsorption.			Tongue.		Correct underlying disorder.
Stomatitis, catarrhal	Poor oral hygiene. Excessive use of tobacco or alcohol. Associated with debilitated persons. Uremia.			Mouth. Mucous membranes erythematous; increased exudate.		As above.
Aphythous ulcer	Unknown.			Vesicle develops, ruptures, and leaves ulcer.		No treatment; heals spontaneously.
Ulceromembranous	Bacillus fusiformis. Borrelia vincentii.	Painful, irregular-shaped ulcer covered with whitish-gray membrane.	Moderate fever, enlargement of submaxillary lymph nodes.	Oral and pharyngeal membranes, particularly gingival tissue. Inflammation and induration surround ulcerations.	Temporarily modifies diet.	Penicillin. Dental hygienic measures to eradicate ulcerations.

Diagnostic Category	Etiological Factors	Incubation Period and Nature of Onset	Severity of Illness and Course	Part of Gastrointestinal Tract and/or Associated Structures Involved and Response	Effect on Adequacy of Nutrition	Major Medical and/or Surgical Treatment
Parotitis	Hemolytic Streptococcus through ducts or blood stream or lymphatics or extension from adjacent structures.	Enlargement of salivary glands associated with pain.	Leukocytosis; rapid pulse; trismus; pressure on gland usually produces purulent discharge from duct.	Acute inflammation of salivary gland; usually parotid but may be any salivary gland.	Temporarily modifies diet.	Antimicrobial agents. Therapeutic doses of irradiation are used if antimicrobials fail.
Regional enteritis	Granulomatous response of submucosa to unknown agent(s).	Acute right-lower-quadrant pain and tenderness; disturbance in bowel motility.	Acute stage can lead to perforation and generalized peritonitis. In nonacute onset, history of intermittent chronic diarrhea fever, weight loss, crampy, pain or distention, anemia. ⅔ develop chronic	Duodenum: usually leads to stenosis. Upper jejunum: usually leads to stenosis. Terminal ileum: encroachment of lumen, scarring of muscle, slow spread to other areas of intestine; beefy-red appearance. Usually leads to ulceration.	Impairment of folic acid, tylose, and iron absorption. "Malabsorption syndrome." Undernutrition.	Surgery: end-to-side ileotransverse colostomy. Provide mental and physical rest. Chemotherapeutics and antibiotics to treat purulent complications. Diet: high-calorie, high-protein (2 gm per kg of ideal

A Survey of Some Disorders of Nutrition and Conditions Involving the Alimentary Canal and Related Structures—Continued

Diagnostic Category	Etiological Factors	Incubation Period and Nature of Onset	Severity of Illness and Course	Part of Gastrointestinal Tract and/or Associated Structures Involved and Response	Effect on Adequacy of Nutrition	Major Medical and/or Surgical Treatment
			enteritis. Eventual obstruction of lumen.			body weight per day), low in seasoning and cold fluids. Therapeutic vitamins. Fluid and elecrolyte balance restoration.
Sprue	Nontropical: adult form of celiac disease; secondary to malabsorption states.	Diarrhea: 2–3 (or more) mushy, light-colored, foul-smelling stools associated with explosive flatus.	Chronic disease, moderate to severe weight loss. Nausea and vomiting may occur. Nocturnal diuresis. Clinical manifestations of malnutrition. Eventually fractures of bones and tetany. Anemia.	Jejunum: villi become short and blunt, width of crypts of Lieberkuhn increases; microville become sparse, blunted, and fused.	Malnutrition results from inability of food products (properly prepared for absorption) to pass through the mucosa. Vitamin A, C, D, B_{12}, K deficiencies. Deficiencies in electrolytes; potassium and calcium. Hypoproteinemia. Progressively reserves of iron, folic acid, and B_{12} are depleted.	Gluten-free diet (do not eat food containing wheat, barley, rye gluten). Takes about 6 months to evaluate this therapy. In presence of nutritional deficiencies, corrective therapy instituted. In presence of malnutrition, adrenocortical hormone therapy initially with diet therapy. Tetany treated with cal-

Diagnostic Category	Etiological Factors	Incubation Period and Nature of Onset	Severity of Illness and Course	Part of Gastrointestinal Tract and/or Associated Structures Involved and Response	Effect on Adequacy of Nutrition	Major Medical and/or Surgical Treatment
					Malabsorption of fats and fat-soluble nutrients. Lowered serum cholesterol and phospholipids, copper, prothrombin.	cium. Electrolyte therapy: potassium chloride 2–3 gm daily. Hemorrhagic complications treated with Menadione intramuscularly, 10 mg daily. Antibiotic therapy when sprue is secondary to diverticula, blind loops, and intestinal strictures. Recognize secondary causes of sprue and institute therapy. Postgastrectomy: small, frequent feedings; addition of pancreatin to diet. Androgens for anabolic effect.
Hepatitis	Filtrable virus A (infectious hepatitis).	20–40 days. 60–160 days.	Icteric stage: jaundice; few days in which anorexia,	Liver: cellular damage ranges from swollen or	Undernutrition as a result of anorexia.	Bed rest. Isolate. Blood and stools considered infec-

A Survey of Some Disorders of Nutrition and Conditions Involving the Alimentary Canal and Related Structures—Continued

Diagnostic Category	Etiological Factors	Incubation Period and Nature of Onset	Severity of Illness and Course	Part of Gastrointestinal Tract and/or Associated Structures Involved and Response	Effect on Adequacy of Nutrition	Major Medical and/or Surgical Treatment
	Filtrable virus B (serum hepatitis).	Preicteric or prodromal phase: gradual or sudden onset. Fever and prostration, transient skin rash, arthralgia, lymph node enlargement. Anorexia, malaise, headache, chilly sensations, nausea, vomiting.	lassitude, and nausea are striking; right upper abdominal pain. This stage may last few days to few weeks, depending on severity. Sudden reappearance of appetite plus sense of well-being indicates beginning of recovery period.	shrunken cells with disintegrating nucleus to massive central necrosis of every lobule of the liver. Küpffer cells are often swollen; edema and cellular infiltration of portal and periportal areas; biliary stasis. Gall bladder is distended; serosa is injected; wall is tense and swollen; mucosa is congested. Frequently small amounts of fibrinopurulent exudate.		tious until fever and jaundice subside. Bland diet and hard candies given liberally. Parenteral feedings if comatose. Removal of calculi after subsidence of acute phase. Symptomatic therapy. Restoration of fluid and electrolyte balance. Low-fat diet. Water-soluble form of vitamins K, A, D, and E. Choledochal exploration. Cholecystectomy. Antispasmodics. Antacids. Laxatives. Rest and sedatives.

Diagnostic Category	Etiological Factors	Incubation Period and Nature of Onset	Severity of Illness and Course	Part of Gastro-intestinal Tract and/or Associated Structures Involved and Response	Effect on Adequacy of Nutrition	Major Medical and/or Surgical Treatment
Cholecystitis						
Acute	Biliary calculi.	Upper abdominal pain, gradual or acute, associated with biliary colic.	Becomes chronic but with severe upper abdominal distress. Fever usually. Nausea and vomiting.			
Chronic	Biliary calculi.		May lead to persistent gall bladder distention as with acute, but having chronic form jaundice.			
	Unknown.		Belching, bloating, and epigastric distress after meals. Variety of digestive and systemic complaints. Symptoms aggravated by ingestion of fats. Insomnia.			
Cirrhosis	Malnutrition. Alcoholism.	Insidious onset.	Anorexia, weight loss, eventually (1)	Liver enlarges and is pale initially;	Malnutrition in terms of essen-	Nutritious diet. Pro-hibition of alcohol

A Survey of Some Disorders of Nutrition and Conditions Involving the Alimentary Canal and Related Structures—Continued

Diagnostic Category	Etiological Factors	Incubation Period and Nature of Onset	Severity of Illness and Course	Part of Gastro-intestinal Tract and/or Associated Structures Involved and Response	Effect on Adequacy of Nutrition	Major Medical and/or Surgical Treatment
			hepatocellular failure, manifested by: ascites, edema, jaundice, pleural effusion, alteration in serum electrolytes, palma errythema, gynecomastia, testicular atrophy, bleeding tendency. (2) Portal hyper-tension manifested by: splenomegaly, esophageal varices (with or without massive hemorrhage), visi-ble venous col-lateral circulation over abdomen, rectal hemor-rhoids; and eventually may have: (3) Hepatic coma.	then fibrosis in portal areas and around central veins.	tial nutrients al-though caloric intake may be adequate or even high.	(where it is etio-logical factor). Regulation of salt and water bal-ance. Prompt control of hemorrhage and replacement of blood loss. Bed rest. Antimicrobial therapy in pres-ence of infection. Prednisone. Diuretics. Para-centesis and/or thoracentesis if needed. Surgery is some-times used: porta-caval shunt. Coma: (1) restric-tion of protein in-take, but calories supplied from fats and carbohy-drates, (2) correc-tion of deficiencies

Diagnostic Category	Etiological Factors	Incubation Period and Nature of Onset	Severity of Illness and Course	Part of Gastrointestinal Tract and/or Associated Structures Involved and Response	Effect on Adequacy of Nutrition	Major Medical and/or Surgical Treatment
						in fluids and electrolytes, (3) Neomycin, (4) administration intravenously of L-arginine mono hydrochloride (25 gm in 500 ml water); frequency depends on response of blood ammonia.
Pancreatitis, acute	Obstruction to outflow of pancreatic juices by gall stones in common duct. Cancer of ampulla of Vater. Secondary pancreatic edema. Epithelial metaplasia in duct. Alcoholism. Peptic ulcer. Trauma.	Severe and prolonged abdominal pain; may be acute or gradual in onset.	Loss of weight although excessive amounts of food are ingested; leading to obstipation; vomiting, distention, and ileus may occur. Tetany may develop. Lead to destructive process in pancreas and fibrotic contracture may cause com-	Destruction of parenchyma of pancreas and ductal obstruction. Varying: edema of head of pancreas to patchy or diffuse necrosis of gland. Extensive fibrosis.	Incomplete hydrolysis of starches, fats, and proteins and hence incomplete absorption. Marked malnutrition. Avitaminosis. Hypocalcemia.	N.P.O. Aspiration of gastric contents. Anticholinergic drugs. Analgesics (opiates sparingly and in small doses). Antibiotics. Restoration of fluid and electrolyte balance.

A Survey of Some Disorders of Nutrition and Conditions Involving the Alimentary Canal and Related Structures—Continued

Diagnostic Category	Etiological Factors	Incubation Period and Nature of Onset	Severity of Illness and Course	Part of Gastro-intestinal Tract and/or Associated Structures Involved and Response	Effect on Adequacy of Nutrition	Major Medical and/or Surgical Treatment
			pression of common duct, producing jaundice. Repeated attacks result in chronic pancreatitis. This, if progresses sufficiently, may result in calcification of pancreas and diabetes mellitus and steatorrhea.			
Appendicitis	Obstruction due to fecalith or stricture. Ulceration. Diffuse phlegmon.	Acute periumbicular or epigastric pain.	Anorexia, nausea, vomiting progressing. Perforation of the appendix and ensuing peritonitis.	Appendix: inflammatory response to cause.	Loss of fluid and electrolytes due to vomiting. Inadequate nutrient intake due to nausea, anorexia, and vomiting.	Surgical removal of appendix. Correction of dehydration and electrolyte imbalance. Restoration of physiological function (in absence of peritonitis).

REFERENCES

Books

Krause, Marie V., *Food, Nutrition and Diet Therapy,* 3rd ed., W. B. Saunders Co., Philadelphia, 1961.

Mayo, Charles W., *Surgery of Small and Large Intestines,* 2nd ed., Year Book Publishers, Inc., Chicago, 1962, pp. 60, 156-70.

Necheles Heinrich and Martin Kirshen, *The Physiologic Basis of Gastrointestinal Therapy,* Grune & Stratton Co., New York, 1957.

Proudfit, Fairfax T., and rev. by Corrine H. Robinson, *Normal and Therapeutic Nutrition,* 12th ed., The Macmillan Company, New York, 1961.

Sherman, Henry Clapp, and Carolyn S. Lanford, *Essentials of Nutrition,* 4th ed., The Macmillan Company, New York, 1957.

Spencer, Richard Paul, *The Intestinal Tract,* Charles C Thomas, Springfield, Illinois, 1960.

Wohl, Michael, and Robert Goodhart, eds., *Modern Nutrition in Health and Disease,* Dietotherapy, 2nd ed. Lea & Febiger, Philadelphia, 1960.

Articles

Aldrich, C. K., "Mechanisms and Management of Obesity," *Medical Clinics of North America,* XLVII, January, 1963, pp. 77-84.

Altemeier, William, and Richard Vilter, "Medical and Surgical Problems in Liver Disease," *Postgraduate Medicine,* XXVI, August, 1959, pp. 167-78.

"Another 'Inborn Error of Metabolism,' Defined?" *New England Journal of Medicine,* CCLXVIII, No. 13, January-June, 1963, March 28, 1963, pp. 737-38.

Astaldi, G., and E. Strosselli, "Biopsy of the Normal Intestine," *American Journal of Digestive Diseases,* V, No. 3, March, 1960, pp. 175-212.

Bachrach, William H., "Anticholinergic Drugs," *American Journal of Digestive Diseases,* III, No. 10, October, 1958, pp. 743-799.

Barker, Wiley F., and Sherman M. Mellinkoff, "Medico-Surgical Teamwork in the Treatment of Ulcerative Colitis," *Medical Clinics of North America,* XLIII, No. 4, July, 1959, pp. 1155-75.

Beeuwkes, Adelia, "Food Faddism—A Growing Threat," *Postgraduate Medicine,* XXVIII, No. 1, July, 1960, pp. 75-81.

Bell, Joseph N., "Want to Lose Weight?" *Today's Health,* December, 1959, pp. 28-31.

Bennett, H. D., "The History and Physical Examination in Hepatic Disease," *Medical Clinics of North America,* XLVI, No. 3, May, 1962, p. 775.

Bercovitz, Z. T., "Recent Advances in the Treatment of Ulcerative Colitis," *Geriatrics,* XVII, No. 8, August, 1962, pp. 507-11.

Brody, Garry S., "Observations on Fecal Continence Mechanisms," *Journal of the American Medical Association,* CLXXIII, No. 3, May 21, 1960, pp. 226-29.

Brown, Charles H., "The Treatment of Acute and Chronic Ulcerative Colitis," *American Practitioner and Digest of Treatment,* IX, No. 3, March, 1958, pp. 405-11.

Child, C. G., III, "Gastrointestinal, Biliary, and Pancreatic Conditions," *Surgery, Gynecology, and Obstetrics,* CXVI, No. 2, February, 1963, pp. 135-38.

Christiansen, P. A., *et al.,* "D-Xylose and Its Use in the Diagnosis of Malabsorptive States," *American Practitioner and Digest of Treatment,* XI, No. 8, August, 1960, p. 677.

Code, Charles F., "The Peptic Ulcer Problem," *American Journal of Digestive Diseases,* V, No. 4, April, 1960, pp. 288-307.

Coffey, Robert J., *et al.,* "Vagectomy, Hemigastrectomy, and Gastroduodenostomy in Treatment of Duodenal Ulcer," *American Journal of Digestive Diseases,* V, No. 4, April, 1960, pp. 324-38.

Cole, Warren H., and William Harridge, "Progress in Gallbladder and Biliary Tract Disease," *American Journal of Digestive Diseases,* IV, No. 2, February, 1959, pp. 93-116.

Coston, Harriet M., "Dining Room Service for Hospital Patients," *Nursing Outlook,* VII, July, 1959, pp. 425-28.

Crosby, William H., and Heinz W. Kugler, "Intraluminal Biopsy of the Small Intestine," *American Journal of Digestive Diseases,* II, No. 5, May, 1957, pp. 236-41.

Crozier, R. E., and H. Jonasson, "Symptomatic Variables of Hiatus Hernia," *Medical Clinics of North America,* XLVII, March, 1963, pp. 407-15.

Cummins, Alvin J., "Nausea and Vomiting," *American Journal of Digestive Diseases,* III, No. 10, October, 1958, pp. 710-21.

Davies, R. E., "The Metabolism of the Acid-Secreting Stomach," *American Journal of Digestive Diseases,* IV, No. 3, March, 1959, pp. 173-83.

Delp, Mahlon, *et al.,* "Physical Signs of Cirrhosis," *Postgraduate Medicine,* XXVII, January-June, 1960, February, 1960, pp. 131-39.

Dericks, Virginia C., "Rehabilitation of Patients with Ileostomy," *American Journal of Nursing,* LXI, No. 5, May, 1961, pp. 48-51.

Dobrushin, Dorothy Jean, "Diaphragmatic Hernia—Nursing Care," *American Journal of Nursing,* LVI, No. 2, February, 1956, pp. 185-86.

Donaldson, G. A., "Current Concepts in Therapy Management of Ileostomy and Colostomy," *New England Journal of Medicine,* CCLXVIII, No. 15, April 11, 1963, pp. 827-30.

Dragstedt, Lester R., "Why Does Not the Stomach Digest Itself?" *Journal of the American Medical Association,* CLXXVII, No. 11, September 16, 1961, pp. 758-62.

Dreiling, David A., "Physiologic Derangements Following Gastric Resection," *American Journal of Digestive Diseases,* VII, No. 3, March, 1962, pp. 209-23.

Dubois, Eoline C., "Hints on the Management of a Colostomy," *American Journal of Nursing,* LV, No. 1, January, 1955, pp. 71-72.

Eisenmenger, William J., "Viral Hepatitis," *American Journal of Nursing,* LXI, No. 11, November, 1961, pp. 56-58.

Farr, Hollon W., "Fluid and Electrolyte Balance—with Special Reference to the Gastrointestinal Tract," *American Journal of Nursing,* LIV, No. 7, July, 1954, pp. 826-31.

Feggetter, G. Y., and R. Pringle, "The Long Term Results of Bilateral Vagotomy and Gastrojejunostomy for Chronic Duodenal Ulcer," *Surgery, Gynecology and Obstetrics,* CXVI, No. 2, February, 1963, pp. 175-79.

Ferguson, Donald J., "The Physiology of Gastric Secretion as It Applies to the Peptic Ulcer Problem," *Surgical Clinics of North America,* XLII, No. 1, February, 1962, pp. 185-200.

Ferguson, L. K., *et al.,* "Colon Resection for Malignancy," *Surgical Clinics of North America,* XXXVII, December, 1957, pp. 1635-51.

Ferguson, L. Kraeer, "Concepts in the Surgical Treatment of Regional Enteritis," *New England Journal of Medicine,* CCLXIV, No. 15, April 13, 1961, pp. 748-51.

Fields, Albert, "William Beaumont: Backwoods Scientist," *American Journal of Digestive Diseases,* XXII, October, 1955, pp. 297-99.

Fisher, Jack, "The Dumping Syndrome," *American Journal of Nursing,* LVIII, No. 8, August, 1958, pp. 1126-27.

Fisk, Jean E., "Nursing Care of the Patient with Surgery of the Biliary Tract," *American Journal of Nursing,* LX, No. 1, January, 1960, pp. 53-55.

Flood, Charles A., "Clinical Features in the Management of Esophageal Hiatal Hernia," *Journal of the American Medical Association,* CLXXII, No. 4, January 23, 1960, pp. 314-19.

General Policy on Addition of Specific Nutrients to Foods. Council Statements, *Journal of the American Medical Association,* CLXXVIII, No. 10, December 9, 1961, pp. 1024-25.

Gilchrist R., and S. Economou, "Acute and Chronic Diverticulitis," *Medical Clinics of North America,* XLII, January, 1958, pp. 229-34.

Gillesby, William, "Gastrointestinal Decompression in Reconstructive Bowel and Biliary Surgery," *Surgical Clinics of North America,* XLII, No. 1, February, 1962, pp. 231-39.

Gilmore, Stuart I., "Rehabilitation After Laryngectomy," *American Journal of Nursing,* LXI, No. 1, January, 1961, pp. 87-89.

Ginsberg, Miriam K., "A Study of Oral Hygiene Nursing Care," *American Journal of Nursing,* LXI, No. 10, October, 1961, pp. 67-69.

Glenn, Frank, and Bjorn Thorbjarnarson, "The Surgical Treatment of Acute Cholecystitis," *Surgery, Gynecology, and Obstetrics,* CXVI, No. 1, January, 1963, pp. 61-70.

Goodhart, Robert S., "Vitamin Therapy Today," *Medical Clinics of North America,* XL, September, 1956, pp. 1473-87.

Goldenberg, Julio, *et al.,* "Diagnostic Value of the Combined Secretin and Cytology Test in Pancreatic Disease," *American Practitioner and Digest of Treatment,* XII, No. 6, June, 1961, pp. 415-19.

Grey, Chester C., and Harry L. Hunter, "Rectal Bleeding," *Surgical Clinics of North America,* XXXVIII, January, 1958, pp. 235-55.

Griffith, Charles A., "Inguinal Hernias: An Anatomic-Surgical Correlation," *Surgical Clinics of North America,* XXXIX, No. 2, April, 1959, pp. 531-56.

Grossman, Morton I., "Regulation of Food Intake," *American Journal of Digestive Diseases,* III, No. 9, September, 1958, pp. 659-68.

Hallburg, Jeanne C., "The Patient with Surgery of the Colon," *American Journal of Nursing,* LXI, No. 3, March, 1961, pp. 64-66.

Halpern, Seymour Lionel, guest ed., "I. Recent Advances in Applied Nutrition" and "II. Obesity," *The Medical Clinics of North America,* XLVIII, September, 1964.

Hansen, Arild E., and J. M. R. Beveridge, "Role of Dietary Fat in Human Nutrition," *American Journal of Public Health,* XLVII, November, 1957, pp. 1367-70.

Hansen, Donald E., "Abdominal Hernias," *American Journal of Nursing,* LXI, No. 3, March, 1961, pp. 102-4.

Hardy, James D., "Cancer of the Lower Left Colon and Rectum: Current Status," *American Practitioner and Digest of Treatment,* X, No. 4, April, 1959, pp. 613-18.

Hashim, Sami A., "Obesity, Drugs and Formula Diets," *Postgraduate Medicine,* XXX, No. 3, September, 1961, pp. 245-50.

Heap, Beth, "Sodium Restricted Diets," *American Journal of Nursing,* LX, No. 2, February, 1960, pp. 206-9.

Heffernon, Elmer, *et al.,* "Irritable Colon and Gallbladder Disease," *Journal of the American Medical Association,* CLXXIII, No. 1, May 7, 1960, pp. 1-5.

Heffernon, E. W., "The Irritable Colon—A Common Mimic," *Medical Clinics of North America,* XLVII, March, 1963, pp. 425-29.

Higgins, John A., "Medical Complications Following Gastric Surgery," *Medical Clinics of North America,* XLVI, No. 4, July, 1962, pp. 979-85.

Hightower, Nicholas C., *et al.,* "Chronic Ulcerative Colitis," *American Journal of Digestive Diseases,* III, No. 12, December, 1958, pp. 931-41.

Hoffmann, C. Rowell, "The Causes and Prevention of Recurrences in Peptic Ulcer Disease," *American Journal of Digestive Diseases,* XXII, January, 1955, pp. 17-20.

Holinger, Paul H., "Cancer of the Larynx," *American Journal of Nursing,* LVII, No. 6, June, 1957, pp. 738-43.
  1. Surgical Treatment, p. 738.
  2. Nursing the Patient After Laryngectomy, p. 741.

Horner, John L., "Natural History of Diverticulosis of the Colon," *American Journal of Digestive Diseases,* III, No. 5, May, 1958, pp. 343-50.

"How Meals on Wheels Help the Shut-In," *Journal of the American Medical Association,* CLXX, No. 4, May 23, 1959, pp. 460-61.

Hunt, J. N., "Some Notes on the Pathogenesis of Duodenal Ulcer," *American Journal of Digestive Diseases,* II, No. 9, September, 1957, pp. 445-53.

Huntington, F. K., and J. T. Sessions, Jr., "The Postgastrectomy Syndrome," *Disease-A-Month,* February, 1963, pp. 11-32.

Ingles, Thelma, and Emily Campbell, "The Patient with a Colostomy," *American Journal of Nursing,* LVIII, No. 11, November, 1958, pp. 1544-46.

Jay, Arthur N., "Colitis," *American Journal of Nursing,* LIX, No. 8, August, 1959, pp. 1133-35.

Jay, Arthur N., "Is It Indigestion?" *American Journal of Nursing,* LVIII, No. 11, November, 1958, pp. 1552-54.

John, Henry J., "Hunger," *American Journal of Digestive Diseases,* XXII, July, 1955, pp. 197-200.

Jolliffe, Norman, "Diagnosis and Treatment of Nutritional Disturbances," *American Journal of Digestive Diseases,* I, No. 8, August, 1956, pp. 323-32.

Judd, E. S., and Meredith P. Smith, "Present Trends in Surgical Treatment of Diverticulitis," *Surgical Clinics of North America*, XXXVII, August, 1957, pp. 1019-27.

Kleckner, Martin S., "The Role of Liver Disease in the Malabsorption Syndrome," *American Practitioner and Digest of Treatment*, XI, No. 8, August, 1960, pp. 661-76.

Klug, Thomas J., *et al.*, "Gastric Resection," *American Journal of Nursing*, LXI, No. 12, December, 1961, pp. 73-76.

Kogan, Edgar, *et al.*, "Management of Patients with Massive Resection of the Small Intestine with Special Reference to the Use of Steroid Hormones," *American Journal of Digestive Diseases*, III, No. 11, November, 1958, pp. 844-56.

Korman, Maurice, and Robert L. Stubblefield, "Definition of Alcoholism," *Journal of the American Medical Association*, CLXXVIII, No. 13, December 30, 1961, pp. 1184-86.

Labecki, Geraldine, and Susan Merrow, "How Wisely Do Students Select Their Diets?" *Nursing Outlook*, VII, August, 1959, pp. 471-73.

Lemmer, K., and S. Watson, "Inguinal Hernia," *American Journal of Nursing*, LIII, No. 12, December, 1953, pp. 1471-75.

Levine, Rachmiel, cons. ed., "Symposium on the Rationale and Clinical Interpretation of Laboratory Tests," *Medical Clinics of North America*, XLIII, No. 2, March, 1959, pp. 339-522.

Lyons, Albert S., "Control of the Colostomy," *American Journal of Digestive Diseases*, I, No. 2, February, 1956, pp. 79-94.

Mackby, M. Judson, "Treatment of Bleeding Esophageal Varices," *Journal of the American Medical Association*, CLXXI, No. 14, December 5, 1959, pp. 1916-22.

Machella, Thomas E., "Medical Aspects of Pancreatitis," *Journal of the American Medical Association*, CLXIX, No. 14, April 4, 1959, pp. 1571-77.

Machella, Thomas E., "What Is the Dumping Syndrome?" *American Journal of Digestive Diseases*, II, No. 5, May, 1957, pp. 278-82.

Machella, Thomas E., "Postsurgical Problems of the Gastrointestinal Tract," *Journal of the American Medical Association*, CLXXIV, No. 17, December 24, 1960, pp. 2111-17.

Magruder, Lucinda, *et al.*, "Gastric Resection—Nursing Care," *American Journal of Nursing*, LXI, No. 12, December, 1961, pp. 76-77.

Matheson, N. A., and H. A. F. Dudley, "Enterotomy and Decompression for Intestinal Distension," *Lancet*, I, March 30, 1963, pp. 695-96.

Matousek, William, "Management of Portal Cirrhosis, Dietary Concepts," *American Practitioner and Digest of Treatment*, X, No. 1, January, 1959, pp. 54-56.

Mayer, Jean, "Nutrition," *Postgraduate Medicine*, XXV, January, 1959, pp. 91-95.

Mayer, Jean, "Obesity: Causes and Treatment," *American Journal of Nursing*, LIX, No. 12, December, 1959, pp. 1732-36.

McHenry, E. W., "Nutrition and Older People," *Canadian Journal of Public Health*, LX, March, 1960, pp. 101-5.

Menaker, Gerald, "The Physiology and Mechanism of Acute Abdominal Pain," *Surgical Clinics of North America*, XLII, No. 1, February, 1962, pp. 241-48.

Mendeloff, Albert I., "Chronic Diarrhea," *American Journal of Digestive Diseases*, III, No. 11, November, 1958, pp. 801-22.

Meyers, Phillip E., "Contamination of Barium Enema Apparatus During Its Use," *Journal of the American Medical Association*, CLXXIII, No. 14, August 6, 1960, pp. 1589-90.

Modell, Walter, "Status and Prospect of Drugs for Overeating," *Journal of the American Medical Association*, CLXXIII, No. 10, July 9, 1960, pp. 1131-36.

Moore, T. C., and H. Baker, "Operative and Radiologic Relief of Gallstone Intestinal Obstruction," *Surgery, Gynecology, and Obstetrics*, CXVI, No. 2, February, 1963, pp. 189-95.

Morris, Ena, "How Does a Nurse Teach Nutrition to Patients?" *American Journal of Nursing*, LX, No. 1, January, 1960, pp. 67-70.

Nardi, G. L., "Pancreatitis," *New England Journal of Medicine*, CCLXVIII, No. 19, May 9, 1963, pp. 1065-67.

Nelburgs, H. E., "Tubeless Gastric Analysis and Cytologic Procedures," *Surgical Clinics of North America*, XXXIX, No. 5, October, 1959, pp. 1213-22.

Palumbo, Louis T., "Present-Day Treatment of Diseases of the Biliary Tract," *American Journal of Nursing,* LX, No. 1, January, 1960, pp. 50-52.

Palumbo, Louis T., *et al.,* "Ulcerative Colitis," *American Journal of Nursing,* LV, No. 3, March, 1955, pp. 311-15.

Pare, C. M. B., "Hypoglycemia Following Partial Gastrectomy," *American Journal of Digestive Diseases,* III, No. 1, January, 1958, pp. 1-11.

Perez-Santiago, Enrique, and C. E. Butterworth, Jr., "Definition and Diagnosis of Sprue," *American Journal of Digestive Diseases,* II, No. 5, May, 1957, pp. 225-35.

Pittman, Adele Corey, and Fred W. Robinson, "Dumping Syndrome—Control by Diet," *Journal of the American Dietetic Association,* XXXIV, June, 1958, pp. 596-602.

Plotz, Milton, "Modern Management of Obesity—the 'Social Diet,' " *Journal of the American Medical Association,* CLXX, No. 13, July 25, 1959, pp. 1513-15.

Point, Walter Warren, "Jaundice," *American Journal of Nursing,* LVIII, No. 4, April, 1958, pp. 556-57.

Pollack, Herbert, C. Frank Consolazio, and Gerhard Isaac, "Metabolic Demands as a Factor in Weight Control," *Journal of the American Medical Association,* CLXVII, No. 2, May 10, 1958, pp. 216-19.

Popper, Hans, "Hepatic Function," *Postgraduate Medicine,* XXIII, April, 1958, pp. 441-45.

Radvin, R. G., "Nutritional Problems in Surgery," *American Journal of Digestive Diseases,* I, No. 8, August, 1956, pp. 350-60.

Randall, H., "Alterations in Gastrointestinal Tract Function Following Surgery. Nutrition and the Dumping Syndrome After Surgery," *Surgical Clinics of North America,* XXXVIII, April, 1958, pp. 585-609.

Ravdin, R., "Inguinal Herniorrhaphy in the Adult," *Surgical Clinics of North America,* XXXVII, December, 1957, pp. 1663-73.

Ravdin, I. S., "Cholecystectomy," *Surgical Clinics of North America,* XXXVII, December, 1957, pp. 1599-1609.

Ray, John E., *et al.,* "Postoperative Problems of Ileostomy and Colostomy," *Journal of the American Medical Association,* CLXXIV, No. 17, December 24, 1960, pp. 2118-23.

"Recent Advances in Gastrointestinal Surgery," *Surgical Clinics of North America,* XXXIX, No. 5, October, 1959, pp. 1149-51.

Reynolds, Mildred, "A Nutrition Program for Older People," *Geriatrics,* XIV, No. 3, March, 1959, pp. 190-93.

Rodman, Theodore, *et al.,* "Reliability of Tubeless Gastric Analysis in Presence of Complicating Diseases," *Journal of the American Medical Association,* CLXVII, No. 2, May 10, 1958, pp. 172-75.

Roth, Harold P., *et al.,* "Patients' Beliefs About Peptic Ulcer and Its Treatment," *Annals of Internal Medicine,* LVI, No. 1, January, 1962, pp. 72-80.

Rumball, John M., "The Emergency Management of Upper Gastrointestinal Hemorrhage," *Medical Clinics of North America,* XLVI, No. 2, March, 1962, pp. 531-35.

Rynbergen, Henderika J., "In Gastrointestinal Disease—Fewer Diet Restrictions," *American Journal of Nursing,* LXIII, No. 1, January, 1963, pp. 86-89.

Sandlow, L. J., *et al.,* "The Use of Tetracycline Fluorescence in the Detection of Gastric Malignancy," *Annals of Internal Medicine,* LVIII, No. 3, March, 1963, pp. 409-13.

Sborov, Victor, "Jaundice," *American Journal of Digestive Diseases,* IV, No. 1, January, 1959, pp. 65-77.

Schevegman, Cletus W., "The Acute Abdomen," *American Association of Industrial Nurses,* XI, February, 1963, pp. 11-12.

Scoggins, Marcella L. Cunningham, "Preparing Patients for X-ray Examinations," *American Journal of Nursing,* LVII, No. 1, January, 1957, pp. 76-79.

Seymour, Charlyne T., and Joseph A. Weinberg, "Emotion and Gastric Activity," *Journal of the American Medical Association,* CLXXI, No. 9, October 31, 1959, pp. 1193-95.

Sherlock, Sheila, " What Is Hepatic Coma?" *American Journal of Digestive Diseases,* II, No. 7, July, 1957, pp. 353-62.

Shoss, Milton, "Re-Evaluation of Oral Cholecystography," *American Practitioner and Digest of Treatment,* XII, No. 8, August, 1961, pp. 582-88.

Shull, Harrison J., "Diet in the Management of Peptic Ulcer," *Journal of the American Medical Association,* CLXX, No. 9, June 27, 1959, pp. 1068-71.

Skillman, Thomas G., George J. Hamwi, and Cecelia May, "Nutrition in the Aged," *Geriatrics,* XV, No. 6, June, 1960, pp. 464-72.

Smith, Ann V., "Nasogastric Tube Feedings," *American Journal of Nursing,* LVII, No. 11, Nov., 1957, pp. 1451-12.

Smith, Hubbard W., and James J. Nordland, "Evaluation of Hepatic Dysfunction," *American Journal of Digestive Diseases,* II, No. 10, October, 1957, pp. 559-76.

Spencer, Richard, "Potassium Metabolism and Gastrointestinal Function; A Review," *American Journal of Digestive Diseases,* IV, No. 2, February, 1959, pp. 145-58.

Stafford, Clarence E., and David B. Hinshaw, "Surgical Indications in Peptic Ulcer Disease," *Medical Clinics of North America,* XLIII, No. 4, July, 1959, pp. 1085-99.

Stare, Fredrick J., "Sense and Nonsense About Nutrition," *Harper's Magazine,* CCIX, No. 1373, October, 1964, pp. 66-70.

Sterling, Julian A., (Editorial), "The Blind Spot in the Bile Duct," *American Journal of Digestive Diseases,* XXII, August, 1955, pp. 241-42.

Storer, Edward H., "The Differential Diagnosis of Jaundice," *Postgraduate Medicine,* XXXI, March, 1962, pp. 225-31.

Stuart, David, "To Depress the Craving for Food," *American Journal of Nursing,* LXII, No. 3, March, 1962, pp. 88-92.

"Surgery of the Biliary Tract, Liver, Pancreas and Spleen," *Surgical Clinics of North America,* XXXVIII, June, 1958, entire issue.

"Surgical Techniques," *Surgical Clinics of North America,* XL, No. 3, June, 1960, entire issue.

Mayo Clinic Number, "Symposium on Abdominal Surgery," *Surgical Clinics of North America,* XXXVII, August, 1957, entire issue, pp. 909-1182.

Rickets, Henry T. and Richard L. Landau, guest eds., "Symposium on Endocrine, Metabolic and Nutritional Disorders," *Medical Clinics of North America,* XLVII, January, 1963, pp. 1-248.

Taylor, Bertha I., "Taking Food and Fluids Through a Tube," *American Journal of Nursing,* LIII, No. 3, March, 1953, pp. 303-5.

Taylor, John C., "Decubitus Ulcers," *Nursing Science,* II, No. 4, August, 1964, pp. 293-310.

Texter, E. Clinton, "Digestive Tract Pain," *American Journal of Digestive Diseases,* III, No. 12, December, 1958, pp. 877-900.

Tisdale, W. A., "Subacute Hepatitis," *New England Journal of Medicine,* CCLXVIII, No. 2, January 10, 1963, pp. 85-89, and CCLXVIII, No. 3, January 17, 1963, pp. 138-42.

Vanamee, Parker, "Nutrition After Gastric Resection," *Journal of the American Medical Association,* CLXXII, No. 18, April 30, 1960, pp. 2072-76.

Wakefield, E., "Treatment of Diverticulitis," and R. Trumbull, Jr., "Surgical Management," *Postgraduate Medicine,* XXIII, June, 1958, pp. 655-60.

Wangensteen, Owen H., "A Critique of Operations for Peptic Ulcer," *Postgraduate Medicine,* XXIII, May, 1958, pp. 466-83.

Wangensteen, Owen H., *et al.,* "Achieving 'Physiological Gastrectomy' by Gastric Freezing," *Journal of the American Medical Association,* CLXXX, No. 6, May 12, 1962, pp. 439-44.

Weber, Robert W., and Jane Elliott, "Needle Biopsy of the Liver," *American Journal of Nursing,* LVI, No. 2, February, 1956, pp. 190-91.

White, Dorothy R., "I Have an Ileostomy," *American Journal of Nursing,* LXI, No. 5, May, 1961, pp. 51-52.

Williamson, Paul, "Hemorrhoids," *American Practitioner and Digest of Treatment,* IX, No. 9, October, 1958, pp. 1579-82.

Wolfman, Earl F., and C. Thomas Flotte, "Carcinoma of the Colon and Rectum," *American Journal of Nursing,* LXI, March, 1961, p. 61.

Zieve, Leslie, "Hepatic Coma," *Medical Clinics of North America,* XLVI, March, 1962, pp. 507-519.

Zollinger, Robert M., "Late Postoperative Problems Following Radical Surgery of the Stomach and Pancreas," *Postgraduate Medicine*, XXIII, March 1958, pp. 297-304.

Zollinger, Robert M., and David L. Kinsey, "The Management of Hernia: All Ages," *Postgraduate Medicine*, XXX, July, 1961, pp. 20-26.

Zuidema, George D., and Marilyn K. Klein, "A New Esophagus," *American Journal of Nursing*, LXI, September, 1961, p. 69.

11 : Nursing the Patient with an Alteration in Body Temperatue

The biologist who investigates the quantitative responses by which organisms self-regulate each property and component of their bodies finds reproducible responses which accurately compensate for the specific property or component suffering disturbance. The specificity applies to hundreds of properties. Apparently the responses are prepared ones and are triggered by specific detectors. The detectors communicate with effectors of varying degrees of specificity; but, in general, the possible non-specific responses appear to have been filtered away in the course of evolution so that the more specific ones remain. The problems of identifying the exact kinds of information used in the effectors are largely unsolved; but the over-all results as seen in compensatory responses can be evaluated now. Organisms compress large numbers of specific response systems into a surprisingly few organs and organelles.[1]

To meet the needs of the patient who has a disturbance in his capacity to maintain his body temperature within the limits described as normal, the nurse requires some knowledge of the homeostatic mechanisms whereby the body controls its temperature. This knowledge is basic to understanding disturbances in temperature regulation as well as to understanding what can be done to increase the patient's comfort or to protect him from the damaging effects of excessive deviations from normal levels. Exposure to either excessive heat or cold can lead to serious bodily harm. Extremes of temperature as causes of cellular injury are discussed in Chapter 3.

Animals are classified as homeothermic (warm-blooded) or poikilothermic (cold-blooded) depending on their ability or inability to regulate their body temperature within well-defined limits, despite changes in the external environment. Homeothermic animals maintain their body temperatures within limits while poikilothermic animals do not. Though this classification is generally useful, it is not completely accurate, because animals that hibernate are homeothermic when they are active and are poikilothermic during periods of hibernation. Their body temperature is subject to homeostatic control when they are active and is determined by the temperature of the environment when they are hibernating.

Although man is homeothermic, this does not mean that the temperature of

[1] Adolph, E. F., "How Specific Are Physiological Regulations," *Perspectives in Biology and Medicine,* III, Autumn, 1959, p. 68.

the blood or of his tissues is the same throughout his body for it is not. What it does mean is that he has the capacity to regulate the temperature of his deeper or core tissues within limits. Thus, it is the temperature of the blood and tissues of the central nervous system, and of the organs in the thoracic and abdominal cavities, that is regulated. According to DuBois,[2] "There is no one body temperature, but a series of gradients." Bard[3] states that even when a person is unclothed, resting, and exposed to a comfortable environmental temperature, the difference in temperature between his rectum and his feet may be as much as 4° C. Even within the interior of the body some organs have higher temperatures than others. DuBois[4] and Bard[5] state that the liver, as a site of much metabolic activity, has a temperature higher than other tissues. Also, as has been indicated, the temperature varies with the location of the tissue. The skin and subcutaneous tissues are cooler than those that are more deeply placed. The fact that the temperature of tissues varies has a bearing on the interpretation of temperatures taken at different sites. Davis[6] states the range for the rectal temperature as 35.9° to 37.3° C. (96.5° to 99.1° F.), with the average being 37.5° C. (99.5° F.). The oral temperature is 0.3° to 0.5° C. (0.54° to 0.9° F.) lower than the rectal temperature. The axillary temperature is 0.5° to 1.0° C. (0.9° to 1.8° F.) lower than the rectal temperature. Whether or not the temperature recorded by the thermometer accurately reflects the temperature of the body also depends on the care with which the procedure is performed. Even for the rectum, the temperature may vary as much as 0.1° to 1.5° F.[7] Whatever site is selected, the purpose is the same; that is, to estimate as accurately as is possible the temperature of the interior of the body. To do this the thermometer should be placed in an area of the body that contains large blood vessels and that is protected in so far as is possible from outside influences. It should be kept in place long enough to register the true temperature. Finally, care should be taken to shake the mercury down before the thermometer is reused.

In Figure 11-2, DuBois indicates that the possible range of body temperatures is greater than that shown in Figure 11-1.[8] In this diagram DuBois attempts to show zones of temperature regulation. It can be seen that between 34° C. (93° F.) and 41° C. (105.8° F.), temperature regulation is efficient. He notes that, except in patients who have brain lesions or heat

[2] Eugene F. DuBois, *Fever and the Regulation of Body Temperature*, Charles C Thomas, Springfield, Illinois, 1948, p. 33.

[3] Philip Bard (ed.), *Medical Physiology*, 11th ed., C. V. Mosby Company, St. Louis, 1961, p. 526.

[4] *Op. cit.*, p. 33.

[5] *Op. cit.*, p. 527.

[6] Harry A. Davis, *Principles of Surgical Physiology*, Paul B. Hoeber, Inc., New York, 1957, p. 259.

[7] J. Mead and C. L. Bonmarito, "Reliability of Rectal Temperatures as an Index of Internal Body Temperature," *Journal of Applied Physiology*, II, 1949, p. 59.

[8] Dubois, *Loc. cit.*, p. 9.

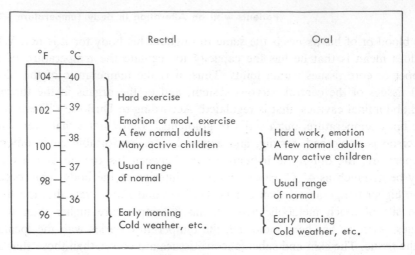

FIGURE 11—1. Thermometer readings, rectal and oral, under various conditions. (Adapted from E. F. DuBois, *Fever and the Regulation of Body Temperature*, American Lecture Series, No. 13, Fig. 233, p. 716, Bard, 1948. Courtesy of Charles C Thomas, Publisher, Springfield, Illinois.)

stroke or are moribund, temperatures seldom rise above 41° C. Then he asks the question, why should the temperature not rise higher? He answers thus:

If in disease a thermoregulatory thermostat can be set quite accurately at 39° or 40° C., why not at 42° C. or higher? From the physical standpoint it is no more difficult to raise body temperature from 40° C. to 42° C. than from 38° C. to 40° C. It is hard to escape the conclusion that there is some sort of secondary temperature regulation in exercise and disease that vigorously opposes any rise in temperature above 40.5° C. Such a mechanism would appear to be absolutely essential to life.[9]

All bodily processes are affected by temperature. Within the limits of the tissue tolerance, biochemical reactions within cells are accelerated by increasing body temperature and slowed by decreasing body temperature. With increased body temperatures, oxyhemoglobin is dissociated more rapidly than at normal temperatures, the heart rate is increased, and wound healing is accelerated. The metabolic rate is accelerated 7 per cent for each degree of elevation.

As with other homeostatic conditions, body temperature depends on a supply of what is needed and the regulation of processes whereby the condition is maintained constant. Unlike some substances that are required by the body economy, heat is one of the products of cellular activity. Though it may be regarded as a by-product, it is necessary to the biochemical activities of the cell. Reference to Figure 11-2 indicates that temperatures in the neighborhood of 24° C. (75° F.) are probably minimal for survival.

[9] *Ibid.,* p. 62.

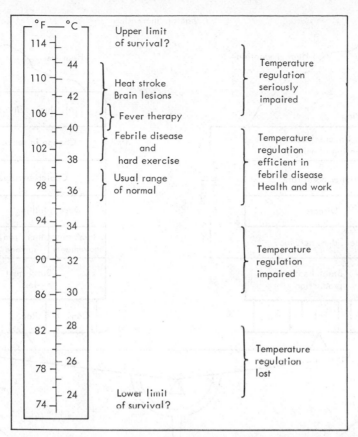

What are some of the elements in heat production?

In Figure 11-3, also taken from DuBois, the factors in heat production are balanced against those causing heat loss. The result of this balance or equilibrium is a relatively constant temperature which ranges from 35° to 39° C. The factors that can be seen to increase production include the ingestion of calorie-containing foods, that is, carbohydrates, fats, and proteins. Food also enhances heat production by its ability to stimulate metabolism. This is known as its specific dynamic action. For some reason protein has a higher specific dynamic action than do carbohydrates or fats. Heat production is also increased by disease, by elevation of the basal rate of metabolism, by the unconscious tensing of muscles, and by exercise, including shivering.

What are some of the factors in heat loss?

On the other side of the balance, basal heat loss is by conduction, convection, radiation, and vaporization. It can be augmented by increasing air

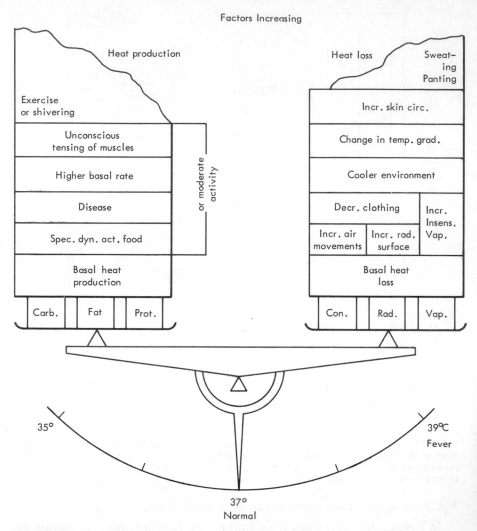

FIGURE 11—3. Balance between factors increasing heat production and heat loss. (Adapted. Courtesy of E. F. DuBois, "Heat Loss from the Human Body," *Bulletin of the New York Academy of Medicine,* XV, March, 1939, Fig. 235, p. 145 Bard.)

movements, by increasing the surface exposed to the air, and by increasing insensible vaporization. Other factors that contribute to the loss of heat include a cool environment, cooling of the skin, increased circulation of blood through the skin, and sweating and panting. Radiation is defined as the transfer of heat by means of waves. These waves are like radio waves in all respects except length. Radiation differs from other means of transferring heat inasmuch as it does not need a medium to pass through space. Convection can be defined simply as the movement of heat from one site to another by currents of air or fluid. As air warms it tends to expand; it becomes less dense and therefore rises. As it rises cooler air takes up its place. It in turn warms, expands, rises and is replaced by cooler air. In conduction, heat is transferred from one molecule to adjacent ones. A good example of conduction is the transfer of heat from a metal coffee pot to its handle. The wall of the pot is heated by the hot water and the heat is transferred directly to adjacent metal in the handle. This movement of heat can be observed by holding the handle and feeling it warm.

Heat loss is primarily through the skin, by radiation, convection, and evaporation. Some is lost in the urine, feces, and expired air. In the deeper tissues and the muscles, blood takes up the heat that is produced in the tissue and transports it to the skin, where it is transferred to the external environment, thereby cooling the blood. The transfer of heat from the tissue to the blood and from the blood to the tissue illustrates one of the laws of thermodynamics; that is, energy travels from an area of greater energy to an area of lesser energy, that is to say, heat moves from the warmer to the cooler tissues. Heat loss may be facilitated by increasing the circulation of blood through the skin, by increasing the amount of skin exposed to the environment, and by increasing the capacity of the air surrounding the body to take on heat or moisture. Body structure also affects the rate at which heat is lost. The apron of fat, the omentum, that hangs in front of the abdominal organs protects them from the loss of heat. A layer of fat under the skin insulates the deeper tissues and reduces heat loss. As was stated earlier, the layer of fat under the skin of the Eskimo plus his short, stocky frame is a type of adaptation to a cold climate, as fat acts as insulating material. Conversely, obesity is a handicap in a tropical climate because the fatty subcutaneous tissue interferes with heat loss. In tropical regions of Africa, adaptation has been in the direction of a long, lean trunk.

Clothing decreases heat loss because it is a poor conductor of heat and it traps air, which is also a poor conductor. Because they trap air in the spaces between fibers, loosely woven woolens are effective under certain conditions (when the air is still) in preventing heat loss. In windy climates close-woven or impervious materials may be more effective than heavy ones, because they trap the body heat air and prevent its dissipation by the wind. Still air limits heat loss, while moving air promotes it by replacing the warm, moist layer of air that surrounds the body with a layer of cooler, drier air. Therefore, an electric fan increases comfort on a hot day, and the wind increases the danger of frostbite on a cold one. Chilling is, therefore, related not only to the temperature, but to the movement of air. Thus, a "windbreaker" coat may offer more protection from the cold on a windy day than a heavier, "warmer" one.

The extent to which the air is saturated with moisture is also a factor in heat loss. One of the ways in which heat is transferred from the skin to the external environment is through the evaporation of the water secreted by the sweat glands in the form of perspiration. Conversion of a liquid to a vapor requires energy in the form of heat to overcome the cohesion of molecules.

Water requires more heat to vaporize than any other liquid. This property is called the latent heat of vaporization, because the heat remains in the steam until it forms water and releases the heat. There is a limit to the amount of water vapor that the air can hold before it becomes saturated. This amount varies with the temperature. The lower the temperature, the lower the absolute amount of water the air will hold before it is saturated. This is demonstrated in hot weather when the humidity is relatively high. During the night and in the early morning when the temperature is low, the capacity of the air to hold moisture is reduced, and though it remains saturated, or nearly so, some of the air vapor is precipitated as dew. As the humidity falls, the grass dries slowly or quickly, depending on the degree of saturation of the air and whether or not there is a wind. For example, this morning the temperature was 63° F. and the humidity was 93 per cent. At noon the temperature was 85° F. and the humidity was 63 per cent. The absolute amount of moisture in the air is as great as or greater at noon than it was earlier in the day. The amount that the air is capable of holding has been increased by the increase in temperature. Another factor in comfort is the relationship of the humidity to the temperature. This is expressed as the comfort index. As the humidity rises in relation to the temperature, comfort declines. Cooling systems are designed differently for use in hot moist and hot dry climates. In hot moist climates an essential feature of a cooling system is a device to remove moisture as well as heat. In fact, unless the temperature is extreme, comfort can be greatly increased by the removal of excessive moisture, despite little or no decrease in temperature. In hot dry climates cooling may be effected by increasing evaporation. Rather than removing moisture, it is added as air is circulated. The windows may be open to supply fresh dry air. Temperature in the room falls due to heat used in evaporation. Persons driving through a hot dry region sometimes utilize a similar device to cool their cars. They hang a wet towel in the car. Cooling is effected by evaporation. The dripping water bags hung on the fenders of cars being driven through the desert are based on the same principle.

In addition to its high latent heat of vaporization, water has other properties that facilitate heat loss and therefore help to protect the tissues from overheating. They include its high specific heat and its high conductivity. Specific heat is defined as the amount of heat required to raise the temperature of 1 gm of water 1° C. Water has a specific heat of one, which is the highest of all liquids. All others have a specific heat of less than one. Defined in terms of numbers, 1 gm of water absorbs 1 calorie of heat in rising 1° C. As a consequence, body fluids are capable of absorbing relatively large amounts of heat with little change in temperature.

Conductivity is defined as the ability to pass from one molecule to another. Since in water heat is conducted rapidly from one molecule to another, water transfers heat from the cells to the blood, from the blood to the skin, and from the skin to the atmosphere.

Although body temperature is regulated, the temperature of the external environment affects the ease with which this is accomplished. Heat loss may be facilitated by cooling the environment, by removing moisture or dehumidifying it, by removing clothing, and by applying fluids that are cooler than the body to the skin. Conversely, heat loss may be diminished by increasing the environmental temperature, by covering the body, by reducing air currents, and by immersing the body in warm water.

Similar to other bodily processes, the temperature of the body is subject to control. Centers for the coordination and integration of those processes that result in a balance between heat produced and heat lost are located in the hypothalamus. There is some evidence indicating that there are heat-regulating centers in the spinal cord. The principal centers are, however, in the hypothalamus. A center in the anterior hypothalamus integrates the responses that prevent overheating, or hyperthermia. Stimulation of this area initiates panting, dilatation of surface blood vessels, and sweating. All these activities promote heat loss. Injury to this area results in elevation of body temperature. A center in the posterior hypothalamus integrates responses that prevent chilling, or hypothermia. Stimulation of this area results in constriction of blood vessels, shivering, and an increase in muscle tone. These activities either prevent heat loss or increase heat production. Messages from the hypothalamus are conveyed to the surface of the body by the sympathetic, or thoracolumbar, division of the autonomic nervous system. It innervates both the sweat glands and the peripheral blood vessels. Though the postganglionic fibers supplying the sweat glands are cholinergic, they respond to stimulation of the sympathetic nervous system.

Because the temperature-regulating centers are not fully developed at birth, temperature regulation is usually less accurate in infants and children than in adults. It is even less well developed in the young premature infant. As a consequence, the premature infant is more sensitive to changes in environmental temperature than is the full-term infant. In infants and children the temperature response in illness is often greater than in adults. They have a higher metabolic rate; therefore, there is more heat to eliminate. Normally they have a larger proportion of their body water in the interstitial fluid space, and their kidneys do not concentrate urine as effectively as do those of adults. Even in a child of school age, temperature regulation may not be as stable as that of an adult. For this reason children with fevers possibly require somewhat more careful observation than do adults.

In contrast to the child and younger adult who respond to a variety of etiological agents by developing a fever, elderly and debilitated persons may have little or even no elevation of temperature when ill. Therefore, other evidence that the elderly person is ill should not be discounted because he does not have a fever. A failure to develop a fever under circumstances when it is usual is generally a poor prognostic sign.

Heat production is also regulated by the hormones thyroxin and epinephrine. Thyroxin augments the rate of cellular oxidation and thereby increases the production of heat. Epinephrine also increases heat production. The female sex hormones have an influence on body temperatures. During the proliferative phase body temperature is low. At the time of ovulation the temperature often falls and then rises. During the period that follows, the temperature remains up and then falls just prior to the onset of menstruation. Fluctuations in body temperature may be used as a basis for determining the so-called safe period in family planning.

How does man adapt to extremes in temperature?

Man is capable of some degree of adaptation to extremes in temperature. As with other adaptations, this takes time. The first hot days of summer cause more discomfort than later hot days, because adaptation has not taken place. According to Bean,[10] even physically fit men are unable to work long or hard when they are first exposed to very hot environments. After they become acclimatized, they may work about as effectively as they did at lower temperatures. They are able to tolerate higher environmental temperatures when the humidity is low than when it is high. When suddenly exposed to temperatures of 120° F. with a relative humidity of 20 per cent or 91° F. with a 95 per cent humidity, the men were unable to work for long periods of time. Among other interesting observations was that adaptation was more rapid when the men worked than when they rested. In fact, they achieved little physiological adaptation when the humidity was high unless they worked. During the period of adaptation the men were miserable and had many of the symptoms that are common in illness such as nausea, vomiting, headache, listlessness, and irritability. Their pulse rates were elevated, blood pressures unstable, faces flushed, nasal mucosas injected, and sweating increased. Some had edema of the feet. Even in physically fit young men sudden exposure to high environmental temperatures and/or humidity places a burden on the circulatory and thermoregulatory mechanisms. Adaptation to the higher temperatures took a period of four or five days. After adaptation the men felt as well and were about as productive as they were at temperate climates. Bean[11] states that since skin temperatures are higher in those who are acclimatized to heat than in those who are not, that acclimatization must depend on either decreased heat production or increased heat loss or both.

Davis[12] states that the changes accompanying adaptation to heat include increased ability to perspire, salt retention, a small decrease in metabolic rate, and, with it, a small weight loss. The ability to retain salt takes longer to develop than the other changes. It is due to alterations in the pituitary-adrenal mechanism. The other changes can be explained on the basis of the setting of

[10] William Bean, "Physical and Toxic Agents," *Pathologic Physiology*, 3rd ed., William A. Sodeman, ed., W. B. Saunders Company, Philadelphia, 1961, pp. 290-93.
[11] *Ibid.*, p. 291.
[12] Davis, *Op. cit.*, p. 263.

the thermostat at a lower level. The circulatory changes are believed to be secondary to this. The reason for devoting attention to the mechanisms by which man adapts to high environmental temperatures is that this knowledge is necessary to understanding the needs of sick, debilitated, and aged patients. In these people the adaptive capacity is either limited or under strain. This is especially true of those with a limited cardiac reserve, as heat places a burden on the circulatory system. This is evidenced by an increase in pulse rate. Also in the adaptive process the tendency to conserve salt may aggravate previous salt and water retention and place an added strain on a limited cardiac reserve.

Persons who are elderly or who have a cardiac disorder should be encouraged to reduce physical activity during hot weather. This is particularly important at its onset. Other measures that reduce the burden on the heart and the thermoregulatory systems include the wearing of light weight clothing, the use of electric fans, and, of course, air conditioning. It is also important for the person to maintain his fluid intake, without exceeding his excretory capacity. When sweating is profuse, it is often difficult to replace the fluid loss by voluntary drinking. When air conditioning is not available, patients who are in congestive heart failure are sometimes placed in oxygen tents in hot weather. Though the increase in oxygen supply may be beneficial, the air conditioning reduces the demands made on the circulatory system to facilitate the loss of heat. When the patient is removed from the tent, he may be called upon to adapt both to a reduction in environmental oxygen and to an increase in the temperature of his surroundings. Consequently, the tent may be removed gradually. When this is done, it is well to take it off during the cooler parts of the day and to replace it when it is hot.

To summarize the physiology of temperature regulation, temperature is one of the conditions that is homeostatically controlled by the nervous, hormonal, and circulatory systems. The heat-regulating centers in the nervous system regulate body temperature primarily by increasing or decreasing the diameter of blood vessels in the skin. The hormonal system influences heat production and salt retention, which in turn increases water retention and in this way aids in the transfer of heat from the interior of the body to the external environment. The temperature that is regulated is that of the deeper, or core, tissues of the body. The temperature of the body varies with such factors as body activity, emotion, environmental conditions, and the method used to measure it. There is also a daily variation in the body temperature from 0.5° to 2.0° F. in all individuals. Body temperatures can be elevated by procedures that interfere with heat loss such as hot baths, hot weather, and strenuous muscular exercise. Children's mechanisms for the regulation of body temperature are less efficient than those of adults. Therefore, they are likely to respond with greater swings in temperature than are adults.

One of the most common findings in disease is some disturbance in temperature regulation. Though temperatures below the lower range of normal do occur, the most common change is an elevation above the upper limits of normal. Because some people normally maintain a temperature somewhat higher than average, the upper limit of normal is difficult to define exactly. However, for persons resting quietly in bed, an oral temperature of 37.5° C. (98.6° F.) is usually accepted as the upper limit of normal. The condition in which the body temperature is elevated above normal in disease is called fever.

What are the two general causes of fever?

Fever is associated with two quite different situations. In the more common and usually less serious one, something happens that causes temperature regulation to be reset at a higher level. Body temperature continues to be regulated, but it is regulated at a level above normal. In the other type of fever, as a result of injury or disease of the hypothalamus, temperature regulation fails and the temperature continues to rise unless external measures are employed to increase heat loss. When the condition that injures the heat-regulating center is temporary and the tissues are protected from excess heat, recovery is possible. For example, in thyroid crises, temperature regulation may fail. If the secretion of thyroid hormones can be restored to normal levels and the body temperature controlled within levels tolerated by the tissues, survival is possible.

Though fever has been recognized as a cardinal sign of disease since the time of Hippocrates, why it occurs or what purpose it serves, if any, is not known. Of the theories that have been advanced to explain the specific cause of fever, the one that appears to have the most support at the present time is that the polymorphonuclear leukocytes liberate a fever-producing substance (pyrogen) which acts on the temperature-regulation centers in such a manner that the thermostat is set at a higher than normal level. Beeson,[13] who was one of the first to isolate a pyrogen from white blood cells, states that all conditions in which fever occurs have one feature in common; that is, there is tissue injury. The body responds to tissue injury with an inflammatory process. The exudate that is formed in inflammation has been demonstrated experimentally to contain a substance that, when injected, induces fever. Wood,[14] in a review of the literature on fever, states that there is considerable evidence to support Beeson's theory. If this theory is correct, then the fever, whether it occurs in the patient with cancer, diphtheria, or an infected wound or following an infarction in the heart or lungs, has a common denominator, that is, a pyrogen released by the polymorphonuclear leukocyte. Attractive as this theory is, it does not explain why fever accompanies tuberculosis and infections from the influenza virus. In tuberculosis, the principal cell found in the

[13] Paul B. Beeson, "Alterations in Body Temperature," in *Principles of Internal Medicine*, 4th ed., ed. T. R. Harrison, *et al.*, The Blakiston Division, McGraw-Hill Book Company, Inc., New York, 1962, p. 62.
[14] W. Barry Wood, "Fever," *Scientific American*, CXCVI, June, 1957, pp. 62-68.

inflammatory exudate is the monocyte, which has not been found to contain a pyrogen. Neither does the lymph cell system, which appears to be the site of action for the influenza virus. Another point of doubt arises out of the fact that, though a fever-producing substance is found in the inflammatory exudate, it has never been isolated from the blood.

Despite lack of knowledge of why fever accompanies many disease states, the mechanisms that are responsible for the actual elevation in temperature are quite well understood. In the fever resulting from elevating the level at which temperature is controlled, heat production is increased much the same as it is in exercise. Heat loss, however, does not increase to the same proportion. In fact, the body responds much as it does when exposed to cold. The peripheral vessels constrict and limit the circulation of blood through the skin. The person shivers and his muscle tone increases. The muscles attached to the hair in the skin contract and elevate the hair; accompanying this are elevations of the skin commonly called goose pimples. The person feels cold and piles blankets over himself or turns the electric blanket on high even when the room is hot. When the temperature of his tissues reaches the new level, shivering stops and the patient may feel warm. Whereas during the chill he was pale, his skin becomes pink. A new equilibrium between heat production and heat loss has been set. Return of body temperature to normal levels is preceded by the regulator being reset at a lower level. The responses that are responsible for the lowering of the body temperature are the same as those accompanying exercises; that is, sweating and vasodilation occur.

The mechanisms responsible for the elevation of the temperature in patients who have a chill are easy to explain. The mechanisms that are responsible in the patient who does not have a chill are not as clear. The elevation in temperature may be brought about simply by a decrease in heat loss. It is also possible that the metabolic processes are stimulated by a specific fever-producing substance.

As was stated earlier, the value of fever is in most instances not known. In certain chronic conditions such as neurosyphilis, some gonococcal infections, and rheumatoid arthritis, fever has been found to be followed by an improvement in the patient's condition. Fever, particularly when it is high or continued for long periods of time, has a number of harmful effects as it accentuates weight loss and the loss of protein. Particularly in patients who have fever for more than a few days, food intake should be increased to prevent the excessive loss of weight. The heart rate is increased in fever. This has a particularly deleterious effect in patients who have a limited cardiac reserve. The extra burden placed on the heart in fever may precipitate heart failure. Sweating increases the loss of salt and water. As much as 3 l of water may be lost in 24 hours by the patient with a fever. The implication to nursing here is that attention should be paid to maintaining the fluid intake of the patient. Insufficient fluid intake is accompanied by an inadequate output of urine and by the development of sordes in the mouth. When the patient gets enough water, he does not develop sordes. In those patients who have drenching sweating (diaphoresis), comfort is increased by giving sponge baths and by replacing wet clothing and linen with dry. Though some patients have little discomfort with moderate degrees of fever, most patients with markedly elevated temperatures suffer from discomforts such as headache, photophobia, general malaise, and an unpleasant sensation of warmth. Of all discomforts, chilling and sweating are probably the most unpleasant. For the relief of headache, applying an ice cap or sponging the patient's face may be helpful. Protection of the patient from bright light is essential when he has photophobia and may be helpful in relief of headache. The doctor may prescribe aspirin to relieve the headache. However, some patients prefer the headache to the sweating that follows the ingestion of aspirin. Unless the patient continues to feel chilly, as sometimes happens in influenza, bathing may increase comfort. When the patient is chilling, he should be covered and protected from drafts. A hot-water bottle to his feet and an ice cap to his head may increase his comfort.

Though the routine varies somewhat, the patient's temperature should be checked at frequent intervals during the chill and frequently enough and long enough following it to determine the height of the fever. For example, during the chill the temperature may be measured every ten minutes, and then after the chill ceases, it may be measured every half-hour until the last reading is no higher or is lower than the preceding one. Whatever the hospital routine is, however, temperature determination may be necessary at more frequent intervals than those prescribed by the physician. When the temperature of the patient is rising very rapidly or it is at a very high level, his safety may depend on more frequent determinations and on the institution of measures effective in its control.

Though instances have been recorded in which patients have survived temperatures as high as 112° F. for a short period of time, a temperature as high as 108° F. for an extended period of time can be expected to do permanent damage. Furthermore, when temperatures exceed 105.8° F., regulatory mechanisms cannot be depended upon to resist further rise. (See Figure 11-2.) Excessively high temperatures endanger the body by irreversibly inactivating essential enzyme systems and by producing permanent alterations in the structure of body proteins. Therefore, when a patient's temperature is elevated to, or approaches, 105° F., measures are often instituted to reduce it. In conditions where the mechanism for cooling the body seems to go out of control or the heat-regulating centers are injured, antipyretics such as aspirin are of no value because they act on the hypothalamus in such a way as to cause it to reset the "thermostat" at a lower level. An example of the first is heat stroke; of the second, tumors or injuries of the hypothalamus.[15] The only measures that are effective are those that increase heat loss by increasing

[15] Louis S. Goodman and Alfred Gilman, *The Pharmacological Basis of Therapeutics*, 2nd ed., The Macmillan Company, New York, 1956, p. 283.

the temperature gradient between the skin and the external environment. To do this, measures are instituted to increase the evaporation of moisture from the skin, or the patient is placed in a cold environment, so that the heat moves from his tissues to the surrounding media. Thus the patient may be sponged liberally with water or alcohol. When his skin is cool, the sponging should be accompanied by rubbing in order to encourage the circulation of blood through the skin. For the patient whose temperature is dangerously high, placing him in a tub of iced water may be lifesaving. When they are available, a patient may be placed between hypothermia blankets. These procedures must be prescribed by the physician. When drastic measures are taken to reduce body temperature, the regular and frequent checking of the patient's temperature is essential. Sometimes the temperature continues to fall after the decline is established. Therefore, the physician should be asked to indicate the level at which the sponge or bath should be discontinued. Another point that is of significance in giving sponge baths is that they should be continued for as long a period of time as is necessary to lower the temperature. A quick "splash" may do more harm than good as it may only stimulate heat production. In young children temperature may be effectively lowered by cooling rectal irrigations.

There are many conditions in which fever is a symptom and may present a problem in the care of the patient. They include most infections, advanced neoplastic disease, including leukemia, Hodgkin's disease and hypernephroma, infarctions, mechanical and crushing injuries, extensive surgery, collagen fiber diseases, and severe anemia. One of the factors contributing to fever in leukemia is the fact that the metabolic rate is elevated. In thyroid crisis, the temperature of the patient behaves as if the temperature-regulating center were out of control. Measures similar to those required in treatment of heat stroke may be required to protect the tissues from the effects of overheating. Some of the conditions in which fever appears to be the consequence of a failure of the homeostatic mechanism to exert control have already been mentioned.

Knowledge of temperature regulation has a bearing on meeting the needs of all patients as well as those with fevers. One general objective in the nursing of patients is to protect the patient from conditions that place strain on the adaptive capacity of the individual. Certainly temperatures outside the range of comfort—either low or high—increase the activity not only of the heat-regulating center, but of the circulatory system. Though the effect of small or moderate changes in environmental temperature may be of no consequence as far as the heat-regulating center is concerned, they may place serious strain on the heart or blood vessels. In heart disease or shock, they may well have serious consequences. Methods that can be used to protect the patient from the consequences of high environmental temperatures have already been suggested. Patients should also be protected from chilling by adequate bed covering and warm clothing. Hot-water bottles to the feet, with attention to the temperature, bed socks, bed jackets, and sweaters help to protect patients from chilling. People, especially the elderly, who are accustomed to wearing their underwear when they go to bed should be permitted to continue the practice when at all possible. Screens in front of open windows or doors may reduce drafts which some patients find chilling. When bathing patients, especially during those times of the year when the environmental temperature is low, care should be taken that the bath water is warm and that the person is kept covered and the skin is thoroughly dried.

The second objective is to make, record, and report observations basic to planning the nursing care of the patient and pertinent to the diagnosis and treatment of the patient's condition. The first, obviously, relates directly to the practice of nursing, the second to the role of the nurse as a co-worker with the physician. Though the physician has the responsibility for establishing the medical diagnosis of the patient, and planning the therapeutic regime, the nurse can and should contribute both by observing signs and symptoms that indicate deviations from health, and by clearly describing her observations. The nurse should keep in mind that fever is not a disease but part of the body's response to tissue injury. The symptoms and signs that accompany it are of three general types. (1) Those that result from the adaptation of the circulatory system to the regulation of body temperature at a higher level include an increase in heart rate and with it a more rapid respiratory rate and alterations in the peripheral circulation. (2) The second group of symptoms and signs include those that result from the body's response to injury. The gastrointestinal tract is very sensitive to injury in any part of the body. Therefore nausea, vomiting, and diarrhea are common accompaniments of injury, particularly in acute illness. A leukocyte count above 12,000 cells or below 5,000 cells per cubic millimeter is indicative of tissue damage. An elevated leukocyte count may also be a nonspecific stress response. An increase in the sedimentation rate also indicates tissue injury. Although patients who have a fever may have few or no subjective symptoms, they may feel warm, have headache and malaise, muscle aching, and photophobia, and be generally miserable. (3) The third group of symptoms that may be observed are those that relate to the factor that is responsible for the tissue injury. For example, if the patient has a pneumococcal pneumonia, his sputum has specific characteristics. Description of the character of the sputum then contributes to the identification of a causative factor. Observation is also important in the detection of changes in the condition of the patient so that his treatment may be adapted to his needs.

A third objective is to promote the comfort and safety of the patient. Some of the measures contributing to the attainment of this objective have been discussed. Some of those mentioned in the accomplishment of the first objective also help in the accomplishment of this objective. Attention should also be given to helping the patient meet his fluid and food needs. Drinking and eating may be difficult for the sick patient. Whether the requirements of the patient are met depends often not only on food or water being placed at his bedside, but on someone giving him the assistance he requires.

A fourth objective relates to the possibility that the cause of the tissue injury may be an infectious agent. This possibility should not be neglected in those patients in whom there is a problem of differential diagnosis. Measures appropriate to the prevention of the spread of infection to personnel and to other patients should be instituted. These measures should take into account the avenues by which organisms leave the host, vehicles whereby they can be transported to others, and portals of entry to others. See Chapter 4.

What mechanisms may be involved in acclimatization (adaptation) to cold?

Just as the tissues can, within limits, tolerate temperatures higher than that of the cells, they can tolerate temperatures that are lower. There is some doubt, however, that man adapts to cold by making physiological alterations as he does in adapting to heat. Rather the adaptation seems to be a decreased perception of cold. Two different types of adaptations to cold have been observed. In one type young Norwegian subjects who were adapted to cold were observed to maintain a relatively warm skin temperature by frequent and severe periods of shivering. Despite the shivering, they were apparently able to sleep restfully. In another type, adaptation is by lowering the body temperature when exposed to cold. Australian aborigines, who sleep out of doors in all kinds of weather, rapidly lose heat. They experience a minimum of shivering.[16]

As implied above, the usual response to cold is shivering and constriction of the peripheral blood vessels. Shivering is accompanied by an increase in the production of heat and by changes decreasing its loss. When these mechanisms are adequate or the environmental temperature is not too low, they may be sufficient to maintain body temperature within normal limits. When, however, heat loss exceeds heat production, hypothermia (abnormally low body temperature) ensues. The most frequent cause of hypothermia is exposure to a low environmental temperature. Although much less commonly associated with pathological conditions than hyperthermia, it does occur.

Hypothermia may result from exposure to the elements or be purposefully induced. As an example, a hunting party is lost in the woods or mountains or on the prairie in freezing or near-freezing weather. The seriousness of their predicament will depend not only on the temperature of the environment, but on the adequacy of their clothing, whether or not it is wet or dry, and their ability to find or construct a shelter for protection from the wind. As indicated earlier, chilling is more rapid when evaporation takes place and/or there are air currents than when clothing is dry and the air is still.

[16] Ralph W. Brauer and Albert R. Behnke, "Hypothermia and Cold Injury," in T. R. Harrison, *Principles of Internal Medicine,* 4th ed., The Blakiston Division, McGraw-Hill Book Company, Inc., New York, 1962, p. 838.

Probably the most common pathological condition in which hypothermia occurs is the depression of the nervous system by drugs such as morphine and the barbiturates. Therapy of the hypothermia is to provide a warm environment. Obviously, any condition contributing to heat loss should be zealously avoided.

As the body temperature falls, the metabolic rate also falls. The most important effect of the decreased metabolic rate is that the oxygen requirements of the tissues are likewise decreased. As an illustration, when tissue temperature is decreased to 25.5° C. (78° F.), oxygen consumption is reduced by approximately 50 per cent. One of the important uses of hypothermia is, therefore, in surgical procedures requiring interruption of the circulation to important structures, such as the brain. By induction of hypothermia, the length of time the circulation is stopped can be prolonged. It is therefore used in open heart surgery and in operations on the aorta to protect the brain from the effects of hypoxia. It is also employed in the therapy of serious injuries to the brain as well as in the treatment of uncontrolled hyperthyroidism.

What methods are employed in the induction of hypothermia?

The method employed to induce hypothermia will depend on why it is used, how long it is to be maintained, and the equipment available. Hypothermia can be induced by immersing the trunk and extremities in a tub of iced water. Although this method is relatively successful with children, it takes several hours to induce hypothermia by this method in adults. In open heart surgery the blood is usually cooled to the desired temperature by circulating it through coils of the cooling system of the pump oxygenator. After the surgical procedure is completed, the patient can be warmed by warming the blood to the desired temperature. The third method of cooling the patient is to place him between hypothermia blankets. These blankets contain coils through which a refrigerant is circulated. With the blanket, hypothermia may be maintained for days.

In the preparation of the patient for hypothermia, a drug such as chlorpromazine may be administered to minimize shivering.

What are some of the nurse's responsibilities in the care of the patient who undergoes hypothermia?

The responsibilities of the nurse vary with the method used and the length of time hypothermia is maintained. When hypothermia is induced by circulating the blood through a pump oxygenator, most of the responsibility is borne by the physician and the technician who runs the pump. When the blanket is used and the patient is maintained in a hypothermic state for several days, much of the responsibility is delegated to the nurse.

To illustrate, Mrs. Molly McRobin was admitted to the emergency room for treatment of a stab wound in her chest. Although she was fully conscious at the time of her admission, she soon lapsed into unconsciousness from which she never recovered. She was rushed to the operating room, where she was found to have cardiac tamponade due to bleeding into the pericardial sac and she experienced cardiac arrest for a period of from five to ten minutes.

Because of the injury to the temperature-regulating centers in the hypothalamus, Mrs. McRobin was unable to control her temperature and it began to rise. To prevent damage to the brain by hyperthermia and to decrease its oxygen requirements, Mrs. McRobin was placed on a hypothermia blanket. At this time Mrs. McRobin was deeply unconscious and she was dependent on the nurse to meet her physiological needs. Observation not only of the status of the patient, but of the functioning of all the different types of equipment, was necessary. Although the only aspect of Mrs. McRobin's care that will be discussed is the hypothermia, she required special attention to maintenance of oxygen supply, fluid intake and output, nutrition, protection of her skin, and attention to position and body alignment. In order to maintain her joints in a functional condition, her extremities were moved through a normal range of motion when she was bathed. Because respiratory insufficiency occurs during hypothermia, maintenance of oxygen supply is an objective in any patient in whom it is induced.

Although the patient may be placed between two hypothermia blankets, Mrs. McRobin was placed on one. The patient may be placed directly on the blanket or it may be covered with a sheet. The latter practice is more esthetic, and may be more comfortable for the patient; when the sheet is tucked under the sides of the mattress, it may also help to keep the blanket in place. In this particular blanket, a 20 per cent solution of alcohol was circulated through an electrically refrigerated cylinder, where it was cooled and then circulated through the coils of the blanket. Since the operation of the system depends on a supply of fluid, the supply tank should be checked regularly and refilled as necessary.

As prescribed by Mrs. McRobin's physician, the thermostat on the blanket was set at 32.2° C. (90° F.). In order to observe her temperature, a rectal probe was introduced and connected to a battery-operated thermometer. Her temperature could be determined at any time by switching on the machine. The blanket operates automatically. Because the patient's temperature drops about 2° after cooling is discontinued, the machine should turn off before the desired temperature is attained. It should also turn on when the temperature starts to rise.

In order to avoid increasing body temperature, Mrs. McRobin was bathed with cool water. Patting, rather than rubbing, motions were used in drying her. When her extremities were exercised, motions were limited to a minimum.

Though not a problem with Mrs. McRobin, the restless patient may move off the blanket. When this happens, either the patient or the blanket must be moved so that the patient is reclining on it.

Conscious patients frequently complain, sometimes bitterly, about shivering. The nurse should talk with the patient. She should try to emphasize the importance of the treatment, but at the same time agree with him that shivering is unpleasant. She should encourage him to try to remain on the blanket, despite his discomfort.

The blanket itself requires some care. Tape rather than safety pins should be used to fasten tubing to sheets. A puncture of the blanket will allow the refrigerant fluid to escape and thereby render the blanket useless. Hot water or strong chemicals should not be applied to the blanket as they may damage the plastic covering. The blanket can be washed with soap and tepid water or a solution of benzethonium chloride. It should not be folded when stored, but it should be rolled loosely and placed on a flat surface.

The purpose of this chapter has been to discuss some of the needs of the patient who has problems in the control of body temperature or in whom hypothermia is induced. As a basis for understandng the nature of these problems, the homeostatic mechanisms utilized by the body in maintaining temperature have been reviewed and related to the mechanisms that are involved in hyperthermia and hypothermia. Suggestions have been made as to how this content applies to the care of patients in general and to those with alterations in body temperature. Students who are interested in pursuing the study of temperature regulation in its various aspects will find references at the end of the chapter.

REFERENCES

Books

Fuerst, Elinor, and Lu Verne Wolff, *Fundamentals of Nursing*, 3rd ed., J. B. Lippincott Co., Philadelphia, 1964, pp. 155-57, 164-72.
Harmer, Bertha, and Virginia Henderson, *Textbook of the Principles and Practice of Nursing*, 5th ed., The Macmillan Company, New York, 1955.

Articles

Benzinger, T. H., "The Human Thermostat," *Scientific American,* CCIV, No. 1, January, 1961, pp. 134-47.
Bogert, C. M., "How Reptiles Regulate Their Body Temperature," *Scientific American,* CC, No. 4, April, 1959, pp. 105-20.
Boba, A., and J. G. Convease, "Ganglionic Blockade and Its Protective Action in Hemorrhage," *Anesthesiology,* XVIII, No. 4, July-August, 1957, pp. 559-72.
British Medical Journal, XVII, No. 1, January, 1961, entire issue, pp. 1-84.
Goldsmith, R., "Use of Clothing Records to Demonstrate Acclimatization to Cold in Man," *Journal of Applied Physiology,* XV, No. 5, September, 1960, pp. 776-80.
Graham, A., and Mary A. MacRestie, "The Case of the Tainted Thermometer," *R.N.,* XX, June, 1957, pp. 45-48.
Graves, Nancy, "Nursing During Prolonged Hypothermia," *American Journal of Nursing,* LX, No. 7, July, 1960, pp. 969-70.
Hoagland, Robert J., and Raymond H. Bishop, Jr., "A Physiologic Treatment of Heat Stroke," *American Journal of the Medical Sciences,* CXLI, No. 4, April, 1961, pp. 415-22.
Hock, Raymond J., and Benjamin G. Covino, "Hypothermia," *Scientific American,* CXCVIII, No. 3, March, 1958, pp. 104-14.

Nugent, G. Robert, "Prolonged Hypothermia," *American Journal of Nursing*, LX, No. 7, July, 1960, pp. 967-69.

Overton, R. C., and M. E. DeBakey, "Experimental Observations on the Influence of Hypothermia and Autonomic Blocking Agents on Hemorrhagic Shock," *Annals of Surgery*, CXLIII, No. 3, April, 1956, pp. 439-47.

Phelps, Elbert T., "Fever—Its Causes and Effects," *American Journal of Nursing*, LVI, No. 3, March, 1956, pp. 319-21.

Postel, A. H., L. C. Reid, and J. W. Hinton, "Therapeutic Effect of Hypothemia Experimental Hemorrhagic Shock," *Annals of Surgery*, CXLV, February, 1957, pp. 311-16.

Sommermeyer, Lucille, and Martin Frobisher, Jr., "Laboratory Studies on Disinfection of Oral Thermometers," *Nursing Research*, I, No. 2, October, 1952, pp. 32-35.

Sommermeyer, Lucille, and Martin Frobisher, Jr., "Laboratory Studies on Disinfection of Rectal Thermometers, *Nursing Research*, II, No. 2, October, 1953, pp. 85-89.

Sosthenesa, Sister M., "New Thermometer Techniques," *Hospital Progress*, XXXVII, No. 9, September, 1956, pp. 80-81.

Vandam, Leroy D., and Thomas K. Burnap, "Hypothermia," *New England Journal of Medicine*, CCLXL, No. 11, September 10, 1959, pp. 546-53, and No. 12, September 17, 1959, pp. 595-603.

Wilson, William J., "Heat Injury," *American Journal of Nursing*, LX, No. 8, August, 1960, pp. 1124-25.

Wood, W. Barry, Jr., "The Role of Endogenous Pyrogen in the Genesis of Fever," *The Lancet*, CCLXXV, July-December, 1958, July 12, 1958, pp. 53-56.

12 : Nursing the Patient Having a Problem Resulting from Failure to Regulate the Proliferation and Maturation of Cells

Cancer is still an unsolved problem. Its incidence has increased in proportion to the aging of the population. Although many early cases can be cured through surgical operations, X ray, and radium, yet a large-scale attack is impossible unless its cause and pathogenesis are known. Biochemistry may solve this problem also, unless we are faced with a biological principle that still escapes us. It is extremely difficult to understand the biology of the cancer cell because it reacts differently from all other cells. In a differentiated organism the cells form a social community. They are specialized and cooperate in a perfect way. The cancer cell is asocial. It goes its own way, has its own metabolism, thrives at the expense of the organism like a parasite, destroys it and in so doing destroys itself. This is against all rules and therefore is difficult to conceive.[1]

In the discussion of homeostasis thus far, emphasis has been placed on the maintenance of the conditions in the internal environment that are favorable to cellular activity. Homeostasis is also dependent on the ability to maintain the structure and function of tissues. The continuity of tissues and the maintenance of function require that cells lost as a result of wear and tear and of injury be replaced. Fundamental to this replacement is the capacity of cells to proliferate (multiply) and to differentiate into mature tissue. As with other homeostatic mechanisms, the usefulness of the capacity of cells to multiply depends on (1) the ability of the organism to regulate the proliferation and maturation of cells and (2) the appropriateness and adequacy of the response. The potential for growth of the different types of tissues varies. Some, such as fibrous connective tissue and reticular cells, are not only able to proliferate but they can differentiate into a number of types of tissue cells. Other types of tissue cells are capable of proliferation, but they can mature only into cells similar to the parent cell. As an illustration, epithelial cells proliferate and mature into some type of epithelial cell. Immature epithelial

---

[1] Henry E. Sigerist, "Civilization and Disease," *Phoenix Books,* University of Chicago Press, Chicago, 1962, p. 176.

cells are capable of differentiating into the different types of epithelial tissue cells. As emphasized throughout, the potential of cells for proliferation varies greatly from one type of tissue to another. In the examples just cited, tissue cells have a great potential for growth. In other types of tissues, such as nervous tissue and striated muscle, the potential for growth is exceedingly limited.

In healthy tissues, the process whereby cells multiply follows a predictable pattern known as mitosis. In mitosis the cell undergoes a complicated series of changes in which each chromosome is divided and two new, or daughter, cells are formed. In a report on the studies being made on cells by radioautography, Baserga and Kisieleski[2] state that only a small proportion of the cells of the adult animal body are capable of dividing at all. In the adult human being only about 3 per cent of the cells are able to divide for the purposes of repairing tissue. By using tritium (the radioactive isotope, H^3), it was found that of the two daughter cells formed during cell division, one remains in the tissue and divides as its parent cell does; the other daughter cell dies. Depending on the potentialities of the cell and environmental conditions, the new cells may be a replica of the parent cell or may differ in some respect from it. The ways in which a daughter cell can differ at maturity from the parent cell are predictable. The daughter cells fit into the over-all organization of the tissue. For example, the type of epithelial cells entering into the formation of a mucous membrane may be altered by exposure of a mucous membrane to an unfavorable environment. Following a tracheostomy, transitional cells in the mucous membrane lining the trachea are replaced by a thick layer of squamous epithelium. The change is adaptive, as squamous cells are better able to survive chronic irritation than are transitional cells. The process by which one type of cell is replaced by another is known as metaplasia. The pattern for metaplasia is predictable and the resulting tissue organized and functional.

As with other homeostatic mechanisms, the multiplication of cells occurs in response to a need or stimulus and ceases when the need is met, which indicates that the potential for growth of cells is subject to regulation. Not all the factors in the regulation of growth are understood. The growth of some tissues is influenced by both intrinsic and extrinsic factors. Among the extrinsic regulators are certain hormones; adjacent cells also appear to exert a growth-inhibiting influence on each other.

Many examples could be cited in which cell proliferation occurs in response to a need and ceases when the need is met. One such example is wound healing. Other examples include the continuous replacement of worn-out erythrocytes and leukocytes. The production of either erythrocytes or leukocytes may be greatly increased in response to appropriate stimuli. The production of erythrocytes is increased following acute hemorrhage or on exposure of the

[2] Renato Baserga and Walter E. Kisieleski, "Autobiographies of Cells," *Scientific American*, CCIX, August, 1963, pp. 106-7.

organism to a lowering of the oxygen tension in the atmosphere. Infection initiated by one of the pyogenic cocci, such as the pneumococcus or meningococcus, is accompanied by an outpouring of neutrophils. When the demand for either erythrocytes or neutrophils is very great, cells may be released from the bone marrow at an earlier stage of development than is usual. Following hemorrhage, the level of not-quite-mature erythrocytes—the reticulocytes— rises from the usual 2 per cent or less to 10 per cent or more. This same response can be observed in the patient who is treated for certain types of anemia. Shortly after the hemorrhage occurs, or the treatment is initiated, the reticulocyte count rises rapidly. The rate at which the level of mature erythrocytes rises is slower. As the normal level of erythrocytes is approached, the reticulocyte count drops to normal. This is, therefore, evidence of a mechanism operating to control the proliferation of erythrocytes. The extent to which the reticulocyte count is elevated, under conditions such as those cited, is an indication of the capacity of the bone marrow to produce blood cells.

In conditions under which the neutrophils are markedly elevated, the proportion of nonfilamented or nonsegmented leukocytes to filamented or segmented leukocytes is increased. Nonfilamented leukocytes are the not-quite-mature form of white blood cells. Like reticulocytes, they represent a normal stage in the development of leukocytes. When the situation calling for the increase in leukocytes is controlled, the normal level of leukocytes is restored.

The process whereby cells multiply and produce cells that are the same type and form as those found in the tissue or organ is known as hyperplasia. It occurs in response to an extracellular stimulus. With the removal of the stimulus the multiplication of cells ceases; that is, in hyperplasia the multiplication of cells is controlled. The cells are typical of the tissue from which they arise and are organized into a normal or healthy pattern, and multiple tissue elements are often involved. For example, in the healing of a wound, macrophages, fibroblasts, epithelial cells, and capillaries participate in the formation of the scar.

How does the normal replacement of tissue cells differ from growth in neoplasia?

The two following statements summarize the principal differences between the normal replacement of cells and abnormal growth. Later in the chapter, the characteristics of abnormal cell growth will be further developed. The proliferation of cells is homeostatic when the multiplication of cells (1) occurs in response to an appropriate stimulus, (2) is adequate to the requirements of the organism, (3) differentiates or matures into normal functioning tissue, and (4) ceases when the need of the organism is met. In contrast, when the proliferation of cells (1) occurs in response to an inappropriate stimulus, (2) is inadequate to, or in excess of, the needs of the organism, (3) results in immature and abnormal cells, and (4) continues without regard for the needs of the organism, the well-being and possibly the life of the individual are threatened.

What is the role of the nurse in caring for the patient who has or who fears that he has cancer?

For many reasons, the nurse has a notable contribution to make in the care of the patient who has or fears that he has cancer (a term generally understood to mean a malignant neoplasm). There are few situations in which a nurse requires more knowledge and understanding or a wider variety of skills than she does in the care of patients with a possible or positive diagnosis of cancer. The knowledge and skills of the nurse need not be limited in their application to patients with a diagnosis of cancer. One of the fears frequently expressed by patients who have other diagnoses is the fear of cancer. The patient who hesitates to make his anxiety known may be encouraged to do so by a "listening and hearing" nurse. The services of the nurse are required and utilized in programs for the prevention and the detection of cancer, in case finding and diagnosis, and in the treatment and rehabilitation of patients. Patients with cancer are from all age and social groups. In terms of degrees of illness, they range from the healthy to those with widespread and progressive disease. The needs of the patient and his family vary from health teaching to detailed physical care and sustained emotional support. Survival of patients following extensive and sometimes mutilating surgical procedures often depends on quality nursing. Whether or not the patient is successfully rehabilitated depends in part on the quality of nursing he receives from the moment he seeks medical attention until his rehabilitation has been completed.

To meet the challenges presented by patients, their families, and the community, the nurse requires an understanding of the following:

1. Hemeostasis of cell proliferation and differentiation
2. The nature of cancer as a disease
   a. Knowledge of past and present trends in incidence
   b. Summary of characteristics of growth in normal and neoplastic cells
   c. System for naming and illustration
   d. Essential differences between benign and malignant neoplasms
   e. Theories of etiology
   f. Natural history (stages in development)
   g. The routes by which cancer spreads
   h. Most common sites
   i. Methods used to express extent and virulence
   j. How neoplasms cause symptoms
3. Prevention, diagnosis, and therapy
4. Factors of particular significance in the nursing of the patient with cancer
   a. The emotional impact of a diagnosis of cancer and its treatment

b. The physical needs of the patient
c. The needs of the patient as related to the site of the lesion and the method of treatment
d. Special problems in the care of the patient with widespread and extensive disease
e. Family and community resources in helping the patient cope with cancer

Before continuing the discussion, several terms will be defined. The first term, "neoplasm," has already been defined as a new growth. The word "tumor" is frequently used interchangeably with neoplasm. Strictly speaking, they do not have identical meanings. A tumor is a swelling which can be due not only to an increase in the number of cells in a tissue, but to inflammation or an accumulation of blood or fluid in a localized area of tissue. Although a neoplasm is defined as a new growth of cells, the growth can be accompanied by a loss as well as an increase in tissue. For example, malignant neoplasms in the stomach are sometimes in the form of ulcers. Despite the differences in meaning, the two terms are commonly used synonymously.

Neoplasms are of two general types, benign and malignant. The words "benign" and "malignant" are adjectives that may be used to describe the character of a wide variety of situations, conditions, diseases, and even people. Benign takes its origin from the latin word *benignus*. *Bene* means *well* and *gnus, kind*. When the word "benign" is used to describe a disease, the implication is that it is relatively harmless. A benign neoplasm is therefore one that is not of itself deadly. It may, however, cause harm by virtue of its location and by the fact that it occupies space. The term "malignant" has its origin from the latin *malignus,* which means *to produce death*. Similar to the adjective benign, malignant may be employed to characterize any type of disease in which death is probable, unless something can be done to halt or alter its course. Some of the significant differences between benign and malignant neoplasms will be discussed in greater detail when the characteristics of neoplasms are presented.

What evidence of neoplasms existed among ancient animals and peoples?

With the current emphasis on cancer as a cause of death, the reader may have the impression that cancer is a new disease and that it is unique to man. Nothing could be farther from the truth. It is neither a new disease nor is it a disease of civilization, per se. Evidence indicating the presence of an osteoma (a benign neoplasm) has been found in the vertebrae of a dinosaur that lived some 50 million years ago. References to neoplasms are found in the earliest medical literature. They were described by the Egyptians in 1200 B.C. Neoplasms were known to Hippocrates. The modern concept of cancer as a disturbance in cellular growth, however, is not much more than 100 years old. It probably had its origin in the work, published in 1838, of Johannes Müller, who is credited with the first description of the cellular nature of cancer. Virchow, some 20 years later, gave impetus to the idea by describing the characteristic changes in cancer cells.

Previous to the discoveries of Müller and Virchow, the relationship of cancer to certain occupations had been observed. In 1775, Sir Percivall Pott reported his observation that chimney sweeps in London had an exceptionally high incidence of cancer of the scrotum. In the sixteenth century, men working in mines in the mountains of Saxony were known to develop a progressive and fatal disease. Not until later, however, was the disease identified as cancer. The discovery that pitchblende was the causative agent did not come until still later. More than 400 chemical agents are now known to be carcinogenic.

Not only is cancer a disease of antiquity, but it is not unique to man; it occurs in both plants and animals. Cows, chickens, parakeets, horses, monkeys, dogs, and laboratory animals such as mice, rats, and rabbits are known to develop neoplasms. Because of the contributions of these animals to the study of disease, they might be included with the dog as best friends of man. When cancer, as well as other types of neoplasms, is viewed as a phenomenon of growth, neither the fact that it is of ancient origin nor that it occurs in species other than man should be surprising. In all living creatures, cancer has the same general characteristics. The organism is unable to control the differentiation, proliferation, and mutation of cells. The result is the unrestricted growth of poorly differentiated cells that are without useful function.

What have been the trends in the incidence of malignant neoplasms since the beginning of the twentieth century?

In the United States, as well as in other countries for which reliable statistics are available, cancer ranks second only to cardiovascular disease as a cause of death. It is known to be the second cause of death in all the countries of the modern world.[3] Besides its importance as a cause of mortality, it is one of the significant causes of morbidity. It is now the leading cause of death among women aged 30 through 54 years. It is second only to accidents as a cause of death in children of school age.[4] Most authorities express the opinion that the incidence of cancer is probably the same all over the world, but the actual occurrence of the disease is difficult to verify because statistics are not reliable in many regions. Furthermore, because of lack of trained medical personnel, many persons who develop cancer may not be identified.

[3] Canada, United States, Germany, Denmark, Finland, France, Norway, Netherlands, England and Wales, Scotland, Northern Ireland, Sweden, Switzerland, Australia. "The Ten Principal Causes of Death in the Modern World," *World Health,* January-February, 1960, XIII, pp. 2-3.
[4] *Progress in Health Services,* VIII, February, 1959, p. 1.

In some countries a smaller proportion of the people die from cancer than in other countries because the average length of life is shorter than it is in countries such as the United States and Canada.

According to *1964 Cancer Facts and Figures* (American Cancer Society, Inc., New York), approximately 284,000 Americans died from cancer in 1963 and in 1962, 278,000 died. The United States Public Health Service has reported that in 1961 273,502 died. The American Cancer Society estimates that 830,000 Americans will be under treatment for cancer during 1964 and that about 540,000 persons will be diagnosed as having cancer for the first time. In a study made by Heller *et al.,*[5] 430 persons per 1,000 were discovered to have cancer some time during the year. The disease was newly discovered in 319 persons, and 149 died as a result of it. On the basis of their findings, Heller and his associates predicted that by 1975 the number of new cases diagnosed each year will increase to 750,000, and that under prevailing conditions, 32 newborn babies out of each 100 can be expected to develop cancer some time during their lifetime. The American Cancer Society states[6] that one in every four Americans now living can expect to have cancer some time during their lifetime. Cancer now causes one out of every six deaths in the United States.

What factors are believed to contribute to the apparent increase in the number of persons having a diagnosis of cancer?

The increase in the number of persons having a diagnosis of cancer is not believed to be due to a significant rise in its actual incidence. The incidence of cancer in certain sites such as the lung is, and has, risen. In other sites, such as the stomach, the incidence is falling, and occurrence of cancer in other sites is leveling off. A number of factors have contributed to the increase in the number of persons diagnosed as having cancer. Part of the increase can be explained on the basis of improved diagnostic methods and facilities. This hypothesis is supported by the finding that the number of persons having a diagnosis of cancer is greater in areas having good medical facilities than in areas with poor facilities. The total is increased by the fact that formerly diseases such as leukemia and Hodgkin's disease were not classified as cancer, as they now are. With the lessening of the infant mortality rate and decrease in mortality from acute communicable diseases, more persons are living to be of an age when the incidence of cancer is highest. Another factor contributing to the increase in the total number of persons having cancer is the fact that the population is rising. The factors listed above are similar to those contributing to the increase in the number of persons having all types of chronic disease.

Although the incidence of cancer tends to rise with age, the disease occurs

[5] John R. Heller, Sidney J. Cuther, and William M. Hoenszel, "Some Observations on the Epidemiology of Cancer in the United States," *Journal of the American Medical Association,* CLIX, December 24, 1955, pp. 1628-34.
[6] *1964 Cancer Facts and Figures, Op. cit.,* p. 3.

in all age groups from infancy to old age. The rate is higher in infancy up through the age of four than it is in childhood. According to *Progress in Health Services,*[7] more than half the deaths from cancer occur in persons over 65 years of age. The common sites in which cancer occurs differ with age. Leukemia and cancer in the brain and nervous system are types most frequently found in children, but leukemia occurs more commonly among persons in older age groups than was once believed. Among persons in older age groups, cancer of the breast, skin, lung, gastrointestinal tract, and genital organs is most common.

Early in the century more women than men died from cancer, but the situation is now reversed. According to *Progress in Health Services,*[8] in 1900 the death rate in women exceeded that of men by 65 per cent. Over the years this ratio has narrowed. By 1947, the mortality rate for the two sexes was equal, and by 1955 the mortality rate for males exceeded that for females by 22 per cent. Two reasons are offered which partly explain the change. One is that the incidence of lung cancer has risen rapidly in men; the other is that cancer in women is generally in more accessible sites than it is in men.

Accessibility of site does not of itself guarantee a reduction in the mortality rate from cancer. The death rate from cancer of the breast remains essentially the same, despite extensive educational programs intended to facilitate early detection of neoplasms in the breast. By way of contrast, the programs for the early detection of cancer of the cervix have been accompanied by a decrease in mortality rate from this cause.

Cancer mortality is greater among nonwhites than among whites. Early in this century the reverse was true. Mortality is also higher in cities and in industrial areas than it is in rural and less heavily populated areas. Possibly the quantity and quality of medical care available to different groups is responsible for some of these differences.

The primary sites in which cancer leads to death have also changed in the last 30 or 35 years. As has been previously indicated, cancer in the lung and other parts of the respiratory system has risen markedly.[9] Furthermore, the increase in incidence in cancer of the lung is real and cannot be attributed merely to an improvement in diagnosis. Leukemia has been increasing in incidence. This increase has been greatest in children and in older people. Mortality from cancer of the breast has remained unchanged. This is true despite the accessibility of the site and an intensive educational program to bring about early detection and case finding. These trends have resulted in one of the paradoxes in modern medicine, that although the rate of cure from cancer is reported to be rising, the mortality rate, that is, the number dying per 100,000 remains essentially unchanged.[10]

[7] *Progress in Health Services,* Health Information Foundation, VIII, February, 1959, p. 2.

[8] *Ibid.,* p. 2.

[9] E. Cuyler Hammond, "The Effects of Smoking," *Scientific American,* CCVII, July, 1962, p. 40.

[10] George Crile, Jr., "The Cancer Problem," *Perspectives in Biology and Medicine,* III, Spring, 1960, p. 358.

Patients with a diagnosis of cancer and who are alive and well at the end of five years are generally described as cured, though cancer can and does recur in the following years. Despite a lack of evidence indicating a decrease in the over-all mortality rate from cancer, progress is being made toward the solution of the problem of cancer. Dr. Heller, as director of the National Cancer Institute, summarized in *Progress Against Cancer 1959*[11] some of the achievements of the last ten years. They include (1) a steady increase in basic knowledge of the nature of cancer, (2) synthesis of knowledge derived from many fields, so that the whole field of cancer research is being unified, (3) advances in knowledge of chemotherapy and virology, (4) the cytological test for cancer of the cervix, and (5) a comprehensive body of knowledge of the epidemiology of cancer.

Two developments of the last 10 to 15 years have a direct bearing on the practice of nursing. They are the use of extensive surgical procedures in treatment of cancer and an increase of interest in, and facilities for the care of, the patient who has widespread and progressive disease. Both of these will be discussed later in this chapter.

How do growth processes differ in neoplastic and healthy cells?

Although the answer in the past has been that the differences are not known, new techniques are making it possible for scientists to obtain information never before known. Possibly by the time this material is published a great deal will be known. Characteristics of the behavior of healthy and neoplastic cells can be obtained by radioautography.[12] From studies on human as well as mouse gastrointestinal mucosa, it has been learned that the speed at which cell division occurs in healthy and neoplastic tissues does not explain the accumulation of cells in a neoplasm. As a matter of fact, the rate of cell division may be slower in some neoplasms than it is in healthy tissues. One of the important elements, however, is that instead of but one cell, each of the two formed by the division of a parent cell goes on to divide again, thus doubling the number of cells. Neoplastic cells differ from healthy cells in their structure and behavior, and they continue their abnormal characteristics in succeeding generations. Neoplastic cells behave as if they were mutants with an impaired sensitivity to the organizing influence of adjacent cells. They disregard the normal regulators of growth; they often continue to multiply without limit or regard for the needs of the organism as a whole, and not infrequently at the expense of healthy cells. The extent to which neoplastic cells differ from healthy cells varies. The structure and organization of cells in a neoplasm may be similar in many respects to that of healthy tissue, or they may be so different that there is little or no resemblance to normal tissue. For example, in glandular structures, goblet epithelial cells are arranged in an orderly fashion around the ducts. In some neoplasms, this pattern may be

[11] *Progress Against Cancer 1959,* U.S. Department of Health, Education, and Welfare, Public Health Service, National Institute of Cancer, January, 1960.
[12] Baserga and Kisieleski, *Op. cit.,* pp. 107-10.

disturbed, but still recognizable. In others, the pattern of organization and the character of cells are so abnormal that most, if not all, resemblance to normal tissue is lost.

Another important characteristic of neoplasms is that they serve no useful purpose. Some neoplasms arising in glands do produce the secretion of the gland, but this usually results in an excess of the secretion. Neoplasms arising in endocrine glands are frequently, though not always, functional. For example, neoplasms in the thyroid gland may secrete the hormones of the thyroid gland thus causing symptoms and signs of hyperthyroidism.

Neoplasms, like other living organisms, require nutrient materials for their growth and survival. They are dependent on the host for their food supply. They grow without regard to the needs of the host and frequently at his expense. Slow-growing neoplasms may exist for extended periods of time without interfering with the nutrition of the host. Rapidly growing ones are likely to be accompanied by severe emaciation and debility of the host. Neoplasms in the alimentary canal may further interfere with nutrition by their mechanical effect. The maintenance of nutrition is one of the common problems in the care of patients with certain types of neoplasms.

As indicated previously, neoplasms are of two different types, benign and malignant. Further, malignant neoplasms are of two general types. Neoplasms arising in tissues having their origin in the ectoderm or entoderm of the embryo are called carcinomas. In terms of mature tissues, a carcinoma has its origin in epithelial tissue. Malignant neoplasms having their origin in tissues that are formed from the mesoderm, or mesenchyme, are known as sarcomas. When the origin of a neoplasm is uncertain, this system of naming may not be very helpful, however. For example, although a melanoma is usually classified as a neoplasm involving the skin (epithelial tissue), it is actually a sarcoma.

For the most part, the system for naming neoplasms is relatively simple. The suffix *-oma* is derived from the Greek and is used to denote a tumor or neoplasm. Benign neoplasms are usually classified as to site of origin. In a few instances, the term for the type of cell is used. In general, the word is formed by adding *-oma* to the combining form, indicating the type of tissue. To illustrate, a benign neoplasm of fibrous tissue is a fibroma. There are some exceptions. Gliomas, which have their origin in the neuroglia, are almost always, if not always, malignant. Malignant neoplasms are also commonly classified as to site of origin. For the purpose of illustration, a brief classification of neoplasms follows. For anyone wishing to examine a complete list, the *International Classification of Diseases*[13] is suggested.

When more than one tissue enters into the formation of a neoplasm, the combining forms for each type are used. For example, the so-called fibroid tumor of the uterus is actually a *leiomyofibroma*, since it contains smooth muscle and fibrous connective tissue.

Many terms are used to describe the character of the neoplasm. The term

[13] *International Classification of Diseases,* U.S. Department of Health, Education, and Welfare, Public Health Service, 1959, pp. 23-40.

Type of Tissue	Type of Neoplasm	
	Benign	Malignant
Connective tissue		
1. Fibrous	Fibroma	Fibrosarcoma
2. Cartilage (chondroblast)	Chondroma	Chrondrosarcoma
3. Bone (osteoblast)	Osteoma	Osteogenic sarcoma
4. Fat (lipoid tissue)	Lipoma	Liposarcoma
Muscle tissue		
1. Smooth muscle	Leiomyoma	Leomyosarcoma
2. Striated muscle	Rhabdomyoma	Rhabdomyosarcoma
Epithelial tissue		
1. Squamous cells	Papilloma or wart	Epithelioma
	Epidermoid cyst	
	Sebaceous cyst	
2. Basal cell	Little adenoma or sweat gland adenoma	Basal cell carcinoma
3. Pigmented layer.	Mole or nevus	Melanoepithelioma or melanoma
4. Gland cells (adeno-)	Adenoma	Adenocarcinoma
Nervous tissue		
1. Nerve tissue	Neuroma	Neurosarcoma
2. Glia		Glioma
3. Meninges	Meningioma	Malignant meningioma
4. Nerve sheath	Neurofibroma	Malignant neurofibroma
Endothelial tissue		
1. Blood vessels	Hemangioma	Hemangioendothelioma
Lymphatic and hematopoietic tissue		Hodgkin's disease
		Leukemia
		Lymphoma
		Lymphosarcoma
Mixed tumors		
Tumors derived from embryonic cells well differentiated	Dermoid cysts	
	Teratoma	Malignant teratoma of the testis

"polyp" or "polypoid" is used to indicate that a neoplasm extends from a mucous membrane into the lumen of a tube. Some polyps have a stem or stalk similar to a cherry. The stalk is called a peduncle and the polyp is said to be pedunculated. Other polyps are attached to the surface by a broad base. The term used to indicate this characteristic is sessile. Some neoplasms grow around the wall of tubular organs, that is, they are annular growths. Annular neoplasms tend to obstruct the tube by constricting or reducing the size of its lumen. Some neoplasms stimulate the production of large amounts of fibrous connective tissue which causes the neoplasm to be firm or hard. A firm, hard neoplasm containing a large quantity of connective tissue is called a scirrhus. There are, of course, many other terms that are used in the description of neoplasms. Satisfactory definitions can usually be found in a medical dictionary.

How do benign and malignant neoplasms differ?

The following represents a number of important characteristics in which benign and malignant neoplasms differ.

FIGURE 12–1

A Comparison of Selected Characteristics of Benign and Malignant Neoplasms

Characteristic	Benign	Malignant
1. Capsule	Usually	Rarely
2. Manner of growth	Expansive	Infiltrative
3. Rate of growth	Usually slow and restricted; extent limited	Rapid and unrestricted; varies greatly from patient to patient
4. Tendency to recur after removal	Rarely	Frequently
5. Characteristic of cells	Fairly normal	Varying degrees of abnormality; immature and abnormal in appearance and organization
6. Mitotic activity	Little	Usually great; mitosis is abnormal
7. Metastasis	Never	Usually
8. Vascularity	Slight	Moderate to marked

The following discussion elaborates on the characteristics outlined in Figure 12-1. The capsule enclosing a neoplasm is formed of fibrous connective tissue as a result of the local tissue reaction to the abnormal growth of cells. Occasionally the cells inside an encapsulated neoplasm are found to be malignant, but this is a rare occurrence. It is not known whether the connective-tissue capsule has its origin in the connective tissue of the organ in which the tissue has arisen or whether it arises from the tumor itself. From the comparison of the capsule characteristics in the figure, it is obvious why benign neoplasms are usually accompanied by a better prognosis than are malignant neoplasms. The capsule tends to confine the neoplastic cells, and the removal of an encapsulated neoplasm is not only easier, but it causes less damage to healthy tissue. Since encapsulated neoplasms grow by expansion rather than by infiltration, their principal effect is pressure. Though some benign neoplasms grow to enormous size, their growth is usually limited. Ovarian cysts occasionally reach great size. Benign neoplasms do not spread to distant parts of the body, and, with rare exceptions, they do not recur. Though some benign neoplasms eventually become malignant, this does not occur very frequently. Few, if any, persons escape having one or more benign neoplasms during their lifetime; most of them are of no significance. One interesting fact is that, according to the U.S. National Health Survey,[14] more patients are hospitalized for the treatment of benign and unspecified neoplasms than for malignant neoplasms.

[14] "Hospitalization," Series B-7, 1958, p. 23.

Because of their manner and rate of growth, malignant neoplasms, as the term implies, will cause death. Some malignant neoplasms, but not all, can be eradicated by present methods of treatment. Furthermore, not all malignant neoplasms behave alike. Some types may be present for many years and never cause any known ill effect. Others are so rapidly progressive that despite what appeared to be prompt diagnosis and treatment, death occurs only a few weeks after their presence becomes known. The differences in the behavior of malignant neoplasms are well illustrated by the different types of cancer occurring in the skin. Three types have been identified. They are: basal cell carcinoma, which tends to remain localized; squamous cell carcinoma, which spreads through the lymphatics to the lymph nodes; and malignant melanoma, which has usually produced systemic disease by the time it is identified. Of the three, basal cell carcinoma seldom causes death, whereas the malignant melanoma is highly deadly.

As commented on previously, malignant neoplasms are seldom encapsulated, with the result that they tend to infiltrate or invade the surrounding tissue as they grow. Despite differences in the rate at which malignant neoplasms grow, the rate of growth is comparatively rapid. Growth usually continues whether or not tissues of the rest of the body are adequately nourished.

Although the cells in some malignant neoplasms are fairly normal in appearance and in organization, they may be so abnormal and immature that there is little or no resemblance to healthy tissues. Cells differ from healthy cells in size, shape, and staining characteristics. Whereas healthy cells are similar in size and shape, neoplastic cells may demonstrate great variability. In normal mitosis, each parent cell divides into two daughter cells, but in tissues taken from a malignant neoplasm, cells can sometimes be seen to be dividing into a number of cells, for example, three, four, or six. Some cells may split by simple fission rather than by mitosis.

Another important characteristic of malignant neoplasms is that instead of being confined to the area where they originate, they tend to disseminate throughout the body, or to metastasize. The studies with tritiated thymidine[15] have also provided some information about the process of metastasis.[16] A single cell or a small group of cells separate from the parent cell and are transported by way of the lymph and blood streams to distant parts of the body. When the cells survive and lodge in a site favorable for their growth, they multiply. The new growth is not detectable, however, until it reaches a size of about 1 cm in diameter, at which time it contains about 500 million cells. The time taken to produce a detectable tumor will depend on the length of the reproductive cycle for the neoplastic cell. If it is ten days, it will take ten months for the original cell to grow into a nodule 1 cm in diameter. If the cycle is 30 days, it will take almost three years for a detectable nodule to develop. This explains why it may take months or even years for a metastatic neoplasm to appear after a surgeon removes a primary growth.

---

[15] Thymidine labeled with tritum, that is, radioactive hydrogen.
[16] Baserga and Kisieleski, *Op. cit.,* p. 110.

The tendency to metastasize varies with the type of cancer and among individuals. When the surrounding tissues recognize the growth as abnormal and considerable amounts of fibrous tissue are formed, it can act as a barrier to spread. In other instances, however, the cancer cells[17] proliferate and overcome the local barriers to spread; they infiltrate or invade the surrounding tissue, and eventually, if left to itself, the malignant neoplasm can be expected to spread to the regional lymph nodes and, via the lymph or blood vessels, to distant points, where it sets up secondary or metastatic growths. Metastasis is now known to take place as easily by way of the blood vessels as through the lymphatics. Because cancer cells have a tendency to separate from the parent growth, large numbers of malignant cells may be found in the venous blood draining the neoplasm. Moreover, the size of the neoplasm bears no relationship to the earliness with which it metastasizes. Extensive metastasis may be found in a patient with a small neoplasm and none in a patient with a large one. In some instances, the primary growth has an inhibiting effect on metastatic lesions. Following the removal of the primary growth, the rate of growth of the metastasis is accelerated.[18] The opposite is also seen; that is, with removal of the primary lesion, metastasic lesions regress.

In addition to the tendency of malignant neoplasms to metastasize, their sites of metastasis may also metastasize. Though the tendency to metastasize is inherent in all malignant neoplasms, whether or not it takes place depends on the individual and the site of origin. For reasons not understood, malignant neoplasms may spread early in one person and late in others.

Certain organs seem to be preferred as sites for metastasis. This suggests that cancer cells are blood-borne and that conditions at the site of metastasis favor growth. Injury to tissue appears to predispose the tissue, or make it more susceptible, to metastasis. The four most common sites of metastasis are the lung, the liver, the bone, and the brain. Cancer in the liver, prostate, and breast metastasizes to the lung; that in the colon, stomach, pancreas, and lung, to the liver; that in the thyroid, prostate, kidney, breast, and lung, to bone; and that in the breast, lung, and kidney, to the brain. From the above, the reader can note that neoplasms in some organs metastasize to a number of organs. For example, cancer in the breast metastasizes to the lung, bone, and brain. The sites of metastasis are summarized in Figure 12-2

All the factors enabling neoplasm to metastasize are not known. One factor, however, is the invasiveness of cells of the neoplasm, or their power to overcome the local barriers to spread. Another is the tendency of malignant cells to separate from the parent growth. The routes by which neoplastic cells are spread throughout the body are the same as those by which any substance can be transported from one part of the body to another. Various terms are employed to indicate the mechanism of spread. Local spread of malignant

[17] The term "cancer," which is also the name of the fourth sign of the zodiac, means crab. The use of the term "cancer" to describe malignant neoplasms is based on the supposed resemblance between a crab and the manner in which the neoplasm invades the surrounding tissue.

[18] Crile, *Op. cit.,* p. 361.

FIGURE 12 – 2

Sites of Metastasis According to The Organs From Which They Most
Frequently Originate

Site of Metastasis	Organs From Which Metastasis Originates								
	Breast	Colon	Kidney	Liver	Lung	Pan-creas	Pros-tate	Stom-ach	Thy-roid
Bone	√		√		√		√		√
Brain	√		√		√				
Liver		√			√	√		√	
Lung	√				√		√		

neoplasms is known as metastasis by the infiltration or invasion of surrounding tissue. When neoplastic cells penetrate and enter blood and lymphatic vessels, and they may grow along the course of the vessel, metastasis is said to take place by lymphatic or vascular permeation. When cells or groups of cells separate from the primary growth and are carried in the blood or lymph to distant points, metastasis is, logically enough, said to be by lymphatic or vascular emboli. During surgery for the removal of a malignant neoplasm, cells may be carried from the original site and be implanted in another area, including the incision. Metastasis is, therefore, by implantation. Cancer of the stomach sometimes metastasizes by sedimentation. For example, cells extending through the wall of the stomach separate from the parent growth and settle on an organ such as an ovary in the abdominal cavity where, if conditions are favorable, they set up a secondary growth.

As has been emphasized, a characteristic feature of malignant growth is its tendency to metastasize, or to set up secondary growths at points distant from the primary site. Some tissues appear to provide conditions that are more favorable to metastasis than do others. Injury to tissue favors metastasis. The routes by which neoplasms spread are, as is to be expected, those by which materials are distributed throughout the body.

No discussion of the characteristics of malignant neoplasms would be complete without a comment about the tendency of malignant neoplasms to recur. As with other characteristics, the likelihood of recurrence varies considerably for different types of malignant neoplasms and from one person to another.

A recently introduced concept to explain the behavior of malignant neoplasms is that of "biological predeterminism." By this term is meant that the course and behavior, or natural history, of a cancer is determined at the time of its inception. A slow-growing neoplasm with little power of invasion can be expected to retain these characteristics, while a rapidly growing and/or highly invasive neoplasm has the potential for rapid growth and invasiveness from the start. The earlier cited example of the different types of malignant neoplasms of the skin illustrates the concept of "biological predeterminism" exceptionally well. (See page 932.)

A point that must be emphasized about malignant neoplasms is that, despite their general characteristics, there is great variability in their behavior in different individuals. For example, cancer cells are found in the prostate without any evidence of invasion to surrounding tissue or spread to distant parts. The fact of their presence may have been unknown to the patient or the attending physician until after death, when the prostate is examined at autopsy. Other neoplasms, such as malignant melanomas, are highly malignant from the start. Despite a small primary lesion, malignant cells may be distributed throughout the body before the primary lesion is known to be active. What appears to be the same type of lesion also behaves differently in different individuals. There is a growing appreciation that each person who has cancer is an individual and that the way in which the disease behaves in each person is also unique.

To illustrate differences in the course of malignant neoplasms in two different people, Mr. Bernard and Mr. Lester will be described. Mr. Bernard, who died last week, had always been a healthy and active man. Five weeks before his death, he complained of feeling ill. When, after a week or so, he continued to feel weak and tired, he consulted his physician who, after appropriate studies, made a diagnosis of acute leukemia. Mr. Bernard did not respond to any of the therapeutic measures and he failed rapidly.

Mr. Lester lives across town from Mr. Bernard. Eight years ago, he was found to have chronic leukemia. Unlike Mr. Bernard, he has responded well to therapy. Although he seldom feels entirely well, he has been able to continue his employment as an accountant and to support himself and his family. Recently he has not been feeling as well as he did in the past, however. How long he will be able to work is a matter for conjecture. Although many elements in the lives of Mr. Bernard and Mr. Lester are similar, the manifestations of leukemia have been quite different.

What are some of the factors in the etiology of cancer?

As in most other chronic diseases, knowledge of the factors in the etiology of cancer is incomplete. Similarly, they can be classified under the general headings of susceptible host, injuring or carcinogenic agents, and the elements in the environment bringing the host and agent together. The concept of necessary and sufficient cause probably applies to some cancers. In the etiology of cancer, no single element is known to be required for its development. Whatever the factors are in the etiology of cancer, they must be of sufficient degree to initiate malignant change and to allow the abnormal growth to continue. The differences in susceptibility of various individuals to the effect of smoking cigarettes appears to illustrate the concept of sufficient causation. Not all individuals who smoke cigarettes develop bronchogenic carcinoma; a few who do not smoke develop it. The length and intensity of exposure are both elements, however, as the incidence of bronchogenic carcinoma rises with the length of time the individual has smoked and as the number of cigarettes smoked increases. Individual susceptibility varies, but bronchogenic carcinoma develops when the injury to the cells is sufficient to overcome the protective mechanisms of the individual. In many cancers multiple factors probably interact to cause the disease.

What is known about host susceptibility?

Among elements presumed to affect the susceptibility of the host are genetic constitution, age, hormone balance, immunity, nutritional status, and precancerous lesions. Data on the possibility that heredity is a factor in cancer are derived from several sources: the occurrence of certain types of cancer among close relatives, so-called cancer families, and the development of cancer strains of experimental animals.

Accurate knowledge of the genetic factors in cancer among human beings is difficult to obtain. Persons who are predisposed to cancer may die from some other cause, before the disease develops. For many reasons, information gained about disease and cause of death among family members tends to be unreliable. Persons may not know what caused the death of members of preceding generations. Some persons withhold information about family members who have had cancer because they believe it is caused by venereal disease or results from an activity that is unclean or sinful. There are undoubtedly a variety of reasons for the unreliability of data reported by persons relative to a history of cancer in the family.

Genetic factors appear to influence the development of cancer either by the effect of a specific gene or as a consequence of the genetic constitution of the individual. Neoplasms for which there is known to be a familial tendency are relatively rare. They include von Recklinghausen's neurofibromatosis, multiple polyposes of the colon, osteochondroma, and pheochromocytoma. There are a few lesions that are not of themselves malignant, but they undergo malignant degeneration when they are exposed to specific conditions. As an example, xeroderma pigmentosa is hereditary, but neoplastic change is dependent on exposure of the skin to sunlight. Besides the disorders in which evidence of genetic factors is reasonably clear, there are studies indicating that a tendency to cancer of the breast is inherited. The transmission of the tendency to cancer of the breast is not consistent enough, however, to make accurate predictions possible. Although a number of cancer families have been identified, the extent to which genetic factors are responsible is not known.

Heredity may predispose to cancer, not by a specific gene or genes, but by the effect of the genetic constitution of the individual. In keeping with this concept, susceptibility to or protection from cancer depends on the effects of these genes on bodily processes. As one example, mutant or abnormal cells are known to be formed by persons who do not develop cancer as well as by those who do. Heredity may be a factor in the efficiency of defense mechanisms against abnormal cells. Theoretically, at least, the genetic constitution of an individual may alter the manner in which his cells respond to or metabolize potentially carcinogenic agents. In one individual the product of the metabolism of a carcinogen may be harmless and in another it may be harmful. Another possibility lies in the ease with which the cells of an individual throw off the restraints on growth. In the vast majority of persons heredity is only one of a number of factors interacting to protect the person from, or to predispose him to, neoplasia. Whether or not a given individual develops cancer depends on the net result of all these factors

Other evidence implicating heredity as a factor in the etiology of cancer is that the neoplasia is universal in nature. Strains of experimental animals, such as mice, have been developed that demonstrate a high degree of susceptibility not only to cancer, but to cancer in certain sites. Even among these animals, in some instances the tendency to the disease requires additional etiological agents to ensure its development. In studies with strains of mice inbred to develop spontaneous tumors of the breast, multiple factors are required for the mice to develop mammary cancers with any degree of consistency. Bittner[19] found three factors to be necessary—hereditary susceptibility, the female hormones required for the growth and development of mammary tissue, and the milk factor. The milk factor is a filtrable substance that is transmitted in the milk and is generally thought to be a virus.

Despite a growing body of knowledge about heredity as a factor in the development of cancer, exact information about how it influences its development is far from clear. For most individuals, their genetic constitution is presumed to protect them from, or to predispose them to, not only cancer, but other diseases. In most instances, additional factors are undoubtedly involved.

Why are hormones believed to be a factor in carcinogenesis?

Hormones have long been suspected of influencing susceptibility to cancer. In 1889, Schinzinger[20] suggested that hormones might be important in the development of cancer of the breast in women. In 1919, Loeb[21] demonstrated that the incidence of cancer of the breast in cancer-susceptible strains of mice could be reduced by removing their ovaries. That cancer of the breast is extremely rare in males and is the leading cause of death from cancer in the female is well known. The exact role of hormones in the induction of cancer is not clear. Knowledge is not available as to whether hormones act as inciting agents or whether they prepare the tissue so that it responds to carcinogenic agents. The hormones found to be carcinogenic in animals are those that have

[19] J. J. Bittner, "The Causes and Control of Mammary Cancer in Mice," *Harvey Lecture,* XLII, 1946-47, p. 221.
[20] James D. Hardy, *Pathophysiology in Surgery,* Williams and Wilkins Co., Baltimore, 1958, p. 169.
[21] *Ibid.,* p. 170.

an influence on the growth of certain tissues. Hormones from the ovaries, testes, and adrenal cortex have been shown to be necessary to the growth of some cancers; that is, the cancers are hormone-dependent.[22] In addition to promoting growth of specific tissues, these hormones are all steroids and their chemical structure is similar to that of the carcinogenic hydrocarbons. The significance of these relationships is not known. That a relationship exists between certain hormones and the development of cancer is supported by animal experiments. Cancer of the breast has been induced in male mice of susceptible strains by the prolonged administration of excessive dosages of female hormones. Some cancers have been induced in animals by upsetting hormonal balance. From the knowledge that is presently available, certain hormones are necessary to the growth of some cancers. Other hormones inhibit for a time the growth of some cancers. After a time, a neoplasm whose growth is inhibited by a hormone adapts to its presence, and it is no longer restrained by it. From this and other evidence, hormones appear to be one of the multiple factors entering into the genesis of cancer.

What are some of the other factors influencing susceptibility to cancer?

Authorities disagree as to the influence of age on susceptibility to cancer. Some interpret the fact that the incidence of cancer increases with age as evidence that age influences susceptibility, while others do not. According to Homburger,[23] evidence obtained from work with experimental animals is contradictory. In general these studies have indicated that younger tissues are more susceptible to carcinogenic agents than are older ones. The age at which the peak incidence for cancer in various sites occurs differs. Although some of these are benign rather than malignant, some types of new growths, such as Wilms's tumors of the kidney, teratomas, neuroblastomas, neurofibromas, chrondromas, hemagiomas, and nevi, are often congenital; that is, infants are born with them. Leukemia, which was once presumed to have its highest incidence in young children, actually occurs more frequently in adults than it does in children, and the rate is increasing.[24] In children, leukemia is more likely to be more acute and the course shorter than in adults.

Certain lesions in the body appear to increase host susceptibility to cancer. The presence of one neoplasm increases the likelihood of developing another. The person who develops cancer in one tissue is more likely to develop another one than is the person who has never had a cancerous lesion. Another type of lesion, the so-called precancerous lesion, may also predispose to cancer. These are lesions which at their inception are not cancerous, but which tend to undergo malignant degeneration. Among the more common

[22] *Ibid.*, p. 170.
Inc., New York, 1957, p. 19.
[23] Freddy Homburger, *The Biologic Basis of Cancer Management*, Paul B. Hoeber,
[24] *1964 Cancer Facts and Figures, Op. cit.*, p. 23.

precancerous lesions are: (1) polyps in the large intestine and stomach, (2) large burn scars, particularly those resulting from third-degree burns, (3) nevi—especially moles near the juncture of the two sides of (midline) the body, (4) senile keratosis—a disease of the epidermis involving the horny layer, and (5) leukoplakia—a disorder characterized by the development of a white patch or patches on the buccal mucosa inside the cheek or on the female vulva.

On the basis of several different types of observations, there has been recurring interest in the role of immunity in cancer. Not all persons require the same degree of exposure to carcinogenic agents to develop cancer. Among those who do there is definitely a host response. Spontaneous regression occurs in 1 of 100,000 cases. Some persons have a desmoplastic, that is, fibrous tissue, reaction. Among others, the disease is manifested by rapid growth and spread. Mutant cells developing in healthy persons are rapidly destroyed. Whether or not each of the above represents immunity or an immune response is not clearly established.

The incidence of some sites of cancer is influenced or determined by sex. As examples, cancer of the breast is common among women, but occurs rarely among men. Cancer of the stomach and lung is more common among men than among women. Not all the reasons for sex differences are known.

What are some of the carcinogenic agents?

In addition to host susceptibility, a variety of chemical, physical, and living agents are associated with neoplasia. According to *Cancer Facts and Figures for 1961,*[25] more than 400 substances have been identified that are carcinogenic; that is, they induce malignant change in cells when applied to tissue for a sufficient period of time. No one knows how carcinogenic agents act. They may overstimulate the cell or release it from the inhibiting influence of growth regulators. Not all persons who are exposed to carcinogenic agents develop cancer. Knowledge of carcinogenic agents is important, however, for many are subject to control. The chances of developing cancer in certain sites can be lessened by reducing or eliminating contact with carcinogenic agents.

Carcinogenic chemicals include a great variety of organic and inorganic substances. Some of them contaminate the air in industrial and urban areas. Among the organic chemicals are aromatic compounds such as tar, soot, asphalt, crude paraffin oil, lubricating and fuel oils, as well as aromatic amines such as benzine and aniline dyes. Inorganic chemicals include nickel, asbestos, and arsenicals.

Physical carcinogens include heat rays, ultraviolet light, and ionizing rays and particles.

Living agents implicated as carcinogens include viruses and *Schistosoma haematobium.*

[25] *Cancer Facts and Figures for 1961, Op. cit.*

Why do the habits and customs of a people influence the incidence of cancer in the group?

Because habits and customs of a people determine to a large extent the carcinogens to which they are likely to be exposed, they are important elements in carcinogenesis. Some of these habits and customs may seem strange because they are unfamiliar. All people, including Americans, have some customs and habits that result in their exposure to carcinogens. From many examples that could be cited, only a few have been selected. In England, the incidence of cancer of the scrotum, which was common among chimney sweeps in the nineteenth century, was reduced by teaching the men to bathe frequently. This form of cancer is absent among similar workers in Japan because they practice meticulous cleanliness.[26] In Kashmir, mountaineers carry charcoal-burning stoves under their cloaks to keep themselves warm. The stoves are supported on the upper areas of the abdomen. Consequently, burns of the abdomen and chest are frequent. There is a high incidence of cancer in the burn scars. Cancer of the cheek is frequent in those who chew betel nuts. Cancer of the lip is more frequent among pipe smokers than among nonpipe smokers. More than 25 scientific studies in ten countries have demonstrated a high degree of relationship between the smoking of cigarettes and the risk of developing cancer.[27] The incidence of cancer of the lung is higher among those who smoke cigarettes than among those who do not. There is also a direct correlation between the number of cigarettes smoked and the risk of developing cancer. In a report in which the mortality experience of nearly 200,000 policy holders of United States government life insurance is summarized, Dorn[28] states that the death rate from cancer of the lung for men who smoke is ten times that for nonsmokers. Men who smoke more than one pack of cigarettes a day have a death rate 16 times that of nonsmokers.

Hammond[29] reports that in the United States between the years of 1935–1960 the standardized death rate[30] from lung cancer increased 600 per cent in men and 125 per cent in women. For the past few years cancer of the lung has been the principal form of cancer causing death in men. Hammond offers several explanations for the differences in incidence between men and women. From his studies he learned that men are more likely than women to inhale cigarette smoke. Women over the age of 40 smoke far fewer cigarettes than do men of the same age. Further, most men who are over 50 and who smoke, started smoking before the age of 20. In contrast, women of the same age averaged over 35 years of age when they started to smoke. The three differ-

26 Homburger, *Op. cit.,* p. 11.

27 American Cancer Society, *Cigarette Smoking and Cancer,* American Cancer Society, Inc., New York, 1963.

28 Harold F. Dorn, "Tobacco Consumption and Mortality from Cancer and Other Diseases," *Public Health Reports,* LXXIV, July, 1959, p. 593.

29 Hammond, *Op. cit.,* p. 40.

30 The term "standardized death rate" means that the death rate has been adjusted for age differences in the composition of the population.

ences in the habit of smoking can be summarized briefly as: men inhale more than women, they smoke more cigarettes, and they start earlier in life. Similar to other investigators, Hammond reported that among men who do and do not smoke there are also significant differences. The total death rate among men who smoke regularly is far higher than among men who do not smoke at all. Men who smoke a pipe or cigars have only a slightly higher death rate than do men who do not smoke. Further, the death rate rises progressively with an increase in the number of cigarettes smoked and falls when men who have smoked discontinue smoking. The difference increases with the passage of time after smoking has stopped. Other environmental factors may contribute to the rise in the incidence of cancer of the lung. They are the exhaust fumes from automobiles and trucks, the smoke from furnaces, dust from asphalt pavements, and dust from tires of automobiles and trucks.

Practices by certain groups may alter the incidence of cancer. As an example, cancer of the penis has a low incidence in Jewish and Moslem men. This is believed to be due to the practice of early circumcision.

Cancer of the skin is more common in persons whose skin is exposed to the rays of the sun, such as farmers and sailors, than it is among indoor workers. Exposure to the rays of the sun probably accounts for the observation that cancer of the skin is more common among persons living in the southern than in the northern part of the United States.

Those who live in cities and industrial areas of the United States have a higher incidence of cancer than those who live in rural areas. Among the factors presumed to contribute to this difference is that those who live in cities are exposed to an atmosphere contaminated by smoke and automobile exhaust gases. From these examples, the conclusion that customs and habits are a factor in cancer appears valid, for they determine to some extent the carcinogens to which the individual is exposed and the degree of exposure.

Certain occupations also increase the likelihood of exposure to chemical and physical carcinogens. A large number of chemical agents of organic and inorganic origin have been implicated as carcinogens. Included among organic chemicals that have been demonstrated to be carcinogenic in animals are the carcinogenic hydrocarbons found in tar and soot. The aromatic amines and benzol as well as many other chemicals are potentially carcinogenic. Among the inorganic chemicals with carcinogenic powers are the arsenicals, chromates, nickel, and asbestos. Many of these chemicals are either used in industrial processes or are products or by-products of these processes. Knowledge of the carcinogenic potential of chemicals is essential to the protection of workers and the members of the community. Protection involves the development of effective procedures for eliminating or minimizing contact and a program to educate workers to use them.

A number of physical agents are known to be carcinogenic. The effect of long-continued exposure to ultraviolet light or to the rays of the sun has already been mentioned. Ionizing radiation, whether produced by X ray or from natural or artificially produced radioactive isotopes, is of increasing significance. The increased use of ionizing radiation in hospitals, in industry, and in national defense increases the amount of and the number of opportunities for exposure. Leavell and Clark[31] emphasize the detrimental effects of increased exposure to ionizing radiation through the following example. Leukemia is four times more frequent among general physicians and ten times more frequent among radiologists than it is among the members of a comparable group in the general population. The incidence of leukemia is also rising and possibly some of the increase is due to an increase in ionizing radiation in the atmosphere.

The role of physical or mechanical injury of the tissues in carcinogenesis has been a subject for debate. The possibility of a single injury being a causative factor in cancer is believed to be remote. When a neoplasm is found following an injury, the probability is that it was there at the time the injury occurred and the injury served to call the attention of the person to it. Following tissue injury, the rate of growth of a neoplasm is sometimes accelerated. This occurs frequently enough that some lay people are aware of the possibility. Some authorities discount the importance of chronic mechanical irritation as a significant etiological factor in cancer. Others regard the fact that cancer develops in old burn scars and in cells forming the walls of draining sinuses as evidence supporting chronic irritation as an etiological agent.

Living agents may also act as etiological agents. Leukoplakia is sometimes, though not always, associated with syphilis. Cancer of the liver is more common in those parts of the world where a type of flat worm, the liver fluke, is ingested in the drinking water. The fluke invades the liver, where it sets up housekeeping.

Of the possible causative agents in cancer none is of greater interest than the possible role of viruses. Interest in the virus as an etiological agent in cancer is not new, for at least 50 years ago Rous demonstrated that a virus caused sarcoma of the breast in chickens. Until recently, however, there was no evidence that a virus acted as a carcinogenic agent in any species except birds and fowl. Since Bittner's discovery in 1936 that the milk factor was a necessary condition to the development of cancer of the breast in mice, a number of neoplastic diseases in animals have been shown to be of virus origin. Included among these are leukemia in mice and papillomatosis in rabbits. Warts and papillomas in man, though nonmalignant growths, are of virus origin. To date no virus has been found in a human malignant neoplasm; until recently this fact has been taken as positive evidence against the virus as an initiating factor in cancer in human beings. In a report on *The Research Program of the American Cancer Society, 1963* (p. 15) the opposite point of view is taken in the following statement: "Cancer-causing viruses have been detected in chickens, frogs, mice, rats, rabbits, hamsters, deer, monkeys, even willow trees. Why not human beings?"

[31] Hugh Rodman Leavell and E. Gurney Clark, *Preventive Medicine for the Doctor in His Community,* Blakiston Division, McGraw-Hill Book Co., New York, 1958, p. 263.

There is a growing body of scientific evidence indicating that a virus or viruses may be the principal cause of leukemia in human beings. Interest in the virus as a causative factor in leukemia has been stimulated by the occurrence of clusters of individuals ill with leukemia in a number of communities. One such instance occurred in Niles, Illinois, where 13 individuals were discovered concentrated in one area; this number is many times the expected incidence.[32]

Even if a virus proves to be a factor in some or all cancers, there is no evidence to suggest that cancer is contagious in the ordinary sense of the word. It is not disseminated in the same manner as measles, chickenpox, or the common cold. It is not transmitted by the blood, as healthy men have been transfused with blood from patients with leukemia without subsequently becoming ill. Mothers with leukemia have healthy babies. Neither a physician nor a nurse has ever been known to develop leukemia after caring for a patient with it.

Despite the possibility that viruses are a factor in the development of some cancers, a number of factors contribute to the difficulty in identifying their presence in tissues even when they are there. Homburger[33] states that there is much evidence to indicate that viruses can be present in the tissues in the absence of morphological evidence that they are there. They are apparently able to assume a latent form and to resume their virulent characteristics when conditions are favorable. In recently reported studies, cells transformed by certain cancer viruses, such as the Rous sarcoma virus, appeared to be able to transmit the genetic material of the virus from one generation of tumor cells to another without producing the virus in the infectious form. For the infectious form to appear, the tumor cells had to be subjected to special conditions.[34] The recent discovery that some viruses that infect animals enter into the genetic DNA is also of more than passing interest.

To summarize, two factors are involved in the development of cancer. One is a susceptible host. The other is an agent or group of agents that are capable of injuring the cell. Except in those rare instances in which cancer appears to result from the action of a specific gene, the induction of cancer depends on the action of multiple factors. In the last ten years or so, knowledge of the epidemiology of cancer has been expanded significantly. Epidemiological studies are directed toward the identification not only of carcinogenic agents and of the characteristics of individuals who develop cancer, but of the characteristics of those who do not. Present evidence points to the conclusion that cancer does not have a single cause and is not really a single disease, but that it is the result of the interaction of multiple factors, some of which have their origin in the host and others in his environment.

[32] *Facts About Leukemia,* American Cancer Society, Inc., New York, April, 1963.
[33] Homburger, *Op. cit.,* p. 78.
[34] "Link Viral Genes to Cancer," *Public Health Reports,* LXXVIII, July, 1963, p. 568.

With what other type of disease can cancer be compared to emphasize its natural history?

To emphasize the natural history of cancer, its course has been compared to that of an infection. Although there are significant differences, the course of cancer has many aspects in common with infectious disease. They both involve a susceptible host, injuring agents, and conditions in the environment bringing the two together. The degree to which host susceptibility and the pathogenecity of inciting agents are significant factors in etiology differs among infectious diseases as well as neoplastic ones. In some infectious diseases, such as measles, the nature of susceptibility is largely a matter of the presence or absence of immune bodies. To date, evidence that immunity plays a significant role in cancer is not clear-cut. Because of the scientific interest in this field, answers may be found to questions about it. In infections such as tuberculosis, factors other than immunity affect susceptibility. This is probably also true in cancer. In neither tuberculosis nor malignant neoplasms are all the factors in etiology understood.

In infection, the causative agent has its origin in the external environment and is a necessary condition of disease; a microorganism is the inciting agent. In cancer, the relationship of the injuring agent to the development of the disease is not as clear and possibly not as direct as in infection. The injuring agent may have its origin in the internal environment as well as in the external environment. It may serve as an inciting or a promoting agent. An inciting agent is one that induces changes in the cell that result in cancer. A promoting agent acts to support or favor cellular growth after cancerous change has taken place.

In both infectious and neoplastic disease a period of time elapses between the moment a microorganism enters the body or a cell is injured and the development of overt disease. In infectious disease, this is known as the incubation period. During the incubation period, the organism establishes itself in a favorable tissue, multiplies, and overcomes the body defenses against its growth and spread. Disease does not occur unless the microorganism is able to proliferate to the point where it can cause some type of cellular injury either directly or by means of its products. In the development of cancer, the period between the time the cell is injured and the overt disease develops is known as the latent, or lag, period. According to Hopps,[35] the latent period is usually not less than one tenth of the life span of the individual. Two theories have been advanced to explain this observation. One is that this is the length of time required by the cell to establish a new metabolic pattern. The other is that time is required for the cancer cell to overcome the restraining influences on proliferation.

In both infectious disease and in cancer, clinical manifestations depend on

[35] Howard C. Hopps, *Principles of Pathology,* 2nd ed., Appleton-Century-Crofts, Inc., New York, 1964, p. 340.

the multiplication of cells—microorganism or cancer cells—to the point where they or their products injure tissue cells. In infection, the body recognizes the microorganism as foreign or alien and mobilizes both specific and nonspecific defense mechanisms. Apparently, the body also recognizes abnormal or mutated cells and destroys them. When the body defenses are adequate, microorganisms or abnormal cells are destroyed and the individual returns to or maintains his health. In addition, in some, though not all, types of infection, the body develops a sort of recognition system that enables it to protect itself against future attacks. Cancer differs from infection in that, once the stage of overt disease is reached, the body does not appear to have an adequate system of defense against it. There have been a few authenticated instances in which cancer in a person with overt disease disappeared, but these are rare. They are, naturally, of great interest. If the reason for the regression of the cancer could be determined, this knowledge might be useful in prevention and therapy of disease in other individuals. When cancer reaches the stage of overt disease, the cancer cells are more or less unresponsive to factors regulating the growth, reproduction, and differentiation of cells. Therefore, unlike an infection, the body is unable to limit the extent of injury or, by itself, to restore health.

In some types of infectious processes, the infection has its origin in a localized site. Whether or not the infection remains localized or spreads to distant points depends on the virulence and invasiveness of the microorganism and the adequacy of the defenses of the body. When the body is unable to localize the infecting microorganisms, it may infiltrate the surrounding tissue or enter the blood and lymphatic vessels. The microorganisms that enter the blood and lymphatic system may be destroyed by cells in the blood or in lymph nodes or they may be deposited in distant tissues. There they may be destroyed or conditions may favor their multiplication. When this is true, a secondary or metastatic infection is established. Cancer cells behave in a similar manner. From the evidence that is available, cancer usually has its origin in a single cell or group of cells. For a more or less extended period of time, it remains localized at the site of origin. It may never go beyond this site and may even regress.

As long as cancer remains localized to the cells in which it has its origin, it is known as cancer in situ. When a biopsy report states that a patient has cancer in situ of the cervix, this means that the growth has not gone beyond the epithelial cells in which it has its origin. Because of the tendency to shed epithelial cells, it is possible to collect and examine cells from the surface of the cervix and to establish the diagnosis of cancer of the cervix while the disease is still localized. In some persons cancer remains a localized disease. Its presence is discovered only at autopsy. To re-emphasize, the comparison between the behavior of microorganisms and malignant neoplasms has been made to clarify the behavior of malignant neoplasms. There is no evidence at this time that malignant neoplasms are infectious in the usual sense of the word. There is considerable evidence that certain neoplasms in animals (Rous sarcoma and certain lymphomas) are of viral origin. This is still not established in man, however.

Where is emphasis placed in cancer research?

Much of the intensive research being conducted today is for the purpose of learning more about the nature of cancer. Among the five principal goals cited in *A Cancer Source Book for Nurses*[36] two relate directly to learning more about the causation of cancer. The other three are concerned with treatment. The five goals of cancer research cited are: (1) "discovery of cellular trigger mechanisms that start malignant cell growth; (2) a means of checking metastasis—the spreading of cancer; (3) chemicals effective in selectively killing, or halting division in cancer cells; (4) understanding the possible immune defense mechanisms that may work against cancer; and (5) learning if viruses are a cause of some forms of cancer in human beings." Although goals 1 and 5 appear to be more directly related to the etiology of cancer than the others, new knowledge throwing light on any aspect of the problem may result in gains in other areas. Moreover, cancer research adds to the fundamental knowledge of the cell and eventually to greater understanding of the human body in health and disease.

Among the broad areas of interest in the study of the cell in health as well as in disease are included the fundamental genetic and biochemical mechanisms controlling the proliferation and maturation of cells; the mechanisms by which hormones control or regulate bodily processes; and the mechanisms by which viruses cause cancer and whether or not they are a cause of some cancers in human beings.

How do neoplasms cause signs and symptoms?

The signs and symptoms accompanying cancer, as well as benign neoplasms, are due to the local mechanical effects of the primary and metastatic growths and to the total biochemical impact of the disease. Except in neoplastic diseases that are manifested as a generalized disease from the beginning (as an example, leukemia), the early signs and symptoms are usually due to the local mechanical effects of the primary lesion. Because of the availability of modern surgical techniques, it is usually possible to remove the primary lesion, so that it is seldom the direct cause of death. Death is usually due to the extensive derangements of normal biochemical functions associated with the systemic or metastatic stage of the disease.[37] The effects observed in late cancer are similar to those seen in generalized sepsis—another point of similarity between infection and cancer.

[36] *A Cancer Source Book for Nurses*, American Cancer Society, New York, 1963, p. 11.
[37] James D. Hardy, "Why Do Cancer Patients Die?" *Surgery, Gynecology, and Obstetrics,* CVIII, 1959, pp. 368-69.

How do neoplasms cause mechanical effects?

The manifestations due to the mechanical effects of a neoplasm result from the neoplasm (1) occupying space, (2) obstructing the lumen of a tube or duct, (3) exerting pressure on overlying mucous membrane, and (4) twisting the pedicle of a polyp. Actually, the obstruction of the lumen of a tube or duct and the pressure on the overlying mucous membrane are due to the space-occupying effect of neoplasms.

The earliness with which symptoms develop, as well as their nature, depends on the anatomical and functional characteristics of the involved organ or structures. Such factors as the size and distensibility of the space containing the neoplasm will influence the period of time likely to elapse before the neoplasm causes signs and symptoms. The location of a lesion in a hollow or tubular organ will also influence its effect. For example, a lesion near the outlet of the stomach will cause symptoms earlier than one in the fundus. A neoplasm growing around a tubular organ causes a greater degree of obstruction than one projecting into it. Each of these points will be illustrated later.

Because neoplasms are formed of masses of cells, they generally occupy space and cause clinical manifestations by (1) interfering with the blood supply of tissue, (2) interfering with the function of an organ, and (3) activating compensatory or defensive mechanisms.

As stated earlier, the size and distensibility of the space or organ containing a neoplasm influence the nature as well as the earliness with which manifestations of disease occur. The examples which follow are intended to clarify the mechanical effects of neoplasms.

Mike Sunny, aged 11, has a rapidly growing neoplasm in his cerebellum. As the neoplasm increases in mass, it occupies space and presses on the tissues of the cerebellum.[38] The earliness with which local pressure is exerted is influenced by the fact that the cerebellum is surrounded by a rigid bony wall, the skull; it does not distend to accommodate the increase in the contents of the cranial cavity. Furthermore, the location of this particular neoplasm is such that it obstructs the drainage of cerebrospinal fluid from the ventricles, causing the fluid to accumulate within the ventricles, and thus further raising the intracranial pressure. Because the size of the cavity containing the brain is fixed, increased resistance to the flow of blood through the brain is a consequence of an elevation in intracranial pressure.

The manifestations presented by Mike are due to an inadequate supply of blood to the cerebellum and other parts of the brain and to the activation of mechanisms to maintain the blood supply of the brain. The signs and symptoms presented by Mike indicate disturbances in the function of the cerebellum as well as evidence of alterations in cardiorespiratory function, which

---

[38] In the cerebellum the space is less confining than that enclosing the cerebrum. Since the neoplasm is malignant, it also invades the surrounding tissue, but at this point the effect of a space-occupying mass is under discussion.

tend to overcome the resistance to the flow of blood to the brain. See Chapter 13B for further discussion of disturbance in the function of the cerebellum and for signs and symptoms of increased intracranial pressure.

In contrast to Mike, who had an expanding lesion within a fixed space, Mrs. Thinly had a neoplasm in a space that was highly distensible. Mrs. Thinly had a benign ovarian cyst which, at the time it was removed, weighed more than 40 lb. It was so large that it overfilled a basin about the size of an ordinary dishpan. The day before Mrs. Thinly was admitted to the hospital she had done the family wash and cleaned the house. For some months previous to seeking medical attention she had noticed a gradual increase in the size of her abdomen which she attributed to the fact that she had had several children and was getting old. Until the tumor reached considerable size, it had little effect on function because the abdominal wall distended to accommodate the increase in contents. As the size of the tumor increased, however, the intra-abdominal pressure rose causing pressure against the diaphragm and decreasing the capacity of her stomach and other abdominal organs. She experienced some shortness of breath, swelling of the feet, and loss of appetite. Because of her loss of appetite she had lost some weight. After the tumor was removed, she weighed 85 lb, but she made a rapid and uneventful recovery. Since the neoplasm was benign, she was cured.

Mike Sunny and Mrs. Thinly have been described to illustrate how the rigidity or distensibility of the space in which a neoplasm grows influences its effects. At the time Mike Sunny's skull was opened, the neoplasm was about the size of a small orange, and it was already threatening his life by its effect on the blood supply to his brain. In contrast, because of the distensibility of the abdominal wall, Mrs. Thinly had a very large neoplasm which had little effect on the blood supply to the tissues in the abdominal cavity. Signs and symptoms observed in Mrs. Thinly were mainly due to the interference with the functions of the respiratory and digestive systems.

Mr. Timothy Thomas illustrates what happens when the diameter of a tubular structure is decreased by a space-occupying mass. Mr. Thomas had a carcinoma of the prostate which, as it increased in cell mass, caused pressure on the urethra, thus increasing the resistance to the flow of urine through the urethra. As shown in Figure 12-3, any tubular structure may be obstructed by

FIGURE   12 – 3

Sites of Neoplasms Which May Obstruct Any Tubular Structure

A. External to structure
B. Internal, arising from lining membrane
C. Internal, arising in and encircling the wall

---

the pressure created by a neoplasm external to it, or by a neoplasm extending from the lining membrane into the lumen of the tube, or by a neoplasm arising in the wall and encircling it as it grows. Both benign and malignant neoplasms may obstruct by creating external pressure on a tubular structure or by extending into its lumen from the lining tissues. Neoplasms arising in the wall and encircling the lumen of a tube, such as the large intestine, are usually malignant.

In the instance of Mr. Thomas, obstruction of the urethra was due to a neoplasm in tissue external to it. Whatever the cause of the obstruction, its primary effect is to interfere with the passage of the tube's contents. When the obstruction of a tubular structure develops slowly enough, the portion of the tube preceding the obstruction dilates, and the muscle layer in its wall hypertrophies. Muscular hypertrophy occurs as a result of the increase in resistance to the movement of the contents of the obstructed tube; it is, therefore, a compensatory mechanism. Eventually, as the degree of obstruction increases, the lumen will be blocked and the tube will cease to function as a passageway. Chronic obstruction, whatever its cause, predisposes to infection of the organ drained by the duct.

To return to Mr. Thomas, who has an obstruction of the urethra due to a carcinoma of his prostate gland—as the neoplasm enlarged, it encroached on the lumen of the urethra, thus impeding the passage of urine. To overcome the effect of the increase in resistance caused by the narrowing of the urethra, the muscle in the neck of the bladder hypertrophied. As the urethra narrowed, Mr. Thomas noted that he had difficulty in starting to void and that the urinary stream was small. He also had a feeling of urgency and seldom felt that he had really emptied his bladder. As time passed and the obstruction increased, the bladder did not empty at the time of voiding. Urine accumulated and became infected. The bladder was distended by the accumulated urine. Eventually, if the obstruction is allowed to continue, the ureters and the pelvis of the kidneys become distended with urine and all the structures— urethra, bladder, and kidneys—become infected. The outcome of unrelieved obstruction along the urinary tract is kidney failure.

The effects of obstruction of the alimentary canal and of the ducts emptying into it have been discussed in Chapters 7 and 10 and will not be pursued further. One effect meriting some consideration is that neoplasms in the alimentary canal usually impair nutrition before those located in other parts of the body. Patients with obstructing lesions in the upper alimentary canal not infrequently experience a rapid loss in weight and are markedly dehydrated and anemic because of impaired intake of food and fluids.

Since the effects of obstruction of ducts forming the tracheobronchial tree and the biliary tract have been discussed elsewhere, they will not be repeated here.

Another mechanical effect of neoplasms results from pressure created by the neoplasm on the overlying mucous membrane. Pressure on any tissue decreases its blood supply. With impairment in its nutrition the mucous membrane atrophies, and if the pressure is severe and unrelieved, it ulcerates. Ulceration predisposes to bleeding in benign as well as in malignant neoplasms. For example, some patients with leiomyofibromas located in the submucosa of the wall of the uterus (fibroids) are predisposed to profuse bleeding or hemorrhage. Tumors located in the deeper layers of the wall of the uterus do not usually result in hemorrhage. To illustrate, Mrs. Beech has a leiomyofibroma located in the submucosa of the wall of the uterus. As a consequence of pressure, the blood supply to the mucosa overlying the tumor was impaired. It atrophied and eventually ulcerated. During her menstrual periods she experienced heavy bleeding, or menorrhagia. Despite the benign nature of leiomyomas, Mrs. Beech's health and possibly her life were threatened by repeated hemorrhage. Since she has multiple fibroids (leiomyomas) and she is bleeding excessively, she has been advised by her physician to have a hysterectomy.

The fourth mechanical effect of a neoplasm results from the twisting of a pedunculated polyp, benign or malignant, on its pedicle. Twisting causes severe pain and it also deprives the polyp of its blood supply. When a polyp is torn from its pedicle, massive bleeding can result.

In the preceding discussion, the manner in which neoplasms cause signs and symptoms by their mechanical effects has been presented. As space-occupying masses, they create pressure on tissues, thus impairing their blood supply; they obstruct the lumen and interfere with the function of tubular organs; and when they are pedunculated, they are likely to twist on their pedicles. All of these are local effects and may be caused by either benign or malignant neoplasms. Specific signs and symptoms will depend on the location of the lesion, the degree to which function is disrupted, and the extent to which compensatory or defense mechanisms are mobilized.

What are some of the possible systemic effects of neoplasms?

Benign and malignant neoplasms may also be accompanied by systemic effects. As stated earlier, neoplasms arising in glands (adenomas) may elaborate the secretion of the gland. When this occurs, symptoms of hyperfunction occur. Functioning tumors may be benign or malignant. At least in the thyroid gland, hyperfunction is more likely to be associated with a benign than with a malignant neoplasm.

As indicated earlier in the chapter, malignant neoplasms differ from benign neoplasms in a number of ways. Whereas benign neoplasms are usually localized to the area where they originate, malignant neoplasms tend to invade the surrounding tissue and to be disseminated throughout the body. Some of the effects of malignant neoplasms are due to the invasion and replacement of healthy tissue at the site of the primary growth or of metastasis. The specific effects of metastasis depend on the site affected. For example, in cancer of the lung, either primary or metastatic, the destruction of lung tissue eventually leads to asphyxia of the patient. In leukemia, the abnormal cells invade and destroy the bone marrow as well as other vital structures. As the bone marrow is invaded and destroyed, its capacity to produce erythrocytes and thrombocytes fails; this predisposes to anemia and bleeding.

A number of the manifestations accompanying malignant neoplasms are due to their tendency to outgrow their blood supply. As in healthy cells, cells in malignant neoplasms die unless their nutritional needs are met. Death or necrosis of cells on the surface of a neoplasm predisposes to ulceration. Ulceration predisposes to infection and bleeding, and is one of the important causes of pain. Ulceration with its concomitant effects can sometimes be observed in the patient with advanced and neglected cancer of the breast. Large, infected ulcerations, often with foul-smelling drainage, occur over the affected area. Signs and symptoms accompanying tissue necrosis and/or infection include fever, leukocytosis, elevation of the sedimentation rate, anorexia, and malaise. Since these symptoms and signs are nonspecific, a patient who manifests them without an obvious cause should be investigated for cancer.

In addition to infections of ulcerated lesions, the patient with metastatic cancer is predisposed to infections of the lung and of the urinary tract. These infections are frequently due to obstruction of a bronchus, a ureter, or the urethra. Curing of the infection depends on relief of the obstruction and use of appropriate antibiotics. Nursing measures which can and should be instituted to prevent obstruction of the airway by secretions in the bedfast patient are discussed in detail in Chapter 7.

Bleeding not only accompanies ulceration, but it can also be the result of the erosion of one or more blood vessels. The amount of blood lost at a time may be micro- or macroscopic. Any abnormal bleeding should be investigated, as it may indicate the presence of a malignant neoplasm. Blood in the stool or urine or any unusual bleeding from the vagina should be investigated for evidence or absence of cancer. Eventually the continued loss of blood leads to anemia, with its characteristic signs and symptoms. Bleeding is not the only cause of anemia in cancer, as anemia occurs in advanced cancer in the absence of any significant loss of blood. Other factors predisposing to anemia include infection and uremia. Metastasis to the liver or bone marrow may reduce the capacity to replace blood cells. Treatment of cancer by radiotherapy or chemotherapy is usually accompanied by some degree of depression of the bone marrow, thus predisposing to anemia. With the exception of pallor, the signs and symptoms are those of circulatory distress. They are tachycardia, palpitation, dyspnea, dizziness, easy fatigability, and weakness.

Malignant neoplasms cause symptoms by utilizing nutritional elements required by normal cells. They continue to grow as long as the host remains alive. This is true even in the most emaciated patient. The rate of growth is sometimes slowed by undernutrition, but growth continues. Why malignant cells have a competitive advantage over normal cells is not known. They seem to require more of some types of amino acids and vitamins than do normal cells, but little more than this is known.

Malignant neoplasms located in the lung, ovaries, and breast frequently are accompanied by the effusion of serous fluid into the pleural and peritoneal cavities. The fluid can be removed by thoracentesis or abdominal paracentesis. When the fluid is formed rapidly, radioactive gold or nitrogen mustard may be introduced into the appropriate cavity to lessen the tendency to effusion; effusion is prevented in about one half of the patients so treated.

One of the most striking effects of advanced cancer is severe cachexia. In lay terms, the individual literally becomes skin and bones. The patient appears to be, and is, suffering from severe starvation. One explanation offered to account for cachexia is that the food intake of the individual is insufficient to support the neoplasm and the individual. Although an inadequate intake of food may be a contributing factor, it is probably not the sole cause of cachexia. Hardy[39] states that forced feeding is often unsuccessful in correcting it. He is of the opinion that cachexia, as well as other manifestations of terminal cancer, is due to derangements in the normal biochemical functions of the body. Whatever its cause may be, every reasonable effort should be made to encourage the patient to eat, particularly protein-containing foods.

What additional considerations about pain are necessary when planning the care of a patient with diagnosis of cancer?

Because pain will be discussed in some detail in Chapter 15, it will be considered here only briefly. Despite evidence that pain is neither as common nor as inevitable as generally believed, it is probably the most feared effect of cancer. The fact that people believe that cancer and pain are synonymous is unfortunate, because it contributes to the dread or fear of cancer that permeates our society. As stated in Chapter 15, the discomfort caused by pain has two sources. One is the pain sensation and the other is the meaning that the pain has for the individual. Studies of persons who are in pain-inducing situations demonstrate that the meaning that pain has for the individual frequently determines the degree of suffering experienced. The belief that pain is inevitable and frequently so severe that it is intolerable can of itself increase the severity of the pain experienced by the patient. When nurses and physicians are convinced that pain is an unavoidable aspect of cancer, it may result in a narrow or unimaginative approach to the care of the patient. The care may be such as to reinforce the fears of the patient, and other causes of discomfort may be missed or neglected. Not only does a morbid fear of pain add to the suffering of the patient who has been diagnosed as having cancer, but it may prevent persons who suspect that they have it from seeking medical attention. Persons who do not have cancer, therefore, experience unnecessary discomfort and those who do may delay until such time as metastasis has occurred. There are undoubtedly other negative aspects of the all-too-common belief that pain and cancer are synonymous.

When pain occurs in cancer, it is usually the result of pressure on, or the involvement of, sensory nerve endings in obstruction, ulceration, or infection. Pain can also be induced by measures employed in the treatment of cancer.

[39] Hardy, *Op. cit.,* p. 180.

For example, the patient who undergoes surgical treatment is likely to experience more or less pain. Radiotherapy, particularly when it induces an inflammatory reaction in tissues in the treated area, may be responsible for pain. Although pain may be present early in the course, it is more likely to be a late symptom. Pain in cancer of the bone is likely to be severe, for the rigidity of the bone allows for little or no expansion. Pressure on sensory nerve endings occurs early.

The prevention and relief of pain are one aspect of the care of the patient with a diagnosis of cancer. Though not all will experience pain, most patients fear that they will. Moreover, there are many other causes of discomfort besides pain which can increase the suffering of the patient or which the patient may perceive as pain. Lack of rest as well as the inevitable discomforts associated with any illness diminish the capacity of the patient to withstand pain and add to his tendency to magnify the degree of pain that he is experiencing. The nurse should be alert to, and try to relieve, whatever is causing the patient discomfort. As an example, Mr. Sands had metastatic cancer involving the ribs and sternum. Even touching his chest with a sheet caused him to cry out in pain. His nurse was able to prevent unnecessary pain by placing a large cradle over his torso as a support for the bed covering. When she moved and turned him she was gentle and moved him slowly. She supported his head and arms in a relaxed position, so that they did not pull on his thorax. Mrs. Lottie had metastatic cancer involving her cervical vertebrae. Although she had a neck brace, she found it uncomfortable. Mrs. Lottie and her nurse worked out a plan for turning her, so that pain was prevented and the brace was not required. Mrs. Lottie supported her head with her hands as she turned. After she was turned, pillow supports were used to keep her head in alignment. Pain was prevented by the identification of the situations causing it and by the utilization of effective nursing measures.

In nursing the patient, gentle handling, attention to his hygienic and physiological needs, intelligent concern for his well-being, an attitude that something constructive can be done to improve his condition, and the sensible use of diversion and occupation—all when appropriately selected and utilized—can contribute to the prevention and relief of pain.

When drugs are required for the relief of pain, they must be prescribed by the physician. In selecting a drug or drugs, the physician usually considers the following points. Even a patient who appears to be seriously ill may live for many months. Furthermore, should the patient become addicted to a drug, then the addiction, not the pain experienced by the patient, takes priority. The evaluation of the symptoms presented by the patient becomes more difficult and his treatment less satisfactory.

To prevent addiction and to provide insurance that drugs with enough potency will be available over a period of many months, the physician usually prescribes the least potent drug in the smallest dosage that is effective. Because of the importance of the meaning pain has for the patient, he may also prescribe a tranquilizing agent. The nurse has the responsibility for preparing the patient so that he is in a comfortable position and condition, and for observing the effects of the drug. Though drugs are usually ordered by the clock, pain does not tell time. The nurse should, therefore, observe the length of time that the patient is relieved. Because of daytime activities, patients often require less medication during the day than at night. In some instances, small doses of a pain-relieving medication given every two hours provide more relief than do large doses given every four hours. Part of the benefit from the drug comes from the faith of the patient in its effectiveness. Nothing should be done to interfere with this, by either word or deed. Occasionally a well-intentioned, though misguided, nurse decides to protect the patient from the danger of addiction by prolonging the time the patient has to wait for his medication, or decides to withhold the narcotic portion of his prescription. The result of the first may well be that the patient receives little or no benefit from his medication because his pain has become intolerable. The result of the second is that the faith of the patient in the power of his medication to relieve his suffering is destroyed.

Unless the patient is presenting evidence of toxicity from the drug, the prescription left by the physician should be adhered to. Any problem related to the drug or drugs the patient is receiving should be discussed with the physician before a change is made. In the use of drugs for the control of pain in the patient with cancer, the objective is to regulate selection and use so that the patient is provided relief over the course of his illness. Callaway[40] summarizes some of the important points in the use of narcotics in patients with cancer by stating that the untimely use of narcotics lessens the chance that they will be effective when they are needed. After addiction has taken place, the complaints of the patient are valueless as a basis for determining his needs. Narcotics cause personality changes which interfere with his relationship with his family. They also reduce his intake of food. Further, an important consideration is that they increase the cost of a not inexpensive illness.

Callaway[41] also emphasizes the importance of using a sympathetic approach to the patient. Mild drugs such as aspirin plus a tranquilizing agent will often give the patient the necessary relief. Every effort should be made to prevent addiction. Once the patient becomes addicted, the problems are multiplied manyfold.

What other measures may be employed to relieve pain in some instances?

In addition to the use of drugs for the relief of pain, surgical procedures to correct conditions causing pain may be instituted. Ulcerated lesions may be excised, obstruction may be relieved by rerouting operations such as colostomy, or pain impulses may be prevented from reaching higher centers in the nervous system by cutting a sensory nerve, nerveroot, or tract in the spinal

---

[40] Enoch Callaway, "The Misuse of Narcotics by Patients Suffering from Cancer," *Ca*, X, January-February, 1960, pp. 33-36.
[41] *Ibid.*, p. 35.

cord. The interruption of sensory nerve pathways is not usually performed unless all other measures fail. With the loss of their sensory nerve supply, tissues are deprived of one of their important defenses against pressure and heat. The patient should be turned and the skin inspected for redness or blanching no less often then every two hours. Protective measures should be instituted such as an alternating pressure mattress or sheepskin under the affected area. The bed linen should be free of crumbs and wrinkles. A cradle should be used to lessen the pressure of the bed covering on the patient.

To control the pain and odors associated with ulcerated lesions, the area may be excised surgically, or the patient may be treated with X ray or chemotherapy. All these measures are utilized because they remove or control the tumor itself. When the lesion remains open, the most important general measure is *cleanliness*. The odors originate from dead tissue and the effects of infection. The agent used to cleanse the lesion should be prescribed by the physician. There is usually no reason for not cleansing the area around the lesion with soap or detergent and water. Moreover, when the patient has a draining and foul-smelling wound, the nurse should take whatever initiative is required to see that it is cleansed. Dressings should be changed when soiled and replaced by clean ones. When wounds are treated by exposure to the air, the patient should be draped and screened so that he is protected from view. Ventilation of the room, with precautions to prevent chilling the patient, reduces the intensity of odors. When deodorizing agents and devices are used, they should not be employed as substitutes for keeping the wound clean.

In some types of malignant neoplasms, the patient may be benefited by the administration of certain hormones. Some patients with metastatic cancer of the breast improve after treatment with androgenic, that is male sex, hormones. Some children with leukemia improve when treated with cortisone or one of its analogues. In contrast, some types of malignant neoplasms regress after the removal of one or more hormone-secreting glands. As an illustration, regression of cancer of the breast occurs after the removal of the ovary, the adrenal gland, and/or the anterior pituitary gland.

In summary, although pain is not inevitable to cancer, it does occur. Even the patients who do not experience pain are almost certain to fear they will. There are few areas in which a kind, gentle, thoughtful, compassionate, and creative nurse can do more to prevent human suffering. The prescription of drugs and treatment by surgical and chemotherapeutic means are the prerogative of the physician. Whether or not the drugs are effective often depends on the quality of nursing care the patient receives. Furthermore, by attention to the hygienic, physiological, and psychosocial needs of the patient, pain and suffering from pain can be alleviated.

What are some of the psychological effects on the patient of a real or imagined diagnosis of cancer?

Not by any means the least important cause of suffering in the patient who has or suspects he has cancer are its psychosocial effects. As mentioned earlier, the psychological effects extend to persons who do not have cancer, inasmuch as many fear that their illness or ill health is due to cancer. The family is also affected by a diagnosis of cancer in a family member. Their response to the diagnosis and to the individual, affects the behavior of the sick person. The psychological effects are those resulting from the manner in which the individual perceives the entire cancer experience, that is, its nature and effects, and outcome, as well as the measures utilized in its diagnosis and treatment. The sociological effects of cancer stem from group attitudes toward it, its nature, effects, and treatment. Each person reading this book has attitudes about cancer, its effects, and curability that were learned from the groups of which he is a part. These attitudes influence how a person feels and behaves when faced with a diagnosis of cancer in himself or in another individual. His behavior toward another individual is also influenced by the way in which the individual defines his role in the situation. The quality of care that a patient receives is affected by the attitude of all who have a relationship to him—his family, his neighbors, his nurses and doctors, and the community. As an illustration, when Mr. and Mrs. Thompkins were driving home from an appointment with her physician where Mrs. Thompkins learned that she had cancer of the breast. Mr. Thompkins asked in a tentative tone, "Don't you think that you would sleep better, if I moved into the guest room?" Mr. Thompkins did not intend to be unkind, rather he was frightened. Despite the fact that the physician had answered his question about the possibility that cancer was infectious in the negative, he was not convinced. Besides, cancer always made him think of suffering and death.

Any person who has a diagnosis of cancer can be expected to be under severe emotional stress. For most persons in the United States, the diagnosis carries with it a threat of a prolonged and painful course, ending in death. Because of the extended course of the illness and the nature of the treatments, cancer is often an economic burden, not only to the patient, but also to his family.

On the discovery of a lesion or symptom that suggests cancer, most persons experience fear. With the fear, the person may have a variety of feelings—a sense of doom, anger, helplessness, shame, and disgrace. He may feel trapped or abandoned. Cameron[42] states, ". . . in general, cancer signifies premature death, supreme physical suffering, abysmal depression, incalculable economic loss, and pathetic family disruption and dissolution." The fear and anxiety experienced by the patient are extended to his family, friends, neighbors, and community.

Nurses also have culturally derived attitudes toward cancer and what nurses ought to be able to accomplish in the care of the sick. To be successful in identifying and meeting needs of the patient, the nurse is helped by knowing what her own feelings are. The aim of the nurse is not to avoid feeling, but to manage her feelings in such a way that she can attend to those of her

[42] Charles S. Cameron, "We Who Are Concerned," *Cancer News*, XIII, Summer, 1959, p. 5.

patients. The nurse should try to take a middle course so that she is able to identify the needs of the patient and to meet them in ways that are helpful to the patient. Neither feeling too strongly with the patient nor isolating herself from him will enable her to achieve this goal with any degree of consistency.

The person who suspects or knows he has cancer can then be expected to experience fear and its attendant feelings. How he reacts to this fear depends on the way in which he customarily behaves when he is under severe stress and the quality of support given to him by his family. If his fear is reasonable, he may be stimulated to seek medical attention and to follow through with recommendations of his physician. In contrast, unreasonable fear leads to denial, disorganization, confusion, and panic. Denial is a very common reaction, and it may be so strong that the patient knows that he does not have cancer. He may know that he does not have cancer even when he has been diagnosed and treated in a center specializing in the treatment of patients with it. When denial is less complete, the patient may grasp at straws, seek new treatments, and ask for constant reassurance. He asks not to know that he has cancer, but to be reassured that he does not. As a result, the patient may delay diagnosis and treatment or consult quacks who promise cures.

Another possible source of stress is that treatment of cancer frequently involves the loss of important functions and organs. These may be important not only to the patient but to the members of his family, his friends, and the community. The lesion, because of its location or the nature of its treatment, may be the cause of psychological stress. Either benign or malignant neoplasms may cause disfigurement. Nevi or birthmarks on the exposed surface of the body may be the cause of more or less psychological stress. One small girl, Mary Lou, had a type of malignant neoplasm in which the skin on the exposed surfaces of her body was covered with wartlike growths. Life was made bearable for Mary Lou when she was given a pretty hat with a veil and encouraged to wear it. The veil served to protect her from the stares and thoughtless comments of bystanders. Because Mary Lou had a widespread and progressive disease and was not expected to live for more than a few months, one of the important objectives in her care was to make her as comfortable as was possible in the time she had. Persons who have benign lesions that are disfiguring must be helped to adjust to the situation. Often a lesion can be made less conspicuous by the use of a covering type of cosmetic.

In addition to the psychological stress caused by a diagnosis of cancer, neoplasms located in certain sites may be responsible for additional stress. Neoplasms located in the head and neck not only cause obvious disfigurement, but the removal of the lesion is usually accompanied by some degree of mutilation and loss of function, including loss of the ability to swallow, to speak, or to breathe normally. After laryngectomy, the patient may feel that because of his loss of speech, he is something less than human. About 70 per cent of persons who have had laryngectomy can learn esophageal speech. It takes about 12 months for the patient to reach the stage of maximum intelligibility. Some patients who cannot learn esophageal speech may be able to use an artificial larynx. It differs from the esophageal speech, which provides an internal source, by providing a sound source external to the human vocal cords.

The loss of the breast causes disfigurement and some loss of function of the muscles moving the shoulder and the arm. It also predisposes to edema of the arm on the affected side. The structural deformity can be corrected by a prosthesis. Because the breast is a symbol of femininity, the woman may feel that she is less of a woman after mastectomy.

The removal of reproductive organs of either the male or female usually is accompanied by some feeling of loss of identity. The man who loses his testes is likely to feel that he is less a man, just as a woman who loses her uterus, breast, or ovaries feels less a woman.

The psychological problems created by a colostomy are discussed later, in the study of Mrs. Wren. The discussion of the needs of the patient who is in the terminally ill phase of the disease is included in Chapter 2.

Some of the factors causing psychological stress in the patient who has a diagnosis of cancer have been presented. Further discussion of psychosocial aspects of care are included in later sections of the chapter. For a more detailed discussion of the effects of severe psychological stress and what the nurse can do to help the patient, see Chapter 6.

Should a patient be told he has cancer?

A problem growing out of the fact that cancer can and often does create a high degree of psychological stress among members of the family, nurses, and physicians is the question of whether or not the patient should be told that he has cancer. In few, if any, other diseases is there any question about withholding the nature of the diagnosis. Often the cooperation of the patient in his treatment requires that the patient know what his diagnosis is. Although physicians may not inform the patient of the nature of his illness, some member of the family is informed. Practice among physicians varies. In cancer, as in other diseases, the physician carries the responsibility for informing the patient of the nature of his diagnosis and the treatment required. At one time the practice not to tell patients unless there was some reason for telling them was general, and some physicians still rarely tell a patient that he has cancer. Others always, or almost always, tell their patients and feel just as strongly that the patient should be told, as do those who feel knowledge of the nature of the diagnosis should be withheld. Many physicians try to make their decision on the basis of whether the patient wants to know and how the knowledge will affect him.

What are some of the possible harmful effects of withholding information about a diagnosis of cancer?

In the past there has been much argument about the harmful effects resulting from the patient's learning that he has cancer; not too much consideration has been given to the harmful effects of his not knowing. Making an issue over whether or not to tell the person who has cancer fosters the urge to secrecy. It also suggests that the situation of the person is hopeless and that there is something mysterious about cancer. The fact that patients know that they may not be told may cause some persons to distrust the information given them by their physician. It is not unusual to hear persons say that they are not certain whether they have or have not been told the truth about their illness. Patients who are not told that they have cancer sometimes obtain this information through questions and statements made to a nurse or doctor. When the patient is not told, this creates the necessity for treating the patient as if nothing were wrong. The patient's questions have to be answered without giving him any information. This, in turn, creates a barrier between the patient and the professional staff. He is cut off from seeking information, help, and comfort from those who, by preparation, should be able to help him. A patient may be told by a visitor or another patient that he has cancer. This can be, needless to say, an exceedingly traumatic experience. Some patients suffer more by not knowing. Uncertainty usually causes more discomfort than certainty. Imagination, unless disciplined by reality, can do terrible things to an individual. According to the accounts of persons writing about their personal experience with cancer, the lives of some persons become richer and more meaningful after they know they have cancer. As emphasized by Mrs. Willis (see Chapter 2), not all persons react in this way. Not knowing that he has cancer may have an adverse effect on the course of the disease, inasmuch as the patient who does not know that he has or has had cancer may fail to keep his appointments for care and for follow-up examinations.

Against telling the patient that he has cancer is the fact that, for many people, the knowledge is very upsetting. In some people it may cause a disruptive panic and possibly lead to suicide. According to some authorities, suicide is actually rare among patients who have cancer.

At the present time, two factors determine whether or not a given patient is told he has cancer. One is the feelings of the physician. The other is the distress of the patient. Unless there is an important reason for telling the patient, he is not told when he indicates that he does not want to know that he has cancer. If he never refers to cancer as a cause of his illness, or if he asks to be reassured that he does not have cancer, this is taken as an indication that he does not want to know. Conversely, when he asks the direct question, "Do I have cancer?" he is answered in the affirmative.

Frequently the intelligent patient who is not using powerful denial mechanisms probably knows that he has cancer by the time the doctor has established the diagnosis. In some of these patients, the condition is worsened by fostering denial mechanisms. They want to know whether or not they have cancer. Doctors who do inform the patient of his status try to do so in a manner that fosters his hope. Though they tell the patient the truth, they do not usually go into all the future possibilities. A friend with cancer of the breast was told by her surgeon that he had removed her entire breast because she had some abnormal cells. Over the course of the next two or three years she learned the extent of her disease. She commented later that in the beginning she did not believe that she could have tolerated knowing the full truth, but by learning it gradually, she had come to accept her situation. With time she was able to accept that she had cancer.

To summarize, whether or not, and how, the patient is told depends on the patient and his situation. The doctor and the family of the patient weigh the factors that enter into the decision. There is not at this time a single answer to the needs of all patients. Decisions should be based on what will, in the long run, make it possible to meet the needs of the patient. One day the problem of telling or not telling the patient will cease to exist. Under all circumstances, every effort should be made to convey to the patient that much can and will be done to promote his welfare.

Through what phases does the person who is susceptible to cancer pass?

In the *Cancer Bulletin*,[43] the life cycle of the cancer patient is depicted as occurring in seven phases. To these seven should be added another, the first, or preventive, phase. The phases as listed include: (1) early diagnosis; (2) recommended treatment; (3) comprehensive treatment; (4) follow-up education for the patient; (5) regular follow-up by the physician; (6) rehabilitation; and (7) adequate terminal care. Not all patients who have a diagnosis of cancer progress through all these phases. Statistics indicate that of 450,000 cases diagnosed each year, 150,000 patients are saved. Three hundred thousand will die. Of these, 225,000 will die within a few years because there is as yet no known means of curing them. Seventy-five thousand could be saved if present-day knowledge were applied soon enough.[44]

The discussion is organized as follows: (1) the elements in primary prevention, (2) the phase of secondary prevention, detection, and diagnosis of cancer, (3) the phase of curative and palliative treatment, (4) the nursing needs of patients, and (5) the phase of terminal illness. Because rehabilitation and instruction begin the moment the individual enters the clinic or doctor's office and continue throughout all phases of the patient's life, they will not be treated separately.

On what information is the general care of the patient with cancer based?

In all phases of the patient's illness, the nurse tries to convey to the patient that something can and will be done to improve his condition. This does not always mean that his life will be prolonged, but that, whatever the probable

[43] *Cancer Bulletin,* XI, May-June, 1959, p. 47.
[44] Daniel Horn, "Public Reaction to Cancer," *Cancer News,* XIII, Spring, 1959, pp. 8-9.

outcome, the quality of his life can be improved. The goals for each patient should take into account the phase of the patient's illness, his psychological and physiological resources, and the nature and extent of treatment. Persons who happen to have cancer are people. They have the same basic needs as do all people. Because of the manner in which cancer and its treatment are perceived, patients with cancer can be expected to be under severe stress. Each patient behaves as an individual. In order to meet the needs of patients, the nurse requires knowledge and competence in all nursing skills. These include skill in making observation, in providing care in such a manner that the patient feels accepted and respected, in teaching the patient and family members, in planning and organizing the patient's care, and in performing the procedures required in his physical care.

Observation is a continuous process directed toward the identification of the patient's physiological and psychological needs. From observation, data are collected that indicate improvement or deterioration of the patient's condition or the development of complications. Instruction of the patient is planned to achieve three goals: first, that the patient continues to have regular medical supervision for the remainder of his life; second, that within the limits of the patient's capacity, he continue as an active and productive member of his family and community; he should not be unnecessarily invalided. The third objective is an aspect of the second—if he can accept in perspective whatever limitations are imposed by his treatment, he can be helped not to allow them to become the focus of his life. The other aspects of nursing will be integrated throughout.

In the control of cancer, prevention is the keynote. As in other chronic diseases, prevention is of two types, primary and secondary. In primary prevention the objective is to eliminate conditions that predispose to its development. In the present state of knowledge evidence points to multiple factors interacting to cause cancer. A problem in prevention is to identify those factors that are controllable. Through the use of epidemiological studies, some of the agents in the external environment have been identified as carcinogenic. As they become known, methods can be developed to eliminate them or to protect persons from their effect. Much has been accomplished in industry to protect workers from carcinogenic chemicals. A familiar example from the health field is the precautions that are taken to protect workers from exposure to ionizing radiation. The basis for, and the nature of, these precautions have been discussed elsewhere. At times knowledge about the significance of a factor is less clear-cut, or the findings of epidemiological studies are difficult to implement. For example, the incidence of cancer of the lung is higher in urban than in rural areas. Many factors may well enter into this difference. Among these is the higher concentration of smoke discharged into the air from all sources—houses, stores, industrial plants, and automobile exhaust gases. Both smoke and exhaust gases contain carcinogenic hydrocarbons. To reduce the pollution of the air by potentially harmful substances, public education is required. The public must accept, demand, and be willing to pay for whatever is required to do this. Further, permanent control of air pollution depends on continued supervision and enforcement of regulations. In the primary prevention of cancer, much has been accomplished to protect workers from the carcinogenic effects of agents used in industry. A beginning has been made in the protection of the general public from known carcinogens.

Equally difficult or possibly even more difficult to accomplish is the primary prevention involving a major change in a custom or habit. As an illustration, despite the Surgeon General's report on the hazards associated with cigarette smoking, many persons continue to smoke. Knowledge of hazards, especially when cause-effect relationships are not immediately observable, is not enough to effect changes in the habits of all people. Many other factors are involved.

A second type of primary prevention is based on the identification and removal of precancerous lesions. These have been discussed previously. One of the reasons cited for the decrease in the incidence of cancer of the cervix is that women receive better obstetrical care than in the past. By preventing injury of the cervix and providing early treatment of lesions that develop, the chances of development of cancer of the cervix are reduced.

Primary prevention of cancer is the ideal method of control. The most extensive and effective applications of the principles of primary prevention have been made in industry in the protection of workers from carcinogenic chemicals. Some cancer is prevented by treatment that eliminates the possibility of development of a precancerous lesion or by the removal of suspicious lesions. Applications of primary prevention, though significant, are limited by knowledge of the direct and indirect causes of cancer.

The nurse assists in primary prevention by (1) supporting research projects, not only those directly related to cancer, but those directed toward understanding the nature of cell growth; (2) supporting community efforts to improve environmental conditions; (3) practicing self-protection in situations in which there is a possibility of exposure to ionizing radiation, and (4) observing and reporting precancerous lesions in herself and others and encouraging others to do likewise.

What is secondary prevention in cancer?

The secondary prevention of cancer is based on the identification of a cancer while it is still a local rather than a systemic disease. In this stage of disease, malignant change has taken place, but cancer cells have not been distributed throughout the body. In terms of the life of the patient with cancer, this is the first phase. The presumption has been in the past that if cancer could be detected, diagnosed, and treated early enough, then its harmful effects could be prevented. Emphasis has been placed on early diagnosis and adequate treatment. In some patients, cancer can be and is detected while it is a local disease. It can be eradicated and the patient cured. In other patients, with the present methods of diagnosis, cancer is a systemic disease by the time its manifestations are evident, and possibly from the beginning. At first sight, this is shocking. It serves to emphasize the fact that cancer is not a single disease with one cause and one method of treatment. Control depends on more knowledge than is now available. Some patients can, however, now be cured by early diagnosis and adequate treatment. Many patients can have their effective lives prolonged. In the American culture the tendency to want one complete answer that works universally appears to be one problem contributing to a person's disappointment when the problem turns out to be complex. In whatever phase the patient is when his cancer is discovered, much can be done to improve his condition. There is also the possibility that some discovery will be made that will reverse the disease process.

In the present state of knowledge, the patient's best hope of cure lies in early diagnosis followed by adequate treatment. Slaughter[45] emphasizes the difficulty in establishing a diagnosis of early cancer. One characteristic of early cancer is that it has not invaded the surrounding tissue. According to the American Cancer Society publications, about one half of the persons who have cancer could be cured, if treatment were initiated early enough.

Ideally, every woman over the age of 35 and every man over the age of 45 should have a physical examination every year. According to Dr. Emerson Day,[46] of the Strang Clinic, the cancer-detection examinations should include the following:

History
    Family
    Environment, habits, illness
    Review of systems

Physical
    Skin and lymph nodes
    Head and neck
    Breasts
    Lungs
    Abdomen
    Genitalia
    Rectum—colon
    Extremities

Laboratory
    Hemoglobin or hematocrit
    White blood cell and differential counts
    Urinalysis
    Chest X ray
    Vaginal and cervical smears
    Tubeless gastric analysis
    Stool guaiac

[45] Daniel P. Slaughter, "What Is Early Cancer?" *Post Graduate Medicine*, XXVII, March, 1960, 271-73.

[46] Emerson Day, "What Is an Adequate Cancer Checkup?" *Post Graduate Medicine*, XXVII, March, 1960, p. 275.

Although the doctor is responsible for making the diagnosis, the nurse should know what constitutes a thorough examination and why it is desirable. This knowledge is of value to the nurse as a person and in her practice as a professional person. In her work with patients, she requires this information in order to prepare them for what to expect and for what is expected of them. The examination is planned to elicit two types of information. One is directed toward identifying any condition or situation that predisposes the patient to cancer; the other, toward determining whether the patient has any signs, symptoms, or tissue changes pointing to the presence of cancer.

The information is utilized in two ways. The more obvious is that it is necessary to the diagnosis of the condition of the patient. The other is that, as data are collected about many patients, the data are subject to analysis and then conclusions are drawn as to their relevance. For example, the conclusion that a relationship exists between cancer of the lung and smoking is based on information obtained from the medical histories of many patients and the statistical analysis of the information.

Most physicians agree that specialized medical training is not required to do a thorough cancer examination. Any physician who is convinced that a thorough examination is important should be able to perform it satisfactorily. The first step is to obtain the family and personal history of the patient. Have other members of the family had cancer? If so, where? Did they recover or die from it? Knowledge of cancer in the family tends to be unreliable. In the personal history, such data as where the person lives, whether or not in his work situation he is exposed to carcinogens, whether he smokes and what he smokes, and whether he drinks alcoholic beverages are pertinent. For women, the menstrual history as well as obstetrical data are desired.

A review of systems is made to elicit any information about previous signs or symptoms that the patient has observed. Unless this is done, the patient may not remember them or may think that observations he has made are insignificant. By the review of each system, one by one, the memory of the patient is refreshed and he is given an opportunity to relate his observations. Patients do not always understand why this is necessary. This is especially true when they seek advice for a symptom or sign in one part of the body. The nurse may help the patient by treating the patient's question courteously and answering it, or by referring it to the physician.

The physical examination consists of the palpation and visual inspection of organs to determine changes in color, texture, contour, and function, and of listening to the heart and lungs. The physician performs the examination systematically so that no part is missed. He often begins by inspecting the skin for evidence of an increase or decrease in tissue and for changes in its appearance. Although the physician examines the entire skin surface, he pays special attention to areas exposed to the sun, to the palms and soles, to the genitalia, and to areas subject to repeated trauma, as these are the sites where cancer of the skin most commonly occurs. The skin is observed for small, scaly lesions, small ulcers or sores, lumps, senile keratoses, nevi, pigmented moles, and burn scars. Basal cell carcinoma usually makes its appearance as a small scale, which later disappears and leaves a sore that increases in size. Squamous cell carcinoma may also start with a scaly lesion or a small lump or an encrusted nodule. It is frequently preceded by senile keratosis, a condition in which there are patches of horny hypertrophy of skin in the aged. They often occur on the face. Nevi, or pigmented lesions, in areas subject to chronic irritation or that have undergone a change in size or color, are ulcerated, or bleed, should be viewed with suspicion. Any person with a lesion that is suspected of being a malignant melanoma should consult or be referred to a surgeon who is experienced in treating melanomas.

The palpation of the superficial lymph nodes is an essential part of any cancer-detection examination. Enlargement of lymph nodes may point to lymphomas or leukemia or to cancer in structures drained by the lymph channels supplying the node. An increase in size in a node or group of nodes may be the first evidence of the disease.

A cancer-detection examination of the head and neck includes the inspection of the skin and the oral and nasal cavities, the visualization of the larynx, and the palpation of the oral cavity, the areas containing lymph nodes, and the thyroid gland.

One of the most publicized cancer-detection examinations is that of the breast. There has been a widespread promotional program to teach women how to examine their own breasts. Many doctors instruct their patients in the procedure. Teaching women to examine their own breasts regularly and systematically each month is based on the expectation that women will be able to detect cancer while the disease is still localized in the breast. Instructions for self-examination of the breast may be obtained from the American Cancer Society or from a local branch of the Society. The woman is instructed to report immediately any findings of lumps or changes in the contour or skin of the breast, or secretions from the nipple. The physician follows essentially the same pattern in examining the woman's breast that he teaches her to follow.

The most essential tool in the detection of lung cancer is the chest X ray. Since the lung is a common site of metastasis, the chest X ray is useful not only in detection of primary cancer but in estimation of its prognosis. In persons who are predisposed to lung cancer by their work or personal habits, cytological examination of bronchial secretions may be performed. The presence of abnormal cells in the sputum is an indication for further examination. Physical examination of the chest is also essential. Partial obstruction of a bronchial tube by a neoplasm may cause a wheezing sound as the air passes through accumulated secretions. Further, the partial obstruction may result in the incomplete expansion of a segment of the lung.

The abdomen is palpated to determine the presence of any lumps or increase in size of abdominal organs. Since the liver is a frequent site of metastasis, it receives special attention.

No examination for cancer in women is complete without a thorough investigation of the female reproductive organs. This includes (1) inspection of the external genitalia, (2) inspection of the vagina and cervix with a speculum, (3) collection and staining of cells from the vagina and cervix (Papanicolaou smear examination), and (4) bimanual palpation of the uterus and adnexa. Day[47] emphasizes the importance of the cytological examination in the detection of cancer of the cervix before it becomes invasive. In a series of 107 women examined at the Strang Clinic, approximately 90 per cent of those with cancer were found to have cancer in situ. Of these, 53 per cent were discovered in a cancer-detection examination and before symptoms had occurred. When cancer of the cervix is discovered in the preinvasive phase, it is almost 100 per cent curable.

In preparation for a gynecological examination, a woman should be instructed not to take a vaginal douche. Immediately preceding the examination, she should be asked to empty her urinary bladder. The bed or examining table should be screened and the patient should be draped, so that the genitalia are exposed, but the surrounding area is covered. The patient should lie on her back with her hips flat on the bed or table. When the patient is on an examining table, the hips should be brought to the edge of the table and the legs and thighs supported by stirrups. When the patient is examined in bed, the thighs should be raised so they are perpendicular with the bed. The feet should be resting with the soles flat on the bed. During the examination, the knees are moved outward.

At the beginning of the examination, the external genitalia are inspected for nevi, leukoplakia, ulcerative lesions, and other abnormalities. The vaginal mucous membrane and cervix are examined. The speculum that is used is moistened with water rather than jelly, as the jelly interferes with the cytological examination. Cells are obtained for the vaginal Papanicolaou smear by aspirating secretions from the posterior lateral fornices with a vaginal pipette. The secretions are then spread thinly on a glass slide. The slide is immediately placed in a jar containing equal parts of 95 per cent alcohol and ether. Material for the cervical smear may be obtained by swabbing the surface of the cervix with a cotton applicator and by inserting the cotton into the cervical os and gently rotating it. Another method is to scrape the cervix with a wooden tongue depressor-like device. Material may be obtained from the cervical os by a specially designed cervical scraper. The material obtained from the cervix is spread thinly on a glass slide, and the slide is immediately placed in the alcohol-ether solution.

The physician also investigates the pelvic organs by means of a bimanual examination. As the prefix bi- implies, two hands are used. One hand is placed on the abdomen, and one or more fingers of the other hand are placed in the vagina. By exerting pressure, the physician can determine alteration in the size and conformation of various structures.

[47] Ibid., p. 280.

When areas of the cervix present a suspicious appearance, biopsy may be done to establish the diagnosis. Some physicians do a punch biopsy of the suspicious tissue. This can be performed in the outpatient clinic or in the office of the physician, as well as in the hospital.

Cancer-detection examinations for men should include an investigation of the male reproductive system. This examination should include the inspection and palpation of the external structures and the palpation of the internal organs. Cytological examination may be made on fluids obtained by aspiration from the testes or from a hydrocele. Prostatic fluid may be obtained by massaging the prostate. Every physical examination on an adult male should include the digital examination of the prostate per rectum. From this procedure the physician can identify changes in the size of a part or the entire gland as well as the presence of nodules. Though the enlargement of a lobe or the entire gland is often a benign condition, unless corrected it can cause serious harm by obstructing the flow of urine from the bladder.

Why is a rectal examination an important part of every cancer detection examination?

The digital examination of the rectum serves a further purpose, in that some 50 per cent of lesions in the large bowel are within reach of the examiner's finger. For this reason the physical examination of every adult should include this procedure. Because some lesions are beyond the reach of the examiner's finger or cannot be felt, the examination of the rectum and colon should include a proctosigmoidoscopy. In the proctosigmoidoscopy, a lighted tube is introduced through the anal sphincter into the rectum and sigmoid. The walls of these structures are directly visualized and abnormalities such as polyps, ulcerations, and narrowing of the lumen are noted. This is a relatively simple and safe procedure that can be performed in the office of the physician or in an outpatient clinic. Some physicians instruct the patient to take an enema the night preceding the morning of the examination. The purpose of the enema is obvious—to cleanse the bowel. The importance of cleansing the bowel to the success of the examination should be stressed. Others prefer to do the examination without any special preparation and remove any feces in the area at the time of the examination. The reason for the omission of enemas is that the solution may injure the mucosa lining the bowel and increase the activity of the intestine. The latter makes the performance of the procedure more difficult.

For the performance of the proctosigmoidoscopy, the patient must be placed in a knee-chest position. The process of assuming this position can be strenuous, and the patient may feel embarrassed. To assist the patient into the knee-chest position, he should lie face down on a table that can be adjusted to the proper position or he may be instructed to assume the proper position on the table. When the patient assumes the knee-chest position, he should turn onto his abdomen with his left arm under his chest. His hips are elevated by bringing his legs up so that he rests on his knees and shoulders. When he is in proper position, his thighs are perpendicular to the table and they form one side of a triangle. The other two sides of the triangle are formed by his back and the table. Since a proctosigmoidoscopy takes about five minutes, the patient should not be placed in position until the physician is ready. As with other procedures, unnecessary exposure of the patient should be avoided by draping and screening. Though the procedure is safe, relatively simple, and leaves no after effects, the introduction and movement of the tube may cause cramping. The patient should be reassured that the discomfort is to be expected, and that it will cease as soon as the procedure is completed.

The laboratory examinations performed as part of a cancer-detection examination are for the purpose of uncovering clues indicating the presence of cancer in the body as well as pinpointing its location. At the present, there is no single test for the identification of early cancer. Some laboratory tests, though not specifically for cancer, should be part of every cancer-detection examination. Every examination should include a hemoglobin or hematocrit determination. An unexplained anemia is often the first symptom in cancer of the gastrointestinal and urinary tracts. A leukocyte count combined with a determination of the types of leukocytes (differential white count) may provide evidence of leukemia or lymphoma. A complete urinalysis may provide information indicating the presence of a neoplasm in the kidney or urinary tract. The finding of microscopic amounts of blood in the urine is especially significant. Occult (hidden) blood in the feces may indicate a malignant lesion somewhere along the gastrointestinal tract.

Since cancer located in the stomach is frequently, but not always, associated with a lack of secretion of hydrochloric acid (achlorhydria), gastric analysis may be performed. Secretions may be removed by a tube passed into the stomach. Because it is more acceptable to patients, a "tubeless" test may be performed. Gastric secretion is first stimulated with caffeine. The patient is then given a cation exchange resin containing the cation quininium, or azure A. When the gastric juice contains hydrochloric acid, the resin exchanges the quininium cation, or azure A, for the hydrogen ion in the gastric juice, and the released cation, or azure A, is absorbed and excreted in the urine. In the absence of hydrochloric acid, the azure A is not released and very little appears in the urine.

When suspicious lesions are discovered during a cancer examination, what is the next step?

The discovery of suspicious lesions, signs, or symptoms may make further investigation necessary. The methods used are those that enable the physician to visualize the lesion either directly or indirectly and to obtain tissue for microscopic examination. X ray, endoscopic, and tissue examinations are made. These procedures have been described in other chapters and will not be repeated. The point that many of these examinations are sources of physical and psychological stress bears repeated emphasis. The patient should be prepared for what to expect and for what is expected of him. When the patient is required to prepare himself for a diagnostic procedure, he should be given written, as well as verbal, instructions.

The location of lesions and their general character may be indirectly visualized by X ray or fluoroscopic examination. The progress of lesions may be followed by either endoscopic examination or X ray or both. For example, a patient is found to have an ulcer in his stomach. At the time of the initial examination, it appears to be a benign lesion on both the gastroscopic and X ray examinations. Though ulcers occurring in the stomach can be benign, they are usually viewed with suspicion. Following treatment, the patient is again examined to determine any changes in the size of the ulcer. Failure of the ulcer to diminish in size and to give other evidence of healing is presumptive evidence that the lesion is not benign.

The diagnosis of cancer is confirmed by the finding of cancer cells by microscopic examination. When tissue is removed for this purpose, the entire procedure is called a biopsy. When the lesion can be reached from the surface of the body either directly or through a small incision, the procedure itself is relatively minor. Cells may be obtained in body fluids by using a needle or by introducing a punch into the tissue or by cutting out a piece. Tissue is removed from the uterus by scraping. At times a body cavity, such as the abdominal or the thoracic cavity, must be opened to obtain the necessary tissue. In the emphasis on the biopsy as the critical procedure in establishing the diagnosis of cancer, the point may be missed that it is equally useful in establishing that a patient does not have cancer. For example, only four out of ten lumps in the breast are cancerous. Neither are all lumps in other organs malignant. When they are, treatment is initiated promptly. When they are not, the patient can be reassured that he does not have cancer.

At the time a diagnosis of cancer is made, the characteristics of the cancer and the extent of its spread are evaluated. This information is useful in estimating the prognosis of a patient. The characteristics of the cancer are determined by macroscopic and microscopic examination. The macroscopic examination yields information about the size, shape, consistency, and location of the neoplasm. From looking at and feeling the growth, information is gained about whether the neoplasm (1) extends into or grows around an organ, (2) is separate from or has invaded the surrounding tissue, (3) is hard or soft, (4) is ulcerating or intact, and (5) has spread to distant points. The microscopic examination provides information about the character of the cancer cells and the degree to which they resemble or differ from healthy cells. It is also useful in determining the extent of metastasis. With few exceptions, the more cells differ from healthy cells in character and organization, the more rapidly they grow and the faster they metastasize. Pathologists have devised a way of classifying neoplasms according to the degree of differentiation and organization of cells. This is known as grading. The scale is from I to IV. Neoplasms in which the differentiation and organization of cells differs from the normal from 0 to 25 per cent are graded as I. Those that differ from 75 to 100 per cent from normal are graded IV. Grades II and III are in between. On this scale, Grade I neoplasms are slow-growing and slow to metastasize. Those of Grade IV are rapid-growing and early to metastasize.

Neoplasms in some organs are also typed according to extent of spread. The organ for which this was done the earliest was the large bowel. The extent of spread of malignant neoplasms in the large bowel is typed as A, B, and C. In a type A neoplasm, the neoplasm involves only the mucosal and muscularis coats. In type B, the neoplasm extends so that it involves, in addition to the above tissues, the serosa. A type C neoplasm not only involves the above tissues, but has spread to the neighboring lymph nodes. At the time typing of neoplasms was introduced, the fact that cancer cells are shed into the venous blood was not known.

The combination of grading and typing provides information used by the physician to predict the prognosis of the patient. In general, poorly differentiated and disorganized cells, combined with extensive spread, indicate a poor prognosis. A slow-growing neoplasm discovered early, that is, while the disease is still localized, offers a good prognosis. The prediction of prognosis is like that of any other prediction; it is based on knowledge of facts as they are known today. Some patients live longer than expected. Others die sooner. New knowledge makes conditions that were untreatable now treatable.

Because the outlook of patients with neoplasms that respond to therapy depends on early diagnosis and treatment, every individual is important in a cancer-control program. Physicians disagree as to the advisability, practicality, and possibility of every person having a yearly or, as some suggest, biyearly cancer-detection examination. Some physicians suggest that efforts be concentrated on patients in high-risk groups. Women over 30 or 35 years of age and men over 40 years of age are encouraged to have yearly examinations. A family history of cancer, a past history of cancer, smoking, and employment in a hazardous occupation (involving exposure to carcinogens) are suggested as indications for a regular checkup.

Every individual has a responsibility in cancer detection. Persons who have regular physical examinations may, however, develop signs or symptoms that indicate the possibility of cancer. Many, for one reason or another, see a physician only when they are obviously ill. In order to help people recognize signs and symptoms that indicate the possibility of cancer, the American Cancer Society has prepared and distributed a list known as the *Seven Danger Signals*. These signs and symptoms are not positive proof that cancer is present any more than smoke in the kitchen is proof that the house is on fire; it may be, or a pan may have been allowed to become dry. In either case, something needs to be done, but the seriousness of the situation varies.

Prompt action is required to prevent unnecessary damage. The seven danger signals are: "(1) any sore that does not heal, (2) any lump or thickening in the breast or elsewhere, (3) unexplained bleeding or discharge, (4) persistent indigestion or difficulty in swallowing, (5) change in bowel habits, (6) any change in a wart or mole, and (7) persistant hoarseness or cough." There are a number of other danger signals. These are, however, the important ones. Prompt reporting of any of these does not necessarily ensure that the cancer is in an early stage. Prompt reporting plus regular medical examination with follow-through on advice given is the best protection available.

There has been some criticism of programs to educate the lay public to have yearly or biyearly examinations, and of techniques of cancer detection. The basis for the criticism is that this may lead individuals to have an unnecessary concern about the possibility of having cancer. Those who disagree say that this happens only in persons who are predisposed to worrying about their health. If they were not concerned about cancer, they would be concerned about some other disease or problem.

Cancer detection depends on people and facilities. The term "people" encompasses everyone, not only the person who suspects or knows he has cancer, but also professional personnel who understand the nature of cancer and its manifestations and have the skills that enable them to identify suspicious lesions or changes. In order for a lay person to participate in cancer detection he must know what to look for and where to go for help. He also needs to know that help is available, if he seeks it. The professional personnel must have the conviction that cancer detection is important and that it makes a significant contribution to the well-being of people. Following the stage of cancer detection, persons with suspicious lesions go on to diagnosis.

With diagnosis, therapy follows. Three types of therapy are available. They are surgery, radiation, and chemotherapy. In the treatment of any patient, any one or a combination may be used. The plan of treatment is based on the condition of the individual patient, the nature, extent, and location of the lesion, and what can be expected from a given therapeutic agent. That is to say, therapy is individually tailored. The initiation of a plan of therapy is contingent on its acceptance by the patient. Occasionally a patient prefers to take his chances with cancer to the treatment that is suggested. This is his right, and must be respected as such. In this event the plan has to be modified, so that it becomes acceptable to the patient. Some patients, given time and support that recognizes their right to make their own decisions, will eventually agree to the original plan. The outcome is not always as bad as anticipated. For example, Mrs. Friend had a malignant melanoma on the sole of her left foot. At the time of diagnosis, the recommendation was made that she have a high leg amputation, but she refused to have the operation. Instead of dying within a few months, she lived for 10 or 12 years. She lived, for the most part, an active life. Sometimes children whose parents refuse amputation for the treatment of melanoma live for a number of years after the diagnosis is made. In other instances where parents allow the amputation to be done, the activity of the disease is increased and death comes soon thereafter. Although patients and parents do not always make what appears to be, at the time, a wise decision, the result is not inevitably bad. Whatever the outcome, however, they have the right to their choice. This right should be respected.

The objective of all types of therapy is to remove or destroy all the cancer cells in the body. To date, no method has been devised that is completely successful. The term "cure" is used cautiously. Though the physician may be reasonably certain that all cancer cells have been eradicated from an individual who has cancer, he cannot be positive. Terms are coined to express this caution in the use of the word "cure." Thus patients who are alive and well at the end of five years are said to have a five-year cure. Those who are alive and well at the end of ten years have a ten-year cure. The patient who is alive and well at the end of five years is presumed to be cured, but this is not a certainty.

In patients with advanced and progressive disease, therapy has as its objective the amelioration of the condition of the patient. The same methods are used as in the curative treatment of cancer. The criterion for success is that the patient is objectively or subjectively improved. Though palliative therapy is sometimes neglected, there is much that can be done to improve the well-being and comfort of the patient for whom there is little chance of cure.

For example, Mrs. Jane Merriweather, who had a large abdominal mass, was short of breath on the slightest exertion, she was anorexic, and when she did force herself to eat, she usually became nauseated and vomited. She was losing weight and strength rapidly. She looked and felt sick and discouraged. Soon after X ray treatment was initiated, improvement was noticeable. On palpation of her abdomen, the tumor could be felt to be smaller in size. Even Mrs. Merriweather had objective evidence that the tumor was regressing as she could again wear dresses with belts. She gained weight. Subjectively she felt better. She was able to carry on moderate activity without becoming short of breath. She felt encouraged and stronger. Her appetite improved and she began to enjoy her meals. The basis for the use of X ray in the treatment of Mrs. Merriweather was palliation. The X ray did not, and was not expected to, cure. Mrs. Merriweather did have, however, several months in which she was relatively well.

What is the history of the use of surgery in the treatment of cancer?

According to *Primer on Cancer for Nurses*,[48] the surgical treatment of cancer goes back some 3,500 years. The Greeks and Egyptians have recorded the surgical removal of tumors. The first successful operation for cancer was

[48] *Primer on Cancer for Nurses,* New York Cancer Committee of the American Cancer Society, New York, 1963.

performed in 1882, when Bilroth removed a cancer of the stomach. The history of the advances that contributed to the development of modern surgery are outlined in Chapter 15. Suffice it to say that as knowledge of ligatures, anesthesia, asepsis, and the physiological needs of man, as well as techniques for meeting his needs, has increased, more and more extensive surgery has been possible. As a consequence, cancer in any body cavity or any part of the body may be removed surgically. Some of the problems that arise as the result of the surgical treatment of cancer are similar to those that arise in the surgical treatment of patients for other conditions. In addition, there are problems that arise out of the fact that the diagnosis is cancer. Then too, the surgical procedure is often, though by no means always, more extensive than it is in the treatment of noncancerous conditions.

What is the objective toward which the surgical treatment of cancer is directed?

The objective on which the surgical treatment of cancer is based is the extirpation of the primary growth and the tissues to which it has extended. In the performance of the operation, the surgeon tries to encircle the growth without cutting into it, in order to prevent its spread. Since learning that cancer cells can be found in the venous blood draining the neoplasm and the surrounding area, some surgeons now tie off these veins before attempting to remove the cancer. The extent of the operation selected depends on the natural history of the cancer, the condition of the patient, and the stage of the disease. For example, a slow-growing cancer that spreads locally by invading the surrounding tissue, such as an early basal cell carcinoma, may be successfully removed by simple excision. In squamous cell carcinoma, however, the lymph channels and nodes are excised in addition to the primary lesion, because it spreads through the lymphatics. In the treatment of malignant melanoma, an entire limb may be removed, because widespread dissemination of malignant cells has occurred by the time the disease is manifested.

Why may surgical therapy be useful in palliation?

Surgical treatment may also be undertaken as a palliative measure. Though it is not expected to prolong the patient's life, it is performed to increase his comfort and well-being. The lesion itself may be removed, or rerouting or short-circuiting operations may be done to relieve symptoms of obstruction. The nerve supply to an area may be disrupted to relieve pain or muscle spasm. The indication for the removal of the neoplasm is that it is necrotic, infected, or bleeding. Ulcerated and infected lesions are the common cause of pain in cancer. When the lesion is at the surface of the body, the control of odors is difficult. Removal of the growth may result in relief of pain and in a general improvement of the patient. The effects of obstruction have been discussed earlier.

Another type of palliative surgery is based on the observation that the growth of some tissues is dependent on certain hormones. Cancer of the breast sometimes regresses after oophorectomy. Castration in the male may be of benefit in cancer of the prostate. Adrenalectomy and hypophysectomy are also of benefit in selected patients. In these operations, the beneficial effect is presumed to result from removing a condition favorable to the growth of the neoplasm. The possibility exists that as more is learned about the factors favoring the establishment of metastatic growths, these and other organs may be removed before, or at the time, the local growth is excised. If this should come to pass, then the operation would be curative.

The same principles apply to the preparation of the patient for a surgical procedure as of other patients, undergoing surgery. The patient requires emotional, physiological, and physical preparation. The patient needs to know what to expect and what is expected of him. He needs to be able to trust those responsible for his care and to know that he can count on them to meet his needs. In patients who are admitted one day and undergo a surgical procedure the following day, there is little time to develop a trusting relationship. Each step or act in the process of the admission of the patient is therefore exceedingly important. When people are under stress, they tend to magnify and personalize behavior that under happier circumstances would pass unnoticed or be dismissed as unimportant.

Patients who require special preparation because of the location of the lesion or because of the need to repair physiological deficits may be in the hospital some days before surgery is scheduled. Improvement in the patient's physiological status may be essential to his survival. The correction of anemia and protein and other nutritional deficiencies, as well as restoration of water and electrolyte balance and/or relief of obstruction, is often a required part of preoperative preparation.

Ionizing radiation is also utilized to eradicate cancer cells or in palliation. In either event, it may be used alone or in combination with surgery or chemotherapy. It may be used previous to operation to reduce the size of the neoplasm or after a suitable period to destroy cells that remain behind. The principle on which the treatment is based is that cells in the process of mitosis are more susceptible to ionizing radiation than are mature cells. The susceptibility of cells to ionizing radiation is greatest when they are proliferating and least when they are well differentiated. Ionizing radiation may be applied over an area or be administered as a radioactive isotope in solution. The latter is useful in the few instances in which the body removes the isotope from the blood and concentrates it in a selected tissue. Radioactive iodine is useful in the treatment of cancer of the thyroid because the thyroid gland removes the iodine from the blood and concentrates it in the gland. In addition, the half-life of iodine is 8.1 days, which makes it suitable and practical to use. Radioactive gold is sometimes injected into the pleural cavity of patients with advanced cancer of the lung to slow the rate at which fluid collects. The effects of ionizing radiation, the measures required for the protection of patient and personnel, and the nursing needs of patients under therapy are discussed in Chapter 3.

New methods for the treatment of cancer are under investigation. Further reduction in the death rate from cancer probably depends on new approaches to the problem. Recently, two surgeons at different meetings stated that new benefits from surgical or radiation therapy could not be expected. The need for new methods for the prevention, identification, and treatment of cancer is emphasized by the following evidence. Goodman and Gilman[49] state that at present only 25 per cent of patients known to have cancer are alive and well at the end of five years. The American Cancer Society estimates that 50 per cent could be cured, were all patients diagnosed and treated early.

How is chemotherapy employed in the therapy of cancer?

Chemotherapy is the newest form of cancer therapy. With rare exceptions, its benefits are largely palliative. Crile[50] summarizes the use of chemotherapy as follows: (1) to prevent the reaccumulation of fluid in the pleural or peritoneal cavities, given locally, (2) to relieve pain, (3) to prevent metastasis, (4) to treat small infants, (5) to enhance the action of radiation therapy by concurrent administration, acting synergistically with it, and (6) to treat certain well-differentiated cancers in the colon, using 5-fluorouracil, which has proved to be useful in their treatment. Crile does not include in his list the use of drugs to induce a remission in leukemia and lymphoma. The use of chemotherapy in the prevention of metastasis is under test at the present time but its value has not been proved. Nitrogen mustard is administered in conjunction with a surgical procedure, in an attempt to lessen the danger of spread of cancer cells at that time.

One value of chemotherapy, or any other new treatment, that is difficult to measure objectively is the hope that it generates in the patient, his family, and those who care for him. During his illness the patient badly needs hope and the feeling that something is being done for him. The patient is often comforted by the knowledge that he may be helping others by participating in the investigation of a drug or treatment. He derives satisfaction from being treated as an important partner in the study. Even when the drug or treatment fails to meet expectations, the psychological benefits to patients and personnel may be considerable. Chemotherapeutic agents are of two general types. One type selectively injures a cancer cell in dosages that are insufficient to injure healthy cells. The other type of agent alters the climate of environment of the cell so that its growth is depressed.

To be ideal, a chemotherapeutic agent would act only on cancer cells and not affect healthy cells. To date no such agent has been discovered. Moreover,

---

[49] Louis S. Goodman and Alfred Gilman, *The Pharmacological Basis of Therapeutics,* 2nd ed., The Macmillan Company, New York, 1955, p. 1414.

[50] George Crile, Jr., "Chemotherapy in Cancer," *Postgraduate Medicine,* XXVIII, September, 1960, 242-47.

as more is learned about the nature of cancer, the expectation of finding a single agent that is effective in all instances seems unrealistic. Goodman and Gilman[51] summarize the difficulties that stand in the way of developing effective chemicotherapeutic agents as follows: (1) unlike microorganisms, neoplastic agents are not foreign invaders; (2) the biological characteristics, particularly with respect to cell growth and differentiation, are similar for healthy and for normal cells; and (3) unlike microorganisms, the defenses of the host are ineffective in destroying cells not killed by the drug. Some authorities are of the opinion that the body has no defense against malignant neoplasms. Others are not sure that this is true. There are some experiments with animals and clinical observations to support the latter view. In the present state of knowledge, however, body defenses against cancer do not appear to be as effective as they are against microorganisms.

Drugs that injure cells are of two types. The alkylating agents have a direct toxic action on cells. Because their effect is similar to that of ionizing radiation, they are said to have a radiomimetic action. Included in this group of drugs are thio-TEPA and the nitrogen mustards. These drugs, like ionizing radiation, are capable of injuring healthy as well as cancer cells. The same general principles apply to both. Cells undergoing mitosis are more vulnerable than are quiescent cells. Their effectiveness appears to be related to the rate of cell division The more rapid the rate, the more easily they are injured. Tissues that are sensitive to ionizing radiation are also sensitive to chemical cytotoxins. The toxic effects result from injury to bone marrow and other sensitive tissues.

The other group of chemicals that injure cells are the antimetabolites. These chemicals simulate and compete with essential components of nucleic acid. They are incorporated into the substance of the cell, but are useless to it. Their action is similar to that of sulfonamides on bacteria. Sulfonamides are more effective against bacteria, because the body defense mechanisms complete the destruction of damaged and remaining cells. Amethopterin (methotrexate U.S.P.) has proved to be effective in the treatment of a rare cancer, choriocarcinoma. The use of 5-fluorouracil in the therapy of certain cancers of the colon has been indicated. One of the uses of the folic acid antagonists, aminoptoroylgutamate sodium (Aminopterin[52]) and methotrexate, is to induce a remission in leukemia. The adrenal glucocorticoids are also useful in the therapy of leukemia. For a complete discussion of these and other drugs used in the chemotherapy of cancer, the student is referred to a pharmacology text or recent periodicals.

To summarize, in our present state of knowledge, drugs that injure cells by their chemical action are primarily useful in palliation. In acute leukemia, appropriately selected drugs may induce a remission lasting up to a year or more. All agents presently available have serious toxic effects. They all de-

[51] Goodman and Gilman, *Op. cit.*, p. 1414.
[52] Trade name.

press the bone marrow. Bleeding and gastrointestinal disturbances are common. Ulcerations in the mouth accompany the use of folic acid antagonists. They add to the discomfort of the patient and make it more difficult for him to eat. Mouth care and selection of bland foods may mitigate the patient's discomfort somewhat. The nitrogen mustards cause irritation of tissues with which they come in contact. They are administered by a physician who makes every effort to prevent the nitrogen mustard from escaping into surrounding tissue.

The main group of chemical agents used to alter the environment of cells are those hormones that affect the growth of tissues. At the present time the effect of hormones is palliative. In estrogen-dependent cancer of the breast, growth of the lesion is temporarily slowed and pain may be relieved by the administration of androgens. One of the curious findings in postmenopausal women who have cancer of the breast is that estrogens may be palliative. Estrogens sometimes are palliative in the treatment of cancer of the prostate. Adrenal cortical hormones, such as cortisone, induce remission in some children with acute leukemia, but the remissions are temporary. In acute leukemia the number of chromosomes in the leukemic cells is abnormal, though the number is constant in all the cells. During a remission the number returns to normal, that is, 46. During a relapse, the number returns to whatever it was before the remission. Since there are now a number of agents that are capable of producing a remission, the fact that the child no longer responds to one does not mean that he will not be responsive to another.

Since hormones are among the growth regulators in the body, as more is learned about the process of cell growth their use may be expanded. Other hormones may come into use. In certain cancers of the thyroid in animals, thyroxin is capable of restoring the tissue to normal. The growth hormone from the anterior pituitary has been recently isolated. Perhaps studies with it will offer clues to more effective treatment.

Despite progress in the control of cancer, much remains to be accomplished. Not all patients with a curable form of the disease are diagnosed early enough to receive maximum benefit from present-day methods. New methods are required for the control of the types of cancer that do not respond to surgery, radiation, or chemotherapy. Further progress awaits greater knowledge of the factors controlling the growth of normal cells. Crile[53] emphasizes this point in a concept that applies to all medicine when he states, "progress comes through understanding the ways of nature rather than from trying to bend them to our will."

How is the patient helped to resume his normal activities?

As the patient recovers, he is helped to resume responsibility for meeting his own needs and to prepare to return to his family and the community.

[53] Crile, "The Cancer Problem," *Op. cit.,* p. 380.

Sutherland,[54] in discussing the psychological impact of cancer surgery, emphasizes the importance of considering every patient in the light of his individual problems. Each person makes his own adjustment to his kind of cancer and its treatment. Sutherland[55] also stresses that the cancer patient is under a special and severe form of stress. The psychological mechanisms of the defense that he utilizes are those he has learned to use in coping with the world. Just as patients use avoidance and denial to defend themselves against anxiety before diagnosis and treatment, they use it after surgery to protect themselves against the anxiety induced by the therapy. They also experience grief, depression, and dependency. Some patients may be so seriously depressed that they cannot recover without help. For most patients, depression is a forerunner of recovery. Instead of becoming depressed, some patients express their anger by projecting their feelings to the members of the family and the nursing personnel.

In cancer and its treatment, many factors may cause psychological stress. The fact that the disease is cancer rather than some other disease is one. Stress is particularly likely to arise out of treatment when the effects of treatment are obvious, or a bodily function is altered in a way that is obvious to the individual and/or to others. The patient often experiences shock when he realizes the extent of the operation or the nature of the change in function. He becomes concerned about how this change in appearance or function will affect his relationship with members of his family, his friends, and his co-workers. His concern extends to how this change is going to affect his ability to make a living.

In the study by Sutherland, et al.,[56] of the problems in living created by colostomy and what patients did to solve these problems, the authors emphasize that one of the most significant factors is a supportive spouse or home situation. The adjustment of the patient was in general more rapid and more satisfactory when the husband-and-wife relationships were favorable. In families where the relationships had been poor before the colostomy was performed, relationships deteriorated after it. These findings point to the desirability of utilizing family members whose feelings toward the patient are positive in his rehabilitation. Nurses are not responsible for the nature of family relationships of their patients, but they can and do observe these relationships. This information can be used in planning to meet the needs of the patient. Recognition of the importance of the family to the rehabilitation of the patient should result in including them in plans made to meet the needs of the patient. Sutherland, et al.,[57] state that the family must understand the needs of the patient and why they are important to him, if they are to give him

[54] Arthur Sutherland, "Psychological Impact of Cancer Surgery," *Public Health Reports*, LXVIII, November, 1952, p. 1143.
[55] *Ibid.*
[56] Arthur M. Sutherland, *et al.*, "The Psychological Impact of Cancer and Cancer Surgery," *Cancer*, V, September, 1952, pp. 857-72.
[57] *Ibid.*, p. 868.

adequate support. The family may require considerable interpretation. To fulfill their supportive role, family members need to have their efforts recognized and appreciated. Perhaps a book is needed to emphasize the fact that families are people, too. There are reasons for their behavior, be it calm, kind, thoughtful, helpful, frantic, neglectful, or unkind. Whatever the behavior of relatives of the patient, they, too, should be treated with courtesy and kindness. Their attempts at being helpful should be guided and appreciated. Relatives can sometimes be of help to themselves and to the patient if they can assist with certain aspects of his care. Since nurses cannot and should not try to be all things to all people, problems with relatives of the patient should be discussed with the physician. The purpose of this discussion should be to find ways of working with the family of the patient more productively. Sometimes the physician can help by talking with one or more of the relatives. In hospitals where social workers are available, the family may be referred to them for help. Another source of help and comfort to the family is their spiritual advisor. The nurse is by no means alone in her efforts to meet the needs of the family for support.

Sutherland, et al.,[58] also reported that patients regarded a warm and supporting relationship with the nurses as important in changing their attitude and aiding in their recovery. The desire of the nurse to be helpful and her willingness to search out measures that improve the feeling of well-being of the patient are imperative. Attention to details that increase the physical comfort of the patient is sometimes neglected. Since lower needs must be met before higher needs can be manifested, the undernourished or dehydrated patient cannot be expected to feel encouraged; neither can the patient whose bed is wet with urine or feces. As an illustration, Mrs. Karlin had an ileostomy in the treatment of chronic ulcerative colitis. She wore an ileostomy bag that was glued to the skin with a type of adhesive. For the seal to be effective, both the skin and the rubber disc that attached to the skin had to be perfectly clean. Any soiling of either meant that the intestinal contents leaked under the rubber disc and out onto the skin of the abdomen, thus soiling her clothing and the bed linen. Since the contents of the ileum are liquid, enzymes contained in them come in intimate contact with the skin, thereby causing irritation. Continuously wet or moist skin also loses its resistance to irritation. Mrs. Karlin was asked to speak to a group of nurses about the quality of care that she received. Her major criticism stemmed from the fact that, until her doctor taught her to care for the apparatus herself, she was never dry. Once she assumed responsibility for her own care, she was never again wet. This patient suffered psychological stress and physical injury not because nurses were unkind or unfriendly, but because a basic physical need was neglected.

To be helpful, the nurse must be able to allow the patient to become dependent without herself becoming unduly anxious. She must also be able to

[58] *Ibid.*, p. 866.

tolerate projection of the negative feelings of the patient and still remain accepting and kindly. This is not always easy to do, especially when the nurse has tried very hard to meet the patient's needs and wants, and he still continues to be critical and dissatisfied. The behavior of the patient is, however, his way of coping with an intolerable situation. If the nurse can accept it as such, she is in a better position to be helpful to the patient. She will have less need to punish the patient or herself for his behavior. One nurse was able to help herself when she was caring for a highly critical patient by saying to herself, "There must be a reason, there must be a reason." To her surprise, when the nurse had convinced herself that the behavior of the patient was reasonable, her relationship with the patient improved.

Another technique that sometimes helps is a group conference in which persons responsible for the care of a patient discuss the nature of the problem presented by the patient. Knowing that others, also, are aware of the problem often is of help. Planning together to develop methods of coping with the patient is most essential.

Observation of the behavior of the patient is also the responsibility of the nurse. Continued disruption in his sleeping and eating patterns after the acute phase of illness or treatment is indicative of depression. Depression may also be accompanied by disturbances in cardiovascular function which is evidenced by tachycardia and palpitation. Patients, especially women, often cry. Though some depression is to be expected, severe or prolonged depression is not.

To summarize, a warm and friendly relationship between the nurse and patient facilitates his recovery. This relationship is characterized by mutual trust. The patient knows that he and his welfare are important to the nurse and that in so far as is possible she will try to meet his needs.

In the restoration of the patient to health, attention must be given to the physiological needs of the patient. If the neoplasm has been in the gastrointestinal tract or has affected its function, the patient may be both dehydrated and undernourished. Loss of weight, fatigue, and weakness may be evident. Anemia present before surgery may be a continuing problem. The ingenuity of the nursing and dietary staff is often taxed in finding ways to improve the nutritional status of the patient. In addition to trying to serve the patient foods that he can and will eat, a number of other activities may be helpful. One is to be sure that he has his dentures and that they are clean. Exercise improves not only muscle tone, but morale and the appetite. Ventilation of the room, and getting the patient into a chair or into a position that facilitates eating may be of help. When possible eating in a community dining room may create a social atmosphere conducive to eating. Continued refusal of the patient to eat may be evidence of depression.

In addition to the psychological and physiological rehabilitation of the patient, the patient is helped to resume responsibilities for the daily activities of living and for his special requirements that result from the fact he has, or has had, cancer and from its treatment. As the patient resumes increasing responsibility for meeting his own needs, the nurse should try to communicate that (1) the shift indicates progress toward recovery, (2) she is standing by to give him assistance, if he really needs it, (3) she has faith in his ability to care for himself, (4) she will not interfere with his efforts unnecessarily, (5) she appreciates the struggle that he is making, and (6) she recognizes his successful efforts.

The nurse should try to avoid any behavior that suggests to the patient that responsibility for his care is shifted to him because the nurse is too busy or does not want to give the care. The nurse should be sure that the patient knows what is expected of him and what he should expect. She is also responsible for supervising his care, so that his needs are met.

Procedures that a patient has to carry out after he goes home should be taught to him, as well as to a member of his family, before he leaves the hospital. The groundwork for the instruction of the patient begins when he first contacts members of the health team with a suspicion of illness and continues throughout all phases of his care. By the time he is ready to be taught to care for his own needs he should have developed confidence in nurses and doctors. The nurses and doctors should also know what the patient wants to know, what he already knows, and something about his home and work situation, as well as his goals. The instructor should know that people learn more slowly when they are excessively anxious. The person instructing should be prepared to repeat over and over, patiently and simply, the instructions to be followed. The nurse who instructs the patient should also be skilled in the performance of the procedure she is attempting to teach the patient; otherwise, the patient will distrust her and may even hold her in contempt. The patient should be helped to practice the procedure using the equipment and materials that are available to him at home, and he should learn how to care for necessary equipment. Enough time should be allotted for practice that the patient has an opportunity to develop some degree of confidence in his ability to cope with the required procedures.

In communities where a visiting nurse service is available, referral of the patient to this agency to provide the assistance required should help the patient to bridge the gap between the hospital and the home. Problems that did not occur to the patient earlier may arise; minor adjustments may assume major proportions. Even patients (and their families) who seem to be well prepared for discharge frequently require some help and emotional support after discharge. In cities where home care programs are available, cooperation between hospital and visiting nursing service often makes possible the early discharge of patients. In some instances a home care program reduces the cost of illness and facilitates the rate at which the patient recovers. When a patient is discharged from the hospital early, supervision of his care and provisions for required assistance become imperative.

In some communities, persons who have had surgical procedures such as colostomy or laryngectomy are organized into a society for the purpose of mutual support. Members of these organizations are eager to assist persons facing surgery and to aid in their adjustment afterward. In some areas, classes are available for laryngectomized patients to learn esophageal speech. Physicians may arrange for a person who has made a successful adjustment to laryngectomy or colostomy to visit each patient who is facing a similar procedure and to continue his visits thereafter. Nurses may also make these arrangements. When they do, they should be acquainted with the wishes of the physician as well as with the nature of the adjustment made by the person called upon to help. Information about local organizations can be obtained from the local division of the American Cancer Society.

In the care of the patient with cancer, in any phase of his life, the objective is to eradicate it and to assist the patient in returning to as normal a life as his condition permits. To meet his needs during detection, diagnosis, and treatment, attention should be given to: (1) his needs as an individual, (2) his needs that result from cancer and its effects, (3) his needs that result from the general method of treatment, and (4) his needs that result from the effects of the treatment on his emotional and physiological condition.

Where is emphasis placed in the care of the patient with widespread and progressive disease?

At the time of diagnosis or at any point thereafter, cancer may be found to be widespread and progressive. Hope for cure or even for prolonging the life of the patient is not expected, that is, death is the probable outcome. For this reason, this phase in the life of the cancer patient is called terminal. It may extend over weeks and months and even, at times, over years. The use of the word "terminal" is unfortunate as it suggests that the patient's situation is hopeless. The result has been that patients in this phase of illness have been and still are neglected. The tendency has been to give preference to those in whom cure is a possibility. Despite the improbability of cure, much can be done to improve the condition and well-being of the patient.

The basic ingredient in the care of the patient with widespread and progressive disease is the firm conviction that something can and should be done to help the patient. Emphasis is placed not on cure, but on what can be done. Hope is encouraged, rather than hopelessness and despair. Objectives for the patient's care include: (1) to encourage and support the patient's efforts to remain independent and useful, (2) to maintain physiological function, and (3) to prevent and relieve suffering. As is often the case, some of the same procedures contribute to the accomplishment of more than one objective. To achieve these objectives the nurse requires some understanding of her own feelings toward death. Most healthy people feel uncomfortable in the presence of the dying and the dead. The words "dead" and "death" are avoided whenever possible. Instead words and phrases such as "passed away," "passed on," and "expired" are used. Until recently little has been available in the medical literature about the care of the dying. See Chapter 2 for a more detailed discussion of the care of the dying patient.

How do patients react to the diagnosis and treatment of cancer? How does the site of the lesion affect the behavior and needs of the patient?

To this point, information that will be useful in understanding the needs of patients with cancer has been stressed. In the section that follows, the needs of Mrs. Robin, who had cancer of the breast treated by radical mastectomy, and Mrs. Alan Wren, who had cancer of the sigmoid colon treated by combined abdominal perineal resection, will be discussed.

During her regular monthly examination of her breasts, Mrs. Robin found a small lump in the upper outer quadrant of her right breast. For a moment she thought that she must be mistaken, but it was there, alright. After a sleepless night, she made an appointment with Dr. Smith, her family physician. He confirmed the fact that there was a lump and suggested that she see Dr. Surgeon for diagnosis. He reminded her that tumors in the breast are frequently harmless. Mrs. Robin asked if there was any hurry about seeing the surgeon. She had not told her husband that she had an appointment with the physician, and their daughter Margery was to graduate from high school in three weeks. Seeking to delay diagnosis and treatment is not uncommon, for the patient reasons that his or her condition cannot be serious, if delay is permitted. Dr. Smith suggested that Mrs. Robin tell her husband that evening. He also stated that if she saw the surgeon within the next week and the lesion proved to be harmless, she would enjoy her daughter's graduation more than if she waited. As a result, ten days after her visit to Dr. Smith, Dr. Surgeon performed a biopsy. A frozen section of the neoplasm was made. It proved to be malignant. Dr. Surgeon then proceeded to perform a radical mastectomy.

Mrs. Robin was admitted to the hospital the afternoon previous to the morning when the biopsy was to be performed. Since the extent of the operation was to be determined by the biopsy, she was prepared for a radical mastectomy. Dr. Surgeon had explained to Mr. and Mrs. Robin that this was a possibility; so she was not surprised. In planning Mrs. Robin's nursing care, four major elements had to be given consideration. First, Mrs. Robin is an individual human being who reacts or behaves in an individual manner; second, at the time Mrs. Robin was admitted, the nature of her illness was uncertain, but following biopsy the diagnosis was established as cancer; third, Mrs. Robin had an extensive surgical procedure; fourth, the operation was a radical mastectomy. The information required to meet the first three is presented elsewhere. The discussion that follows relates principally to meeting Mrs. Robin's requirements arising from having radical breast amputation. All elements, had to be taken into account in meeting her needs for nursing.

In the postoperative period the nursing care required by Mrs. Robin was accomplished by planning to meet the following objectives: (1) to facilitate her emotional adjustment to the removal of her breast, (2) to heal her wound, and (3) to maintain the function in her right arm.

When Mrs. Robin recovered from the anesthetic she was overwhelmed by the extent of the procedure. Her entire breast had been removed along with lymph channels, axillary lymph nodes, and the pectoral muscles. Her chest and the upper part of her right arm were swathed in dressings.

In a radical mastectomy a large area of tissue is removed and many blood vessels are disrupted. This results in the formation of a large amount of fluid exudate in the wound area. Although some fluid in the wound is to be expected, large amounts delay healing, and the fluid must be removed before healing takes place. Surgeons meet this problem in different ways. One is, as was done for Mrs. Robin, to apply a large pressure dressing over the area to lessen the exudation of fluid and to prevent it from accumulating in the wound. This fluid drains from the wound into the dressings. When the dressings become saturated, they may be reinforced by the nurse. Because hemorrhage is always a possibility, the nurse must decide when the quantity of drainage is excessive. In general, the wound exudate is a straw-colored fluid that is blood-tinged. Obvious bleeding is bright red in color and should be immediately reported to the physician. Changes in vital signs, such as a fall in blood pressure and an increase in pulse rate, are also indicative of hemorrhage. When there is external evidence of bleeding, the nurse should not wait for the pulse and blood pressure to change before reporting the bleeding to the physician. A point to remember when checking dressings for blood or other fluids is that water runs downhill. Therefore, the part of the dressing next to the bed should always be checked. This same principle is also used to facilitate drainage from a wound.

A second method employed by some surgeons to remove the wound exudate is to insert catheters into the wound to which gentle suction is applied by a suction machine or a commercial device known as a Hemovac. (See Figure 12-4.) As wound exudate is suctioned into the Hemovac, pressures are gradually equalized. To maintain suction, the drum must be emptied of drainage and the negative pressure re-established as illustrated below. The inside of the Hemovac is sterile; great caution must be taken to maintain this sterility when the drum is emptied, as the serosanguineous exudate being suctioned from the wound provides an ideal medium for the proliferation of microorganisms.

Characteristics of drainage are easily observed through transparent walls of the drum; all pertinent facts about drainage are reported and recorded when the drum is emptied.

Because of materials used in its construction, the Hemovac cannot be resterilized. It is discarded after use for a single patient. No dressing, or only a small dressing, is applied. The catheters may be left in place for three or four

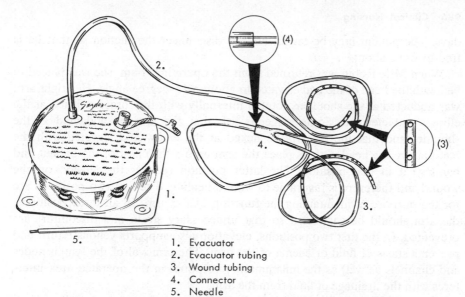

1. Evacuator
2. Evacuator tubing
3. Wound tubing
4. Connector
5. Needle

FIGURE 12—4-A. The Snyder Hemovac, a light, simple commercial device with gentle suction used for the removal of fluid exudate of extensive wounds. All wounds, clean or septic, are completely closed. Wound suction is continuously applied from the insertion of the tubes, through the wound closure, and until the tubes are removed. Drip and suction for closed circulation is started as soon as the tubes are placed and before wound closure is started. Drip and suction never cease during wound closure, during transportation of the patient from surgery, or until the permanent attachment to the mechanical pump is made for continued use. (Adapted. Courtesy of Snyder Laboratories, Division of Snyder Manufacturing Company, Inc., New Philadelphia, Ohio.)

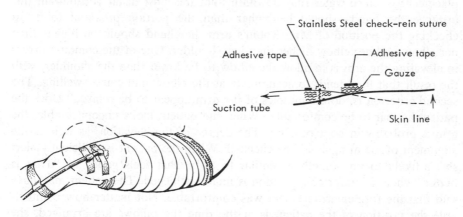

FIGURE 12—4-B. The Snyder Hemovac tube inserted in leg wound. Schematic of dressing: If tubes are to be in for some time as in cases of circulation, the check-rein suture is used. Otherwise no suture is used. In either instance it is a great convenience to have the wound dressing completely separated from any attachment to the tubes. Manipulation, inspection, and removal of tubes can then be done without disturbing the wound dressing. Keep tubes in line with their skin exits. Do not curl them to put pressure on the skin holes or the skin will become irritated or slough. Pad lightly between skin and tube but put adhesive directly against and over the tube to anchor it firmly to the skin. Circle denotes area before gauze and tape. (Adapted. Courtesy of Snyder Laboratories, Division of Snyder Manufacturing Company, Inc., New Philadelphia, Ohio.)

days. The patient may be taught how to disconnect the suction so that he is free to walk about.

When Mrs. Robin was returned from the operating room, she was placed in bed with the head of the bed elevated to about a 15-degree angle. Her right arm was abducted at the shoulder, rotated internally with the forearm flexed at the elbow, and elevated. Some surgeons ask that the arm be abducted at the shoulder and that the forearm be flexed at the elbow and elevated with the hand above the head. Others place the arm across the chest of the patient and bandage it in that position. The latter position reduces the tension on the wound and therefore is favorable to wound healing. The first two positions are for the purpose of maintaining the function of the arm. In all three positions, the arm should be supported so that unnecessary strain and discomfort are prevented. In the first two positions, elevation also supports venous return and prevents stasis of fluid or edema of the arm. The removal of the lymph nodes and channels as well as the inflammatory response in the operated area interferes with the drainage of fluid from the arm.

Whatever the position of the arm, it should be supported so that there is no unnecessary pull on the muscles. A pillow should be placed along the side of the chest and under the arm that is strapped over the chest, as well as under those parts requiring elevation. The pillows or supports should be placed so that they support the arm of the patient rather than the reverse. Because the patient can and should move about, the supports tend to become disarranged and require readjustment. The first criterion to be used in checking their placement is, since water runs downhill, that the most distal portion—in this instance the hand—should be higher than the portion proximal to it. In checking the position of Mrs. Robin's arm, her hand should be higher than her elbow and her elbow higher than her shoulder. One of the common errors in elevating the arm is to allow the elbow to be lower than the shoulder, with the result that fluid tends to accumulate at the elbow and cause swelling. The second criterion is, do the muscles of the arm appear to be relaxed? Does the patient appear to be comfortable? When the patient looks uncomfortable, the arm is probably in poor position. The degree of the elevation, as well as the alignment of the arm, should be checked. When the patient is sufficiently alert she is likely to say something similar to "My, that feels good" or "That is better" when a comfortable position is finally achieved. The patient may have said that the former arrangement was comfortable. Not matter how comfortable the position of the patient is at the time the pillows are arranged, she does not stay comfortable. Even if she does, one position soon becomes fatiguing. Therefore, the plan for the nursing of the patient should include provision for regular checking and changing of the patient's position.

At the same time, the hand and arm should be checked and any evidence of swelling of the hand or interference with the circulation noted. You will remember that the dressing extended over the upper part of Mrs. Robin's arm. As was emphasized in an earlier chapter, when swelling is allowed to continue in a part surrounded by a fixed or nondistensible wall, first the venous return and then the arterial circulation are interrupted. With a loss of the arterial blood supply, death of tissue follows.

In addition to hemorrhage and swelling of the hand and arm, pneumonia is a possible complication in the early postoperative period. This can usually be prevented by encouraging the patient to move about in bed and to deep-breathe and to cough. Mrs. Robin was encouraged and assisted to move and to cough, and she recovered without developing respiratory complications.

Mrs. Robin had some pain in her incision which was controlled by Meperidine Hydrochloride (Demerol) 75 mg, on request, but not oftener than every four hours. Dr. Surgeon had informed Mrs. Robin that she could have a pain-relieving medication when she needed it. She required meperidine hydrochloride only twice.

One of the objectives following radical breast amputation is to restore the arm on the affected side to full usefulness. Two problems require control to achieve this objective. One is the prevention of limitation of motion of the arm by the scar tissue formed in healing of the wound. The other is to prevent or limit edema of the hand and arm. The restoration of the arm to full usefulness, by preventing disability due to contractures, is accomplished by arm exercise. When exercises are to be started and what type are to be used at a given point are decisions made by the surgeon. Some surgeons start exercises early, while others prefer to wait until wound healing is well under way. When the quantity of tissue that has been excised is extensive, the amount of skin left to close the wound may be marginal, and additional tension on the incision may interfere with healing. In the early postoperative period Dr. Surgeon asked that Mrs. Robin's arm be put through the normal range of motion without forcing abduction. Mrs. Robin was fearful, and arm movement was painful. Dr. Surgeon reassured her that the movement of her arm would not produce harmful effects and was necessary to her recovery. The nurse reinforced Dr. Surgeon's statements. The first few times that Mrs. Robin exercised her arm, the nurse supported it and abducted and adducted it slowly and gently. She also encouraged Mrs. Robin to alternately flex and extend her elbow as well as her wrist and fingers. Because movement of the arm is painful, arm movements should be started slowly. As soon as the physician's prescription permits, the patient should be encouraged to carry on her usual activities with her arm. These include feeding herself, washing her face and hands, brushing her teeth, and combing her hair. These activities serve a double purpose. They not only exercise the arm, but they improve the morale of the patient. They are more effective than countless words in convincing the patient that the arm will in fact be restored to usefulness. The fact that the use of the arm is painful at the beginning should be recognized. The patient can be assured, however, that within a relatively short period of time pain on use will disappear and by exercising she is helping with her own recovery. As the nurse cared for Mrs. Robin, she tried to communicate to Mrs. Robin the fact that she did appreciate her discomfort, but that movement of the arm was necessary if she were to recover its full use.

In preparation of Mrs. Robin for discharge from the hospital, the nurse asked that she be given the booklet, "A Handbook for Your Recovery."[59] Mrs. Robin was taught to do wall-climbing, pendulum, pulley, broom-raising, and rope-turning exercises. Dr. Surgeon told Mr. and Mrs. Robin that, as her strength returned, she should resume full activity. Household activities that involve reaching and stretching and full movements of the arm are especially helpful.

To do the wall-climbing exercise, Mrs. Robin was taught to stand with her feet about 8 in. apart and facing the wall, and as close to it as possible. Both hands are placed against the wall at shoulder level. Then, using the fingers, the hands parallel to each other climb the wall until the arms are completely extended. When this exercise was started, Mrs. Robin was unable to fully extend her right arm. This is to be expected. The nurse made a small mark on the wall, so that Mrs. Robin could check her progress. In the beginning the nurse encouraged Mrs. Robin to take her time as she performed the exercise, and to repeat it ten times.

In the performance of the pendulum exercise, Mrs. Robin was taught to stand with her feet 8 in. apart and to bend forward, allowing her arms to hang toward the floor. At first she allowed her arms to dangle and then she swung them back and forth. Eventually, she was able to swing them in circles.

To perform the pulley exercises, an 8-ft. length of rope is placed over a door, a shower curtain rod, or a suspended pulley. The patient then alternately raises and lowers each arm. The arms are in adduction and extended.

To perform the broom-raising exercise, any horizontal bar similar in weight to a broomstick may be used. The stick or broom handle is grasped by both hands with the hands about 2 ft. apart. The broom is then raised until the arms are fully extended. Then it is brought down behind the head of the patient. This exercise is somewhat harder to do than some of the others. The patient should therefore be encouraged to try it only once or twice the first few times and to gradually increase the number of times that it is performed.

The rope-turning exercise is performed by turning a rope, ribbon, or string that has been tied to a doorknob or other suitable object. The patient holds the rope in the hand on the affected side with the arm straight in front of her and places the other hand on her hip for balance. Then she moves the rope in a circle without turning her elbow or wrist. As the function of her arm improves, she will be able to form larger and larger circles.

In instruction of the patient, emphasis should be placed on the objective— to return the arm to its normal function. Although some patients require support and urging to return to full activity, others need to be cautioned against overuse of the arm. This is true especially in the beginning. As the patient returns to normal activity, the need for special exercises is lessened.

[59] Helen B. Radlee, *A Handbook for Your Recovery*, Society of Memorial Center, New York, 1955.

One of the expressed or unexpressed problems of the patient who has a radical mastectomy is the loss of the breast and the resulting disfigurement. The patient should be encouraged to discuss with her surgeon the earliest time that she can start wearing a brassiere and then to shop for the type that is suitable and comfortable for her. Mrs. Robin was very much concerned about the extent of her operation and its effect on her appearance. The surgeon and nurse both tried to reassure her that the operation was similar to what is usually done. The nurse told Mrs. Robin about the types of brassieres now available. They are sold in department stores and at specialty shops. They are made with a variety of fillers and in different sizes. Fillers contain fluid or are made of sponge rubber and other similar materials. For the patient who feels lopsided, the filler containing fluid may be preferred; the shape of the breast also changes with position. The patient should be encouraged to select a brassiere that is comfortable and fits her individual requirements.

Patients should be encouraged to resume normal activities after they return home. There is some evidence that patients tend to regress immediately after they go home and to be more dependent than they were in the hospital. If the family accepts the behavior of the patient, the increase in dependency is usually short-lived and the patient soon begins to assume more responsibility Actually, there is some evidence that the patient who is permitted to be dependent recovers more rapidly than the one whose family is not as accepting.

Before the patient is discharged, plans should be made with her and a family member about when she will visit the doctor. If X ray therapy is planned and the patient knows this, she may have questions, some of which the nurse may answer. Others may need to be referred to the physician. Some increase in anxiety at this time can be expected.

The family may require some instruction and support. They should know what is to be expected of the patient and how they can be helpful. They should know that the patient may not be very active for a week or so after she goes home. Though the equipment required for the exercises is not very complicated, a husband or son may get satisfaction from preparing it. They can be helpful to the patient by making a conscious effort to note and comment on the progress and efforts made by the patient.

The patient who faces, or who has, a radical mastectomy has special problems. To most women, the breast has significance as a symbol of femininity. The operation itself involves the removal of a large amount of tissue and the disruption of many blood vessels. The nursing care has among its goals to preserve and strengthen the self-esteem of the patient as well as to contribute to the accomplishment of the medical goals—to heal the wound and to restore the function of the arm. The accomplishment of these goals depends on application of knowledge of the patient, the effects of cancer, and the nature of the operation to the care of the patient.

Mrs. Alan Wren—an active, vivacious, charming, fastidious, intelligent, and well-educated woman of 65—and Mr. Wren had been married for 39 years. Their position as substantial and contributing members of the community was well established. Mr. Wren's income was sufficient so that they had both a country estate and an apartment in town. Mrs. Wren was active in community affairs.

The day after her sixty-fifth birthday Mrs. Wren called her family physician to make an appointment for her annual physical examination. She had seen her physician about six months previously when she had an attack of influenza. She had always been a healthy woman who took good health for granted. She was neither overly concerned about her health nor neglectful of it.

At the time of the examination, she told Dr. Olds that she had had some discomfort in her abdomen, but that she found it difficult to describe. She had had some flatulence which she considered to be embarrassing. She also had recently been constipated. On physical examination Dr. Olds found that Mrs. Wren's general state of health was good. Her weight, 125 lb. was the same as for the previous year. Her hemoglobin level was 13.8 gm, which was also unchanged. Her leukocyte count at 7,500 cells per cubic millimeter was within normal limits.

The proctoscopic examination revealed a narrowing of the bowel at the junction of the rectum and sigmoid. At one point there was an ulcerated area. On X ray of the large bowel, Mrs. Wren was found to have an encircling, or annular, lesion. As the result of these findings, Dr. Olds referred Mrs. Wren to Dr. Surgeon, who recommended and performed a one-stage combined abdominal perineal resection with a colostomy.

In Mrs. Wren, cancer was located in one of the common sites. The large intestine is among the five common sites for cancer, and the rectosigmoid is the most common site for the large intestine. According to *1964 Cancer Facts and Figures* 41,900 persons were expected to die from the effects of cancer in the colon and rectum in 1964, and 76,000 persons were expected to be diagnosed as having cancer of the colon and rectum for the first time. The incidence of cancer of the rectum is higher in men than in women, while the reverse is true in cancer of the colon. One of the hopeful aspects of cancer of the rectum and colon is that some of these cancers start out as rectal polyps. If the polyps are discovered early by rectosigmoidoscopy, they can be removed. Harkins, *et al.*,[60] state that discovery and removal of polyps in the rectum and colon offer the best opportunity for cancer prevention of any part of the body. Harkins also states that the chance of cure by surgery is greater for cancer of the colon and rectum than it is for other common sites.

Symptoms that accompany the development of cancer of the colon and rectum vary with the location of the lesion. Symptoms of obstruction are more commonly associated with lesions on the left than on the right side. Water is absorbed from the feces as they pass through the large intestine, and the narrowing of the lumen of the intestine offers more resistance to the semisolid

[60] Henry Harkins, *et al.*, "Tumors of the Colon and Rectum," *Surgery, Principles and Practice*, 2nd ed., J. B. Lippincott Co., Philadelphia, 1961, p. 959.

feces than to liquid feces higher in the intestine. Symptoms include, as in the instance of Mrs. Wren, vague abdominal distress and a change in the bowel habit including constipation, obstipation, and diarrhea. Especially in low left-sided lesions, the shape of the stool changes and becomes smaller in diameter; ribbon-shaped stools are not uncommon. Hemorrhoids not infrequently accompany left-sided lesions. They may, in fact, be an early warning sign. Bright-red blood can be observed in the stool in left-sided, but not in right-sided, lesions. Anemia accompanies lesions located on either side. Anemia of unexplained origin may be the first indication of cancer of the cecum. Weakness and general debility occur as the cancer progresses. Mrs. Wren had not experienced any of these effects.

The treatment of cancer of the large intestine, like treatment of cancer in other parts of the body, is directed toward the eradication of all cancer cells. The same methods—surgery, ionizing radiation, and chemotherapy—are used. Treatment of cancer on the left side often, though not always, includes a colostomy. Cancer of the right bowel can usually be treated without a permanent colostomy; the diseased portion of the bowel is removed and the ends are anastamosed (joined).

Bowel resections with or without colostomy may be performed for conditions other than cancer. A permanent or temporary colostomy may also be constructed for the treatment of a number of noncancerous conditions. For example, a patient with colitis may have a portion of his bowel resected or a colostomy made to allow the diseased portion of the bowel to heal. Resection of the bowel may be required in the treatment of diverticulitis. Diverticuli are saclike outpouchings that occur along the gastrointestinal tract, usually in the esophagus or colon. They may become inflamed as the result of food or feces accumulating in the pouch. A colostomy may also be used as a palliative measure to relieve obstruction.

The purpose of the colostomy in all instances is to provide an avenue for the discharge of intestinal contents. It may have a single opening, as in the instance of Mrs. Wren; it is then called a single-barreled colostomy. When the proximal and distal loops are brought to the surface, it is known as a double-barreled colostomy. Occasionally there is difficulty in identifying the proximal loop for irrigation; the surgeon should be asked to identify it, when this is the case. When the distal loop is irrigated, the patient discharges the fluid via the rectum.

As mentioned previously, Mrs. Wren was treated by a combined abdominal perineal resection. In this operation, a left hemicolectomy is performed. All of the bowel distal to the splenic end of the transverse colon is removed. In Mrs. Wren's case, the distal end of the remaining bowel was brought through the abdominal wall to form the colostomy. During the performance of this operation, Mrs. Wren had three incisions: a stab wound for the formation of the colostomy; an anterior incision for the exposure, exploration, and preparation of the area for the removal of the lesion; and, finally, a perineal incision for the completion of the removal of the tumor and the surrounding tissue. Readers who are interested in the details of the operation are referred to the References.

The surgeon had two objectives that related to the nature of the cancer and its site. His first objective was to remove all of the tumor-bearing tissue, including the lymph channels and nodes draining the area. The second was to prevent the dissemination of cancer cells in the lumen of the bowel or through the veins draining the area. Dr. Surgeon also had in mind a third objective, which he was unable to achieve, that is, to preserve, if possible, the anal sphincters.

Throughout all phases of Mrs. Wren's experience as a patient with cancer, the objectives on which her nursing care was based took into account: (1) Mrs. Wren's needs as an individual human being, (2) the fact that she was diagnosed as having cancer, (3) the fact that she had had an extensive surgical procedure, and (4) her resultant colostomy.

Factors considered in meeting Mrs. Wren's needs for nursing as they relate to the first three points have been previously discussed. The discussion will be limited to the steps in the eventual adjustment of Mrs. Wren to the fact that she had a colostomy. The time span over which she made adjustment was about a year.

Time is required to adapt to major changes in one's way of life. Though the social, psychological, financial, and health factors were favorable, she required time to adjust to the fact of the colostomy and to develop confidence that she would be able to control its behavior. During the ensuing months Mrs. Wren was to experience more or less emotional turmoil, but her adjustment began when Dr. Olds told her that, though her symptoms were vague and mild, she did have a lesion in her intestine. He suggested that he make an appointment for her to see Dr. Surgeon at her earliest convenience. Mrs. Wren's immediate reaction was a common one—to seek to delay diagnosis. Could not this appointment with Dr. Surgeon be deferred until she returned from Florida? Mr. Wren had made reservations for them to leave on Thursday. They would be gone only three months. Certainly nothing bad could happen in that time. Dr. Olds was firm, but kindly, as he urged her to delay the trip. She was quiet a moment, and then said, "You think that I have cancer, do you not?" Dr. Olds had known Mrs. Wren for a number of years and he did not evade the question. He answered her by saying, "Yes, I think so, but I think that it is an early cancer. If it is removed now, there is a good chance that it can be entirely removed. Dr. Surgeon is a competent surgeon. You will be in good hands." Mrs. Wren then said, "I never thought about it happening to me. I'd like to talk to Alan before I decide. Would it be satisfactory with you if I call you tomorrow?" Dr. Olds agreed that she should talk it over with her husband. He recognized Mrs. Wren's need to maintain some control over her situation and her reliance on her husband. Furthermore, in the difficult days ahead she would need the help, support, and understanding of her husband as well as the knowledge that she had made her own decision.

Sutherland, et al.,[61] emphasize the importance of a supportive spouse in the eventual adjustment of the patient to the colostomy. In his studies of families where rapport was poor before the operation, the relationship deteriorated afterwards; in a series of patients, 4 out of 57 patients who had colostomies had to live away from home because they were unacceptable to their families. Both patients and family members studied tended to hide the fact of the colostomy from others. Of the 57 patients referred to above, 25 had not allowed even other family members to see the colostomy. Even when the patient was willing to allow family members to see the colostomy, they sometimes refused to view it. Mrs. Wren was fortunate because Mr. Wren was a kindly and dependable man who gave her understanding and support through the months that followed the diagnosis and treatment of her disorder.

To return to Mrs. Wren, who had just learned that her family physician was of the opinion that she had cancer of the colon, though she was feeling shaken, she waited until that evening after dinner to tell Mr. Wren about the outcome of the visit to Dr. Olds. After talking, they decided to visit Dr. Olds together. At this time Dr. Olds urged them not to delay treatment. They decided to follow Dr. Olds's advice, and an appointment was made with Dr. Surgeon for the following day. To give Mrs. Wren support, Mr. Wren went with her to see Dr. Surgeon. After examining Mrs. Wren, Dr. Surgeon confirmed Dr. Olds's suspicions and explained to both Mr. and Mrs. Wren, the need for prompt surgery as well as the type of procedure that would probably be required. He explained that the left half of the bowel would have to be removed and that a colostomy would have to be performed. Despite her expectation that an operation would be necessary, she felt overwhelmed and confused when Dr. Surgeon stated that she should prepare to go to the hospital without delay. Later she told members of the family that she felt that she was in a fog. She went through the necessary motions, but they were automatic. Mr. Wren was also upset, but tried to hide his feelings and to comfort Mrs. Wren. He assumed the responsibility for making the arrangements for her admission to the hospital.

For the first two or three days following the operation, Mrs. Wren's needs were similar to those of other patients who have had extensive abdominal surgery. Dr. Surgeon had reassured both Mr. and Mrs. Wren that, as far as he could tell, all of the tumor had been removed. Mrs. Wren's postoperative progress was most satisfactory. On the morning of the third postoperative day, Mrs. Wren passed flatus through the colostomy. Though this indicated that normal physiological functioning of the gastrointestinal tract was returning, it also reminded Mrs. Wren that she was no longer capable of controlling defecation. This aroused the fear that she could never again leave her home because of the danger of involuntary defecation. Her anxiety was to become more severe and to plague her for months. As Mrs. Wren recovered physically, she became more and more aware of the physiological alterations in her alimentary canal. As the function of the bowel returned, flatus and liquid

[61] Sutherland, et al., Op. cit., p. 864.

feces were discharged through the colostomy stoma. When irrigations were started, Mrs. Wren found the procedure exceedingly distressing. Her discouragement and depression deepened and she was unable to eat or to sleep. Her general attitude was one of hopelessness.

Mrs. Wren's behavior was by no means unusual. Some degree of depression usually accompanies serious illness and treatment by a major surgical procedure. Furthermore, the patient who has a colostomy may suffer additional shock from seeing the colostomy for the first time, from the involuntary discharges, and from the irrigations. A more or less severe emotional reaction is to be expected, because of what a colostomy means to many individuals. Some of these meanings stem from the fact that one of the important achievements in the life of a child is the attainment of control of the sphincters. Removal of the rectum with the ensuing loss of the ability to control defecation has consequences that go beyond the physiological aspects. These consequences are largely emotional. In a few instances they may be so serious that, despite thoughtful and careful management, the life of the patient is permanently disrupted. In most instances, however, patients can be helped so that unnecessary restriction is prevented.

Two weeks postoperatively, Mrs. Wren was discharged from the hospital. She had made a good physiological recovery, but she was still depressed and fearful. Her fears were centered around her ability to control the behavior of the colostomy and to perform the irrigations. There was nothing unusual about those fears. In fact, studies made on patients having colostomies indicate that these are the common areas of concern. Because she feared spillage, she was concerned with the effect of what she ate on the activity of the bowel. Although the patient may find that certain foods, especially those that are high in roughage, such as raw cabbage and fresh fruits, or very rich foods, do stimulate peristalsis, he should be encouraged to eat a variety of foods. Foods such as cabbage and rich desserts can be avoided without threatening the nutritional status of the individual. Most authorities emphasize that no special diet is required. A well-balanced diet in amounts necessary to maintain the desired weight and strength should be the objective. Mrs. Wren required support and encouragement to maintain an adequate food intake. As her physical and psychological status improved, she gradually added different foods to her diet. Eventually she found that by limiting the amount, she could eat almost anything but highly seasoned foods. She rarely had diarrhea, but when she did, she selected foods that are low in residue. She used as a reference "Care of Your Colostomy."[62]

Because she was afraid of spillage, Mrs. Wren felt that she should wear a colostomy bag. She was, however, fearful lest the bag would be noticeable and draw attention to the colostomy. Despite the reassurance of her surgeon that in time the colostomy would become regulated and that she would not require a bag, she found this difficult to believe. As is usual, in the early postoperative

---

[62] *Care of Your Colostomy,* American Cancer Society, New York, 1959, pp. 18-19.

period Mrs. Wren had many liquid stools from her colostomy. As time passed, the number of defecations diminished and the contents became less fluid or more formed. In the early postoperative period, the bowel responds by increasing its activity and allowing less time for the absorption of water, resulting in liquid feces. As the activity of the bowel diminishes, water is absorbed and the stool becomes formed. The period in which her bowel was adapting to the artificial opening was a very trying time for Mrs. Wren, as it is for most patients. When a colostomy bag is applied soon after the colostomy starts to function, the patient is protected from spillage of intestinal contents on the wall of the abdomen—provided, of course, that it is properly applied. When absorbent dressings are used, they should be changed as soon as they are soiled. The skin around the colostomy should be washed and dried and a water-repellent powder applied. Low-lying areas such as the groin should be checked and washed as necessary. In the reapplication of dressings, the fact that water runs downhill should serve as a guide to their placement. Dressings should be fluffed to increase the surface for absorption and placed around the colostomy forming an encircling mound. They have little value when they are piled on top of the colostomy. When the bed linens are soiled, they should be changed. After the patient is clean and dry, the room should be aired.

At the time the dressing is changed, the skin around the colostomy should be checked for signs of redness or excoriation. The colostomy itself should be observed for any changes in appearance. When the patient has an anterior abdominal incision, the dressing should be protected from, and checked for evidence of, soiling. Any abnormalities should be discovered and reported to the surgeon.

An early decision that Mrs. Wren had to make was whether or not to irrigate her colostomy. Her surgeon had recommended that she irrigate her colostomy daily, but Dr. Olds had suggested to her that she might prefer to regulate the colostomy without irrigation. She decided after several weeks to irrigate. After some trial and error, she also decided to irrigate at night as this allowed time for any solution left in the intestine to be discharged. During her first few weeks at home Mrs. Wren had the help of a practical nurse, who was under the supervision of a visiting nurse who came in three times a week. In time Mrs. Wren was able to assume full responsibility for herself, including the irrigation of her colostomy, which took about an hour each evening. After about a year, Mrs. Wren had developed sufficient confidence that she and her husband took a trip around the world. She took a bottle of paregoric and the names of physicians that she could consult with should she need their services. Though she took a colostomy bag, she had graduated to wearing a piece of soft tissue lubricated with a small quantity of petroleum jelly over the colostomy. She wore an elastic girdle to hold it in place. During the entire trip, she spent only one day in her hotel room because of diarrhea. This was the only time that she needed her colostomy bag. When she returned home, she resumed her social and community activities.

Not all patients make as complete an adjustment to a colostomy as did

Mrs. Wren. She was fortunate in that, as a person, she had the inner resources that made it possible for her to recover from the emotional shock created by having a colostomy. She was most fortunate in having an understanding and supporting husband as well as the financial resources to provide for her needs. Her medical and nursing care also contributed to her recovery. As a result of these and other factors, Mrs. Wren made a complete recovery.

Not all patients make as complete a recovery as Mrs. Wren. This is reflected in some degree or curtailment of their activities. Reasons given include fear of spillage, feelings of being unacceptable to others, the fear of being offensive because of odor, the fear of gas escaping, and the time required for irrigation. An occasional patient spends his entire day irrigating his colostomy. The problems that confront the patient are those illustrated by Mrs. Wren. They include: (1) acceptance of the colostomy as necessary and manageable, (2) irrigations—if required, (3) what is worn over the colostomy, and (4) diet—to the end that the food intake is adequate in quantity and quality. The over-all objective should be to help the individual with a colostomy learn to manage it so that, although it is necessary to his remaining alive, it does not become the focus of his life.

Some of the factors in the patient's acceptance of the colostomy have been presented in the discussion of Mrs. Wren. To these might be added that patients regard a warm and supporting relationship with nurses as important in changing their outlook and aiding in their recovery. Moreover, an operation such as a colostomy lowers the self-esteem of the patient. Attention should be paid in the care of the patient to preventing further decrease in his self-esteem by the way in which care is given.

Patients who have a natural bowel movement at a regular time each day do not require colostomy irrigations. The patient who does not, or who, like Mrs. Wren, feels more secure if he irrigates his colostomy, is taught to irrigate it.

When irrigation is required, the patient and, if possible, a member of the family should be taught the procedure to be followed, before the patient leaves the hospital. The equipment that the patient expects to use should be procured and the patient should use it when he is learning to irrigate his colostomy. Such factors as whether the patient has a bathroom that he can use and the time of day that it is available should be considered in selecting the time to irrigate the colostomy. The nurse who instructs the patient should be competent and skillful. The patient can be expected to be highly anxious, and his anxiety decreases his ability to learn. As a result, instruction may need to be repeated over and over. Learning is also easier when the person providing the instruction is understanding and supporting. Persons under stress are likely to interpret the behavior of the nurse in terms of himself. If the nurse is incompetent or appears to find the performance of the procedure distasteful, her behavior is likely to increase the anxiety of the patient and impair his ability to learn.

What procedure should be followed when irrigating a colostomy?

Many hospitals have developed a procedure which they have found to be satisfactory. For hospitals lacking such a procedure, The American Cancer Society has a booklet, *Care of Your Colostomy*[63] which may prove helpful; it outlines a procedure for colostomy irrigation adapted for use at home. This same procedure can also be followed in the hospital. The instruction of the patient should be based on the fact that the purpose of the colostomy irrigation is the same as that of an enema. The same general principles apply in both instances. There is one important difference. The anal sphincters normally prevent the fluid that is introduced from returning immediately. Since there is no sphincter at the opening of the colostomy, fluid may return as rapidly as it is introduced. A guard is required to prevent the backflow of fluid while it is introduced. A guard can be made by cutting off the tip of a rubber bulb syringe (ear syringe) and making an opening in the opposite end. The catheter is then introduced through the upper part of the bulb and down through the tip of the syringe. The position assumed by the patient during colostomy irrigation usually differs from that suggested for an enema. The patient sits on the toilet or a low stool and uses the toilet or a pail to catch the return. A plastic sleeve or conduit placed over the colostomy is helpful to direct the flow of the contents of the colon into the appropriate receptacle. Before the catheter is introduced, the air should be removed and the catheter lubricated as for an enema. When there is resistance to the passage of the catheter, force should not be used as the bowel can be perforated by forcible introduction of the catheter. Rather, the clamp on the tubing should be opened and water allowed to flow into the intestine as the tube is introduced; the water opens the lumen of the bowel. Because the opening into the colostomy may narrow with the passage of time, some surgeons teach patients to dilate the colostomy by inserting a finger into its opening and gently rotating it.

The amount of solution required to effectively cleanse the bowel varies. Some patients use as little as a pint, while others use a quart or more. Some doctors advise patients to use warm water, while others suggest that 2 teaspoons of salt or 1 teaspoon of baking soda be added to a quart of water. The frequency with which different individuals require irrigation also varies. Occasionally an individual has a regular evacuation and remains clean and dry in between. Some patients irrigate daily. Others irrigate only every second or third day. Timing is something that the patient has to learn by experience. After the patient becomes adept in the performance of the procedure, the total length of time required should not be more than one half to three quarters of an hour. If he consistently takes more than an hour, he should be encouraged to discuss this problem with his physician. The patient should aim toward

[63] *Ibid.*

the development of a regular routine and schedule which he follows. The patient should be assured that once he is adjusted, the schedule does not have to be followed slavishly. Moreover, the time selected for the irrigation should take into account the needs of other members of the family as well as those of the patient. The time selected should be one that enables the patient to be comfortable and relaxed. The colon is sensitive to the feelings of the person. Feelings of pressure or tension have an adverse effect on the activity of the bowel.

The patient should be prepared for the difficulties that are encountered in the performance of the procedure. Painful cramping is caused by the too rapid introduction of fluid into the intestine or by too large a volume; the flow of water should be stopped and the height of the irrigation lowered.

Just as with an enema, the results obtained from a colostomy irrigation may be inadequate. This may be due to constipation or to fatigue or nervous strain. When the fluid does not return after a suitable interval, it may be siphoned back. If the flow is just slow to return, massage of the abdomen may hasten its return.

Because the mucous membrane lining the colostomy is fragile, irritation may cause a small amount of bleeding; a small amount of blood staining the gauze covering the colostomy usually is indicative of irritation.

Doctors vary in their recommendations to patients about what type of covering to wear over the colostomy. Some recommend that a colostomy bag be worn. Others prefer that a small, flat dressing—gauze, paper tissue, or cloth—be worn. A small amount of petroleum jelly placed over the colostomy lessens irritation. A girdle or supporter is worn to hold the dressing in place.

With the exception of odors caused by escaping flatus, odors can be controlled by attention to scrupulous cleanliness. The skin around the colostomy should be thoroughly washed with soap and water, and any equipment used must be kept clean. Equipment includes not only the colostomy bag, if one is worn, but girdles and irrigating equipment. There are deodorizing agents that can be taken by mouth or inserted into the colostomy, but those taken by mouth often cause diarrhea.

Despite careful instruction of the patient and a member of his family before his discharge from the hospital, the patient frequently requires, or benefits from, some assistance in adjusting to his home situation. In communities where a visiting nurse service is available, referral of the patient for this service should be considered. Patients are seldom fully recovered at the time of discharge. The home situation and family relationships may differ from those perceived by nurses and physicians who care for the patient in the hospital. For example, Mrs. Wren required continuing help and support for several months. The fact that it was available to her undoubtedly contributed to her eventual recovery. During the period of adjustment, the family frequently requires help in understanding the needs of the patient and their role in helping him. The visiting nurse is accustomed to working with patients and their families in the home situation. She can guide them in working out practical and acceptable solutions to problems as they arise.

In communities where there are colostomy clubs, some persons gain comfort and help from other members of the club. They learn that they are not alone, as many others have a similar problem. They have an opportunity to learn from each other and to give each other mutual support.

The successful management of a colostomy by an individual requires knowledge, skill, and confidence that it can be managed without its being an undue burden. Whether or not the patient eventually achieves success depends on the patient, his family, and the quality of professional service that he receives during the entire period of his illness and recovery. There are a few patients who are, despite excellent management, unable to adjust successfully to a colostomy, but most patients will adjust successfully with appropriate assistance. The adjustment of the patient is facilitated by all of the members of the health team working with the patient and the members of his family to meet the needs of the patient at each stage of his recovery.

Why do people consult cancer quacks?

No discussion of the problems created by neoplasms is complete without some consideration of why people consult cancer quacks and of the kinds of information useful in distinguishing between a quack and a bona fide physician. First, quacks are not unique to cancer. They seek out people who have a health problem that is not easily solved by available methods of treatment. Any long-term and disabling illness offers the quack an opportunity to offer sick people hope and to exploit their feelings to his own ends. Sometimes a quack treats many types of disease including arthritis, cancer, diabetes mellitus, and gout.

Possibly cancer offers a more fertile field for the quack than many other diseases because people all too often regard cancer as a mysterious and hopeless disease having a poor prognosis. Knowledge or even a suspicion that cancer is a possibility may cause the person and his family to go into a state of panic. This may result in the person grasping at straws and seeking help from someone who promises cure—the cancer quack.

When a person consults a cancer quack for diagnosis and treatment, he may be "cured" because he does not have cancer. Persons who do have cancer may lose valuable time or undergo treatments that spread rather than eradicate the growth. Persons who are in the terminal phase of cancer may experience an extended period of declining health. As the patient and members of his family observe his failure to respond to treatment, their anxiety increases as they wonder whether all that can and should be is being done. When they are told or read about a "doctor" who not only promises, but is able to cure persons who are seriously ill with cancer by injections of a magic solution or rays of a mysterious light, they may be sorely tempted to consult him.

One form of protection of the patient and his family is the kind of supportive care that convinces them that all that can be done will be done. Among the values to patients who participate in studies of drugs and other treatments for cancer is that they are offered hope that they will be benefited in time. Perhaps at least as important is the interest that medical and nursing personnel express in their behavior and progress. Many patients take pride in knowing that they may die making a contribution to knowledge of the prevention and treatment of cancer.

To help people avoid cancer quacks, the American Cancer Society has prepared a group of criteria which the public can use in the selection or rejection of a doctor to diagnose and treat cancer. They are:[64]

1. Be suspicious of a doctor who promises a sure cure when other doctors will not;
2. Beware of the doctor who says that he has an *exclusive method;*
3. Be on guard against the doctor who tells you that organized medicine is against him;
4. When in doubt about a man who says he is a cancer specialist, ask your family doctor to investigate.

The American Cancer Society and the local county medical society are sources of information about many quacks.

In addition to the role of the nurse in public education, the nurse also helps to prevent patients from seeking attention from quacks by the practice of her supportive role. Patients and their families desperately want to have something done that offers hope. They want evidence that something is being done. They want to feel that those who care for them care about what happens to them. The quack offers this hope and exploits the feelings of the patient and his family to his own ends.

In all phases in the life of the patient with cancer, the nurse contributes to the care of the patient through her use of her supportive and therapeutic roles. She has a part to play in prevention and in detection of cancer, as well as in the phases in which the patient has overt disease. Although prevention is superior to cure, many are cured. According to the American Cancer Society,[65] of every six persons who develop cancer today, two will be saved and four will die. One additional person will die who might have been saved by proper treatment. Three will die from cancers that cannot yet be controlled. The cure of these patients awaits the discovery of new knowledge. In whatever stage of illness, the nurse has much to offer the patient. This is true even, and particularly, in the care of patients who have widespread and progressive disease. To paraphrase Oliver Wendell Holmes's injunction to physicians, "Nurses participate in cure seldom, relieve often, and comfort always."

[64] "Cancer Quacks," *Cancer News,* XII, Spring, 1958, p. 10.
[65] *1963 Cancer Facts and Figures, Op. cit.,* p. 4.

REFERENCES

Books

A Cancer Source Book for Nurses, American Cancer Society Inc., New York, 1963.

Aldrich, C. Knight, *Psychiatry for the Family Physician,* Blakiston Division, McGraw-Hill Book Co., New York, 1955, Chapters 1-4, pp. 20-21.

American Cancer Society (Mass. Division), *Cancer: A Manual for Practitioners,* 3rd ed., American Cancer Society, Boston, 1956, pp. 1-53 and 251-301.

. . . *The Physician and the Total Care of the Cancer Patient.* A Symposium presented at the 1961 Scientific Session of the American Cancer Society, Inc., Biltmore Hotel, New York, N.Y., October 23-24, 1961. Published by the American Cancer Society, Inc.

Cancer Manual for Public Health Nurses, U.S. Department of Health, Education and Welfare, Public Health Service, Division of Chronic Diseases, Washington, D.C., 1963.

Field, J. B. (ed.), *Cancer: Diagnosis and Treatment,* Little, Brown & Co., Boston, 1959.

Fuerst, Elinor V., and LuVerne Wolff, *Fundamentals of Nursing,* 3rd ed., J. B. Lippincott Co., Philadelphia, 1964, pp. 619-35.

Homburger, Freddy, *The Biologic Basis of Cancer Management,* Hoeber-Harper Co., New York, 1957.

Homburger, Freddy (ed.), *The Physiopathology of Cancer,* Medical Book Department of Harper & Brothers, New York, 1959.

Leavell, Hugh R., and E. Gurney Clark, *Preventive Medicine for the Doctor in His Community,* The Blakiston Division, McGraw-Hill Book Co., 1958, pp. 260-75.

Scheinfield, Amram, *The Human Heredity Handbook,* J. B. Lippincott Co., Philadelphia, 1956.

Schiffrin, M. J. (ed.), *The Management of Pain in Cancer,* Yearbook Medical Publishers, Inc., Chicago, 1956.

Simmons, Harold, *The Psychosomatic Aspects of Cancer,* Peabody Press, Washington, D.C., 1956.

Snyder, Lawrence H., and Paul R. David, *The Principles of Heredity,* 5th ed., D. C. Heath & Co., Boston, 1957.

Standard, Samuel, and Helmuth Nathan (eds.), *Should the Patient Know the Truth?* Springer Publishing Co., Inc., New York, 1955.

Articles

Adams, Theodore, "The American Cancer Society," *Public Health Reports,* LXXII, January, 1957, p. 81.

Alexander, Sarah, "Nursing Care of a Patient After Breast Surgery," *American Journal of Nursing,* LVII, December, 1957, pp. 1571-72.

Alston, Frances, *et al.,* "Perfusion," *American Journal of Nursing,* LX, November, 1960, pp. 1603-7.

Barckley, Virginia, "What Can I Say to the Cancer Patient?" *Nursing Outlook,* VIII, June, 1958, p. 316.

Beierwaltes, William H., "Radioisotopes in Clinical Medicine," *Medical Clinics of North America,* XLV, July, 1961, pp. 1055-67.

Berk, J. Edward, and Sheldon M. Kanton, "Demethylchlortetracycline-Induced Fluorescence of Gastric Sediment," *Journal of the American Medical Association,* CLXXIX, March 31, 1962, p. 997.

Biehusen, Irma, "Cancer Nursing Is Expensive," *Nursing Outlook,* IV, August, 1956, pp. 438-41.

Brauer, Paul H., "Should the Patient Be Told the Truth?" *Nursing Outlook,* VIII, December, 1960, pp. 672-76.

Brewer, Lyman, *et al.,* "Carcinoma of the Lung," *Journal of the American Medical Association,* CLXVI, March 8, 1958, pp. 1149-55.

Britton, Richard C., "Causes and Treatment of the Postmastectomy Lymphedema of the

Arm," *Journal of the American Medical Association,* CLXXX, April 14, 1962, pp. 95-102.

Hardy, James D. and Curtis P. Artz, guest eds., "Cancer Management—Current Knowledge," *Surgical Clinics of North America,* XLII, April, 1962, pp. 271-558.

Cancer News, American Cancer Society, New York, published quarterly.

Cole, W., *et al.,* "Current Trends in the Treatment of Cancer," *Postgraduate Medicine,* XXIII, March, 1958, pp. 231-41.

Crile, George, Jr., "The Cancer Problem: A Speculative Review of the Etiology, Natural History, and Treatment of Cancer," *Perspectives in Biology and Medicine,* III, Spring, 1960, pp. 358-82.

Crile, George, "Chemotherapy of Cancer," *Postgraduate Medicine,* XXVIII, September, 1960, pp. 242-47.

Daland, Ernest M., "Palliative Treatment of the Patient with Advanced Cancer," *Journal of the American Medical Association,* CXXXVI, February 7, 1948, pp. 391-96.

Davies, Dean F., and Alice H. Davies, "Cancer: Cigarette Smoking as a Cause," *American Journal of Nursing,* XLI, April, 1961, pp. 65, 68-69.

Day, Emerson, "What Is an Adequate Cancer Check Up?" *Postgraduate Medicine,* XXVII, March, 1960, pp. 275-80.

Dericks, Virginia, "Rehabilitation of Patients with Ileostomy," *American Journal of Nursing,* LXI, May, 1961, pp. 48-51.

Dorn, Harold F., "Tobacco Consumption and Mortality from Cancer and other Diseases," *Public Health Reports,* LXXIV, July, 1959, pp. 581-93.

Emerson, Kendall, "The Endocrine Management of Breast Cancer," *Medical Clinics of North America,* XLIV, September, 1960, pp. 1393-1409.

"Evaluation of Early Diagnosis of Cancer," *Postgraduate Medicine,* XXVII, March, 1960, special issue.

Evang, Karland, and Einar Perderson, "Public Health Aspects of Cancer Control," *Journal of Chronic Diseases,* II, February, 1960, pp. 149-69.

Fitzpatrick, Genevieve Manfredonia, and Jane McDonald Shotkin, "Pelvic Perfusion," *American Journal of Nursing,* LXI, June, 1961, pp. 79-81.

Gilmore, Stuart I., "Rehabilitation After a Laryngectomy," *American Journal of Nursing,* LXI, January, 1961, pp. 87-89.

Golbey, Robert B., "Chemotherapy of Cancer," *American Journal of Nursing,* LX, April, 1960, pp. 521-25.

Grace, James T., and Tatsuhei Kondo, "Investigations of Host Resistance in Cancer Patients," *Annals of Surgery,* CXLVIII, October, 1958, pp. 633-41.

Grove, William J., *et al.,* "Cancer: Prevention of Dissemination," *Postgraduate Medicine,* XXX, August, 1961, pp. 157-63.

Hall, Thomas C., "Chemotherapy of Cancer," *New England Journal of Medicine,* CCLXVI, January 18, January 25, and February 1, 1962, pp. 129-33, 178-84, and 238-45.

Hammond, E. Guyler, "Trends in Cancer Death Rates and Cure Rates," *Annals of Internal Medicine,* L, February, 1959, pp. 300-12.

Hatcher, Sara Lou, "Life Experience of Cancer Patients in Tennessee Tumor Clinics," *Public Health Reports,* LXXII, April, 1957, pp. 348-54.

Heller, John R., Sidney J. Cutler, and William M. A. Haenszel, "Some Observations on the Epidemiology of Cancer in the United States," *Journal of the American Medical Association,* CLIX, December 24, 1955, pp. 1628-34.

Higginbotham, Sarah, "Arm Exercises after Mastectomy," *American Journal of Nursing,* LVII, December, 1957, pp. 1573-74.

Hislop, Rhoda, "Nursing Care of Patients with Mouth or Throat Cancer," *American Journal of Nursing,* LVII, October, 1957, pp. 1317-19.

Hueper, W. C., "Carcinogens in the Human Environment," *Archives of Pathology,* LXXI, March, 1961, 237-67, and April, 1961, pp. 355-80.

Hueper, William C., "Lung Cancer, air pollution as a cause," *American Journal of Nursing,* LXI, April, 1961, pp. 64, 66-67.

Hynes, John J., and Eleanor Jansson, "Hodgkin's Disease," *American Journal of Nursing,* LVIII, March, 1958, pp. 371-72.

Ivy, Horace K., "Treatment of Breast Cancer with 5-Fluorouracil," *Annals of Internal Medicine,* LVII, No. 4, October, 1962, pp. 598-605.

Jessiman, A. G., D. D. Matson, and F. D. Moore, "Hypophysectomy in the Treatment of Breast Cancer," *New England Journal of Medicine,* CCLXI, December 10, 1959, pp. 1199-1207.

Kaiser, Raymond, "Cancer Control Activities of the National Cancer Institute," *Public Health Reports,* LXX, October, 1955, pp. 1029-33.

Kaiser, Raymond F., and Alexander G. Gilliam, "Some Epidemiological Aspects of Cervical Cancer," *Public Health Reports,* LXXIII, April, 1958, pp. 359-67.

Kalaycioglea, M. V., and H. C. Myers, "Results of Earlier Treatment of Cancer," *Southern Medical Journal,* LIV, January, 1961, pp. 43-47.

Karnofsky, David, "Cancer Quackery," *American Journal of Nursing,* LIX, April, 1959, pp. 496-500.

Kennedy, B. J., and Athanasios Theologides, "The Role of 5-Fluorouracil in Malignant Disease," *Annals of Internal Medicine,* LV, November, 1961, pp. 719-29.

Knapp, Margaret, "Cancer—A Review," *American Journal of Nursing,* LVI, April, 1956, pp. 440-43.

Kurihara, Marie, "The Patient with an Intestinal Prosthesis," *American Journal of Nursing,* LX, June, 1960, pp. 852-53.

Kutner, Bernard, Henry B. Makover, and Abraham Oppenheim, "Delay in the Diagnosis and Treatment of Cancer: A Critical Analysis of the Literature," *Journal of Chronic Disease,* VII, February, 1958, pp. 95-119.

Lahey Clinic, *et al.,* "Symposium on Results and Prognosis in Cancer Therapy," *Surgical Clinics of North America,* XXXIX, June, 1959, entire issue.

Levin, Morton L., *et al.,* "Cancer Incidence in Urban and Rural Areas of New York State," *Journal of the National Cancer Institute,* XXIV, June, 1960, pp. 1243-57.

Lombard, Herbert L., and Leonid S. Snegireff, "An Epidemiological Study of Lung Cancer," *Cancer,* XII, March-April, 1959, pp. 406-13.

Louis, John, "Management of Reticuloendothelial Malignancies," *Medical Clinics of North America,* XLVI, January, 1962, pp. 171-215.

Lubic, Ruth W., "Nursing Care After Adrenalectomy or Hypophysectomy," *American Journal of Nursing,* LXII, April, 1962, pp. 84-86.

Lyons, Albert S., "Control of the Colostomy," *American Journal of Digestive Diseases,* I, February, 1956, pp. 79-94.

Macklin, Madge T., "Inheritance of Cancer of the Stomach and Large Intestine in Man," *Journal of the National Cancer Institute,* XXIV, March, 1960, pp. 551-71.

Manfredonia, Genevieve, "Radiation Therapy for Cancer of the Cervix," *American Journal of Nursing,* LIX, April, 1959, pp. 513-17.

Medical Clinics of North America, XLVI, May, 1961, entire issue devoted to medical treatment and aspects of cancer.

Miller, Opal, "Nursing Care After Pelvic Exenteration," *American Journal of Nursing,* LXII, May, 1962, pp. 106-7.

Monterio, Lois, "The Patient Had Difficulty Communicating," *American Journal of Nursing,* LXII, January, 1962, pp. 78-81.

Moore, George E., Avery A. Sandberg, and Alvin L. Watne, "Spread of Cancer Cells," *Journal of the American Medical Association,* CLXXII, April, 1960, pp. 1729-33.

Mullan, John F., and Mildred Van Schoik, "Intractable Pain," *American Journal of Nursing,* LVIII, February, 1958, pp. 228-30.

Paulson, Elmer E., and Donn G. Mosser, "Clinical Applications of Radioisotopes," *Postgraduate Medicine,* XXIII, May, 1958, pp. 493-98.

Pearson, Olaf H., "Adrenalectomy and Hypophysectomy," *American Journal of Nursing,* LXII, April, 1962, pp. 80-84.

Perese, Dogan M., "How to Manage Pain in Malignant Disease," *Journal of the American Medical Association,* CLXXV, January 14, 1961, pp. 75-81.

Perlia, Charles P., and Samuel G. Taylor, "Hormonal Treatment of Breast Cancer," *The Medical Clinics of North America,* XLVII, No. 1, January, 1963, p. 159.

Perrin, George M., and Irene R. Pierce, "Psychosomatic Aspects of Cancer," *Psychosomatic Medicine,* XXI, May, 1959, pp. 397-421.

Peterson, Rosalie I., "Federal Grants for Education in Cancer Nursing," *Nursing Outlook,* IV, February, 1956, pp. 103-5.

Popma, Alfred M., "Cancer of the Breast," *American Journal of Nursing,* LVII, December, 1957, pp. 1570-71.

Reagan, James W., "Cyotological Studies," *American Journal of Nursing,* LVIII, December, 1958, pp. 1693-95.

Rhoadas, Cornelius P., "Cancer Control—Present and Future," *American Journal of Nursing,* LVIII, April, 1958, pp. 516-19.

Schilling, Robert F., "Principles of Management of Patients with Leukemia," *Postgraduate Medicine,* XXVI, July, 1959, pp. 55-58.

Shingleton, William W., *et al.,* "Studies on Abdominal Organ Perfusion for Cancer Chemotherapy," *Annals of Surgery,* CLI, May, 1960, pp. 741-49.

Skaggs, Lester S., and Rosemary Haughey, "Radio Active Isotope Therapy," *Nursing Outlook,* IV, April, 1956, pp. 214-16.

Slaughter, Danely P., "What Is Early Cancer?" *Postgraduate Medicine,* XXVII, March, 1960, pp. 271-73.

Stehlin, John S., *et al.,* "Regional Therapy for Cancer," *Annals of Surgery,* CLI, April, 1960, pp. 605-19.

Sutherland, Arthur, "Psychological Impact of Cancer Surgery," *Public Health Reports,* LXVII, November, 1952, pp. 1139-43.

"A Symposium: Cancer," *Journal of Chronic Diseases,* VIII, July, 1958, entire issue.

Taren, James A., and Edgar A. Kahn, "The Surgical Relief of Intractable Pain," *Surgical Clinics of North America,* XLI, October, 1961, p. 1159.

Addie, Thomas, "Typical Patient and Family Attitudes," *Public Health Reports,* LXVII, October, 1952, pp. 960-62.

"Unproven Methods of Cancer Treatment," *Cancer,* XI, January-February, 1961, pp. 17-18, and March-April, 1961, pp. 67-68.

Westberg, Granger E., "Advice to the Family on Being Given a Diagnosis of Cancer," *Medical Clinics of North America,* XLII, March, 1958, pp. 563-68.

White, Dorothy Ruth, "I Have an Ileostomy," *American Journal of Nursing,* LXI, May, 1961, pp. 51-52.

Wolfman, Earl F., and C. Thomas Flotte, "Carcinoma of the Colon and Rectum," *American Journal of Nursing,* LXI, March, 1961, p. 60.

13 : Nursing the Patient Having a Problem Resulting from Disorders in Regulation

PART A : Chemical Regulation

> Living things, including people, go to a considerable amount of trouble to stay alive. Some of the work and effort involved in staying alive is expended at the level of consciousness, but fortunately much of it is carried on automatically under the direction of the two great communication systems of the body—the nervous system and the endocrine system. In any multicellular organism which consists of cooperative clusters of highly differentiated cells there are systems of signals and mechanisms for the transmission of messages from one part of the organism to another.

Although notable progress has been made, the mechanisms regulating and integrating physiological and psychological processes are only beginning to be understood. This should not be surprising, as regulation takes place on many levels and is highly complex. The general function of regulation is to enable the organism to modify its behavior so that it adapts to its environment and/or adapts the environment to its needs. Most adaptive behavior is of one of the following types: (1) the defensive escape, and avoidance reactions that serve to protect the organism from injury, (2) the reactions that are concerned with providing materials for energy, for the maintenance of protoplasm, and for growth, and (3) the responses that are required for the perpetuation of the species. In a broad sense all these reactions contribute to the maintenance of physiological and psychological homeostasis. Any disturbance in homeostasis acts as a stimulus which initiates activity resulting in its restoration.

Adaptations to the environment involve all aspects of function from those taking place within individual cells to the integrated functioning of the organism as a whole. Within the cell, biochemical activities are regulated so that controlled amounts of energy are released and the structure and function of

---

[1] Jay Tepperman, *Metabolic and Endocrine Physiology,* Yearbook Medical Publishers, Inc., Chicago, 1962, p. 13.

the cell are maintained within limits. This is accomplished despite differences in the supply of nutrients and the demands placed on the cell by the organism. Metabolic activities are regulated so that anabolism and catabolism are kept equal. If equilibrium is disturbed, adjustments are made so that balance is restored. Proteins are synthesized to maintain the protoplasm of the cell. The growth potential of the cell is controlled so that cells grow and divide only in response to specific stimuli.[2] Growth ceases when the need of the organism has been met. The physical and chemical structure of the cell is maintained. The differences in the chemical composition and volume of intracellular fluid of individual cells are maintained with remarkable accuracy. In multicellular organisms, the composition and volume of extracellular fluid are also accurately controlled.

Adaptations of multicellular organisms depend on structures and processes whereby messages can be communicated from one area of the body to another. Activities in which the entire organism participates to a greater or lesser degree include those involved in the maintenance of physiological and psychological homeostasis, locomotion, sensation, and psychic processes. All these activities depend on the function of individual cells, tissues, organs, and systems, but no part of the organism functions independently of other parts. Through regulation, structure and function of the parts are maintained within limits, so that the needs of the entire organism are met. Priority is usually given to basic needs. When the basic needs are met more or less automatically, attention can be devoted to higher needs.

Regulatory agencies are of two general types—chemical and neurochemical, or neurohumoral. Formerly the regulation of intracellular activities was thought to be entirely chemical. Recent findings support the belief that the nervous system probably also participates. Chemical regulators within the cell include genes, enzymes, and vitamins. Scientists are not certain about whether homones act within the cell or at its surface. Possibly they act at both sites. Products of metabolism, such as carbon dioxide, also influence the activity of the cells; consequently, they are regulatory. Two types of agencies are involved in the communication of messages from one part of the body to another. The older and more primitive type is the hormones; the other is the nervous system.

Before discussing specific regulatory structures and functions and the effects of injury or disease of specific structures, the general implications of disturbances in regulation will be presented. To reiterate, regulation enables the organism to maintain the function of cells, tissues, organs, and systems within the central range described as normal. Regulatory mechanisms prevent the excessive excursions of function that are incompatible with the safety and survival of the individual. They do this despite changes in the internal or external environment. A change in the internal or external environment acts

    [2] Renato Baserga and W. E. Kisieleski, "Autobiographies of Cells," *Scientific American*, CCIX, August, 1963, pp. 103-10.

as a stimulus which sets into motion a change or series of changes that correct the effects of the disturbance, or remove the individual from it.

What are some of the etiological factors in disorders of regulation?

The same general causative agents produce malfunction, injury, and disease of regulatory structures as of other structural facilities. These include infectious agents, trauma, vascular disturbances, poisons, neoplasms, developmental defects, and psychogenic disorders. Particularly in the brain, disturbance in the blood supply is a frequent source of injury. Traumatic injury to the brain and other parts of the nervous system is not infrequent. Neoplasms involving endocrine glands differ from those in other parts of the body inasmuch as they sometimes secrete the hormone of the parent gland, thus causing signs and symptoms of hyperfunction. Regulatory facilities are also subject to defective development which may be of genetic origin, or they may result from a lack or excess of required materials, or injury at a critical point in the process of development. Disturbances may also result from the failure of a regulatory structure to respond to agencies controlling its function. For example, in some instances hyperactivity of the adrenal cortex appears to result from the failure of the gland to respond to the governing influence of the adrenocorticotrophic hormone (ACTH).

Disturbances in regulation with alterations in physiological or psychological behavior may arise out of the manner in which the individual perceives his situation. Thus harmless things or situations may be the source of malfunction. Six-year-old Bobby Tears presented an extreme example of this type of causation of disturbed function. When he was two years old, he had been knocked down by the dog of a family with whom his parents had left him for a week end. Except for an abrasion on his elbow, he was not hurt physically. However, for years, if even the most sedate and harmless old dog approached him, he became terrified and developed nausea and vomiting, which was frequently followed by prolonged anorexia. In contrast, disturbances in regulation can result in effects that are interpreted as being of psychological origin when they actually have a physical basis. As a result, they may be ignored or misinterpreted. For example, Mr. Heron had physiological manifestations which were thought to be of psychological origin, but were actually due to a neoplasm causing pressure on his spinal cord. One of the major manifestations experienced by Mr. Heron was a lack of desire to void until his urinary bladder contained approximately 3,000 ml of urine. The nurse can contribute to the identification of the nature of the patient's medical problem by a careful description of her observations including the circumstances under which the signs and symptoms presented by the patient occur.

The general consequence of failure of regulation is an inability of the organism to adapt appropriately to its environment. Except at the time of death, failure of adaptation is not complete, but there is an inability to maintain one or more functions within the central range referred to as normal. Function may be hypo-, hyper-, or disorganized. Since most important physiological processes are subject to more than one regulatory mechanism, a disturbance in one is likely to unbalance others. Sometimes this is useful to the organism; at other times it may be harmful. Depending on the nature of the offending agent and the site of its action, the condition may be temporary or permanent. When a disturbance is of limited duration, the care of the patient is directed toward protecting him from the effects of his adaptive failure until such time as he is restored to health. When a disability is of a long-term or permanent nature, the patient and his family require instructions and support so that the patient can learn how to live as fully as possible within the limits imposed by the disorder. Since a long-term illness involving one member of a family usually affects the lives of the others, any assistance to the patient is likely to have a beneficial effect on the family as well.

The nurse has an important role in the care of patients with disturbances in regulation. Attention should be given in the nursing plan of care to modifying the environment of the patient so that the effect of the regulatory disability is minimized. This may be done by modifying the environment of the patient so that his needs are met with a minimum of effort on his part, or by supporting a defective adaptive mechanism. For example, Mr. Olena is admitted to the hospital in an unconscious state as the result of a cerebrovascular accident. His capacity to protect himself from injury is minimal. His survival depends on identifying the sources of injury and protecting him from them. One of the most immediate and serious threats to his well-being is the inability to maintain a clear airway. Measures must be instituted and carried out regularly to promote drainage of the tracheobronchial tree and to prevent aspiration of pharyngeal and gastric secretions. Since Mr. Olena is unable to protect his tissues from the effects of pressure, this must be done for him. His future recovery also depends on his extremities being maintained in good alignment and position, so that joint and muscle function is preserved. Passive exercise of extremities is essential to preserving joint and muscle function.

In contrast to Mr. Olena, whose survival depends on others modifying his environment so that his needs are met, Mr. Esbo requires care directed toward supporting a failing adaptive mechanism. Mr. Esbo, who is obese, secretes insufficient insulin to utilize normal amounts of glucose. If his requirements for insulin can be reduced, his own insulin-secreting capacity may be adequate to his needs. One of the objectives in his care is, therefore, to lessen the demands on his islet cells to secrete insulin. The methods employed are a diet limiting the quantity of carbohydrates as well as the number of calories. By reduction of the carbohydrates in his diet, his insulin requirement is lessened. The reduction is his calories should lead to a loss of weight and, with it, further diminishment of his insulin requirement. Should these measures be inadequate to maintain the level of glucose in his blood within physiological limits and to prevent the excessive use of fat and protein for fuel, insulin may be prescribed to supplement his own supply.

With the preceding overview of some of the general aspects of regulation, attention will be directed first to a brief summary of the roles of chromosomes, genes, enzymes, and vitamins in regulation of intracellular activities and to some of the results of failure of these regulators. A more detailed presentation of the role of hormones and the nervous system in integration of bodily processes will be made.

What are genes and how do they act?

Modern genetics can be traced back to the work of Mendel. In 1866 Mendel published his work in which he demonstrated that certain characteristics of peas are transmitted in an orderly and predictable pattern from parent to progeny. Despite the accuracy of his observations, Mendel did not know how or by what means hereditary characteristics were transmitted. In 1869, Miesche isolated from the nucleus of the cell a substance that he called nuclein; today this nuclein is called DNA. He knew that it contained nitrogen and phosphorus, but he had no idea about what it was or how it functioned. The specific question "What are genes and how do they act?" has been asked for about 50 years. Since approximately 1913 it has been known that genes— the individual units of heredity—are strung along chromosomes, which are threadlike structures in the nucleus of the cell. In 1953 James D. Watson and Francis H. C. Crick first described the information giving part of the cell as a giant molecule of desoxyribonucleic acid, or, as it is commonly called, DNA.[3]

From studies made over the past few years DNA has been demonstrated to be present in the nuclei of all cells. It is the chemical control system that governs heredity. Not only does it transmit information from one generation to the next, but it directs all the processes within the cell. Though DNA remains in the nucleus of the cell, it regulates the activities of all its parts. It has the capacity to divide into two parts in such a way that each new part is an exact copy of the original.

The DNA molecule is a helix, or spiral, that is sometimes described as a coiled ladder. Crick[4] describes DNA as being made by joining four kinds of nucleotides to form a backbone to which four kinds of side groups, called bases, are attached at regular intervals. In the DNA molecule the amino acids are paired, and can be compared to the rungs in a ladder.[5] Although the bases are attached at regular intervals, their order is not regular. It is the sequence of the bases that is believed to carry the genetic message. More specifically,

---

[3] Marshall W. Nirenberg, "The Genetic Code: II," *Scientific American,* CCVIII, March, 1963, p. 80.

[4] F. H. C. Crick, "The Genetic Code," *Scientific American,* CCVII, October, 1962, pp. 66-74.

[5] Nucleotides are formed from a combination of a purine or primidine base with a sugar and phosphoric acid. In DNA, the sugar is desoxyribose. The four bases in the DNA molecule are the amino acids adenine, guanine, cytosine, and thymine.

the order in which the bases are attached to the backbone of the nucleic acid determines the sequence of the amino acids in the proteins. They therefore determine whether the protein that is synthesized is that of a man, mouse, or tree. Within an individual the sequence and arrangement of the amino acids within the DNA molecule determines whether the protein synthesized is muscle or insulin or whether either is formed at all. Proteins contain most or all of the 20 common amino acids. Each amino acid is directed to its proper place in the protein chain by the sequence of bases in the DNA molecule. When the fact that a typical protein molecule contains approximately 200 subunits linked together in a specific sequence is considered, the possibilities for mistakes in sequence would appear to be large.

Among the questions puzzling geneticists and biochemists has been how the information incorporated in the genetic units is transmitted from the nucleus of the cell to the ribosomes in the cytoplasm where proteins are synthesized. Since DNA remains in the nucleus of the cell at all times, some means is required to transfer its instructions to sites of synthesis in the cytoplasm. Apparently another nucleic acid, ribonucleic acid (RNA), is required for this purpose. RNA differs from DNA inasmuch as the sugar in its molecule is ribose rather than desoxyribose and uracil is substituted for thymine. Brachet[6] states that DNA directs the formation of RNA, and RNA which is present in both the nucleus and the cytoplasm acts as an intermediary arranging the amino acids in the proper sequence in the synthesis of protein. There are actually two kinds of RNA. One is called messenger, or template, RNA. The order of the bases in template RNA specifies the sequence of amino acids in the protein to be synthesized. The other RNA is called transfer RNA. It transports the amino acids to the proper sites on messenger RNA. According to Nirenberg,[7] for each amino acid there is a specific enzyme; each cell contains a specific enzyme that functions to attach a specific amino acid to its particular RNA. The functions of DNA and RNA in the synthesis of protein have been compared to those of the architect and contractor or builder. The DNA is the architect who makes the blueprints or plans for the building. The RNA is the contractor who, following the directions of the architect, constructs a building of bricks and mortar. The size and function of the building depend on the original directions and how they have been executed.

Nirenberg[8] states that the number of proteins required by a typical cell to perform its functions is not known, but it is probably several hundred. Most, if not all, proteins act as enzymes within the cell to direct the hundreds of chemical reactions going on continuously within each cell. As a consequence of the lack of or the presence of an abnormal protein or enzyme, there may be a failure in one or more chemical reactions in the cell which can result in the synthesis of an abnormal substance or the failure to use one or more metabolites.

6 Jean Brachet, "The Living Cell," *Scientific American*, CCV, September, 1961, p. 52.
7 Nirenberg, *Op. cit.*, p. 83.
8 *Ibid.*, p. 80.

Knowledge of the function of the genetic material in the activities of the living cell has developed enormously over the last few years. Much of this has been made possible by the use of the electron microscope and of radioactive materials. Undoubtedly refinements of the use of radioactive substances as well as of other techniques will enable man to learn more about the biochemical activities within his cells. With greater understanding, some of this information may be useful in the prevention and treatment of disease. For readers who have an interest in this area, *Life Magazine* as well as *Scientific American* has carried an interesting series of articles. References from these as well as other journals will be included at end of chapter.

Although there is great interest in the regulatory activities of DNA, its functions in the transmission of the so-called hereditary traits are also important in health, in disease, and probably in the process of aging. It is only within the last ten years that the normal number of chromosomes in the human being has been established as 46, or 23 pairs. Two chromosomes, the X and Y chromosomes, are known as the sex chromosomes. The X chromosome is called the female chromosome and the Y chromosome the male chromosome. The sex of the individual is determined by the type of sex chromosome contained in the sperm fertilizing the ovum. If it is an X chromosome, the individual will be a female, as each cell in the new individual contains two X (XX) chromosomes. If it is a Y, then the individual will be a male, as each cell contains an X and a Y (XY) chromosome. Gametes, male or female reproductive cells, contain only 23 chromosomes. All female gametes contain X chromosomes. One half of the male gametes contain X chromosomes and one half contain Y chromosomes. As a cell prepares to divide, each chromosome as well as each gene divides into two in such a way that the daughter chromosome or gene is an exact copy or replica of the original. Since the gene, though a part of a chromosome, is the unit of hereditary material, the remarks which follow will be related to the gene, rather than to the entire chromosome.

One of the principles of genetics is that each gene comes from a preexisting gene. Each daughter cell contains exactly the same number of chromosomes and genes as did the parent cell. Genes are self-reproducing inasmuch as they copy themselves as they multiply. A gene may, however, change its character, or mutate. The rate of mutation can be speeded up by even a single exposure to X ray. Each gene has a specific position or locus on the chromosome. The gene occupying that same relative position on a corresponding chromosome is known as an allelomorph, or allele. This is true of a gene whether it is in the same or in other cells. Although a gene usually stays on the same chromosome, it may exchange with its allele by a process known as crossing over. Crossing over makes the recombination of genes possible. Chromosomes can also break and recombine.

If both genes of a pair influence a given trait in the same way, the individual is said to be homozygous for that characteristic. If one member influences a character differently from the other, the individual is said to be heterozygous. For example, if both genes influence growth in such a way that tallness results, then the individual is said to be homozygous for tallness. If, however, one gene is for tallness and the other is for shortness, then the individual is heterozygous for height. The trait exerting its influence over the other one is said to be dominant. The one that is hidden is recessive. Thus, if the person is heterozygous for height and at maturity he is tall, tallness is dominant over shortness. At one time dominance was thought to be complete. Now it is known that this is not necessarily true. For example, sickle cell anemia is a disorder in which a defective gene produces an abnormal form of hemoglobin. The person who has one normal gene and one sickle cell gene synthesizes two kinds of hemoglobin, one normal or hemoglobin A and the other abnormal or hemoglobin S. Through the use of appropriate methods both types can be identified. Whether the person evidences sickle cell disease depends on the proportion of normal to abnormal hemoglobin. Only a slight excess of abnormal to normal hemoglobin is sufficient to cause sickle cell disease. Persons who have some abnormal hemoglobin but do not have sickle cell disease are known as carriers. Though they do not have the disease, they can transmit the tendency to their offspring. The gene for sickle cell anemia illustrates a point made earlier; that is, genes direct the synthesis of proteins, and the specific character of a protein depends on the instructions relayed to the ribosomes by a specific gene. Sickle cell hemoglobin differs from normal hemoglobin in only one respect; the amino acid valine is substituted for glutamic acid at a specific point in the hemoglobin molecule. Hemoglobin S, when deoxygenated, tends to form rod-like particles in the erythrocytes and causes distortion of the red cell.

When genes for different traits are carried by the same chromosome, this condition is known by the term "linkage." Linkage is the basis for certain hereditary disorders that are associated with sex. The X chromosome carries genes for traits other than those that affect sex differentiation. Since the Y chromosome does not carry as many genes as the X chromosome, some of the genes on the X chromosome may not be matched by a corresponding gene on the Y chromosome. If the unopposed gene is defective, its effect will be evident in the individual. As a consequence of linkage, the genes for sex-linked diseases such as hemophilia pass from father to daughter. Since the daughter has two X chromosomes, the defective gene is opposed by a normal allele and the daughter carries the trait for, but does not develop, the disease. The affected father's sons are free from the defective gene, as they get their Y chromosomes from him and their X chromosomes from their mother. The sons of the carrier daughter run a 50-50 chance of receiving a defective gene and her daughters have the same chance of becoming carriers. A famous example of a sex-linked disease transmitted by female carriers is that of Queen Victoria. Several of her great-grandsons were hemophiliacs because her grand-daughters were carriers of the gene for hemophilia.

As carriers of the hereditary characteristics of the individual, genes have an important influence on the health potential and longevity of the individual.

There is some evidence to support the belief that heredity determines the reserve capacity of the tissues and organs of individuals and, as such, has a positive aspect. It also predisposes individuals to diseases such as the ones previously mentioned. Whether certain other diseases in which heredity appears to be a factor develop, depends on the interaction of the individual with his environment. For example, a person who inherits a limited reserve of insulin-secreting cells may protect himself from diabetes mellitus by avoiding obesity. Conversely, a combination of a hereditary tendency, overeating, and underexercising favors its development.

Since genes direct the synthesis of proteins and proteins act as enzymes or catalysts in chemical reactions, an abnormal gene may result in the failure to metabolize some substance. For example, a disorder which has been receiving considerable attention in popular as well as scientific literature is phenylketonuria. Phenylketonuria results from the failure of the individual to metabolize one of the common amino acids, phenylalanine, due to the absence of an essential enzyme. In the absence of this enzyme, phenylalanine accumulates in the blood and other body fluids. Unless the defect is discovered early in infancy, the phenylalanine injures the brain, causing mental retardation. If the condition is discovered early enough in the life of the child, the damaging effects to the child can be prevented by a diet low in phenylalanine. There is one negative aspect: any offspring of an individual with phenylketonuria will carry the trait.

One of the problems facing the individual who may be a carrier or who has a hereditary defect is whether or not he should marry. Despite the inability of the nurse to give the patient a definite answer to his questions, she can be of help by encouraging him to seek advice from his physician. In some instances the family physician will be able to provide the person with the desired information. In others, he may be referred to a physician who specializes in medical genetics. Not all persons who fear that they are carriers of hereditary disease can be proved to be. Some, such as sons of fathers who have a sex-linked disease, will not be. In others, even when they are carriers of a defective gene, the chances of their having defective offspring is remote. In some individuals, with appropriate control of other predisposing factors, the chances of developing a disease can be minimized or the effects of the disease lessened.

Summary

Genes, as the units responsible for the hereditary characteristics of the individual, may transmit abnormal as well as normal traits. Though a person carries one or more abnormal genes, he is not certain to develop a hereditary disorder. A variety of factors influence the expression of hereditary diseases. These include: (1) the character of the gene—dominant or recessive, (2) the effects of heredity on the reserve capacity of tissues or organs, and (3) the conditions in the environment of the individual. Each of these points has been discussed and illustrated.

The chromosomes may also be responsible for congenital malformations. Despite the involvement of the material of inheritance, they are not hereditary in the usual sense of the word. Neither are these disorders environmental. They arise from a defect in the mechanism by which the hereditary material is transmitted from parent to offspring. In the process of maturation of germ cells, the number of chromosomes is reduced by a process known as meiosis from 23 pairs to 23 chromosomes; each new cell contains one of each pair. The reduction in number prevents the doubling of chromosomes in each generation thus keeping the number of chromosomes constant. Meiosis differs from mitosis, in which each daughter cell receives a quantity of genetic material equal to that of the parent cell. In meiosis, the reduction in the number of chromosomes is accomplished during the last two cell divisions. The parent cell divides twice, while the chromosomes divide only once.

Abnormalities in development may result from nondisjunction (failure of chromosomes to segregate) or from translocation of chromosomal material. Translocation results when parts of two dissimilar chromosomes break off and are relocated. During meiosis the abnormal pairing of the anomalous chromosomes is likely.[9]

A number of disorders have been demonstrated to be due to one or the other of the above. Mongolism results when an ovum containing two number 21 chromosomes (a small somatic chromosome) is fertilized by a sperm containing one 21. The resulting zygote contains three chromosomes, instead of a normal pair. Most patients with Klinefelter's syndrome who have been studied have two X chromosomes in addition to a Y chromosome. The resulting individual is a male who is tall, has enlarged breasts, and produces few, if any, sperm. In this instance, the individual may inherit the abnormality, that is, nondisjointed chromosomes, from either his father or his mother.

There are a number of other disorders known to result from a failure in the process whereby the hereditary material is passed from the parent to his child. The type of resulting abnormality depends on the nature of the defect. These disorders are not hereditary nor are they environmental in the usual sense of these terms. They may result from the effect of an illness, for example a virus infection, at a critical stage in the development of a gamete. In mongolism the age of the mother appears to be a predisposing factor, as the incidence of mongolism rises steeply as the age of the mother increases. The nurse may be able to reinforce the assurance given by the physician that anomalies due to an abnormality in the process of meiosis are not hereditary. Children born later are likely to be normal. Healthy individuals do not have to be concerned about the possibility of having abnormal children.

What are enzymes and how do they affect health and disease?

Enzymes are proteins that are synthesized under the direction of the genes. They function as organic catalysts in biochemical reactions in the body. Simi-

---

[9] A. G. Bearn and James L. German III, "Chromosomes and Disease," *Scientific American,* CCV, November, 1961, p. 71.

lar to inorganic catalysts, they do not initiate, but they affect the speed of, chemical reactions without themselves appearing in the final product. Organic catalysts have the advantage of being effective at lower temperatures than inorganic catalysts are. During a chemical reaction in which catalysts are involved, they combine momentarily with the substance whose reaction they are speeding. In the absence of enzymes or other catalytic agents, the rate at which many chemical reactions would occur at body temperature would be so slow that life could not exist. The actions of most enzymes are specific; that is, they act on a single substance or a closely related group of substances. Some enzymes are concentrated in a particular type of tissue. For example, among the enzymes found in the cells of lung are those that catalyze the conversion of the bicarbonate ion to carbon dioxide. Enzymes in the kidney catalyze the reabsorption of glucose and the excretion of urea. The synthesis of enzymes is not unique to human beings as all living cells produce them. Some of the products of bacteria, such as exotoxins, may be enzymes. One factor in bacterial resistance to penicillin is that bacteria synthesize an enzyme, penicillinase, that destroys penicillin. Frieden[10] quotes the biochemist Ernest Borek as follows: "We live because we have enzymes. Everything we do—walking, thinking, reading these lines—is done with some enzymic process." And in the words of Frieden himself, "Life is essentially a system of cooperating enzyme reactions."

The variety of biochemical reactions catalyzed by enzymes in human beings is illustrated by the following reactions: (1) the hydrolysis of foods ingested into the alimentary canal; (2) the movement of substances across cell and other membranes; (3) the transformation of carbohydrate, fat, and protein into energy; (4) the synthesis of proteins; (5) the synthesis and degradation of hormones; (6) the formation of a blood clot; and (7) the digestion of tissue and other debris associated with inflammation. The above list of body processes in which enzymes are involved is in no sense complete, as all biochemical processes in the body require the presence of enzymes. The variety of chemical reactions listed does not emphasize the importance and extent to which enzymes participate in regulating biochemical activities. Anything that interferes with the activity of one or more enzyme systems can be expected to have widespread effects.

As knowledge of the nature and actions of enzymes has grown, interest in them as causative agents in disease as well as in the diagnosis and treatment of disease has been stimulated. In the last 30 years or so, knowledge of enzymes has increased at a phenomenal rate.

As indicated earlier, the presence of a mutant gene may deprive the organism of an enzyme required by the cell to catalyze a step in a biochemical reaction. This can result in the accumulation of partly utilized materials in the tissues or in the formation of an abnormal or defective protein. It can result in failure to digest or to absorb nutrients, or in the failure to clot blood. It also

[10] Earl Frieden, "The Enzyme-Substrate Complex," *Scientific American*, CCI, August, 1959, p. 125.

leads to the possibility that enzymes may be involved in disorders of growth. One recurring and as yet unsubstantiated theory relating to cancer is that the enzyme pattern in malignant neoplasms differs from that of healthy tissue. What actually happens in the absence of an enzyme depends on the process that is blocked by the lack of the required enzyme. Because the rate of a multitude of biochemical processes is dependent on enzymes, the variety of disorders having their origin in some disturbance in the enzyme system would appear to be great.

Since enzymes appear to be dependent on the physical and chemical conditions in their environment, many disorders may have adverse effects on the functioning of enzyme systems. Most enzymes function at a narrow range of temperature and hydrogen ion concentration. The injury to tissue in hyperpyrexia may result from the effect of elevated temperature on enzyme systems. Failure to convert the hydrogen ion to water when oxygen is deficient may be the cause of death in shock.

Certain poisons, such as salts of cyanide, are highly lethal because they inactivate respiratory enzymes. Without respiratory enzymes, oxidation-reduction reactions proceed at such a slow rate that insufficient energy is released to carry on the activities of the cell. Death occurs within a matter of minutes.

The removal of a glandular organ either by disease or by surgery may also be responsible for a deficiency of one or more enzymes. For example, when the pancreas is surgically removed in the treatment of cancer, the enzymes secreted by the pancreas are not available for the digestion of fats, proteins, and carbohydrates. Since the pancreas is the principal source of lipase (fat-digesting enzyme), the individual has a problem in the digestion of fat unless lipase is replaced. The most serious problems that arise following pancreatectomy do not stem from a lack of insulin, but from the absence of the digestive enzymes secreted by the pancreas.

How is knowledge of the sources of enzymes employed in the diagnosis of disease?

Knowledge of the action of enzymes is employed in the diagnosis and treatment of disease. Their use in diagnosis is based on the hypothesis that enzymes produced by a cell remain in the cell until the cell disintegrates, or until there is sufficient alteration in energy-producing pathways to alter the cell membrane and increase the permeability of that membrane to the point where enzyme leakage occurs. As the cell breaks up, enzymes are released into the blood. Through the use of appropriate laboratory tests, the increase in the level of the particular enzyme in the blood serum can be demonstrated. Some examples include the elevation of serum amylase in acute pancreatitis, the elevation of the serum *acid* phosphatase in cancer of the prostate, and the elevation of lactic dehydrogenase in acute myocardial infarction. In all these disorders, cells undergo necrosis and the cell membrane is disrupted, releasing enzymes into the blood.

How are enzymes utilized in the therapy of disease?

Not only are enzymes useful in establishing the site of a disease process, but they have a variety of uses in therapy. They may be administered to replace enzymes that are deficient or to modify the effect of a disease or treatment. For example, pancreatic enzymes may be given to the patient who has had a pancreatectomy. Hyaluronidase, an enzyme that digests hyaluronic acid, may be administered with subcutaneous fluids or local anesthetics to facilitate absorption. Agents containing protein-digesting enzymes are sometimes applied to wounds to aid in their débridement. An enzyme, fibrolysin, is being studied to determine its effectiveness and safety in the treatment of intravascular clotting.

Besides the introduction of enzymes into the body, treatment may involve the inhibition of enzymes already present. For example, a number of modern diuretics are effective because they block an enzyme system. The organic mercurial diuretics are believed to interfere with the enzyme systems which are required for the reabsorption of chloride anions. Diuresis occurs because an equivalent amount of sodium is excreted with the chloride ion. Acetazolamide (Diamox) inhibits carbonic anhydrase, an enzyme catalyzing the conversion of carbon dioxide to the bicarbonate ion. Similar to the chloride anion, the bicarbonate anion is matched by an equivalent quantity of cation, principally sodium, for its excretion. With an increase in the excretion of sodium, water is excreted.

The problems arising in the nursing of patients who have a deficiency or lack of essential enzymes are related to the fact that many of these disturbances have a genetic basis and continue throughout the life of the individual. In these conditions the capacity of the individual to adapt on the biochemical level is in some way deficient. In some instances, as in phenylketonuria, the nature of the disturbance is known and, if discovered early enough, can be controlled. In others, control is not yet possible.

The objective relating most specifically to the nursing of these patients is to assist the patient and his family to gain the knowledge and skill required to control the progress of his disease, when this is possible. When the course of the disease cannot be altered, the nurse should direct the attention of the patient and his family toward living as full a life as is compatible with his disorder and toward preventing unnecessary disability. For the nurse to be of maximum assistance to the patient and his family, she should have some understanding of the cause and nature of disorders of enzyme systems, and be familiar with the objectives and means of therapy. Because of the nature and prognosis of these disorders, she will undoubtedly require competence in the expressive role of nursing.

The field of enzymology and its applications to health and disease is rapidly expanding. The literature in the field is enormous. Since enzymes function in regulation on the biochemical level, their effects are widespread and profound. By their action or lack thereof, they influence the capacity of the organism to adapt to its environment. Lack of, or alterations in, the activity of enzymes may be the cause of disease. Likewise disease may alter the activity of enzymes. Without enzymes life does not exist.

What mechanisms are available for the communication of information from one part of a multicellular organism to another?

The importance of the regulation of the biochemical processes within the cell to its health and survival cannot be overestimated. Life will not long continue, however, unless favorable conditions in the environment of the cell are maintained. Since these conditions have been discussed earlier, they will not be enumerated here. The maintenance of homeostasis depends on the regulation of cells, tissues, organs, and systems so that the organism functions as a whole. To achieve the integration of all the processes used by the organism to meet its needs, structural facilities are required whereby information about conditions in the internal and external environment can be perceived and communicated from one area to another. Large multicellular organisms have two mechanisms for accomplishing these functions. The older and more primitive mechanism is the endocrine system. The newer and more sophisticated mechanism is the nervous system. Nowhere are the interrelationships among the various regulatory agencies clearer than in the relationship of hormones to the other regulators. The genes determine the adequacy of the hormone-secreting tissue. They also direct the formation of enzymes catalyzing reactions involved in the formation of hormones as well as those involved in their degradation.

There are many overlapping functions between the nervous and endocrine systems. The adrenal medulla is part of the sympathetic nervous system and its products, epi- and norepinephrine, are secreted by other portions of the system as well.

Recent findings indicate that the production of most hormones is directly or indirectly under the control of the nervous system. Since hormones are important in the regulation of physiological homeostasis, deficiencies or excesses in their production may have profound effects on the functioning of enzymes and of the nervous system, and often do.

As implied in the preceding discussion, hormones are chemical regulators synthesized by specialized organs, the endocrine glands. They are carried by the blood and other body fluids to the cells of the body. Specific structures on which they have a marked effect are called target tissues, or organs. Despite seeming specificity, the action of hormones is not limited to their target organs; rather they all probably have widespread effects. The actions of hormones influence the rate not only of energy metabolism, but of mineral metabolism, as well as the growth and development of the organism.

How can hormones be classified?

One way in which hormones can be classified is by their chemical structure. They are of three general types—steroids, proteins and polypeptides, and phenolamines.[11] The sex hormones and the adrenal cortical hormones are steroids. At one time the process by which each of these hormones was synthesized was thought to be unique. They are now known to have a common precursor. The glands that synthesize steroid hormones have many common enzymes. There is some overlapping of functions of adrenal cortical and sex hormones. As an example, women patients receiving or secreting large quantities of adrenal cortical hormones undergo masculinizing changes.

Hormones from the anterior and posterior hypophysis, the parathyroid hormones, insulin, and glucagon are proteins or polypeptides. Of these, oxytocin and insulin have been synthesized. Insulin is a relatively simple protein consisting of 51 amino acids. One of the most recent accomplishments has been the identification of the complete molecular structure of ACTH (adrenocorticotrophin).[12] Although most naturally occurring hormones are more effective when administered parenterally, proteins and polypeptides must be administered this way; otherwise they are destroyed by digestion.

The phenolamines include epinephrine and norepinephrine, which are secreted by the adrenal medulla, and the thyroid hormones. Thyroxin was the first hormone to be isolated in pure form. The study of the effects of hormones has been facilitated by advances in knowledge of their chemical nature. Until a hormone is isolated in pure form, scientists cannot be certain about its action.

Besides the grouping of hormones chemically, they may also be classified according to how they produce their effects on tissues. Some hormones, such as insulin and the thyroid hormones, act directly on target tissues. Others, such as thyrotrophin and adrenocorticotrophin, act by stimulating another gland to produce its hormones.

Certain hormones have what is referred to as a permissive action. They condition the animal to adapt to or respond to his environment. In other words, they affect the manner in which the organism responds under a given set of circumstances. To illustrate, the adrenal cortical hormones are essential for the organism to respond to any form of stress, be it physical, chemical, or emotional. In intact, fasting rats, adrenal cortical hormones are required for

[11] Polypeptides and proteins are similar inasmuch as they are both composed of amino acids. The principal difference between them is in the size of the molecule. Protein molecules are larger than those of a polypeptide.

[12] Choh Hao Li, "The ACTH Molecule," *Scientific American*, CCIX, July, 1963, p. 46.

estrogenic hormones to increase liver glycogen. In the human being, the thyroid hormones sensitize the individual to epinephrine. The patient whose thyroid gland is hypersecreting thyroxin is hypersensitive to epinephrine. A therapeutic dose for a person who is euthyroid may cause ventricular fibrillation in a person who is suffering from hyperthyroidism. Hypothyroidism increases the sensitivity of the nervous system to depressant drugs such as codeine, morphine, and meperidine. A single dose of any depressant drug may result in profound depression of the nervous system. The actions of other hormones are also determined by conditions in the body. Desoxycorticosterone predisposes to nephrosclerosis, provided the individual also ingests sodium chloride. In hyperthyroidism, the possibility of liver injury can be reduced by an adequate intake of the vitamin thiamine.

Hormones may also be classed as those that are essential to life and those that are required for normal growth and development. For example, the adrenal cortical hormones are necessary to life. The same is true for insulin. Although the thyroid hormones are required for normal growth and development and for healthy physical and mental functioning, their absence does not result in the death of the individual.

Where and how do hormones act?

Three theories have been advanced to explain the site or locus of action of hormones.[13] The first and older theory is that hormones control the action of enzymes. This theory was proposed after the discovery was made that vitamins enter the cell and act as coenzymes.

A second and newer theory is that hormones control the permeability of the cell membrane. Insulin brings about a great increase in the permeability of the cell to glucose. Possibly all the effects of insulin may be explained on this basis. One of the effects of thyroxine on metabolism in the mitochondria[14] may be due to changes in permeability of the cell membrane. Action of thyroxin, however, is not considered to be primarily on membrane permeability. Even in the instance of the steroid hormones, the possibility that they act by altering cell permeability has been considered.

The third and newest theory proposed to explain some of the actions of hormones is that they alter the activity of genes. One factor in achieving maturity is that genetic information comes into play in the correct order and at the proper time. Karlson[15] states that, because hormones reach all the tissues, they may well act as a timing device for the development of peripheral organs.

Finally, there is a possibility that the site of action differs for different

[13] Peter Karlson, "New Concepts on the Mode of Action of Hormones," *Perspectives in Biology and Medicine*, VI, Winter, 1963, pp. 203-14.

[14] Mitochondria are the power plants in the cells of both plants and animals. From the mitochondria, energy is released for the energy-producing processes within the cell.

[15] *Op. cit.*, p. 208.

hormones. Some may act by influencing the activity of enzymes, others by altering the permeability of membranes, and still others by their effects on the genes.

What are the shared characteristics of hormones?

One of the common characteristics of hormones is that none are believed to initiate functions. They alter the rate of reactions, usually by augmenting them, but they do not start them. Thus the cells metabolize glucose in the absence of insulin. In the presence of insulin, the rate at which glucose is removed from the blood is accelerated.

A second common characteristic of hormones is that none are secreted at a precisely uniform rate. Some hormones, such as the adrenal steroids, are secreted according to a daily (diurnal) rhythm. Others, such as the gonado-trophins and the female sex hormones, maintain a cyclical rhythm. Still others, such as insulin, are secreted in response to the level of a constituent in the blood. Some, such as insulin, are secreted somewhat in excess of the quantity required. As a consequence, after the blood glucose is raised, its level in the blood may drop slightly lower than it was before glucose was ingested. It then returns to normal.

A third common characteristic of hormones is that they are effective in relatively small amounts. The effective dose of some, such as tri-iodothyro-nine and aldosterone, is in the microgram range.

A fourth common characteristic is that hormones are continuously lost from the body either by excretion or by metabolic inactivation, and they must be replaced. Effects of hypersecretion may, therefore, be due to oversecretion by a particular gland or to failure of a mechanism by which a particular hormone is inactivated. For example, aldosterone is inactivated by the liver. One of the factors in edema in diseases in which there is functional failure of the liver is believed to be an elevation in the level of aldosterone.

A fifth common characteristic of hormones is that a latent period exists between the administration of a hormone and the time its effects become apparent. In the case of epinephrine or insulin the length of the latent period is relatively short. Thyroxin, on the other hand, has a long latent period as it takes from 8 to 14 days to act.

For reasons that are not understood, individuals tend to be hypersensitive to hormones that they lack. The patient who is hypothyroid requires a smaller dosage of thyroxin to cause symptoms of hyperthyroidism than the one who is euthyroid.

There are a number of other generalizations that may be made about hormones. Each hormone has widespread effects on the organism. Few, if any, functions are exclusively dependent for regulation on one hormone. Most functions are dependent on a number of hormones in adequate balance and sequence. Several hormones may act at the same time or in a series. A hormone may oppose or supplement the action of another. For example, insulin lowers blood sugar; the adrenal glucocorticoids oppose the action of insulin by elevating it. The growth and thyroid hormones have synergistic effects on growth. Some hormones have overlapping actions. Oxytocin and vasopressin have long been known to have some common pharmacological properties. This is also true of the mineralo- and glucocorticoids secreted by the cortex of the adrenal gland. Their actions are quantitatively, but not qualitatively, different. Since hormones do not initiate functions but only modify them, other elements may be responsible for disturbances in functions regulated by particular hormones. To illustrate, growth depends not only on adequate secretion of thyroid and growth hormones, but on the genetic background and nutrition of the individual. A serious or a prolonged illness at a critical period in the life of a child may also serve to stunt growth. Although thyroid hormones regulate the rate of energy metabolism, other factors contribute to it. This is demonstrated by the fact that in the absence of the thyroid gland, the basal metabolic rate falls about 35 per cent. Expressed in the usual terms for reporting, the metabolic rate of an athyroid individual is about −35. Other factors are responsible for the remaining 65 per cent of the metabolic rate.

In health, the level of each hormone is maintained within physiological limits as well as in a state of equilibrium with other hormones by at least two types of regulatory mechanisms. One type is a negative feedback relationship between the regulator and the target gland. (In negative feedback, there is a regulatory relationship between two factors or elements in which the increase in one results in an increase in the activity of the second, but the increase in the activity of the second results in a decrease in the activity of the first.) In the other type, no feedback relationship between two glands has been demonstrated. Rather, stimulation or depression of secretion results from the level of a component of the blood such as glucose, water, or the sodium cation. An example of a negative feedback is the relationship of the anterior pituitary to the adrenal cortex. The level of production of the adrenal glucocorticoids is increased by adrenocorticotrophin (ACTH) from the anterior pituitary. As the concentration of the glucocorticoids rises, the secretion of ACTH is depressed. As the level of the glucocorticoids falls, the secretion of ACTH rises. Where no feedback mechanism is known to exist, the rate of hormone production is presumed to be controlled by some mechanism at the site of the formation of the hormone. This may be nervous, chemical, or physical in origin.

What kinds of processes are regulated by hormones?

As implied above, hormones participate in the regulation and integration of all important bodily activities. The functions in which hormones play a significant role are summarized as follows:

1. Hormones are important to reproduction and all the activities related to it.
2. Hormones are essential to growth and to structural and biochemical differentiation.
3. Hormones are required for the adaptation of the individual to environmental and nutritional circumstances threatening his life or health.[16]

Although it would be appropriate to do so, this chapter does not include a discussion of the role of hormones in reproduction. The content of the chapter will be limited to points two and three, with particular emphasis on three.

Another way to indicate the variety of processes influenced by hormones is to list some of them. Some of the metabolic (biochemical) reactions regulated by hormones include: (1) energy metabolism—that is, the rate of oxidation-reduction reactions in the mitochondria in the cytoplasm of cells, (2) calcium-phosphorus balance between body fluids and bony structures, (3) water balance, (4) electrolyte balance, and (5) metabolism of carbohydrates, proteins, and fats. Not only are these reactions regulated in relation to supply, but they are regulated in relation to conditions in the internal and external environment. Furthermore, hormones not only modify the rate of bodily functions in health, but they integrate many responses of the organism to injury or threats of injury. They also modify the course of some diseases. For instance, some breast cancers appear to be dependent on ovarian and adrenal cortical hormones for their growth. In hormone-dependent cancers of breast, regression of the growth may follow removal of the ovaries and adrenal glands. In contrast, the growth of some malignant neoplasms is inhibited by the adrenal cortical hormones. Some children with acute leukemia improve for a time when they are treated with adrenal cortical steroids.

The level of hormones in the body fluid is influenced by the rate at which they are destroyed or excreted. Any mechanism interfering with their destruction or elimination could be presumed to result in malfunction. Whatever type of mechanism regulates the production of hormones, little doubt exists at the present time that the release of a number of them is under the control of the nervous system. Regulatory mechanisms can be viewed as parts of one system, organized in a hierarchy with the nervous system as the head. In some instances the exact means by which the nervous system controls the secretion of hormones is not clear. In others, the relationship of the chemical regulator to its neural counterpart is so intimate that they appear to be part of the same mechanism. For instance, the relationship between the sympathetic nervous system and the adrenal medulla is so close that some authorities speak of them as the sympathoadrenal system. There is an embryological, anatomical, and functional basis for this hypothesis. The adrenal medulla arises in the embryo from the same structures forming the nervous system. Adrenal medullary cells appear to be modified, or secreting, nerve cells. They are supplied by

[16] Tepperman, *Op. cit.*, p. 15.

preganglionic rather than postganglionic fibers from the sympathetic nervous system. As in other sympathetic ganglia, the chemical mediator is acetylcholine. On stimulation, the cells in the adrenal medulla secrete epinephrine and norepinephrine. The chemical mediators formed at the endings of the postganglionic sympathetic fibers are norepinephrine and epinephrine. The results of the action of epinephrine and norepinephrine and of sympathetic activity are indistinguishable. Although knowledge of how the hypothalamus regulates the sympathetic nervous system is far from complete, it is generally conceded that it does. Since there are numerous connections between the hypothalamus and other centers in the brain, there is little doubt that the sympathoadrenal function is under the control of the nervous system.

The neurohypophysis (posterior pituitary) is generally described as an anatomical and functional extension of the nervous system. Like the adrenal medulla, the neurohypophysis originates from embryonic structures in common with the nervous system. There are also clearly defined nerve pathways between nuclei (groups of cells) in the hypothalamus and the neurohypophysis. The hormones released by the posterior pituitary, the antidiuretic hormone and oxytocin, are believed to be synthesized in nuclei in the hypothalamus, after which they travel down to the gland, where they are released on stimulation.[17]

The control of the adenohypophysis (anterior pituitary) by the hypothalamus has been much more difficult to establish. From the location of these two structures, the hypothesis that there should be a functional relationship appears to be reasonable. The anatomical connection seems to be by way of a hypophyseal portal system rather than by nerve fibers. The regulation of the secretion of the adenohypophyseal hormones will be discussed with greater detail later.

No discussion of the functions of the endocrine system is complete unless the relationship between the nervous system and the secretion of hormones is emphasized. Best and Taylor[18] state that the hypothalamus stands in the key position between the nervous and endocrine systems. Either directly or indirectly the hypothalamus serves as a center for the exchange of messages between higher centers in the nervous system and endocrine glands. The hypothalamus receives messages from the higher centers that it relays to the appropriate endocrine gland. It also sends messages to the higher centers apprising them of conditions within the organism.

Endocrine glands are subject to the same types of pathology as other structures in the organism. Structures and function are impaired when a gland is deprived of its blood supply. Infection and autoimmune disorders may have a similar effect. Unfavorable genetic and/or environmental conditions may result in an absence of, or insufficient, tissue to secrete an adequate supply of

[17] *Ibid.*, p. 26.
[18] Charles H. Best and Norman B. Taylor, *The Physiological Basis of Medical Practice,* 7th ed., The Williams & Wilkins Company, Baltimore, 1961, p. 953.

a hormone or hormones. Failure to control the growth potential of the secreting or supporting cells of a gland may result in a benign or malignant neoplasm. When secreting cells are involved, alterations occur in the level of secretion of the hormone(s) elaborated by the affected gland. Either hypo- or hypersecretion may result. The effects of neoplasms as space-occupying and metastasizing lesions depend on the location of the gland involved. A neoplasm of the thyroid gland may obstruct breathing or swallowing.

A disturbance in the functioning of an endocrine gland may result from malfunction in the regulating mechanism or from failure to respond to regulation. To illustrate, Cushing's syndrome is a disorder resulting from hyperactivity of the adrenal cortex. The hyperplasia of the gland, along with its hypersecretion, could be the result of excessive stimulation due to oversecretion of ACTH or to failure of the adrenal cortex to secrete only in response to an increase in the level of ACTH. According to present theory, the adrenal cortex does not respond appropriately to the controlling mechanisms. It continues to secrete despite a decrease in the secretion of ACTH.

Because hormonal disturbances are usually characterized by the hypo- or hypersecretion of a hormone or result from the imbalance between or among hormones, the first objective in the therapy of patients with hormonal disturbances is to restore hormone balance. When a disorder is characterized by hypofunction, one or more of the following approaches may be used to maintain function. The first and most frequently employed is the replacement of the deficient hormones. In some instances, the individual's requirements for the hormone may be lessened. Finally, measures may be utilized to stimulate the production of the hormone by the individual. For example, among the factors in the etiology of diabetes mellitus is a deficiency in insulin supply. Diabetes may be treated by replacing the deficient insulin, by reducing the individual's insulin requirements, or, if he is middle-aged or older and his diabetes is not too severe, by stimulating his islets cells to secrete insulin.

In patients with conditions characterized by hyperfunction, therapy is, of course, directed toward returning secretion to normal levels. This may be accomplished by the surgical removal of all or a part of the secreting tissue or by blocking of the production of the hormone. When all the tissue is extirpated, or destroyed, the individual is treated by the same general methods employed in the therapy of persons with hypofunction.

When patients require continued therapy with hormones, they should be observed for symptoms and signs indicating over- and underdosage. They should also be taught why they require the hormone, what effects are to be expected, and what to do should untoward symptoms develop; sensitivity to hormones differs from person to person and in the same person from time to time. Symptoms of over dosage are comparable to those found in disease states characterized by hyperfunction. In addition to the factors mentioned, patients also should be instructed about how to administer their own medication and why a regular schedule is required. Some endocrine disorders make it necessary for the person to modify one or more aspects of his life. Emphasis in the instruction should be on helping the patient to develop the knowledge and competence that he requires to manage his disease. Success in management of some of the more common endocrine diseases frequently depends on the willingness and ability of the patient and his family to assume responsibility for the management of the disease. Physicians and nurses can and should act as teachers and consultants. Instructional plans should, therefore, help to prepare the patient to assume the necessary responsibility. To be successful, the instruction should take into account what the patient can and will be able to do. A highly elaborate teaching plan may not be effective unless it makes provision for the individual patient's home and work situation.

To summarize, hormones are essential for the communication of information from one area of the body to another. They are produced by the glands comprising the endocrine system. Each gland in the system is an individual organ. There exists, however, among the endocrine glands a complicated relationship and a complex yet unified working together toward a common goal—the maintenance of homeostasis.

Although there are many disorders involving hormones, only diabetes mellitus, hyper- and hypothyroidism, and hyper- and hyposecretion of the adrenal cortex will be presented in detail. For detailed information about other disorders of the endocrine system consult the References at end of chapter.

Anterior Pituitary (Adenohypophysis)

Introductions to a discussion of the anterior pituitary frequently include a statement to the effect that it is the master gland of the body. It is a small structure, about the size of a pea, in man, and it is located along with the neurohypophysis just below the center of the brain in the sella turcica. As stated earlier, because of its close proximity to the brain, it is possible that the anterior hypophysis is under the direct control of the brain, but to date evidence of this is only fragmentary. Despite its small size, the anterior hypophysis secretes at least seven different hormones. These hormones control growth, sexual development, reproduction, and thyroid activity, and they have an important effect on the general response of the body to stress.[19] Of the seven hormones secreted by the anterior hypophysis, the two most important are the growth hormone (GH) and adrenocorticotrophin (ACTH). Of the other physiologically active hormones three are gonadotrophins—the follicle-stimulating hormone (FSH), the luteinizing hormone or interstitial cell-stimulating hormone (LH or ICSH), and prolactin or lactogenic hormone (LTH) in some species. The thyroid-stimulating hormone (TSH) and the melanocyte-stimulating hormone (MSH) are the other two physiologically active hormones known to be secreted by the anterior pituitary.

The hormones secreted by the anterior pituitary induce their effect in two

[19] Choh Hao Li, *Op. cit.*, p. 46.

different ways. They affect tissues directly, and they regulate the output of hormones of other glands such as the adrenal cortex, thyroid, and gonads (ovaries and testes). Although the function of the trophic hormones was formerly believed to be limited to their target glands, these hormones can produce effects in the absence of their target glands.[20] Because of the difficulty of discussing the trophic hormones without also including the hormones secreted by their target glands, they will be considered with the gland that they stimulate.

What are the effects of the growth hormone as well as of hypo- or hypersecretion?

The growth hormone increases the rate of growth of the skeleton. With the increase in growth, there is a gain in body weight. Absence of the growth hormone before the maturity of the organism is accompanied by a marked slowing of the rate of growth. Tepperman[21] states that growth continues, but it is greatly reduced in rate. He also states that the failure in growth of the hypophysectomized animal is due not only to the lack of the growth hormone, but probably to other factors as well. The growth hormone, or a closely related substance, inhibits the action of insulin. Hypophysectomized and pancreatcctomized animals have little, if any, diabetes. Disorders characterized by hypersecretion of the growth hormone are frequently accompanied by glycosuria.

Hypersecretion of the growth hormone in an immature animal leads to overgrowth of the skelcton, that is, to giantism. Hypersecretion after growth has ceased leads to a condition known as acromegaly. A characteristic fcature in acromegaly is an enlargement of flat boncs such as those of the hands, feet, and head. The lower jaw enlarges and the face takes on a coarse appearance. There is also an enlargement of all viscera except the brain. Acromegaly may be accompanied by symptoms of hyperthyroidism and of diabetes mellitus. Many patients can be cured by irradiation of the pituitary gland. The skeletal changes are permanent, however.

A brief discussion of the implications of panhypopituitarism follows. According to Tepperman,[22] the anterior hypophysis is not essential to life. Hypophysectomized animals not given any hormone substitution therapy may live for months or years provided they are protected from environmental stress. They must be kept in a warm, air-conditioned room, protected from infections and from very much physical exercise. In panhypopituitarism, whether induced by disease or by the complete removal of the gland, the manifestations result from a deficiency of the antidiuretic, the thyroid, the adrenal cortical, and the gonadal hormones.[23] Of these the first three are of the most significance

[20] *Ibid.*, p. 46.
[21] *Op. cit.*, p. 29.
[22] *Ibid.*, p. 28.
[23] The antidiuretic hormone is released by the posterior hypophysis.

to survival and health, and they must therefore be replaced. Because the thyroid gland contains a supply of hormones, after hypophysectomy a patient may not require an exogenous supply of thyroid hormones for as long as three months. The other hormones, however, are necessary immediately. In most instances the patient will require hormonal replacement therapy for the remainder of his life.

What hormones are secreted or released by the posterior pituitary (neurohypophysis)? What are their effects?

Modern theory postulates that antidiuretic hormone (ADH) and oxytocin are synthesized by the neurons of the supraoptic and paraventricular nuclei. They are stored in and released by the neurohypophysis. The principal effects of these hormones are to increase the reabsorption of water by the renal tubules, to stimulate uterine contraction, and to enhance the secretion of milk by the lactating mammary gland. In anesthetized animals, they have a blood pressure-raising effect. The adrenal cortical hormones appear to antagonize the action of the antidiuretic hormones. Newer theory postulates that the secretion of ADH is increased as one of the responses of the organism to traumatic injury.

The disorder with which the hypofunction of the neurohypophysis is most commonly associated is diabetes insipidus. In diabetes insipidus the patient voids a large volume of urine of low specific gravity. There may be as many as 15 to 28 l of urine per day, and its specific gravity ranges from 1.001 to 1.005. With this large loss of water, dehydration with dry skin and intense thirst occurs. The polyuria is not lessened by depriving the patient of water, nor is the specific gravity of the urine increased. Polydipsia is secondary to the polyuria. Thirst may be so intense that unless the patient is continuously supplied with water, he will drink whatever fluid is available including, in extreme cases, his own urine.

When the cause of polyuria and polydipsia are in doubt, the patient may be deprived of water for a period of time. When water is withheld from a patient, he should be closely observed for signs indicating the development of vasomotor collapse. Changes in the rate and volume of the pulse as well as any decrease in the blood pressure should be reported immediately. Because polyuria and polydipsia may have psychogenic causes, the patient should also be observed to be sure that he does not have access to water and other fluids.

The treatment of diabetes insipidus has two aspects. When a pituitary lesion is responsible, it is corrected. Until this is done and in those persons who have a permanent loss of function, replacement therapy with ADH is indicated. This usually is required throughout the life of the individual. The antidiuretic hormone may be administered by subcutaneous or intramuscular injection or by nasal insufflation. In the latter, a solution containing pituitary hormones may be applied by placing small cotton pledgets that have been soaked with a solution containing the hormone against the nasal mucosa or by snuffing posterior pituitary powder into the nares. When replacement is in the form of pitressin tannate in oil, it is administered intramuscularly. It is best given at night to prevent polyuria and thus to insure the patient of a good night's sleep. The patient (or nurse) should be instructed to warm the vial of pitressin tannate and to shake it repeatedly and thoroughly, as the active material has a tendency to precipitate out of the oil.

Disorders arising out of hyperfunction of the neurohypophysis have not been described. Although hypersecretion of the neurohypophysis can occur, when it does, it is an appropriate or inappropriate response to injury or threat thereof. Secretion returns to normal when the crisis is past. As an example, some authorities ascribe the retention of water after major surgery or a serious injury to an increase in the secretion of the antidiuretic hormone. A factor in edema in heart failure may be the inappropriate secretion of the antidiuretic hormone. Neither of the above can in any sense be considered to be due to a disordered function of the neurohypophysis.

In addition to disorders due to abnormal secretion, tumors of the pituitary gland are occasionally responsible for pressure on related structures. The usual cause is an adenoma (tumor originating in gland cells). The most serious effect of enlargement of the pituitary gland is blindness as a result of pressure on the optic chiasm. The optic chiasm is formed by the fibers of the optic nerves which pass over the pituitary gland on their way to the visual areas in the occipital lobes of the brain. Fibers from the retina on the lateral side travel to the same side of the brain. Those on the inner, or nasal, side of the retina cross and go to the opposite side of the brain. As the lesion enlarges, pressure on the optic tracts leads to the loss of one or more fields of vision and eventually to complete blindness. Because of the proximity of the floor of the brain, there may be disturbances in vegetative functions. Depending on the nature of the lesion, removal may be by irradiation or by surgical means. Irradiation is used when at all possible, because of the difficulties involved in exposing the area.

The Adrenal Gland

Adrenal Medulla

The adrenal gland consists of two parts, the medulla and the cortex. The medulla arises along with the sympathetic nervous system from the neural crest. It secretes two hormones, epinephrine and norepinephrine. The latter is also released at the nerve ending of the sympathetic nervous system. Both hormones are secreted continuously in small amounts. The adrenal medulla along with the sympathetic nervous system appears to regulate functions that enable the organism to adapt to emergency situations. It responds readily to stimulation by the sympathetic nervous system in a wide variety of conditions, with the result that a message borne by a preganglionic fiber of the sympathetic nervous system is converted to a blood-borne one. The release of the hormones epinephrine and norepinephrine by the adrenal medulla contributes to the massiveness of the reaction induced when the sympathetic nervous system is activated. As emphasized elsewhere, the action of the sympathetic nervous system and the hormones secreted by the adrenal medulla are similar. Emergency conditions activating the sympathoadrenal system include hemorrhage, hypoglycemia, hypoxia, pain, strenuous exercise, fear, and anger, as well as various pharmacological agents.

The physiological effects of the two hormones are different. Norepinephrine increases both diastolic and systolic blood pressure by increasing the peripheral resistance. Epinephrine does not increase peripheral resistance, but it increases the systolic blood pressure by increasing the cardiac output. It also causes increased contractility and excitability of the heart muscle. It facilitates the flow of blood to the muscles, brain, and viscera and increases the basal metabolic rate. It enhances the blood sugar by stimulating the conversion of glycogen to glucose by the liver and by decreasing the uptake of glucose by muscle. The adrenal medulla is not necessary to maintain life but contributes to the ability of the organism to cope with stress.

What is the principal cause of hyperfunction of the adrenal medulla?

A neoplasm known as a pheochromocytoma is associated with hyperfunction of the adrenal medulla. A pheochromocytoma is characterized by hypertension which may be either paroxysmal (periodic attacks) or continuous. The character of the hypertension depends on whether the tumor secretes constantly or intermittently. The clinical manifestations depend on whether the tumor secretes epinephrine, or norepinephrine, or both. Mrs. Lanera presented a classical picture of a patient with the paroxysmal type of hypertension due to pheochromocytoma. Between attacks she lay quietly in bed. During an attack she appeared to be acutely anxious. She thrashed about in bed, she complained of her heart pounding (palpitation), felt nauseated, and vomited and perspired profusely. Her blood pressure rose to 200 systolic and 135 diastolic. According to Thorn and Goldfien,[24] about 50 per cent of patients with pheochromocytoma have the classical syndrome with paroxysmal hypertension.

Since there is a possibility for cure, and patients having this condition are frequently young, the diagnosis of pheochromocytoma in patients who have this disorder is important. In patients whose blood pressures are below 170 systolic and 110 diastolic, a drug such as histamine or methalacholine hydrochloride may be administered to provoke symptoms. Following the administration of histamine the healthy person's blood pressure falls, his skin flushes,

[24] George W. Thorn and Alan Goldfien, "Diseases of the Adrenal Medulla," in *Principles of Internal Medicine*, T. R. Harrison (ed.), McGraw-Hill Book Co., Inc., New York, 1962, p. 630.

and he is likely to have a headache. In the patient with pheochromocytoma, the blood pressure, usually though not always, rises. Methacholine chloride, likewise, causes a rise in blood pressure. To prevent overreaction to metacholine chloride, atropine sulfate, 1 mg, may be administered before it is given.

In patients whose blood pressures are above 170/110, drugs that block the effect of norepinephrine on the blood vessels may be employed to establish the diagnosis. The best known is phentolamine hydrochloride (Regitine[25]). When a dose of 5 mg of Regitine hydrochloride is administered intravenously to a patient with pheochromocytoma, the blood pressure falls immediately. The maximum decrease is reached in from two to five minutes and lasts for ten minutes or longer. A fall of 35 mm systolic and 25 mm diastolic or more is considered to be positive; that is, it indicates the presence of pheochromocytoma.

The treatment of pheochromocytoma is the surgical removal of the tumor. Since the manipulation of the lesion during the operative procedure may cause the release of epinephrine and/or norepinephrine, the blood pressure of the patient may rise to critical levels. Since the patient can be protected from an excessively high blood pressure by the administration of Regitine, the blood pressure of the patient should be checked frequently. In the immediate postoperative period the patient may have episodes of hypotension, and occasionally a patient suffers severe shock. Authorities are not agreed about whether this is due to an excessive release of epinephrine into the blood or to a lack of it. Phenylephrine hydrochloride (Neo Synephrine[26]) may be prescribed by the physician to elevate the blood pressure. The blood pressure of the patient should be observed frequently until it is stabilized. Since stabilization may not occur for two or three days after surgery, the patient requires frequent observation for a longer period than most postoperative patients. When the patient gets out of bed, he should be cautioned to change from the supine to the upright position slowly so that the blood vessels have time to adapt. Dizziness and a feeling of faintness are indicative of hypotension. Depending on the severity of these symptoms, the patient may have to be returned to bed. Certainly he should be protected from falling. In the absence of irreversible shock, patients usually make an uneventful recovery. Unless both adrenal glands are removed, adrenal steroid therapy usually is not required. Adrenal medullary secretions do not have to be replaced, regardless of whether one or both glands are excised. As far as can be determined, the adrenal medulla is not essential to life. When both adrenal glands are removed, the adrenergic response to stressing situations is somewhat lessened, but the sympathetic nervous system still reacts as a whole.[27]

[25] Trade name.
[26] Trade name.
[27] Tepperman, *Op. cit.*, p. 128.

*What hormones are secreted by the adrenal cortices and
what are their effects?*

The adrenal cortex, unlike the adrenal medulla, is essential to life. In the
absence of adrenal cortical secretions the individual has difficulty in adapting
to even mild degrees of stress. This includes all types—variations in temperature, exercise, changes in position, infections, burns, and emotional stresses.
The degree of susceptibility varies somewhat from individual to individual.
Exposure to severe stress, however, can be expected to induce a shocklike
state characterized by prostration and peripheral circulatory failure. Death
follows unless the deficient hormones are replaced.

According to Cahill, Jenkins, and Thorn,[28] many steroids have been isolated from the adrenal cortex, but only a few appear to be of major metabolic
significance. Of the steroids that have been identified, hydrocortisone, cortisone, corticosterone, and aldosterone are the most abundant. In man hydrocortisone predominates over corticosterone. In addition to the above, some
biologically active androgens are also secreted. The actions of all adrenal
hormones are similar in quality, but they differ in the quantity or in the extent
of their effect on different functions. For example, all biologically active
adrenal hormones increase the retention of sodium and the elimination of
potassium by the renal tubules. The potency of their action, however, varies
considerably.

Adrenal cortical hormones are classified into three groups according to
their major effects. They are: (1) cortisol (glucocorticoids), (2) mineralocorticoids, and (3) adrenosterones (adrenal androgens). Examples of
glucocorticoids are cortisone and hydrocortisone. In man the principal glucocorticoid is hydrocortisone. Mineralocorticoids are aldosterone and desoxycorticosterone. Aldosterone is secreted by the adrenal cortex; desoxycorticosterone
is a synthetic analogue. The mineralocorticoids, as their name implies, regulate the reabsorption of the sodium cation and the excretion of the potassium
cation by the renal tubules. All adrenal steroids affect sodium retention and
potassium and chloride excretion to some degree.

The glucocorticoids such as cortisone and hydrocortisone have a number of
effects which are not exhibited to any degree by the mineralocorticoids.
These include the following:

1. They reverse the delay in water diuresis seen in the adrenalectomized
   animal.
2. They enhance protein catabolism and inhibit protein synthesis.
3. They antagonize the action of insulin.
4. They affect the metabolism of glucose.
   a. They increase the synthesis of glucose by the liver—the source of
      glucose is mobilization of amino acids by the hormone from the

[28] George F. Cahill, Dalton Jenkins, and George W. Thorn, "Diseases of the Adrenal
Cortex," in *Principles of Internal Medicine,* 4th ed., McGraw-Hill Book Co., Inc., New
York, 1962, pp. 609-30.

peripheral supporting structures such as connective tissues. The amino acids are deaminized in the liver and converted to glycogen. The glycogen is converted to glucose, which is released into the blood, thereby elevating the level of glucose in the blood.

5. The glucocorticoids influence the defense mechanisms in the body. High concentrations act to suppress inflammation, inhibit the formation of scar tissue, and block certain allergic responses. They are also believed to have a significant role in adaptation to many kinds of stresses, such as traumatic injuries (surgical or accidental, burns, severe infections) and other similar challenges to the organism. The mechanisms by which the adrenal cortical hormones participate in these complex events have not been elucidated. Other hormonal, neural, and nutritional factors also influence the response of the individual to injury. Current and future studies will undoubtedly contribute to an understanding of all the factors involved in the response of an individual to stress. Although some animals can be maintained on aldosterone, man requires hydrocortisone or corticosterone for his survival.[29]

6. Hydrocortisone participates in the regulation of melanin metabolism.

7. The secretion of ACTH is regulated by the level of hydrocortisone in the blood.

8. The glucocorticoids appear to play a permissive role in metabolism. Many cells appear to respond to other influences such as neural or homoral stimulation only when there is a certain basic level of adrenal cortical hormones.

9. The glucocorticoids influence (directly or indirectly) emotional functioning. In adrenal insufficiency patients are often depressed and anxious. With adequate replacement therapy, these effects are ameliorated. The long-term administration of large dosages of adrenal steroids in the therapy of patients with rheumatoid arthritis may result in euphoria (an unrealistic optimism or cheerfulness) or even in a frankly psychotic state in persons who are predisposed to this condition.

The secretion of the glucocorticoids and adrenal androgen is controlled by ACTH (adrenocorticotrophic hormone), secreted by the anterior pituitary gland. A decrease in the level of hydrocortisone, either directly or by way of the hypothalamus, results in an increased release of ACTH. As the level of adrenal cortical hormones rises, the production of ACTH by the anterior pituitary declines. Although ACTH may have some effect on the secretion of aldosterone, it appears to be regulated by the concentration of sodium and potassium in the body fluids. After the removal of the pituitary gland, secretion of aldosterone is maintained. In some instances, it is increased over prehypophysectomy levels.

Manifestations of disorders of the adrenal cortex result from the effects of

[29] *Ibid.,* p. 614.

hypo- or hypersecretion. Adrenal insufficiency may result from atrophy, destruction by a disease such as tuberculosis, hemorrhage into the gland, or surgical removal of both adrenal glands. It may be secondary to failure of the anterior pituitary gland. Although tuberculosis was formerly a more common cause of adrenal insufficiency than it is now, it still is responsible for a significant number of cases. Secretion of hormones by the adrenal cortex is depressed by the administration of exogenous hormones; withdrawal of hormone therapy may leave the patient in a state of relative deficiency. During the period immediately following withdrawal, the person is likely to be more susceptible to infection than usual. At one time adrenal insufficiency and other disorders of the adrenal cortex were believed to be extremely rare. With improved methods of diagnosis, disorders of the adrenal cortex are being identified with greater frequency. Where they were once believed to be rare, they can no longer be considered to be. Most of the effects of adrenal insufficiency are due to a deficiency of the mineralo- and glucocorticoids.

The clinical manifestations of adrenal insufficiency were described by Thomas Addison more than 100 years ago and were as a result called Addison's disease. It was not, however, until the adrenal cortical steroids were isolated and synthesized that marked progress was made in understanding their role in the regulation of bodily activities or in controlling the manifestations of the disease. Before the introduction of adrenal cortical extracts, the prognosis of a person with Addison's disease was extremely poor. Since they have become available, it is much improved. The change in the outlook for the patient with chronic adrenal insufficiency is well illustrated by an uncle and his nephew, both of whom had Addison's disease. In 1926 John Seebon, aged 17, died from the effects of Addison's disease. Thirty years later his nephew, James, aged 14, developed symptoms which his mother recognized as being similar to those experienced by her brother. Medical examination revealed that her suspicions were justified. Seven years later James is living and well. He works every day on his father's farm.

Untreated adrenal insufficiency is characterized by weakness (asthenia), easy fatigability, and hypotension. Weakness is one of the most outstanding symptoms in adrenal insufficiency. In the beginning it tends to be worse on some days than on others. Eventually, it becomes so severe that the patient is confined to bed. Eventually, even bed rest does not afford relief. Hypotension is also a common finding. The majority of patients have blood pressure readings of less than 110/70. In extreme cases it may be as low as 80/50 or even lower. A change in the color of the skin to brown, tan, or bronze is the most striking physical change that can be observed directly. The pigmentation may be diffuse involving exposed and unexposed areas of the body, or it may appear in patches or freckles. Bluish-black or slate-gray discoloration of the mucous membranes may also occur. Disturbances in the function of the gastrointestinal tract may give rise to anorexia, nausea, vomiting, diarrhea, constipation, and abdominal pain. Weight loss is a common finding. As might be expected, mental changes may be prominent. Depression, irritability, lethargy, apprehension, and anxiety are common.

What methods are used in evaluating the functional status of the adrenal cortex?

Adrenal cortical function is evaluated directly for the signs and symptoms listed above and by observing the patient for evidences of failure of metabolic processes regulated by the adrenal cortical steroids. One direct method employed to determine the functional capacity of the adrenal cortex is the measurement of the level of 17-hydroxycorticoids in the blood plasma or urine in response to the administration of ACTH. ACTH is administered intravenously over an eight-hour period on two consecutive days. Twenty-four-hour urine specimens are collected for two days preceding and during the administration of ACTH, and examined for 17-hydroxycorticosteroid. Cahill, Jenkins, and Thorn[30] state that by one method of assay a person with normal adrenal cortices should show an increase in the plasma and urine levels of 17-hydroxycorticoid over control levels of 1 to 10 mg to 5 to 25 mg the first day after ACTH is administered and 15 to 40 mg the second day. In patients whose adrenal cortices fail to respond, the test may be continued for a third and fourth day. Patients with adrenal insufficiency fail to respond, or respond very minimally, to ACTH. Since the test is administered over a period of eight hours, attention should be given to the comfort of the patient. Since ACTH preparations are essentially foreign proteins, the danger of an allergic response exists, particularly in patients who lack endogenous corticoids. A potent steroid such as 1 mg fluorohydrocortisone may be prescribed to be given orally on the days that ACTH is administered by intravenous infusion to minimize the danger of a serious hypersensitivity reaction. The patient who has adrenal insufficiency is also predisposed to an acute febrile reaction when ACTH is administered in a solution of glucose and water. During the period when the urine is being collected, the patient, his relatives, and all nursing personnel should be instructed regarding the importance of saving all urine. The loss of even one voiding of urine can delay diagnosis, be responsible for unnecessary discomfort to the patient, and increase the cost of his illness.

Another less specific, but simpler, test of adrenal cortical function is the determination of the number of eosinophils in the blood before and after the administration of ACTH. In a person whose adrenal cortical function is normal, a decrease in the number of eosinophils of 70 per cent or more is expected. A lesser decline may indicate adrenal insufficiency.

Indirect tests of adrenal function have been developed to identify inadequacies in metabolism accompanying adrenal insufficiency. They include tests to determine: (1) the rate at which water is excreted following the ingestion of a given volume in a fixed period of time; (2) the capacity of the kidney to

[30] *Ibid.,* p. 613.

conserve sodium and to excrete potassium when the supply of sodium is restricted; and (3) the effect of fasting on the level of glucose in the blood. The patient with adrenal insufficiency tends to develop hypoglycemia with fasting. Although any of these tests may precipitate adrenal crisis, fasting and the withholding of sodium combined with the administration of potassium are most likely to do so. Because of the dangers associated with these tests, since ACTH has become readily available, they are seldom used. When they are performed, evidence of increasing weakness or hypotension should be reported to the physician immediately. No time should be lost in so doing.

What measures are available for the treatment of adrenal insufficiency?

Patients with chronic adrenal insufficiency can be compared in a number of respects to those with diabetes mellitus. Hormones are available which can be employed to replace those that are lacking. Whether or not the patient is maintained in a satisfactory state of health frequently depends on himself. As in other disorders in which there is a permanent deficiency state, the patient must understand that he must continue therapy for the rest of his life. He must follow a prescribed routine and remain under medical supervision. Since he requires more hormones when he is under the stress of illness or other severe stress he must understand this and know what to do. He should carry a card providing information such as his name, address, diagnosis, and the medications he is taking.

In some patients, adrenal insufficiency can be controlled by the administration of cortisone (5 to 25 mg twice daily) by mouth. In other patients a potent salt-retaining steroid such as fluorohydrocortisone or desoxycortisone is required in addition to cortisone to maintain electrolyte balance. The first is administered orally in small dosages of from 0.1 to 0.3 mg daily. The administration of desoxycorticosterone is more complicated. The dosage is first established by determining the effects of daily intramuscular injections on blood pressure and serum electrolyte concentration. After the requirements of the patient have been determined, desoxycorticosterone may be administered by deep intramuscular injection once every three to four weeks or by intraoral tablets or buccalets placed in the mouth two or three times a day. Since absorption is less complete from the mucosa of the mouth than when the drug is administered intramuscularly, the daily requirement is two to three times that established for intramuscular injection. The patient who receives desoxycorticosterone should be instructed to weigh himself regularly as overdosage causes edema as a consequence of retention of the sodium cation. In marked overdosages of desoxycortisone, hypertension and congestive heart failure may be induced.

Adrenal cortical failure secondary to failure in anterior pituitary function differs in a number of respects from primary adrenal insufficiency, as there usually are disturbances in thyroid and gonadal function as well. Disturbances in electrolyte balance, though present, are often less severe. As in primary adrenal insufficiency, the characteristic features are weakness, inability to cope with stress, poor resistance to infection, and the tendency to spontaneous hypoglycemia. These effects can usually be controlled by small doses of cortisone.[31]

The most serious event in adrenal insufficiency is the development of acute adrenal insufficiency or crisis. In this condition all the signs and symptoms of adrenal insufficiency are intensified. Although prevention is to be preferred to therapy, the survival of the patient in acute adrenal insufficiency depends on prompt and vigorous treatment. Because an increased supply of adrenal cortical hormones is required to cope with stress, any condition that makes extra demands on the individual can be anticipated to predispose to adrenal crisis. The dosage of hormones should be increased during infection, gastrointestinal upsets, trauma, surgery, and any other condition that is likely to increase the need of the individual for adrenal hormones. When the condition occurs, all signs and symptoms of adrenal insufficiency worsen. Unless it is corrected promptly, the patient goes into vascular shock and dies. The nurse should be alert to and report any evidence of an intensification of signs and symptoms such as increasing weakness or a lowering of the blood pressure.

Therapy in adrenal insufficiency has three objectives: (1) to raise the level of adrenal hormones in the circulation, (2) to support the heart and vascular system, (3) to control infection.[32] To raise the level of hormones in the circulation, the patient is given 100 to 150 mg of hydrocortisone in 1,000 ml of 5 per cent glucose in physiological saline. The first 250 ml is administered quickly. The remainder is administered slowly over a four- to eight-hour period.

Objectives on which to base the nursing care plan include: (1) to contribute to the accomplishment of the medical objectives including the protection of the patient from infection, and (2) to maintain conditions of the physical, emotional, and social climate so that demands made on the patient to adapt are reduced to a minimum. The contribution of the nurse to the medical objectives includes the supervision of the treatments and observation of their effects on the patient. The patient should not be left alone. Observation and reporting of vital signs are important. Blood pressure readings may be ordered as often as every 15 minutes. Any drop in the blood pressure of the patient is likely to be significant because it may be at a critical level at the time treatment is initiated. Since hyperthermia is a problem in some patients, hourly recordings of temperature may be requested by the physician.

The importance of eliminating inasmuch as possible all form of stimuli is based on the fact that the patient who is in adrenal crisis is unable to adapt to

---

[31] Raymond V. Randall and Edward H. Rynearson, "Clinical Aspects of Anterior Pituitary Failure," *Postgraduate Medicine*, XXIX, January, 1961, p. 25.

[32] Thorn and Jenkins, in Harrison, *Op. cit.*, p. 614.

even minor stresses. As a consequence, a situation that might be of no importance to a healthy person or one who is experiencing other types of illness may worsen the condition of the patient experiencing acute adrenal insufficiency. Attention should be given to details such as maintaining the temperature of the room between 70° and 75° F., protecting the patient from drafts and from bright lights, and providing a comfortable bed. The room should be quiet. Loud noises and talking should be prevented. Until the crisis is past, physical care should be kept to the minimum required for the comfort of the patient. He should do nothing for himself. Whatever care is required should be administered. This includes moving and turning as well as activities such as mouth care and feeding. When the patient is vomiting, he should be given assistance. Mouth care after an emesis is recommended. Conversation should be kept to the minimum required to give directions to the patient or for brief explanations of what is to be done. The patient should be protected from all sources of infection including members of his family and hospital personnel who have colds or other infections. The condition of the patient is of an emergency nature. As with other patients who are in a state verging on shock, shock blocks should be in the room ready to use if necessary. The recovery of the patient depends on prompt and effective treatment. An environment that limits the demands made on him to adapt contributes to his recovery.

What determines the manifestations associated with hypersecretion by the adrenal cortex?

The adrenal cortex secretes a number of hormones each of which have different physiological effects. Consequently the clinical manifestations in disorders characterized by hypersecretion will depend on which hormones are oversecreted. In either hyperplasia or adenoma of the adrenal cortex, oversecretion of one hormone may predominate, or there may be a variable mixture of hormones. Three different clinical syndromes of hyperfunction are usually described. They are Cushing's syndrome, adrenogenital syndrome, and primary aldosteronism. Cushing's syndrome results largely from the hypersecretion of hydrocortisone. In primary aldosteronism, as the name implies, synthesis of aldosterone is excessive. The adrenogenital syndrome includes all the disorders of sexual development that can be attributed to abnormal adrenal cortical function.

Cushing's Syndrome

Cushing's syndrome is a state manifested by a group of signs and symptoms resulting from the hypersecretion of hydrocortisone. The disorder may be due to an adenoma, to a highly malignant neoplasm of the adrenal cortex of one gland, or to the diffuse hyperplasia of both glands. In some instances no abnormality of the adrenal gland is readily identifiable. At one time hyperplasia was thought to be due to overstimulation of the adrenal cortex by

ACTH, but there is some evidence that the adrenal cortex fails to respond to the regulating effects of ACTH.

The characteristic features of Cushing's syndrome are a peculiar type of obesity in which fat is distributed in pads between the shoulders—buffalo hump—and around the waist—girdle obesity; moon face; hypertension; easy fatigability and weakness; hirsutism; purplish striae over the obese areas; thin and fragile skin which is subject to ecchymosis; acne, the face and neck often being ruddy in color; amenorrhea in women or impotence in men; edema; glycosuria as a result of disturbances in carbohydrate metabolism; osteoporosis; and increased susceptibility to infection. The patient is frequently irritable and changeable in mood. In addition to his clinical manifestations, almost all persons with this disorder have a high level of 17-hydroxycorticosteroid in the plasma and urine.

Medical therapy is directed toward reducing the level of adrenal cortical secretion. Some patients respond favorably to irradiation of the pituitary gland. Others require surgical treatment. In addition to the above the patient requires potassium chloride, 4 to 6 gm daily, to supplement that obtained in his diet. Potassium is given as enteric-coated tablets with meals, or as a 25 per cent solution of potassium chloride. Testosterone may be prescribed to facilitate the replacement of protein lost as a result of the disease.

The objectives on which the nursing care plan is based include: (1) to make observations that will be helpful to the physician in establishing an accurate medical diagnosis and medical plan of treatment, (2) to provide the patient with a physical, emotional, and social climate that is safe and supporting, and (3) to assist the patient in acquiring the knowledge and skill that he will need to maintain physiological functioning should this be required.

One of the simplest and at the same time most difficult responsibilities in the care of the patient with Cushing's syndrome is the collection of urine specimens. Because adrenal hormones are excreted in the urine and some of the effects of the disease or its therapy are reflected in the composition and quantity of the urine, accurate and complete measurement and collection of all urine voided by the patient are important. Besides the collecting and recording of urine output, the intake of water and food should also be recorded. Despite the apparent obesity of the patient, he usually suffers from effects of the loss of protein and potassium, as an excess of adrenal cortical hormones increases protein catabolism. Excessive potassium is lost in the urine and sodium is retained. The patient should be encouraged to eat the diet that has been prescribed for him. When a low-sodium, high-potassium diet is prescribed, the nurse should check the patient's tray to be sure that he has received the appropriate food.

The patient with Cushing's syndrome has a tendency toward emotional lability (fluctuation in mood). Depression and moodiness are common. The nurse should identify the types of situations that are disturbing and record them on the nursing care plan. The patient should be observed for evidence of depression, as suicide is not an uncommon occurrence. Some patients continue to be depressed after surgical removal of the adrenal gland. Observations made by the nurse indicating a depressed state should, of course, be reported promptly to the physician.

The tendency toward masculinization with hirsutism in women and obesity are frequent sources of emotional stress. Patients in whom the disorder is caused by a benign adenoma or hyperplasia of the adrenal cortices can be given reasonable reassurance that following treatment they can expect to be restored to their former selves. Weakness, accompanied by the frustration of not being able to carry on their usual activities, is also distressing to patients. At times weakness is the most outstanding symptom. Friends, as well as members of the family, often have little sympathy for the patient. They do not see how anyone who is fat can be as weak as the patient says he is. Nurses who meet these patients in the community should encourage them to seek medical attention. The family should be helped to understand that weakness and obesity are, in fact, compatible.

Patients undergoing adrenal surgery require adrenal hormones before as well as after surgical therapy. When some adrenal cortical tissue remains, the dosage is tapered off after recovery from the operation. Patients undergoing total adrenalectomy must continue under competent medical supervision for the rest of their lives. A therapeutic plan identical with that of the patient with Addison's disease is indicated.

Another disorder due to hypersecretion of the adrenal cortex is primary aldosteronism. It is usually due to a tumor of the adrenal cortex that secretes aldosterone. The principal features of this disorder are hypertension, renal and electrolyte abnormalities, muscle weakness, and an increase in the concentration of the salt-retaining hormone in the urine.[33] This substance leads to the retention of sodium. Potassium is lost from the body in excessive quantities. Aldosteronoma is treated by surgical removal. Recovery when the condition is due to a neoplasm is complete. The nursing care of the patient is essentially that of any patient undergoing adrenal surgery.

To recapitulate, adrenal cortical hormones have widespread effects on the metabolism of protein, carbohydrates, lipids, and the electrolytes sodium, potassium, and calcium. They also affect and are affected by hormones elaborated by other glands. They are essential to survival. In the absence—either absolute or relative—of adrenal cortical hormones, the capacity to cope with stress of all types is lost. Hypersecretion of adrenal cortical hormones leads to serious defects in the adaptive capacity of the individual. Clinical manifestations of disorders involving the adrenal cortex depend on which hormone predominates or is hypersecreted. The nursing of patients with disorders in which there are abnormalities in the secretion of the adrenal steroids should be based on the knowledge that they have difficulty in coping with stress of all

[33] James D. Hardy, *Pathophysiology in Surgery*, The Williams & Wilkins Company, Baltimore, 1958, p. 578.

types. Their increased susceptibility to infection should be kept in mind. Other nursing responsibilities include the making of observations that contribute to the medical diagnosis and carrying out of that part of the medical regime usually assigned to nursing. When the disorder experienced by the patient is incurable, the nurse has an important role in assisting the patient to acquire the knowledge and skills that he needs to maintain life and health.

What are the actions of the thyroid hormones?

Although the exact mechanism of action of the thyroid hormones is not known, they play an important role in the regulation of the speed of biochemical reactions in cells. They increase the rate of heat production in the mitochondria of cells. In hypothyroidism cellular oxidation as measured by oxygen utilization is below normal limits. In hyperthyroidism it is above. In hypothyroidism heat production by cells can be restored to normal by the administration of thyroid hormones. In hyperthyroidism reduction in the rate of energy metabolism can be restored by suppressing thyroid function by destroying or removing a portion of the gland.

The thyroid hormones affect the rate of metabolism of proteins, lipids, and carbohydrates, as well as of water, minerals, and vitamins. In hyperthyroidism the increased secretion of thyroid hormones is reflected by an increase in the loss of nitrogen in the urine and by a lowering in the level of cholesterol (a lipid) in the blood. In hypothyroidism the concentration of cholesterol in the blood rises. Thyroid hormones also have an influence on calcium metabolism, as osteoporosis is a not uncommon finding in severe hyperthyroidism.

The thyroid hormones are essential to the normal physical and mental growth and development of the child. A child who is born without functioning thyroid tissue or who develops this condition soon after birth fails to develop either physically or mentally. Maturation of his skeleton and other body structures is delayed. Hypothyroidism in a child results in a characteristic type of dwarfing known as cretinism. Mental development is also retarded. Idiocy is common. In older children and adults hypothyroidism is evidenced by physical and mental slowing. These effects can, however, be reversed by the ingestion of adequate amounts of thyroid hormones.

A number of biologically active substances have been isolated from the thyroid gland. Two of the best known are thyroxin and tri-iodothyronine. Thyroid hormones are transported in an unstable combination with the globulin fraction of the serum proteins. The concentration of the thyroid hormones in the blood serum can be determined by precipitating the protein to which they are attached. The laboratory test by which this is done is known as the protein-bound iodine (PBI). The normal level is from 4 to 8 μg of protein-bound iodine per 100 ml of blood serum. In hypothyroidism the level may drop to less than 1 μg. In hyperthyroidism it may rise to as much as 20 μg.

Another method of determining the functional activity of the thyroid gland is by the administration of a tracer dose of iodine, I^{131} (radioactive iodine). The patient is given I^{131} mixed with water to drink. The iodine is absorbed into the blood from the alimentary canal. As the blood circulates through the thyroid gland, iodine (include the I^{131}) is trapped in it. The rate at which I^{131} is concentrated in the thyroid gland is measured by monitoring with a counter of radioactivity, and it is frequently indicative of the functional capacity of the gland. The I^{131} not trapped by the thyroid is excreted in the urine. Testing the functional capacity of the thyroid with I^{131} is possible because the cells of the gland are unable to distinguish between radioactive and non-radioactive isotopes. Increased trapping of iodine occurs in hyperthyroidism and decreased in hypothyroidism. Because the rate of uptake of iodine may be influenced by the previous ingestion of iodine by the patient, the physician will want to know whether the patient has been taking iodine-containing drugs before the test is undertaken. Drugs that depress thyroid activity also inhibit the removal of iodine from the blood and will therefore influence the outcome of the test.

What are the effects of the thyroid hormones?

The effects of thyroxin and tri-iodothyronine are similar. They differ inasmuch as tri-iodothyronine is three to five times more potent than thyroxin. Its action is more rapid but is less sustained than that of thyroxin. Thyroxin has a long latent period and a prolonged action. It takes about eight to ten days for it to cause its maximum effect and the effect lasts for five to six weeks.

How is the secretion by the thyroid gland regulated?

The thyrotrophic hormone secreted by the anterior hypophysis regulates the activity of the thyroid gland. The relationship of the anterior hypophysis to the thyroid gland is not one of a simple feedback system. The need for an increase in the rate of cellular oxidation is transmitted to the hypothalamus by nerve fibers. It responds by releasing neurohormones that are transmitted to the anterior hypophysis via the pituitary portal system. The anterior hypophysis reacts by increasing the output of the thyrotrophic hormone, which increases the activity of the thyroid gland. The thyroid hormones suppress the activity of the anterior hypophysis. Therefore, as their level rises, the activity of the anterior hypophysis diminishes. As a consequence of a system of balanced stimulation and suppression, the organism is protected from either hypo- or hypersecretion. This also protects the person who, though not hypothyroid, ingests exogenous thyroid hormone. As the level of ingested thyroid hormone rises, his own production of thyroid hormone falls.

In addition to the regulatory effects of the thyrotrophic hormone, the synthesis and release of the thyroid hormones involve at least six major enzyme systems. Preparatory to the formation of the hormone the thyroid removes iodine mostly in the form of iodine from the blood and concentrates it in the gland. Specific enzymes are required to catalyze these reactions as well as those in the formation of the hormone proper. A defect in any one of these systems will interfere with the capacity of the organism to form hormones. Defects in one or more of the required enzyme systems are among the causes of congenital hypothyroidism.[34]

Disorders of the thyroid are manifested by changes in the size and structure of the gland and by an increase or decrease in the production of hormones. The condition in which the size of the gland is increased is known as goiter. Goiter may be accompanied by normal, hypo-, or hypersecretion of thyroid hormones. Locally, as a space-occupying mass, a goiter may interfere with swallowing or breathing by causing pressure on the esophagus or trachea. In our culture, the enlargement of the neck is considered unsightly. And as such it may be cause of psychological stress. In areas of the world where goiter is endemic and common, it has been accepted as evidence of health and beauty. In the Andean Mountains in South America, where goiter was the rule, dolls were made with enlarged necks such as was observed in the person with a goiter.

As a result of epidemiological studies, scientists have learned that the incidence of goiter is high in the areas of the world where the soil has been leached of its supply of iodine. Its incidence is low where the diet includes iodine-containing foods. For example, in mountainous and inland areas of the world the incidence of goiter is found to be high. In those parts of the world where the land was sprayed by sea water or where an appreciable part of the diet is from the sea, the incidence of goiter is low. Goiter may also have a genetic basis. A defect in any one of the enzyme systems involved in the synthesis of thyroxin may result from the presence of a mutant gene. As in other disorders, multiple factors influence whether or not goiter develops. It is much more common in females than in males. It is more likely to develop during those periods in the life of the individual when the iodine requirement is increased. Thus goiter is more likely to appear during puberty or pregnancy and in individuals whose protein intake is excessive. In some women who develop goiters during pregnancy, the condition disappears at the termination of the pregnancy. Infections, especially those in the gastrointestinal tract, may contribute to the development of goiter by interfering with the absorption of iodine.

Goiters caused by a lack of an adequate intake of iodine can be prevented by the regular intake of water or salt to which iodine has been added. When the addition of iodine to water or salt was first proposed, the furor was no less than it is today over the introduction of fluorides into public water supplies. Nurses have a responsibility to instruct homemakers to use iodized salt. The addition of iodine to the salt is one of the simplest forms of primary prevention available.

[34] Lawson Wilkins, "The Thyroid Gland," *Scientific American*, CCII, No. 3, March, 1960, p. 126.

Enlargement of the thyroid gland may be diffuse or nodular. Though not very common, goiter may also be caused by a malignant neoplasm. In all types of goiters, hormone production may be within normal limits, deficient, or excessive. The general effects that result from disorders of the thyroid depend on the extent to which the output of thyroid hormones is below or above the normal range. Conditions characterized by hypofunction include cretinism and myxedema. Cretinism characteristically occurs in infants and young children, myxedema in older children and adults. Hypothyroidism may be present in the absence of either. In disorders characterized by alterations in the secretion of the thyroid gland, there is a tendency to classify them as hypo- or hyperthyroidism rather than by name, such as cretinism or myxedema. Hypothyroidism may be due to failure of the thyroid gland to develop as a consequence of a genetic defect or from a pre- or postnatal immunological disturbance. Infection or surgical removal of the gland or therapy with iodine I^{131} reduces the quantity of tissue below that required for normal functioning. Hypothyroidism may also be secondary to failure of the anterior hypophysis to produce TSH.

Conditions characterized by hyperfunction include exophthalmic goiter or Graves's disease and toxic nodular goiter. Whether these are two distinct disorders or two different stages of the same disease is a moot point. In exophthalmic goiter disease, the thyroid gland is diffusely enlarged. In nodular goiter, parts of the gland are increased in size. In exophthalmic goiter, the eyes protrude and the disorder is usually more severe than in nodular goiter. The question of why the thyroid gland hyperfunctions has not been answered. All the signs and symptoms observed in hyperthyroidism except the exophthalmos can be produced by excessive dosages of thyroid hormones. Some authorities contend that the exophthalmos results from overstimulation of the thyroid by the thyrotrophic hormone. Because the onset of the hyperthyroidism is frequently precipitated by an event causing emotional stress, some authorities attribute it to emotional factors. One explanation of the relationship of emotion to hyperthyroidism is that persons who develop thyrotoxicosis are emotionally dependent individuals who become hyperthyroid at the time of an emotional crisis, particularly from the loss of a person who is important to them. Not all authorities agree, however. At least one study points to the emotional status of the patient being due to, rather than causing, the disorder. Robbins and Vinson[35] discovered that thyrotoxic patients do not differ from patients with known structural and physiological changes in the brain. Moreover when patients studied were adequately treated, they did not differ from normal controls. As a consequence of their studies, Robbins and Vinson define thyrotoxicosis as a "metabolic disease manifested by impaired psychologic integration, involving particularly the autonomic nervous system." This

[35] Leonard R. Robbins and David B. Vinson, "Objective Psychologic Assessment of the Thyrotoxic Patient and Response to Treatment," *Journal of Clinical Endocrinology*, XX, January, 1960, pp. 120-29.

definition emphasizes that there are changes in psychological and biochemical reactions of the individual. Many of the manifestations result from the alterations in the functioning of the autonomic nervous system.

The individual who is in a hypothyroid state has inadequate capacity to adapt to changes in his environment. The individual with hyperthyroidism makes inappropriate adaptations to his environment. The hypothyroid individual complains bitterly when he is in a cool environment. The one who is hyperthyroid behaves as if it were hot even when the environmental temperature is cool as judged by a person who is euthyroid. Some of the differences between the effects of hypo- and hypersecretion of the thyroid hormones are summarized below.

	Hypothyroidism	Hyperthyroidism
Conditions with which associated	Cretinism—infants, young children	Exophthalmic goiter or Graves's disease
	Hypothyroidism without myxedema (atrophy or destruction of the thyroid gland). Surgical extirpation	
	Myxedema—older children, adults	Toxic nodular goiter
Basic physiological disturbance	Decreased production in thyroid hormones at some stage of their production	Increased production of thyroid hormones
Effects of alteration in level of thyroid hormones	1. Reduction in heat production 2. Failure of mental and physical growth in infants and children 3. Disturbances in the metabolism of proteins, lipids, carbohydrates, water, and minerals with abnormal collections of water, salt, and protein in tissues	1. Production of heat rises 2. Deranged carbohydrate metabolism with glycosuria 3. May be increased use of fat and protein as fuel
Characteristic laboratory findings	Elevated blood cholesterol, 300-700 mg/100 ml	Lowering of level of blood cholesterol
Basal metabolic rate (BMR normal —20 to +15)	—20 to —40	+15 to +60
Uptake of I^{131} in % of uptake	Less than 15%	Greater than 50%
Protein-bound iodine in μg per 100 ml	Less than 4	Greater than 8
Red cell count	May be severe anemia	
Signs and symptoms related to speech	Swelling of tongue and larynx—a halting, slurred, hoarse speech	Rapid and excited. May be hoarse from local pressure on recurrent laryngeal nerves.

	Hypothyroidism	*Hyperthyroidism*
Skin	Thick, puffy, dry	Warm, moist, and flushed
Hair	Dry, brittle, sparse. May be alopecia of outer third of eyebrows. May be premature graying	Increased sweating. Hair soft and silky
Nervous system and mental and emotional state	Often apathetic and lethargic. May be hyperirritable. Cerebration slow. In older children and adults intelligence is retained. Condition returned to normal when hormones are replaced. Patients with myxedema may develop psychosis. Infants and young children, mental retardation	Hyperactive. Emotionally labile. Mood labile. Tears are caused by trivialities. Hypersensitive, hyperirritable. Tense, jittery, restless. Has forebodings of disaster. Occasionally depressed, but is agitated and restless at the same time. Fine tremor of extended hands or tongue.
Body fat and weight, appetite	Increased weight. Weight may not increase because appetite usually decreases	Loss of weight depends on relationship of food intake to metabolic rate
Susceptibility to cold	Increased	Decreased—susceptible to heat
Circulatory system (includes heart and blood vessels)	Increased capillary fragility. Bruises easily. Heart may be enlarged and fail. Cardiac output decreased. Blood pressure decreased. Weak heart beat. Increased circulation time	Tachycardia. Increased cardiac output. Palpitation. Increased systolic blood pressure. Decreased circulation time. Paroxysmal arrhythmia. Cardiac failure is not infrequent. Wide pulse pressure. Dyspnea
Gastrointestinal tract	Constipation. Hypophagia. Low glucose absorption rate	Anorexia, nausea, vomiting, and diarrhea. Hyperphagia
Muscle	Weakness. Hypotonia	Weakness. Muscle fibrillary twitching, tremors
Eyes		Protruding eyeballs (proptosis). Infrequent blinking, lid lag. Failure of convergence. Failure to wrinkle brow on looking upward
Immune mechanism	Infection-susceptible. Subnormal phagocytic capacity of leukocytes	Infection-susceptible
Menstruation	Prolonged	Oligomenorrhea. Amenorrhea
Subjective symptoms	Vague aches and pains. Cramps, arthralgic pain. Some have constant rhinorrhea or coryza	

	Hypothyroidism	*Hyperthyroidism*
Therapy	Thyroid U.S.P. or some other form of thyroid hormone	1. Inhibit the activity of thyroid tissue (lessen the synthesis of thyroid hormones) (goiterogens)
		a. Propylthiouracil
		b. Methylmercaptoimidazale (Tapazole[1])
		c. Iodine
		2. Reduce the amount of functioning thyroid tissue
		a. Radioactive iodine (I^{131})
		b. Surgical removal

[1] Trade name.

To illustrate the problems of the patient who is experiencing severe hyperthyroidism, Mrs. Thinis, aged 28, sought medical attention after her husband gave her the alternative of seeing a physician or a lawyer. Patients with hyperthyroidism frequently find their way to an internist by way of a psychiatrist or a lawyer. For some time she had been increasingly irritable, tense, and jittery. She screamed at her husband and children at the slightest provocation, accused her husband of being unfaithful, and was upset for hours over insignificant things. Though she had always eaten moderately, she was continuously hungry. Despite eating huge meals and frequent between meal snacks she did not gain weight.

During her visit to her doctor, Mrs. Thinis sat on the edge of her chair, jumped at a slight noise, and talked rapidly and in an excited manner. At one point she burst into tears. Mrs Thinis told her physician that she was certain that her husband planned to leave her. On examination her hands were found to be wet, her pulse rapid, and there was some lid lag (the eyelid moves more slowly than the eyeball) and widening of the palpebral fissures of her eyes. She stated that her mother had recently commented about her looking popeyed.

After examining Mrs. Thinis, her physician decided to hospitalize her for further study and to initiate a plan of therapy. In less acutely ill patients, many of the diagnostic tests can be made in the clinic or office of the physician. In the instance of Mrs. Thinis, the physician felt that she needed to be placed in a quiet, nonstimulating environment, where she could get as much rest as possible. He arranged for her to be in a private room for a few days and prescribed the following: (1) preparation for a basal metabolic rate the day following admission, (2) protein-bound iodine test, (3) diet—high-calorie, high-carbohydrate, and high in vitamins, (4) thiamine chloride, and (5) phenobarbital, 30 mg. four times a day.

From the description of Mrs. Thinis and knowledge of the effect of hyperthyroidism, it should be clear that Mrs. Thinis' capacity to adapt to her environment was impaired in a number of respects. Among those that are of immediate importance in making the nursing care plan were disturbances in her capacity: (1) to adapt to increases in environmental temperature, (2) to control her emotional and muscular responses, and (3) to maintain a food intake that was adequate in quantity and quality to her needs. Other factors to be considered in the making of the nursing care plan include the fact that Mrs. Thinis sweated continuously and her heart rate was rapid. Both sweating and tachycardia were adaptive. The sweating protected her from an excessively high body temperature, by increasing the heat loss. Her heart rate also contributed to heat loss by circulating the blood through the skin. It served further to increase the supply of oxygen and nutrients to the cells and to remove the products of metabolism. The increase in the rate of metabolism and the associated tachycardia placed a burden on the heart. When tachycardia is continued over a long period of time, or the patient has a previously damaged heart, it may precipitate heart failure.

The objectives on which the nursing care plan for Mrs. Thinis were based were:

1. To modify her physical and emotional environment so that her need to adapt would be minimized.
2. To provide her with food adequate in quantity and quality to her needs.
3. To replace fluid lost from the body.
4. To provide the family with the knowledge and support they needed to be helpful to the patient.

The most important modifications of Mrs. Thinis' physical surroundings are those that were directed toward facilitating the loss of heat and preventing unnecessary stimulation. In the instance of Mrs. Thinis the radiator was shut off and the window opened. In hot, humid weather an air-conditioned room will add much to the comfort of the patient and reduce the strain on the heat-eliminating mechanisms. The severely thyrotoxic patient may be placed in an oxygen tent. He benefits not only from the higher than normal concentration of oxygen, but from the low environmental temperature. Sponging the patient's face and hands and arms several times a day adds to his comfort.

Mrs. Thinis' bed was prepared by removing the blanket and spread, leaving only the top sheet. The rubber sheet was removed. When this is contrary to hospital policy, the rubber sheet should be placed under the mattress pad. A contour sheet was placed over the mattress in order to facilitate keeping the bottom sheet free from wrinkles. The nurse suggested that Mrs. Thinis might find pajamas more comfortable than a gown, as a top sheet would be unnecessary should she be too warm. Because Mrs. Thinis was restless and perspired profusely her bed required straighteneing and changing rather frequently. Every effort was made to convey to Mrs. Thinis that these procedures were being done to add to her comfort and to minimize her feeling that she was in some way responsible.

Because Mrs. Thinis overreacted to emotional and physical stimuli her need for rest was greater than that of many patients. The nature of her illness contributed to the difficulty in providing conditions favoring rest. Every effort was made to prevent sudden and loud noises. Talking and laughing outside her room were avoided, particularly as Mrs. Thinis tended to be suspicious. When she heard voices outside her room, she would get out of bed and go to the door to check on the talkers. The fact that the conversation had nothing to do with her did not alter her disquiet. Mrs. Thinis was found to be less restless and more relaxed in bed when she had some nonstimulating activity to do. Since she liked to knit, her husband brought her needles and yarn. She was encouraged to select a relatively simple pattern and to alternate periods of rest and activity. When rest is an important objective and the condition of the patient interferes with his resting, his program should be adapted so that he obtains as much rest as possible.

The fact that Mrs. Thinis was hyperirritable and easily upset for extended periods of time by minor incidents contributed to the difficulty in securing rest for her. Mrs. Thinis was given her bath and assisted with all aspects of her care despite her apparent ability to do many of these things for herself. Because Mrs. Thinis' frustration level was low, her light was answered promptly and every effort was made to get her medications to her on time. Topics that were disturbing to her were avoided in conversation, and this information was relayed to all the personnel in the unit. As is not infrequent, some of her visitors were upsetting to her. As a result all visitors with the exception of her mother and husband were asked not to stay more than ten minutes. The method of dealing with this problem will, of course, differ with the wishes of the patient and his family. The objective is to protect the patient from unnecessary stimulation. The nurse who was responsible for Mrs. Thinis was well suited to her requirements. She had a quiet, low-pitched voice. Her manner was unhurried and relaxed. Since tension tends to be communicable, a tense nurse is likely to add to the tension of the patient. The same nurse was assigned to care for Mrs. Thinis over a period of time. This enabled her to learn what was important to the patient and to utilize this information in meeting her needs. The patient also had an opportunity to develop confidence in the nurse. As the nurse identified Mrs. Thinis' needs and ways of meeting them, she recorded this information on Mrs. Thinis' nursing care plan so that it was available to others as required. Because of the severity of Mrs. Thinis' clinical manifestations and her need for rest, her physician ordered phenobarbital, gr 0.5 four times a day. Not all patients with hyperthyroidism need sedation. It is necessary only in those who are seriously ill.

One of the most important responsibilities of the nurse who cared for Mrs. Thinis was to make certain that all personnel—professional and nonprofessional—and the patient's family understood that Mrs. Thinis' behavior was part of her illness. Adjustments should be made by the person caring for the patient, rather than by the patient. If Mrs. Thinis' behavior was accepted as part of her illness, then attention could be given to modifying her environment in such a way that stimuli inducing the behavior were avoided. Reactions to the patient's irritability and hypersensitivity with anger or irritation only act to intensify her symptoms.

Mrs. Thinis was similar to many patients with hyperthyroidism in that her appetite was enormous. To satisfy it and to provide her with the extra calories she needed, she was given a diet high in calories, carbohydrates, and vitamins. The high carbohydrate and high vitamin content of the diet also help to protect the liver from damage. Liver glycogen tends to be depleted in hyperthyroidism. Mrs. Thinis ate well. She disliked soft-boiled eggs and became upset when they were served to her. Therefore her nurse made a point of checking her breakfast tray before it was served. Because she was hungry between meals, she was served sandwiches and milk mid-morning and afternoon and before retiring. Fresh iced water was kept at her bedside at all times.

Some years ago the author cared for a man with thyrotoxicosis who consumed a triple serving of food at each meal. In that institution between-meal nourishments were distributed to the patients by the dietary department. In the evening these were left at the bedside of the patient soon after dinner was served. As soon as the patient received the food, he would begin to eat it. By bedtime the several sandwiches and the fruit would have long since disappeared and he would ask for a lunch. Needless to say, he did not lose weight. Neither did he gain any.

Occasionally a patient will have a poor appetite despite hyperthyroidism. Under these circumstances, particular attention should be paid to increasing the patient's food intake. This may be done by providing him with food that he likes. Between-meal feedings, unless they result in a decrease in appetite, may increase his intake of food. The patient should be helped to understand that his food requirements are increased by his illness. Personal remarks about the enormity of his appetite may make the patient self-conscious and cause him to eat less than he needs.

With this review of the needs of Mrs. Thinis and other thyrotoxic patients, we will return to the time of her admission. As stated earlier, her room and bed were prepared to meet her needs. The personnel who were to be responsible for her care were also acquainted with the nature and effects of her illness. During the admission process, each procedure was explained and modified in terms of Mrs. Thinis' behavior. Since she was to have a basal metabolic rate the following morning, she was asked if her doctor had explained the test to her. She replied that he had, but that she was too upset to understand much about it. After checking the knowledge of the patient, the nurse explained to her that the test was for the purpose of determining the rate at which her cells utilized oxygen and that during the test she would be asked to breathe through a tube placed in her mouth. Because the purpose of the test is to determine the rate at which cells utilize oxygen at rest, food is withheld after the evening meal and until after the test has been performed the following morning. In addition, she was to remain in bed in the morning until after the test had been performed. In order to ensure that Mrs. Thinis got a good night's sleep, the physician prescribed seconal gr. 1.5, at ten o'clock that night. The next morning Mrs. Thinis was again reminded to stay in bed and to rest. The shades on the windows of her room were drawn and a sign was placed on the door not to disturb the patient.[36] Arrangements were made for her to have the test early so that her breakfast would not have to be unnecessarily delayed.

Mrs. Thinis' basal metabolic rate was found to be +65 per cent. The basal metabolic rate is reported in the percentage to which it deviates from the average person of a given age, sex, height, and weight. Rates below the average are reported as minus and rates above average as plus. Mrs. Thinis' metabolic rate was therefore 65 per cent greater than for the average person.

When a patient does not require hospitalization for some other reason, he may have the test in the office of a physician or in a clinical laboratory. The patient must then be given specific directions for his preparation at home. After he arrives at the laboratory, he is instructed to lie on a cot for about an hour. A period of rest helps to ensure that he will be physically relaxed at the time the determination is made. Some patients, such as those who must arrange to be away from work or employ a baby sitter, may require information about the approximate length of time required for the test.

Another test that is useful in confirming a diagnosis of either hyper- or hypothyroidism is the determination of the level of protein-bound iodine in the blood. In the instance of Mrs. Thinis, the findings were compatible with hyperthyroidism. The clinical manifestations as well as the results of the BMR and the protein-bound tests confirmed the provisional diagnosis that Mrs. Thinis was thyrotoxic (hyperthyroidism). Following diagnosis a therapeutic plan best suited to Mrs. Thinis' needs was made. The objective was to restore Mrs. Thinis to a permanently enthyroid state as quickly and safely as possible, by reducing the amount of hormone secreted by the thyroid gland. No therapeutic measure does all of the above equally well. Often a number of therapeutic measures are used in combination.

In the selection of the method of therapy, the physician considered the degree of hyperactivity of Mrs. Thinis' thyroid gland, the status of her cardiac function, as well as her age, and her personal preference. He also considered the possibility of each possible therapeutic method effecting a cure, and what, if any, harmful effects it might have. Among the therapeutic methods to be considered were drugs suppressing the synthesis of thyroid hormone, surgical

[36] For a complete description see Bertha Harmer and Virginia Henderson, *Textbook of Principles and Practice of Nursing,* 5th ed., The Macmillan Company, New York, 1955, pp. 592-95.

removal of the thyroid gland, and treatment with radioactive iodine. Because Mrs. Thinis was only 28 years of age and still in the childbearing period, radioactive iodine was eliminated as a possible choice. In patients who are 40 years of age or older, iodine[131] (radioactive iodine) is frequently employed in the treatment of hyperthyroidism.

The plan finally decided upon for Mrs. Thinis was to prepare her for surgical removal of a part of the thyroid gland at a later date. To decrease the synthesis of thyroid hormone, propylthiouracil 100 mgm, and minims 10 of Lugol's solution were prescribed to be administered three times a day. To maintain the concentration of these drugs at constant level they were administered at eight-hour intervals—8:00 A.M., 4:00 P.M., 12:00 midnight.

The observation that iodine is useful in the treatment of disorders of the thyroid has been known since antiquity. During the Middle Ages, persons with enlargement of the neck were treated with burnt sponge or seaweed. Not until 1916 did the now classic experiments of Marine and Kimball prove that iodine could be used in the prevention of goiter. Simple goiter is endemic in areas where iodine is deficient in the soil and water supply. When it is administered to patients with the form of hyperthyroidism associated with a diffuse enlargement of the thyroid gland (Graves's disease), the thyroid gland undergoes involution and the storage of colloid is promoted. Maximum effects are obtained in from 10 to 15 days after therapy is initiated. The effects of iodine on the thyroid gland are reflected in a lowering of the basal metabolic rate as well as in the pulse rate and in an improvement in the general condition of the patient. The effects of iodine therapy are temporary, as the patient returns to his hyperthyroid state. In fact, the degree of hyperthyroidism may be intensified. The mechanism by which iodine acts in hyperthyroidism is not known.

The introduction of thiouracil, followed by its safer analogue, propylthiouracil, made it possible to induce a more or less permanent remission of hyperthyroidism. Thiouracil and related drugs are classified as goitrogens. A goitrogen, as defined by Goodman and Gilman,[37] is a "chemical agent which lowers the BMR by interfering with the synthesis, release, or peripheral action of the thyroid hormone." The pulse rate is slowed and the other effects of hyperthyroidism are reversed. Therapy is initiated by administering 225 to 300 mg of propylthiouracil daily. The total dosage is divided into three so that the patient receives 75 to 100 mg three times during the 24 hours. After the patient becomes euthyroid, the dosage is reduced until the maintenance dosage is achieved. This may be as little as 25 mg daily. In about 50 per cent of persons treated for hyperthyroidism with propylthiouracil a permanent remission of the disease is induced. In patients in whom remission does not occur, signs and symptoms diminish and the general state of health improves.

Mrs. Thinis responded rapidly after therapy was initiated. After three days of treatment she was discharged from the hospital with the expectation that

[37] Louis S. Goodman and Alfred Gilman, *The Pharmacological Basis of Therapeutics,* 2nd ed., The Macmillan Company, New York, 1955, p. 1543.

she would continue drug therapy and a high-calorie diet for six or eight weeks. After her hyperthyroidism was controlled and her general health status was improved, she was to have a subtotal thyroidectomy. When she returned to the hospital eight weeks later her BMR was +2, pulse was 74, and she had gained 10 lb. in weight. She was more relaxed and less easily upset than she had been on her first admission.

Before discussing the needs of the patient who is treated surgically, the use of radioactive iodine, or I^{131}, in the diagnosis and treatment of thyroid disease will be presented. Of the radioactive isotopes, I^{131} is the most valuable in the therapy of disease. Because the thyroid gland removes iodine from the blood and concentrates it in itself, radioiodine is useful in the diagnosis and treatment of disease of the thyroid. Since iodine is readily absorbed from the gastrointestinal tract, it is administered by mouth. The amount of iodine concentrated in the thyroid gland can be tested with a Geiger or similar counter. In hypothyroidism little iodine will be concentrated in the gland. In hyperthyroidism the quantity will be excessive. Iodine not absorbed by the thyroid gland is excreted in the urine. Because the quantity of radioiodine used in diagnosis is very small, no precautions are required to protect the nurse or others giving care to the patient. Because larger quantities are used in therapy, the patient should be isolated. (See Chapter 3.) Therapy with I^{131} has several important advantages. It is easy to administer and it results in the highest rate of cure of all forms of therapy. Though there may be some increase in symptoms on the fourth or fifth day, radioiodine is less likely to cause a serious exacerbation of the hyperthyroid state than other forms of treatment. The increase in the degree of hyperthyroidism is explained as follows: radioiodine produces some degree of thyroiditis with necrosis of thyroid cells. With the disintegration of cells of the gland, there is an increase in the release of the thyroid hormone stored in the gland.

Radioiodine has three disadvantages. It requires special equipment for its storage and handling. As a consequence it is available only in medical centers. It may have an adverse effect on the germ plasm, and it may be carcinogenic. To avoid the possibility of either of these effects some physicians prefer not to treat patients younger than 40 or 45 years of age with I^{131}.

Although surgery is employed less frequently in the treatment of hyperthyroidism than it once was, it is still the treatment of choice for some patients. Furthermore some of the hazards accompanying surgery on the thyroid gland have been lessened since introduction of the goitrogenic drugs, as most patients will become euthyroid after therapy with them. As a result of the use of the goitrogenic agents, there has been a marked reduction in the incidence of thyroid crisis following operation and a marked improvement in the mortality rate. Since these drugs reduce the metabolic rate and improve the general status of the patient, time can be taken to improve his nutritional state. Furthermore, emotional calm and confidence that his needs will be identified and met promptly have positive effects.

The basic principles underlying the care of the surgical patient are presented in Chapter 15. Following any operation the site and nature of the operative procedure have an important bearing on the needs of the patient and the complications that are most likely. On return from the operating room Mrs. Thinis was placed in low semi-Fowler's position with her head well supported. In her preoperative preparation she had been taught that she should avoid either extending or flexing her head or her neck. She had also been taught to brace her head with her hands when she moved. This action served to prevent unnecessary pain and strain on the suture line. Until she was up and about she was turned every two hours. Deep breathing and coughing were encouraged at the same time. Her vital signs were checked every 15 minutes for two hours, then every four hours for 24 hours. She was gotten out of bed the evening of the day of surgery. In preparation for getting up she was instructed to brace her head and assisted to the "dangling" position. After a few minutes she was assisted off the edge of the bed and to walk.

As soon as Mrs. Thinis was able to swallow, she was encouraged to drink high-carbohydrate fluids. She was given glucose in water intravenously. As is usual in patients following thyroidectomy, she complained of discomfort on swallowing.

post op Complications to which Mrs. Thinis was particularly predisposed were hemorrhage, paresis or paralysis of the vocal cords, tracheitis, parathyroid failure, and thyroid crisis or storm. The fact that the thyroid gland has a rich blood supply increases the possibility of hemorrhage. Although external hemorrhage is possible, bleeding into the tissues is more common and more dangerous. To detect external bleeding, dressings should be checked each time the patient is seen. Since fluids tend to flow downhill, the back and lower portions of the dressings are likely to be stained first. To detect bleeding early, she was asked if her dressing felt comfortable each time she was observed. Had she had a feeling of fullness or tightness in her neck, the physician should have been called immediately. If hemorrhage is allowed to continue, the patient can be expected to become dyspneic and to have other symptoms indicating respiratory obstruction. When the symptoms progress rapidly, the nurse may loosen the dressing before the physician arrives. Because hemorrhage into the tissues surrounding the trachea can be expected to cause respiratory obstruction, a tracheotomy tray was placed in Mrs. Thinis' room before she returned from the operating room.

The recurrent laryngeal nerves which supply the vocal cords may be injured during the surgical procedure. When one nerve is injured, the sole effect is hoarseness, which improves with time. Should both nerves be injured or severed, a tracheotomy may be required for the relief of respiratory obstruction. Because of the possibility of traumatizing the recurrent laryngeal nerves at the time of surgery, some surgeons check the condition of the vocal cords immediately after the operation by observing the vocal cords. When they are in good condition and the patient develops hoarseness within 24 to 48 hours after surgery, it is almost certainly due to swelling in the region of the glottis and can be expected to subside. Following thyroidectomy, hoarseness should, of course, be reported promptly to the surgeon.

A third complication following thyroidectomy is hypoparathyroidism. It may be caused by the removal of all or some of the parathyroid tissue or by the combined effect of edema and swelling of the remaining tissue. According to Hardy,[38] evidence of this complication is not likely to be present before 24 or to develop after 48 hours.

A complication once common in patients who were severely thyrotoxic was thyroid crisis or storm. Thyroid crisis or storm can and does occur before surgical therapy as well as in the immediate postoperative period. In either event, it is a serious condition and is accompanied by a high mortality rate. In thyroid crisis all the symptoms of hyperthyroidism are exaggerated. The pulse rate rises to 140 or 200 beats per minute. There is also a rise in the rate of respiration and in the body temperature. In severe thyrotoxicosis, the temperature-regulating center loses control of body temperature and the temperature continues to rise until the time of death. Treatment during thyroid crisis is directed toward supplying cells with oxygen and glucose and preventing hyperpyrexia. To accomplish these objectives the patient is placed in the oxygen tent and given fluids high in glucose by mouth and by intravenous therapy. Heat loss can be facilitated by continuous sponging with cool water or the application of ice packs. When a hypothermia blanket is available, it may be employed to increase the loss of heat. Whatever method is used must be sufficiently vigorous and continued long enough to prevent the exposure of the cells to the effects of prolonged hyperpyrexia.

A source of stress for some patients is the scar resulting from the incision. Mrs. Thinis was concerned lest she be left with an unsightly scar. She was reassured that she could expect that the scar would, after a time, be no more than a fine line. The incision is usually made so that it follows that lines of the neck. Some surgeons use skin clips to further decrease scarring. Although the newly formed scar can be expected to be red, it will shrink and fade with the passage of time. Women who wish to cover the scar may do so by wearing a necklace or scarf.

A complication accompanying hyperthyroidism in some patients is exophthalmos. It is associated with the disease and is not a complication resulting from surgical or other forms of treatment. In exophthalmos the eyeballs protrude or appear to do so. The mechanism that is responsible remains unsettled. In some patients it may be due to hypersecretion of TSH (thyroid-stimulating hormone). Apparently the mechanism responsible for the apparent protrusion is not the same in all individuals. In some patients there is no forward displacement of the eyeball. In others there is. When there is true forward

[38] *Op. cit.*, p. 549.

displacement, it is due to edema and fibrosis of orbital tissues. It does not appear to be related to the severity of the hyperthyroidism nor is its progress affected by thyroidectomy. In fact, in some instances, exophthalmos seems to get worse following thyroidectomy. Though progressive exophthalmos is a self-limiting process, the eye may be lost before a remission occurs. If the eye is to be saved, it is imperative that the cornea be protected from drying. The patient should be taught to consciously close his eyes at regular intervals to moisten the eyeball with tears.

What are some of the disorders of the thyroid gland in which glandular secretion is within normal limits?

One not uncommon disorder of the thyroid gland is simple goiter. In the early stages of simple goiter, the thyroid gland is diffusely enlarged. There is usually no change in function, though occasionally hypofunction occurs. Simple goiter is most likely to develop during periods when additional thyroid function is required, such as puberty or pregnancy. Although the enlargement tends to disappear, it may persist; it then almost always becomes nodular. When the gland is greatly enlarged, it may cause compression on the surrounding structures. Simple goiter is treated with Lugol's solution, minims 15 three times a day for two or three months. Desiccated thyroid, 30 to 180 mg, may also be prescribed.

Mrs. Grivin, aged 50, illustrates fairly well the pattern by which simple goiter develops into a nodular goiter. She was born and reared in a large city in the Great Lakes region. Her mother had been thyrotoxic in 1918. At age 13, Mrs. Grivin had an enlarged thyroid gland that was diagnosed as a simple goiter of the thyroid-deficiency type. She was treated with 15 drops of potassium iodide three times a day for three months. Though the gland decreased in size, she continued to have some asymmetrical enlargement of the gland. At age 30 her BMR was -17. At age 41 it was $+1$. At age 45 it was $+3$.

At the time of Mrs. Grivin's admission to the hospital for a thyroidectomy, she had an extensive nodular goiter. Study with I^{131} indicated that thyroid function was normal. There was no clinical evidence of hyperthyroidism, though for the three months previous to her hospitalization her thyroid gland had been progressively enlarging. During the three weeks immediately preceding her admission to the hospital, she had had difficulty in swallowing and had been hoarse. Total thyroidectomy was performed to relieve pressure on the esophagus and the recurrent laryngeal nerves.

With the exception of developing parathyroid tetany, Mrs. Grivin made an uneventful recovery. The manifestations and treatment of hypoparathyroidism are discussed in relation to the parathyroid gland. Because it was necessary to remove all of her thyroid gland, she will have to take thyroid hormone for the remainder of her life. Should she neglect this for a period of time, signs and symptoms of hypothyroidism could be expected to develop.

The clinical manifestations of hypothyroidism have been summarized on pages 1045-46. Not all persons with hypothyroidism develop a full-fledged picture of cretinism or myxedema. In mild hypothyroidism the patient may complain of mild aches and pains, easy fatigability, inability to control emotions, and, in women, menstrual disturbances. The patient may be pale in appearance. Since the symptoms experienced by the patient are common to many disorders, the fact that he is suffering from hypothyroidism may be missed. The most serious consequence of hypothyroidism is a type of heart failure known as myxedema heart. It can be prevented by continued and adequate dosages of thyroid hormone. Probably the most important reason for the correction of hypothyroidism and maintenance of the euthyroid state is that it is essential to the feeling of well-being and productivity of the individual. Patients who complain of symptoms or whose appearance suggests hypothyroidism should be encouraged to seek medical attention. Patients such as Mrs. Grivin should be helped to understand why they should take their medication every day for the rest of their lives. Because the effects of thyroid hormones are initiated slowly and continued for some weeks, the patient may feel well for a time after he discontinues his medication and conclude that he no longer requires it. The patient should be encouraged to continue under regular medical supervision.

When making a nursing care plan for the patient with hypothyroidism, the ways in which he fails to adapt to his environment should be identified. Plans should then be made to modify his physical and emotional environment. Unlike the patient with hyperthyroidism, the one with hypothyroidism is intolerant to cold. He is comfortable only when the temperature is relatively high. At night he sleeps in a flannel gown and bed socks and has three or four woolen blankets on his bed. If he has an electric blanket, the heat is turned on high. When in the hospital, despite the complaints of his roommates that the room is too warm, he desires several blankets on his bed.

Because the patient with hypothyroidism has a dry skin, soap should be used sparingly, and cream or oily lotion may add to his comfort. To prevent bruising the patient, care should be taken when handling him. Furniture should be placed so that the chance of bumping into it is minimized.

Though patients are often apathetic and lethargic, they may be hyperirritable, and their ability to maintain their emotional control may also be disturbed. As in the care of other patients, the nurse should adapt her behavior to the needs of the patient. When the patient is apathetic and lethargic, he cannot be hurried or stimulated to move quickly. When he is hyperirritable, this too is part of his illness. Fortunately, the patient can be approached with optimism. When he is treated with thyroid hormones, the condition can be corrected. Depending on the form of drug prescribed, improvement of the patient should not be expected immediately. It may take as long as ten days to two weeks for signs of definite progress to be evident. The dosage of hormone has to be adjusted to each patient. As stated earlier, patients with a hypofunctioning gland are more sensitive to the thyroid hormones than are those with normally functioning glands. Signs and symptoms of overdosage are those of hyperthyroidism. One precaution relates to the increased sensitivity of hypo-thyroid individuals to drugs such as morphine or codeine. When they are prescribed by the physician, dosages should be lower than they are for persons who are euthyroid.

To recapitulate, the manifestations of disorders of the thyroid have their origin in the effects of the expanding lesion on the tissues in the vicinity of the thyroid and in alterations in the level of production of thyroid hormones. Mrs. Grivin illustrated two of the effects of a goiter on the surrounding tissue. She was hoarse (pressure on the recurrent laryngeal nerve) and she had dysphagia or difficulty in swallowing. Had the condition been allowed to continue she might have developed respiratory obstruction.

She also exemplified one of the causes of hypofunction of the thyroid gland, as she had a total thyroidectomy. She should not develop signs and symptoms of hypothyroidism if she continues to take thyroid hormone for the rest of her life. The manifestations of hypothyroidism are the result of a lack of the thyroid hormones. The manifestations of hyperthyroidism, as exemplified by Mrs. Thinis, arise from an excess of these hormones. Patients with either hyper- or hypofunction of the thyroid gland are unable to adapt appropriately to certain aspects of their environment.

What is the function of the parathyroid hormone?

Among the regulators of the stability of the composition of the internal environment is the parathyroid hormone. This hormone has been separated from beef parathyroid glands by Rasmussen.[39] It is protein in nature. The molecule is rather small, though it is larger than insulin. Now that the hormone has been obtained in pure form, physiologists and biochemists are able to study its mode of action. For some time there has been a considerable body of knowledge about the effects of the parathyroid hormone which was obtained by observing the consequences of disease or by removing the parathyroid glands and by administering to animals crude extracts containing the hormone. The parathyroid hormone regulates the level of calcium and phosphate ions in the body fluids so that their product is maintained constant. Calcium and phosphate ions are regulated so that when the level of one or the other rises, the other falls. A rise in the level of calcium ions in the blood, therefore, is accompanied by an increase in the excretion of the phosphate ions in the urine with the result that their product, that is, $Ca^{++} \times HPO_4 = C$. Conversely, a rise in the level of the phosphate ions results in an increase in the excretion of the calcium ions.

In the past scientists have not been agreed as to whether the effect of the parathyroid hormone was primarily on the kidney or on the bone. Those who supported the first view thought that the hormone regulated the rate of excretion of the phosphate ions in the urine and that other effects of its action were

[39] Howard Rasmussen, "The Parathyroid Hormone," *Scientific American,* CCIV, No. 4, April, 1961, pp. 56-63.

secondary. Others contended that its primary effect was to regulate the rate of release of calcium from bone.

According to Rasmussen,[40] studies made with the purified parathyroid hormone show that it acts both on the bone and on the kidney and on absorption from the gut. It increases the activity of bone-destroying cells or osteoclasts with the result that calcium is released from the bone to be utilized elsewhere. The hormone also acts to increase the excretion of phosphate in the urine. Both actions are essential to the homeostasis of calcium and phosphate ions. With the release of calcium ions from the bone, phosphate ions are also liberated. Without some mechanism for their removal, the level of the product of the two ions would be endangered. Recent studies using the purified hormone indicate that it also regulates the rate of exchange of calcium in the lactating mammary gland and in the gastrointestinal tract.[41] In brief, then, the level of calcium ions in body fluids as well as their relationship to phosphate ions is regulated by the parathyroid hormones. Parathyroid hormone increases the rate of release of calcium from the bones, the excretion of phosphate by the kidney, and the reabsorption of calcium by the kidney and absorption from the alimentary canal. This complicated regulating mechanism provides for both rapid and slow responses to changes in the level of the parathyroid hormone. The kidneys and the gastrointestinal tract are sensitive and respond rapidly to small changes in its level. Bone, on the other hand, is much less sensitive and responds slowly.

Unlike the thyroid hormones and certain other hormones, the secretion of the parathyroid hormone is not under the control of the anterior pituitary gland. Secretion is regulated by the concentration of calcium in body fluids. With a fall in the level of calcium in the blood, secretion is increased. Conversely, as the level of calcium rises, secretion of the hormone is decreased.

As in other homeostatic conditions, the concentration of calcium in body fluids is maintained by several regulatory agencies. The parathyroid hormone appears to regulate bodily processes so that the relationship of calcium to phosphate ions is maintained constant. The level of calcium ions in body fluids is also maintained constant. The principal regulator of this function appears to be vitamin D. As long as man wore few clothes, ingestion of vitamin D was unnecessary, as the skin manufactures vitamin D when it is exposed to sunlight. From the time most of the skin surface was covered with clothing, the addition of vitamin D from exogenous sources has been necessary.

What are some of the significant functions of calcium and phosphate ions?

Calcium and phosphate ions are important in the formation of new bone. The source of these ions to the newly forming bone is the circulating fluids of

[40] *Ibid.*, p. 59.
[41] *Ibid.*

the body. They are considered to be in simple equilibrium with the new bone; that is, calcium and phosphate ions move into and out of the bone depending on their level in the body fluids. When the level of vitamin D falls, the level of calcium and phosphate falls. These minerals are, therefore, unavailable for deposit in the collagen of the newly forming bone. As a consequence the bones stop growing and bend out of shape. The resulting disorder is known as rickets.

Other functions that are dependent on the level and ratio of calcium to phosphate include (1) the normal transmission of nerve impulses, (2) the contraction of muscles, and (3) the coagulation of blood. When the level of calcium and phosphates in body fluids falls below a critical level, the irritability of nerve and muscle fibers increase. The patient suffers from tetany, which is characterized by painful muscle spasms. An outstanding feature of the condition is carpopedal spasm. The muscles of the hands and feet contract powerfully and painfully. The hands assume a characteristic position. Spasms of the muscles of the face can be precipitated by tapping over the facial nerve. This is known as Chvostek's sign. Tetany can be relieved by the intravenous injection of calcium gluconate.

The action of digitalis is enhanced by calcium. The size of the dose and the rate of administration of calcium to a patient who is digitalized should be less than in those who have not been digitalized. Patients who have been digitalized and who are given calcium should be observed for evidence of digitalis toxicity.

Besides the parathyroid hormone and vitamin D, other hormones also play a role in the regulation of the calcium phosphate balance. These include the sex and the adrenal cortical steroids, the growth hormone from the anterior pituitary, insulin, and the thyroid hormone.

The level of calcium and phosphate ions in body fluids depends not only on the integrity of the regulatory mechanisms, but on the adequacy of the supply of calcium in the diet, and the health of the gastrointestinal tract, the bones, and the kidney.

The parathyroid glands are also subject to disease and to injury; disturbances in the structure of the parathyroids may be accompanied by disordered function. Benign neoplasms are the most frequent cause of hyperparathyroidism. Inadvertent removal of the parathyroid gland during surgery of the neck, particularly thyroidectomy, and idiophatic atrophy are the most frequent causes of hypoparathyroidism. In both hyper- and hypoparathyroidism homeostasis of calcium and phosphate is disturbed. Specific effects depend on the direction of the change in secretion.

According to Nordin,[42] the clinical manifestations of hyperparathyroidism are so diverse that they defy classification. This disorder, though by no means rare, is often discovered accidentally. Frequently the disturbance that causes

[42] B. E. C. Nordin, "Primary Hyperparathyroidism," *Postgraduate Medicine*, XXIX, January, 1961, pp. 65-74.

the patient to consult a physician is bilateral renal lithiasis (kidney stones or calculi).[43] With the increased secretion of the parathyroid hormone, the activity of the osteoclasts in the bone is enhanced. If the quantity of calcium phosphate stored in the bone is decreased and the concentration of calcium in blood is elevated as calcium is removed from the bone, its density is reduced (osteoporosis). Occasionally the loss of mineral from the bone is so great that there are areas of cystic degeneration resulting in a disorder known as osteitis fibrosa cystica. With the demineralization of the bone, they become fragile, thus predisposing to fractures. Hyperparathyroidism can, however, exist without changes in the bones provided the intake of calcium is sufficient to prevent excessive demineralization of bone.[44]

With an elevation in the level of calcium in the blood, its excretion in the urine is increased. When conditions favor precipitation, such as concentration or alkalinity of the urine, stones form.

Symptoms experienced by patients with hyperparathyroidism include bone pain, particularly in the back, muscular weakness, anorexia, and vomiting. The high level of calcium and phosphates in the blood results in increased excretion of these substances by the kidney. Polyuria follows as water excretion increases with the loss of calcium. With polyuria, polydipsia is to be expected. A vast number of other signs and symptoms may occur, especially in patients in advanced stages of hyperparathyroidism.

When hyperparathyroidism is caused by a benign neoplasm, the disorder is cured by surgical removal of the neoplasm. Because the glands are small and the neoplasm may also be small, the surgeon may have difficulty in finding it. Hyperplasia of the parathyroid glands is a possible, though less frequent, cause of hyperparathyroidism. It may be either primary or secondary to some other disorder. For example, in advanced kidney disease in which the kidney no longer reabsorbs normal amounts of calcium, the parathyroid gland undergoes hyperplasia.

Much of the nursing of the patient with hyperparathyroidism is similar to that of any sick person who is undergoing diagnosis and possible surgical treatment. In the care of patients in whom bone changes are evident, care should be taken to prevent placing stress or strain on bones when the patient is being moved either in bed or from the bed to the wheel chair. Attention should also be given to providing the patient with an adequate supply of water.

Hypoparathyroidism occurs occasionally as a complication following thyroidectomy, either as a result of removal of all of the parathyroid tissue or from edema and swelling of remaining tissue. For example, about 24 hours after Mrs. Grivin had a thyroidectomy she began to complain of a tingling sensation in both legs which she said awakened her from sleep. She later

---

[43] Hyperparathyroidism is not, however, the sole cause of this condition.
[44] Daniel S. Bernstein, Alan Goldfien, and George W. Thorn, "Diseases of the Parathyroid Glands," in Harrison, *Op. cit.*, p. 604.

complained of paresthesia (abnormal sensation) of her hands and mouth and that her feet and legs seemed to fall asleep. Though laryngeal stridor, forced breathing due to obstruction of the glottis, may occur, Mrs. Grivin did not experience it. Chvostek's sign was positive. To elicit this sign, the facial nerve is tapped in front of the ear. When the test is positive, muscles of the face and around the mouth twitch. Carpopedal spasm was induced by placing a blood pressure cuff around her arm and inflating it to the level of the systolic blood pressure for 30 seconds. The urine Sulkowitch test was elevated (a test for calcium in the urine). To control her symptoms she was given calcium gluconate, 4 gm six times a day, and Dihydrotachysterol (A.T. 10), or vitamin D_3, 10 mg daily. When treatment was discontinued a week later, her symptoms did not recur, indicating that the condition was due to edema of parathyroid tissue.

The management of patients with chronic hypothyroidism is directed to the objective of increasing the level of calcium in the blood and reducing the amount of phosphate ion. To increase the level of calcium, vitamin D or Dihydrotachysterol (A.T. 10) is prescribed. The latter, a derivative of ergosterol, more closely simulates the action of the parathyroid hormone. To further reduce the level of phosphates in the blood, the patient may be placed on a low-phosphorus diet. Foods high in phosphorus include milk products, cauliflower, and molasses. Aluminum hydroxide, 0.6 gm three times a day, may be administered to decrease the absorption of phosphates from the intestine.

In nursing the patient with acute hypoparathyroidism, or the one who is predisposed to it, attention should be directed toward detecting signs indicating increased neuromuscular irritability. Treatment should then be given promptly. Should the patient have a convulsive seizure, care of the patient during the seizure is no different from that of convulsions of other causes. The seizure can be terminated by the administration of calcium gluconate intravenously. This should, therefore, be done promptly.

Summary

One of the important factors in the maintenance of each homeostatic condition is regulation of one or more processes. In order for regulation to be effective, a receptor or sensing body must be affected by disturbances in the environment of a cell or of an individual. Some means must be available to communicate information gained by the receptor to all parts of the body and finally to effector (muscle or gland) cells. One of the most important systems of communication is the endocrine system. Hormones secreted by the endocrine glands are distributed throughout the body, where they regulate the responses of cells to changes in their environment. Some hormones, such as those secreted by the thyroid gland, alter the activities of all cells. Others appear to influence some but not all.

Though exactly how hormones act is not known, they all regulate activities having to do with the adaptation of the individual to his environment. In cooperation with the nervous system, hormones act to integrate the total behavior of the individual. Like other service facilities, endocrine glands are subject to disease and injury. As they are regulating mechanisms, disturbances in endocrine structure and function are likely to be reflected by increased or decreased activities of cells or structures regulated by a particular hormone. Disturbances in the secretions of one endocrine gland are likely to lead to dislocations in others. Often many, if not all, bodily functions are affected.

In nursing the patient with an endocrine disturbance, the nurse should have an understanding of the physiological effect of hormones as well as the effects of hyper- or hyposecretion. Since the patient with an endocrine disorder is unable to adapt to certain aspects of his environment, the nurse should be prepared to appropriately modify the demands made on him. In controllable, but not curable, disorders the nurse has a responsibility to assist the patient and the members of his family to learn to manage his disease.

PART B : Neural Regulation[45]

Any complex multicellular organism requires means by which its activities can be controlled. Organisms with highly elaborate differentiated systems demand means for relating these to one another, for adjusting to varying demands. Part A of this chapter has discussed various regulatory systems which facilitate these adjustments. The nervous system, which will be the concern of this section, stands in position to integrate, direct, and control them all. With a mature and functionally perfect nervous system the bodily life of the organism goes on smoothly, meeting exquisitely, in the environment to which it is suited, its needs as an individual. When there are defects in the nervous system, the organism may be handicapped only slightly and able to compensate quite satisfactorily, or, as is the case in any complex organization with a highly elaborate administrative system, when departments are absent or ineffective, chaos can result.

Embryogenesis.

The history of the nervous system reaches far back in evolution; and the basic patterns of the simpler forms of animal life have been used, built upon, and elaborated until it is hard to see in the healthy adult the simple beginnings of so complicated a structure. By returning to the early life of the embryo and following the first weeks of its development, it may be seen that certain principles of growth will hold as well for the nervous system, within the body, as for the body as a whole. Here is a single example: Growth proceeds in cephalocaudal direction.

The earliest aggregation of cells which will shortly be delegated to undertake the elaboration of the nervous system is seen first at the anterior dorsal part of the embryo. As development proceeds, it is at the cephalic end that evaginations and foldings occur that indicate the primitive brain. The simpler cord, growing caudally, retains for some time an appearance reminiscent of the nervous system of segmented animals such as worms, the nerves growing out from it seeming to pursue the primitive muscles which develop earlier.

Organization of the central nervous system.

There are other principles, less familiar than the one above, which are more specific for understanding the nervous system. They will be stated here and referred to or applied in discussion later on.

[45] This part of the chapter was contributed by Esther H. Read, Associate Professor of Nursing, College of Nursing, Wayne State University, Detroit, Michigan. Miss Read acknowledges her gratitude to Dr. John Stirling Meyer, Professor of Neurology, Wayne State University, for his reading of the manuscript of this part of Chapter 13, and for his helpful suggestions.

1. The more important an organ or system is to the economy of the body as a whole, the more provisions there are for protecting its structure and blood supply.
2. The more highly specialized a tissue, the less able it is to survive severe and sudden deficits in supply.
3. After destruction of nerve cells, those remaining are unable to replace those that are lost.
4. Within the nervous system there is a hierarchy of control. No single part functions separately from other parts.
5. The nervous system imposes regulation and control not only on organs and systems of the body but on itself.
6. In general, higher centers inhibit lower and phylogenetically newer parts inhibit older.
7. The later in embryonic life a part of the nervous system develops, the more susceptible it is to injury.

As the system responsible for the control and regulation of all others, the economy of the body dictates that the nervous system be well shielded (Principle 1). While this armor lies outside the nervous system, its structure needs to be appreciated nevertheless, because a break in the integrity of the protectors may constitute a threat to the nervous system they guard. Example: A compound fracture of the skull may be serious not so much on its own account as for the hazard of brain injury or infection it presents to the contents within.

The nervous system in man is well protected. The brain, after the period of rapid growth in infancy is over, is enclosed in a relatively rigid cranium of bone which is shaped by its inner tables to conform to and support the friable tissues which lie within the several fossae of the skull. In like manner, the spinal cord is guarded by a chain of vertebrae, rigid in themselves but held into a flexible tunnel for the cord by means of the heavy cartilaginous discs between their bodies and by powerful tendinous and muscle attachments. The safety of parts of the cord is enhanced by additional fixation offered from the shoulder and sacral girdles, although the thoracic section of the cord does not profit from such an additional shield.

Within the skull and vertebral column are three membranous coverings, the meninges. The outermost, the *dura mater,* is a heavy, nonelastic tissue which forms a cloaklike covering for brain and cord and is reflected at two points to form deep folds: one, the *falx,* between the two cerebral hemispheres, and the second, the *tentorium,* between the cerebral hemispheres and the cerebellum. Like that of the skull, the protection offered by the dura is mechanical, and the partition erected by the falx tends to cut down on the transmission of pressure, or force, from hemisphere to hemisphere. The tentorium affords a comparable shield between forebrain and the more vital structures of midbrain and medulla below.

The second meninx, or *arachnoid,* is thin and made up of a delicate, fibrous, weblike tissue which both separates it from and joins it to the *pia mater,* the third membrane. Filling this mesh is the cerebrospinal fluid, which eventually will be returned to the blood by way of specialized structures of the arachnoid called arachnoid villi, or granulations, or the pacchionian bodies.

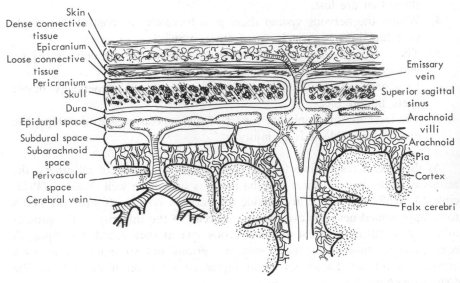

F I G U R E 13—1. Diagrammatic coronal section through the head, including the layers of the scalp and the superficial cerebral cortex. This shows the emissary veins and the relations of the arachnoid villi to the dural sinuses. (Adapted from *A Functional Approach to Neuroanatomy* by Earl Lawrence House and Ben Pansky. Copyright 1960. McGraw-Hill Book Company. Used by permission.)

The *pia mater* is a most delicate covering of the nervous system to which it is closely applied at every point, following the curvatures of every sulcus and gyrus. It can hardly qualify as a protector to the nervous system on a mechanical basis but rather on the richness of the blood supply, a matter which will be discussed briefly further on. The pia and arachnoid together are referred to as the *leptomeninges.*

Cerebrospinal fluid.

The *cerebrospinal fluid* found circulating in the subarachnoid space has its origin largely from the choroid plexuses in the ventricles of the brain. These are fluid-filled cavities which serve as another means for absorbing shock. The ventricular system is rather like a short series of little lakes, spring-fed, which are connected to one another by canals of greater and lesser width to reach a marsh which spreads wide to cover the brain and which eventually drains, by way of the arachnoid granulations, into the great channels of the dural sinuses. Thus the brain floats on a fluid cushion; and since the specific gravities of the brain and cerebrospinal fluid are about the same, a blow to the head moves all the cranial contents together so that contortion is at a minimum.

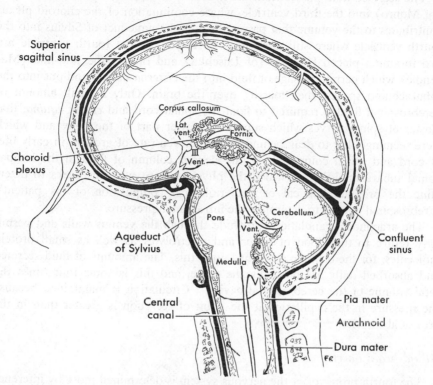

FIGURE 13—2. Diagram showing relationship of brain and cord to meninges. The choroid plexus forms the cerebrospinal fluid. (Modified with permission of The Macmillan Company from *The Principal Nervous Pathways*, 4th ed., by Andrew T. Rasmussen. Copyright 1952 by The Macmillan Company.)

In the analogy, the "springs" are the *choroid plexuses,* which are little clusters of blood vessels, rather resembling a raspberry, which project into the lateral, third, and fourth ventricles. Cerebrospinal fluid is extravasated from them continuously at a rate estimated to be 400 to 800 ml a day.[46] Nothing

Average	Blood Plasma	Cerebrospinal Fluid
Protein, mg/100 ml	7,500	20
Na, MEQ/1	137	141
Cl, MEQ/1	101	124
K, MEQ/1	4.9	3.3
Glucose, mg/100 ml	92	61

[46] Arthur C. Guyton, *Textbook of Medical Physiology,* 2nd ed., W. B. Saunders Co., Philadelphia, 1961, p. 74.

is found in cerebrospinal fluid which is not found in blood, but the concentrations are quite different, which implies that the fluid is a secretion rather than a filtrate.

The secreted fluid passes from the lateral ventricles through their foramina (of Monro) into the third ventricle, where continuation of the choroid plexus contributes to the volume that passes through the aqueduct of Silvius into the fourth ventricle where still more fluid is formed. In the fourth ventricle are two foramina placed laterally (of Luschka) and one in the mid-line (Magendie) which permit passage of fluid into the *cisterna magna* and out into the subarachnoid spaces, the "marsh" over the brain. Only a small amount of cerebrospinal fluid is required to float the spinal cord and *cauda equina,* that cluster of spinal nerves which supply the lower part of the body and which were seemingly left to drag behind by the uneven rate of growth, in early life, of cord and spinal column. It is this slender column of fluid in the lumbar spinal subarachnoid space which the physician taps when he seeks to determine the present chemical or bacteriological composition of his patient's cerebrospinal fluid or to determine the intracranial pressure.

The arachnoid granulations protrude through the venous walls and permit easy return to the blood of water and electrolytes as well as small protein molecules, for the osmotic gradient favors this. The amounts of fluid secreted and absorbed daily are normally the same, and this is some four times the total volume of the cerebrospinal cavity.[47] Circulation is maintained because the pressure in the capillaries at the point of secretion is greater than in the area of absorption.

Blood-brain barrier.

The fourth protector of the nervous system is determined more by inference than by vision: this is the "blood-brain barrier." All substances that circulate freely in the blood stream and pass into interstitial spaces of the body cells will not pass into the cerebrospinal fluid or brain parenchyma under normal circumstances. Whatever the nature of this "barrier," it tends to protect the central nervous system from being affected by many agents that are potentially harmful. While the circumstances which lower this barrier and permit molecules ordinarily excluded to pass through have been extensively studied, there is still no consensus of opinion on this point. The student who wishes to read further on the subject is referred to references listed at the end of the chapter. The presence of the barrier is important to appreciate in drug therapy. When a drug is prescribed to treat an infection in the nervous system, meningococcus meningitis, for example, it is necessary to use one which penetrates the barrier, such as sulfadiazine. Many other forms of sulfa do not, and would be ineffective.

[47] *Ibid.*

Blood supply of brain.

The tissue of the nervous system, which will be discussed shortly, is the most specialized of any tissue of the body and as such demands and receives a rich blood supply, about 750 ml per minute.[48] This is provided both by the carotid arteries, which enter at the base of the skull and divide to form the middle and anterior cerebral arteries, and by the two vertebral arteries, which branch off the subclavian and enter through the foramen magnum to form the basilar artery. These great vessels deliver to the brain blood which has only recently left the heart and is rich in oxygen and nutrients. Both the carotid and vertebral arteries variously coalesce, branch, and subdivide to assure excellent blood supply to all areas, the smallest arteries eventually forming capillaries from which veins arise which return to the subarachnoid spaces, and finally to the dural sinuses through which the brain is drained at last into the internal jugular veins which return to the superior vena cava.

A test frequently performed in the course of a diagnostic spinal tap illustrates some points discussed in the foregoing paragraphs. With a manometer attached to a lumbar puncture needle free in the spinal canal, the cerebrospinal fluid will be noted to oscillate in direct relation to both the patient's pulse and respiration. If pressure is then applied to the patient's neck over the jugular veins, there will be a prompt rise in the column of cerebrospinal fluid in the manometer. Partial occlusion occasioned by jugular vein compression has temporarily interfered with blood leaving the cranium, but the arterial inflow continues. This increases the volume of the intracranial blood and hence increases the intracranial pressure which is reflected at once in the height of the fluid column in the manometer.

Cerebral metabolism.

It will be well here to discuss in some detail the histological structure of the nervous system. Brain tissue demands much for its nourishment and respiration to meet its large energy requirements. Cerebral oxygen utilization is about 3.5 ml per minute for each 100 gm of brain.[49] In the absence of oxygen, cerebral function can be supported for only ten seconds before symptoms result. Glucose consumption of the brain is 5.4 mg per minute for each 100 gm of brain. The brain can survive for only one to one and a half hours in the absence of glucose, before symptoms of hypoglycemia appear. (Principle 2: the more specialized a tissue, the less able it is to survive severe and sudden deficits in supply.) While nerve cells have certain features in common and are quite unlike cells of other tissues—muscle, bone, and blood, for instance—these nerve cells vary greatly from one another, for they are well adapted in form to the special activities they carry on. In discussing "a typical nerve cell," one needs to understand that many nerve cells will be structurally quite different in appearance from the "typical" one used for illustration.

[48] *Ibid.*, p. 398.
[49] *Ibid.*, p. 399.

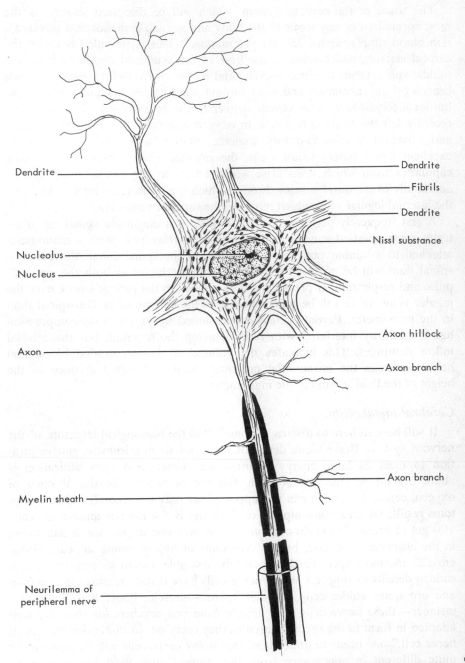

Dendrite

Dendrite

Fibrils

Dendrite

Nissl substance

Nucleolus

Nucleus

Axon hillock

Axon

Axon branch

Axon branch

Myelin sheath

Neurilemma of
peripheral nerve

FIGURE 13—3. Diagram of a nerve cell with processes. (Adapted. Courtesy of Charles H. Best and Norman B. Taylor, *The Living Body*, 4th ed., Henry Holt and Co., New York, 1958, p. 508.)

Microscopic structure of brain.

A nerve cell and all that is contained within it together with the processes of the cell are termed a *neuron*, the structural unit of nerve tissue. The processes which convey impulses to the cell are termed *dendrites* and referred to as *afferent processes* (*ad* meaning to, *ferre* meaning to bring). Those that convey impulses away from the cell to deliver to a muscle or gland or to the dendrites of another nerve cell are *axons* and are referred to as *efferent processes* (*ex* meaning from). When an axon of one cell delivers its message to the dendrites of another, the point of transfer is a *synapse* (*syn* meaning together, *aptein* meaning clasp). It is believed that the synapse offers some resistance to passage of nerve impulses and that the frequency with which impulses are sent along a pathway may influence this resistance so as to reduce it, a factor which may well be a part of perfecting manual or mental skills. Certain drugs, of which strychnine is an example, act at the synapse.

Inside the nerve cell will be found all the activities in any cell, with the exception of those having to do with cell division and replication. Since nerve cells cannot replace themselves, there will be no centrosome and no mitotic activity to be seen. (Principle 3. After destruction of nerve cells, those remaining are unable to replace those that are lost.) There are structures found only in nerve cells, of which only one will be mentioned here. *Nissl bodies* appear as heavily stained granules scattered plentifully about the healthy nerve cell. They are nucleoprotein in nature, are concentrations of RNA (see page 1009), and respond promptly to illness of the cell by breaking up and largely disappearing, a situation referred to as *chromolysis*. This is a reversible process, and if the cell recovers, Nissl substance returns as before.

Structure of nerve.

The description of nerve fibers to follow applies to both afferent and efferent fibers of the peripheral nerves and to efferent within the central nervous system. The only difference that needs to be mentioned is that nerve fibers within the central nervous system lack a *neurolemma* (sheath of Schwamm), the cellular sheath of the peripheral nerve which permits successful regrowth after destruction of the fiber within, a privilege not accorded to nerve fibers lying within the central axis. These nerve fibers are probably very long protein molecules lying parallel to the long axis of the axon (or dendrite). They are sheathed in an insulating coat of *myelin*, a fatty material, in greater or lesser amount. Although some nerve fibers are referred to as "unmyelinated," this is really not the case;[50] all fibers have some, and for many fibers the myelin sheath is far heavier than the fiber it insulates. It is myelin which makes the "white matter" of the nervous system, for nerve cells, or "gray matter," have no glittering fatty covering to reflect light.

[50] H. Chandler Elliott, *Textbook of the Nervous System*, 2nd ed., J. B. Lippincott Co., Philadelphia, 1954, p. 113.

Figures 13-3 (page 1070) and 13-4 (page 1073) will show that the nerve fiber itself, in this instance the axon, emerges naked from the cell but, as it proceeds, is very soon wrapped in myelin and covered over by a thin neurolemma. The myelin sheath, however, is broken at short intervals, and the neurolemma appears to be nipped in at this point. Each interruption is termed a *node of Ranvier*. The continuity of the nerve fiber and that of the neurolemma remain; only that of the myelin is broken. Myelin acts to insulate the contained fiber. Nerve fibers which conduct rapidly and for which discreteness of function is important, as, for instance, that of discriminating touch, are heavily insulated by myelin. The neurolemma of each node of Ranvier has a single flattened cell which is vital to repair of a damaged fiber, a process which, when comprehended, will make clear some points of importance for the care of patients who have suffered damage to a peripheral nerve.

When rapidly growing, skinny Sarah stumbles up the back steps, she trips, falls, and knocks over a milk bottle. As she and the bottle tumble down the steps, the bottle breaks and Sarah cuts her forearm deeply on a fragment of the heavy glass bottle. In addition to incising skin, blood vessels, and muscle, Sarah severs the radial nerve, which is a *mixed peripheral* nerve that supplies a part of her hand. It is a *peripheral* nerve because it lies outside the central nervous system and supplies peripheral areas, and it is *mixed* because it contains, bound up in its structure, many nerve fibers each with more or less myelin, each with a neurolemma, some of which carry information from Sarah's hand to her spinal cord and brain (afferent fibers) and some of which, the axons of cells located in her spinal cord (efferent fibers), are responsible for delivering directions for action to the muscles and glands of her hand. The mixed nerve is like a telephone cable in some respects, containing many insulated wires each with assigned work to perform.

In such an injury, the patient cannot feel anything in the parts once supplied by the now severed nerve: the area supplied is *anesthetic,* or without feeling. The afferent fibers are cut. She cannot move the parts either, and, very shortly, the muscles will begin to atrophy. If an appropriate electric current is supplied, there will be a failure to respond to galvanic current although there continues to be a response to faradic current: the so-called "reaction of degeneration." This paresis of the parts must follow the break in continuity of the efferent fibers. The muscles are present but they have now lost their innervation: they are *denervated* and cannot act.

Sarah has excellent surgical care, no infection, and good health. Her well-repaired wound heals cleanly. She is careful to follow the directions given her to protect the partly anesthetic hand from thermal or mechanical injury and, a few months later, notes curious prickly sensations, pain, and tingling in her hand. These abnormal sensations, or *paresthesias*, continue to herald the fact that nerve repair is progressing, and eventually Sarah may regain much of what she lost when the radial nerve was severed by the fragment of glass.

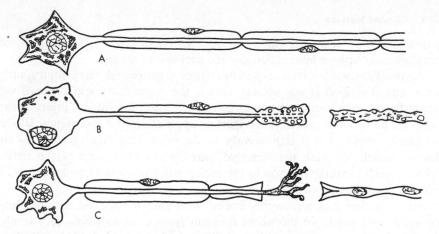

FIGURE 13—4. Diagram of nerve regeneration. A, A normal neuron with its axon enclosed in myelin and a nuerilemma sheath. Two nodes are shown, B, A neuron two or three days after section of the axon. Retrograde degeneration back to first node proximal to cut; swelling and chromolysis of the cell body, with displacement of the nucleus. Wallerian degeneration in the distal stump; the axon disintegrates, the myelin breaks down into droplets and only the neurilemma survives. C, Beginning of regeneration. The axon sprouts into profuse branches. The cell body reverts towards normal. If a branch of the axon reaches the surviving neurilemma sheath of the distal stump, it will grow down it and restore functional continuity. (Adapted. Courtesy of H. Chandler Elliott, *Textbook of Neuroanatomy*, J. B. Lippincott Company, Philadelphia, 1963, p. 47, Fig. 4—9.)

The process of reinnervation of the partly denervated hand can be understood by following what goes on in a single fiber of the patient's radial nerve. This fiber originates as the axon of a motor cell in the anterior horn of the spinal cord. It is a very long fiber and was cut well toward the end. After such an injury, the distal fragment of the axon becomes swollen, the myelin disintegrates, and both are disposed of by phagocytosis. The neurolemma remains and survives. On the proximal side of the cut nerve as well there are changes. The cell body within the cord may demonstrate profound shock due to the damage to its process far away. The Nissl substance undergoes chromolysis, and the nucleus of the cell itself loses its central position. At the cut end of the axon, degeneration occurs comparable to that which is happening in the distal fragment, but this proceeds only as far as the next node of Ranvier. In a few days' time, when the cell has recovered its normal healthy state and the injured fiber fragments have been carried away, new little nerve fibrils begin to emerge from the node. They wave about seeming to seek guidance and a path. There are many of them, but it is obvious that only a few will find the waiting neurolemma of the distal stump which is essential both to guiding them to the muscles they should supply and also to provision of myelin needed for efficient performance.

Many of the new fibrils find no way and eventually disappear. If the break between proximal and distal fragments is great, more than a few millimeters, the regenerating fibrils will not find the distal neurolemma at all and, although they will continue to grow for some time, will ball themselves up in a little

1073

matted tumor, or *neuroma,* which can be a source of pain. The hand will, of course, remain without innervation and the part will be useless.

The most favorable outcome possible from a peripheral nerve injury such as the one described is not by any means the commonest and depends on circumstances only partly subject to control. At the time of the injury great care must be taken to prevent overvigorous application of a tourniquet. Blood lost can be replaced if it is necessary to do so; a little free bleeding is an effective douche to wash the damaged parts; and compression of the nerve higher up with resulting hypoxia to the entire arm from a tight tourniquet will seriously insult already damaged tissues.

Sarah's mother took a smoothly ironed linen guest towel, laid Sarah's forearm on it, and bandaged the whole forearm from wrist to elbow very firmly with a strip torn from an old sheet, before driving her to the hospital. The towel was reasonably clean having been ironed and stored in a linen drawer probably free of pathogenic bacteria. Firm pressure exerted over the length of the forearm checks but does not stop bleeding and in no way interferes with arterial supply. The emergency treatment provides gentle pressure to the bleeding points locally and does not cause additional pain to the patient and thereby increased demand on her mechanisms for adaptation to stress which the original trauma has already activated. (Chapter 5.)

Infection cured but with resultant scarring may leave a barrier which no newly regenerating axon fibril can cross. It is, therefore, important for everyone to do everything possible to prevent infection from occurring. Everyone needs be his brother's keeper; and while the gentlest and most skillful surgery is indicated, it will not bring the best possible results if there has been a lack of respect by anyone for bacteria, for the vulnerability of injured tissue, or for the person of the injured patient.

The second principle given at the beginning of the chapter stated that the more highly specialized a tissue, the less likely it is to survive deficits in supply. A neuron, nerve cell and fiber, has been described, and the effects of injury discussed. Although all nerve tissue is specialized, the specialization varies in degree. We have seen in the foregoing that even the most homogeneous part of the neuron, the fiber, suffers actual dissolution at its point of injury for a measurable distance toward its cell (up to the next node of Ranvier), and that the sensitive cell itself, though many inches away, reflects the shock when serious injury to the fiber is sustained. However, recovery of the shocked cell is prompt as is the cell's immediate attention to repair its fiber. But this regeneration is not a simple process even in the fiber. It is one that demands no interference with the prescribed sequence, is possible only in the peripheral nerves, and has been lost to the nerves within the cord and brain.

Reflex arc.

As the neuron is the unit of nerve structure, the *reflex arc* is the unit of function. Since nervous structures exist to direct, control, and integrate all parts of the organism, discussion of the reflex arc involves end organs and nerves as well as neurons. In the broadest sense, these are: a structure to receive a stimulus and one to react to a stimulus, which may be referred to simply as *receptor* and *effector* end organs. Thus, in simplest form, one may see the reflex arc illustrated when the patellar tendon, the receptor end organ, is stretched by a sharp blow upon it and the leg, the effector end organ, extends in response. This reaction implies the presence of an afferent nerve to convey the impulse to the spinal cord, intact synapses within the cord, and an efferent nerve to take the message for contraction out to the muscles of the leg. All parts of the circuit are needed. Any break in the circut results in loss of the reflex. Each reflex, whenever elicited, is invariably repeated in the same pattern. It represents a pathway which has become useful to the animal over generations and, as it were, brooks no interference with its habits. A little thought will recall many familiar reflexes: the blink of the eye in response to threat, withdrawal of the finger from a flame, etc. In the case of peripheral nerve transection, described previously, both afferent and efferent fibers were cut by the injury, so the hand was neither aware of the injury nor could it move to react. In poliomyelitis, however, the reflex will be lost because the motor cell in the spinal cord is destroyed by disease; and although the message from the struck tendon can be conveyed to the cord, there is no longer a motor cell within to activate an impulse to be conveyed out to the muscle of the leg.

This cell in the anterior horn of the spinal cord has many dendrites. All directions for the control of motion which are coming from the brain above by way of the descending tracts will eventually end at the synapses on these dendrites. This cell with its processes is therefore called the *lower motor neuron*. The axons which proceed from it to form the spinal and then peripheral nerves are called the *final common path*. In other words, all motion, consciously planned or not, must in the end be effected through these large motor cells and be carried out through these axons, a pathway which, while it may begin as far away as the cortex of the brain, is the last segment in the road on the way to the effector end organ (muscle or gland), and is common for all travelers. The name is a good one; it is the final pathway, to be used by all.

The simple cord reflex used to illustrate a reflex arc requires no planning on the part of the individual, but ordinarily, he is aware that it has occurred. He may see it; he may be aware of the coldness or heat of the instrument that struck his knee; he may even inhibit the reflex by an elaborate play of higher activities on these simple ones which have not actually required any involvement of his brain at all.

Spinal cord.

Since this chapter is concerned with the over-all administrative system of the body, it is necessary to understand more than the last and simplest unit of action, to appreciate the main channels of communication, some of the lower and higher administrative branches, and how they influence one another. The discussion has referred already to the spinal cord and structures within it, the motor cells with their many dendrites around which axons synapse bringing impulses from the brain above. Much of the cord is devoted to conveying information up and down its length and also to delivering some of the messages at appropriate stops along the way. The remainder of the cord is concerned with its relations to the periphery of the body. Structurally, the cord

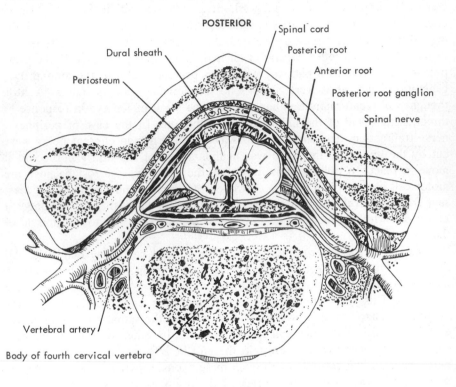

POSTERIOR

Dural sheath

Periosteum

Spinal cord

Posterior root

Anterior root

Posterior root ganglion

Spinal nerve

Vertebral artery

Body of fourth cervical vertebra

ANTERIOR

FIGURE 13–5. Cross section of vertebral column at the level of the fourth cervical vertebra, showing spinal cord in position. (Adapted. Courtesy of Ellen E. Chaffee and Esther M. Greisheimer, *Basic Physiology and Anatomy*, J. B. Lippincott Company, Philadelphia, 1964, Fig. 136, p. 203.)

reflects these functions. Only slightly larger in diameter than a pencil, it is somewhat elliptical in shape with some increase in size at the thoracic and sacral enlargements. Neatly suspended in the spinal foramina of the vertebrae, two roots emerge on each side, one dorsal and one ventral, and pass through foramina in each vertebra. These roots presently join, and from this point on belong to the peripheral nervous system, which has just been discussed briefly in considering the reflex arc.

Looked at in cross section, the cord shows a central, H-shaped portion made up of cells, or gray matter, lying within a heavy border of fiber masses, or white matter. Many of the cells are those of neurons which are responsible for intercommunication within the cord: these are connectors which constitute a large part of the bulk of nervous tissue and are termed *internuncial* neurons. The white matter or nerve fibers of the cord tend to be grouped according to function; each group of fibers which is fairly discrete is called a *tract* and has a name. The form of the name usually indicates the direction of the tract, the point of origin being stated first and destination second. Thus, the *spinocerebellar tract* names a group of nerve fibers which conveys from the spinal cord to the cerebellum, which may be required to act upon this knowledge, information about the state of contraction of muscles. A tract, then, represents a group of nerve fibers all of which have the same function.

Ascending Tracts

The first neuron implicated in conveying a sensation to the brain is the neuron whose cell is located in a small swelling in the dorsal root just outside the spinal cord, called the *dorsal root ganglion* (see Figure 13-5). The processes of this cell extend in two directions: the shorter one centrally to enter the cord in the dorsal part and the other extending to the periphery to end in muscle, in skin, or around a hair follicle. This process extending to the periphery should be recognized as a single afferent unit in the cable of the peripheral nerve. It will terminate in one or another of a specialized nerve ending, peculiarly adapted to its place and function. Fibers which carry pain are nearly naked and end in little brushes which cover a considerable surface, a square centimeter,[51] and may overlap one another, whereas touch, for which the animal requires far more discrimination than for pain, is provided with a better myelinated fiber and three different kinds of specialized endings. Cold, heat, pressure—each is represented by its own ending adapted to meet the need. (Figure 13-6.) Each specialized ending, on stimulation, sends the message along the sensory nerve fiber to the cell in the dorsal root ganglion whence it proceeds into the dorsomedial part of the cord. If this sensation was one of pain or temperature, the fiber, on entering the cord, ascends a segment or two and ends on the dendrites of a second neuron which immediately *decussates* (crosses over to the other side), to travel in the *spinothalamic* tract in the lateral part of the spinal cord to the thalamus.

The *proprioceptive* pathway accounts for the conveyance of those sensations which are peculiarly one's own, within oneself (*proprio* meaning own). These are the muscle-tendon-joint sensations and vibration. It is by means of these columns that one is aware of his position in space. It is not, for example, necessary to look at one's foot to know where it is and whether or not the knee is bent. These fibers enter the cord by way of the dorsal root and sweep upward into the great wedge-shaped columns which occupy the whole dorsum of the cord. These columns are variously named, and the student should recognize *dorsal* or *posterior columns, fasciculus gracilis* and *fas-*

[51] *Ibid.,* p. 118.

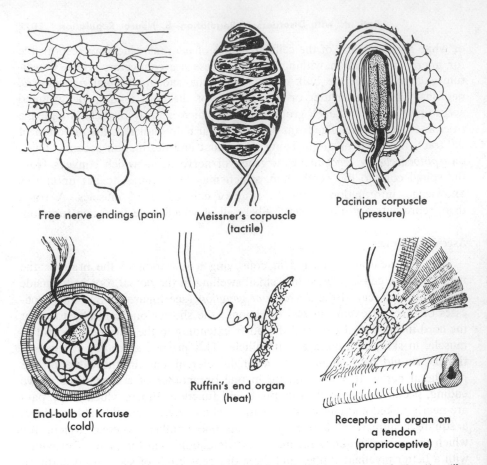

Free nerve endings (pain)   Meissner's corpuscle
(tactile)

Pacinian corpuscle
(pressure)

End-bulb of Krause
(cold)

Ruffini's end organ
(heat)

Receptor end organ on
a tendon
(proprioceptive)

FIGURE 13–6. Specialized nerve endings. (Adapted with permission of The Macmillan Company from *Anatomy and Physiology*, 14th ed., Fig. 169, p. 202, by Diana Clifford Kimber, Carolyn E. Gray, Caroline E. Stackpole, and Lutie C. Leavell. Copyright © The Macmillan Company, 1961.)

ciculus cuneatus, and *dorsal fasciculus* as terms that indicate these tracts which proceed without decussation to the medulla, where the fibers end on secondary neurons. These fibers decussate at once and proceed as the *median fillet* to the thalamus.

Reference has been made earlier to the spinocerebellar tract, another afferent pathway of the spinal cord, but this one goes to the cerebellum. This tract lies at the periphery of the cord in two distinct divisions. The fibers conduct with great rapidity and are heavily myelinated. They ascend for a considerable way before they synapse with secondary neurons which are scattered along in the dorsal columns. Since the cerebellum is responsible for rapid adjustments of posture it requires quick and accurate information. This spinocerebellar tract keeps the cerebellum continuously informed of the state of contraction of muscles and of any change in tension. A disease which is not commonly seen today, tertiary syphilis, may result in degeneration of the dorsal columns which, it will be recalled, convey also part of touch as well as proprioception

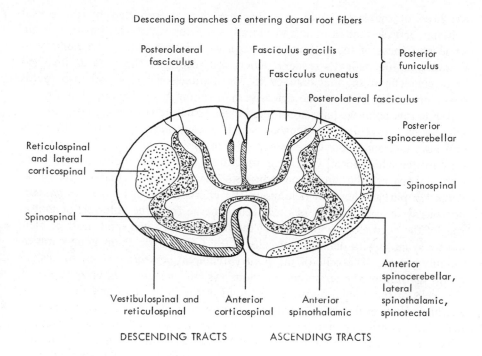

POSTERIOR

Descending branches of entering dorsal root fibers

Posterolateral fasciculus

Fasciculus gracilis

Fasciculus cuneatus

Posterior funiculus

Posterolateral fasciculus

Posterior spinocerebellar

Reticulospinal and lateral corticospinal

Spinospinal

Spinospinal

Anterior spinocerebellar, lateral spinothalamic, spinotectal

Vestibulospinal and reticulospinal

Anterior corticospinal

Anterior spinothalamic

DESCENDING TRACTS   ASCENDING TRACTS

ANTERIOR

FIGURE 13—7. The main tracts of the spinal cord. Afferent, ascending tracts on the right side; efferent, descending tracts on the left. It must be remembered, however, that both ascending and descending fibers are present on each side. (Adapted. Courtesy of Ernest Gardner, *Fundamentals of Neurology*, 4th ed., W. B. Saunders Company, Philadelphia, 1963, Fig. 128, p. 223.)

and vibration. Patients with this disease suffer many disabilities of which loss of position sense, *ataxia* (without order), and awkward, faulty coordination (cerebellar adjustment) are conspicuous. This condition is called *tabes dorsalis* (*tabes* meaning decay, *dorsalis* meaning of the back).

Ascent of the sensation of touch is less simple to detail, and no attempt will be made here to do so to any extent. Some of the touch axons ascend in the dorsal columns and others end on the secondary neurons which decussate and form the ventral spinothalamic tract. The whole inflow of touch is widespread, an arrangement which permits considerable damage to the spinal cord in one area or another without utterly obliterating this extremely important sensation.

It will be noted by now that: (1) sensations all land in the thalamus, and (2) all afferent pathways have decussated once on the way to the brain. Knowledge of where that decussation occurs is helpful on occasion to understanding a patient's symptoms and complaints. If Mr. Samuelson has a lesion which has obliterated the function of his spinal cord at a low thoracic level on the right side, one may expect that he will lose sensations of heat and cold and pain on the opposite side of the body, his "good," or left, side, below the level of the lesion; will lose the sensations transmitted by the dorsal columns, muscle-tendon-joint and vibration, on the right side; but will retain some awareness of touch, however defective, on both sides. The nurse who is aware of the patient's sensory deficit will recognize the hazards involved in mechanical or thermal damage to Mr. Samuelson's legs and also to his peace of mind if he notes the defective perception in his "good," left leg.

Up to this point we have considered these structures in the spinal cord: the afferent pathways and the neurons which convey messages within the cord; and have mentioned the large motor cells of the anterior horn of spinal cord gray matter which form, with their processes, the "lower motor neuron" and whose axons are the "final common path." A third cell found in the *thoracolumbar* part of the cord belongs to the efferent system of the *sympathetic* nervous system. The axons of these cells emerge from the anterior, or motor, root of the cord along with those of the anterior horn cell, and most of them have a synapse with dendrites of cells in the sympathetic chain lying paravertebrally outside. The cells of the *parasympathetic nervous system*, or *craniosacral* division of the autonomic nervous system, are quite differently placed. The cells of the cranial division are found in the brain stem and those of the sacral division in the sacral cord, in two compact masses and some scattered cells. The autonomic nervous system has been discussed to some extent in Chapter 5 in respect to the responses of the body to injury. There will be here no further extended consideration, but a few reminders to the student. Hormones are chemicals, and chemicals act diffusely; even chemicals which act quickly may not be at hand at the right moment unless there is something authoritative that reacts quickly to call them forth. The autonomic nervous system and the other regulators, hormones, enzymes, etc., work closely together, but it is the nervous system which responds promptly when, for instance, there is a need to speed up the heart in an emergency, and sees to it that epinephrine is produced promptly and a supply maintained.

The remaining parts of the spinal cord consist chiefly of the descending or efferent tracts. These tracts constitute the rest of the white matter of the cord. They are concerned with bringing to the lower motor neuron the results of the concerted and integrated work of the higher centers: the cortex, various subcortical cell masses, and the cerebellum which have worked and planned together on the information presented to them by the afferent pathways. These tracts are now bringing the result of the brain's planning to deliver to the anterior horn cell. This cell will send it out by way of the peripheral nerves to the final performers, the muscles and glands. It will be simpler, since the student has by now the outlines of the circuit traced, to learn about these descending tracts from their sites of origin in the brain, rather than working backwards from their termination, which is the same for all anyway, the anterior horn cell of the gray matter of the spinal cord, or the lower motor neuron. Therefore, discussion of the descending tracts will be delayed for the present.

Integration of brain function.

It is now time to re-examine the cranial cavity to discuss the brain, which is itself responsible for originating much of that which is carried out by the cord and peripheral nerves as well as all that goes on in respect to the special senses, vision, hearing, etc., and everything that we think of as "brains," e.g., higher thought, emotion, learning, and memory.

As the brain developed in higher animals from the simple linear structure seen in worms, and tended to concentrate at the anterior end of the animal, it bent back upon itself, and, in higher mammals and man, developed and enormously enlarged certain parts, notably the cerebral hemispheres. These great hemispheres, which bubble over and obscure almost all else seen by the casual viewer, cover up the evidence that remains of the curves and bends in the structure of the brain which is finally crammed into a space and maintained at a weight (1400 gm) that a man can support and still not be top-heavy. Study of the brain's development in the embryo does demonstrate these changes, and even in the cut adult brain one can easily note that the lower parts, *medulla oblongata*, or *bulb*, and *midbrain*, are in direct linear continuity with the cord and are smaller, less complicated in physical form than are other much larger, evolutionarily newer, parts. These newer parts, some of the cerebellum, and the cerebral hemispheres show, even on gross examination, much greater bulk than bulb and midbrain, and reveal an enormous surface area which has been achieved by wrinkling and folding of the surface layers. Even a cursory view of the cut brain should demonstrate two other points which are helpful in looking at the structural basis for control and integration of function from a developmental point of view and which recall principles stated early in the chapter. (Principle 4: Within the nervous system there is a hierarchy of control. No single part functions separately from other parts. Principle 5: The nervous system imposes regulation and control not only on organs and systems of the body but on itself. Principle 6: In general, higher centers inhibit lower centers and phylogenetically newer parts of the brain inhibit older or lower centers.)

On examination of the brain two things are striking: (1) heavy bands of white matter are evident running between various recognizable parts of gray matter; and (2) while it is obvious that the surface of cerebrum and cerebellum is gray matter, e.g., made up of nerve cells, there are a good many other masses of cells lying embedded in white matter paired up along the central axis. These clumps of gray matter, literally covered up, and to an extent metaphorically as well, by the cerebral hemispheres, are referred to as "nuclei."[52] They were present and more completely dominant in simpler animals

---

[52] This use of the word "nuclei" may confuse the student. The term as used in this paragraph, and to be used considerably in the text that follows, means a group of nerve cells and does not refer to the central structure of a single cell. Examples: (1) The *red nucleus* (group of cells) is in the midbrain. (2) The two major parts of a cell are the *nucleus* (the central organizing part of a single cell) and the *cytoplasm.*

before the cerebral cortex developed and overwhelmed them. We shall make frequent reference to these cell masses from now on, for although in man they are by no means at the top of the hierarchy of control, they are of great importance to him; and when any of these structures are damaged directly, or thrown out of kilter by being poorly informed, integrated performance is handicapped.

What one sees, hears, smells, tastes, or feels must involve anatomically many parts if it is to be physiologically useful. One must not simply see or hear the car coming round the corner but retreat to the curbing to avoid being struck, an act which utilizes many nervous connections from the instant the eye or ear perceives the threat until the muscles of trunk and leg effect the lifesaving backward steps. This activity involves sense organs, cerebral cortex and cerebellum and subcortical cell masses, reticular formation in the brain stem, and efferent tracts in the cord. All of these will be considered in their turn. Before going further it may be well to review, restating somewhat differently and adding a bit.

Above the cord, the relatively simple form of an H-shaped mass of cells surrounded by fiber tracts becomes modified. Centrally, from bulb to thalamus, there is the reticular formation, a loose-appearing network of cells and nerve fibers in which some quite discrete cell masses are seen. From the bulb to the *pons* (bridge) the pairs of cranial nerves branch off; the cells of these nerves form nuclei which are embedded in pairs along the way. Still larger masses of cells are to be found as one moves upward, and all are surrounded by the great masses of white matter, tracts carrying their messages from one area to another, connecting, projecting, and associating the work of their cells. The greatest bulk of white matter will be found in the cerebral hemispheres, and there too are the greatest number of nerve cells, spread in the thin wrinkled layers of the *cerebral cortex* (*cortex* meaning bark). It is these millions of cells which initiate; and it is their fibers, their axons and dendrites (some so short that they run only between cells of the cortex itself and some so long that they pass all the way to the spinal cord) that make possible those activities which are most characteristically human, complex thinking, memory, judgment, and highly developed learned skills. These cells are at the top of the hierarchy: they are newest in evolutionary and embryological development. Although the most human, they are least vital in a biological sense and the most intolerant of hypoglycemia and anoxia. (Principle 7: The later in embryonic life a part of the nervous system develops, the more susceptible it is to injury.)

Looking at the nervous system from a developmental point of view and at the cerebral hemispheres as very late comers, one will realize that control and integration of everything of a biological nature must have been possible for the organism before the cerebrum was there at all. These structures, which are both dominated by the cerebrum in man and yet important to the integrity of cerebral function, are: the vestibular nuclei belonging to the eighth cranial

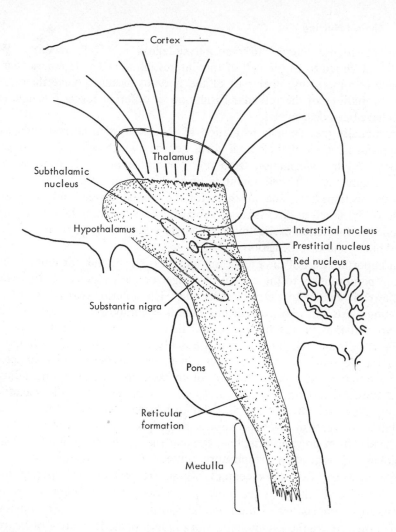

FIGURE 13–8. The reticular formation and its relationship to adjacent structures of the brain stem and cerebrum. (Adapted. Courtesy of Arthur Guyton, *Textbook of Medical Physiology,* 2nd ed., W. B. Saunders Company, Philadelphia, 1961, Fig. 595, p. 773.)

nerve, thalamus, cerebellum, basal ganglia, reticular formation, and a number of cell masses enclosed within it.

Reticular formation.

Some of these cell masses, or nuclei, just referred to, seem in the course of evolution to have condensed from a more diffuse-appearing substance made up of scattered cells and fibers which extend along the central axis from the bulb through the pons to the posterior part of the hypothalamus and into the ventral thalamus. This diffuse nerve cell-fiber system is called the *reticular formation* (*reticulum* meaning net). The reticular formation has become a subject of intense interest to neurophysiologists relatively recently. While there is still much to be learned of this interesting area (a statement that can be made of almost any other part of the nervous system), nevertheless, certain contributions of the reticular formation at different levels throughout its length have been determined.

Functionally the reticular formation of the brain stem corresponds to the internuncial neurons of the spinal cord, neurons which work like the Senate pageboys, taking information from one committee of the legislature to another, committees which will facilitate or inhibit action. In it a vast number of reflex connections are made, all those for the cranial nerves, and many others which will be noted in discussion of subcortical nuclei. Stimulation of parts of the reticular formation excites muscle activity and of other parts inhibits it—a sort of brake-and-throttle action.

An important part of the life of any animal is sleep; and, for animals which must respond quickly to the advent of danger or the presence of approaching prey, a ready change to alertness is as vital. The anterior part of the reticular formation alerts the whole cerebrum. This is accomplished by connections to the hypothalamus, to the thalamus, and thence to both the cortex and basal ganglia. The brain, thus made alert, is quickly cleared for action whether this be for the sleeping cat to waken and run across the lawn and leap into the grape arbor to escape the collie dog or to develop a strategy and adjust its entire muscular system in order to catch a field mouse in the meadow at evening. When this area of the reticular formation is destroyed by disease or mutilation, the patient gives the appearance of sleep and cannot be wakened.

Already, from previous chapters, the student has become familiar with the physiology of respiration (respiratory center) and with factors which affect arterial pressure (vasomotor center). These are part of the reticular formation. The needs of the body for more or less pulmonary ventilation are mediated through connections in the reticular formation, as are other homeostatic mechanisms; so are the sympathetic and parasympathetic control of heart and vascular system and relays from the hypothalamus for control of temperature and other affairs of metabolism. The hypothalamus itself is essentially a development of the reticular formation at the forward end, and, as such, it is to be expected that the relations with the reticular formation itself would be close.[53]

Thalamus

Anatomically, the thalamus lies above the brain stem and beneath the cortex, seeming to push up against the floor of the lateral ventricles. It is bounded on its sides and below by the fibers of the internal capsule which are wedged between the thalamus and basal ganglia. While the most primitive part of the thalamus has no connections to the cortex because it developed in

[53] Guyton, *Op. cit.,* p. 775.

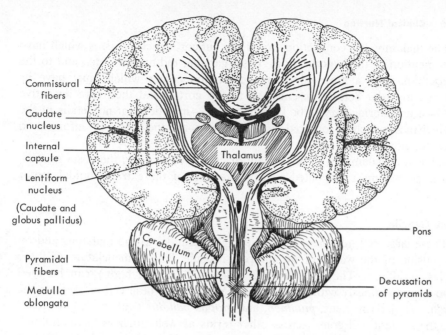

Commissural fibers

Caudate nucleus

Internal capsule

Lentiform nucleus

(Caudate and globus pallidus)

Pyramidal fibers

Medulla oblongata

Thalamus

Cerebellum

Pons

Decussation of pyramids

FIGURE 13–9. Vertical transverse section through the brain. (Adapted. Courtesy of Charles H. Best and Norman B. Taylor, *The Living Body*, 4th ed., Henry Holt and Co., New York, 1958, Fig. 12-16, p. 538.)

simple animals that had none, the rest of the thalamus is organized into large nuclei, cells onto which specific sensory tracts discharge and from which the information they bear is sent on to the cortex to be associated with different information coming from other thalamic sources, appreciated, integrated, and acted upon. The cerebral cortex, in turn, reports to the thalamus. The trip by the sensations to the cortex and back seems by some means to have modified and refined the traveler, for the thalamus itself has a sort of coarse, undisciplined, conscious awareness which can be demonstrated when the cortex of an animal is removed. The creature reacts excessively: the decorticated cat will spit and snarl in response to a stimulus at which a normal cat would simply rise, stretch, and walk away. The cat with the mutilated nervous system has no means by which to evaluate the stimulus: if it is of a noxious nature, no matter how minor, he "gives it all he has" in response. The normal cat, on the other hand, has all his integrating mechanisms intact and, evaluating the minor nature of the annoyance for just that, simply moves away and conserves himself for a real emergency.

The absence of the cortex results in dementia with impaired memory, speech, judgment, and insight and *intensity of affect* (an emotional response out of relation to the stimulus). This intensity of affect is due to loss of the disciplining effect of the intact cortex on the thalamus and is an illustration of the sixth of the principles stated at the beginning of the chapter: that higher centers inhibit lower and phylogenetically newer parts inhibit older.

The thalamus has connections to all the subcortical cell masses which have been mentioned, the hypothalamus, basal ganglia, red nucleus, etc., and to the cerebellum. It is a most important correlation center which must have its material in order before presenting it to the cortex and then take an active part—as an intermediary to be kept informed—in order that no details of the performance which is ordered by the cortex on the basis of information received should go astray.

While the thalamus is to be thought of chiefly as sensory, the basal ganglia, also large cell masses situated nearby, are part of the extrapyramidal motor system.

Basal Ganglia

These large cell masses or nuclei lie slightly caudal to the thalamus and on the outside of the wedge of the internal capsule. The nomenclature of these bodies is difficult. The term "corpus striatum" (striped body) can be used almost synonymously with basal ganglia. Separately, these cell masses are the *caudate* (tailed) nucleus, *putamen*, and *globus pallidus* (pale body). In reading, the student will come across other terms as well, such as "neostriatum" and "paleostriatum." In this chapter the parts will be discussed simply as a unit and called the basal ganglia; but the student should recognize the other terms and also realize that not all parts of the basal ganglia have identical functions.

In general terms, the basal ganglia are concerned with the control of automatic associated movements of the body (example: the swing of the arms in alternation to the legs in walking). They work togther with the cerebellum, thalamus, and cortex and have many connections with the reticular formation. The red nucleus in the reticular formation of the mid-brain is the origin of a main efferent descending tract, the *rubrospinal*, which carries directions for control to the lower motor neuron and thence to muscles or glands.

Some of the motor tracts originating in the brain stem are short and completely contained within the brain itself (example: for eye movement), while others run in close proximity to the voluntary motor tract, the pyramidal, down the cord. All these tracts decussate and therefore exert control on the side of the body opposite their origin. The student can easily determine their origin and destination simply by their names: reticulospinal, reticulobulbar, etc. Their great responsibility for the perfection of motor control can be grasped best by observing the problems of those who have disease in any of the nuclei from which they rise.

When there is injury or disease referable to the basal ganglia and nearby nuclei in the reticular formation, the individual is greatly handicapped. Depending on the part involved, he not only loses his automatic associated control but is beset with a variety of nuisance movements which plague him, and also by alteration in muscle tone, a rigidity which makes every move more difficult. The student can easily learn to recognize these aberrations.

Athetosis is a writhing, wormlike squirminess. In *chorea,* there are contractions of muscles occurring without control so that the sequence of movement is interrupted and the patient accomplishes nothing effectively, for he is repeatedly thrown off by jerks of interrupted patterns. The *tremor* of basal ganglia disease is most obvious in the hands, which tend to be held pointing medially, fingers rather close, moving against the thumb in what is called a "pill-rolling" tremor. *Hemiballismus* is a violent jerking of large parts of the body. Like other abnormal movements of basal ganglia disease, hemiballismus may be provoked or made worse by voluntary efforts for controlled movement on the part of the patient. The rigidity seen in damage to basal ganglia is of a plastic type. When the individual is quite at ease, he may seem free of it, but on effort or with anxiety, the stiffness returns to resist the smooth accomplishment of every act. Parkinson's disease and some types of cerebral palsy are diseases wherein the basal ganglia are affected.

Vestibular nuclei and cerebellum.

Vestibular Nuclei

That portion of the eighth cranial nerve which comes from the vestibular, or labyrinthine, portion of the ear and is concerned with informing the brain of the position and change of direction of the head in order that appropriate adjustments can be made to maintain equilibrium is called the vestibular portion of the eighth, or auditory, nerve. It has four nuclei in an irregular line along the floor of the fourth ventricle at the level of the caudal portion of the pons and upper portion of the medulla oblongata. As the vestibular fibers coming from the peripheral sense organ, the ear, enter the central nervous system, they bifurcate. Some of the branches go to a fifth vestibular nucleus in that part of the cerebellum which is phylogenetically the oldest, having arisen in animals (fishes) whose most important problem in coordination is maintaining appropriate swimming position. (You will recall noting that the dying goldfish keeps losing this position and slips over onto its side.) The other branches go to one or another of the four pair of vestibular nuclei more centrally located. The bulk of the fibers of secondary neurons collect to form a tract, the vestibulospinal, which descends in the cord and ends on cells many of which control extensor muscles of the limbs.[54]

The whole vestibular apparatus, from ear, to brain stem, to cerebellar nuclei, to efferent cell in the cord, helps to keep the animal on an even keel. When the horse is galloping round the ring, his legs on the inside must take up more sharply or he will topple on the curving track. The horse's vestibular apparatus contributes to maintaining perfection of gait even though this demands continuous adjustment due to the constant curve of the riding ring.

[54] When the brain stem is cut across just above these nuclei, the decerebrated animal goes into a state of "extensor rigidity." This state may be seen in human beings when, through disease, the brain stem and cord are functionally cut off from control of higher parts, as with any large intracerebral mass which compresses the upper brain stem. This is called in man "decerebrate rigidity."

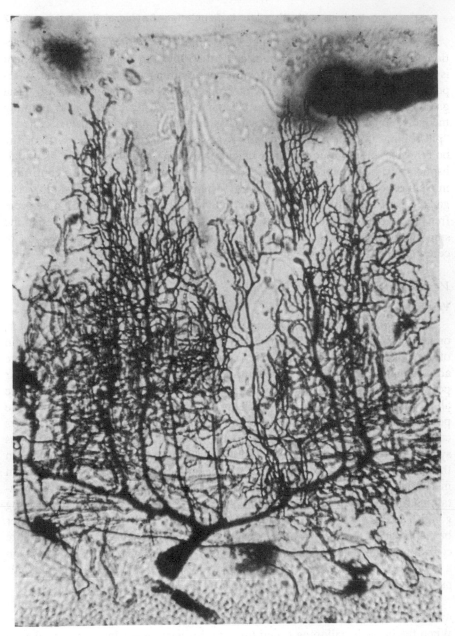

FIGURE 13—10. Purkinje cell with branching dendritas, greatly enlarged, in the cerebellar cortex.

Cerebellum

This is the largest division of the brain after the cerebral hemispheres. Situated posterior to the central axis, it is connected by three large masses of white matter, the cerebellar peduncles, to the pons, mid-brain, and medulla oblongata. The cerebellar cortex consists of two layers whose cells are provided with an enormous number of processes. The Purkinje cell, which is the effector cell, has so extensive a provision of branching dendrites that it looks like a microscopic Japanese barberry bush. The cellular structure and arrangement of the cerebellar cortex is such that incoming stimuli will excite a wide cortical area.

The cerebellum has evolved with the increasing complexity of the animal, as has the rest of the brain, and several divisions can be recognized that are correlated with phylogenetic age. We have spoken of one, the most primitive, which is simply an outgrowth of the vestibular system, but shall here, as was done in the case of the basal ganglia, discuss briefly the function of the cerebellum not in parts but as a whole.

In reviewing the material to this point the student will recall that:

1. The afferent tracts to the cerebellum report to it the existing state of contraction of muscles and changes in tension; that the fibers are heavily myelinated and conduct with great rapidity.
2. The basal ganglia, concerned with control of associated movement and acting on information received from thalamus and cortex, report to mid-brain centers.
3. The reflex connections of the cranial nerves, vestibular included, whose nuclei are in bulb and pons, take place in the reticular formation.
4. There are connections of these structures to thalamus and cerebral cortex.

It must, then, be evident with mention of the large peduncles of white matter which bind the cerebellum to all these structures by way of their connections to the brain stem that the cerebellum works with them all; and this is the case. Its work is in association with others, not independent. There is, for example, no tract running from cerebellum to cord. In its function the cerebellum illustrates especially well the second part of the fourth and the fifth principles. (No single part of the nervous system functions separately from other parts. The nervous system imposes regulation and control not only on organs and systems of the body but on itself.)

Cerebellar function.

Specifically, the cerebellum accepts on many dendrites the motor impulses discharged from the various centers we have just reviewed and spreads them widely in the cerebellar cortex. Although these incoming impulses, which represent a plan for action to be undertaken, have already been organized to some extent, they need a final revision with correction of errors. This is the work of the cerebellum. If more impulses for a given movement have been initiated than will be required, the cerebellum can arrange to have them cut down; if too great speed has been undertaken, this will be inhibited by instruc-

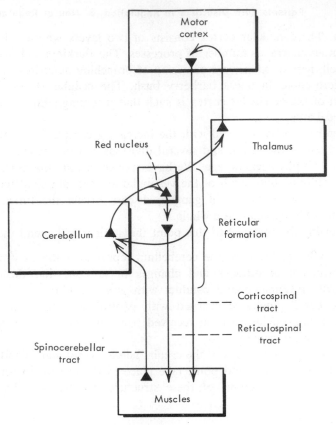

FIGURE 13—11. Pathways of cerebellar "error" control of voluntary movements. (Adapted. Courtesy of Arthur Guyton, *Textbook of Medical Physiology*, 2nd ed., W. B. Saunders Company, Philadelphia, 1961, Fig. 600, p. 782.)

tions to the motor cortex to excite antagonist muscles and inhibit agonists. The revisionist activities of the cerebellum are accomplished by very efficient and extremely rapid feedback mechanisms, which Guyton, terming it a servomechanism, compares to the control system of an automatic pilot in an airplane.

When the cerebellum is diseased and this servomechanism breaks down, the individual no longer is able unconsciously to make the necessary corrections. He does not predict very well how a sequence of planned motions will come out, and the results are worse the faster the motions. A common test of this is to ask the patient to rotate the forearm and hand rapidly. It is a simple thing to do with an intact cerebellum, but results in a futile jumble of uncoordinated moves when there is cerebellar disease. This inability to perform rapidly coordinated movements is called *adiodochokinesia*. Talking demands rapidly coordinated sequential movements. When these cannot be effected, speech may become nearly unintelligible. Some syllables are too loud or too soft, held too long or not long enough, and the patient is said to have *dys-*

arthria. Cerebellar disease results also in *dysmetria*, a faulty ability to measure. The individual over- or undershoots his mark. *Asynergia* is also a problem for the patient with defective cerebellar function. The student will recognize the meaning from remembering its use in pharmacology. Synergistic drugs work together effectively to enhance each other; but the cerebellar patient's activity is asynergic—nothing works together. Hypotonia, tremor, nystagmus, ataxia may all be noted in disease of the cerebellum. The patient, being competent intellectually, will make conscious attempts to compensate for errors which his previously intact cerebellum would not have permitted. Some efforts are more successful than others. He can make his ataxic gait safer by walking with his legs far apart, thrusting his pelvis forward, and holding onto the furniture. No amount of intelligence, or conscious planning, or years of experience in the act will enable him now to perform neatly an act such as cracking and emptying a soft-boiled egg.

This is, perhaps, a good place to stop and illustrate in a small way a basic reason for a professional nurse's having some understanding of the nervous system. One is taught that, ordinarily, a patient should be permitted to undertake independently or with assistance all the activities of daily living that he can. This is better for his morale than having them done for him. It may help him to recover. Like all generalizations, this one must be accepted with wariness, and the knowledge that generalizations do not always hold true. The nurse who understands the basis for the awkwardness of her cerebellar patient knows that he will be nothing but worse off for the attempt to open his own eggs, being left frustrated, humiliated, and hungry. She will see that this and like little services are performed for him.

Cranial nerves.

In an early paragraph the statement was made and has since been referred to that the reflex connections for cranial nerves were centered in the reticular formation; little, however, has yet been said about the cranial nerves themselves other than the vestibular portion and nuclei of the eighth and a statement that the nuclei of the cranial nerves are paired along either side of the center, in bulb and pons. There are several points by which it is interesting to compare cranial with peripheral nerves. (1) They are specialized, in that some are sensory, some motor. Although some have both, or a sensory and a motor component, these have their own nuclei and are quite discrete. (2) Their fibers are without neurolemma and cannot regenerate. They seem in some respects rather more like tracts than nerves. The cranial nerves are very frequently referred to by number instead of name in speaking and in designation on the patient's chart. It is convenient to know the names that belong to the Roman numerals, but some persons find the task of learning them difficult. There is a mnemonic which has helped students for generations to learn the names.[55] A brief discussion of arrangement may also help. The sense organ right out in front in animals is the snout; so the *olfactory* nerve is the most anterior, number I. Eyes come next; so *ocular* is II, large nerves whose fibers cross at the optic chiasm above the pituitary and proceed as "optic tracts" to the visual cortex. These two cranial nerves are sensory. But eyes need to be moved; and III, *oculomotor*, IV, *trochlear*, and VI, *abducens*, provide this control. III includes parasympathetic fibers to constrict the pupil of the eye. Eyes are set in a face which is both above and below them; the Vth nerve, *trigeminal*, emerges between IV and VI. This great nerve, with three branches, is sensory (pain, temperature, touch, proprioception) to face and scalp and motor to muscles of mastication. The slender VIIth nerve, the facial, supplies motion to the muscles of expression of the face and taste to the anterior two thirds of the tongue. It pursues a circuitous route intracranially and fans out to supply a large area extracranially, and not infrequently is damaged either centrally or peripherally. Sadly collapsed muscles of the face result. Ears are double organs set to deal with hearing and to assist with balancing. Cranial nerve VIII has two divisions, auditory and vestibular, each coming from the appropriate portion of the ear. Not much below the ears, the throat begins; so IX, the glossopharyngeal (tongue-pharynx) is largely sensory, supplying taste to the posterior third of the tongue and feeling to upper pharynx. X is the vagus, the main outflow for the cranial division of the parasympathetic fraction of the autonomic nervous system. It is sensory to auricle, pharynx, larynx, and viscera of chest and abdomen, and motor to pharynx, larynx, base of tongue, and autonomic ganglia of chest and abdomen. The maintenance of homeostasis (see Chapter 2) depends heavily on the activities of the parasympathetic, and the largest bulk of fibers of the vagus goes to visceral organs which are assisted by its activity to maintain their normal vegetative functions or to regain these when they have been disturbed by stress on the animal. The XIth is the spinal accessory nerve, motor supply to the pharynx and palate and to the trapezius and sternomastoid muscles; and the hypoglossal, or XIIth cranial nerve, provides the motor supply to the tongue and muscles of the neck.

Long before this point in discussion of brain stem and subcortical nuclei, the student must have become clearly aware of the validity of Principle 4, the interdependence of various parts. Everything that has been described or illustrated so far, however, has been concerned with patterns of activity and mostly with immediacy, and not with individuality or originality. We are human beings, and although other animals share with us ability to store experiences, to learn, and to modify behavior in terms of learning, this is

[55] *On*	*Old*	*Olympus*	*Topmost*	*Top*
olfactory	optic	oculomotor	trochlear	trigeminal
A	*Finn*	*And*	*German*	*Viewed*
abducens	facial	auditory	glossopharyngeal	vagus
Some	*Hops*			
spinalaccessory	hypoglossal			

limited and more stylized than for man. Only in man can the life experiences of one individual or group be transmitted to the next generations so that they can be appreciated and used. However great the genius of an individual, even though he may be a true innovator, his works are never completely his own creation. His human heritage, the effects on his consciousness of work and techniques of artists who preceded him, have been received and integrated. While what he builds or paints may be quite unlike anything that has been done before, the unique product of the creative genius of one man, it could not have been built or painted so had other artists not left him their buildings, paintings, musical scores, and poetry.

In this respect, the oriole's nest hanging in perfect level and balance from the elm branch is different. We admire it and say "It is a work of art." But the beautiful structure perfectly adapted to the needs of orioles would not satisfy all definitions of a "work of art." Orioles have built nests like these for many generations of both orioles and men. It is true that, even in our lifetimes, we may see some modification in the nests if the American elm has only a few more years to live. But the adaptations will be of a mechanical nature, in terms of the type of tree the bird selects when the elm which it prefers is no longer there; and they will be the same for all orioles.

With these last paragraphs on structure and function of the nervous system we have reached the top of the ascent from the cord and peripheral nerves and shall remain at this height long enough to gain a view, though cursory, of the activities of the human cerebral cortex. Then, with a quick descent on the motor tracts, the circuit will be completed.

The cerebral cortex and its function.

The activities of the cerebral cortex are intimately and inextricably tied to the thalamus. The connections in both directions, thalamus to cortex and cortex to thalamus, are innumerable, constituting most elaborate feedback situations whereby impressions arriving at the thalamus by way of afferent pathways are relayed to appropriate parts of the cortex for analysis. Since analysis may demonstrate the need of appreciation from other parts of the cortex before final actions are taken, this factor may require another trip to the thalamus and relay by still other neurons to different parts of the cortex. These cortical-thalamic relays may have both immediate and long-lasting effects, relatively simple and quite complex. The sensory stimulus may cause a *motor response,* and the total experience may provoke new thoughts and also be stored in *memory* perhaps to be useful in the future, three results differing from each other considerably but all necessary for men.

The student who wishes to learn any considerable amount of what is known today of the functions of the cerebral cortex is referred to a contemporary medical or neurophysiology text. The knowledge is incomplete at best, and this author unqualified to impart more than an over-all summary. Structurally, the cortex is a very thin, layered structure, the thickest part not more than 4 mm. The area is enormous, however. If one could flatten out its convoluted surface, it would cover more than 2 sq yds. Considering the size of a single cell, this surface, even though only a few millimeters deep, provides a large acreage for a human being to manage and direct the work of his body, to think, plan, act rationally or not, communicate with others, and develop cultural, and ethical behavior. This thin sheet of cells shows histologically six layers wherein one can detect not only communication between the layers of cells in a given area, but a veritable matting made up of the processes which connect regions of the cortex itself, nearby and remote—in the same or opposite hemisphere—or are part of the afferent and efferent systems to the brain and cord below.

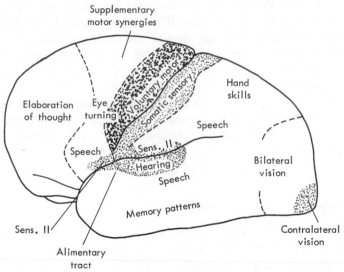

FIGURE 13—12. Functional areas of the human cerebral cortex as determined by electrical stimulation of the cortex during neurosurgical operations and by neurological examinations of patients with destroyed cortical regions. (Adapted with permission of The Macmillan Company from *The Cerebral Cortex of Man*, Fig. 117, p. 221, by Wilder Penfield and Theodore Rasmussen. Copyright 1950 by The Macmillan Company.)

The cerebral cortex looks quite homogeneous, yet certainly there are parts which are specialized in function. Considerable areas seem not to have a single function but only to reinforce by presenting wider areas for activity. Figure 13-12 shows broad areas of cortical localization. One of the most interesting of these for human beings is the surface of the temporal lobe and angular gyrus. This small region bears responsibility for interpreting sensory experience from whatever source. Complex and elaborate memories are stored here,[56] and any damage to the area has serious effect on intellectual competence. Even though the entire visual and auditory apparatus from eye

[56] Guyton, *Op. cit.*, p. 792.

and ear to visual and auditory cortex may be intact, if there is loss of the interpretive area no proper use can be made of the sensory experience; it will not be integrated with previous experiences and so is valueless. Example: On walking toward a railroad crossing the individual might see the flashing red light and hear the noise of the approaching train but even though, before his damage occurred, the meaning of this sight and sound was clear to him and his behavior appropriate in terms of the correct interpretation and recollection, now he walks on, for the meaningless signals have no value to him any more.

The most anterior parts of the cerebrum in front of the motor areas are termed the prefrontal lobes. There are connections from these to the hypothalamus which evoke responses associated with anger and distress and other responses mediated by the autonomic nervous system. For the most part, however, the prefrontal lobes seem to have a disciplinary function to perform. Without specialized function themselves, they provide a considerable area for reinforcement. In their presence, the individual has the means to work at complicated problems, resist distraction, deal with abstract thought, and weigh the relative merits of one line of behavior against another. If they are cut off from their influence on the rest of the brain, the individual is unable to discipline himself to any of these complex activities. He is incapable of abstract reasoning although he can follow concrete patterns of behavior. He may perform correctly the arithmetical tasks involved but be unable to solve a problem which, indeed, presents no interesting challenge to him for he is too easily distracted to grasp its import. His social behavior may be quite unorthodox and unsatisfactory to others for he responds directly to his impulses without evaluation of consequences. This apparent isolation of the braking, inhibiting, or disciplinary effect of the frontal lobes is sometimes one of the unfortunate consequences of encephalitis, an inflammation of the brain.

Human beings can talk; it is their most important means of communication. They read and write and use symbols to express themselves by these means. These activities are very complicated, utilizing many areas of the cortex, some highly specialized. These are sometimes selectively destroyed by hemorrhage, tumor, or disease, and the patient may have any of the following disabilities resulting: he may be unable to form words although he knows what he wants to say, *motor aphasia*; he may be unable to comprehend by word or gesture what is said to him, *sensory aphasia*; one variety of sensory aphasia is an inability to attach meaning to words heard, *auditory agnosia*, or *word deafness*; and there may be a similar problem with words read, *visual agnosia, or word blindness.*

It is common knowledge that in right-handed persons the left hemisphere has ascendency over the right after early childhood. Motor speech for these persons is largely handled by the appropriate area—low in the premotor cortex—of the left hemisphere. One of the frequent and most trying disabilities of those who suffer a cerebral accident or "stroke" resulting in damage to this hemisphere is not the weakness of arm and leg so much as the maddening inability to express, in words, the thought that the mind can formulate. The student has probably noted that, in right-handed persons, the cerebral accident which occurs in the right hemisphere does not have this unhappy result.

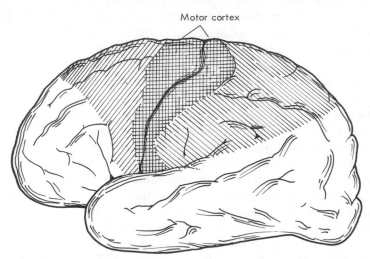

Motor cortex

FIGURE 13—13. Areas of the cerebral cortex from which corticospinal fibers originate. (Adapted. Courtesy of Arthur Guyton, *Textbook of Medical Physiology*, 2nd ed., W. B. Saunders Company, Philadelphia, 1961, Fig. 587, p. 762.)

Mention of these difficulties with communication brings us at last to the parts of the cortex concerned with the control of motion and appreciation of sensations. There are large areas of the surface of the brain which, if stimulated, will result in movement of one or another group of muscles. These must all be included under the term "motor cortex" although some parts considerably overlap areas which are sensory (see Figure 13-13). The cortical region right around the central sulcus is purely motor. The numbers of cells which are present and responsible for initiating volunatry control of a part relate to fineness of control expected of that part: thus, there are more cells in the cortical area concerned with voluntary control of the fingers than in the region devoted to control of the muscles of the thigh. Neurophysiologists have mapped the cortex out in irregular plots and given them numbers. The strips of motor cortex students are most likely to find referred to by number are 4g, 4s, and 6. The region just referred to is 4g; 4s is a narrow strip just anterior to 4g which is regarded by some neurologists as having a suppressing influence on 4g. In the monkey, this is so; destruction of 4s results in spasticity, a state of constant contraction, of the muscles controlled by 4g.[57] Area 6 works together with 4, assisting to organize movements serially.[58]

Figure 13-12 demonstrates the considerable surface devoted to sensory

[57] Elliott, *Op. cit.*, p. 240.
[58] *Ibid.*, p. 241.

functions, for the special senses, and for body sensations of temperature, proprioception, etc. While, for example, the primary auditory cortex recognizes sounds, and bilateral oblation of this area of cortex will result in deafness, the sounds are not analyzed into useful forms until they have undergone switchbacks to the brain stem and again to the cerebrum where, in the angular gyrus of the temporal lobe, they are correctly interpreted, having been correlated with other experiences, and can be intelligently acted upon. Example: The auditory motor cortex is stimulated by the train whistle, the sound coming to it from the eighth nerve by way of the thalamus. Switchback to the reticular formation results in alerting the necessary cortical areas so that when the cortex and angular gyrus put everything together, the man will note the flashing red lights, and stop his car. (Sound was used here as an example. A like process occurs with other sensations.)

A curious example of sensory defect is not uncommonly seen in children who have cerebral palsy with spastic hemiplegia of a type wherein there is cortical damage and includes the somatosensory areas just posterior to the central sulcus. These children have an *astereognosis,* an inability to identify a familiar object by the feel and form in the affected hand. With eyes closed they will accept a key and say that it is cold and that it has weight, but until they open their eyes they cannot identify the key. Such a damage can occur later in life but it is not then so much of a handicap as to the child, who is so active a learner.

Earlier in the chapter, under discussion of the cerebellum and subcortical nuclei, something was said about the coordination of unconscious muscle activity and automatic associated motion and the efferent tracts which arise from them. With this brief discussion of the cerebral cortex, there has been mention of voluntary control. It will be evident now, if we regard critically a simple activity of daily living, that these work together. The motor systems of the brain are very complex and, as yet, by no means completely understood or worked out.[59] In a very general way the *pyramidal* or *corticospinal* system is largely concerned with the control of voluntary motion, and those pathways which have to do with the coordination of unconscious adjustments and with the control of automatic associated movements are termed "extrapyramidal" or "extracorticospinal" (*extra* meaning outside of). A perfectly executed "voluntary" act implicates not only the pyramidal and extrapyramidal but sensory systems as well. The student is asked here to seat himself in a chair from a standing position paying the most alert attention he can to all that goes on the while. Although he will not note everything, nevertheless, he will realize that the strictly voluntary, consciously willed part of the act is only a small fraction, and that the sensory awareness of his initial position and the shifts that were made as he neatly lowered himself to the chair were coordinated and adjusted with an exactness impossible for him had they depended on conscious planning alone.

[59] *Ibid.,* p. 217.

The voluntary part of the controlled act of sitting down originated in cells of the motor cortex just anterior to the central sulcus. There are large cells there, the cells of Betz, whose heavy axons form a conspicuous fraction of the pyramidal tract. But the entire sensory motor cortex contributes to this tract whose fibers gather together first in the *internal capsule*. (The internal capsule is a massive band of white matter which contains the bulk of all fibers running to and from the cortex. It forms a sharp angle and appears to be squeezed in between thalamus and basal ganglia.) The fibers of the descending pyramidal tract give off collaterals to basal ganglia, reticular formation and nuclei therein, and indirectly to the cerebellum as they continue through the pons to the medulla oblongata. Here they appear on the surface, and, as they continue caudally, most of the fibers descussate. The few that do not are found in the ventral part of the spinal cord, but the major number which decussate form the lateral *pyramidal tracts* that occupy a considerable fraction of the lateral

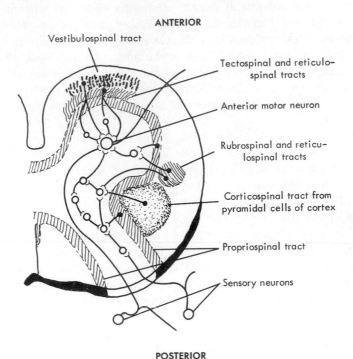

ANTERIOR

Vestibulospinal tract

Tectospinal and reticulo-
spinal tracts

Anterior motor neuron

Rubrospinal and reticu-
lospinal tracts

Corticospinal tract from
pyramidal cells of cortex

Propriospinal tract

Sensory neurons

POSTERIOR

FIGURE 13 — 14. Convergence of all different motor pathways on the anterior motor neurons. (Adapted. Courtesy of Arthur Guyton, *Textbook of Medical Physiology*, 2nd ed., W. B. Saunders Company, Philadelphia, 1961, Fig. 594, p. 771.)

white matter of the cord, running just anterior to the important extrapyramidal tract, the rubrospinal. As the text indicates, these two systems, pyramidal and extrapyramidal, are repeatedly in communication with one another through brain stem nuclei. The term "extrapyramidal" is not a good one; the interplay is too close. As is the case with all efferent tracts, the termination is on the lower motor neuron. It is the anterior horn cell there which will send the impulse to muscle or gland along the final common path. Interference with the tract at any point or with the cortical cells from which it arises will necessarily result in some measure of weakness and inadequacy of voluntary control, especially in fine discriminative movements.

The origin of the pyramidal tract is higher than for the extrapyramidal pathways, and Principle 6 reminds us that higher centers tend to inhibit lower. When a patient has damage to the pyramidal pathway, these inhibiting forces are released and one sees activity which the wholly intact nervous system has under disciplined control after babyhood. There is constantly increased muscle tone, spasticity, with increased tendon reflexes and a marked tendency to develop contractures, and absence of surface reflexes (abdominal and cremasteric), and the Babinski reflex is present (upturning of the big toe and fanning of the others when the plantar surface of the foot is gently stimulated). Any number of pathological states in the nervous system will in some way encroach on the pyramidal tract so that testing for its integrity by eliciting abdominal reflexes and a normal plantar response (clenching of the toes and withdrawal on plantar stimulation) are commonly part of any general physical examination. If the person's responses to these are normal and he has no obvious signs of central nervous system disease, the physician will often assume that no further neurological testing is necessary.

Nurses may observe the signs of involvement of the pyramidal tract in the course of daily care of a patient after a cerebrovascular accident, or stroke. The abnormal reflex responses are demonstrated in the course of the bath, and the others will be noted during range of motion exercises.

With the act of sitting down in the chair perfectly performed, we have involved nearly everything that has been discussed in this chapter on the nervous system.[60] An effort has been made to increase the student's knowledge of the nervous system beyond that gained in her basic course in anatomy and physiology and so to provide a basis for understanding difficulties patients may have which relate to involvement of the nervous system. Then it is easier to observe intelligently, to analyze the patient's needs for nursing care more specifically, and thereafter to meet them wisely. The nervous system is not a thing apart even though shut up in a boney box. It is nourished by the same blood supply and suffers insults from many of the same agents as injure the rest of the body. Whatever types of patients the nurse cares for, she will inevitably find some with complications involving the nervous system. Often, it is the nurse who is present when these signs first manifest themselves, and the professional nurse should be prepared to recognize their import. The remaining paragraphs of this chapter offer suggestions for rational care to meet the needs of patients troubled by some of the everyday problems of neurological origin one encounters in nursing.

[60] Students working in pairs should make a complete analysis of this by way of review exercise. It will take some time to do and requires a chair, a good text with diagrams, and, if possible, a third person as critic; but the exercise will consolidate learning.

Care of persons with increased intracranial pressure.

In the adult, there is no potential for expansion of the skull when the need arises. The skull has many foramina in it provided for the entry or emergence of blood vessels and nerves, but they are well sealed off. The fontanels have long been closed, and the suture lines are too tight to be split open again. There can be no increase in bulk of any element within the head except at the expense of something else (Monro-Kellie doctrine).[61] Therefore, increase in intracranial pressure must occur with increase in intracranial bulk from any cause, and if this is long continued, there will be cell death.

Increased intracranial pressure may develop slowly, as in the case of a tumor growing above the tentorium, or very rapidly after a head injury with intracranial bleeding which frees a high-protein fluid eager to attract and hold water in a box that is already full. Intracranial pressure rises in inflammatory diseases of the nervous system such as encephalitis. In any condition where there is arteriolar spasm, the volume of blood circulating in the capillaries is reduced, and they become highly permeable. This sometimes occurs in acute nephritis and in malignant hypertension, and results in an edematous brain. Anything which blocks, partly or completely, the normal course of cerebrospinal fluid will cause pressure to rise. This could be a tumor which presses on the channels, or gluey inflammatory exudate from meningitis which seals the foramina of Magendie and Luschka or absorptive areas in the meninges over the cortex. Whatever the cause, the patient is likely to demonstrate some characteristic signs. Although some signs may be due to local pressure, they depend much more on the fact that the more crowded the nonexpansible space becomes within the cranium, the more limited will be the blood supply, and hence the oxygen, to each cell. The point of no return for the cells of the cerebral cortex in respect to lack of oxygen comes quickly, and for the cells of the brain stem a little later, but none can stand starvation for long; and the patient's symptomatology reflects their faltering.

Persons with increased intracranial pressure have headache. They need to have their heads elevated somewhat and often to be given acetylsalicylic acid compounds and caffeine. Elevation assists with venous return from the head, and caffeine is a cerebral vasoconstrictor agent and so decreases the headache. The nurse will find no orders to give opiates which decrease respiratory rate and efficiency, already depressed by the disease process. As congestion increases, the blood pressure will rise and the rate of pulse will slow down, due to ischemia of vasomotor centers. The patient, who may have been restless and irritable earlier, becomes lethargic and slow in his verbal responses. Later he may be stuporous. In stupor the individual is not alert to the stimuli to which he would ordinarily respond but can be roused with some effort. As pressure continues, respirations may become arrhythmical with periods of apnea, and the patient falls into a coma from which he cannot be roused; and

[61] Elliott, *Op. cit.,* p. 287.

at last, unless relieved, the hard-pressed bulb can no longer send forth stimuli to produce any respiration.

At any point in this sequence of events the nurse may note signs referable to involvement of cranial nerves other than X and should be alert to these and report them: a dilated pupil which fails to constrict on exposure to a light, drooping of one eyelid (III), and facial weakness (VII) should not only be recorded but also the time should be noted at which they were first observed. These signs, and others, are not necessarily results of the increased intracranial pressure itself but are indicative of changes going on and of further involvement which the nurse, being present, may be the first to note.

Patients with increased intracranial pressure are required to have pulse, respiration, and blood pressure recorded frequently and regularly. Whoever may be assigned the task, it is the professional nurse's duty to know the trend of the record so that the physician may be notified if this trend becomes adverse. A record of vital signs which shows a consistent slowing of pulse and respiration accompanied by a rising blood pressure should be called to the physician's attention and not just left for him to find for himself.

When patients have surgery for some difficulty which lies intracranially below the tentorium and within the confines of the posterior fossa, the bone which is removed is not replaced. Often the dura is not resutured at the end of the operation. Several blood vessels will have been clipped during the surgery, and the blood supply may be temporarily somewhat less than normal. Edema may build up in the area in the hours after operation and endanger the patient's respiration temporarily, for he may be subjected to considerable compression of the bulb thereby. It is safest always with patients who have had craniotomies of this sort to keep the head in alignment with the body at all times including those moments when he is being turned. The rules are simple: (1) have as many persons as are necessary to turn the patient without twisting him, and (2) leave him supported on his side so that his nose is in line with the xiphoid process. If the patient is an infant, one nurse can accomplish the turning safely alone; but if he is a man, this may require four, with one person whose sole duty is control of the head. The infant's large head and narrow shoulders usually permit lining up nose and xiphoid very simply, securing the position by a small folded pad under the side of the chin. A child's head, being relatively smaller in relation to his shoulders than the infant's, will need one or two folded pillowcases; and the athlete with heavy broad shoulders will need to have considerable height to the support under the head to bring it in line. When the work of adjusting the patient's position has been well done, he should be so perfectly balanced that there is no need for a pillow at his back although there is no objection to this if the patient wants it, after correct position has been attained.

Care of patients subject to seizures.

Many times disease in the nervous system is accompanied by seizures, convulsions, or fits, three terms which should be equally useful, although the shortest one seems, nowadays, to be regarded as undignified. Until the nurse has had some experience with patients who are subject to seizures, she may fail to recognize those of a minor nature (petit mal) which often have no, or only a slight, motor component. The experienced person will recognize the momentary lapse of focus, the fading out of the voice, and the little meaningless movements of a part as manifestations of a seizure, and record the occurrence. No one can fail to note or recognize a major convulsion, but the inexperienced may be frightened and rendered incompetent when first seeing one. Fear reduces effectiveness, and the patient who has seizures may need some assistance from his nurse. His physician too, may need a careful description of the attack.

While the patient may be in bed when the attack starts, it is quite likely that he is not and that he falls down wherever he is. In a large percentage of major (grand mal) attacks, the person is immediately unconscious and in a state of generalized tonicity, with teeth clenched, body stiff, and no respiratory exchange occurring at all. Although this phase lasts only a few seconds, it is long enough for the face to become very turgid in appearance and for saliva to collect in great quantity. Shortly, the fit shifts to rhythmical jerking, the clonic phase, the patient breathes adequately, and his color clears. This clonic phase lasts from moments to many minutes. Gradually, the rhythmical jerking becomes slower and slower and finally stops, and the patient shows signs of returning consciousness, often making random movements accompanied by attempts at verbalization, but he seems confused and still incompetent. Complete recovery from the attack is usual after he has slept for a period, although headache for a few hours is not uncommon.

Since clenching of the jaws occurs at once, there is no possible way to prevent the patient's biting his tongue if it was between his teeth when they clamped together. Neither is there any way to prevent the patient from "turning black in the face and foaming at the mouth," for he is not breathing. No attempt should be made to force a wedge between the teeth. To do so results in bruising the gums and has been known to break a tooth. These few moments can be employed more usefully in loosening the collar and belt. After this, one cannot do better than to drop to the floor, kneeling at the patient's head, and, taking it firmly in hand, prop it either on one's own thighs or on a jacket or sweater placed underneath it, turning the head so that saliva can run out and the tongue drop forward away from the airway. It is now possible to insert a padded wedge, but this is rarely useful. By this time the convulsion will be in the clonic phase and one can protect the patient's head from pounding up and down on the floor or pavement throughout the attack. While a postseizure headache may be the rule, it is certainly not made less severe by preventable banging. It is neither useful nor advisable to restrain the patient during the attack other than to control the head. Urinary incontinence often occurs during the seizure and sometimes fecal as well. No attempt should be made to move the patient till the seizure is over unless attendant circumstances make this imperative. Furniture or other encumbrances should be moved away from him. When the attack is over, he should be helped to a quiet place and permitted to sleep until he wakes, when he may resume his activities as before, if he feels able.

Certain convulsions are focal in nature. They start at a point and spread. This type of seizure may indicate a localized lesion in the brain and is often immediately preceded by paresthesias in the part which will shortly begin to twitch. Patients subject to such attacks often have time to walk to a bed and lie down and even to put a wadded face cloth or handkerchief between their teeth before the attack begins. They are usually conscious for the early part of the seizure, but, when it spreads to become generalized, are likely to go unconscious briefly.

These attacks should be carefully and completely described by the nurse especially if one has not already been observed by the patient's physician. This is not easy to do the first time, and a nurse should not be chagrined if she has failed to note everything, so long as she is sure she is accurate in reporting what she has seen. The following will illustrate a description.

Patient came to me looking scared and said, "Rub my left hand." I did so and walked with her to her bed where she lay down, and immediately the fingers of the left hand began rhythmical twitching. This spread to involve wrist, whole arm, and then left leg. The patient seemed to watch the jerking until the attack became generalized, at which time she was apparently unconscious. I did not time the attack but estimate it to have been altogether about a minute and a half, with the period of unconsciousness about 15 seconds. The patient was alert again shortly after the attack. Her left hand grip was weak and remained so for an hour.   [Signature]

Care of the patient who is subjected to lumbar puncture, pneumoencephalogram, and ventriculogram.

These diagnostic procedures are not always accorded the seriousness they deserve and are needlessly uncomfortable. One who is to have a lumbar puncture should be helped to the appropriate position on his side with thighs flexed on the abdomen, head flexed (not pleasant if one has increased pressure), and the spinal column parallel to the edge of the treatment table. The patient must keep his "up" shoulder from falling forward or his spine will rotate. If the nurse will slip her arm under the patient's neck, stoop, and oppose her shoulder to the patient's, it will make this easy for the patient, and secure the shoulder.

Patients who are to have air or oxygen injections into the ventricular system either directly or by the lumbar subarachnoid space should have forewarning of postprocedure headache and know that they will be asked afterward to turn from side to side. The injected air, being light, tends to pocket in the uppermost ventricle. There is no mechanism for absorption in the ventricle; the gas will have to go the regular route (see page 1068). Recovery from the procedure is slow if the patient refuses to roll, and rolling over hurts for the first day.

Both these procedures have hazards. Gases such as air or oxygen are foreign bodies to these tissues and produce cellular reaction. Sudden withdrawal of considerable fluid from below may cause dislocation downward of the medulla into the foramen magnum and respiratory death; therefore, encephalogram is not done when there is any considerable increase in intracranial pressure. It is especially hazardous if the cause of pressure lies below the tentorium, as in cerebellar tumor. If visualization of the ventricles is important, the ventriculogram may be safer, for the tentorium provides a roof between, and the pressure changes incurred by the procedure are less likely to produce medullary compression. Uncomfortable and unfavorable responses may occur in response to these air injections whether or not the report is "negative." Every patient subjected to these examinations deserves intelligent observation and thoughtful care, which will necessarily include watching for signs of generalized increase in intracranial pressure, as a response to the irritation from the injected gas, and, especially, for depressed respirations.

Nutrition: care in feeding the physically dependent patient.

In normal healthy existence, one ordinarily swallows while in a sitting or standing position when the head is in line with the body. It is not difficult, however, to swallow when the head is flexed forward, as one does in using a drinking fountain; but to twist the head sharply to the side and eat is so difficult that one always returns his head to the mid-line, or nearly, before swallowing. Persons who are recumbent in bed are therefore at a disadvantage in respect to ease of swallowing. The position is unnatural. If the nurse remains aware of her own behavior in respect to this normally automatic act, she will be careful to make eating as easy as it can be for the patient in bed. This will always include having the patient's head in line with his body and, unless specifically contraindicated, somewhat elevated. If this elevation cannot be allowed, the patient should be carefully placed in a side-lying position, for it is very difficult for a small nurse to assist a large patient, who is lying perfectly flat on his back, quickly enough to avoid serious aspiration if he chokes in an attempt to swallow. If the patient has a neurological problem, he may be trying to cope not only with a position that is mechanically unfavorable but with an organic difficulty in the act of swallowing, too.

In some clinics, after craniotomy no patient is permitted anything by mouth until "tested for swallowing" by the surgeon. The observant nurse will note that the doctor who is doing this has put the patient well over on his side, has made sure the patient's mouth is clear, and has the suction tip in one hand and a teaspoon of water in the other. The doctor then introduces the water carefully and watches intently to see how successfully this act of swallowing is completed. If swallowing is impossible for the patient at this time, it is easy for the doctor to suction the fluid back. Even when a patient is permitted feedings after a successful test, the nurse need appreciate his recent difficulties, and act to make eating as safe and as easy as it can be.

Neurological patients often have trouble with vomiting, both those with lesions in the appropriate areas in the brain stem and those with generalized intracranial pressure (see Chapter 10). If the reasons for this vomiting cannot be remedied promptly, the individual's nutrition suffers. Careful observation of time and circumstances which provoke emesis is needed. The patient's observations about himself in this regard may be helpful and should be sought. There are often patterns of serving food to the patient which will result in more calories being retained than just by giving the three meals a day in the routine manner at the routine hours. If, for instance, radical change of posture provokes trouble, it may be advisable to get the patient out of bed before breakfast so that the episode will be over some time before breakfast is served. If the man has had trouble after his regular full meals but manages successfully a dry ham sandwich at three-thirty every afternoon, it will be worth trying to give him only solids at meals and his fluids in between. There are no rules for guidance except those of careful observation, resourcefulness, and concern for the patient's welfare. Remember that the patient's trouble is in his brain and not his digestive tract; and if the nurse either withholds food because of vomiting or fails to meet the basic nutritional needs of the patient through supplying again the calories he loses—and chlorides along with them as well—there may arise problems of electrolyte balance to add to those already present. (See Chapter 8.)

Care of the patient with spinal cord damage (acute).

Chapter 16 considers rehabilitation of the patient with spinal cord damage. Since, in these days of street accidents, many persons suffer injury to the spinal cord, nurses not infrequently have such patients to care for on general wards. There are few patients who so promptly and devastatingly reveal poor care as these; but, on the other hand, nurses who can maintain in good shape the bodies and spirits of their patients with pathology in the spinal cord may well feel proud.

Everything one has learned of the structure and function of the spinal cord and peripheral nervous system can be put to use. Everything one knows of normal development of the personality and the effects of sudden helplessness upon it will be invaluable knowledge to the sensitive nurse. If transection is functionally complete, one knows that afferent impulses cannot ascend from below the level of the lesion to the brain or efferent descend to parts below the break in continuity of the cord. There will be paralysis, necessarily, and there will be anesthesia and vasomotor instability of the body beginning a little higher up than the level of the lesion (see page 1077). The patient will be unaware of his distended bladder and unable to empty it, or his bowel, voluntarily. Sooner or later he will be aware of inadequacy of sexual function. If the lesion is in the thoracic cord, or above, his breathing will be affected, and his weak chest movements keep him continuously in danger of pneumonia. Only isolated cord reflexes, cut off from any inhibiting control from above, remain. These, if they occur, have nuisance value only.

The helpless patient lies dead weight in gravity position on his bed and quickly begins to develop contractures and foot drop. The muscles, whose nerves are no longer supplied by axons coming from anterior horn cells constantly excited by the stimuli coming to them from above, lose tone, and will atrophy. A soft atrophic muscle supports poorly; the veins are not well pumped by vigorous muscle contractions any more, so the circulation is not brisk, and the patient's tissues are prepared to break down easily.

If the patient has a badly fractured spinal column, he may have to be immobilized. But if the cord is damaged either traumatically or by disease without significant fracture of bone, effective nursing care seems to hinge largely on cleanliness and movement. A good rule for the nurse to have for herself is: "I must see every square inch of this patient's body every day."

There are mattresses which are made in cells and so inflated by circulating fluid that the pressure is continuously changing under the weight of the motionless body and limbs of the patient. These are excellent, but one may not always have such a mattress and, even with one, there is need for meticulous care.

The patient needs be washed with soap and plenty of water daily, rinsed with clear water, and dried by brisk friction with a Turkish towel. This, of itself, exercises the tissues as well as cleaning the skin. The clean, dry patient needs a perfectly smooth, dry bed. He will not feel the wrinkle or the bread crumb which injures the skin of his buttock. The supports of his flail feet must be kept clean and smooth as well as those pads arranged to prevent hyperextension of his knees. All the movement that can be provided is to his advantage: joints stay mobile; skin and muscle, which is of poor tone, are relieved of pressure; vital capacity remains higher than otherwise; the often cheerless and disheartened person gets a little change of view.

Although drugs for control of urinary-tract infections are excellent today, the paralyzed patient is at risk. High fluid intake which provides for a copious output of dilute urine is less likely to become infected and to burn tissues than the meager output of concentrated urine of the dehydrated incontinent. Whatever may be the eventual pattern of bowel and bladder evacuation of the chronic patient with a damaged spinal cord, it is not established at once. The newly incontinent invalid demands great sensitivity on the part of his nurse, and this includes awareness that prevention of fecal impactions is accomplished best through knowing what is taking place from day to day and seeing that this preventable complication does not occur. The fluid fecal seepage which keeps the bed damp and soiled indicates both impaction and inattentive nursing, and will be followed by tissue breakdown.

Skin surfaces that lie on top of one another are not shifted in the paralyzed. Moving the patient tends to separate the skin surfaces, remove pressure, and permit air to bathe them. Often a patient, even one quite acutely ill, can be moved about a good deal if the nurse understands the need of it. A litter provides different pressures on the body from a mattress on a bed; a wheel chair has a firm surface, and an upholstered chair a more resilient one. These little changes are helpful and supplement the absolutely essential ones of daily complete bath and toweling repeated at night for back, sacrum, and buttocks at least. Moving, shifting body position, and providing a high water intake are things that can be done to try to prevent renal calculi, which so frequently occur when bones decalcify as a result of continuing immobility. These renal stones compound the danger of stasis in the urinary tract.

A mere "ounce of prevention" is not enough in nursing the patient with spinal cord injury; there are too many issues at stake. Each one of them, the integrity of lungs, skin, urinary tract, etc., needs its own ounce if the patient is to be accorded even a chance for his "pound of cure."

REFERENCES

Part A—Endocrine

Books

Gardiner-Hill, Harold, ed., *Modern Trends in Endocrinology,* Paul B. Hoeber, Inc., New York, 1958.

Greenberg, David M., and Harold A. Harper (eds.), *Enzymes in Health and Disease,* Charles C Thomas, Springfield, Illinois, 1960.

Harris, G. W., and B. T. Donovan, "Section VII—The Ductless Glands or Endocrines," *The Physiological Bases of Medical Practice,* 7th ed., in Charles H. Best, and Norman B. Taylor (eds.), Williams & Wilkins Co., Baltimore, 1961.

Lucas, Colen C., and Jessie H. Ridout, "The Vitamins," in *The Physiological Bases of Medical Practice,* 7th ed., Charles H. Best, and Norman B. Taylor (eds.), Williams & Wilkins Co., Baltimore, 1961, pp. 899-939.

Scheinfeld, Amram, *The Human Heredity Handbook,* J. B. Lippincott Co., Philadelphia, 1956.

Scheinfeld, Amram, *The New You and Heredity,* J. B. Lippincott Co., Philadelphia, 1950.

Selye, Hans, *Textbook of Endocrinology,* 2nd ed., Acta Endocrinologica, Inc., Montreal, 1949.

Sinnott, Edmund W., L. C. Dunn, and T. Dobzhansky, *Principles of Genetics,* 5th ed., McGraw-Hill Book Co., Inc., New York, 1958.

Snyder, Lawrence H., and Paul R. David, *The Principles of Heredity,* D. C. Heath & Co., Boston, 1957.

Sorsby, Arnold, *Clinical Genetics,* Butterworth & Co., Ltd., London, 1953.

Turner, C. Donnell, *General Endocrinology,* 3rd ed., W. B. Saunders Co., Philadelphia, 1960.

Wagner, Robert P., and Herschel K. Mitchell, *Genetics and Metabolism,* John Wiley & Sons, Inc., New York, 1955.

Articles

Adams, H. D., and R. Murphy, "The Management of Primary Hyperparathyroidism," *Surgery, Gynecology, Obstetrics,* CXVI, January, 1963, pp. 45-52.

Adams, Ralph, and Norman Siderius, "Postoperative Acute Adrenal Cortical Insufficiency," *Journal of the American Medical Association,* CLXV, September, 1957, pp. 41-44.

Albright, Edwin C., "Thyroxin Analogs and Their Place in Therapy," *Postgraduate Medicine,* XXIX, January, 1961, pp. 51-56.

American Journal of Clinical Nutrition, IX, July-August, 1961, entire issue.

August, J. Thomas, Don H. Nelson, and George W. Thorn, "Aldosterone," *New England Journal of Medicine,* CCLIX, November 6, 1958, 917-23, and November 13, 1958, pp. 967-71.

Bissell, Grosvenor, and Patrick Goseglia, "Endocrine Emergencies," *Medical Clinics of North America,* XLVI, March, 1962, pp. 495-507.

Byrd, Benjamin F., Fr., "Treatment of Hyperthyroidism—A Comparison of Surgery, Versus Other Modes," *Annals of Surgery,* CLI, May, 1960, pp. 669-74.

Caspo, Arpad, "Progesterone," *Scientific American,* CLVIII, April, 1958, pp. 40-55.

Centerwall, Willard R., and Siegried A. Centerwall, "Phenylketonuria (Fölling's Disease) The Story of Its Discovery," *Journal of the History of Medicine and Allied Sciences,* XVI, July, 1961, pp. 292-96.

Cluxton, Harley E., Jr., "ACTH and the Corticosteroids in Surgery," *Surgical Clinics of North America,* XXXIX, February, 1959, pp. 31-40.

Coursin, David Baird, "Present Status of Vitamin B₆ Metabolism," *American Journal of Clinical Nutrition,* IX, May-June, 1961, pp. 304-14.

Crandon, John H., Bernard Landau, Stanley Mikal, James Balmanno, Mildred Jefferson, and Norman Mahoney, "Ascorbic Acid Economy in Surgical Patients as Indicated by Blood Ascorbic Acid Levels," *New England Journal of Medicine,* CCLVIII, January 16, 1958, pp. 105-13.

Crick, F. H. C., "Nucleic Acids," *Scientific American,* CXCVII, September, 1957, pp. 188-203.

De Groat, Leslie J., "Physiology of the Thyroid Gland," *Postgraduate Medicine,* XXIV, August, 1958, pp. 170-78.

Dreyfus, Pierre M., and Victor Maurice, "Effects of Thiamine Deficiency on the Central Nervous System," *American Journal of Clinical Nutrition,* IX, July-August, 1961, pp. 414-25.

Engbring, Norman H., and Edward Lennon, "The Diagnosis and Treatment of Toxic Nodular Goiter," *Postgraduate Medicine,* XXIX, January, 1961, pp. 57-64.

Fernandez-Herlihy, Luis, "The Structure and Biologic Activity of the Corticosteroid Hormones and ACTH," *Medical Clinics of North America,* XLIV, March, 1960, pp. 509-19.

Forland, Marvin, and Theodore N. Pullman, "Electrolyte Complications of Drug Therapy," *Medical Clinics of North America,* XLVII, January, 1963, p. 113.

Fowler, Edson F., "Physiologic Considerations in the Diagnosis and Treatment of Thyroid Disease," *Surgical Clinics of North America,* XLII, February, 1962, p. 151.

Frohman, I. Phillips, "The Steroids," *American Journal of Nursing,* LIX, April, 1959, pp. 518-21.

Fry, William J., *et al.,* "Cancer of the Thyroid," *Surgical Clinics of North America,* XLI, October, 1961, pp. 1191-1201.

Ganam, John F., "The Unpredictable Thyroid," *G.P.,* XX, December, 1959, pp. 136-40.

Goldsmith, Richard, "Classification, Diagnosis and Treatment of Hypothyroidism," *Postgraduate Medicine,* XXIX, January, 1961, pp. 46-50.

Gray, George W., "The Organizer," *Scientific American,* CXCVII, November, 1957, pp. 79-91.

Greenblatt, Robert B., and James C. Metts, "Addison's Disease," *American Journal of Nursing,* LX, September, 1960, pp. 1249-52.

Griffith, Wendell H., "The Physiologic Role of Vitamins," *American Journal of Medicine,* XXV, November, 1958, pp. 666-72.

Hamolsky, Milton W., and A. Stone Freedberg, "The Thyroid Gland," *New England Journal of Medicine,* CCLXII, January 7, 1960, pp. 23-27, and January 14, 1960, pp. 70-78, and January 21, 1960, pp. 129-37.

Hardinge, Mervyn G., and Hulda Crooks, "Lesser Known Vitamins in Foods," *American Dietetic Association Journal,* XXXVIII, March, 1961, pp. 240-45.

Horowitz, Norman H., "The Gene," *Scientific American,* CXCV, October, 1956, pp. 77-88.

Howard, John Eager, and Richard J. Meyer, "Intoxication with Vitamin D," *Journal of Clinical Endocrinology,* VIII, November, 1948, pp. 895-909.

Hurxthal, Lewis M., and Marios C. Balodimos, "Limited Adrenocortical Reserve: Recognition and Methods of Detection," *Medical Clinics of North America,* XLIV, March, 1960, pp. 349-62.

Ingram, Vernon M., "How Do Genes Act?" *Scientific American,* CXCVIII, No. 1, January, 1958, pp. 68-74.

Jacob, Francois, and Elie L. Wollman, "Viruses and Genes," *Scientific American,* CCIV, June, 1961, pp. 92-110.

Jailer, Joseph W., and Julian I. Kitay, "Some Aspects of Adrenocortical Function," *Postgraduate Medicine,* XXIV, December, 1958, pp. 674-80.

Kaplan, Ervin, "Thyroid Function," *Medical Clinics of North America,* XLIII, March, 1959, pp. 483-95.

Kinsell, Laurance W., "Clinical Physiology of the Pituitary Gland," *Postgraduate Medicine,* XXIV, October, 1958, pp. 407-18.

Knowlton, Abbie I., "Endocrine Relationships," *New York State Journal of Medicine,* LX, November, 1960, pp. 3442-51.

Lanes, Phyllis, "Primary Aldosteronism," *American Journal of Nursing,* LXI, August, 1961, pp. 46-47.

Lerner, Aaron B., "Hormones and Skin Color," *Scientific American,* CCV, July, 1961, pp. 98-112.

Levitsky, John, "Heredity and the Blood Dyscrasias," *Medical Clinics of North America,* XLVI, January, 1962, pp. 295-302.

Li Choh Hao, "Anterior Pituitary Hormones," *Postgraduate Medicine,* XXIX, January, 1961, pp. 13-23.

Lloyd, Christopher, "The Introduction of Lemon Juice as a Cure for Scurvy," *Bulletin of the History of Medicine,* XXXV, March-April, 1961, pp. 123-32.

McKusick, Victor A., "Medical Genetics—1960," *Journal of Chronic Diseases,* XIV, July, 1961, entire issue.

Montgomery, Max, *et al.,* "Relationship of ACTH and Cortisone to Infection," *Medical Clinics of North America,* XXXIX, January, 1955, pp. 81-94.

Osborne, Richard H., and Frances De George, "The Nature of Inheritance," *American Journal of Nursing,* LVIII, June, 1958, pp. 824-26.

Postgraduate Medicine, XXIX, January, 1961, special issue, "Endocrinology."

Randall, Raymond, and Edward H. Rynearson, "Clinical Aspects of Anterior Pituitary Failure," *Postgraduate Medicine,* XXIX, January, 1961, pp. 24-39.

Rasmussen, Howard, "The Parathyroid Hormone," *Scientific American,* CCIV, April, 1961, pp. 56-63.

Reich, Barbara Hoffman, and Leilee Powell Ault, "Nursing Care of the Patient with Addison's Disease," *American Journal of Nursing,* LX, September, 1960, pp. 1252-55.

Reynolds, Frank W., "Hormonal Alterations with Aging," *Postgraduate Medicine,* XXIV, December, 1958, pp. 624-26.

Richtsmeier, Anthony J., "The Symptoms of Hypercalcemia Associated with Sarcoidosis Masquerading as Peptic Ulcer," *Annals of Internal Medicine,* LI, December, 1959, pp. 1371-78.

Schwartz, Bernard M., "Hypercalcemia Nephropathy," *Journal of Mount Sinai Hospital,* XXV, September-October, 1958, pp. 460-63.

Selye, Hans, "The Physiopathology of Stress," *Postgraduate Medicine,* XXV, June, 1959, pp. 660-67.

Simpson, D. P., and W. P. Vanderlaan, "Treatment of Hyperthyroidism with Antithyroid Drugs," *Postgraduate Medicine,* XXIX, January, 1961, pp. 86-93.

Smith, David W., Robert M. Blizzard, and Harold E. Harrison, "Idiopathic Hypercalcemia," *Pediatrics,* XXIV, August, 1959, pp. 258-69.

Lahey Clinic Number, "Symposium on Surgery of the Endocrine Glands," *Surgical Clinics of North America,* XLII, June, 1962.

Taylor, S. Herbert, "Duplication of Chromosomes," *Scientific American,* CXCVIII, June, 1958, pp. 36-50.

Thomas, William C., *et al.*, "Diagnostic Considerations in Hypercalcemia," *New England Journal of Medicine,* CCLX, March 19, 1959, pp. 591-96.

Thomas, William C., *et al.*, "Some Observations on Patients with Hypercalcemia Exemplifying Problems in Differential Diagnosis Especially in Hyperparathyroidism," *Journal of Laboratory and Clinical Medicine,* LII, July, 1958, pp. 11-19.

Van Rymenant, Marc, and Henry J. Tagnon, "Enzymes in Clinical Medicine," *New England Journal of Medicine,* CCLXI, December 24, 1959, pp. 1325-30, and December 31, 1959, pp. 1373-78.

Wagner, David H., "The Function of the Parathyroid Glands and Their Disturbances," *Surgical Clinics of North America,* XLII, February, 1962, pp. 171-84.

Wilkins, Lawson, "The Thyroid Gland," *Scientific American,* CCII, March, 1960, pp. 119-29.

Williams, Carroll M., "The Juvenile Hormone," *Scientific American,* CXCVIII, February, 1958, pp. 67-75.

Woodward, John D., "Bivtin," *Scientific American,* CCIV, June, 1961, pp. 139-50.

Wroblewski, Felix, "Enzymes in Medical Diagnosis," *Scientific American,* CCV, August, 1961, pp. 99-107.

Zuckerman, Sir Solly, "Hormones," *Scientific American,* CXCVIII, March, 1957, pp. 76-89.

Part B

Books

Elliott, H. Chandler, *Textbook of the Nervous System,* 2nd ed., J. B. Lippincott Co., Philadelphia, 1954.

Gardner, Ernest, *Fundamentals of Neurology,* 4th ed., J. B. Lippincott Co., Philadelphia, 1963.

Guyton, Arthur C., *Textbook of Medical Physiology,* 2nd ed., W. B. Saunders Co., Philadelphia, 1961.

Articles and Periodicals

Floodmark, S., and O. Steinwall, "A Method for Study of the Interrelation Between EEG and Blood Barrier Phenomena," *Acta Physiologica Scandinavia,* LVI, No. 2, October, 1962, pp. 112-19.

French, J. D., "The Reticular Formation," *Scientific American,* CXCVI, No. 5, May, 1957, pp. 54-60.

Rahman, A. N., and C. N. Luttrell, "Pathogenesis of Meningoencephalitis: Enhancement of Viral Penetrance into the Brain," *Bulletin of The Johns Hopkins Hospital,* CXII, No. 1, January, 1963.

Robertson, J. D., "The Membrane of the Living Cell," *Scientific American,* CCVI, No. 4, April, 1962, pp. 64-72.

Tizard, J. P. M., R. S. Paine, and B. Crothers, "Disturbances of Sensation in Children with Hemiplegia," *Journal of the American Medical Association,* CLV, No. 7, June 12, 1954, pp. 628-32.

Treherne, J. E., "Transfer of Substances Between the Blood and Central Nervous System in Vertebrate and Invertebrate Animals," *Nature,* CXCVI, No. 4860, December 22, 1962, pp. 1181-83.

14 : The Relationship of Illness to the Maturational Level of the Individual[1]

> *There is a tide in the affairs of men*
> *Which, taken at the flood, leads on to fortune;*
> *Omitted, all the voyage of their life*
> *Is bound in shallows and in miseries.*
>
> *Julius Caesar* IV: 3, Shakespeare

In the preceding chapters man has been presented from many views: his basic needs, physiological, psychological, and sociological; his major systems, such as the circulatory system as the transporter, and the nervous and endocrine systems as the coordinators and integrators of all levels of response from the simplest to the most complex. Every human being has these major systems, minor systems, organs, tissues, and cells which present needs that must be met so that the total body may function harmoniously in health. They may be altered in illness, with all the protective and adaptive mechanisms coming to the fore to re-establish a harmonious balance or homeostasis and restore man to health. In this chapter the nurse is asked to keep all of those factors to which she as been introduced previously in mind, but to regard them now synthesized as they are in one complex whole—a human personality whatever his age or constitution may be.

The complexity of the human organism is so great that, in order to understand its different aspects, systems, organs, and needs, each must be studied separately. As one part, system, or need is studied, it becomes readily evident that even study of one system is difficult because it does not function alone. Each part is dependent on every other part if it is to survive and accomplish its functions. Furthermore, no part is static, but it is changing, moving, growing, or developing. Thus too, the whole is an ever-changing, dynamic, moving force. John Henry Cardinal Newman put it more aptly when he said, "Growth is the only evidence of life."

Let us begin at conception, wherein man is endowed with a complex of genetic potentialities or constitution. One accepted definition is:

Constitution is currently conceived as the sum total of the structural, functional, and psychological characters of the organism. It is in large measure, an integral

[1] This chapter was contributed by Jane Frances Ronan, Assistant Professor of Nursing, College of Nursing, Wayne State University, Detroit, Michigan.

of genetic potentialities influenced in varying degrees by internal and external environmental factors. It is not a biological given, a structure destined to function in a predetermined manner. Rather it is a process, a series of operative questions that even by the time of birth have not become final declarative answers.

What is given is the genotype, the complex of genetic potentialities with which the organism is endowed. Each individual's genotype is a unique physicochemical system comprising particular kinds of potentialities that have definite limits. . . . The genes, self-duplicating giant protein molecules of great complexity, are organic catalysts that accelerate essential chemical reactions, the original builders of the body, which they serve to differentiate according to the type of medium or other conditions that surround them in their interactive chemical relations. . . .

The manner in which the genotype functions depends in part on the environment in which it undergoes development. . . . Heredity, accordingly, is not constituted merely by the genotype, but by the genotype as modified by the environment in which it has developed. It is the resultant of the dynamic interaction between the two.[2]

From the definition it is clear that this complex of genetic potentialities is not static but ever changing and developing according to the environment, internal and external, in which man lives. Therefore, throughout life man reflects both his constitution and his environment through his total being. Consequently, if we are to look at a human being, child or adult, at a given time we must consider his genetic endowment and his total experiences from conception, as well as those of the present.

In this great complex and ever-developing organism with its dynamic interrelationship of activity there is not chaos, but great order. Laws have been identified which govern the growth and development of man. They are:[3]

1. Growth is both quantitative and qualitative.
2. Growth is a continuous orderly process.
3. The tempo of growth is not even.
4. Different aspects of growth develop at different rates.
5. Both rate and pattern of growth can be modified from within and without the body.
6. Each child grows in his own unique way.
7. Growth is complex—all of its aspects are interrelated.[4]

The above laws, more specifically the implication of them, apply to full maturity of the organism, and continue to govern and affect the development of the organism throughout the life span. For example, growth is a continuous and orderly process. What happens to the fertilized ovum in utero affects the individual positively or negatively throughout his life. Another example of this

---

[2] Helen Witmer and Ruth Kotinsky, *Personality in the Making,* Harper and Brothers, New York, 1953, p. 30.

[3] Marian Breckenridge and E. Lee Vincent, *Child Development,* W. B. Saunders Company, Philadelphia, 1955, p. 4.

[4] For further study of the laws of growth see Marian E. Breckenridge and E. Lee Vincent, *Child Development,* 4th ed., W. B. Saunders Company, Philadelphia, 1960, Chap. 1.

same law is: the relationship that the mother and infant establish in early infancy is the infant's basis for making relations with all persons the rest of his life. Granted the individual's relationships with others can be changed or modified to some extent by later experiences, nevertheless the early mother-infant relationship is the basis or the raw material the infant has for the development of relationships with others throughout his life. The law that reads both rate and pattern of growth can be modified from within and without the body is very evident in molecular diseases with reference to the degree of expressivity of the genetic defect.

The laws governing growth and development are simply stated, but their implications are far-reaching. In studying and contemplating these laws it becomes evident that age alone means little. There are norms of development available that are stated in terms of age alone, e.g., a baby sits at six months. These norms are averages; they do not imply that an individual is not within the range of normalcy if he does not reach a maturational level at this given age. Evaluation of developmental progress must be made in terms of normal range rather than the precise age norm. The use of ranges in preference to ages is cumbersome, but the individuality of man is greatly maligned if ranges are not used. A baby seven months old may or may not be able to sit alone; or a woman of 48 may or may not be going through the menopause. Whether the infant is sitting or the woman has reached the maturational level of menopause will depend on the law of individual difference. A given individual may be on a fast or slow developmental schedule based on the dynamic interrelationship of his constitution and his past experiences. Although each individual grows and develops in his own way, each goes through a life cycle of development that, in a broad framework, is similar to that of all other human beings. Therefore, human development is generally predictable passing from one state or level of development into the next from conception to death. Consequently it is more meaningful to ask in which stage of development is this individual rather than to ask how old is this individual.

In perusing the literature one can find examples of the great authors defining different stages of development of man. Probably the most classic examples are those found in the Bible and in the works of Shakespeare. These two examples will be given because they are interesting to read and to compare with the contemporary scheme of development that will be presented. Both are in some aspects akin to twentieth century living.

In Shakespeare's *As You Like It,* he says:

> *. . . All the world's a stage*
> *And all the men and women merely players.*
> *They have their exits and their entrances,*
> *And one man in his time plays many parts,*
> *His acts being seven ages. At first the infant,*
> *Mewling and puking in the nurse's arms.*
> *Then the whining schoolboy with his satchel*

And shining morning face, creeping like snail
Unwillingly to school. And then the lover,
Sighing like furnace, with a woeful ballad
Made to his mistress' eyebrow. Then a soldier
Full of strange oaths and bearded like the pard,
Jealous in honor, sudden and quick in quarrel,
Seeking the bubble Reputation
E'en in the cannon's mouth. And then the justice,
In fair round belly with good capon lin'd,
With eyes severe and beard of formal cut,
Full of wise saws and modern instances:
And so he plays his part. The sixth age shifts
Into the lean and slipper'd pantaloon,
With spectacles on nose and pouch on side;
His youthful hose well sav'd, a world too wide
For his shrunk shank, and his big manly voice,
Turning again toward childish treble, pipes
And whistles in his sound. Last scene of all,
That ends this strange eventful history,
Is second childishness and mere oblivion—
Sans teeth, sans eyes, sans taste, sans everything.[5]

Ecclesiastes III (Verse 1-8) reads:

For everything there is a season
and a time for every matter under the heaven:
A time to be born, and a time to die;
a time to plant, and a time to pluck up
what is being planted;
A time to kill, and a time to heal;
a time to break down, and a time to build up;
A time to weep, and a time to laugh;
a time to mourn, and a time to dance:
A time to cast away stones, and
a time to gather stones together;
A time to embrace, and a time to refrain
from embracing;
A time to seek, and a time to lose;
a time to keep, and a time to cast away;
A time to rend, and a time to sew;
a time to keep silence, and a time to speak;
A time to love, and a time to hate;
a time for war, and a time for peace. . . .

This chapter was introduced by a quotation from Shakespeare,

There is a tide in the affairs of men
Which, taken at the flood, leads on to fortune;
Omitted, all the voyage of their life
Is bound in shallows and in miseries.

[5] Scarlett, in his article (see number 9 of References at the end of the chapter), presents excerpts from other works of Shakespeare which expound on each of these stages.

This Shakespearean quotation is identical in essence to Havighurst's definition of a developmental task, which reads: "A developmental task is a task which arises at or about a certain period in the life of the individual, successful achievement of which leads to his happiness and to the success with later tasks, while failure leads to unhappiness in the individual, disapproval by the society, and difficulty with later tasks."[6] Shakespeare's observation and Havighurst's definition are similar to that which Erik Erikson, in his ground plan of the life cycle of man, describes as the central tasks or core problems of each developmental stage. (The student may well be reminded of the same concept from her study of embryology: each organ has its time of origin; if missed, not only is the organ doomed as an entity, it endangers the whole hierarchy of organs.)

Erik Erikson's thesis of human development will be the contemporary one presented in this chapter.[7] His scheme of development was chosen because it shows clearly the flow of development during the entire life span. It gives the beginning student the major stages of human development and how each stage is built on the previous ones, and is at the same time the foundation stone for the successive ones. From this approach the student is able to grasp an over-all view of development from birth to death. As the student grows in personal and professional life her grasp of human development will take on greater meaning. She then will be able to add depth and understanding to this broad framework learned as a beginning student.

Erikson divides the life cycle of man into eight stages each with a core problem or crisis which the individual struggles to master during these specific stages. Each core problem or central task has a positive and negative component, e.g., trust-mistrust, which must be fought through successfully by the individual so that he can move to the next stage. In addition to these central tasks are innumerable other tasks (developmental, e.g., walking, talking) to master. Each is distinct in itself but, when mastered, aids in the accomplishment of the central task or problem. For example, the core problem of the toddler age is autonomy. Some of the developmental tasks of this maturational level are walking, talking, and bowel and bladder control. It is easy to see how these play an important role in the over-all task of autonomy.

Although Erikson's is primarily psychosocial development of man, much more is included. Concerning this factor Erikson[8] says, "For the eight stages of psychosocial development are, in fact, inextricably intwined in and derived from the various stages of psychosexual development that were described by Freud, as well as from the child's stages of physical, motor, and cognitive development. Each type of development affects the other and is affected by

---

[6] Robert J. Havighurst, *Human Development and Education,* Longmans, Green and Company, New York, 1953, p. 2.

[7] Erik Erikson, *Childhood and Society,* W. W. Norton and Company, New York, 1963.

[8] Kathryn Close, "Youth and the Life Cycle," *Children,* VII, No. 2, March-April, 1960, p. 45.

it." The following is an overview of Erikson's eight stages of the life cycle of man.

The eight stages in the life cycle of man.

"Personality," Erikson has written, "can be said to develop according to steps predetermined in the human organism's readiness to be driven toward, to be aware of, and to interact with a widening social radius, beginning with a dim image of a mother and ending with an image of mankind . . ."

Following are the steps he has identified in man's psychosocial development, and the special crises they bring. In presenting them, he has emphasized that while the struggle between the negatives and positives in each crisis must be fought through successfully if the next developmental stage is to be reached, no victory is completely or forever won.

I. Infancy: Trust Versus Mistrust

The first "task" of the infant is to develop "the cornerstone of a healthy personality," a basic sense of trust—in himself and in his environment. This comes from a feeling of inner goodness derived from "the mutual regulation of his receptive capacities with the maternal techniques of provision"—a quality of care that transmits a sense of trustworthiness and meaning. The danger, most acute in the second half of the first year, is that discontinuities in care may increase a natural sense of loss, as the child gradually recognizes his separateness from his mother, to a basic sense of mistrust that may last through life.

II. Early Childhood: Autonomy Versus Shame and Doubt

With muscular maturation the child experiments with holding on and letting go and begins to attach enormous value to his autonomous will. The danger here is the development of a deep sense of shame and doubt if he is deprived of the opportunity to learn to develop his will as he learns his "duty," and therefore learns to expect defeat in any battle of wills with those who are bigger and stronger.

III. Play Age: Initiative Versus Guilt

In this stage the child's imagination is greatly expanded because of his increased ability to move around freely and to communicate. It is an age of intrusive activity, avid curiosity, and consuming fantasies which lead to feelings of guilt and anxiety. It is also the stage of the establishment of conscience. If this tendency to feel guilty is "overburdened by all-too-eager adults" the child may develop a deep-seated conviction that he is essentially bad, with a resultant stifling of initiative or a conversion of his moralism to vindictiveness.

IV. School Age: Industry Versus Inferiority

The long period of sexual latency before puberty is the age when the child wants to learn how to do and make things with others. In learning to accept instruction and to win recognition by producing "things" he opens the way for the capacity of work enjoyment. The danger in this period is the development of a sense of inadequacy and inferiority in a child who does not receive recognition for his efforts.

V. Adolescence: Identity Versus Identity Diffusion

The physiological revolution that comes with puberty—rapid body growth and sexual maturity—forces the young person to question "all sameness and continuities relied on earlier" and to "refight many of the earlier battles." The developmental task is to integrate childhood identifications "with the basic biological drives, native endowment, and the opportunities offered in social roles." The danger is that identity diffusion, temporarily unavoidable in this period of physical and psychological upheaval, may result in a permanent inability to "take hold" or, because of youth's tendency to total commitment, in the fixation in the young person of a negative identity, a devoted attempt to become what parents, class, or community do not want him to be.

VI. Young Adulthood: Intimacy Versus Isolation

Only as a young person begins to feel more secure in his identity is he able to establish intimacy with himself (with his inner life) and with others, both in friendships and eventually in a love-based mutually satisfying sexual relationship with a member of the opposite sex. A person who cannot enter wholly into an intimate relationship because of the fear of losing his identity may develop a deep sense of isolation.

VII. Adulthood: Generativity Versus Self-absorption

Out of the intimacies of adulthood grows generativity—the mature person's interest in establishing and guiding the next generation. The lack of this results in self-absorption and frequently in a "pervading sense of stagnation and interpersonal impoverishment."

VIII. Senescence: Integrity Versus Disgust

The person who has achieved a satisfying intimacy with other human beings and who has adapted to the triumphs and disappointments of his generative activities as parent and coworker reaches the end of life with a certain ego integrity—an acceptance of his own responsibility for what his life is and was and of its place in the flow of history. Without this "accrued ego integration" there is despair, usually marked by a display of displeasure and disgust.[9, 10]

In studying the stages of development of man whether stated in a classic or contemporary form it becomes evident that each stage with its problem must be mastered by the individual himself. Meaningful people in his environment assist him in his development. The members of his immediate family are the persons who generally are the most meaningful, but the nurse is in a very singular position to assist the patient in his development regardless of the level of his maturation. It is also evident that these problems in mastery take considerable effort and time on the part of the individual to accomplish.

Although there are definite and progressive stages of development, how the individual develops will depend on his genetic inheritance and his environ-

[9] From "Youth and the Life Cycle." An interview with Erik Erikson by Kathryn Close, March-April, 1960, issue of *Children,* interprofessional journal published by the Children's Bureau, Department of Health, Education and Welfare.
[10] For further study see, Erik Erikson, *Op. cit.*

ment. Environment includes the culture in which he lives, the age in which he lives, and how his own family views the development of their own children in accordance with their own philosophy. It includes as well how he, as an individual, perceives his own growth, his own family, and the society and the age in which he is living.

It is interesting to note that nowhere in the schemes of development presented nor in other developmental schemes is there an allotted time for illness. (One of the verses from Ecclesiastes might be interpreted by some to mean illness.) In reality man does become ill and illness does demand much energy and effort on the part of the individual to return to health. The individual's total being is affected by his illness and he uses his total development to overcome his illness.

The reader at this point may well be saying, "This chapter is all about the growth and development of children—even Erikson's scheme of development deals more with childhood than adult life. We'll learn that in the nursing care of children. Now, we want to learn about the nursing care of adults." These stages of development are not just acquired for the individual to have permanently—they must be reinforced or reaffirmed throughout life. An example will help to clarify this. Mr. Smith comes into the hospital to have elective surgery, i.e., a herniorraphy. Mr. Smith, like most people, was reared in a family that encouraged the development of trust in other people, but Mr. Smith has lived some three decades and has learned that all people are not to be trusted. He must, therefore, discover if his nurse and the other hospital personnel are trustworthy. Until he is assured of this, his relationship with his nurse will be tentative and superficial. He must develop faith in her. He does this in the same ways that he used to establish his basic sense of trust, i.e., testing, questioning, looking for behavior that says to him, "She thinks I'm worthy, she respects me as a human being, she knows I'm demanding but she likes me anyway; she will comfort me." What happens to Mr. Smith's sense of autonomy at this time? When he is given a general anesthesia, he surely loses his autonomy and his ability to control himself and his environment because he loses all consciousness and therefore all control over himself. In order to survive and go on to full recovery, he must reaffirm his autonomy. How does the nurse help him to gain self-control? How does the child acquire autonomy? Think of the toddler! His stock answer to most things is "No!" Another statement he uses frequently is "Me do!" These are ways the toddler tells of his desire and need to be in charge of himself and his environment. Frequently, when the adult patient is in a stressful situation, i.e., asked to cough or ambulate postoperatively, he replies with a negative statement. And just as the toddler says, "Me do," the adult patient desires to be a participating member of the health team—not just a blank entity for whom procedures are being performed by many people. If the nurse permits him to participate and to really be an active member of the team, she will find she has more time for actual care because it takes less time to win his confidence and cooperation in his care. A cliché that is heard around sick people too often is, "He seems to have no will to live." How is this related to these central tasks or problems that we have been talking about?

The other two stages of development dealing primarily with childhood, i.e., initiative and industry, could be explored and shown to play important roles throughout life. A very practical manner of studying and learning in these areas is to observe and study children as they go about their daily activities— then compare their behavior with the behavior exhibited by adults. The student will find that much of the behavior is in essence the same—perhaps a bit more veneer or social tact but basically the same. Watch especially how preschool children establish relationships with each other. Watch, too, how the school-age child initiates conversation with his peers and with persons in authority.

The first four phases of development, trust, autonomy, initiative, and industry, have been discussed on the preceding pages. They are primarily tasks of infancy and childhood. These tasks, like all others in life, are not simply acquired at specific times in one's life and therefore a permanent acquisition for the rest of the individual's life; they continue to be threatened and must be reaffirmed if the individual is to maintain his homeostasis. Take an example of a developmental task; around a year an infant learns to walk, but if as an adult he is confined to bed or chair over an extended period of time because of illness, he must struggle again through the steps in learning to ambulate independently just as he did when he was a small child. If this is true in this elementary task, it is equally true in the entire realm of development; the human being strives to maintain the development he has gained and continues to further its growth.

The next stage of human development is the period of adolescence. In years this period extends over a longer period than do any of the first four. Therefore, it is usually divided into three phases, prepubescence, pubescence, and postpubescence, each of these phases contributing to the total growth and each initiating specific needs. It is the time in life when the youngster moves from being a child to being a man or a woman. This is the time when sex differences begin to play a major role in the total developmental patterns of the human being.

Adolescence is not a gray vague interim, but a period of accelerated growth and development in all areas, physical, social, emotional, intellectual, and spiritual. Postnatally, there is more rapid growth in this period than in any other period with the exception of infancy. There are tremendous physical changes accompanied by great hormonal changes that introduce new and demanding biological urges. At the same time the psyche is undergoing an upheaval so that this individual may move from childlike reactions to adult reactions that society demands of its mature citizens. Is it any wonder that the adolescent is continuously complaining of one trouble or another? Equally true, it is easy to understand why so many adults stereotype the adolescent as the chronic hypochondriac. Adolescents are not hypochondriacs; they are simply asking, "Is this normal?" With the tremendous changes going on in their bodies they do not know what is normal and what is abnormal. They are asking for help to understand the rapid change in their bodies and psyches. With so much growth in so short a period, many things can go wrong. It is the adolescent's birthright to have an excellent evaluation of his total health.

The central task of this developmental stage is identity. The development of the sense of identity points up many questions the adolescent must meet and answer if he is to develop a sense of who he is. Some of the more obvious questions are: Who am I? Where am I going? What is the purpose of life? Where do I fit in society? Will I be able to select, win, and hold a mate for life? Will I be able to be a parent? Will I be able to get a job—to hold it? The negative component of this stage of development is diffusion. This is seen in all adolescents as they struggle for identity—they are erratic and vacillating, unable to grasp or take hold. If they receive help from meaningful adults, the positive component, identity, takes over and they are less and less diffuse in their actions and beliefs.

With all these bodily changes and psychic upheaval that are going on, the adolescent is struggling valiantly to establish his identity. Add to this struggle an illness such as diabetes mellitus, or a fractured leg when he has just made the varsity team, or the orthopedist's decision at this time to correct the scoliosis that resulted from the poliomyelitis that he had at age four! What effect does one of these conditions have on this individual youngster and his struggle for identity? He overreacts to all stimuli very much like the toddler in the period of autonomy. He probably is the most demanding, erratic, vacillating patient to be found. Right in the middle of a procedure he may change from adult behavior to childlike behavior, demanding, questioning, resisting, screaming, and crying. Today he may be very knowledgeable about his condition and have a sound approach to his illness. Tomorrow he may be able to use very little of his knowledge and have an entirely different idea of what this illness is, why he has it, or what it means to him. Will you punish him for his behavior by demanding that he act as an adult or even that he act as a child? Or will you use your knowledge of this developmental stage and support him through this illness.

Regression often accompanies illness or great stress at any age. This intensifies the problems to be met in illness, perhaps more—at least more dramatically in the adolescent than for any others. All too often we find the adolescent or youth in the adult hospital ward. Remember he is no longer a child, but he is not yet an adult. An example will be helpful. The female adolescent patient may well be as big as or bigger than the nurse; the male adolescent may well be 6 ft. tall and weigh 180 lb. Physically they are more adult than child, but under this frightening stressful situation of illness and hospitalization they may well regress and act very much like the toddler. The behavior of a toddler is understandable and acceptable; you simply pick up the youngster and cuddle him; show you love and accept him; and help him with his own controls. Physically you cannot pick up this big adolescent; furthermore it would be inappropriate behavior. How do you, the nurse, show your affection, acceptance, and love for this adolescent? Will you as a nurse remember his valiant efforts toward achieving identity or will this be the patient you avoid as much as possible because his behavior is so aggressive? Will the patient's aggression be met with aggression from you with accompanying increase in anxiety and guilt feelings on his part and with resulting increase in pulse, respirations, and blood pressure? Or, through your understanding of his struggle for identity, can you help him to achieve at least a small measure of identity through his relationship with you?

Another factor plays an important role here, especially with the male adolescent. Around 16 to 18 years of age, or in postpubescence, the male youth experiences stronger sexual drives than he will throughout the remainder of his life. Most nurses are female. Keep this in mind when you come in close physical contact with your young male patient, do not add burdens to his already great struggle for control by unwitting, but nevertheless seductive behavior. This factor demands that you use your ingenuity and imagination to the utmost when you are seeking ways to comfort and support this young male as he experiences stressful situations, and he must borrow from your strength to maintain himself through the experience.

It is not only the adolescent who is struggling for identity, but all adults, sick or well, continue this struggle in a more or less intense manner the rest of their lives. They continue to seek their place in the flow of history, to realize themselves as individuals. For the adult who is critically ill or who is hospitalized over a long period of time the intensity of the struggle for maintaining his identity is heightened by simply being cut off from normal family life, job situation, and normal social intercourse with peers. The struggle may be heightened because of the illness itself, loss of control over bodily functions, loss of privacy, procedures which involve exposure of the body, and intrusion into bodily orifices and cavities. It may be heightened by the attitudes and behavior of the nurse and other hospital personnel, i.e., failure to gain the explicit consent of the patient, autocratic treatment, depersonalized care, or failure to prepare the patient for what to expect and what is expected of him. An empathetic attitude in the nurse will do much to help the patient maintain his identity, thereby being a more contributing member of the health team and better prepared to resume his place in the family, job, and society.

In our culture when the individual has reached physical maturity and has developed a considerable sense of identity, a relatively consistent pattern of reactions to stimuli which meets with society's approval emerges, and we say this individual is now an adult. The central task or problem of this stage of development is intimacy. If the individual has met and resolved the conflicts inherent in the other stages of development as he grew up, he is now ready to move into this stage. When the young person is quite sure of his identity (who he is—where he fits into society), he seeks friendships of a closer or more intimate nature. He desires to know himself better and share the essence of his being with others on a reciprocal basis. This eventually leads to a love-based, mutually satisfying sexual relationship in marriage. The culture in which the individual lives affects the stages of development: the American culture, on the whole, does quite well in contributing to the earlier stages of development; but it gives little help even in its literature and music to the development of this stage of intimacy. Our family life and its institutions, including the church and school, give little help to the young adult striving for a mature sense of intimacy. Youngsters coming through our school systems are reared on an age-grading system, and essentially the same pattern is carried on at home, e.g., the ten-year-old can stay up an hour later in the evening than the eight-year-old. The young adult soon becomes aware that the adult society functions on a social status system and not on an age-grading system. He soon realizes he stands alone and is expected to function as a full-fledged adult as soon as he embarks on his life's work. He needs help, but he is also acutely aware that there are not many resources to help him; he must depend on his own inner strengths. Owing to the mobility of our society many young people do not even have the emotional support that comes from living close to one's family. It is as though this period of young adult life were the final examination for his childhood.

In all phases of development society has specific expectations for the individual; e.g., during late childhood, in the period of industry, society expects the child to learn his basic intellectual skills. This is also true of the stage of intimacy. The specific tasks or expectations that society dictates are the establishment of oneself in a career and in marriage. These are two very demanding tasks closely related to the central task of intimacy—the ability to commune with oneself and relate effectively to others in a job situation as well as in a more personal way in courtship and marriage. And yet society really offers little help to our young adults.

These tasks are demanding not only physically but also psychically. They are demanding financially too, at a time in the life of the individual when he has had little time to accrue much in the way of savings. What does it cost physically, psychologically, and financially to establish oneself in a profession such as pharmacy, or to start a small business, or to furnish the first home following marriage? All of this puts great stress on the person. Here society fails too! We offer little to the young male in the way of adequate, much less excellent, medical supervision. The young female in our society, in a way, is better cared for medically because these are her childbearing years, and she is under the care of a physician more often than her spouse or the rest of the young male society. We know these people do succumb to illness as they are seen on the hospital wards. What does illness mean to them? Separation from their spouse, an interruption in their career, a missed chance for advancement, a pay check or two lost, a baby cared for by someone other than its mother? The implications of these questions are great, but do we think about this as we see the young adult on the ward or do we think and act toward him as we do toward the 50-year-old adult who is likely to be established in his career and marriage?

There is another factor about young males which is of importance to those in the health fields. The young male (18 to 25 years of age) overreacts to illness. Given the same illness, the same virulence of organism, the young female adult will usually return to health more quickly with fewer sequelae than her male counterpart. Clinical evidence supports this well, but there is less scientific support for this observed phenomenon. We do know that in convalescence there is a less pronounced metabolic and endocrine change in the female than in the male. It is thought to be related to the smaller tissue mass in males; it may well be sex-associated.

What do illness and hospitalization do to the young adult male or female who is struggling for the attainment of intimacy over isolation? Do we give him an opportunity to relate to us or do we treat him in a formal, stereotyped manner cutting off a very good opportunity for him to release tension through giving him the opportunity to relate effectively with his nurse and doctor?

As the young adult increases in his sense of intimacy, he has more and more meaningful relationships and experiences in the adult world. Out of these intimacies in adult society his concern and interests gradually move from those of just the present generation to the nurture of the coming generation, also the nurture of all products of creativity or productivity. He then moves into the next stage in the life cycle of man, which is the period of generativity, or the development of the parental sense. He is not only concerned about having children of his own but about nurturing or caring for children of others. He is ready to take on greater responsibilities—not just those of providing for himself and spouse, but of guiding a new life to maturity. He is able now to give of himself in a more profound way. The parental period of development extends over a span of many years. It flows out of intimacy and extends up to senescence.

Society expects much of the individual as he goes through this period of his life. For most people it is their entire period of productivity—the years they make a place for themselves in the flow of history. The two tasks that society expects of the individual in the period of intimacy are brought to fruition—he matures in his career and he watches his children grow in wisdom and strength. This too is a very demanding and taxing stage of development. To succeed in one's career, to be a good spouse and a good parent, demands great energy and effort on the part of the individual. It means giving of oneself and in turn being able to receive much from colleagues, spouse, and children. Society demands not only that he succeed in his career and his family life, but also that he have energy, creativity, and interest left over so that he can serve the community on a voluntary basis. At the beginning of this period and during the preceding period he was establishing himself in the adult world;

now he is helping to run the adult world and shape history for the oncoming generations.

This is not only an age of great activity, but because most people in this developmental period hold responsible positions, many other persons are dependent on them in a variety of ways, i.e., for emotional support, for financial support and for important decisions. Think for a while what it means to this individual who recognizes and accepts these responsibilities to be hospitalized for a week, a month, or longer. Reflect on what it means to the hospitalized female patient who has four school-age children at home. She may well be anxious, demanding, or depressed, or perhaps have a rise in blood pressure around three o'clock in the afternoon. What might these behaviors mean; are they always the result of the disease process? Also consider the effects of this mother's hospitalization on her children, on her spouse!

There are many cartoons depicting the busy executive frantically answering the three or four telephones that are on his bedside table as the attendant stands patiently waiting to take him to surgery or X ray. Funny, yes! Sad, yes! Perhaps his subordinates need this kind of help and support from him to function and he knows it. Perhaps not! This may well be his way of saying to you, "Don't take my autonomy from me!" "Don't let me lose my identity in this maze of strange and frightening activity; I'm frightened." "Help me!" Do you, as a nurse, have a responsibility to this patient with reference to this kind of behavior?

One of the major health concerns in the early part of this period, and extending as far back as late adolesence, is that this is the period of life when many of the chronic degenerative diseases (e.g., multiple sclerosis) begin to manifest themselves. What does the diagnosis of multiple sclerosis mean to the young man just established in his profession? What does it mean to the young woman who has just married or perhaps has been married for five years and has three preschool children? What does it mean to the spouse of this patient? What does it mean to the small children of this parent? Let your imagination work for you! Chronic degenerative diseases are not curable, but only manageable. These individuals and their families (colleagues too) need much help to understand and resolve the conflicts surrounding a diagnosis such as multiple sclerosis, tuberculosis, or diabetes mellitus. It is not only the immediate adjustment that causes strain on personal and family relationships but the continuing adjustment that is required as the disease process progresses. Families or individuals not only need help to adjust psychologically to this kind of condition, but need very practical kinds of help, i.e., equipment, household help, nursing care, and financial help. Do you know the resources in your community so that you can refer them to the right people? Or do you say, "That's none of my business; I can't afford to get involved." Isn't it? Can't you?

At the end of the generativity period, a biological maturational task occurs that is of concern to all people in the health fields: that is, the climacteric. A very simple explanation of the climacteric is an altered hormonal balance primarily concerned with reduction of gonadal function. In the male this is a very slow, gradual process beginning as early as 30 years of age in some males and later in others. There is usually no sharp demarcation of beginning or end as there is in the female. In fact, if men experience acute overt manifestations of the climacteric (e.g., vasomotor symptoms, emotional instability), it is taken out of the realm of normality and considered pathological. In females it is different. It is one of the three fundamental biologically determined maturational crises in womanhood. The other two are puberty and pregnancy. These three maturational crises are different from other maturational tasks. The difference lies in the intense and specific interdependence between the psychological and the biophysiological changes, and the fact that they are all remorselessly irreversible. In all three of these periods, a number of new, specific libidinal and adaptive tasks confront the individual. Often these tasks are diametrically opposed to the central tasks and activities of the preceding stage. Each one of these stages seems to revive and unsettle psychological conflicts of earlier development, each one requiring new and different solutions. In all three the mastery of this biologically initiated phase depends on the solution and maturational reorganization of this disequilibrium, i.e., adulthood in puberty, motherhood in pregnancy, and aging in menopause. It is this factor which adds to the adaptive process the quality of the inevitable, emphasizing it as the point from which there is no return. Once an adolescent you cannot be a child again; once a mother you cannot be a single unit again; and once beyond the menopause you cannot bear a child again. The demands, psychological and biophysiological, that are placed on the woman's body as she goes through this maturational task are surely important factors to consider when caring for a patient at this stage in development. How do these demands affect the management of her diabetes mellitus, hypertension, or convalescence from a thyroidectomy?

The final stage in the development of the human being is old age or the development of the sense of integrity. It is the culmination and integration of his entire development. The child and youth who has come through the various maturational levels satisfactorily is ready and eager for adulthood. The adult who has enjoyed the intimacies of the adult world with his spouse and colleagues, who has enjoyed and adequately met the responsibilities of parenthood and also his work responsibilities, arrives at the end of his life with ego integrity. Erikson describes this as:

Integrity thus means a new and different love of one's parents, free of the wish that they should have been different, and an acceptance of the fact that one's life is one's own responsibility. It is a sense of comradeship with men and women of distant times and of different pursuits, who have created orders and objects and sayings conveying human dignity and love. Although aware of the relativity of all the various life styles that have given meaning to human striving, the possessor of integrity is ready to defend the dignity of his own life style against all physical and economic threats. For he knows that, for him, all human dignity stands or falls with the one style of integrity of which he partakes.[11]

The adult in senescence who has not or does not develop integrity is the adult who feels he has been cheated in his life and wishes he could relive it. If you carry this to the extreme, he is the adult who experiences despair and disgust. Despair conveys the feeling that life was too short to develop integrity; he has been cheated! Disgust is a cover-up for despair, chronic complaining of how poorly life is run. The sense of integrity is a part of human nature that must be reaffirmed over and over with the help and comfort of faith, the arts, and wisdom which offer proof of the integrity of humanity.

Although aging begins at birth (the aorta is the body structure to show initial aging) and continues very gradually throughout life, senescence is the period of life when the greatest amount of the aging process takes place. Today with the great strides in all health fields, we have more and more people living to old age.

The laws of growth that were presented earlier in this chapter seem to deal primarily with the growth and development (anachronobiology) of the organism, but they are also applicable in the aging process (catachronobiology). For example, each child grows in his own way—each adult ages in his own way—some fast, some slow. Another example, the tempo of growth is not even—the tempo of the aging process is not even; some of the structures of the body age rapidly and others more slowly. The law which states that growth is a continuous, orderly process is one of which we see clinical evidence every day on hospital wards—the 85-year-old woman's hip does heal; the suture line of the operation in the 80-year-old man does grow together. Probably the fact that all aspects of growth are interrelated is seen most dramatically in the elderly person. It is quite easy to relate his emotional, social, psychological, and physical needs to his illness. He may well be ill because he was physically or financially unable to nourish himself or just not interested in eating or too lonely to eat. The interrelatedness of the body brings problems of duplicity and multiplicity to illness in the aged. For example, poor nutrition leads to poor resistance, which may lead to contracting pneumonia, which may lead to cardiac difficulties, which may lead to renal failure. Another related problem in illness in the aged is the chronicity of the illness.

The period of senescence is long for a good many people. The aging process itself varies with individuals. These two statements are very much related to nursing care. Just because a patient is 65, 75, or 85 years old does not mean that he cannot hear, think adequately for himself, or be a contributing member of the team that is engaged in his health care. His total behavior will dictate his nursing needs.

The material in this chapter was presented to help the nurse bring into

[11] Witmer and Kotinsky, *Op. cit.,* p. 25.

sharp focus her knowledge of human development and to show how she can relate this knowledge to her day-by-day care of her patients. It was presented to remind the young student that each patient is an individual member of society, each struggling to further his development in order that he may be a better or more complete human being, thus fulfilling his destiny as he understands it, to remind the student, too, that each of her patients is an individual, with his own genetic endowment, his unique past and present experiences, as well as an individual with a pathological condition.

It is hoped that, from reflecting on the material presented, the student may see the art in nursing as well as the science. Generally a young person comes into nursing more knowledgeable and interested in the art rather than the science of nursing. She comes in wanting to commit or dedicate herself to the nurturing of mankind through the practice of nursing. It is hoped that through practicing nursing as presented in this chapter she may further develop her appreciation and knowledge of the art and bring it into sharp focus with her knowledge of nursing science, thereby gaining greater satisfactions for herself and better care for her patients. Only as the nurse is able to fuse the art and science of nursing will she be able to give excellent care, because man has a psyche as well as a body—each of which needs to be nurtured.

Reactions to illness at various maturational levels.

In the following paragraphs a common medical condition and a simple surgical procedure will be explored to show how they affect an individual at various phases of his development. The medical condition to be explored is simple diarrhea and the surgical procedure is circumcision.

Diarrhea is a common condition at any age. In the newborn and in early infancy it is a dread disease accompanied by severe fluid and electrolyte problems. Unless the infant is treated promptly by physicians who understand the significance of fluid and electrolyte balance in infancy, he may well die. Most infants, well treated, go on to live with few sequelae even to their development of trust because they are hospitalized such a short time.

Diarrhea in the toddler age (period of autonomy) is physiologically not a severe disease. The greater problem of diarrhea to this child is psychological (precisely with his psychosocial and psychosexual development). He has just acquired bowel and bladder control, which is very much a part of his total autonomy or his will to control himself and his environment. With diarrhea the toddler has little or no control over bowel evacuation. The toddler's intellectual development is not such that he has any appreciable concept of time or ability to understand diarrhea; consequently, he cannot say to himself, "Oh, this will only last a few days and I'll be in control again." He can only think, "I've failed! Will Mama scold? Mama doesn't love me anymore. That's why I'm here." (Of course his language development is not this great—but his thinking and feeling are.) His loss of control, so hard-won, and his separation from his mother are overwhelming problems to the small child and must be taken into consideration when planning and giving his nursing care. Diarrhea may cause the same problems for the child in the next period of development, preschool, but this child has a bit more intellectual and ego development to help him.

From this stage of development until late in senescence, diarrhea is more a nuisance than anything else. In the elderly again the problem arises of fluid and electrolyte balance.

Regarding the surgical procedure, circumcision in the newborn period is a very safe, simple surgical procedure. The baby is not upset by the procedure in the least. A little older infant will object strenuously while the procedure is being performed but then is not bothered by it.

Circumcision in the toddler age (one to three years old) is something different. Ordinarily the child is given a general anesthetic and experiences considerable discomfort and pain following the procedure. It is ordinarily done in a hospital setting, and this usually means separation from his mother. This is the age when the child is struggling for autonomy. The discomfort is quite localized to his penis and becomes very clearly related to control of his bladder. Separation is one of the most threatening experiences a toddler or a preschool child can experience. It can have a very real effect on his total development.

As the child moves from a toddler to a preschooler (three to six years old), he is sure he is a separate person in his own right. He spends considerable time and effort exploring the various kinds of people there are in the world. This is the period that the youngster learns whether he is a boy or she is a girl and what it means to be a boy or a girl. He is developing considerably in his self image and is threatened by activities concerned with bodily mutilation. It is very easy to understand, from a child's point of view, that circumcision represents mutilation of his body. What does it do to his self image? Do not be surprised if the child wonders whether he is still a boy. This age child, too, will be given a general anesthetic and hospitalized, which usually means separation from his mother.

Let us move to the period of adolescence with all of its turbulence surrounding sexual growth accompanied by new and powerful biological drives. What does a circumcision mean to a youngster aged 13 or 15? In his quest for identity he is questioning all authority. Two powerful authority figures, i.e., parents and physician, say he must have a circumcision now. It is not just a medical or surgical treatment but a procedure closely related to his masculinity. What is his reaction to this? How will he react to this at the time of the surgery?

Compare the adolescent to the young adult aged 23 or 24 who is preparing for marriage and whose physician recommends that he be circumcised before marriage. Difficult as it for the young male, it is his choice. The decision to have surgery holds tangible rewards.

Many other medical conditions or surgical procedures could be explored to point up the significance of the relationship between reactions to illness and the stage of development of the patient. Some are anatomical in nature, such as the short, thin omentum in infants and small children, which is ineffectual in walling off intra-abdominal infections. Others are related to physiological reactions, i.e., the encephalopathy (usually followed by mental deterioration) in the lead poisoning of children as compared to polyneuritis commonly found in adults. One of the major physical factors to keep in mind when dealing with an adolescent who is growing with great rapidity is that growth must always be considered with maintenance, whether it be in nutrition or with a long term drug such as insulin. Maintenance alone is not sufficient. Still others are more related to the psychological, e.g., the differences in reaction to a radical mastectomy for a malignancy in a newlywed young woman, a young matron of 30 years, and a woman 65 years old.

It is evident from the above discussion that individuals react to illness differently at various maturational levels. This phenomenon is equally true with respect to invasion of the body by particular organisms, e.g., hemolytic *Streptococcus:* a toddler overreacts with a temperature of 105° F. which may well be accompanied by convulsions; an adult is sick but rarely develops such exaggerated symptoms. Specific kinds of illness, e.g., infections and anomalies in infants and small children and chronic degenerative diseases in the middle years, are common at certain levels of maturation. If the nurse is to meet the individual patient's needs she must consider his genetic endowment, his total life experiences, and the pathology of the illness.

REFERENCES

Books

Bourne, Geoffrey (ed.), *Structural Aspects of Aging,* Hafner Publishing Company, New York, 1961.

Breckenridge, Marian, and Margaret Murphy, *Growth and Development of the Young Child,* 7th ed., W. B. Saunders Company, Philadelphia, 1963.

Breckenridge, Marian, and E. Lee Vincent, *Child Development,* 4th ed., W. B. Saunders Company, Philadelphia, 1960.

Duvall, Evelyn, *Family Development,* 2nd ed., Lippincott Company, Philadelphia, 1962.

Engel, George, *Psychological Development in Health and Disease,* W. B. Saunders Company, Philadelphia, 1962.

English, Spurgeon, and Gerald Pearson, *Emotional Problems of Living,* 3rd ed., W. W. Norton Company, New York, 1963.

Erikson, Erik, *Childhood and Society,* 2nd ed., W. W. Norton and Company, New York, 1963.

Haimowitz, Morris, and Natalie Haimowitz (eds.), *Human Development, Selected Readings,* Thomas Y. Crowell Company, New York, 1960.

Havighurst, Robert, *Developmental Tasks and Education,* 2nd ed., David McKay Company, New York, 1952.

Stuart, Harold, and Dane Prugh (eds.), *The Healthy Child,* Harvard University Press, Cambridge, Massachusetts, 1962.

Witmer, Helen, and Ruth Kotinsky (eds.), *Personality in the Making: The Fact-Finding Report of the Midcentury White House Conference on Children and Youth*, Harper and Brothers, New York, 1952.

United States Veterans Administration, *Research in Aging VA Prospectees*, Report of the transactions of a meeting of the Veterans Administration Advisory Committee for Problems of Aging and their guests, May 16, 1958, U.S. Government Printing Office, Washington, D.C., 1959.

Articles

Aasterud, Margaret, "Explanations to the Patient," *Nursing Forum*, II, No. 4, Fall, 1963, p. 37.

Donovan, Helen, "Creativity and the Nurse," *Hospital Progress*, XLV, No. 6, June, 1964, p. 98.

Engel, George, "A Unified Concept of Health and Disease," *Perspectives in Biology and Medicine*, III, No. 4, Summer, 1960, p. 459.

Erickson, Janet, "How Nurses Feel About Their First Work Experience," *Nursing Outlook*, XII, No. 5, May, 1964, p. 62.

Goldfarb, Alvin, "Patient-Doctor Relationships in Treatment of Aged Persons," *Geriatrics*, XIX, No. 1, January, 1964, p. 18.

Gould, Grace, "A Philosophy of Personalized Care," *Hospital Progress*, XLV, No. 5, May, 1964, p. 148.

Henderson, Cynthia, "Can Nursing Care Hasten Recovery?" *American Journal of Nursing*, LXIV, No. 6, June, 1964, p. 80.

Kastenbaum, Robert, "Multiple Personality in Later Life—A Developmental Interpretation," *The Gerontologist*, IV, No. 1, January, 1964, p. 16.

Scarlett, E. P., "Doctor Out of Zebulun: The Case History of Man," *Internal Medicine*, CXIII, No. 5, May, 1964, p. 769.

Shock, Nathan, "The Physiology of Aging," *Scientific American*, CCVI, No. 1, January, 1962, p. 100.

Skipper, James, Daisy Tagliacozzo, and Hans Mauksch, "Barriers to Communication Between Patients and Hospital Functionaries," *Nursing Forum*, II, No. 1, Winter, 1963, p. 14.

Smith, Sydney, "The Psychology of Illness," *Nursing Forum*, III, No. 1, Winter, 1964, p. 35.

Tryon, Phyllis, "Patient Participation vs. Patient Passivity," *Nursing Forum*, II, No. 2, Spring, 1963, p. 48.

Wolanin, Mary, "They Called the Patient Repulsive," *American Journal of Nursing*, LXIV, No. 6, June, 1964, p. 73.

15 : The Requirements of Patients Treated Surgically

"Notice"

As of today, May 15, 1847, every doctor or student who comes from the dissecting room is required, before entering the maternity wards, TO WASH HIS HANDS thoroughly in a basin of chlorine water which is being placed at the entrance. This order applies to all, without exception.

I. P. Semmelweis, M.D.[1]

With the development of modern surgery many conditions that have plagued man since the beginning of time have been brought under control. Though the list is much too long to enumerate, examples include such conditions as acute appendicitis, cholecystitis, hernia, compound fractures, and even defects in the structure of the heart. Much of the knowledge on which modern surgical treatment of disease is based has been acquired in the last 100 to 150 years. Since the early nineteenth century the science of surgery has been developed so that an increasing number of surgical procedures can now be performed with reasonable safety and with the expectation that the patient will be benefited. Actually the treatment of disease and injury by surgical methods probably goes back to the beginning of mankind. The earliest records of surgical procedures left by man are found in burial grounds where bones or pieces of bones and the tools that were used to open the skull and to treat fractures of bones have been uncovered. Other early records include writings and drawings on stone tablets and on the walls of caves and houses. Records may also have been made on perishable materials such as bark or bamboo, but if they were, they have been destroyed by the elements and are no longer available.

What types of surgical procedures were performed by primitive man?

A variety of surgical procedures were performed by primitive man including the setting of broken bones and the treatment of wounds. Trephining, a procedure in which a hole is made in the skull, was performed by primitive surgeons in many parts of the world. Skulls, eight to ten thousand years old, have been found bearing marks of trephination in France and other parts of Europe. In the New World, Peru is the site where trephining was practiced

[1] J. Thornwald, *Century of Surgery,* Pantheon Books, Inc., New York, 1959.

most extensively, but it was performed as far north as Alaska. As far back as 4000 B.C., the Egyptians did circumcisions as well as ophthalmic surgery. The Homeric legends refer to regimental surgeons as fighters and physicians.[2] Histories of other civilizations contain reference to surgical treatment, but much of the early surgery was both cruel and crude. Its use was hampered by inadequate knowledge of effective and humane ways to control hemorrhage and to prevent pain and infection. Some of it was done, not for the purpose of removing diseased tissue or of correcting anatomical defects, but to allow evil spirits to escape. By modern standards, making an opening in the skull to provide an avenue for the escape of a demon seems strange, but in relation to the knowledge of the time, it was logical.

Some of the knowledge essential to the practice of surgery was discovered and then lost, to be reintroduced at a later time. For example, the use of ligatures was known and described by Celsus shortly before the beginning of the Christian era. It was not until Ambroise Paré (1510–1590) reintroduced them that ligatures were again used as the method of choice in hemostasis.

Through what phases has surgery gone in its development?

Modern surgery has gone through two phases in its development. In the first, the objective was to make surgery safe for the patient. In the second, the objective has been to make the patient safe for surgery. Both are important to the welfare of the patient. The first phase has its origins in the sciences of anatomy, chemistry, bacteriology, and pathology. The second phase is based on knowledge derived from biochemistry, physiology, psychology, sociology, and anthropology.

What three elements are fundamental to the development of safe and humane surgical treatment?

The three elements that are essential to safe and humane surgery are hemostasis, asepsis, and anesthesia. Without an adequate method for the control of bleeding, the patient dies from hemorrhage. Before the development of the science of bacteriology, he frequently died from infection. Since anesthesia made possible the prevention of pain, the surgeon can take time to handle tissues gently and to develop skill in the performance of surgical procedures. Knowledge of anatomy and of the factors that influence wound healing was also important to the development of surgical methods.

Trace the development of the methods used in the control of bleeding.

Since man has always been faced with bleeding following disruption of body tissues, the development of methods of stopping the flow of blood oc-

[2] Otto L. Bettmann, *A Pictorial History of Medicine,* Charles C Thomas, Publisher, Springfield, Illinois, 1956, p. 15.

curred early. Methods used to control hemorrhage developed in three stages. As might be anticipated, pressure and bandaging were the first known methods of hemostasis; the second was the cauterization of wounds; and the third was use of some type of material to occlude by tying the ends of blood vessels. As in many other fields of knowledge, the introduction of new methods did not entirely replace the old, but each new procedure increased the ability to control hemorrhage. All these methods are used today in hemostasis. The causes, effects, and treatment of hemorrhage will be discussed later in the chapter.

Trace the development of the modern concept of asepsis.

The modern concept of asepsis is based on two premises, neither of which is really new. One is that the environment contains something which, when it is introduced or it enters into a wound or individual, can cause harm. The other is that something can be done to prevent the harmful agent (spirit or microbe) from entering the body or its harmful influence can be nullified. As an example, some primitive people isolated the sick by placing them outside the village walls or abandoned their houses when someone died in them. Others made loud noises or practiced some kind of ritual to frighten the evil spirit or immobilize him.

Asepsis as it is known today developed in three stages, the first was the stage of isolation and cleanliness; the second, the stage of antiseptic surgery; and the third and present stage, the stage of asepsis. The value of isolation and cleanliness was demonstrated in the 1840's by Semmelweis, a young Hungarian physician who practiced in Vienna.[3] Despite lack of precise knowledge of microorganisms, Semmelweis instituted measures that were successful in the prevention of puerperal fever. These measures were based on the observation that the incidence of puerperal fever was much lower in a ward where the women were delivered by midwives than in a ward where the women were examined by medical students who had come from dissecting rooms. Next he instituted techniques to control the factor he believed to be responsible. He insisted that physicians and medical students wash their hands before they examined patients. Despite active opposition to this rule, the lives of many mothers were saved by it. Semmelweis died a depressed and disappointed man; although he had proved over and over the soundness of his ideas, they were not accepted by his colleagues. As happens even today, there was a considerable lag between knowledge and the use of this knowledge in practice.

The work of many men, some who preceded Semmelweis and some who followed him, contributed to the development of modern aseptic surgery. Among those usually mentioned is the seventeenth-century Dutch lens grinder, Leeunwenhoek. He is credited with being the first to see what we now

---

[3] About the same time Oliver Wendell Holmes published an essay, "On the Contagiousness of Childbed Fever."

know as protozoa and bacteria. It was not until 1850–1865, or nearly 200 years later, that the foundation was laid for antiseptic and, soon thereafter, aseptic surgery. A French chemist, Louis Pasteur, was employed by the wine growers of France to identify the cause of the souring of wine and to devise techniques for preventing it. A result was that the theory of spontaneous generation was disproved for all time and the germ theory of disease was firmly established. According to the germ theory, disease is caused by a living agent. After it is introduced into an individual, the agent establishes itself, grows, and multiplies, and causes disease.

Other men, notably Lister and Koch, added to the body of knowledge which contributed to the acceptance of the germ theory. Lister, a physiologist and surgeon, read reports of the studies made by Pasteur on the cause and prevention of the souring of wine. If microorganisms present in the air caused wine to sour, might not microorganisms infect wounds? To remove microorganisms from the air, Lister had the operating room sprayed with a dilute solution of carbolic acid previous to the start of the operation. Following the operation he placed a disinfectant bandage over the incision. He had some success with the latter, for he found that he could prevent the infection of compound fractures, that is, fractures in which the skin is broken and there is a direct communication between the broken bone and the external environment. Compound fractures treated in this manner healed as well as simple ones, that is, those in which the skin remained intact. Lister reported his experiments and clinical trials in 1867.

The third stage, or the stage of asepsis, quickly followed the stage of antisepsis. In 1877 Robert Koch published *The Cause of Infection in Wounds*. In what has come to be known as Koch's postulates, he stated the conditions that must be fulfilled for a microorganism to be established as the cause of a disease. Further, the work of Semmelweis, Pasteur, Lister, Koch, and others demonstrated that the pus which was formed in a wound resulted from the introduction of an outside agent and was not an essential part of the healing process. With this knowledge as a basis, methods were developed to prevent microorganisms from gaining access to the wound.

Previous to the discovery of the necessary knowledge and the development of techniques for the practice of asepsis, wounds were so regularly infected that pus was considered an essential aspect of wound healing. The type and quantity of pus present in a wound depended on the infecting microorganism. The character of the pus provided a clue to prognosis. Thus abundant, creamy pus was usually associated with recovery and was therefore called laudable. A thin, watery or serous pus, such as is present in a hemolytic streptococcal infection, implied a poor prognosis. Presently, it is known that any type of infection in a wound delays healing and may also threaten the life of the individual.

Despite a large body of knowledge acquired over the last 100 years or so indicating that the environment external to the individual does contain agents

—microorganisms—capable of causing disease, wounds continue to be infected. Among the elements contributing to the incidence of wound infection is that some individuals either lack understanding of existing knowledge or fail to accept prescribed techniques as necessary and valid. For example, Miss Smith, a nurse in the operating room, awakens in the morning with a sore throat or she has a boil on her neck. A heavy operative schedule is planned for the day. Should she go to work or should she remain at home? If she goes to work, she may be able to rationalize her behavior by saying, "I'm not very sick. I'll wear a mask. It's on the back of my neck. I'm needed." But she will be demonstrating that she does not know what, as an operating room nurse, she should know or that she does not accept her knowledge as having validity. Other considerations take precedence in influencing her behavior. Among the additional elements contributing to the continued problem of wound infection are susceptibility of the host and the ecological balance between or among microorganisms. It is likely that there are others as well.

Fundamentally, the practice of asepsis depends on two factors:

1. Knowledge of the factors to be controlled and development of suitable techniques.
2. The conviction of practitioners that the knowledge is valid and that the techniques will accomplish their purpose and are practical.

Semmelweis failed, not because his observations or techniques were unsound, but because his colleagues refused to accept them as valid and necessary.

The third element required, if surgery is to be safe and humane, is some means of preventing pain during the performance of surgery. Thus, the discovery and acceptance as safe of a variety of chemical agents has been important to the development of surgery. The discovery of anesthetic agents preceded their actual use by many years. According to Goodman and Gilman,[4] the first anesthetic, nitrous oxide, was discovered in 1776 by Priestly. In 1799 Sir Humphry Davy reported that it prevented pain and suggested that it might be used in surgical operations. Though others experimented with nitrous oxide and ether as anesthetic agents, the regular use of anesthesia in surgical operations did not come about until Morton, in October, 1846, successfully anesthetized a patient with ether.

Today a great variety of anesthetic agents are available. Some are suitable to use to induce unconsciousness; others may be used to anesthetize a region of the body or a small area of the skin or mucous membrane. Methods used in their administration are also varied and are related to the state in which the agent occurs. For example, gaseous anesthetics are administered by way of a face mask or through a tube introduced into the trachea. Liquid anesthetics that evaporate rapidly effectively anesthetize the skin by freezing it. Other

[4] Louis S. Goodman and Alfred Gilman, *The Pharmacological Basis of Therapeutics,* 2nd ed., The Macmillan Company, New York, 1955, p. 21.

liquids produce anesthesia when applied to mucous membrane. Liquids may also be injected into the skin, sensory nerves, spinal canal, and even intravenously. Because of the variety of agents now available, an anesthetic agent can be selected which suits not only the desired method of administration, but also the condition of the patient. The discovery and development of anesthetics made elective surgery not only possible, but humane.[5]

Previous to the discovery of effective and safe anesthetics, speed was one of the essential features in the performance of a surgical procedure. As a consequence, incisions were often crudely made and tissues suffered unnecessary damage. One of the most significant contributions to modern surgery was made by Halsted who correlated surgical technique with wound healing. He also introduced the use of small hemostats, so that damage to tissue was minimized. The care taken by the surgeon in making and closing a surgical incision is one of the important factors in recovery of the patient.

In less than 200 years, surgery as a method of treatment has been developed to the point where it can be performed with relative safety in the treatment of a wide variety of disorders. Its indications and limitations are reasonably well established. Surgery is employed in the treatment of disease, injury, of structural defects occurring in all organs of the body. The discoveries making surgery safe for the patient—hemostasis, asepsis, anesthesia, and the treatment of wounds—have been reviewed in an historical perspective.

As the above accomplishments have become a reality, and knowledge of psychology, biochemistry, and physiology are advancing, surgeons are directing their attention toward making patients safe for surgery. Knowledge of physiological and biochemical processes has led to the discovery of methods which can be used to support patients during prolonged surgical procedures. As the relationship between the capacity of the patient to adapt physiologically and psychologically and his recovery has come to be appreciated, methods to evaluate his status and to correct abnormalities have been developed. With greater understanding of the physiological and psychological needs of people and the effects of surgery on structure and function, the care of the patient can be better regulated, so that recovery is facilitated.

Many discoveries and refinements of technique have contributed to the development of modern surgery—some, such as surgery on the heart as well as that involving the transplantation of organs, has been the subject of interest to the lay public. All surgical procedures require attention to the prevention of bleeding and infection as well as to the prevention and relief of pain.

What elements should be considered when planning the nursing care of a patient who is treated surgically?

Among the elements to be considered is that every patient is an individual. For most persons some aspect of surgical therapy is tantamount to a crisis

[5] For detailed information about various anesthetic agents, the student is referred to the references.

situation. The psychological, social, and physiological behavior of the patient can be expected to be similar to his behavior in any other highly stressful situation. (See Chapter 6.) Because of their familiarity with the risks and other aspects of surgical treatment, physicians and nurses may not be sufficiently aware of the uniqueness of the experience to each patient. Furthermore, their perception of the proposed procedure and its consequences may be quite different from that of the patient. Unless they are aware of the possibility of differences in perceptions and are alert to cues indicating the emotional state of the individual, they may not be as helpful as they could be.

As an illustration, 15-year-old Jesse is to have a wart removed from the sole of his foot. Though his physician has tried to reassure him that removal of the wart is a relatively simple procedure, Jesse fears that he will lose his leg or at least his foot. Physicians and nurses know that a removal of this wart is a minor procedure, and they cannot understand why Jesse continues to turn on his light and to make unnecessary demands for service. About three o'clock in the morning, when the night nurse was answering his light for the fifteenth time, she said, "Jesse, you are having trouble getting to sleep, aren't you? It's hard to sleep when you are away from home. Would you like me to stay with you for a little while?" She sat quietly beside his bed. In a few minutes Jesse asked, "Are they going to cut my foot off, tomorrow?" When the nurse knew what was troubling Jesse, she was able to reassure him by saying, "My goodness, no," and then explained in some detail what was actually planned.

Besides the individuality of the patient, a variety of other factors should be considered. In each phase of therapy—preoperative, operative, postoperative, and convalescence—definite objectives are to be accomplished and the patient is exposed to a variety of risks or threats to his well-being. As a basis for planning nursing action, additional factors should also be known: *the site of the incision, the function of the organ or tissue*, as well as the *disease or condition being treated*. For example, to remove the thyroid gland an incision is made in the neck. Extension of the neck causes strain on the incision, as well as pain. The patient's head should be supported in such a manner that it is kept in a desirable anatomical position and strain on the incision is prevented. The location of the scar is a possible source of psychological stress particularly among women. Since the thyroid gland is a highly vascular organ, it is important to observe the patient for evidence of bleeding in the tissue surrounding the operative site. Because the parathyroid glands are located in the region of the thyroid gland, they may be accidentally removed (a rare event) or become inflamed. Consequently, the patient may experience parathyroid deficiency (see Chapter 13A). One of the more common complications is due to the anatomical relationship of the thyroid gland to the recurrent laryngeal nerves and to the trachea. Breathing can be obstructed by closure of the glottis by the vocal cords, by edema of the trachea, or by pressure on the trachea by blood. Knowledge of the state of thyroid function is important in all phases of surgery. Though less frequent today than in the past, symptoms of hyperthyroidism may be intensified during the immediate postoperative period. The prognosis of the patient and his future needs will depend on many factors such as the nature of the cause and whether or not enough, and not too much, tissue was removed to secrete adequate quantities of thyroid hormones.

Although the example cited above is limited almost entirely to the factors to be considered during the post operative phase, the same general points have relevance to the other phases of surgery. To summarize and to emphasize the points to be considered in planning nursing care, the nurse should give attention to the following:

1. The patient as an individual person.
2. The risks to which the patient is exposed during this period.
3. The relationship of the route of approach to the organ or tissue to the needs of the patient for nursing.
4. The involved organ or region of the body.
5. The disorder under treatment and the effects of therapy.
6. The patient's perception of the nature of his disorder, the therapy, and his prognosis.

What are the needs of the patient during the preoperative period?

The preoperative period may be defined as the period of time beginning with the moment the patient recognizes that something is wrong and ending when he arrives in the operating room. During this period the nature of the patient's illness is determined and a therapeutic plan is made. For example, Mr. Thome has had symptoms of indigestion periodically for the last six months. For the most part, his symptoms have been mild and he has been able to explain them to his satisfaction and secure relief by drinking soda water. One morning he awakened feeling nauseated and with a pain in his upper abdomen. He reviewed what he had eaten during the last 24 hours to determine what might be responsible for his symptoms. He took two anti-indigestion pills. Instead of his feeling relieved, however, the symptoms increased and he began to feel frightened. When his wife suggested that she call a doctor, he agreed. Mr. Thome had entered the preoperative period, which did not end until he was transferred to the operating room, where he expected to have a partial gastrectomy for the removal of a portion of his stomach.

During the early preoperative period the nurse may act as a case finder and a health educator by encouraging the patient who is in the "Is it or isn't it" stage to seek medical attention. Delay in the treatment of some disorders increases the danger of serious complications and may lessen chances for recovery. As an illustration, acute appendicitis, when operated on early, is accompanied by only a small risk. The death rate following appendectomy is less than 0.3 per cent when the operation can be performed before perforation. The complication rate after perforation has been shown in at least one study to be seven times that of the preperforation rate.[6]

At the time Mrs. Thome called the family physician, Mr. Thome entered the phase of diagnosis. He still had moments of "Is it or isn't it?" He also felt relief that at last he was under medical care, but his relief was mixed with anxiety about the nature of the cause of his symptoms and the treatment that would be required. At this time Mr. Thome was subjected to a series of investigations directed toward answering two questions: What was the nature and extent of his illness? What was his physiological and psychological status? Answers to the first question determined whether or not surgery was indicated in his treatment and the type of procedure that would be of benefit to him. Answers to the second question provided information about any abnormalities that required correction before he was operated on and his capacity to adapt to surgical therapy.

What are some of the causes of psychological stress to the patient in the preoperative phase of surgery?

Many of the sources of psychological stress are similar to those to which any sick person is likely to be exposed. There are some, however, that are peculiar to, or more likely to occur among, surgical patients. During the period of diagnosis, the patient may be subjected to a variety of procedures some of which are strenuous, embarrassing, and even painful. At the time surgery is performed the diagnosis may be uncertain, or the patient may believe that it is. Even when the diagnosis has been established as something relatively benign, it is not unusual for a patient to fear that he has cancer. The patient may not understand the nature of the procedure to be performed or believe that it will be more extensive than it is actually planned to be. Uncertainty about the diagnosis and required treatment can be the source of severe stress. Jesse was under psychological stress because he did not understand the extent of the planned surgical procedure. Another example is Mrs. Thomas, who had a small lump in her breast. Although her physician tried to assure her that the tumor was almost certainly benign (harmless), Mrs. Thomas was sure that it was malignant and that she would have a radical mastectomy. Previous to the removal of the tumor for examination, she was in a state of near-panic. During the period of recovery from the anesthetic, she wept and referred over and over to loss of her breast. Not until she was fully recovered from the anesthetic could she be assured that her breast had not been removed.

Among other sources of concern to some patients are the anesthetic, its effect, and its effectiveness in preventing pain, as well as the possibility that they may behave in an embarrassing manner. Mr. Thome wonders whether he

---

[6] Henry N. Harkens, Carl A. Moyer, Jonathan E. Rhoads, and Garrott Allen, *Surgery Principles And Practice*, 2nd ed., J. B. Lippincott Company, Philadelphia, p. 856.

will be awake or asleep during the operation. He has heard that people sometimes reveal secrets or say foolish or embarrassing things as they go to sleep. The man in the room next to him was awake while he was operated on, but he is not sure that he would like that, either. Is it really possible to prevent pain when one is awake? How does one lie awake and allow someone to cut into one's abdomen? If he is awake, will the time of the operation pass quickly or will it be endless and seem to go on and on? Will he have pain after the operation?

In some types of surgery, organs having special meaning to the patient may have to be removed. Although any organ can have some special significance to a given individual, certain ones are more likely to have special meaning than others. Since the heart is essential to survival, surgical procedures on the heart are likely to be associated with death. Surgery on the organs of reproduction may affect the individual's self-concept, so that he or she feels that he or she is less a man or woman. In the American culture, the breast is a symbol of femininity. A woman may therefore feel less a woman after losing a breast. When a surgical procedure either temporarily or permanently prevents a husband and wife from having sexual relations, it may affect the stability of the marriage or the individual may fear that it will. When the loss of a part of the body necessitates changes in the way of life of the patient or in his role at work or in the family, the patient usually experiences more or less anxiety.

Another source of anxiety is the risk to which the patient exposes himself by undergoing surgical therapy. The nurse should be aware of the fact that every operation, no matter how minor, is accompanied by some risk. The risk may be very slight or it may be great. When a new procedure or an exceptionally hazardous one is performed, the patient may be aware of the nature of the risk. He may also know that if surgery fails, his chances for living are negligible. Some of the above continue to be sources of anxiety during the period of recovery following the operation. Attention is given to provide the patient with sufficient care of good quality to assure him that his needs will be met. Possibly too little consideration is given to the effects of what the patient regards as too much care. For example, during the period when Mr. Norman was being prepared for, and immedidately following, the introduction of an aortic prosthesis (artificial aortic valve), he received more attention than he had possibly experienced over his entire life span. The effect was not to assure him, but to frighten him, for he said, "Who am I to receive all this care? No one has ever cared this much about me before. Why should they do so at this time? I must be terribly sick, or people would continue to ignore me as they have in the past." Following the immediate postoperative period, Mr. Norman became deeply depressed. Though some depression is common, Mr. Norman was unusually depressed. During an interview with a psychiatrist, he expressed his feelings. The nurse who cared for him before and immediately after the operation remembered that he had made a similar comment to her but she had not recognized its significance. Possibly, if he had had an opportunity to express his feelings previous to surgical therapy his depression would have been less severe.

What can be done to minimize anxiety among patients in the preoperative period?

Despite the virtual impossibility of eliminating all psychological stress, much can be done to minimize it. Among the various factors contributing to a lessening of psychological stress is a climate in which the patient feels that nurses and doctors are concerned for his welfare. Some of the actions that contribute to this include: (1) being kind and courteous, (2) preparing him for what to expect and for what is expected of him, (3) respecting his rights as an individual, (4) protecting his patterns of modesty, (5) determining his level of knowledge and what he wants to know, (6) personalizing his care by modifying those aspects of his care that are important to him, insofar as these modifications do not interfere with his recovery, (7) attending to his physiological and physical needs, and (8) utilizing other sources of support for him, such as arranging for him to talk with his spiritual advisor or a social worker.

Most of the points enumerated above are discussed in Chapter 6. Essentially their implementation does not differ for the patient undergoing surgical therapy from that required by any seriously ill patient.

In most situations, stress can usually be minimized by creating a climate in which the patient feels free to raise questions that are troubling him. To help to prevent misconceptions and misunderstandings, the patient requires information about the nature of the illness, why the surgery is needed, and what can be expected from the anesthetic and the surgical procedure and experience. He should be provided with information about hospital routines, the recovery room, and postoperative procedures. The patient wants to be assured that those who are responsible for his care are competent and will be available when he needs them. Though some of the above are the responsibility of the surgeon, nurses are frequently faced with questions which the patient asks for information and reassurance. Even when the surgeon provides the patient with a detailed explanation, the patient may be so overwhelmed and confused by the fact that surgery is necessary that he comprehends very little of what he is told. In addition, the patient may stand in awe of the surgeon and hesitate to ask questions. Later, when the patient has had an opportunity to think about his situation, he may have questions which should be answered. The nurse has an obligation to secure answers to the question or questions the patient is asking. Whether she answers the questions herself or refers them to the physician and how she answers those she does not refer depends on the nature of the questions and of her own competence.

When the patient has questions that the nurse cannot or is not permitted to answer, she can still be helpful to the patient. She can express her interest in the patient by listening to him and, if required, initiating action. Someone who is willing and able to listen may be all the patient wants or needs. She can also help the patient to clarify his questions and can encourage him to ask the surgeon for information. She can also determine the urgency of the need of the patient to have his question answered. Miss Elder had been in the hospital for some weeks for the treatment of a fractured hip. The fracture was treated by open reduction following which Miss Elder was encased in a double spica cast. About a week previous to the incident related below, she had been told that she might go home on the following Tuesday and all the arrangements had been made. The day before she planned to leave the hospital, the surgeon made a window in the cast in order to examine and dress the wound. After the required equipment was delivered to the room, the surgeon explained what he was going to do. Because Miss Elder was unprepared for the procedure, she heard nothing. Though her wound was healing nicely, she quickly concluded that it was not healing and that she would not be discharged from the hospital. She was so upset that she could not ask the surgeon for an explanation. Shortly after the surgeon left, a nurse found Miss Elder in tears. Although the nurse knew that Miss Elder was to be discharged as planned, she was sure that reassurance of the patient depended on direct word from her physician. She immediately called him and he assured her that Miss Elder was to be discharged the following day. This information was relayed to Miss Elder so that she could relax and complete her plans for leaving the hospital.

In some hospitals the problem of what patients can be told about the nature of their illness, why surgery is needed, and what can be expected during all phases of illness is met by the preparation of two types of manuals which the patient may be given to read and the nursing staff given to use as a guide in answering questions. One type includes essential information about the nature of a particular disease and its therapy, or its content may deal primarily with the surgical aspects of therapy. For example, one manual might cover the disease diabetes mellitus and its treatment. Another might be prepared for the use of the patient having a colostomy or thoracic surgery. These manuals emphasize what the patient needs to know to help himself recover and answers frequently asked questions. They are usually prepared by a committee of physicians and nurses.

A second type of manual provides information about hospital routines such as admission procedures, visiting hours, and special facilities such as the recovery room. The guide may also include suggestions about how the patient and his visitors can help to facilitate the recovery of the patient as well as what they can expect from the hospital personnel. It may be given to the patient before admission by the physician or at the time he is admitted. Any material preparing the patient for what to expect and for what is expected of him should be helpful. In addition to well-prepared written explanations, the patient needs oral instruction as to what to expect. Admission to the hospital is accompanied by emotional stress and, at the time, the patient is likely to be more or less confused. Some attention should be given to the family of the patient. Relatives should know the time the patient is expected to be taken to the operating room and whether or not he is expected to return to his room immediately after his operation or will be cared for in a recovery room or an intensive care unit. For example, a patient may remain only until he has regained consciousness and major physiological derangements have been corrected, or for 24 to 48 or more hours. Whatever the practice is, the patient and his family should be prepared for what to expect. They should know that the recovery room or intensive care unit is a service provided for the welfare of the patient.

Summary

The psychological status of the patient is an important factor in his capacity to withstand the stress imposed by surgery. How the patient regards the surgical procedure that is to be performed, as well as its possible effects, influences his chances for survival and for recovery. The nurse may be helpful to the patient and to his family by providing a climate in which the patient feels free to express his feelings and in which he feels accepted and esteemed as an individual human being. She can also be helpful to the patient by relaying any concerns that he has to the physician, so that the physician can more accurately assess the psychological status of the patient and plan to correct his misconceptions and misinformation. To paraphrase Fielding (see Chapter 2), when fears are hidden, they grow until they become overwhelming, but when they are taken out and examined, they can be put into their true perspective and confined.

What are some of the physiological factors that are evaluated in the preoperative period?

Just as surgical therapy places a strain on the capacity of the patient to maintain emotional homeostasis, it also places a burden on his capacity to maintain physiological homeostasis. An important aspect of making the patient safe for surgical therapy is, therefore, the evaluation of his physiological status. The results of this evaluation are used as a basis for a regimen for the prevention or correction of abnormalities in physiological homeostasis. The investigation of the status of the patient includes: (1) an evaluation of all homeostatic conditions with particular emphasis on his nutritional state, (2) the identification of any diseases or disorders that increase the risk of surgical therapy, and (3) an estimation of the capacity of the patient to tolerate additional stress and to respond favorably. All of the above are, of course, interrelated.

Because there is a relationship between age and the capacity of the individual to maintain physiological homeostasis under stress, the age of the patient has some bearing on the risks to which he is exposed during surgical therapy. Very young children tolerate the trauma of surgery remarkably well and recover quickly. They are, however, easily upset, and they are particularly sensitive to chilling, exposure, and rough handling. Gius[7] states that the loss of an ounce of blood by an infant is equivalent to the loss of a pint of blood by an adult. The infant should therefore be closely observed for evidence of blood loss, since seemingly small losses represent a relatively large part of his blood volume. With proper care, an infant survives surgical therapy very well. He must be protected from conditions in the environment predisposing to chilling. These include a low environmental temperature, drafts, and wet clothing.

At the other end of the life span, the elderly patient has generally been believed to tolerate surgical therapy poorly. Although modern surgical management has greatly reduced the hazards of surgery to the elderly patient, some surgeons have known for many years that old age, by itself, is not a contraindication to surgical therapy. One surgeon who is frequently quoted on this point is Sir James Paget.[8] He wrote:

Years, indeed, taken alone are a very fallacious mode of reckoning age: it is not the time but the quality of a man's past life that we have to reckon. . . . The old people that are thin and dry and tough, clear-voiced and bright-eyed, with good stomachs and strong wills, muscular and active, are not bad; they bear all but the largest operations very well. But very bad are they, who looking somewhat like these are feeble and soft skinned, with little pulses, bad appetites, and weak digestive powers; so that they cannot in an emergency be well nourished.

Moyer,[9] in a summary of a review of the literature on the influence of age on operative mortality, concludes that: (1) the operative mortality is higher among the aged in disorders accompanied by pus formation or other complications such as perforation of a viscus, (2) the operative mortality rate is the same for all groups in disorders that are seldom accompanied by complications, and (3) the death rate from burns is higher among the aged than among younger persons.

In more general terms, the elderly person's capacity to respond to the stress of a single surgical procedure of short duration is satisfactory, but he is less able to tolerate prolonged stress and multiple stresses than are younger persons. The elderly person is less able to tolerate disorders accompanied by prolonged physiological disturbances. Because he has less reserve than the younger person, the old person's capacity to maintain and to restore homeostasis in the presence of continued strain is less than that of a younger person. He is more likely to have one or more chronic diseases which decrease his reserve or place a burden on his capacity to adapt. When the strain placed on

---

[7] John Armes Gius, *Fundamentals of General Surgery,* 2nd ed., Year Book, Inc., Chicago, 1962, p. 260.

[8] Sir James Paget, *Clinical Lectures and Essays,* London, 1877, quoted in U. H. Eversole, "The Anesthetic Management of the Elderly Patient in Surgery," *Surgical Clinics of North America,* XXXIV, June, 1954, p. 622.

[9] Earl A. Moyer, in Harkens, *Op. cit.,* p. 188.

his adaptive capacity is within his reserve, he responds favorably. As in the care of the very young, attention should be given to preventing unnecessary demands on the adaptive capacity of the elderly person.

When planning and implementing the nursing care of the elderly patient, the nurse should be mindful of the fact that as people age, their renal, cardiovascular, and pulmonary reserves diminish. As a consequence, these structures are less able to cope with conditions placing stress on their functional capacity, and they are more likely to be sites of complication than they are in young persons. As implied, among the elderly, the exact chronological age of the patient is of less significance than his outlook and physiological status. A hopeful optimistic attitude combined with a good nutritional status and reasonable cardiovascular, renal, and pulmonary reserve makes an elderly person quite safe for surgery.

In addition to age, what other kinds of disorders reduce the capacity of the individual to adapt to surgery?

Any disorder that reduces the capacity of the individual to adapt and to maintain homeostatic conditions increases the risk of surgery. Among the many disorders increasing risk are shock; hemorrhage; disorders in water and electrolyte balance; acidosis and alkalosis; anemia; pulmonary, cardiac, and renal disorders; undernutrition; hypoproteinemia; obesity; adrenal insufficiency; pregnancy; alcoholism; hyperthyroidism; diabetes mellitus; disease of the liver; and psychic and emotional disturbances. All these disorders lessen in some manner the capacity of the individual to maintain homeostasis. Some, such as disturbances in water and electrolyte balance, indicate impairment of one or more homeostatic conditions. Most of the disturbances increasing surgical risk are discussed elsewhere. Comments that follow will be limited to the relationship of a few of the above to surgical risk. When the life of the patient is not immediately threatened, surgical treatment is usually delayed until the physiological and psychological condition of the patient is such that he is relatively safe for surgery. In the investigation of the patient, the surgeon is interested in uncovering any condition that will make the development of a complication more likely or to reduce the capacity of the person to adapt to stress.

Among the important factors influencing response to surgery is the nutritional state of the patient. Since the various factors in nutrition have been covered in Chapter 10, they will not be reviewed here. Among the nutritional factors that are of greatest significance to the surgical patient are undernutrition, with or without hypoproteinemia, and obesity. Adequate nutrition is essential to the general response of the patient and to wound healing. The nutritional elements that are of the most importance in wound healing are protein and vitamins B and C.

Of the patients who are treated surgically, some are more likely to be undernourished than others. Chronically ill and aged persons are more likely to be malnourished than are previously healthy children and adults. Persons who have disturbances in the functioning of the alimentary tract are predisposed to malnutrition, from failure to either ingest, absorb, or retain food in the alimentary canal long enough for it to be digested and absorbed. The patient who has lost protein-containing body fluids, including blood, is likely to suffer from hypoproteinemia. One often neglected aspect relating to nutrition is the effect on the patient's nutritional status of diagnostic examinations which require the withholding of food and purging. For example, examinations of the alimentary canal usually are preceded by withholding of food and fluids, sometimes for an extended period of time. In the already dehydrated and undernourished patient, both conditions are aggravated. For these patients, it is essential that food and fluids be served, unless contraindicated, between meal feedings and bedtime snacks; this will also aid in increasing the food and fluid intake. All these measures require a thoughtful concern for the welfare of the patient and appropriate planning. All the measures suggested in Chapter 10 may be required to improve the nutritional status of the patient sufficiently to make him safe for surgery.

Obesity is also a problem in many patients. Since it cannot be corrected quickly, excessively obese patients may be placed on a weight-reduction regimen and surgery delayed until the patient reaches a satisfactory weight. Obesity burdens the patient with a number of handicaps. Since fat has a poor blood supply, it is more susceptible to infection than are tissues with a larger blood supply. Large amounts of fat increase the difficulty of exposing organs in the abdominal cavity, and may reduce the pulmonary vital capacity by pressure on the diaphragm. The problems associated with weight reduction have been presented in Chapter 10.

Some disorders that are associated with undernutrition are also responsible for the loss of water and electrolytes. In addition to insufficient water and/or electrolytes, water may accumulate in body cavities or in the interstitial spaces in the form of edema. Since water and electrolyte balance is treated in another chapter, other than to say that it is a significant factor in surgical risk, it will not be further discussed.

Since conditions in the lung and tracheobronchial tree affect and are affected by the response of the patient to anesthesia, unconsciousness, and bed rest, correcting—or minimizing the effects of abnormalities in these structures—is imperative. X ray examination of the chest is an essential part of the assessment of the status of the respiratory system. It is useful in detecting tuberculosis and emphysema as well as many other disorders of the lung. Among the disorders that aggravate the problem of cleansing the airway in the immediate postoperative period are tracheobronchitis and emphysema. Tracheobronchitis is more common in persons who smoke than in nonsmokers. When tracheobronchitis is present and the person smokes, he is usually encouraged to stop or to reduce the amount he smokes.

The patient who has a large accumulation of secretions in the tracheo-bronchial tree may be instructed to perform postural drainage. This has been described in Chapter 7. The patient who has a disorder that makes keeping the tracheobronchial tree clean more difficult will require more attention to this function in the immediate postoperative period than the patient who has no such disorder.

How is the cardiovascular system evaluated?

In the evaluation of the cardiovascular system, the condition and reserve capacity of the heart and blood vessels are investigated. When there is evidence of pathology, the physician then tries to estimate the adequacy of the cardiac reserve, as this knowledge provides him with evidence that the patient will or will not be able to tolerate the strain of surgery. Contrary to popular opinion, the patient may have considerable pathology and the heart still be able to tolerate a surgical procedure with little or no difficulty.

In the evaluation of the state of the blood vessels, two factors are reviewed. One is the capacity of the body to adapt the diameter of the blood vessels to the changing needs of the organism. The other is the adequacy of the blood supply to the tissues which will be operated on. The level of the blood pressure of the patient provides information about the first factor. In a patient with a blood pressure below 90 systolic or above 120 diastolic, the capacity of the patient to adapt to the stress of surgery is likely to be inadequate. The patient with an excessively low systolic blood pressure may be suffering from adrenal insufficiency or from shock. The one with the high diastolic pressure is bordering on renal failure. Both require special care to survive surgery. Since healing is dependent on the adequacy of the blood supply, an estimation of the capacity of blood vessels to deliver sufficient blood to the tissues is essential in any condition where there is a question. Pallor and coldness of extremities and blanching on pressure with slow return of color are indications that the amount of blood being delivered to the tissue is less than adequate.

The capacity of the circulatory system to deliver supplies to the tissue depends not only on the competence of the heart as a pump and the adaptability and patency of the blood vessels, but on the quantity and quality of the blood. Following an acute hemorrhage both the quality and quantity of the blood may be diminished. In longstanding nutritional deficiencies or those associated with the chronic loss of blood, the quality of blood may be poor. The most commonly used measure of the quantity of blood in relation to the size of the vascular system is the blood pressure. The quality of the blood in relation to its red cell content may be measured by either the hematocrit or the hemoglobin content, or both. A reduction of either indicates a decrease in the oxygen-carrying capacity of the blood. Because the adequacy of the oxygen-carrying power of the blood and the blood volume both directly affect the chances of the patient for survival, surgery is seldom scheduled until arrangements have been made to replace needed blood. If the surgical procedure is one entailing a large loss of blood, additional blood may be required to replace that which is lost at the time of the operation.

How is renal function evaluated?

In any condition in which the body is placed under increased physiological stress, the capacity of the kidney to function is of great significance. It functions in homeostasis to eliminate or conserve water and electrolytes and it eliminates the wastes of protein metabolism. In the absence of evidence to indicate that the kidney reserve is limited, or that the kidney is diseased, the urine is tested for sugar, acetone, and albumin. The presence of sugar and acetone in the urine are not tests of kidney function but they are important because they are presumptive evidence of diabetes mellitus. Albumin in the urine, on the other hand, indicates the presence of some condition that limits blood flow through the kidney or of injury to it. In a woman, albumin may not be significant unless the urine specimen is obtained by catheter. In order to estimate the adequacy of kidney function, the level of the urea or of nonprotein nitrogen in the blood is determined. Other tests of kidney function include the capacity of the kidney to concentrate phenolsulfonphthalein in the urine or to increase its specific gravity when water is withheld.

Evaluation of renal function is important not only because it influences operative risk, but because it affects the capacity of the patient to handle the parenteral fluid and electrolytes administered during the postoperative period. Although output should be compared with intake in all patients, in the patient with limited renal reserve this is essential.

During the preoperative period, disorders affecting operative risk are identified and treated so that their effect can be minimized. In addition to corrective therapy, attention is paid to preventive care, one aspect of which is ambulation. Attention to ambulation is most important for the patient who is admitted to the hospital for diagnosis and preparation for surgery. Patients who remain at home during this period are less likely to be able to remain in bed. Though the patient was once kept in bed because it was thought that rest conserved strength, recent studies indicate that bed rest results in a loss of strength, as well as of proteins and other nutrients. Exercise within the limits tolerated by the patient improves his psychological as well as his physiological status. When the patient feels unwell, he may have to be encouraged to be up and about, while the patient who feels reasonably well may require some protection from overactivity. The patient should have the help that he needs to get out of bed and to walk. In order to make certain that he does ambulate, there should be a plan to ensure it. Because most people eat better when they are out of bed, part of the plan might include getting the patient into the chair for his meals. Depending on how the patient feels, he might then have a rest period followed by a bath, then another rest period followed by a walk down the hall. When he is in bed, he should be encouraged to do deep-breathing exercises and to flex and extend his feet and legs. By alternating periods of activity with rest, the patient builds up his strength and is at the same time protected from overactivity.

How is the gastrointestinal tract prepared for surgery?

In addition to the correction of conditions adding to the hazards of surgery and the general psychological and physiological preparation, which may take several days or longer, the gastrointestinal tract and the skin are prepared during the hours just preceding surgery. Regardless of whether or not the gastrointestinal tract is directly involved, preparation of the patient for surgery almost always includes emptying the gastrointestinal tract. Food and fluids are withheld and the lower bowel is emptied by the administration of one or more enemas. In the past, to make sure that the stomach was empty at the time of surgery, food and fluids were withheld from midnight until the surgery was performed the following day. Many surgeons have modified this procedure in terms of the time it takes the stomach to empty, for prolonged abstinence from food and fluid is of no general value and increases the likelihood of dehydration. Unless there is an obstruction, no food remains in the stomach after six hours. Liquids remain in the stomach much less time. In fact, they may pass immediately from the esophagus to the duodenum. To make sure that the stomach is empty, food intake is restricted for four to eight hours and fluids are prohibited for four hours before surgery. An empty stomach is important, because it reduces the likelihood of the patient's vomiting and aspirating gastric juice into the lung; when gastric juice is inhaled, it produces a serious type of pneumonitis. However, dehydration of the patient is not necessary to prevent aspiration.

In preparation for many major abdominal operations such as gastric surgery, intubation of the stomach may be performed to remove the secretions and to empty the stomach. When the patient has an obstruction of the intestinal tract, decompression of the bowel may be necessary before he can be operated on with safety. The cause and effects of obstruction of the alimentary canal are presented in Chapter 10. Gastric or intestinal intubation with suction may be employed during the postoperative phase of surgery as well as in the preparation of the patient for surgical treatment. Following surgery, the purpose is usually to relieve physiological or mechanical obstruction.

Decompression is accomplished by the introduction into the stomach or intestine of a tube to which suction is applied. Removal of fluids and gas from the stomach can be accomplished by a single-lumen Levin tube. Removal of the contents from the intestine requires a long tube with either a single or double lumen. A device is required at the end of the tube to facilitate its movement after it enters the duodenum. When a single-lumen tube is used, a bag filled with mercury is attached to the tip before it is inserted. When a double-lumen tube is used, one lumen opens into a balloon which is distended with water, air, or mercury; the other lumen provides for the removal of fluid and gas. Either type tube is passed through a nostril, the pharynx, and the esophagus to the stomach. After the short tube (Levin) reaches the stomach, it is taped to the face. No tube should be taped to the nose and above the eye, because when the tube is taped in this position it presses on the underside of the nostril and may cause pressure necrosis. Rather it should be taped to the upper lip or otherwise anchored in the position that it takes naturally. See Figures 15-1, 15-2, and 15-3.

The long tube is passed from the stomach through the pylorus and into the duodenum. The passage of the tube through the pylorus may be facilitated by having the patient lie on his right side. After the tube enters the duodenum, the physician inflates the balloon; peristalsis will then carry the balloon and tube through the intestine. To hasten the movement of the tube toward the site of the obstruction, the physician may leave an order for the nurse to advance the tube a specific distance at regular intervals of time. If the patient is able, he can assist in this by swallowing as the tube is pushed forward. The act of swallowing also helps to suppress the gag reflex. During the procedure the physician can check the location of the tube by X ray or by fluoroscopic examination. When the tube reaches the desired site, it is then taped in a manner previously described.

After either the short or long tube has reached the stomach, suction is applied. There are a number of methods of producing suction. The principle

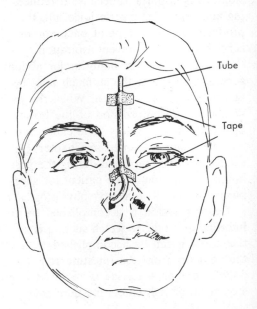

FIGURE 15-1. NO. This technique will soon produce pressure necrosis on the underside of the nostril.

on which suction devices are based is that energy runs downhill, or, in terms of the contents of the alimentary canal, fluids and gases move from an area of greater pressure to one of lesser pressure. The method that is selected depends

Suggested Techniques for Anchoring Nasal Tubes with Tape.

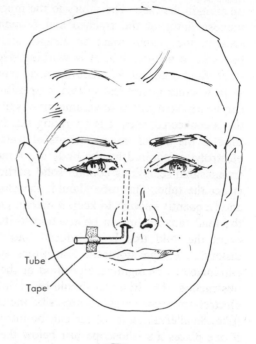

FIGURE 15—2. YES. When this technique is used, adherence of the tape must be checked frequently; when the patient perspires, the upper lip soon becomes moist, and the tape is dislodged.

FIGURE 15—3. YES. When this technique is used, adherence of the tape to the nose must be checked frequently. Perspiration and skin oils cause the tape to loosen. The tape is split half its length, and the split ends are wrapped securely in opposite directions, around the tube after the broad end has been taped to the nose. The free end of the tube can then be taped over the zygomatic arch or secured to the clothing of the patient, to prevent pulling on the tube.

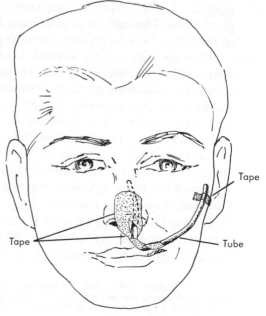

on the wishes of the physician and the equipment provided by the hospital.[10] Whatever method is utilized to secure suction, the force should be gentle; usually not in excess of 1.5 lb. of negative pressure. When excessive suction is applied, the mucosa lining the intestine or stomach may be sucked into the opening in the tube. The injury to the mucosa is similar to that induced in the mucosa lining of the trachea and bronchi by excessive suction. To secure suction, the system must be airtight and the device should be checked at intervals to be sure that it is working. However, since secretion is not constant, fluid does not flow continuously from the tube. Should there be doubt as to whether or not the system is operating, the tube leading to the stomach can be irrigated with a small amount of saline. If fluid returns when the apparatus is connected, then it is operating satisfactorily. Frequent irrigations of the tube or the use of large amounts of water should be avoided, as water and electrolytes required by the body are removed in the process. However, gastrointestinal secretions contain solid particles which may accumulate and obstruct the tube. The tube should, therefore, be irrigated at regular intervals and frequently enough to keep it patent. Occasionally when a tube is irrigated, the fluid runs in, but an obstruction to its return acts as a ball valve. In this event the fluid that is introduced into the stomach contributes to further distention of the stomach. Sometimes the obstruction of the tube can be eliminated by changing the position of the patient. If this does not relieve the obstruction, the physician should be notified. To prevent the loss of fluids and electrolytes, some surgeons prescribe the use of air to check the patency of the tube. Smaller amounts of air can be introduced, and thus distention avoided, if one places a stethoscope just below the xiphoid process and listens for the muffled "woosh" which accompanies the passage of air through a patent gastric tube. The amount of air required varies with the length and diameter of the tube; with a Levin tube, for example, 15 to 25 ml. is usually adequate.

When the outlet of the stomach is obstructed, a large tube with multiple openings may be required to remove the food particles and other debris that accumulate. Cleansing of the stomach may be furthered by pouring water into the tube and then removing it. The procedure is repeated until the solution that returns is clear. Because of the size of the tube, it is passed through the mouth and is removed at the completion of the procedure.

Gastrointestinal intubation is frequently accompanied by psychological stress in the patient. Many patients regard this as one of the most disagreeable aspects of the entire operative experience. Mrs. Repeat illustrates this point very well. Two and a half years ago, she had abdominal surgery. She says, "The thing that I dread the most is having all those tubes. Worst of all is that tube they put into my stomach." When gastric intubation is a part of a patient's preoperative preparation, he should be helped to understand how

[10] For students who wish an extensive review of intubation and drainage of the alimentary canal, see Bertha Harmer, and Virginia Henderson, *Textbook of the Principles and Practice of Nursing*, 5th ed., The Macmillan Company, New York, 1955, pp. 823-39.

intubation contributes to his recovery. He should also understand how the tube is passed and what he can do to help and what will be done to assist him. He should know that the tube will be lubricated to make it pass more easily. He should also know that he will be able to help by swallowing as the tube is passed and that he will be reminded to swallow at the appropriate times. The patient who has had the symptoms that accompany obstruction may welcome the relief which the introduction of the tube brings.

Although the physician usually passes the tube, the nurse may be required to learn to do it. Before the nurse does this, she should prepare herself by studying the anatomy of the area and acquaint herself with the possible difficulties she may encounter. In addition to preparing the patient for what to expect and for what is expected of him, she also prepares the patient physically. The patient may be in either the recumbent or the sitting position. In either event, the head should be hyperextended. Because the patient is likely to gag and may vomit and secretions are increased, he should have a supply of paper tissues and an emesis basin within easy reach. The required equipment and supplies should be at hand and in working order before the procedure is started. Thorough lubrication of the tube makes for ease in passing it. If oil is used, any excess should be removed to decrease the danger of aspiration of oil into the lungs. Because of this possibility some physicians prefer to use glycerine or a water-soluble substance to lubricate the tube. As the tube is passed the patient should be reminded at appropriate intervals to swallow. Some patients find swallowing easier, if they are allowed sips of water as the tube is passed. Patients should be kept apprised of the success of their efforts and they should know when the tube reaches the stomach. The nurse should be mindful of the fact that the tube cannot be passed through the upper alimentary canal without the cooperation of the patient who is conscious. Each patient should know what his role is and be helped to carry it out.

The mouth of the patient who is undergoing gastric or intestinal decompression requires the same care as does that of any patient who is not taking food and fluid by mouth. The patient should have an opportunity to brush his teeth and rinse his mouth with mouthwash three or four times a day. Mouthwash, if not overused, is refreshing. Too frequent rinsing of the mouth contributes to dehydration by loss of saliva. The flow of saliva may be stimulated by encouraging the patient to chew gum, or to suck lemon or orange slices or sour lemon balls. The saliva helps to keep the mouth moist and clean. It also washes out the ducts leading from the parotid gland and decreases the possibility of surgical parotitis. Free drainage from any gland is essential to its health. Blocking of the duct from a gland favors the development of infection in the gland.

When the tube is left in place for some days, the throat may be irritated by it. The patient may be allowed sips of water or anesthetic troches to relieve the soreness. When he is allowed water, attention should be given to limiting the amount of water taken to that prescribed by the physician. Any water that is taken returns through the tube bringing with it electrolytes that are secreted into the stomach. The relief that the patient obtains is therefore at the expense of his body's electrolytes. Some surgeons remove the tube after two or three days and allow the patient to have a period of rest. The tube is then reinserted 12 or 18 hours later, if the patient continues to require it. After the tube has been removed, the nurse should observe the patient for signs and symptoms that indicate that the gastrointestinal tract is not functioning. These include a feeling of fullness, vomiting, and distention. The sensation of fullness is often the earliest symptom to indicate that the stomach is failing to empty. It, along with any other symptoms, should be reported promptly. Instead of removing the tube, the degree to which the function of the alimentary canal has been restored can be tested by clamping the tube for a period of time. When the tube is clamped, the patient should be checked for the symptoms just listed above. When the tube is unclamped, the amount of fluid escaping from the tube should be measured. Any accumulation of fluid indicates that gastrointestinal function has not yet been restored.

Because the nostril through which the tube is passed may be irritated by the tube and the secretions that are encrusted on it, the tube may be passed through the opposite nostril when it has to be reintroduced. Sometimes structural abnormalities make it difficult if not impossible to use the other nostril, however.

As long as the tube is in place, the nurse should observe the amount and character of fluid that is returned through it. Any abnormality of color or odor is important. Since the effectiveness of the procedure depends on the equipment being in working order, it is the duty of the nurse to check at regular intervals to make sure that the system is airtight and operating.

As peristalsis resumes or the obstruction is relieved, the surgeon removes the tube or clamps it. The removal of a tube from the stomach is relatively simple. The removal of the long tube is more complicated. If the tube has passed the ileocecal valve, the surgeon will cut the tube and allow it to progress through the gastrointestinal tract, as the forcible return of the tube and balloon through the valve will damage it. Hardy[11] cautions that the tube should not be released at the nose until it has been secured below. Otherwise a laparatomy may be required to retrieve the tube. The patient may need to be reassured that the tube will progress through the alimentary canal just as the normal contents do. When the tube is returned through the mouth, the doctor pulls gently and allows the intestine time to release its attachment to the tube.

Because fluids and electrolytes are removed by the suction, the oral fluid intake of the patient is restricted, and fluids are administered by intravenous infusion. In order to have a basis for determining the adequacy of the fluid intake of the patient, his urine output should be measured as long as the gastric or intestinal tube is in place.

[11] James D. Hardy, *Pathophysiology in Surgery,* The Williams & Wilkins Company, Baltimore, 1958, p. 332.

In addition to the preparation of the upper alimentary canal for surgery, the colon and rectum are usually emptied by the administration of one or more enemas. The reason generally advanced is that the practice lessens the possibility of soiling on the operating table. Not all surgeons, however, agree that enemas are either necessary or desirable. Harbison[12] condemns the routine practice of giving an enema in the preoperative preparation of patients. He states that since most people defecate early in the day, an enema is unphysiological and it also subjects most people to unnecessary psychological stress. According to Harbison,[13] the omission of the enema prior to a general anesthetic does not increase the incidence of soiling of the operating room table. There are, of course, other reasons for cleansing the lower bowel before an operative procedure. When the intestine itself is the site of surgery, it is cleansed to lessen the likelihood of spillage of its contents into the peritoneal cavity. In surgical procedures involving organs in the pelvic cavity, an empty bowel is essential to the exposure of the operative site and to its protection from injury. When barium studies have been made of the gastrointestinal tract, enemas may be required to remove the barium in order to prevent it from forming an impaction postoperatively. In some disorders such as acute appendicitis, enemas are contraindicated in the preparation of the patient for surgery as the fluid introduced into the intestine raises the pressure within the intestine and stimulates peristalsis. When the solution contains soap or some other irritating agent, peristalsis is further intensified, and the danger of perforation of the appendix is enhanced.

In surgery on the large intestine, prevention of contamination of the wound and the peritoneal and pelvic cavities by feces requires that special measures be taken to lessen the volume of feces. Bacteria are responsible for more than half the weight of the dried stool. These organisms are harmless and may even be helpful as long as they remain in the intestine. However, when they escape into the peritoneal or other body cavities, they may cause serious morbidity. Since the introduction of antibiotics and chemical antiseptics that are not absorbed from the intestine, the intestinal contents can be sterilized, and repeated irrigations are no longer necessary. Because of the variety of bacteria as well as yeasts and molds in the intestinal contents, a number of agents may be required. The use of antibacterial agents has simplified the preparation of the patient for bowel surgery. Previous to their introduction, the patient was subjected to the stress of repeated purging and bowel irrigations.

What measures are employed in the preparation of the skin at the site of the incision?

An important aspect of the immediate preparation of the patient for surgery is the thorough cleansing of the skin. Both the skin and mucous

---

[12] Samuel P. Harbison, "Unnecessary Routine Surgery," *Journal of the American Medical Association,* CLII, May 30, 1953, pp. 396-98.

[13] *Ibid.,* p. 396.

membranes have large numbers of bacteria on their surfaces. These organisms are usually harmless unless they are provided with a portal of entry, such as a break in the skin. Despite differences in details or routines, the objective toward which the preparation of the skin is directed is to reduce the number of microorganisms on it to a minimum and at the same time protect it from injury. The skin must be thoroughly cleansed but not broken or damaged in the process. In some hospitals patients who are able are asked to shower or take a tub bath, and those who are not able are given a bath in bed. In other hospitals, only those patients whose skins can be seen to be dirty are bathed. When showering or bathing is part of the preoperative preparation, the patient should understand that this requirement is not a reflection on his standard of cleanliness or hygiene. When a sudsing agent containing a germicide is employed, the germicide must have time to act. Varco[14] suggests that part of the skin preparation should be repeated sudsing of the skin with an agent containing hexachloraphene. He[15] also states that, in theory, the skin should not be shaved the day or evening before the operation is scheduled, because if the skin is broken, bacteria have an opportunity to enter the lesion and to multiply. If the incision crosses the area where bacteria have entered the tissue, they may be carried deep into the wound.

Whether or not the entire body is showered or bathed, the region surrounding the projected site of the surgery should undergo special cleansing to remove microorganisms and materials that may harbor microorganisms. Two procedures, washing with a sudsing detergent and shaving, are usual. When cationic surface active agents such as benzalkonium chloride solution U.S.P., (Zephiran Chloride[16]) are employed in preparation of the skin, soap should not be used as the lathering agent previous to the operation. Because soap is anionic[17] it antagonizes the action of the cationic agents. Care should be taken to remove all the hair and to avoid nicking the skin. The size of the area to be shaved depends on the nature of the proposed surgical procedure and the directions of the surgeon. Crile[18] states that pubic hair should be shaved only when necessary. The discomfort suffered by the patient as the hair grows outweighs any advantage of its removal. For this reason some surgeons do not require the pubic hair to be shaved preceding a dilatation of the cervix and curettage of the uterus. Harbison[19] states that larger areas are often shaved more than is necessary. He agrees that the pubic hair does not require removal previous to abdominal surgery. Eyebrows should not be removed. Though Harbison blames outdated nursing texts for extensive skin preparation, some surgeons are of the opinion that it is necessary. Perhaps one implication

[14] Richard Varco, "Principles of Preoperative and Postoperative Care," in Loyal Davis (ed.), *Christopher's Textbook of Surgery,* 7th ed., W. B. Saunders Co., Philadelphia, 1960, p. 104.
[15] *Ibid.,* p. 105.
[16] Trade name.
[17] Goodman and Gilman, *Op. cit.,* p. 1110.
[18] George Crile, Jr., and Franklin L. Shively, Jr., *Hospital Care of the Surgical Patient,* 2nd ed., Charles C Thomas, Springfield, Illinois, 1946, p. 125.
[19] *Op. cit.,* p. 397.

of the questions raised about the validity of some routine practices in pre-operative preparation is that nurses as well as physicians should examine what they do in terms of its value and effects.

Because of the serious nature of bone infections, some orthopedic surgeons order that the skin be specially prepared. In preparation for surgery on a bone, the skin is washed with a detergent and shaved and covered with sterile towels; this procedure may be repeated twice daily for several days. Particular attention should be given to preventing nicks in the skin. The towels should be anchored so that they stay in place, and the equipment and materials used should be sterile. Attention should be paid to principles essential to the maintenance of asepsis.

Preparation of the scalp for a surgical incision also requires some modification of the ordinary procedure. Before the hair can be cut and the scalp shaved, a permit from the patient or a responsible member of the family is usually required. As a rule, arrangements are made to have a barber cut the hair and shave the scalp. Particularly for women, the removal of the hair is a source of considerable psychological stress. Members of the family, such as the husband or mother, may also be understandably distressed. For a not inconsiderable number of women, their hair is truly their crowning glory. Before the hair is removed, the nurse should make sure that the patient is not facing a mirror and that a head scarf or cap is ready to cover the head as soon as it is shaved. Some hospitals provide wigs for female patients. The hair should be placed in a paper bag and given to a relative. When a woman or girl has long hair, she may want to have a headpiece made from it. Now that headpieces and fancy caps are available to disguise the head, they should be used.

How is the patient sedated before surgery?

To ensure that the patient sleeps well and to reduce the apprehension of the patient, the surgeon usually prescribes a sedative for the patient the night preceding and the morning of surgery. The specific drug selected varies with the surgeon, but is often one of the barbiturates such as Pentobarbital (Nembutal), 0.05 to 0.1 gm, or secobarbital (Seconal), 0.1 to 0.2 gm. When the patient has been prepared for sleep, he should know whether or not the nurse expects to visit him during the night. Nothing can be more frightening to a person who sleeps in a room by himself at home than to go to sleep and to be awakened by someone opening the door and coming into the room. For example, Miss Tee was admitted to the hospital in the late afternoon for diagnostic surgery the following day. About nine in the evening she was given secobarbital (Seconal), 0.2 gm, and prepared for sleep. The door to her room was closed. At midnight an aide opened the door and entered her room to remove the water glass. Miss Tee awakened frightened, and, needless to say, she had difficulty returning to sleep.

The morning of surgery the same drug that was administered the preceding night is repeated. In addition, morphine, 8 to 15 mg, or meperidine hydro-chloride (Demerol), 50 to 100 mg, may be administered an hour before the operation is scheduled. Currently, there appears to be disagreement among physicians about the necessity and desirability of using either morphine or meperidine hydrochloride preoperatively. Some surgeons are of the opinion that they serve no useful purpose because, previous to the operation, patients do not have pain and the barbiturates are at least as effective as morphine in relieving preoperative apprehension. Morphine has some undesirable effects which are avoided by its omission. In some patients, it causes nausea and vomiting. It also depresses respiration, the cough reflex, and the activity of cilia in the tracheobronchial tree and increases the tone of the tracheobron-chial musculature. Although the latter effect is not usually of importance in man, it can be in the patient who is asthmatic. All these effects decrease the capacity of the patient to cleanse the tracheobronchial tree and to aerate the lung. The influence of morphine on mechanisms for cleansing the tracheo-bronchial tree is particularly undesirable in patients having thoracic and upper abdominal surgery.

Certain disorders or circumstances alter the patient's response to morphine. For example, the patient with hypothyroidism often becomes stuporous and suffers respiratory depression following small doses of morphine. According to Goodman and Gilman,[20] infants are not especially sensitive to morphine, if the dosage is adjusted to their body weight. In contrast, there is evidence that elderly persons are. Because morphine depresses the respiratory center and increases the cerebrospinal fluid pressure, it is contraindicated in patients who are undergoing brain surgery or who have had surgery of the brain. It is contraindicated after, as well as before, the operation.

To encourage an "I don't care" attitude on the part of the patient toward surgery and to counteract the tendency toward increased tracheobronchial secretions, atropine sulfate or scopolamine hydrobromide is frequently pre-scribed to be administered to the patient about one hour before the operation is scheduled. When the tranquilizing effects are desired, scopolamine is more likely to be selected than atropine. It normally causes drowsiness, amnesia, euphoria, and fatigue.[21] Occasionally it produces excitement, talkativeness, restlessness, and even delirium and hallucinations. Goodman and Gilman[22] point out that the patient who is given scopolamine when he is in pain is more likely to respond with excitement than if given it when he is free of pain. The nurse should anticipate this possibility when a patient who is in pain is given scopolamine. The more important action of both atropine and scopolamine is the depression of the effector cells of organs enervated by postganglionic cholinergic fibers. The effect desired is a decrease in secretions in the tracheo-bronchial tree. Because one of the results of the action of the alkaloids or

[20] *Op. cit.*, p. 235.
[21] *Ibid.*, p. 544.
[22] *Ibid.*, p. 544.

belladonna is dilation of the pupil, their use is contraindicated in patients who have glaucoma.

What are the responsibilities of the nurse in the immediate preoperative period?

In most hospitals the patient or a responsible relative signs a permit for the patient to undergo the contemplated surgery. While there is usually a time limit on the validity of the permit, the patient should sign it before he receives his preoperative medication. Practice varies as to who secures the signature of the patient, the physician or the nurse. Even when the physician is responsible, the nurse should ascertain whether or not the permit has been signed before administering the preoperative medication.

To prevent overdistention of the urinary bladder during the operative period and, with it, the danger of injury to the bladder or the soiling of the operative table, the urinary bladder should be emptied just before the patient is transferred to the operating room. To facilitate exposure of pelvic organs and to lessen the possibility of injury of the bladder during surgical procedures in the pelvic cavity, an indwelling catheter is usually introduced previous to surgery in this region.

Because of the danger of aspiration into the airway or dentures or removable bridges, they should be removed before the patient is transferred to the operating pavilion. Occasionally a patient has very strong feelings about having others see him without his teeth. In rare instances, when the psychological stress created by removing dental prostheses is very great, the nurse should explore the possibility of the patient keeping them in place until he arrives in the operating room. They can then be removed and returned to the patient's room or ward. Care should be taken to prevent the loss of dentures. Their loss or damage subjects the patient to inconvenience and psychological stress and the hospital and patient to added expense.

If the patient does not already wear some form of identification such as an identification bracelet, an identification tag should be prepared and attached to him before he is transferred to the operating room. On it should be his full name, his hospital number, the name of the surgeon, and any other information that is required. The chart of the patient should be complete. The following should be included: (1) his morning temperature, pulse, and respiration, (2) the results of the blood tests, hematocrit or hemoglobin, and the urinalysis, (3) the drugs that were administered preoperatively, and (4) any significant observation that relates to the patient's emotional or physiological status. Should any of the above be found to be abnormal, the abnormality should be drawn to the attention of the physician.

Though the practice varies from hospital to hospital, the patient may be transported to the operating room in his bed, on a cart, or in a wheel chair. Even if an orderly is responsible, when possible the nurse should accompany the patient. In some hospitals relatives are encouraged to accompany the patient as far as the entrance of the operating suite. Throughout the entire preoperative period every effort should be made to convey to the patient and his family: (1) that the welfare of the patient is the prime consideration in his care, and (2) that all persons who participate in his care are competent and trustworthy.

Summary of Essential Points in the Preoperative Preparation of Patients

In the preoperative preparation of the patient, the care of the patient is planned and organized to meet the objectives: (1) to prepare the patient psychologically, (2) to prepare him physically, and (3) to prepare him physiologically for the operative experience. The time available to accomplish each of these varies. One patient is admitted the afternoon of the day before he is to undergo surgery; another may have been in the hospital for weeks or months. Unless emergency surgery is contemplated, the patient who is in the hospital for only a short period of time receives much of the preliminary preparation for his operation in the physician's office and/or clinic. The way in which nurses in the office or clinic treat him and his problems contributes to his preparation for his hospital experience. Courtesy and thoughtfulness on the part of everyone from the doorman to the nursing personnel contribute to the feeling of the patient that he is welcome and that everyone is interested in his welfare.

What are some of the significant aspects of the care of the patient during the operative phase of surgery?

The operative period begins the moment the patient enters the operating room and ends when the last stitch is in place. During this time the needs of the patient are met by a team of individuals each of whom has a well-defined role and tasks and on whom other members of the team depend. Some members of the team are removed from direct contact with the patient, but every member acts in behalf of the patient. The surgeon is the leader of the team, but certain circumstances may make it necessary for him to temporarily relinquish his leadership role.

Throughout the operative phase the surgeon also gives attention to the prevention of serious physiological disturbances. He ties blood vessels before he cuts them, and he tries to prevent excessive loss of fluid by covering exposed organs with moist towels. He handles organs and tissues gently. He estimates blood loss, or when procedures are long and there is the possibility of considerable loss of blood, he has the sponges weighed. He takes time to identify structures so that the blood supply to the tissues in the area is maintained and injury to important structures is prevented. He also attends to the nature of the response of the patient and modifies the surgical procedure in terms of the reaction of the patient. During the operative phase, the complications that are most troublesome and frequent are those of hemorrhage, shock, and hypoxia. Since these complications may also be problems in the post-operative phase, they will be discussed later. During the operative phase of surgical therapy, the purposes of the operation are, hopefully, accomplished, and the dangers to which the patient is exposed are controlled. When the last suture is in place, the postoperative phase begins. Many of the problems encountered by the patient during the postoperative phase depend on the care and attention the patient received in earlier phases of treatment.

A second member of the surgical team is the anesthetist. In some hospitals, the anesthetist visits the patient and acquaints him with what to expect from the anesthetic experience. During the operative procedure the anesthetist has several important responsibilities. One is to induce a sufficient degree of anesthesia to prevent the patient from having pain and to secure the degree of relaxation necessary to the performance of the operation. The anesthetist is also concerned with the observation and maintenance of the physiological status of the patient. He pays particular attention to:

1. Maintenance of a clear or patent airway. In addition to the usual problems encountered in the maintenance of an open airway, the patient must be protected from aspirating secretions from the gastrointestinal tract into the airway. The danger of aspiration may be a problem in patients who have emergency surgery, because time may not be sufficient to allow the stomach to empty itself.
2. Maintenance of adequate breathing and exchange of gases (oxygen and carbon dioxide) in the lungs.
3. Maintenance of an adequate supply of oxygen to the tissues.
4. Maintenance of the systemic circulation.

Throughout the entire operative period the anesthetist is charged with the responsibility of observing the general condition of the patient and reporting the results of his observation to the surgeon. He observes and records the pulse, respiration, and blood pressure of the patient at regular intervals. Should an abnormality occur, he calls this to the attention of the surgeon so that appropriate measures can be taken.

The third member of the surgical team is the nurse and her assistants. The nurse has two general responsibilities. One is to anticipate and meet the needs of the surgeon for instruments and supplies during the operative procedure. The other is the general management of the operating room so that all those who are participating in the surgical procedure have what they need and the safety of the patient is protected. Obviously, these two different functions require two nurses. The first nurse is usually called a scrub, or instrument, nurse because she scrubs her hands and arms before donning a sterile gown and gloves; the second is called the circulating nurse. Though the activities of the nurse who handles instruments may appear to be the more difficult and responsible role, it is not. The circulating nurse has multiple responsibilities, as she must anticipate and plan to meet the needs of each member of the operating team; she must be alert to threats to the patient's safety; she watches for breaks in technique or for conditions which, if allowed to continue, will lead to a loss of asepsis; she saves and counts discarded sponges and instruments; she controls the number and behavior of visitors in the operating room; and she reminds the surgeon and others that the patient is awake when this reminder is necessary. In general she manages the environment of the patient, so that the progress of the procedure is furthered and the safety of the patient is protected. Few activities of the circulating nurse are glamorous or exciting. Yet the smooth running of the operating room depends on having a circulating nurse who has initiative and intelligence and who exercises sound judgment. All members of the team are important. Each member of the team contributes to the success of the surgical procedure the patient undergoes.

What are the three objectives of the surgical team during the operative phase?

They are: (1) to achieve the purpose of the surgical therapy, (2) to keep the patient safe during the operative procedure, and (3) to keep the surgery safe for the patient. Each of these objectives is important. Failure to achieve any one of them may result in injury or death to the patient.

The purposes for which surgery is performed are several. One is to observe the gross or microscopic structure of an organ or tissue. When tissue is removed for the purpose of microscopic examination, the procedure is called a biopsy. The word "biopsy" comes from the Greek. *Bio* is derived from the Greek *bios,* which means life. *Opsy* comes from *opsis,* which means sight or vision. The term "biopsy" means not only the taking of tissue, but its microscopic examination. Biopsy is useful in confirming diagnosis and in estimating prognosis and in following the course of disease and the effectiveness of treatment. To illustrate, Mrs. Stubby has a lump in her breast. The surgeon removes the lump and the pathologist examines it microscopically. He reports to the surgeon that the tumor is benign or that it is malignant. Should it be malignant, the surgeon removes the breast and surrounding lymph nodes. From the examination of the breast tissue and the lymph nodes, the nature of the neoplasm can be determined and the extent to which it has spread can be estimated. If the lesion is benign, Mrs. Stubby's prognosis is excellent and she should make a complete recovery. Should the lesion be malignant, both the nature and extent of spread will be important in predicting her chances for recovery.

Tissue may be removed for study by various methods. The method used depends on the nature and location of the lesion. In the instance of Mrs. Thomas, her breast tumor was removed by surgical excision. A patient with a tentative diagnosis of myelogenous leukemia had bone marrow removed from his sternum by means of a punch. A punch is a hollow instrument similar in appearance to a large needle; it is introduced into, and removes, a piece of tissue. Tissue may also be obtained by aspiration, a method useful when the lesion contains fluid or when fluid is formed in a serous cavity. Tissue may be procured by a number of other methods which include: (1) curettage, or the scraping of the surface of a lesion, (2) dragging of a sponge over the surface of tissue, usually a mucous membrane, (3) irrigation or washing of a serous cavity, and (4) examination of materials such as sputum or other secretions from an organ or part. The latter, which is known as the Papanicolau technique, is based on the fact that cells are shed into secretions. The first organ from which Papanicolau obtained cells was the cervix. Secretions are obtained by placing a wooden spatula into the cervical os. The material thus obtained is placed on a slide and stained. This procedure enables the physician to identify the presence of cancer of the cervix while the lesion is still localized to its point of origin.

After the surgeon removed the tumor from Mrs. Thomas, it was sent to the pathological laboratory for examination. The pathologist examined its gross appearance and then he gave it to a technician who prepared slices of tissue from the tumor for examination by two different methods. One is called a frozen and the other a paraffin section. Each has its advantages and disadvantages. In this instance the surgeon wished to have an immediate report and a frozen section was made at once. Later another portion of the tumor was treated by a slower method. The specimen was placed in paraffin after it had been fixed in a suitable preservative. Although the latter method is more accurate, either method can be utilized with good results by experts. When the results obtained by frozen section indicate that the patient requires additional surgery, it can be instituted without delay.

Besides biopsy, exploratory surgery with or without the removal of tissue may be performed for the purpose of establishing diagnosis. At times, despite the best efforts of the physician and the use of modern diagnostic devices, a diagnosis cannot be confirmed or rejected, nor can the extent of a disease process be known for sure. For example, Mr. James has bronchogenic carcinoma. His surgeon is not certain that it is inoperable. He therefore performs exploratory surgery just preceding more definitive surgery. Mrs. Smith has had periodic attacks of severe pain in her abdomen. Despite inconclusive evidence as to its cause, the surgeon operates and finds the source of her pain, which is corrected.

In addition to its use in the diagnosis of disease, surgery is performed to effect a cure by the removal of diseased tissue or organ. Organs such as the kidney or lung may be removed provided the other organ of the pair is healthy. Some organs such as the stomach or large intestine may be removed in part or in entirety. The resection of most or all of the stomach is usually followed by some impairment in health. A tumor may be removed with or without the removal of surrounding tissue. Cure can sometimes be effected by the drainage of an abscess that is well walled-off. Following the removal of the contents of the abscess, the tissues are then able to complete the process of repair.

Surgery may also be performed to restore normal functional relationships after the normal continuity of structures has been disrupted following the removal of an organ or a part or as a result of disease or injury. For example, Mr. Brave has the distal two thirds of his stomach removed following repeated hemorrhage from a peptic ulcer located in the proximal portion of his duodenum. A new connection between the remaining portion of the stomach and the intestine is required. Following fractures in which the ends of the bone are displaced, surgery may be required to restore and maintain the normal alignment of the bones. In the treatment of hernia, the contents that have escaped from a body cavity are replaced and the opening through which they escaped closed. Deformities resulting from failures in development or from disease may be corrected. One of the major triumphs of modern surgery is that, in the abnormal heart, openings may be closed, valves opened or reconstructed, and blood vessels rerouted so that the effects of deformities are overcome.

Surgery may also be performed to relieve symptoms, even when there is no expectation that the patient can or will be cured. Operations that are performed to relieve symptoms and to increase the comfort of the patient are said to be palliative. Palliative surgery is of several types. Infected and necrotic tissue may be removed in order to lessen odors and to relieve pain, detours may be established around obstructing neoplasms, pressure on vital structures may be relieved, and pain may be eliminated. For example, in advanced cancer of the breast in which ulceration of the skin and superficial tissues has occurred, the breast may be removed, not because the removal of the breast is expected to cure the patient, but to relieve the pain that accompanies ulceration.

In conditions accompanied by obstruction of a body tube, surgery may be performed so that the contents of the tube are rerouted around the obstruction. For example, in cancer of the head of the pancreas, the common bile duct may be obstructed by the expanding neoplasm. The obstruction can be relieved by connecting the gall bladder or a portion of the common duct to the duodenum or jejunum. In cancer of the urinary bladder, the ureters may be transplanted into the ileum or sigmoid colon or opened onto the abdominal wall. A colostomy is performed to relieve a bowel obstruction. A gastroenterostomy, a new opening between the stomach and jejunum, may be made to relieve the symptoms accompanying the blocking of the pyloric end of the stomach. Many of these same procedures are also used in the treatment of disease in which the outcome is expected to be curative. Any treatment whose primary objective is to relieve symptoms is palliative.

Expanding lesions in the cranial or spinal cavities cause symptoms by pressing on brain, spinal cord, or nerve tissue and by increasing intracranial pressure. Relief of symptoms can sometimes be secured by removing a portion of the skull or of a vertebra. In the latter instance, the lamina and the spinous process are most likely to be removed.

Under certain circumstances the nerve supply of an organ or part may be interrupted to relieve muscle spasm or pain. In some patients whose spinal cords have been transected, muscle spasms may be severe. By cutting of the motor nerve root a spastic paralysis is converted into a flaccid, or limp, one. In patients with severe and intractable pain, such as that associated with trigeminal neuralgia, sensory nerve fibers may be cut. Occasionally a patient suffering from advanced cancer may have severe pain that is not relieved by the usual methods. The surgeon may then cut the lateral spinothalamic tract in the spinal cord whose fibers carry pain impulses from the affected part to higher centers. When any tissue is deprived of its sensory nerve supply, it loses one of its important defense mechanisms. The involved area should be inspected regularly for redness, pallor, and other evidence of impending tissue injury, and when they occur, measures should be instituted to protect the area. For example, the eye of a patient who has had the ophthalmic branch of the trigeminal nerve interrupted is deprived of its sensory nerve supply. He should be taught to protect his eye from dust and other foreign bodies and to inspect it regularly, as well as after he has been out of doors or in a dusty area, for redness. The patient who has a transection of the sensory pathways in the cord should be instructed to change his position regularly and to keep his bed and clothing free from crumbs and wrinkles. He should also inspect the involved areas regularly. When the patient is unable to do these things for himself, they should be done for him.

As indicated above, when the patient arrives in the operating room, the surgical procedure that has been planned can be expected to accomplish one or more purposes. It may establish the nature and extent of his illness or how well he is responding to therapy. It may effect cure or relieve symptoms.

At the time the patient arrives in the operating suite he is likely to be awake, but drowsy. Operating room personnel should keep the fact that he is awake foremost in their minds and remind each other that the patient is awake. Conversation other than that directed to the patient should be avoided. He should be greeted by the surgeon or told that the surgeon will arrive shortly. Until he is anesthetized, he should be apprised of what to expect and he should also be protected from physical harm. Since he is drowsy, he should not be left alone on a cart in a corridor or operating room.

After the patient arrives in the operating room, he is transferred from the cart or bed to the operating room table. (He may or may not have been previously anesthesized.) The position in which he is placed on the table depends on the organs to be exposed during the operation. Sometimes the position in which the patient is placed during the operative phase contributes to his discomfort in the postoperative period. In order to prevent the patient from moving and/or from falling during the period of surgery, he is strapped to the table. Straps should be well padded and loose enough to allow adequate circulation to the extremities. The elbow should be padded to prevent ulnar nerve palsy. Care should be taken not to let the arms of the anesthetized patient dangle over the side of the table. The table should be well padded. This is of particular importance during a lengthy operation.

Another important aspect of the safety of the patient as he is prepared for surgery, as well as during the operative phase, is the maintenance of asepsis. In fact, the preparation of an aseptic environment and materials forms a large part of the preparations that are made before the patient arrives in the operating room. Because of its importance, every member of the team is responsible for securing and maintaining asepsis in all phases of surgery.

Upon what kind of knowledge is the protection of the wound from infection based?

One of the important factors in the safety of the patient is the prevention of infection of the wound. As in the prevention of any infection, the following types of information are essential: (1) the reservoirs of sources of microorganisms, (2) the vehicles by which they are spread, (3) the resistance of the microorganisms to environmental conditions including their susceptibility to physical and chemical agents, and (4) the conditions favoring the spread and growth of the microorganism.

The reservoirs of sources of microorganisms are usually people who are carriers or are infected by the offending organism, but they may be animals or contaminated objects or materials. Not only are other persons possible sources of microorganisms, but the skin and mucous membrane of the patient may be. Vehicles for the transmission of microorganisms from the reservoir to the wound include the hands, the air, instruments, linens, sutures, and any other material coming in contact with the wound. In the practice of asepsis, attention is given to preventing the escape of microorganisms from the reservoir and to ridding vehicles of them. The methods employed depend on the character of the object to be disinfected and the susceptibility of the microorganism to destruction.

Since the incision through the skin or mucous membrane provides a portal of entry, measures are instituted to prevent the introduction of microorganisms into it. The site of the incision, skin or mucous membrane, is thoroughly cleansed. When time permits, cleansing procedures are usually initiated some time before the patient is transferred to the operating room. In the operating room the final skin preparation is made and the area is draped with sterile materials.

To isolate members of the surgical team from the wound, they remove clothing worn in the other areas of the hospital or on the street and don special clothing. The hair is covered with a cap or turban and the mouth and nose with a mask. The mask should be discarded before it becomes wet. One of the factors in the effectiveness of a mask is that it is dry. The maximum length of time the mask should be worn is from 60 to 90 minutes. The purpose of the mask is to prevent the spread of microorganisms from the nasal and pharyngeal mucosa to the wound of the patient. Even when masks are properly constructed and worn, they do not trap all of the microorganisms carried by the droplets of moisture during talking. Because masks are only partly effective, some surgeons discourage all but the most necessary conversation in the operating room.

Following the thorough scrubbing of the hands and arms, a sterile gown is donned and rubber gloves are placed on the hands. The gown and gloves act as a barrier between the member of the surgical team and the wound. Before gloves were introduced, various chemicals were utilized to reduce the number of microorganisms on the hands. Semmelweis dealt with the problem by insisting that persons examining patients wash their hands in a solution containing chlorine. Lister introduced the use of carbolic acid, or phenol. Interestingly, the introduction of rubber gloves did not come about as the result of a brilliant idea, but was the result of evolution. Gloves were introduced by Dr. William Halsted, who had them made to protect the hands of a nurse who assisted him. She had developed a mercury dermatitis which made working in the operating room impossible. Because he valued her services, he had a pair of rubber gloves made for her. Later, members of his operating team wore them, first to protect their hands and then to protect the wound.

In addition to the above, all materials and instruments coming in contact with the wound are sterilized before they are used in the operative procedure. A variety of physical and chemical agents are now available for this purpose. They can be selected not only on the basis of being effective against organisms in either the vegetative or spore state, but according to the type of material to be sterilized.

Maintenance of asepsis is one of the important elements in making surgery safe for the patient. Each and every member of the surgical team is responsible not only for his own conduct, but for that of other team members. Thus, the nurse reminds the surgeon that he is in danger of, or has, contaminated his gloves, gown, a drape, or an instrument. The surgeon likewise reminds the nurse. Every team member is asepsis-conscious and acts to protect the safety of the patient.

A second factor in making surgery safe for the patient was the introduction of anesthetic agents that were both safe and effective. Prior to the middle of the nineteenth century, surgery was limited to emergency procedures or at least to those procedures absolutely essential to life. Agents used to prevent painful sensations were limited to belladonna, hemp, opium, and alcohol. Most of these drugs lessened the patient's perception of pain or his memory of it. In some instances the patient was rendered unconscious by a blow on the head. When the condition of the patient was believed to contraindicate the administration of large doses of alcohol or opium, the patient was held or tied and the operation performed with all possible speed. After the introduction of safe and effective anesthetic agents, time was no longer the prime consideration.

Before the operative procedure is begun, the patient is anesthetized. The type of anesthetic used and the method by which it is administered will depend on the type and length of the procedure to be performed, the condition of the patient, his preference, the equipment available, the skill and the training of the anesthetist, and the preference of the surgeon. When an operation is performed under local or spinal anesthesia, everyone in the operating room should also be fully aware that the patient is awake. Conversation that may be disturbing to the patient should be avoided.

What is accomplished during the postoperative phase and and how is this phase promoted?

The postoperative period begins the moment the surgeon completes the last stitch and continues until repair of the metabolic and tissue changes resulting from the surgical procedure has occurred. One of the major goals during this period is to anticipate, prevent, and, if necessary, treat postoperative complications. When this goal is accomplished, the patient can utilize his resources for recovery. Whether or not complications are prevented frequently depends on the quality of nursing that the patient receives. Many nurses enjoy the care of patients in the postoperative phase of surgery because the results of their efforts are immediately evident. The patient fulfills the expectations of the nurse by getting well promptly. Changes indicating progress toward recovery can be seen from one day to the next and are sources of satisfaction to the nurse. There are, of course, disappointments, because not all patients do get well and some develop complications, but these patients are overshadowed by those who do.

To anticipate and prevent complications the nurse requires some knowledge of: (1) the effects of anesthesia on the capacity of the patient to function, (2) the site of the incision and its effects on function, (3) the organ and tissue operated on and the general nature of the surgical procedure, and (4) knowledge of the manner in which the body responds, locally and generally, to trauma. This knowledge will influence: (1) the preparations that are made for the patient who is in the immediate postoperative phase, (2) how he is transported from one area to another, (3) the care he receives in the period that follows the completion of the operative procedure until he is ambulating, and (4) the care he receives until he is fully rehabilitated. Knowledge of the patient and his status is also necessary. The psychological and physiological status of the patient are not only important in the preparation of the patient for his operation and in assessing his ability to withstand the actual procedure, but they influence his recovery from the operation. His age predisposes him to, or protects him from, certain hazards. Personal habits, such as smoking, make him more vulnerable to certain complications, particularly those involving the tracheobronchial tree.

A few generalizations that can be used as guides in the care of the patient during the early postoperative phase of surgical treatment are: (1) the periods of induction and recovery from anesthesia are the most critical of the operative experience, (2) the patient can be expected to have some disruption or depression of his defense mechanisms, (3) his capacity to adapt physiologically or psychologically is lessened, (4) the functions of organs and systems may be stimulated or depressed, (5) not only does the patient experience physiological changes, but there are also evidences of metabolic changes, (6) disturbance in one function can be the cause of disturbances in others, and (7) therapeutic measures may have adverse effects.

As stated above, the periods of induction and of recovery from anesthesia are the most critical in the entire operative experience. Gius[23] compares the induction and recovery from anesthesia to the take-off and landing of an aircraft. In both situations human and mechanical failures occur. Many of the hazards to the patient and the circumstances contributing to accidents are known, and should therefore be preventable. The principal complications during the period of anesthesia are circulatory collapse, cardiac arrest, respiratory complications, and injury or death due to fire and explosions. The nurse shares in the responsibility for the care of the patient during both periods, but the extent of her responsibility is usually greater during the period of recovery. Nowhere, however, is the identification and control of unsafe acts more important than in the care of the patient who is in one of the stages of anesthesia.

When the operation is completed, the patient is transferred to the recovery room or to his own room. The recovery room has the advantage of having a trained and experienced staff who know what to expect and how to prevent and treat conditions predisposing to complications. The recovery room is also equipped to meet the emergencies likely to arise. When it is located in or adjacent to the operating suite, equipment from the operating room is readily available. Physicians are likely to be nearby should their services be required.

What preparations are made for the patient who is in the immediate postoperative period?

Preparations for the care of the patient following surgery should be begun as soon as he is transferred to the operating room. The bed or frame on which he is to be placed should be secured and prepared. In this preparation three criteria should be met. First, the bed should be made so that the patient can be easily transferred into it. In general, the transfer of the patient is facilitated if the top bedding is not tucked in at the foot, but placed neatly folded to one

[23] Gius, *Op. cit.,* p. 305.

side. Second, the mattress and pillows should be protected from emesis and drainage as necessary. For example, for a patient having a general anesthetic or a procedure involving the gastrointestinal tract, or the head and neck, the pillow under the head should be protected by a plastic cover. However, the patient who has had a local anesthetic and the drainage of an abscess of his tibia is not likely to stain the pillow under his head. The mattress and pillow under his leg are in danger of being contaminated by drainage from his leg and should therefore be protected. Last, the bed or frame on which the patient is to be placed should be selected and equipped so that the needs of the patient can best be met. To illustrate, if the patient is expected to have a general anesthetic, or to have his eyes bandaged following eye surgery, or is elderly, side boards may be placed on the bed to remind the patient of the edges of the bed. A patient having surgery on his back may be placed on a frame so that turning from face to back is facilitated. If the patient is to be encased in a cast, a board may be placed under the mattress to provide a firm support for the cast. Though most hospitals are now equipped with beds having Gatch frames to elevate the head of the bed, few have the type that make elevation of the foot of the bed easy.[24] The necessity for elevating the foot of the bed should be anticipated when the patient goes directly from the operating room to his room following a prolonged and difficult operation or when there is any other reason for anticipating that he may be unconscious or in shock. Some surgeons prefer to have their patients in the Trendelenburg position to facilitate drainage from the airway and to prevent the aspiration of vomitus.

In the past the warming of the bed was considered to be essential. Though warming of the bed probably does no harm, unless the room and bed are cold, it probably is unnecessary. If hot-water bottles or other heating devices are used, they should be removed before the patient is transferred to the bed to protect the patient from burns and from overheating. Overheating causes sweating and contributes to the dehydration of the patient. The aim should be to maintain the temperature of the room so that the patient is comfortable.

In addition to the preparation of the bed to meet the requirements of the patient, the equipment and supplies that will be required in the care of the patient should be assembled. Provisions take into account the kind of anesthetic used and the nature of the surgical procedure. Since the number one problem in the immediate postoperative period of patients having a general anesthetic is the maintenance of respiration and the prevention of blocking of the tracheobronchial tree, provisions should be made to remove secretions and to prevent saliva and vomitus from being aspirated. With some patients this can be accomplished by positioning the patient, but suction apparatus should be available to be used as required. Suction apparatus should also be available and in working order for patients who have gastric or other tubes.

---

[24] Some carts or stretchers used in recovery rooms are adjustable and a patient can be placed in almost any position desired.

A tracheostomy tray should be secured and placed at the bedside of patients who have undergone head and neck surgery, including thyroidectomy, in anticipation of the possibility of acute obstruction of the airway. Other equipment such as that required for the administration of oxygen and drainage bottles and irrigation sets and solutions should be obtained and prepared as required. Since practice varies, no attempt will be made to list all the types of equipment or supplies that may be required in the care of the patient; however, whatever is necessary should be obtained and tested to make certain that it is working before the patient is returned to his room.

What problems are most likely to be encountered in the first six to eight hours after surgery?

The problems in the care of the patient during the first six to eight hours following the completion of the surgical procedure are: maintaining a clear airway, preventing aspiration of vomitus, maintaining his blood pressure, and preventing injury due to falling. Depending on the type of anesthesia used and the stage of anesthesia he is in, the patient may be deeply unconscious or fully awake. During the first six to eight hours after surgery, the patient's cardiovascular system does not adapt well to rapid changes in position. Even when his blood pressure is stable at the completion of the surgical procedure, movement or jarring of the patient is likely to cause it to fall. Care should be taken to handle him slowly and gently and to avoid bumping the cart or bed. To prevent obstruction of the respiratory tract by secretions and aspiration of saliva and gastric juice, the patient should be placed in a position favoring drainage. Varco[25] recommends that the unconscious patient be transported and maintained in a position in which the head and shoulders are lower than the legs and buttocks. Though he does not so state, the head should be turned to one side, in order to keep the posterior portion of the tongue and soft tissues from blocking the glottis. This position not only favors the drainage of fluid from the tracheobronchial tree and the mouth, but it prevents blood and fluid from pooling in the lower extremities. Return of fluid and blood to the general circulation is important for maintaining cardiac output. If this position is not appropriate for a particular patient, then the patient should be placed in a lateral position. When the patient is placed in the lateral position, two points should be kept in mind. One is that the weight of the body should not be allowed to rest on the dependent arm. The other is that the weight of the body should be distributed so that the body holds itself on the side. To prevent pressure on the arm, the body may be turned on the side with the lower arm parallel to the side. The arm on the dependent side is then pulled through so that it lies posterior to the trunk. The nurse then stands behind the patient and places one hand under the iliac crest and the other under the trochanter of the femur and pulls his body toward herself. The upper leg and

[25] *Op. cit.,* p. 107.

thigh may be flexed at the knee and be carried forward over the dependent leg. The side-lying position not only facilitates the drainage of secretions, but it helps to maintain the tongue and soft tissues forward so that they do not block the larynx. In the event that this should happen, the mandible should be raised and moved forward. If the mouth can be opened, the tongue can be grasped with a gauze square and pulled forward so that the obstruction of the airway is relieved. When the patient must of necessity be transported on his back, his head should be turned to the side. During the period that the patient is unconscious and well relaxed by the anesthetic, an oropharyngeal airway placed in the mouth may be helpful in keeping the tongue and soft tissues from falling back into the pharynx.

Though precautions are taken to prevent obstruction of the tracheobronchial tree and aspiration of gastric secretions and saliva while the patient is being transported from one area to another, he should be observed for signs indicating an obstruction. Because the period immediately following the operation is a hazardous one, the patient should be accompanied by a professional person.

When the patient arrives in the recovery room, he may be fully awake or in any stage of anesthesia including the third. If he is unconscious, he may have an oropharyngeal airway in place. It should not be removed until the swallowing reflexes of the patient return and the patient tries to remove it. The oropharyngeal airway should not be confused with an endotracheal tube. As may be deduced from its name, an endotracheal tube is placed in the trachea and its primary purpose is to administer inhalation anesthetics. Because of the sensitivity of the larynx to stimulation during the second stage of anesthesia and the danger of laryngospasm, the endotracheal tube is removed either in the third stage of anesthesia or after the patient has fully recovered. It should always be removed by a physician, because the tube may have to be reinserted.

Through what stages does the patient who has been anesthetized pass, and what are his needs during each stage?

As the patient recovers from the effects of a general anesthetic, he passes through the same stages that he did in its induction, except that the order is reversed. In the induction of the anesthetic, the concentration of the anesthetic gas or mixture of gases is higher in the alveoli than it is in the blood. Therefore, the gas moves from the alveoli into the blood at a more rapid rate than it moves out of the blood into the alveoli. When the desired level of anesthesia is reached, the amount of gas inhaled by the patient is adjusted, so that the amount entering the blood equals that leaving the blood. At the termination of the operation or at some suitable point previous to it, the administration of the anesthetic gas is terminated. In the period of recovery, the process is reversed. As the patient inhales air or oxygen, the concentration of the anesthetic gas in the alveoli is diluted and, as a consequence, its partial pressure is reduced. With the reduction in the partial pressure of the gas in the alveoli, the gas in the blood escapes into the alveoli, where it is mixed with inspired air and exhaled. This process continues until all the gas is removed from the body.

The degree of general anesthesia may be divided into four stages. Since stage IV is the stage of respiratory paralysis, it is more likely to occur in the patient in the operating room. In stage IV, respiratory paralysis of central origin occurs. Death occurs as a consequence of heart failure, unless artificial respiration is instituted.

Stage III is known as the stage of surgical anesthesia. The patient is unconscious and reflexes are repressed or paralyzed. Because the degree to which reflexes are repressed or paralyzed varies, this stage is divided into four planes, with plane 1 being the lightest and plane 4 being the deepest. Most surgical procedures are carried out on plane 2.

As the patient eliminates the anesthetic, he goes into the second stage or the stage of excitement or delirium. This stage, as the name implies, is accompanied by a number of hazards to the patient. In stage II, the patient is unconscious. There is great variability in the degree of excitement manifested by patients, as some patients pass through this stage relatively quietly while others may be so disturbed that they are difficult to control. As a result of the use of modern drugs and anesthetics, the length of the stage of excitement has been shortened and decreased in severity. The nurse should, however, be alert to the possibility of the patient's becoming excited. She should take appropriate steps to decrease the likelihood of his becoming excited and to protect him from injury if he does. Bedside rails should be raised, and someone should be in constant attendance on the patient. The environment of the patient should be regulated so that all sources of stimulation such as noise, drafts, and loud talking are eliminated. The patient should be handled gently. In the past, efforts were sometimes made to increase the rate at which the patient regained consciousness by stimulating him by shouting at him or shaking him. Since the rate of the recovery of the patient depends on the rate at which the anesthetic agent is eliminated, these procedures cannot be counted on to be very effective and they may be harmful. In addition to increasing the likelihood of the patient's becoming excited during stage II, the capacity of the patient to adapt the functioning of his cardiovascular system to rapid changes in position is reduced and as a result his blood pressure may fall.

During stage I, the patient is drowsy. He can be awakened and will respond to questions, but then he lapses back into sleep. He may waken and complain of pain and in a moment or two return to sleep. At this time the nurse must assess the need of the patient for a pain-relieving medication. She must estimate the severity of the pain experienced by the patient and the extent of his recovery from the anesthetic and preanesthetic medications. Questions the nurse should be able to answer before she administers an analgesic medication include: Has the patient recovered sufficiently from the effects of the anesthetic to require a pain-relieving medication? Is the respiratory status of the patient such that it is safe to administer a drug to him that depresses respiration? What evidence indicates that the patient does or does not require an analgesic? The objective is neither to give nor to withhold medication; too great delay in the administration of an analgesic can cause as much harm to the patient as administering one too soon. The objective should be to minimize the pain experienced by the patient and at the same time protect him from the hazards of overmedication. For example, the writer recently spent the afternoon with a friend who had had a general anesthetic earlier in the day. She was drowsy and slept for extended periods of time. At one point she roused and complained of pain. In a moment or so she went back to sleep and continued to sleep for an hour or more. When she awakened at this point, she again complained of pain. This time she did not go back to sleep and she was obviously uncomfortable and restless. Since her respiratory rate was within normal limits and there were no other contraindications, she was given a pain-relieving medication.

During the period in which the patient recovers from the effects of the anesthetic, the problems in his care continue to be (1) the maintenance of a clear airway, (2) the prevention of the aspiration of saliva and gastric secretions, and (3) the maintenance of cardiovascular stability. Until he regains consciousness, the head down or lateral position is favored, unless there is some reason contraindicating it. The child who has had a tonsillectomy under general anesthesia is usually placed face down. Since blood and saliva will be drained from the mouth by gravity, aspiration into the tracheobronchial tree is avoided and the extent to which the patient is bleeding can be determined. The patient having intracranial or head and neck surgery is not placed in the head-down position. No matter where a part is located, if that part is placed in a dependent position gravity decreases venous return and increases swelling and the possibility of hemorrhage. The position of the patient may also be modified by the presence of other disorders. The obese patient or the one with emphysema may be placed in a sitting position as this facilitates breathing. The position of the patient who has received a spinal anesthetic is modified in respect to the effects of this type of anesthesia. Since spinal anesthesia lessens the ability to adjust the diameter of the blood vessels to position, it predisposes to severe postural hypotension (the blood pressure falls as the individual rises to sit or stand). A less dangerous effect is headache (spinal headache), which is thought to be due to a reduction in the pressure of the cerebrospinal fluid.[26] To prevent either or both of these complications the patient is usually kept in the supine or recumbent position for a longer time than the patient having a general anesthetic.

As stated earlier, equipment should be available to remove secretions from the mouth and pharynx as necessary. The patient should be observed for signs

[26] Hardy, *Op. cit.,* p. 523.

of airway obstruction, that is, noisy respirations and/or labored breathing. The movements of the chest as well as the use of the accessory muscles of respiration should be observed and abnormalities reported. Cyanosis is a relatively late sign of oxygen deficiency or hypoxia, as it depends on the presence of 5 gm or more of reduced (unoxygenated) hemoglobin in the arterial blood and dilatation of the peripheral blood vessels. Other evidence of obstruction should not be ignored until the patient becomes cyanotic. Treatment should be promptly instituted to prevent and to relieve obstruction and to lessen the possibility of a serious degree of hypoxia. (See Chapter 7 to review the effects of a lack of oxygen to the brain and other tissues.)

To prevent obstruction of the airway, secretions and vomitus should be removed from the mouth as they appear. The patient should be turned at regular intervals from side to side. As soon as he responds, he should be encouraged to perform deep-breathing exercises and to cough at hourly intervals. An upright position increases the effectiveness of coughing and increases the vital capacity. When the condition of the patient permits, some surgeons direct that the patient be placed in the sitting or standing position to cough and to do breathing exercises. Although either position increases the effectiveness of mechanisms for cleansing the tracheobronchial tree, the patient who has so recently experienced a major operation may become very anxious when the suggestion is made that he is to sit up or get out of bed. He should, therefore, be given appropriate psychological and physical support.

Should the unconscious patient develop signs indicating a respiratory obstruction, the nurse should check the tongue to make certain that it is not responsible. In prolonged unconsciousness, obstruction can be due to the lodging of a foreign body transversely in the oral pharynx. One source of foreign bodies is crusting which frequently develops on the hard palate of the mouth breather and subsequently becomes dislodged. Conscientious mouth care and an adequate fluid intake can prevent this complication. The condition of not only the anterior but of the posterior part of the mouth should be regularly determined. Movement of the patient from side to side may promote coughing and expulsion of a mucus plug. In the patient having head and neck surgery, including thyroidectomy, the area around the incision should be checked for signs of hemorrhage. When the obstruction cannot be relieved by procedures within the province of nursing, the physician should be notified immediately so that the cause of the obstruction can be determined and the appropriate remedy initiated. The therapy prescribed by the physician will be determined by the factors contributing to the hypoxia and to the severity of the hypoxia.

When laryngospasm is responsible for obstruction of the airway, action must be taken promptly to relieve it or the patient will die from the effects of hypoxia. The nurse can recognize this condition by the characteristic crowing sound occurring during respiration. The sound is caused by tension placed on the vocal cords by spasm of laryngeal muscles. The patient appears to be struggling to breathe and uses his accessory muscles of respiration. While the simplest method used to treat laryngospasm is to administer oxygen under pressure by way of a tight-fitting mask placed over the face, laryngospasm can also be relieved by the introduction of an endotracheal tube by a physician. A nurse must *never* attempt this procedure. The administration of oxygen under pressure is usually successful. Enough oxygen gets by the adducted vocal cords to reduce the degree of hypoxia sufficiently to cause the cords to relax. When the proper equipment is not readily available, a tracheotomy may have to be performed to establish an open airway. Other indications for tracheotomy such as pressure on the trachea and excessive secretions, as well as the care of the patient with a tracheotomy, are discussed in Chapter 7.

In addition to the observation and maintenance of respiratory function, the nurse should check all the vital signs. These include the pulse and blood pressure as well as the depth, rhythm or pattern, and rate of respiration. Vital signs should be checked every 15 minutes for the first four hours and then hourly until they are stable. When evaluation is made of the condition of a patient, all evidence should be taken into consideration. The fact that the blood pressure of a patient is within the range expected for the patient should not cause the nurse to discount other evidence that the patient is in trouble.

A second and relatively frequent complication occurring during the operation and early postoperative phase of surgery is shock. In serious states of shock, life may be threatened unless the disorder is treated promptly and effectively. As defined elsewhere, shock is an abnormal physiological state in which there is a serious disproportion between the capacity of the blood vessels and the circulating blood volume. Any disorder resulting in a marked increase in the capacity of the blood vessels or noticeably decreasing the volume of circulating blood therefore causes shock. The objective effect of the disparity between blood volume and the capacity of the blood vessels is a fall in the blood pressure. The consequence, in terms of cells, is failure to deliver to the cells oxygen required for oxidation, that is, the release of energy.

What factors are responsible for the maintenance of blood pressure? What are the causes of shock in the surgical patient?

In a closed system such as the vascular system, the maintenance of the pressure of the fluid within the system above simple hydrostatic pressure is due to three factors. They are: (1) an effective pumping mechanism, (2) fluid to pump, and (3) a resistance to pump against. Although any one of these factors may be involved in development of shock in the surgical patient, the latter two are probably the most frequent. In the patient who is treated surgically or who suffers serious physical trauma or is burned, fluid volume is decreased by loss of blood by hemorrhage and loss of body fluids from the vascular system. Dehydration may be an initiating or sustaining factor in shock because it contributes to a reduction in circulating blood volume. Shock due to the reduction in the circulating blood volume is classified as hemorrhagic or oligemic.

What is the role of the nervous system in shock?

Since the nervous system regulates the contraction and relaxation of the muscles in the blood vessels, shock may result from the effect of injury or drugs on the nervous system. Shock due to the vasodilatory action of the nervous system is classified as neurogenic shock. It is usually transitory. The nervous system itself does not have to be directly injured. The result of the involvement of the nervous system is vasodilation due to decreased tone of the muscles of the blood vessels. Fainting or syncope was formerly considered a form of neurogenic shock. Spinal anesthesia, as a consequence of its depressing effect on the nerve supply to the anesthetized area, also predisposes to neurogenic shock.

What is a possible relationship between sepsis and shock?

The third type of shock associated with surgical and other forms of trauma is septic shock. This type of shock is called septic because it results from the action of toxic substances on blood vessels. Bacteria and their products and histamine absorbed from the injured tissue may be responsible. Like neurogenic shock, it results in an increase in the capacity of blood vessels to hold blood. In both neurogenic and septic shock, resistance to the flow of blood is decreased by the increase in the capacity of the blood vessels to hold blood.

All the above factors contribute to the development of shock in patients who are treated surgically and who suffer traumatic injuries. The loss of blood, the anxiety, the absorption of bacteria and bacterial toxins from the alimentary canal, and the release of histamine from injured tissue combine to create a disparity between the volume of circulating blood and the capacity of the vascular chamber. Besides these factors, other conditions such as pain, dehydration, heat, cold, and hunger can be initiating or sustaining factors in shock. Many of the responsibilities of the nurse in preventing and minimizing shock have been previously presented.

The care of any patient who is in or who is predisposed to shock should be guided by the following objectives: first, to control conditions in the environment tending to predispose to or to intensify shock; second, to detect evidence that shock is developing or increasing in intensity; and third, to protect the tissues from the effects of inadequate circulation.

The physical, psychological, and social environment of the patient should be regulated so that no unnecessary demands are made on the patient. The environmental temperature should be regulated so that the patient is protected from undue loss of heat. Neither should he be overheated, as this leads to peripheral vasodilation. Loud, sudden noises as well as loud or unnecessary talking should be avoided. Gentle handling, and the avoidance of jarring of the bed, as well as unnecessary hurry or tension are recommended.

Since efforts to prevent shock are sometimes unsuccessful, an important aspect of the care of the patient is to observe him for evidence that it is developing. Once the patient is in shock, continued observation is required to determine the effectiveness of the corrective measures that have been instituted. It is well to remember that shock is a dynamic, not a static, process. The condition of the patient in shock is either improving or deteriorating. Therefore, careful observation accompanied by the prompt reporting of signs and symptoms indicating impending or worsening shock is imperative. Regardless of whether or not the physician has requested that a given patient be observed for evidence of shock, the nurse should nevertheless assume responsibility as indicated, for example, with all patients who: (1) undergo major surgery or are seriously injured by physical trauma or burning, (2) bleed from a hollow organ or continue to hemorrhage, and (3) have an acute myocardial infarction. This list is suggestive rather than exhaustive. The significant question that the nurse should ask herself is: "Does this patient have a disorder or treatment that is likely to cause a serious disparity between the capacity of the vascular system and the volume of blood?" If the answer is yes, the patient should be investigated for signs and symptoms indicating impending or fully developed shock. When they occur, they should be brought to the attention of the physician immediately.

What are the principal signs of shock?

The principal signs of shock are a falling blood pressure; usually, though not invariably, a rising pulse rate; and evidence of decreased peripheral circulation. Among the signs of decreased peripheral circulation are a cold, clammy skin (sweating) and an ashen or cyanotic skin as well as weak or absent radial, pedal, and popliteal pulses.

What are the principal symptoms of shock?

Many of the symptoms of early shock result from the effect of the inability to adapt the circulation to the brain with changes in position. Others result from the initiation of protective mechanisms. Vasoconstriction occurs in organs not of immediate importance to survival. Eventually as shock develops, centers in the brain are hypoxic, even at rest. Some of the early symptoms of shock can be elicited from the patient before there is a change in his appearance. They include: dizziness, weakness, thirst, apprehensiveness, restlessness, nausea, vomiting, and the feeling of impending death. Because the patient is apprehensive and restless, there is danger of ascribing them to pain, rather than to their true cause, shock. Another sign of considerable import is a reduction in the hourly urine output. The significance of the early detection of signs and symptoms of shock to the welfare of the patient cannot be overemphasized. Neither observation nor recording of them is of any value to the patient unless they are brought to the attention of the physician as early as possible. The patient requires treatment, and the earlier it is instituted, the better the patient's prognosis. The status of shock does not stand still; the patient either improves or deteriorates.

What are some of the measures that are useful in protecting the tissues from the effects of inadequate circulation?

One measure that is useful in protecting the tissues from an inadequate supply of blood is to decrease their activity. Consequently no unnecessary demands are made on the patient. As stated earlier, the head of the bed can be lowered, so that the blood in the lower extremities is returned to the heart. With an increase in the circulating blood volume, cardiac output is increased and with this increase blood supply to vital organs is improved. In mild shock, this procedure may be sufficient to restore the blood pressure to safe levels. As a rule, the nurse is permitted to lower the head of the bed about 10 in. on her own initiative. Lowering the head is contraindicated in patients with head injuries, brain surgery, or chest injuries.

When hemorrhage or other conditions causing a decrease in blood volume are causative factors, measures are instituted to restore blood volume. Blood, plasma, plasma expanders, or other fluids may be infused for this purpose.

In addition to measures directed toward correcting the cause of shock, attention should be given to maintaining a patent airway and adequate ventilation. Unless the blood circulating through the lungs can be adequately oxygenated, other measures are not likely to be fully effective.

When the degree of shock is severe and the blood pressure cannot be maintained at a safe level, a vasoconstrictor drug may be prescribed by the physician. Vasoconstrictor drugs counteract shock by increasing peripheral resistance. Among the drugs in use are metaraminol bitartrate (Aramine Bitartrate[27]) and levarterenol bitartrate (Levophed[27]). There are, of course, other vasoconstrictor drugs. The use of these drugs in inducing vasoconstriction has been discussed elsewhere. Unless they not only elevate the blood pressure, but improve blood flow to the tissues, they are ineffective.

To summarize, shock is a most important complication in any disorder in which there is a disparity between the blood volume and the size of the vascular chamber. It may be due also to a failure in the pumping action of the heart. In the care of any patient who is predisposed to shock, the nurse has the responsibility to initiate measures to minimize the likelihood of its developing. Second, the patient should be observed regularly and conscientiously for signs and symptoms pointing toward its development. Last, the patient in shock requires care directed toward correcting its cause and protection from the effects of hypoxia on vital tissues.

What factors predispose to hemorrhage?

As indicated in the discussion of shock, hemorrhage is one of the more common causes of shock. Moreover, it is a possibility in all phases of surgery. In the instance of Mr. Brave, bleeding from an eroded blood vessel located in a peptic ulcer caused him to seek medical attention. Mrs. Smith lost approxi-

[27] Trade name.

mately 3 pt of blood during the removal of her uterus (hysterectomy), and Sunny Day bled profusely from the tonsillar fossa in her pharynx after tonsillectomy. Johnny Hopper suffered an open or compound fracture (a break in a bone in which one or more fragments protrude through the skin) when he fell from a tree. In all these patients the primary factor causing hemorrhage was a disruption in the continuity of one or more blood vessels.

Although physical or chemical injuries are usually responsible for breaks in the continuity of blood vessels, the condition of the wall of the blood vessel influences its ability to withstand trauma or chemical destruction. Examples of disorders weakening the walls of blood vessels include arterial aneurysms or venous varicosities. In an arterial aneurysm, the wall bulges as a result of disease or structural defect. As it bulges, the wall thins and becomes less resistant to the pressure of the arterial blood. Sooner or later it is likely to rupture and result in arterial hemorrhages. When varicosities—elongated, tortuous, thin-walled veins—are located in the esophagus, food passing over them causes erosion of the already thin wall and causes serious hemorrhage. In addition to localized areas of weakness in the wall of a blood vessel, deficiency of vitamin C is accompanied by a generalized fragility in the walls of capillaries.

Following the destruction of a blood vessel, the body responds to protect itself from the excessive loss of blood. Among these responses are the self-sealing mechanism, the elevation of interstitial fluid pressure created by the escaping blood, and the immobilization of the injured area by muscle spasm. In the self-sealing mechanism, the muscle in the cut end of the blood vessel contracts and thereby reduces the diameter of the lumen, and the intima curls inward to further occlude the vessel. Muscle contraction occurs whether the blood vessel is large or small and may be sufficient to control bleeding from even large arteries. Sealing of the remaining lumen is accomplished by the formation of a blood clot within the terminal portion of the cut end of the blood vessel. As the clot matures, it, too, contracts and forms a tight plug in the end of the blood vessel. The self-sealing mechanism is usually successful in limiting blood loss from small wounds and from areas where the surface tissue has been removed, as in an abrasion or burn.

When a large area of tissue has been denuded or for some other reason the self-sealing mechanism is ineffective, sufficient blood may be lost to form a soft clot over the site of bleeding. The clot, instead of contracting and sealing the underlying blood vessels, remains soft and the vessels behind it continue to bleed. Before blood loss can be checked, the soft clot must be removed, so that clotting within the ends of the blood vessels will be stimulated.

To illustrate, after the surgical removal of the tonsils, the surgeon dries the denuded area by gently patting the surface with a sponge. He continues this process until the cut ends of the blood vessels have constricted and the blood has clotted within them. Should bleeding recur, a clot forms external to cut ends of the blood vessels and bleeding continues underneath it. One theory advanced to explain continued bleeding is that the blood clot probably releases fibrolysin, which prevents clotting in the ends of the blood vessels. Control of bleeding usually requires that the blood clot be removed and the area be again dried. Pressure is often applied to control bleeding until the self-sealing mechanism becomes effective.

Following prostatectomy, bleeding from the lining of the bladder usually occurs. Because of its anatomy, pressure over the bleeding sites is difficult, if not impossible, to apply. Continued bleeding is usually the result of a soft clot adhering to the lining of the bladder and interfering with the formation of clots within the disrupted blood vessels. Bleeding can usually be prevented or stopped by the removal of blood and clots from the bladder by irrigation. When irrigation of the bladder is prescribed following prostatectomy, sufficient fluid should be introduced to remove blood and blood clots, and the procedure should be performed frequently enough to prevent clot formation.

Besides the self-sealing mechanism, blood loss into a closed space is opposed by the rise of tissue pressure caused by blood accumulating in the space. As tissue fluid pressure rises, it exerts pressure against the wall of the bleeding vessel. Blood flow ceases when the interstitial pressure exceeds the blood pressure. Conversely, bleeding into a body cavity where blood can escape is sometimes severe, because the blood is removed from the cavity; it does not create a counterpressure to counteract the blood pressure. Thus bleeding from the nose or into the alimentary canal or other hollow organ is likely to be profuse. Muscle spasm in the affected part contributes to immobilization and also increases the pressure exerted against the exterior of the blood vessels. All these factors combine to lessen the quantity of blood lost.

What are the effects of hemorrhage?

Hemorrhage has one effect, it decreases the capacity to deliver blood and oxygen to the cells. It lessens circulation of blood by decreasing blood volume. When a large quantity of blood is lost quickly, the blood pressure falls. As much as 10 per cent of the blood volume can be lost without any appreciable effect on the blood pressure. A loss of 30 per cent or more is associated with a considerable drop in blood pressure. As stated above, if the fall in blood pressure is not too great, it is beneficial, as blood flow through the severed blood vessels is diminished. The effect of the decrease in the blood volume is counteracted by: (1) the constriction of blood vessels, which lessens the size of the vascular bed, (2) constriction of the arterioles, which increases peripheral resistance, and (3) transfer of fluid from the tissues to the blood. All these mechanisms decrease shock, by reducing the disparity between the size of the vascular bed and the blood volume.

In addition to a decrease in the volume of circulating blood, hemorrhage causes a reduction in the oxygen-carrying capacity of the blood due to a loss of erythrocytes and hemoglobin. Serious as the loss of hemoglobin is, it is not of as much immediate importance in acute hemorrhage as it is later on in chronic blood loss. The effects of the loss of hemoglobin are discussed in Chapter 9.

When arteries are disrupted, a third problem is created because the tissues supplied by the artery are partly or completely deprived of their blood supply. For example, in an accident with an electric saw, Jim Green's lower leg was severed, so that only about one fourth of the tissue remained intact. Whether or not his foot can be saved will depend in part on whether the arterial blood supply is sufficient or, if not, whether it can be re-established.

What signs and symptoms accompany hemorrhage?

Besides the signs and symptoms due to the effects of hypoxia and reduction of blood volume, the site of hemorrhage influences some of the other effects of hemorrhage. The site of bleeding determines whether blood increases pressure within an organ or tissue or escapes to the outside. In tissues or organs where the escaping blood is trapped, such as in the cranial or spinal cavity, the signs and symptoms may be due primarily to increased pressure on the brain or cord or to the irritation of the brain or nerves by the blood. Though some blood is lost, the quantity is not sufficient to affect the blood volume.

When bleeding is in an organ or tissue from which it can escape to the external world, blood as well as the consequences of a reduction in blood volume can be observed. Blood escaping from an artery is bright red and comes in spurts; blood from a vein generally has a dusky hue and flows steadily; and capillary bleeding is characterized by seepage.

How is hemorrhage treated?

In instances in which bleeding is not self-limiting, therapy of hemorrhage is directed toward two objectives. The first is to stop the hemorrhage. The second depends on the extent of blood loss and the effects of the accumulation of blood on involved structures. When the loss of blood is sufficient to affect the blood volume, a second objective is to replace the blood volume. When blood has accumulated in a tissue or organ in sufficient quantity to impair its function, then an objective is to remove the blood or to relieve the pressure created by it. Before bleeding can be treated, it must be detected. Any patient who is predisposed by the nature of his illness or treatment to hemorrhage should be under an intelligent program of surveillance. Dressings should be inspected regularly for evidence of fresh blood. Like other fluids, blood runs downhill; parts inferior to the dressing should be inspected. Fluids drained or discharged from affected organs should be examined for blood. When the incision or injury is in an organ or tissue from which blood cannot escape, the patient should be observed for signs and symptoms indicating pressure on an organ or surrounding tissues.

Though bleeding may occur in any incision, it is most likely to take place in large wounds, in those in which the operated surface is exposed, and in highly vascular areas. Internal bleeding may also result from the failure of a ligature to hold a large artery severed during the operative procedure; large amounts of blood can be lost in a very short period of time. Traumatic injuries are a frequent cause of hemorrhage, and certain blood dyscrasias are associated with a tendency to bleed. Formerly operations on patients with obstructions in the biliary tract were likely to be associated with hemorrhage because of failure to absorb vitamin K. Now, these patients can usually be prepared so that they are not subject to any special hazard.

In some surgical procedures the tendency of the patient to bleed can be controlled by appropriate care. As previously indicated, patients having intracranial and head and neck surgery are usually placed in a position with the head and back up. In patients who have surgery on an extremity, the limb is elevated to improve the venous return and to lessen the tendency to bleed into the wound. The extremity is also immobilized until the danger of hemorrhage has decreased. As discussed earlier following prostatectomy, bleeding from the bladder is controlled by bladder irrigation. In the control of bleeding from any organ, the location of the structure and the nature of its function have to be considered. In general, measures are used to immobilize the part, or to overcome the force of the blood pressure, or to support or to assist the self-scaling mechanism.

One of the most common, and perhaps the oldest, method of controlling hemorrhage particularly in the emergency situation is the application of pressure. The points at which bleeding may be stopped by applying pressure are those where large blood vessels overlie bony prominences. The vessels which meet this criterion, and therefore are most effectively compressed, include the temporal, facial, carotid, brachial, and femoral arteries. Pressure should be applied with the cleanest available material. Although tourniquets have long been used to control bleeding from an extremity, they often do more harm than good. Their use is not advocated. If a tourniquet is applied, it should be tight enough to prevent blood from entering the affected limb and it should be left in place until the patient is examined by a surgeon. The patient should be treated as soon as possible to protect the tissue that is deprived of its blood supply from injury from a lack of oxygen. A properly applied tourniquet should be left in place only one or two hours; if prolonged, this method of hemostasis may extend tissue injury.

Pressure is often applied over a bleeding point to control hemorrhage from an accessible organ or cavity such as the uterus or the nares by packing the organ with sterile gauze. The gauze is usually left in place until the self-sealing mechanism controls bleeding. Occasionally, bleeding is renewed after the packing is removed, and packing may have to be replaced. Patients should always be observed following the removal of packing for evidence of hemorrhage.

Although the application of pressure is frequently lifesaving when utilized to control bleeding from a large artery or vein, large vessels often must be ligated before hemorrhage is actually checked. As soon as the pressure is removed, bleeding recommences. Bleeding from small vessels differs, inasmuch as the self-sealing mechanism is usually successful in curbing blood loss. Pressure applied over an area in which there is bleeding from small vessels may be of value until the self-sealing mechanism is effective in controlling bleeding.

Another old, but probably newer, method of controlling the loss of blood is cauterization of the wound. In its earliest use, cauterization was not the carefully confined and controlled application of heat to a limited area of tissue that it is today. One old method of cauterizing tissue was to pour boiling oil into the wound. Styptics, astringents, and a hot iron were also used. Although the techniques used in cauterizing wounds have changed and it is less frequently utilized than it once was, it still has its uses. Not only is it useful in controlling hemorrhage, but it is employed to destroy tissue. For example, it is used in brain surgery to destroy tissue and to prevent bleeding. Cautery is employed to open the type of colostomy in which a loop of the colon is brought above the surface of the skin and allowed to remain closed until the second or third day after the initial surgical procedure. This procedure is not painful because the tissues of the intestine do not have nerve endings that are sensitive to heat. The patient may be frightened, however, because he does not believe that it will not hurt. To lessen his fear, his eyes should be covered with a small towel and he should be informed about the successful progress of the procedure. Through the use of heat enough tissue is destroyed to provide an opening into the intestine and the blood vessels in the affected tissue are sealed.

Though pressure and cauterization are of value in hemostasis, neither method provides an adequate means of controlling the loss of blood during a major operative procedure. It was not until materials were selected or developed that could be used to tie the ends of blood vessels that the prevention of blood loss during surgery became a practical reality. Early materials to be used in tying off blood vessels were silk or linen thread. As was noted earlier, ligatures have been known for centuries, but their regular use is of relatively modern origin. Today the surgeon has the choice of many materials, some of which are absorbable and some of which are not. During an operative procedure he also has instruments, hemostats, which he can use to close the ends of vessels before he severs them or to grasp and occlude bleeding points.

A variety of methods are available to prevent and to limit the loss of blood. The method selected depends on a variety of factors. Among them are the urgency of the situation, the rate at which blood is being lost, the extent to which blood volume has already been diminished, the site of bleeding, as well as the facilities at hand. As in shock, the safety of the patient depends on the earliness with which hemorrhage is detected and appropriate measures are instituted.

In addition to stopping of the bleeding, blood volume must be restored if it has been significantly decreased. When the loss of blood is within the limits to which the patient is able to adapt, no special measures may be required, but when the loss of blood seriously threatens the blood volume, measures such as intravenous fluids, plasma, volume expanders, and blood transfusion may be required.

What discoveries have made the transfusion of blood relatively safe?

Although attempts have been made to transfuse blood for at least 400 years, the ability to transfuse blood with reasonable safety to the patient is an accomplishment of the twentieth century. In some of the early experiments, blood taken from one dog was successfully transfused into another. Transfusion of human blood from one person to another was less successful, as about half of the recipients died. Because of the frequency with which death occurred, laws were passed prohibiting blood transfusions in England, France, and Italy. Before blood can be safely transferred from one person to another, three types of information are required. They are: (1) knowledge of blood groups and the Rh-Hr System, (2) the function of calcium in blood clotting, and (3) the diseases transmitted by blood.

What is the basis for blood grouping?

In 1900 Landsteiner made an observation that was to serve as the basis for the discovery of why about one half of those who were transfused with the blood of another died. He noted that when the red blood cells of one person were exposed to the serum of another, they sometimes clumped or agglutinated. During the next two years Landsteiner and his associates investigated this phenomenon more fully. From these studies they learned that all human beings could be placed in one of four blood groups. The blood group to which any individual belongs is determined by the presence or absence in his erythrocytes of one or both of two antigens or isoagglutinogens. Landsteiner called these antigens A and B. Persons whose erythrocytes contain neither antigen A nor antigen B were classified as belonging to blood group O, the most common blood group among caucasians, as 40 to 45 per cent of the population have type O blood. Those who have isoagglutinogen A in their erythrocytes belong to blood group A; this is the next most frequent type, as about 40 per cent of the population belong to group A. Those who have isoagglutinogen B in their erythrocytes belong to group B; about 10 per cent of the population are in group B. About 4 per cent of the population have both isoagglutinogen A and B in their erythrocytes and are in group AB.

Agglutination depends on the presence in the serum of an antibody agglutinin that reacts with the antigen in the erythrocyte. The agglutinin reacting with isoagglutinogen A is named anti-A and the one reacting with B is called anti-B. The blood serum of a person does *not* contain the agglutinin that reacts with the isoagglutinogen in his red cells. Thus type A blood contains anti-B but *not* anti-A agglutinin. Persons in blood group O do not have either antigen A or B in the red cells, but they do have both anti-A and anti-B in their serum. Persons in blood group AB have antigens A and B in their erythrocytes, but they do not have either agglutinin in their serum. Because the blood of the donor is diluted as it enters the blood of the recipient, there is little concern about the effect of the antibodies in the serum on the red blood cells of the donor. Some authorities question the dilution factor as an explanation of why the donor's isoagglutinins do not agglutinate the erythrocytes of the recipient. Whatever the reason, the antibodies in the donor's serum do not usually adversely affect the recipient's red cells. Since erythrocytes of group O blood do not contain either antigen, they can be transfused into persons with other types of blood. For this reason a person with group O blood is said to be a universal donor; theoretically his blood can be transfused into all other individuals. Though group O blood can often be transfused into persons of other blood groups without causing a reaction, it can cause a reaction because of a high titer of anti-A and anti-B in the serum of the donor. When the titer of antibody is high, the agglutinin in the blood serum of the donor reacts with the isoagglutinogen of the recipient to produce hemolysis of the erythrocytes of the recipient. Persons with group O blood must be transfused with group O blood. Despite their ability to give to other groups, they can take only from their own group.

Because antibodies are absent from the serum of persons with group AB blood, they can theoretically receive blood from persons of all blood groups. They can give blood only to persons with type AB blood. Because not all persons react as expected on receiving blood, cross matching is an essential part of the preparation for blood transfusion. In cross matching, the erythrocytes of the donor are exposed to the serum of the recipient and the erythrocytes of the recipient are treated with the serum of the donor.

As Landsteiner and his associates studied the factors influencing the agglutination of erythrocytes, they learned that there were more antigens and isoagglutinogens than A and B. Perhaps the most important of these are those belonging to the Rh-Hr system. There are six cell characteristics that have been identified with this system. These factors have two sets of names, the American and the British. They are Rho, rh', rh", Hro, hr', hr". The corresponding British nomenclature is D, C, E, d, c, c_1. The red cells of each person contain at least one member of each of the three groups of antigens. In some persons the red cells contain four, five, or six of them. The number of possible combinations is therefore great.

Rh-Hr antigens differ from A and B antigens in that the antibody that acts against them is not normally found in the blood serum. It is formed when an Rh-negative person is given Rh-positive blood. This happens under two circumstances. In one, a person who is Rh-negative is transfused with Rh-positive blood. Although there is no obvious reaction, the individual reacts by producing antibodies in his blood serum against the Rh factor. Should this person receive a transfusion of Rh-positive blood at a later date, a serious reaction occurs. In the second situation an Rh-negative woman who is pregnant with an Rh-positive child is sensitized to the Rh factor. Usually nothing obvious occurs during the first pregnancy, and often during the second pregnancy, to indicate that the woman is becoming sensitized to the Rh factor. In many instances a number of normal children can be borne before the mother becomes sensitized to the Rh factor. Apparently, the sensitization comes about because the red cells of the Rh-positive baby escape through the placenta and stimulate the production of anti-Rh antibodies in the mother. These antibodies pass from the mother through the placenta into the blood of the baby causing hemolysis of the red cells of the baby. The condition in the baby is known as erythroblastosis fetalis. Some of these babies are born alive, and if the condition is not too severe, their lives may be saved by an exchange transfusion in which the blood of the baby is removed and replaced by Rh-negative blood.

In 1926 another type of agglutinin was described by Landsteiner and Levine.[28] The agglutinin in the blood plasma of an individual coagulates his erythrocytes when the temperature of the blood plasma is reduced below normal body temperature. Because the activity of the agglutinins depends on temperature, they are called cold agglutinins. According to Allen,[29] cold agglutinins are present more frequently in the blood of Negro donors than in Caucasians. They are also frequent in persons who have cirrhosis of the liver, severe anemia, hemolytic anemia, and many other chronic diseases. Cold agglutinins were not of much significance when blood was administered soon after it was drawn. It has assumed more importance now that blood is stored under refrigeration in blood banks. When patients are known to have cold agglutinins, blood is warmed before it is administered. After the blood is warmed, its temperature may be maintained by placing hot-water bottles at a temperature of 37° C. (98° F.) around the tubing through which it passes. Blood should be warmed slowly over a period of several hours to 37° C. Since the blood proteins can be altered by heat, care should be taken not to overheat the blood. Any mixing of the blood should be gentle, as hemolysis of red cells is increased by mechanical stress. Because of the increased possibility that the blood plasma of the patient with chronic illness may contain cold agglutinins, when he is transfused with cold blood he should be observed regularly and frequently for symptoms indicating hemolysis of cells. Hemolysis may result from the action of cold agglutinins in the serum of the donor on the red cells of the recipient or from the action of cold agglutinins in the serum of the recipient on the red cells of the donor.

[28] K. Landsteiner and P. Levine, "On the Cold Agglutinins of Human Serum," *Journal of Immunology*, XII, 1926, p. 441.
[29] Harkins, Moyer, Rhodes, and Allen, *Op. cit.*, p. 136.

Besides the antigens and antibody systems just presented, there are other rare antigens which may be present in erythrocytes. In certain diseases, such as hemolytic anemia, the red cells of the person become sensitized to an antibody in his own serum. The cells of these patients, as well as those of persons who are Rh-negative and who have been sensitized to the Rh-factor, react with Coombs's serum. Since Coombs's serum reacts only with the red blood cells that are sensitized in the living organism, the test is useful in determining the presence of hemolyzing antibodies in the blood serum of the patient. One of the important uses of the Coombs test is in determining the presence of antibodies against the Rh factor in a person with Rh-negative blood. When the test is performed by treating blood cells from an individual with Coombs's serum, it is called the direct Coombs's. In the indirect Coombs's, the cells of the donor are exposed to the serum of the recipient in order to identify antibodies in the recipient's serum.

Second in importance to the discovery of blood groups was that sodium citrate could be used to prevent the clotting of blood. Before this discovery, blood had to be transferred immediately from one person to another, usually by direct transfusion. When sodium citrate is added to blood, it prevents blood clotting so that the transfer of the blood from the donor to the recipient is delayed and the procedure is simplified.

A more recent innovation, the development of methods for the refrigeration and storage of blood, has made even greater delay possible. Because the life span of erythrocytes is from 100 to 120 days, the oxygen-carrying capacity of blood continues for some time. However, blood that is three weeks old or older is considered to be aged. White blood cells and platelets die within a few hours after blood is drawn. Therefore, when their action is desired, the blood must be freshly drawn. Freshly drawn blood can be used to restore any of the elements of the blood. Stored blood is satisfactory for restoring the blood volume, the oxygen-carrying power of the blood by replacing erythrocytes, and the blood proteins, but it is of no value in the replacement of thrombocytes or leukocytes. In the seriously undernourished patient, blood is sometimes administered for its nutritive value. Just as an example, each pint of blood contains approximately 35 gm of protein in the form of plasma protein. Cellular elements are further sources of protein, as well as of other nutrients.

In addition to the previously cited uses of blood in therapy, blood transfusion makes certain forms of treatment possible. Many surgical procedures could not be performed today were it not for the availability of human blood and the ability to transfuse it safely. Most patients undergoing prolonged surgical procedures require from 2 or 3 to 10 pt or more of blood to maintain blood volume and oxygen-carrying capacity. The more extended the operation and the greater the loss of blood, the more blood that is needed. Some surgical procedures could not be started without blood. Although the newer types of pumps used in heart surgery require little or no blood for priming, a large quantity of blood may be used before the procedure is completed. As much as 500 to 700 ml of blood is required to prime an artificial kidney. Some treatments such as total-body irradiation could not be performed were it not for the ability to replace the cellular elements of the blood.

What are some of the problems and hazards associated with blood transfusion?

Despite the values and uses of blood transfusion, there are also problems and hazards. One is the problem of obtaining sufficient blood to meet the demand for blood. A second problem is to protect the recipient from the hazards attending the transfusion of incompatible blood. The third is to prevent the transmission of blood-borne diseases. The first problem becomes obvious when one knows that, according to one estimate, 1 person in 80 will require a blood transfusion within the next year, and some of these individuals will require as many as 40 pt of blood. In fact, a patient who is dialyzed weekly on an artificial kidney may use as much as 416 pt during a year. Where does all this blood come from and how is it obtained? Obviously blood is obtained from individuals who either donate or sell it. In the past, most of the blood was donated, but because too few people give blood, more and more blood has to be purchased. In addition to the cost and the possibility of the price rising greatly, blood that is purchased from a commercial agency is much less reliable than donated blood, as the blood donors are more likely to misrepresent their medical histories. Blood-borne diseases for which there is no ready method of identification include hepatitis and malaria. The protection of the patient depends on the honesty of the donor in reporting that he has had either or both of these diseases.

Blood is obtained by two different types of agencies; one is voluntary and the other commercial. Voluntary agencies include the Red Cross, hospital blood banks, and community blood banks. Commercial blood banks, located in large cities, collect, process, and distribute blood for the purpose of making a profit. They depend on paid donors for blood, and the risk that the blood will carry organisms of one or more of the blood-borne diseases is therefore greater.

Why are less people donating blood than did formerly?

There are a number of explanations for the decrease in blood donations, despite an adequate number of persons who meet the criteria for blood donors. According to *Changing Times*,[30] if every eligible person gave blood, the supply would be ten times the need. That there are actually more people who are eligible to give blood than are needed is demonstrated by the experience in Delaware. In Delaware, there is a nonprofit blood-replacement program covering 40 per cent of the people of the state. Persons participating in

[30] July, 1963, p. 26.

this plan agree to donate blood when they are called upon. Although this plan has been in operation for eight years, some persons are now only being asked to contribute their second pint of blood. Through the organization of the community, the needs of persons requiring blood have been met without any individual being required to make a great sacrifice.

Multiple factors, mostly psychological and cultural, account for the failure of people to donate blood in proportion to the need and their capacity to give. In some communities two or more agencies may work cooperatively or vie with each other to collect blood from willing and available donors. The Red Cross is the largest single agency collecting blood, but it does not have centers in some communities and does not completely fill the need in others.

Many persons who have not donated blood hesitate to do so because they fear the consequences to themselves or the unpleasantness of the procedure. There are altruistic and selfish reasons for donating blood. There is no more personal way of helping one's fellow man than by donating blood. Many voluntary agencies encourage individuals to donate blood by promising that should they or a member of their families need blood within a specified period of time, it will be available. In terms of safety, a healthy person who is between the ages of 18 and 59 can give blood every eight to ten weeks for an indefinite period of time without his health being threatened.[31]

In the previously cited article in *Changing Times,* a manager of a nonprofit blood-collecting agency is quoted as saying that giving blood is not a status symbol. In factories, proportionately more blood is donated by the men on the assembly line than by union stewards or office personnel, and the executive class gives least of all. Because blood for transfusion is essential to save lives, nurses have a responsibility to help to interpret to the public why it is needed and why the donation of blood is safe and is a source of satisfaction to the donor.

As indicated above, blood transfusion can be a source of danger as well as of benefit. The dangers result from: (1) the possibility of the transfer of blood-borne diseases, (2) the transfusion of incompatible blood, (3) the too rapid infusion of blood into the individual, and (4) the introduction of pyrogenic substances. Under appropriate circumstances all of the above can be life-threatening.

In the prevention of transmission of diseases by blood, those that are of the greatest concern are syphilis, malaria, and homologous serum jaundice, or serum hepatitis. Persons who have syphilis can be identified by one of a number of serological tests. Each of these tests is named after the man who originated it (Kline, Kahn, and Hinton). These tests depend on the presence of an antibodylike substance (sometimes called reagin) in the blood serum. It

[31] The Red Cross has a well-organized plan for blood donors. They accept as a donor any healthy adult 18 through 59 years of age who weighs at least 110 lbs. Those under 21 years of age must have written consent of a parent or guardian, unless they are married. Donors are allowed to give blood every eight weeks, but not more than five times in a calendar year.

appears in the patient's blood serum soon after the onset of the disease. Those who have a history of having had malaria or who have been in a malarious area within a two-month period are not used as blood donors.

Though persons having a history of jaundice are not used as blood donors, this condition still develops in persons having blood transfusions. In the United States, hepatitis is probably the most common disease to be transmitted by transfusion. Because of the possibility of serum hepatitis, some physicians avoid the administration of blood unless it is absolutely essential. Serum hepatitis is associated with a high mortality and morbidity rate. For example, four months ago Mrs. Seven was delivered by caesarean section of a 6-lb baby boy. She required a blood transfusion. Two months after delivery she became ill. Because she was acutely ill and jaundiced, she was admitted to the hospital for diagnosis. Though her progress has been satisfactory, she had to spend six weeks in the hospital. Until there are methods of identifying carriers of the virus that produces jaundice, this condition will be one of the risks that attend the transfusion of blood.

A second danger, the infusion of incompatible blood, is present in every blood transfusion. That it does not happen more often is a tribute to the care that is taken to prevent any unsafe act at any point from the moment blood is taken from a donor until it is infused into a recipient. As indicated above, the transfusion of incompatible blood results in the agglutination and hemolysis of the erythrocytes of the donor by isoagglutinins in the blood plasma of the recipient. Should the blood plasma of the donor have a high titer of isoagglutinins, the erythrocytes of the recipient can also be agglutinated. Such cells tend to be hemolyzed more readily than normal. Signs and symptoms are due to the blocking of blood vessels by agglutinated cells and possibly are aggravated by the hemolysis of cells. Among the usual signs and symptoms are severe lumbar pain, tightness in the chest, and a sensation of burning of the face. There may be some degree of collapse, chilling, fever, and a rapid pulse. Hemoglobin may appear in the urine and anuria may develop. There are differences of opinion about the cause of anuria. Some believe that it is due to a blocking of the renal tubules by hematin which is released on hemolysis of red cells; others believe that it is due to reduced blood flow through the kidney.

*What are some of the precautions taken to prevent
transfusion reactions?*

Though not all transfusion reactions due to the infusion of incompatible blood are accompanied by serious effects, they may be. In addition, mild reactions in seriously ill or depleted patients may have grave consequences. In order to make sure that the patient receives properly matched blood, hospitals have rules regulating the collection and labeling of blood, the removal of blood from the blood bank, and the identification of the patient who is to receive the blood. All regulations are for the purpose of protecting patients from receiving mismatched blood. They should be meticulously followed.

All labels for blood taken from a patient for typing and cross matching should include the full name of the patient, address, and diagnosis, the name of his physician, and his hospital or clinic number. This information should be printed or written legibly. The possibility always exists that two patients with identical names and diagnoses may be present in the hospital at the same time. An added precaution to the complete labeling of all slips is to have the slips made at the bedside at the time the blood is drawn. In some hospitals only the physician is allowed to remove blood from the blood bank. As a further precaution, only one unit may be removed at a time. Blood taken from the bank should be labeled with the name both of the patient and of the donor, the date the blood was drawn, the blood group, and the hospital where the blood is to be administered. The safety of the patient depends on all persons paying strict attention to details, so that unsafe acts are prevented.

What should be done when a patient has manifestations indicating a transfusion reaction?

Despite the precautions instituted to protect the patient from incompatible blood, transfusion reactions do occur. At any time the patient evidences any of the signs or symptoms attributable to incompatible blood, blood flow should be discontinued at once. Even small amounts of mismatched blood can cause a serious reaction. The remaining blood should be saved to be returned to the laboratory, where it is checked for type and for bacterial contamination. Following a transfusion reaction the urine output of the patient should be measured and at least the first specimen should be saved. When there is a decline in urinary output, the patient should be weighed daily and his fluid intake adjusted to his output. (See Chapter 8.) Infusions of blood are frequently administered by a "double setup." One tube is attached to the bottle of blood and another to a bottle of physiological saline or glucose in water solution. The two tubes join leading to the patient by means of a Y tube. The flow of blood or fluid into the patient can be regulated by opening or closing the tubing leading from one or the other of the bottles. Unless care is taken, air can be taken into the system and infused into the patient. (See Chapter 8.)

A third hazard to the patient is the too rapid infusion of blood. Too much blood, or blood given too rapidly, predisposes to right heart failure, pulmonary congestion, and edema. Judgment as to the rate at which blood is to be administered is the responsibility of the physician. At times, when a large volume of blood has been lost in a short period of time, the life of the patient may depend on blood volume being restored quickly. In other instances, blood must be administered slowly to protect the circulation from overload. The responsibilities of the nurse are two: one is to maintain the rate of flow as prescribed by the physician and the other is to observe the patient for evidence indicating the development of any type of reaction to transfusion—in addition to the rate of flow of blood, vital signs including temperature, pulse, and respiration, and symptoms reported by the patient such as apprehension, feeling overly warm, or back pain. Although the temperature is not routinely checked during the administration of a transfusion, a rise in temperature frequently occurs earlier than most other signs and symptoms. Elevation of the temperature is not limited to the reaction to pyrogenic agents. Should any of these occur, blood flow should be terminated until the physician has had an opportunity to check the patient. The physician should be notified immediately.

Besides the dangers cited above, the blood or equipment used may contain a variety of substances which cause varied types of reactions. Before the introduction of plastic disposable sets, the tubing used for blood transfusion sometimes contained pyrogenic materials causing a febrile reaction. This type of reaction is not usually serious, though it may be in debilitated patients. Urticaria sometimes occurs during a transfusion reaction. Although the cause is not known, it may be due to the sensitivity of the patient to some substance in the blood of the donor.

Certain patients are more likely to develop one or another type of reaction to transfusion than others. For example, some blood dyscrasias, as well as repeated blood transfusions over a period of time, appear to predispose to reaction. Though all patients should be conscientiously observed during blood transfusion, those who are predisposed to reaction should be even more carefully observed.

In addition to the transfusion of whole blood, some fraction of the blood such as plasma, packed erythrocytes, or platelets may be administered. In place of plasma, a plasma expander may be used. Plasma or a plasma expander is utilized when the requirements for blood replacement are very large or, more importantly, when the plasma portion of the blood is diminished out of proportion to the red cells. For example, Mrs. Norman has second- and third-degree burns over two thirds of her body. She had attempted to light a wood stove by throwing gasoline on smoldering wood. It had blazed up and ignited her clothing. Shortly after she was admitted, her hematocrit was elevated to 75 per cent. The increased concentration of her blood was the result of the loss of plasma into the burned area. Saline and blood plasma were infused in addition to whole blood. Plasma and plasma expanders are more effective than solutions of glucose or electrolytes because they remain in the blood vessels longer and contribute to the osmotic pressure of the blood. Because blood is pooled in the preparation of plasma, plasma is more likely to be contaminated with the virus of hepatitis than is whole blood. Packed red cells are administered to increase the oxygen-carrying power of the blood without causing a comparable increase in the blood volume.

Despite the hazards that are associated with blood transfusion, it has many indications. As stated earlier, extensive and prolonged operations, such as are involved in open heart surgery, would not be possible without large amounts of blood being available. The uses of blood transfusion, whatever the nature of the patient's illness, can be summarized as follows:

1. To restore the volume of blood following hemorrhage or the loss of body fluids such as occurs in burns.
2. To restore the oxygen-carrying power of the blood by replacing erythrocytes.
3. To provide the elements required to support the body's self-sealing mechanism.
4. To provide the nutritive elements in the blood.

Of the above, the first two are the most common purposes of blood transfusion. The need for either may arise out of conditions that are treated medically or surgically. Despite the frequency with which blood transfusions are administered, they are always attended by the possibility of a serious complication. The patient should always be under the surveillance of a doctor or a nurse.

By virtue of the nature of surgical treatment, the patient always experiences some degree of shock and he always loses some blood. The significance of shock and bleeding, in terms of their threat to the survival of the patient, depends on the degree to which the circulation to the cells is maintained. Although shock can and does exist in the absence of hemorrhage, hemorrhage predisposes to shock.

How is the gastrointestinal system affected by surgery?

Not only are the functions of the respiratory and circulatory systems threatened by the various aspects of surgical therapy, but the functioning of the gastrointestinal system is also affected. As emphasized earlier, the gastrointestinal tract is very sensitive to the state of health of an individual. Furthermore, the sympathoadrenal system, which is activated by the physical and psychological stress of surgery, depresses the activity of the alimentary canal. Some disturbance in the functioning of the alimentary canal is, therefore, to be expected in patients who have been anesthetized and have undergone surgical treatment. The effects are usually manifested as anorexia, nausea, and vomiting. Because of the inactivity of the alimentary canal, bowel sounds are usually absent.

With the exception of patients having surgery on the gastrointestinal tract, vomiting does not usually last for more than a few hours. Soon after vomiting ceases, fluids are tolerated and gastrointestinal function returns promptly. In patients who have surgery on the gastrointestinal tract, function returns more slowly. It usually takes two or three days for the patient to be able to tolerate fluids and for the normal bowel sounds to appear. All the above effects are normal accompaniments of surgical treatment and do not constitute complications, unless they are prolonged or unusually severe. In order to prevent overdistention of the bowel and to increase the comfort of the patient whose gastrointestinal functioning is expected to be slow in returning, nasogastric suction may be instituted. Since the responsibilities of the nurse in the care of the patient treated with nasogastric suction were discussed earlier in the chapter, they will not be repeated here. After nasogastric suction has been discontinued, symptoms such as a feeling of fullness and vomiting indicate that the gastrointestinal tract of the patient is not ready to tolerate fluids.

When the bowel sounds are returning, but before water is tolerated, other fluids such as ginger ale or a similar carbonated beverage may be tried. Some patients find tea more acceptable than water or coffee. Dry crackers or toast may be better tolerated than fluids. Simple nursing procedures such as providing the patient with mouthwash after he vomits and emptying and washing the emesis basin promptly help to increase the comfort of the patient. Since suggestion sometimes plays a part in the continuance of vomiting, the emesis basin, while placed within easy reach, may be placed out of sight. When vomiting continues and there does not appear to be an organic basis for it, the physician may order a drug such as dimenhydrinate U.S.P. (Dramamine), or chlorpromazine (Thorazine). Just as the character and amount of fluid removed in gastric suction should be observed and recorded, the characteristics of emesis such as odor, color, consistency, and the type or description of solid particles should be noted and recorded. The circumstances under which the patient vomits are sometimes significant and should be observed. Should vomiting continue longer than is expected, a search should be made for its cause.

Since nausea and vomiting are frequent accompaniments of disease, by themselves these symptoms mean little more than that the patient is sick. Persistent nausea and vomiting in the postsurgical patient can be due to a great variety of disorders. They are, however, more likely to be due to an idiosyncrasy to drugs, emotions, pain, shock, uremia, disturbances in water and electrolyte or acid-base balance, or obstruction somewhere along the alimentary canal. As stated above, this list is by no means inclusive of all the disorders in which nausea and vomiting occur.

Perhaps the simplest cause of vomiting in the postoperative patient is idiosyncrasy to a drug. Often the observing nurse notes that after the administration of a drug, such as morphine or meperidine hydrochloride, vomiting occurs. It is most severe soon after the drug is administered and recedes as the time for the next dose approaches.

Though disturbances in function are more likely to be prolonged when a surgical procedure involves the gastrointestinal tract, the peritoneum, or the abdominal organs, they may follow any operative procedure. The three most serious complications are acute gastric dilation, paralytic ileus, and obstruction somewhere along the gastrointestinal tract. Both acute gastric dilatation and paralytic ileus result from failure to restore function of the gastrointestinal tract in the expected period of time. Obstruction may result from functional failure, or it may be the consequence of organic changes involving the wall of the digestive tube. Obstruction may occur soon after surgery or years later. Functional disturbances along the gastrointestinal tract tend to be self-perpetuating; that is, they act like a positive feedback system. As the activity of the digestive tube decreases, secretions and air accumulate causing distention. Distention further inhibits activity. With the distention of the wall of the stomach or intestine, the wall thins and lessens the capacity of blood vessels to deliver blood. A vicious circle ensues: inactivity → distention → thinning → decreased blood supply → inactivity. When functional disturbances are accompanied by vomiting or the need for continued suction, they may also lead to dehydration and serious disturbances in water and electrolytes.

Symptoms indicating that the function of the gastrointestinal tract is not returning as expected include: (1) nausea and vomiting after 12 to 24 hours —may persist longer in patients having surgery on the gastrointestinal tract or in those with peritonitis, (2) distention of the abdomen, (3) pain in the abdomen (gas pain), (4) silent abdomen, and (5) evidence of obstruction on X ray.[32]

In the patient who develops an acute gastric dilatation, prodromal symptoms may include a feeling of fullness, hiccoughs, and retching. Overflow vomiting may also occur. The patient vomits small amounts of dark-colored, foul-smelling fluid. Gastric dilatation may develop rapidly with the patient presenting a picture of acute shock. Unless the stomach is emptied and kept empty until function returns, death is a possibility. The nurse assists in the prevention of acute gastric dilatation by maintaining the function of the gastric suction apparatus and by regulating the amount of fluid which the patient ingests orally until the capacity of the gastrointestinal tract to tolerate fluids has been tested. The manner in which this is done was presented when the problems in the care of the patient having nasogastric suction were considered. The nurse also helps to prevent the gastric dilatation from becoming serious by reporting early signs and symptoms indicating that gastrointestinal function has not been re-established.

In paralytic ileus the normal motor activity of the gastrointestinal tract is not re-established in the expected time after surgery. The tract is characterized by both impairment and disorganization of function. As a result, the normal bowel sounds do not return as expected. Loops of the bowel fill with gas, but neither gas nor feces are passed by rectum. Gastric suction and the insertion of a rectal tube will often relieve the symptoms. When distention is not relieved by gastric suction, a long tube may be necessary to decompress the bowel.

Another common discomfort following major surgery or trauma is gas pains. Like vomiting, gas pains are expected. They differ from vomiting in that they indicate that gastrointestinal function is returning but that its activity is not yet coordinated. Since the introduction of nasogastric suction and early

[32] Gius, *Op. cit.,* pp. 316-17.

ambulation, few patients have severe gas pains. When a patient does have severe gas pains, the insertion of a rectal tube or a small enema may provide relief. Both must be prescribed by the physician. Since analgesic drugs such as morphine reduce the activity of the alimentary canal, they favor the development of gas pains. They should therefore be administered only as required to prevent pain in the postoperative patient.

Although it does not usually cause difficulty during the first hours after surgery, fecal impaction is another problem that arises from disturbances in the function of the gastrointestinal tract. It may result when a patient has had barium introduced into the alimentary canal previous to surgery and not all of the barium was removed. As the water is absorbed from the barium, it forms a hard mass similar to a plaster cast. Barium impactions can usually be prevented by the removal of the barium after the examination is completed. This can be accomplished by the administration of a mild laxative and cleansing enemas. Both of these must be prescribed by the physician. Identification of the need for such a prescription is a responsibility of the nurse. She should also be alert to signs and symptoms indicating that a barium impaction has been formed. Should the enema fail to remove the barium, this should be reported and recorded. Aged patients may also develop fecal impactions either following surgery or in the course of an illness. Symptoms that suggest the presence of an impaction include painful defecation, a feeling of fullness in the rectum, pain in the rectum, and constipation or a diarrhealike stool.

To lessen the possibility of fecal impactions, some surgeons prescribe mineral oil for the patient the day before surgery and for a few days after gastrointestinal function is resumed. Some surgeons also prescribe an enema for the patient on the second or third day postsurgery or after there is evidence that gastrointestinal activity has resumed. Others do not believe that enemas are necessary. When enemas are given, the extent of their effectiveness should be reported. Especially in elderly patients, not only should the fact that feces were evacuated be noted, but also the size of the stool should be described. Symptoms indicating the possible development of a fecal impaction should be reported and recorded.

As soon as the gastrointestinal tract begins to function normally, that is, vomiting ceases and bowel sounds are evidenced, fluids and food are prescribed by the surgeon. The length of time that oral food and fluids are withheld varies with the nature of the surgical procedure, the type of anesthetic used, and the response of the patient. Thus fluids may be started immediately postnausea and the patient progress rapidly to a full diet, or fluids and food may be withheld for several days. Usually patients having operations on the alimentary canal are not able to tolerate food as early as those having surgery on other parts of the body. When fluids are first administered, the volume may be restricted to 15 to 30 ml per hour and increased gradually to fluids as desired. Fluids should be discontinued and the physician notified if the patient vomits or complains of a feeling of fullness. (See Chapter 10.)

When a patient was reasonably healthy before surgery, his appetite can be expected to return within a few days. Except in those patients who have special requirements, patients are returned to a full diet as soon as they are able to tolerate it. Patients having surgery on the stomach usually require some reduction in the volume of food eaten at one time. The consistency may also be modified by reducing the amount of roughage contained in it. The objectives are to prevent distention of the stomach with strain on the sutures and to meet the nutritional requirements of the patient. Thus the patient is fed four to six small meals each day. Foods having a high cellulose content, such as cabbage and cucumbers, are eliminated.

All patients require an adequate intake of protein and vitamin C. Since the nutritional requirements of persons undergoing severe stress are discussed in Chapter 10, they will not be further elaborated on here.

What effects does surgery have on the function of the urinary system?

In the period immediately following surgery, or a traumatic injury, the formation of urine by the kidney is depressed. Oliguria is generally believed to be due to an increase in the production of the antidiuretic hormone (ADH) by the posterior pituitary gland.[33] Accompanying the retention of water is sodium retention, which may be the result of an increase in the production of the adrenal cortical steroids. Because of this tendency to retain salt and water after injury (surgery), the urine output of the patient is likely to be decreased below normal levels for the first 12 to 24 hours after operation. Following a period of oliguria, the patient may have a period of diuresis. In patients who have been in severe shock for an extended period of time, oliguria or even anuria may continue for days or even weeks. Unless the fluid intake of the oliguric or anuric patient is balanced against his fluid output, he may die from overloading with water. Because of the possibility of continued suppression of urine following surgery, the accurate measurement and recording of the urine output and the fluid intake for the first days following surgery are of great importance.

In addition to the possibility of oliguria or anuria, a considerable number of patients experience retention of urine; that is, they are unable to void during the early postoperative period. Failure to void, or retention of urine, can be a troublesome condition. In some patients who undergo surgery in the region of the bladder, such as gynecological surgery, or in operations on the large bowel, the ability to empty the bladder may be temporarily depressed.

One not uncommon cause of urinary retention is that some patients cannot void in bed. The position is abnormal and psychological conditioning against it may be very strong. When a patient cannot void in bed, the surgeon may permit the male patient to stand beside the bed or the female patient to use a

---

[33] Hardy, *Op. cit.*, p. 12.

bedside commode. One or more of a variety of nursing measures can some-times be employed successfully to induce voiding when a patient finds it difficult. Since tenseness of the patient aggravates the problem, the approach to the patient should be relaxed and the patient protected from anxiety-provoking situations. A screen around the bed or in front of the door will help to shield the patient from unexpected visitors. A warm bedpan is a necessity. Relaxation is sometimes encouraged by placing the feet of the patient in warm water. Suggestion sometimes works. Water is allowed to run from the tap, or warm water is poured over the vulva of a woman. When the bladder is not overly full, the patient may be urged to try to void and, if he is not able, to try at a later time. One thing to be avoided is to encourage the patient to try too hard, as he then becomes overly tense and is unable to relax the sphincters in the urethra.

When other measures are ineffective in encouraging the patient to void, or the nature of the surgical procedure is such that the bladder should not be allowed to become distended, catheterization may become necessary. When catheterization is required, it must be prescribed by the physician, and he makes the decision about whether the patient is to be catheterized when the bladder is full, at regular intervals, or whether an indwelling catheter be inserted. Two objectives should guide the nurse in her preparations for, and performance of, catheterization. The first is, obviously, to remove urine from the bladder. The second is no less important than the first and is more difficult to achieve. It is to prevent infection of the urinary tract. To prevent infection, all equipment and materials should be sterile, the procedure itself should be clean, and trauma to urethra and bladder should be avoided. To prevent trauma to the bladder, it should not be permitted to become overdistended. Overdistention predisposes to breaks in the continuity of the mucosa and diminishes the blood supply to the wall of the bladder. The danger of trauma to the bladder and urethra by the catheter can be lessened by lubricating the catheter well and encouraging the patient to relax. The lubricant lessens fric-tion by preventing the catheter from coming in direct contact with the wall of the urethra. Relaxation can usually be achieved by asking the patient to take a deep breath at the moment the catheter is introduced. The patient should, of course, have been prepared for what to expect and he should be adequately covered, so that his modesty pattern is observed. Should an obstruction to the passage of the catheter be encountered, the catheter should not be forced. It will usually slip into the bladder if the pressure on the catheter is reduced and the patient is asked to take a deep breath. When the catheter is in place, it must be held there, as the pressure of the urine in the bladder is likely to carry it out. Should the catheter escape from the urethra, another sterile catheter must be introduced.

To minimize the number of microorganisms introduced into the bladder, a number of precautions should be taken. The catheter and lubricant should be sterile; the area around the meatus should be well cleansed. In order to adequately expose the meatus, the patient should be in the recumbent position, with the knees flexed and the legs separated. A good light placed to illuminate the area is essential. Unless the patient is in a position that permits adequate exposure of the meatus, and the nurse can see what she is doing, the catheter is likely to be contaminated before it is introduced and the prevention of urethral trauma is more difficult to prevent. If the catheter becomes contaminated before it is introduced, another sterile catheter should be obtained.

Unnecessary discomfort to the patient should be prevented. In patients who have surgery on the perinum, exposure of the meatus may be painful. This discomfort can be minimized by preparing the patient for what to expect and by assuring the patient that every effort will be made to handle the tissues with gentleness. When the patient to be catheterized is a male, the female nurse should still provide the same instruction and precautions for him as she does for a female patient. In relation to the procedure itself, she is responsible for setting up the equipment and obtaining the doctor or a qualified male attendant to catheterize the patient. Catheterization can usually be performed with a minimum of distress to the patient. Time must be taken to prepare the patient for what to expect and for what she can do to assist the nurse. She should know that she will be told when her assistance will be needed, that her feelings are recognized and appreciated, and that the nurse expects to perform the procedure with carefulness. Since the introduction of early ambulation, catheterization for the retention of urine is less frequently required than in early preambulation days.

When an indwelling catheter is left in place, attention should be given to the maintenance of continuous free drainage. The tubing should be free of kinks, twists, or bends, and from pressure of resting body parts. It should be arranged so that the urine flows downhill into the drainage bottle. When prescribed by the physician, the catheter should also be irrigated at regular intervals to ensure its patency; this procedure should be carried out according to strict surgical aseptic principles. One way to irrigate the catheter, which is equally as effective and which eliminates the possibility of introducing microorganisms, is to make certain that the patient has an adequate fluid intake. Ansell[34] suggests that, when possible, the fluid intake should be sufficient to produce a flow rate of 50 ml of urine an hour, thus preventing the upward migration of motile bacteria in the collection tubing. He further urges the use of "bacteriologically sealed drainage systems with antiseptic in the collecting bottle to prevent growth of any possible contaminant." Figure 15-4 demonstrates dangerous and effective bladder-drainage systems.

When the catheter is removed, the quantity of each voiding should be measured accurately so that retention with overflow is detected should it occur. Frequent voiding of small amounts of urine is indicative of retention with overflow. In the care of patients who are catheterized for retention of urine,

[34] Julian Ansell, "Some Observations on Catheter Care," *Journal of Chronic Diseases,* XV, July, 1962, pp. 675-82.

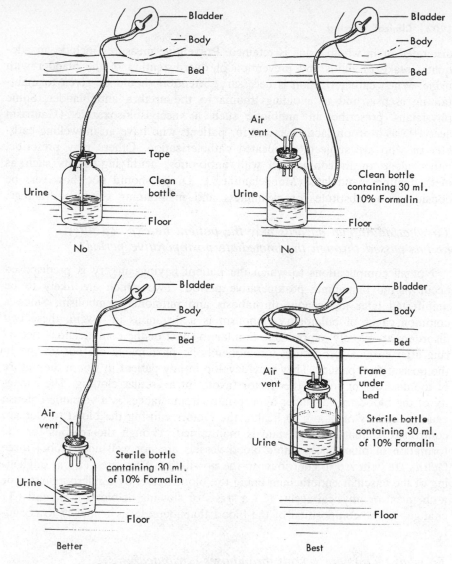

FIGURE 15—4. Gravity bladder drainage systems.

the bladder should not be allowed to become overdistended, as overstretching of the mucosa predisposes to breaks in its continuity and diminishes the blood supply to the wall of the bladder. Both disorders predispose to infection of the urinary bladder. This applies to patients who are catheterized for retention with overflow. Overdistention may result in injury to the mucosa and thus render it liable to infection. The overstretching of the muscle wall may also delay the return of normal function.

Urinary-tract infection is a possibility in any patient who is subject to repeated catheterization or in whom the bladder is allowed to become overdistended or in whom urine is retained. Preventive measures include an adequate intake of fluids and prevention of overdistention of the bladder with urine. When catheterization is necessary, attention should be given to maintaining asepsis and to avoiding trauma to the urethra and bladder. Some physicians prescribe an antibiotic such as acetylsulfisoxazole (Gantrisin acetyl[35]) as a prophylactic measure for patients who have an indwelling catheter or who are subject to repeated catheterization. Others may prescribe, either alone or in conjunction with antibiotics, acidifying agents such as methenamine mandalate (Mandelamine[35]). Drugs should not, however, be considered a substitute for cleanliness and maintaining effective drainage.

To what additional hazards may the patient be exposed after he has passed through the immediate postoperative period?

Not all complications to which the patient having surgery is predisposed occur in the immediate postoperative period. Two which are likely to be manifested later are venous thrombosis and pulmonary embolism. Since a common cause of pulmonary embolism is a thrombus in a vein, these two disorders are closely interrelated. Similar to most of the complications occurring after surgical procedure, thromboembolic phenomena are not unique to the postsurgical patient. They may develop in any patient in whom the nature of the disorder or some other factor favors intravascular clotting. The capacity of the blood to clot under appropriate circumstances is a valuable defense against the loss of blood. In health, the factors causing the blood to clot are controlled so that its fluid state is maintained. Though the reasons for the formation of blood clots within blood vessels are not well understood, three factors are believed to contribute to the possibility. They are: (1) a roughening of the vascular endothelium lining the blood vessel by a microorganism or a chemical or physical agent, (2) a stasis or slowing of blood flow, and (3) changes in the composition of the blood that increase its tendency to coagulate.

To what factors are venous thromboses attributed?

In health, damage to platelets and other elements in the blood is minimized by the smoothness of the vascular endothelium. Further protection is offered by the probability that a single layer of negatively charged molecules of protein repels negatively charged platelets and prevents the platelets from coming in contact with the vascular endothelium. Incident to surgery, as well as to disease, the vascular endothelium can be injured by microorganisms, trauma, or chemical agents with the result that it becomes roughened. The roughened surface increases the likelihood of thrombocytes being broken down. When the wall of a thrombocyte is ruptured, it releases thromboplastin which, in the presence of calcium ions, reacts with prothrombin to form

[35] Trade name.

thrombin. Thrombin then interacts with the blood protein, fibrinogen, to form fibrin. The fibrin forms a network of long, sticky threads or strands which entraps, in a manner similar to sticky flypaper, platelets (thrombocytes), and red cells and forms a blood clot.

The second factor favoring the formation of blood clots in blood vessels is stasis, or slowing of the flow of blood. Inactivity combined with the supine or sitting position favors stasis in the veins of the legs. With a normal rate of blood flow, cells are concentrated in the center of the blood vessel and are separated from the intima by a layer of plasma. As the rate of blood flow slows, cells tend to leave the center core and move toward the periphery, where they come in contact with the intima. Thus stasis of blood is believed to increase the likelihood of venous thrombosis in patients who are predisposed by other factors to it.

One aspect of the response to surgical or other trauma and to disease is an increase in the tendency of the blood to clot. Inasmuch as this response contributes to the effectiveness of the self-sealing mechanism, it is homeostatic. Like other homeostatic mechanisms, it can also be the source of problems. A number of changes in the blood contribute to its increased tendency to clot. Thrombocytes increase in number and become sticky. Instead of repelling each other, they tend to adhere one to another. Leukocytosis also occurs. When dehydration is allowed to develop, all the solid elements, including platelets and fibrinogen, increase in proportion to plasma and further increase the tendency of the blood to clot. In the absence of an adequate clotting mechanism, the individual faces the possibility of hemorrhage. When it is too active or clotting occurs in inappropriate sites, the clotting mechanism is also a source of danger to the individual.

As was stated previously, knowledge of why intravascular clotting occurs following surgery or trauma is incomplete. Although blood clots may form in any vein, deep veins in the lower extremities are most commonly affected. Something, perhaps a roughening of the endothelial lining of the vein, causes a disintegration of blood platelets. They release thromboplastin, which initiates the process of blood clotting. Guyton[36] emphasizes that once a clot is formed, it continues to grow, provided the clot does not obstruct the flow of blood. The continued growth of the clot depends on blood flowing over it to provide the materials from which the clot is formed. Growth usually ceases when the clot reaches a site where the vein in which it is formed joins another vein. The rate of blood flow is increased at the point where two vessels unite; the thromboplastin in the blood from the vein containing the thrombus is diluted and its clotting effect is reduced. Gius,[37] however, states that clots formed in the deep veins in the calf of the leg may propagate into the femoral and iliac veins.

As the clot forms, the fibrinogen within the clot is converted into fibrin. If

[36] *Op. cit.*, p. 210.
[37] John Gius, *Op. cit.*, p. 319.

there are thrombocytes in the clot, the fibrin threads within the clot fold and pull the clot together resulting in clot retraction. The clot is also invaded by macrophages which digest the red blood cells and release their hemoglobin into the body fluids. Later fibroblasts enter and organize the clot, so that within a few weeks it becomes a firm, fibrous mass. After a period of months, all that may remain of the thrombus is a small fibrous band.

Not only are the factors that are responsible for intravascular clotting unclear, but authorities disagree about the relationship of phlebothrombosis and thrombophlebitis. Some believe that these two conditions are phases of the same condition. Others state that they are two different conditions. Be that as it may, the predominating feature in phlebothrombosis is the formation of a blood clot. In thrombophlebitis the predominating characteristic is inflammation of the wall of the vein which may extend to the surrounding tissue and involve lymphatic channels as well. In phlebothrombosis, the problem is to prevent the detachment of a portion of the clot. The floating clot, or embolus, in a vein is dangerous because it causes pulmonary infarction. Venous emboli always are trapped in the lung. Veins increase in size as they approach the heart. Clots originating in the leg veins reach the right atrium and ventricle of the heart by way of the inferior vena cava. From the right ventricle, the embolus enters the pulmonary circulation via a pulmonary artery. It continues to move forward until it is trapped in, and plugs, an artery through which it cannot pass. If the clot is large enough to obstruct the entire pulmonary circulation, or the pulmonary arteries go into a severe spasm, the patient may die without warning or go into a severe shocklike state. Smaller clots continue in the pulmonary circulation until they reach a point which is too narrow for them to pass. They then obstruct the flow of blood to the area supplied by the occluded artery. The tissue undergoes necrosis, that is, infarction.

The symptoms and signs that accompany small emboli vary. Pain in the chest, which is similar to the pain of pleurisy and which may be described by the patient as a "catch in his chest" when he breathes, is common. Hemoptysis (blood in the sputum) occurs less frequently than the above. When there is hemoptysis, the sputum is brick red at first, but later it becomes dark red or brownish black. Small clots may also be expectorated. Although the patient usually has some fever, according to Chapman[38] it rarely exceeds 101.5° F. and lasts only four or five days. Chapman states that the treatment of pulmonary embolism is basically that of treating the phlebothrombosis or thrombophlebitis that causes it.

Unlike phlebothrombosis, a massive embolus is not likely to be formed in thrombophlebitis.[39] Thrombophlebitis is more likely to be followed by disturbances in venous and lymphatic drainage with the development of lymphedema.

[38] John S. Chapman, "Diseases Primarily of Circulatory Origin," in Harrison *et al.*, 2nd ed., *Principles of Internal Medicine*. The Blakiston Company, Inc., 1954, p. 1491.
[39] Leo Zimmerman and Rachmiel Levine, *Physiologic Principles of Surgery*, W. B. Saunders Co., Philadelphia, 1957, p. 455.

Although patients with phlebothrombosis may have little in the way of signs or symptoms to indicate the presence of a clot, they may have slight increase in temperature over normal levels. In some patients the temperature remains slightly elevated longer than is usual and there may be a small elevation in the leukocyte count. Mild pain in the calf of the leg is not infrequent. Should the patient mention the pain, he is likely to ascribe it to the fact that he is wearing slippers with heels that are lower than those to which he is accustomed. According to Julian and Dye,[40] the patient may suffer only mild symptoms and go on to complete recovery or he may develop a severe form of thrombophlebitis or a pulmonary embolism. Pulmonary embolism may occur before the local symptoms are manifested.

In the patient who has a thrombophlebitis, symptoms may range from mild to exceedingly severe. At the site of the thrombus, the cardinal signs of inflammation may be marked. The concern of the surgeon in the care of the patient is the prevention of the changes that lead to lymphedema.

As with other complications, prevention is preferred to cure. Authorities, however, do not agree as to the value of the various methods that are employed in prevention. With few exceptions the following are stressed: early ambulation, leg exercises while the patient is in bed, avoidance of pressure against the leg and thigh by a pillow or knee roll, maintenance of sufficient fluid intake to prevent dehydration, and prevention of hypotension. Zimmerman and Levine[41] state that while these procedures have not reduced the incidence of phlebothrombosis and thrombophlebitis, their incidence has not increased. That the magnitude of surgical procedures has been extended would seem to indicate that they have some preventive value. Other authorities also state that the incidence of these complications continues to be considerable.

For the patient who is predisposed to intravascular clotting or who has already developed phlebothrombosis or thrombophlebitis, the physician may prescribe an anticoagulant such as heparin or bishydroxycoumarin or one of its substitutes. Goodman and Gilman[42] state that the action of heparin in preventing coagulation of the blood is complicated and that it involves at least four interrelated effects. These are: (1) It acts as antiprothrombin to prevent the conversion of prothrombin to thrombin. (2) It antagonizes the action of thromboplastin, by a mechanism not fully understood. (3) It prevents the conversion of fibrinogen to fibrin. (4) It prevents the agglutination or clumping of platelets. The mechanism by which bishydroxycoumarin produces its effect is by inhibiting the synthesis of prothrombin. Because heparin interferes with the action of substances already present in the blood, its action is prompt. Since bishydroxycouramin inhibits the synthesis of prothrombin, its maximum effect does not occur for from two to four days and its action continues for some days after it has been discontinued. In patients in whom

[40] Orman C. Julian and William S. Dye, in Henry Harkins, *et al., Surgery, Principles and Practice,* 2nd ed., *Op. cit.,* p. 1126.
[41] *Op. cit.,* p. 459.
[42] *Op. cit.,* p. 1502.

the anticoagulant effect is immediately required, heparin may be administered by intravenous or deep intramuscular injection until the bishydroxycoumarin has had an opportunity to be effective. Bishydroxycoumarin is almost always administered orally. All patients who are being treated with anticoagulant therapy should be observed for evidence of bleeding. Should it occur, the condition should be reported immediately. The physician may discontinue the drug or decrease the daily dosage. To reduce the danger of hemorrhage in the patient who is receiving bishydroxycoumarin or one of its substitutes, the prothrombin time is checked either daily or every other day. The objective is to keep it between 25 and 15 per cent of normal.[43]

To prevent the clot from becoming an embolus, venous ligation may be performed. Bed rest with elevation of the affected leg is also prescribed. Though elevation of the leg is a simple procedure, its effectiveness in promoting venous return and the comfort of the patient depend on its being properly done. Since water runs downhill, distal parts should be higher than proximal parts. Support of the leg should extend along its entire length. Pillows should be placed so that they form a firm base under both the leg and thigh, and after they are in place, the muscles of the leg and thigh should appear to be relaxed. The pillows should look as if they are supporting the leg rather than the leg the pillows. Moreover, pillows have a way of becoming disarranged. Any position, no matter how comfortable at the beginning, becomes tiring. The obvious conclusion is that the nurse should check the patient regularly. He should have an opportunity to change his position and to have the supporting pillows rearranged, so that they continue to be supporting.

The physician may prescribe heat to be applied locally to the area. When warm, moist packs are used, they should be kept warm and some method should be employed to keep the bed dry. Chilling increases vasospasm and aggravates the condition.

Should the patient develop signs and symptoms indicating the possibility of a pulmonary embolism, the doctor should be notified immediately. In addition to anticoagulant therapy, the patient is placed on absolute bed rest and oxygen therapy is usually prescribed. Drugs to relieve the apprehension of the patient and to relax smooth muscle spasm may also be ordered. These include morphine, atropine, and papaverine. The development of a pulmonary embolism, especially a large one, is a frightening event for the patient, his family, and those responsible for his care. An embolism may occur during sleep or it may be associated with some ordinary activity such as getting out of bed or using the bedpan. Should the patient be out of bed at the onset of symptoms, he should be returned to bed and supported in a comfortable position. Should he be short of breath, he is likely to be more comfortable in a sitting than in a supine position. If at all possible, someone should remain with the patient until he is comfortable and his acute symptoms are relieved.

One aspect of postoperative care that has changed greatly over the last 20

[43] *Ibid.*, p. 1513.

or 25 years is the shift in emphasis from rest to exercise. As recently as 25 years ago, any patient who had major abdominal surgery was kept in bed for from ten days to two weeks postoperatively and then he was permitted to gradually resume activity over a period of six weeks to three months.

What is the rationale governing rest and exercise in the care of the patient who has undergone surgery?

The rationale on which bed rest was based in the postsurgical treatment of patients was that rest was conducive to healing and that the wound was liable to disruption should strain be placed on it. Men such as Dr. Daniel Leithauser noted that patients who refused to stay in bed did as well as or better than those who remained in bed and that the incidence of wound disruption was no greater. Though the practice was recommended by Reis more than half a century ago,[44] early ambulation did not receive widespread acceptance until Leithauser[45, 46] reintroduced it.

Some of the general effects of rest and exercise on the response of the patient to surgical and other trauma will be reveiwed before discussing the general types of exercise employed in postoperative treatment of patients. A more extensive discussion of the nervous, hormonal, and metabolic response of the individual to stress is included in Chapter 5. One of the immediate responses to acute injury or threat of injury is activation of the sympatho-adrenal medulla system. Many of the effects of its increased activity, such as increased sweating, vasoconstriction, and inactivation of the alimentary canal, have been previously described. According to Leithauser, this response is intensified and prolonged by bed rest and can be minimized in degree and shortencd in length by the early mobilization of the surgical patient.

Following surgery, the patient undergoes a metabolic response similar to that of the general response to injury. It is more severe in the young healthy individual than it is in the debilitated and elderly and it is intensified by bed rest. In the early stages, it is characterized by an increase in the catabolism of protein and a negative nitrogen balance. Later, protein anabolism takes place and the nitrogen balance becomes positive.

Among the positive effects of exercise following surgery is the reduction in the loss of nitrogen. According to Coller and DeWeese,[47] simple bed rest leads to a loss of nitrogen and a depression in the appetite. It also leads to a loss of muscle tone and to muscle weakness. Not only is nitrogen lost from muscles, but calcium is lost from bones during rest. In active healthy young

[44] Varco, *Op. cit.*, p. 120.

[45] D. J. Leithauser, *et al.*, "Prevention of Embolic Complications from Venous Thrombosis After Surgery," *Journal of the American Medical Association*, CXLVII, No. 4, September 22, 1951, pp. 300-3.

[46] Daniel J. Leithauser, "Early Ambulation," *American Journal of Nursing*, L, No. 4, April, 1950, pp. 203-6.

[47] Frances A. Coller and Marion S. DeWeese, "Preoperative-Postoperative Care," *Journal of the American Medical Association*, CXLI, November 5, 1949, p. 641.

persons, especially young men, who are suddenly and completely inactivated, loss of calcium may be so great that it forms kidney stones. This tendency can be counteracted by standing the patient on a standing board and by encouraging a high fluid intake. Return to physiological functioning of the respiratory, circulatory, gastrointestinal, and nervous systems is earlier in patients who exercise. Although exercise out of bed has more positive effects on function, exercise in bed is also beneficial and has its indications. Exercise improves the psychological status and morale of the patient. To the extent that exercise is accompanied by relaxation of the patient, it lessens pain and, as a consequence, less postoperative medication is required. Exercise also promotes relaxation. Mrs. Hammer illustrates the latter point. During a recent pregnancy Mrs. Hammer was found to have a marked elevation of her blood pressure. At the time of delivery, she went into hypovolemic shock as a result of severe hemorrhage. Despite reasonably prompt replacement of blood loss, she became anuric and remained so for about ten days. After this time her kidneys formed some urine of low and fixed specific gravity, but renal function did not approach that required to maintain the homeostasis of water and electrolytes. Because potassium and urea levels had risen to a critical level, peritoneal dialysis was initiated and Mrs. Hammer was instructed to lie still. What the physician meant was that Mrs. Hammer should not toss about or get out of bed. What Mrs. Hammer perceived was that she must not move a muscle. In fact, she was so fearful that she contracted her muscles so strongly that she developed muscle soreness that persisted for a week.

Because Mrs. Hammer was being "specialed" by a physician, she was given little attention by a nurse. When a nurse finally asked her how she felt, she said, "Awful, nobody does anything for you; no one talks to you." The nurse gave Mrs. Hammer a bath and, as she did, she put her extremities through their normal range of motion. She showed Mrs. Hammer how she could wiggle her toes and exercise her arms and legs without disturbing the tubing. Except for giving directions and instructions, the nurse did not talk very much. When she had completed Mrs. Hammer's care, she asked her how she felt. At this time Mrs. Hammer said, "Oh so much better. I had just about given up." Although there were other factors in Mrs. Hammer's improvement, exercise was one.

For the purpose of this discussion exercise following surgery will be considered under three headings: (1) mobilization or exercise of the patient in bed, (2) mobilization or exercise of the patient out of bed, and (3) exercises for the restoration of specific functions. All types of exercise have a common goal, the restoration of function. The effects of exercise can be summarized as a law of nature; parts develop in proportion to the stresses and strains placed on them. The branch of the tree attached to the trunk is larger than the twig at the end of the branch holding a leaf.

Many of the exercises performed in bed have been previously presented in other chapters. Mobilization of the patient in bed, while not as effective as exercise out of bed in preserving and restoring function, is essential for patients who for some reason cannot get out of bed. In bed, exercises are essential to the protection of respiratory, circulatory, and joint function and to the prevention of the loss of muscle strength and tone. Depending on the condition of the patient, exercise can be passive, that is, performed by the nurse, or it can be active, that is, performed by the patient. Exercise can also be assistive, inasmuch as the nurse helps the patient to exercise.

What exercises improve respiratory function?

The exercises performed by the patient to protect respiratory function have been discussed in some detail in Chapter 7. They include turning the patient from side to side, deep breathing, and coughing. Deep-breathing exercises can be made more effective by exhaling against resistance after inspiring deeply. A simple device for this purpose is a set of blow bottles. (See Chapter 7.) As a result of these exercises, the patient cleanses his airway, improves his vital capacity, and strengthens his respiratory muscles. Complications such as atelectasis and postoperative pneumonia are prevented.

How can circulatory function be improved by exercise?

Not only do the exercises that have been described improve respiratory function, but they also aid in promoting circulation. With inspiration the pressure within the thoracic cavity falls. Blood in the veins in the abdomen moves from the area of higher to lower pressure, that is, from the abdominal to the thoracic cavity. Circulation in the lower extremities may be further stimulated by foot and leg exercises. These should be taught to the patient during the preoperative period. They are based on the principle that the muscles of the feet and legs act as secondary hearts in the legs and move the blood toward the heart. Valves in the veins support the column of blood so that it can move only in the direction of the heart. As these muscles relax and lengthen, pressure against the wall of the vein is reduced and the blood flows into larger veins from the smaller distal veins. Inactivity leads to venous stagnation and congestion. The effects of venous congestion can be seen in the person who sits quietly for an extended period of time. Examples include the person who takes a long bus ride and the elderly person who sits in a chair from morning until night without moving. Because of inactivity and relaxation of blood vessels as a consequence of the depressing effect of anesthesia, congestion of blood develops in the leg veins during the operative and early postoperative phases of surgery. It is particularly marked in spinal anesthesia, and the problem is created by the loss of the mechanism for constricting the vessels in the extremities. Because of the tendency to pool blood in the lower extremities during anesthesia, some surgeons wrap the lower extremities from the toes to the knee or to the groin with elastic bandages.

Unless there is a specific contraindication, patients undergoing surgical procedures should perform foot and leg exercises regularly. These exercises consist of dorsiflexion alternating with hyperextension of the feet. The knee and the thigh should also be flexed and then extended. The movements of the leg and thigh may be referred to as bicycle exercises, because the movements are similar to those used in riding a bicycle. Though foot and leg exercises are more beneficial when the patient is able to perform them himself, they may also be performed by the nurse as passive exercises. Until the patient is up and walking, they should be initiated at one- or two-hour intervals, depending on the condition of the patient and the prescription of the surgeon. As with the deep-breathing exercises, most patients require reminding and, in the beginning, assistance.

Many physicians discourage the use of pillows or rests under the knees for two reasons. One is that a localized area of pressure tends to interfere with the venous return from the lower extremities and predisposes to venous stasis and thrombosis. The other is that it tends to reduce the mobility of the patient, because the pillow or knee rest helps to hold the patient up in bed. Without the pillow or the knee rest, the patient slides down in bed. When he becomes uncomfortable, he boosts himself up in bed to increase his comfort and in the process stimulates his circulation, respiration, and muscle activity.

For patients who are confined to bed over a period of time a variety of simple devices are available to increase the mobility of the patient as well as to enable him to assist with his care. One such device is the overhead swing, which, when used, strengthens the arm muscles and enables the patient to move about in bed and to assist with his care. A rope or sheet tied to the foot of the bed may be used by the patient to pull himself into a sitting position. The arms and shoulders may be strengthened by the patient placing his hands palms down on the bed and raising his buttocks from the bed. This exercise is useful in the preparation of the patient for crutch walking.

Exercise should be a part of the care of the patient. When a patient is treated by bed rest, the nurse should include range of motion exercises as an aspect of morning and evening care and the bath. When the patient is able, he may perform these exercises himself, or the nurse may assist him with them or perform them by herself. As the term "range of motion" implies, extremities are moved at the joints within the limits of the usual range of motion for the patient. One precaution should be observed; in the performance of these exercises, the nurse should never force a part beyond the point at which it moves freely nor should pain be caused by the movement.

Valuable as exercises mobilizing the patient in bed are, they are not as effective as mobilizing the patient out of bed. Although patients do get out of bed and sit in chairs, the discussion that follows will concentrate on ambulation as a form of therapy. The term "to ambulate" means to walk, not to get up and sit in a chair. This is a point emphasized by Leithauser in his writings and lectures about ambulation. In fact, he stresses the point that patients should be discouraged from sitting in a chair. They should either be walking or in bed. Leithauser opposes the sitting position because the dependent position of the legs and the weight of the body on the thighs interferes with venous return from the legs. Venous stasis predisposes to the development of thrombophlebitis, which, in turn, predisposes to pulmonary embolism. Varco[48] states that, particularly in elderly patients who fall asleep in the sitting position, hypotension may develop. This may lead to syncope (fainting) and the falling of the patient. Varco[49] summarizes the benefits to the patient from ambulation, including less pain in the operative site, the earlier disappearance of pain, the reduction in certain postoperative sequelae, the improvement of the patient's morale, and the earlier discharge of the patient from the hospital.

Coller[50] emphasizes some of the physiological effects of ambulation. He states that ambulation has a protein-sparing action. The catabolic phase of metabolism is minimized by exercise. The length of the period in which the patient feels weak and asthenic is reduced, and his vital capacity is more quickly restored.

The earliness with which patients treated surgically are ambulated varies with the surgeon, the surgical procedure, and the patient. Leithauser, who was one of the more vigorous proponents of early ambulation, advocated that patients be ambulated as soon as they had recovered from the depressing effects of the anesthetic. The only exceptions were patients in profound shock, experiencing severe uncontrolled hemorrhage, in thyroid crisis, or who were dying.[51] Varco[52] adds sepsis to this list of exceptions. He is of the opinion that bed rest is probably indicated in patients who have an infection, as exercise can promote the spreading of an infection.

Particularly when early ambulation was first introduced, patients, nurses, and physicians were fearful that harm might come to the patient. All had been indoctrinated with the belief that bed rest was necessary to healing of the wound and that exertion on the part of the patient was dangerous. Patients entering the hospital expected to have a good rest. Instead they were forced out of bed to walk. They, too, were frightened. Today patients are likely to be prepared to ambulate. They know that the neighbor across the street was out of bed a few hours after he returned from the operating room. Despite previous warning, however, the patient who gets out of bed for the first time after undergoing a major surgical procedure is frequently frightened and anxious lest he be harmed. Enough competent assistance should be available to assure the patient that he will not be allowed to fall. When a patient is large or heavy, a male nurse or orderly can make a real contribution not only to the patient's feeling of safety, but to his actual physical safety. In the actual process of getting the patient out of bed, the patient should be allowed time to adjust to each change in position.

---

[48] *Op. cit.,* p. 121.
[49] *Ibid.,* p. 120.
[50] Coller, *Op. cit.,* p. 644.
[51] Leithauser, *Loc. cit.,* p. 301.
[52] Varco, *Op. cit.,* p. 120.

If the method suggested by Leithauser[53] is followed, the patient starts from the supine position. Preparatory to getting the patient out of bed, when the height of the bed can be easily adjusted, the bed should be lowered. Then the patient turns on his side and, as he starts to sit up, swings his feet over the edge of the bed. By the time he is in the upright position, his feet are over the edge of the bed. At this point the patient may wish to rest with his hands on the edge of the bed or on the shoulders of a nurse standing in front of him. Then the patient should be assisted to the standing position. In those hospitals where the height of the bed is fixed, the simplest way to get the patient out of bed is to let him slide off the edge of the bed until his feet touch the floor. He should be supported and encouraged to cough, so that secretions are eliminated from the tracheobronchial tree. He should then be encouraged to walk to the foot of the bed and return to the center of the bed. He is assisted into bed, where he assumes the supine position. After a period of rest, he is again encouraged to get up and walk. With each period out of bed his strength and courage return.

Following chest surgery, ambulation offers some difficulties. However, they are not insurmountable. If the patient has chest drainage tubes, attention should be given to preventing tension on them. If the bottles are moved, they should be kept below the point where the tubes enter the thorax to prevent fluid from being sucked into the pleural cavity. Suction is discontinued and tubes are clamped only when prescribed by the physician or when they are approved policy of the institution. Ambulation of the patient receiving intravenous fluids can be accomplished if the arm into which the needle is introduced is stabilized. When the needle is introduced into a vein over a joint, the joint must be immobilized with a splint. Attention should be given to the prevention of tension on the tubing. In patients with indwelling catheters, the catheter can often be clamped while the patient is up and about. If there is some contraindication to clamping the catheter or the patient is to be up for some time, then the catheter may be attached to a bag strapped to a leg or to a leg urinal, or the bag may be carried with the patient.

With exercise, rest is also important in the care of the patient. Despite Leithauser's contention that patients will not overdo, some patients do require protection from overactivity. As the patient begins to recover, he may feel that he is farther along in his convalescence than he is. He should be encouraged to exercise, but to stop before he becomes fatigued.

Another source of exhaustion of patients is the number of procedures performed on them. Frail or seriously ill patients are sometimes exhausted by the continuous activity. Mr. Watts had open heart surgery and the replacement of his aortic valve with a prosthesis. For the first three days postoperatively, he continued to be in incipient shock. On his first postoperative day, he was to be turned from side to side, to do deep-breathing exercises, and to cough each hour. All the above are required to prevent postoperative atelecta-

[53] Leithauser, *Loc. cit.*

sis and to promote the re-expansion of the lung. However, because Mr. Watts was frail, these took the better part of an hour. At one point when his care had just been completed and he was prepared to rest, his surgeon and his assistants came in. The patient was then raised to a sitting position and moved so that his chest could be examined. Shortly after the physicians departed, the patient vomited without any warning nausea and soiled the bed with emesis. The bed required changing; Mr. Watts required rest. His nurse felt that there was another requirement—that is, some planning between the surgeon and the nurse so that the visit of the physician could be substituted for one of his exercise periods. The nurse has the responsibility for taking initiative to protect the patient from too rigorous exercise and to make sure that he gets needed rest.

A third type of exercise is prescribed to protect or restore the functions of a specific structure or part. For example, the loss of muscle tone in an extremity can be lessened by the performance of muscle-setting exercises. To prevent the loss of strength in a leg encased in a cast the physician sometimes prescribes the setting or contraction of the quadriceps muscles. Since these muscles are inserted into the kneecap, the nurse can practice performing this exercise on herself as preparation for teaching patients. As the quadriceps muscles shorten, the kneecap can be felt to move. Before encouraging a patient to exercise a muscle or muscles of an extremity that has been incised, the nurse should consult with the physician about the time the procedure should be instituted.

Following a radical mastectomy, exercise of the arm and shoulder on the affected arm may be prescribed by the physician to maintain motion in the joint in the affected side and the tone of the muscles in the area. Surgeons differ as to the time exercises are to be started. When the resection has been extensive, closure of the wound may be difficult and healing of the wound may depend on immobilization of the area. The nurse should always consult the surgeon before initiating exercises. Allen[54] states that exercise should be begun as early as the first postoperative day. Specific exercises that are used are described in Chapter 12.

When patients are treated by physical therapy, the nurse should know what the purpose of the therapy is and how the nurse can extend the work of the therapist in her care of the patient. Though this discussion has been related to the needs of the postsurgical patient, it is no less relevant to the care of any bedfast patient, whatever his diagnosis or treatment.

In achieving the objective to restore the person to health, exercise is one of the very necessary requirements. Whether exercise is performed in bed or out of bed, it improves the psychological as well as the physiological status of the patient.

[54] *Op. cit.*, p. 556.

How can wound infection be prevented?

Perhaps the most nearly unique aspect of the surgical patient is the incision that is made to provide a route of approach to the organ to be operated upon. Many additional aspects of wound healing are discussed in Chapter 5. As emphasized earlier in this chapter, the incision disrupts one of the individual's most important defenses against infection. All patients who undergo surgical treatment are predisposed to wound infection.

The prevention of wound infection depends on the application of the principles of asepsis from the moment the patient is admitted to the hospital until the time of his discharge. Other factors contributing to its prevention include a good state of nutrition. Overweight predisposes to wound infection. Adipose tissue is more vulnerable to infection than many other tissues because it has relatively poor blood supply. The problem of wound infection is further considered in the section on wound healing.

What is one of the most serious consequences of impaired
wound healing? What are the nurse's responsibilities?

Disruption of the wound is one of the serious sequelae of impaired wound healing. Separation of the wound may occur at any time following the closure of the incision. It may occur immediately after the wound is closed and before the patient has been transferred from the operating room or at some later time. A common time is about the seventh day.[55] The degree to which the wound separates varies. When the skin as well as the underlying tissue separates and the contents of the abdominal cavity extrude, the condition is known as evisceration. Although disruption of any wound may occur, the most common site is in mid-line abdominal incisions.

Although wound disruption is possible in any patient, certain conditions in the various phases of surgery predispose to it. In the preoperative phase, obesity, undernutrition particularly of protein and vitamin C (ascorbic acid), conditions associated with metabolic disorders such as diabetes mellitus, Cushing's syndrome, and uremia, and advanced cancer appear to predispose to impaired wound healing. Weight reduction, when a patient is obese, and attention to the nutritional status of patients during the preoperative period are important preventive measures. During the operative phase, many of the activities of the surgeon are directed toward making and closing the incision in such a manner that wound healing is favored or, conversely, is protected from disruption. Thus attention is given to the site and direction of the incision. Long mid-line abdominal incisions are avoided. Wound healing is a consideration in the selection of sutures and in the suturing technique. Careful hemostasis and the maintenance of asepsis are also important. With the exception of asepsis, all the above preventive measures are the responsibility of the surgeon.

[55] Varco, *Op. cit.,* p. 113.

During the postoperative phase a variety of conditions predispose to separation of an abdominal incision. Perhaps the most frequent cause is some disorder that places strain on the incision by increasing intra-abdominal pressure. Thus separation of the wound is associated with abdominal distention, retching, unrelieved coughing, sneezing, hiccoughs, or uncontrollable motor activity. When any of the above disorders exist, attention should be directed toward their relief. The nurse has a responsibility to report any of the above to the physician and to carry out measures for their relief. Should the surgeon believe that the patient is seriously predisposed or that separation of the wound is imminent, he may apply a spica bandage of tape to the abdomen of the patient.

What signs and symptoms indicate some degree of wound disruption?

Staining of the dressing over the incision with a serosanguineous material is a warning sign that wound disruption will possibly occur. At the time the wound separates a large amount of serosanguineous material may escape. The patient may feel something give or burst. He may call attention to the fluid by saying that the area around the wound felt as if warm water had been poured over it. He may have pain in the wound, which may be severe. In addition, he may vomit, have symptoms of abdominal distention and paralytic ileus, and develop signs of shock. When evisceration occurs, coils of intestine may protrude from the wound or escape into the bed, an extremely hazardous situation.

What are the responsibilities of the nurse when wound dehiscence or evisceration is impending or has occurred?

When there is evidence that wound dehiscence or evisceration is impending or has occurred, the physician should be immediately notified. At best, these sequelae to impaired wound healing are extremely serious. As little time as possible should be lost between the event and the initiation of treatment. The patient should be instructed to lie quietly on his back in a horizotal position. If coils of intestine can be seen, they should be covered with a sterile towel or other sterile materials. Since wound disruption predisposes to shock, the patient's blood pressue should be determined and his pulse and respirations counted. When at all possible, a nurse should remain with the patient until he is seen by his physician. To assure the patient that all is being done that can be, he should be told that the physician has been notified and is coming. For most patients who are suddenly faced with a serious threat to their physical well-being, evidence that measures are being taken to correct the condition is in itself reassuring. They rightly interpret action as the appropriate activity. Preparations should be made for the physician. A nasogastric tube and suctioning equipment should be secured and the tube should be ready to insert. Since retching increases intra-abdominal pressure, a local anesthetic should be ready for use to anesthetize the pharynx. A mask and a sterile gown and gloves, as well as sterile towels, should be obtained for the surgeon. Sterile saline should be warmed and available. When the surgeon arrives, he will decide on the place and type of therapy. When the condition of the patient permits, most surgeons prefer to have the patient transferred to the operating room for treatment. In the process of transferring the patient, enough help should be available to move the patient without increasing his intra-abdominal pressure. Depending on the extent to which the tissues are separated and on the condition of the patient, the surgeon may support the incision by taping the abdomen or return the patient to surgery for a secondary closure.

What other signs and symptoms may the patient exhibit
related to the effect of surgical trauma or function?

Among the signs and symptoms accompanying the surgical state that have not been discussed in relation to the effect of surgical trauma on function are pain, fever, and hiccough. Although pain and fever always occur, the incidence of hiccough of a severe degree is not very great. None of the above are at all unique to the surgical patient. The discussion of pain and hiccough will, however, be presented here.

One of the most common manifestations of illness is pain and fear of pain. In the minds of many people some illnesses, such as cancer, as well as certain treatments, such as surgery, are practically synonymous with pain. The nurse has a significant role in both the prevention and relief of pain. This role may be summarized as:

1. To make the necessary observations which serve as a basis for making a judgment as to whether or not a patient is in pain and for arriving at an appropriate course of action.
2. To institute appropriate action to prevent or to alleviate pain.
3. To observe the effects of measures used to relieve pain.

To fulfill her role with understanding, the nurse requires some knowledge of: (1) the nature of pain, (2) the anatomy and physiology of pain, (3) what constitutes the pain experience, (4) the factors in the suffering caused by pain, (5) the physiological and emotional responses to pain, (6) the observations that are significant in pain, and (7) the measures useful in the therapy of pain.

The fact that pain is a private and personal experience is not to be denied. No one except the person who is in pain knows how much pain he has, or its exact nature, or what the pain means to him. There is a poverty of words in the English language to describe pain. The words used by the patient to describe his pain are chosen on the basis of what he thinks is happening. He uses words such as crushing, boring, burning, prickling, or gnawing. For many centuries and until recently, pain was not classified as a sensation, but as the antithesis of pleasure. Despite extensive study, pain had never been defined to the satisfaction of all scientists. Most definitions, however, include the following points: (1) pain is a sensory perception, (2) pain has a psychic component, (3) pain is unpleasant, (4) pain, even when it is localized, involves the whole person, and (5) pain is useful to the extent that it causes the individual to seek help in determining its cause and in securing relief. Fear of pain may, however, cause a person to delay seeking necessary treatment.

Knowledge of pain as a sensation has come about during the last hundred years or so. Keats and Lane[56] state that most of the progress in the treatment of pain has been made in the therapy of specific pain. Nonspecific pain is one of the unsolved problems in clinical medicine. To illustrate the magnitude of the problem these authors state that the *Physician's Desk Reference* for 1963 lists 156 systemic analgesics. Until relatively recently the anatomy of pain has been described in terms of specific pain receptors, pain fibers, and pain centers in the central nervous system. Melzak[57] states that the modern view of pain is not that it is a single sensation, but that it is a complex experience that involves the total individual. The anatomy of the sensory perception of pain is fairly well known; that of the complex experience is just beginning to be identified. Knowledge of the latter is at the point where there is sufficient knowledge to make hypotheses, but not enough to be sure that the hypotheses are correct. Haugen[58] states that there are two pathways that carry pain impulses to the central nervous system, one conducting impulses rapidly and the other conducting them slowly. Like other sensory perceptions, pain impulses are transmitted from receptors to spinal tracts by way of mixed peripheral nerves. Keats and Lane[59] also state that pain impulses are transmitted over two sets of nerve fibers, both of which are present in all peripheral nerves. In one system, known as the A delta fibers, the fibers are large and myelinated. They conduct impulses rapidly. In the other, or the C fibers, the fibers are small and unmyelinated and they conduct pain impulses slowly. The two systems contribute somewhat differently to the pain experience. The A delta fibers alert the individual to the presence of pain and localize it. The C fibers contribute to the suffering in pain. Keats and Lane summarize the pain pathways in Figure 15-5. The A delta fibers, which are myelinated, pass more or less directly to the thalamus and the sensory areas in the cerebral cortex. The collateral system connects with the reticular formation and provides for slower conduction than does the main pathway. In addition, it has many diffuse connections with many centers in the brain. These fibers are unmyelinated. The suggestion has been made that the role of the collateral system

[56] Arthur S. Keats and Montagne Lane, "The Symptomatic Therapy of Pain," *Disease a Month,* Yearbook Medical Publishers, Inc., Chicago, June, 1963, p. 3.
[57] Ronald Melzak, "The Perception of Pain," *Scientific American,* CCIV, February, 1961, pp. 41-49.
[58] Frederick P. Haugen, "Current Concepts of the Pain Process," *Journal of Chronic Diseases,* IV, July, 1956, 4-10.
[59] *Op. cit.,* p.4.

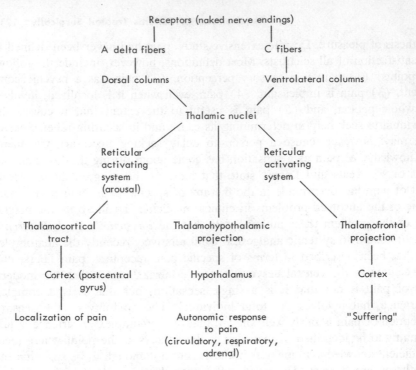

Receptors (naked nerve endings)

A delta fibers   C fibers

Dorsal columns   Ventrolateral columns

Thalamic nuclei

Reticular activating system (arousal)   Reticular activating system

Thalamocortical tract   Thalamohypothalamic projection   Thalamofrontal projection

Cortex (postcentral gyrus)   Hypothalamus   Cortex

Localization of pain   Autonomic response to pain (circulatory, respiratory, adrenal)   "Suffering"

FIGURE 15—5. Schema of pain pathways. (Adapted, with permission, from Arthur S. Keats and Montague Lane, "The Symptomatic Therapy of Pain," *Disease-A-Month*, p. 7. Year Book Medical Publishers Inc., Chicago, June, 1963.)

is to integrate information from many sources and to modify the reaction of the individual to pain. Melzak[60] states that fibers have been identified that go from the brain to message-carrying nerve pathways in the spinal cord. These fibers modify impulses coming into the spinal cord over sensory fibers. As a consequence, impulses may be suppressed and never get beyond the level of the spinal cord, or be altered so that the message which is delivered is different from the one that originated the impulse. According to Melzak,[61] a portion of the sensory nerve impulse entering the spinal cord or brain stem passes over a dense network of interconnecting internuncial neurons. Though not proved, this may be the point at which memory, thoughts, and emotion modify sensory messages after injury. There is experimental and psychological evidence to support the assumption that higher centers in the brain do modify sensory nerve impulses at various lower levels. In time, the pathways whereby higher centers influence lower centers will undoubtedly be identified.

Sensation of any type requires not only pathways for the conduction of impulses and centers for their interpretation and integration, but receptors that are sensitive to painful stimuli. Formerly it was believed that there were specific pain receptors in the skin. The current view is that the skin contains

[60] *Op. cit.*, p. 44.
[61] *Ibid.*, p. 44.

1218

widely branching bushy networks of receptors that overlap one another and are stimulated by noxious stimuli, including stretching of the tissue. When the stimulus approaches the point of tissue damage, the sensation that results is interpreted as pain. The point at which the individual interprets sensory stimulation as pain is known as sensory pain perception. In our present state of knowledge, the thalamus appears to function in the awareness to pain. The thalamus has, however, connections with many areas of the brain. The cerebral cortex is presumed to function in the localization of pain and in the recognition of its nature, severity, and significance.

The integrity of sensory mechanisms is essential to the perception of pain. occasionally a child is born who lacks pain and temperature receptors in his skin. Though this deficit does not interfere with the survival of the child, he lacks one of the mechanisms for learning to protect himself from injury. More common is the individual who, because of disease, injury, or therapy, is deprived of structures or functions enabling him to perceive or interpret pain sensations. The individual then must learn how to protect the tissues thus deprived from injury and to inspect them for evidence of injury. For example, Melvin Gale suffered a transection of his spinal cord at the level of the first lumbar vertebrae. He was completely paralyzed below the point of injury. For the remainder of his life, measures must be instituted for the protection of the paralyzed parts of his body from the effects of pressure and other injury. As soon as his physical condition permitted, he was taught the importance of moving and turning himself regularly, of checking the temperature of bath water with his hand or a thermometer, and of inspecting his skin for evidences of pressure or injury. In contrast, Mr. Roberts, who was paralyzed as a result of acute anterior poliomyelitis, did not have this problem. Despite his flaccid paralysis, he was sensitive to painful stimuli. In fact, during the acute stage of his illness, his skin was so sensitive that his nurse was frequently reminded of the princess who could feel a pea though it was covered by seven mattresses.

A third example is that of Mr. Westwind, a 68-year-old man with trigeminal neuralgia. As a result of this disorder, Mr. Westwind suffered paroxysms of excruciating pain. To relieve him of his pain, the surgeon cut all the sensory branches of the trigeminal nerve. The distribution of the sensory branches of the trigeminal nerve can be seen in Figure 15-6. The trigeminal nerve is sensory to the skin and mucosa of the head, to the teeth, and to the cornea of the eye. Mr. Westwind was therefore deprived of the ability to detect foreign bodies in, or injury to, the eye, or to detect stimuli indicating the possibility of injury to the skin of his head or to the buccal mucosa. In his care, provisions were made to protect the structures thus deprived of sensation and to teach Mr. Westwind what he needed to know and do to protect himself from injury. Part of his instruction was to inspect his eye at least three times a day for evidences of irritation. He was also taught to inspect the inside of his mouth and tongue after each meal for food remaining in his mouth and for evidences of injury, and to protect the affected side of his face from

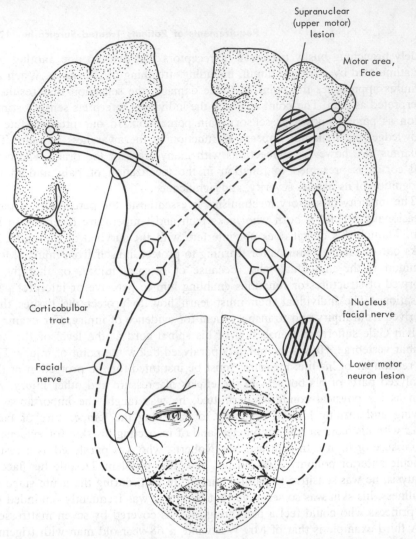

FIGURE 15–6. The shaded areas of the face show the distribution of facial muscles paralyzed after a supranuclear lesion of the corticobulbar tract, and after a lower motor neuron lesion of the facial nerve. (Adapted. Courtesy of John T. Manter and Arthur J. Gatz, *Essentials of Clinical Neuroanatomy and Neurophysiology*, 2nd ed., F. A. Davis Company, Philadelphia, 1961, Fig. 24, p. 59.)

overexposure to cold. Fortunately most patients with trigeminal neuralgia do not require that all branches of the trigeminal nerve be cut for relief of pain. The branch supplying the cornea of the eye can usually be saved, and when it is, special protection of the eye is unnecessary.

Mr. Gale and Mr. Westwind have been used to illustrate some of the problems that arise when an individual is deprived of his sensory nerve supply. Tissues are no longer warned that they are being exposed to noxious stimuli. Plans for the nursing of the patient should include provisions for the protection of the tissue from injury and for the instruction of the patient in how to protect himself. The basic protective measures are those that prevent injurious agents from coming in contact with the tissue or that limit the length or degree of exposure. Since there is always a possibility of injury, the affected area should also be subjected to regular inspection for evidence of inflammation.

In addition to the perception of pain, the pain experience has a second aspect, or the psychic component, which is also known as the reaction to pain. It includes what the person thinks and feels about his pain as well as what he does about it. Interest in the psychic component in the pain experience has been stimulated by the observation that, despite similar bodily injuries, the degree of pain varies from individual to individual or even in the same individual at different times. Melzak[62] illustrates this point by quoting the studies of Beecher. During World War II, Beecher was surprised to find that among seriously injured soldiers admitted to a combat hospital, only one in three complained of pain severe enough to require morphine. Moreover, many of these men denied having any pain at all. After the war, he studied a group of civilians who had incisions similar to the wounds received by the men in battle. In this group, four out of five stated that they had severe pain and wanted something to relieve it. From these findings, Beecher concluded that factors other than the extent of the wound determine the degree of pain experienced by an individual. One of the most fundamental factors is the meaning that the pain has for the person. The soldiers were grateful for having escaped from the field alive. In contrast, civilians regarded their situations as a serious misfortune or even a catastrophe. Instead of being saved from death, they were facing the possibility of serious injury, pain, and even death. On the battlefield, injury results in the relief of anxiety. The patient facing surgery or some other painful experience has an increase in anxiety. In the words of Crowley,[63] three factors contribute to the production of anxiety in the patient in pain: "They are the threat to the self, the loneliness of pain, and the element of the unknown in pain."

Contributing to the meaning that a pain-eliciting situation has for an individual are his past experiences and his memories of them. Apprehension, with the resulting tension, is likely to be increased when a patient fears that he is going to be hurt. The tension resulting from fear and anxiety can be expected to increase the degree of pain suffered by the patient. When the patient knows that those who are responsible for his care will be gentle, that they will not allow him to suffer unnecessarily, and that when pain is unavoidable he will be warned so that he can prepare himself, he is less likely to be unnecessarily apprehensive.

Since culture influences the way in which people view the various events in

[62] *Ibid.*, p. 42.
[63] Dorothy M. Crowley, *Pain and Its Alleviation,* University of California, Berkeley, 1962, p. 61.

life, it also influences what the individual regards as painful and how he reacts to pain. Mark Zborowski's studies of the cultural components in responses to pain were cited in Chapter 6. In the United States, the groups of people who place a high value on health regard pain as an indication for seeking medical attention. They expect that the cause of the pain can be determined and the condition treated successfully. The behavior of the patient in pain is in part due to culture and training. In many American families, girls may cry when in pain, but boys are told that men do not cry and that they should bear pain like a man. In some cultures, such as certain tribes of American Indians, children are taught from infancy to bear pain without giving evidence of suffering. Procedures such as hypodermic injections that cause the ordinary child to cry out are tolerated without any display of emotion. Other patients are also seen who, as a result of culture and training, bear pain silently. The only evidence that they are in pain may be a drawn facial expression, beads of perspiration on the brow, or a quickened respiratory or pulse rate. Others express their pain for all to hear and see. Patients with deep religious faith may tolerate conditions that are ordinarily associated with severe pain with little evidence of pain. This is explained by the meaning that the religious faith of the patient gives to his pain. He firmly believes that pain has a spiritual purpose and that suffering should not be wasted. Care should be taken to make sure that patients who have pain receive attention. Patients who do not express their pain freely may be overlooked. Those who are noisy and demanding may also be neglected, because of the tendency to regard them as overdemanding, neurotic, or childish.

Any condition or event that distracts the attention of a person from the pain or pain-provoking stimuli tends to lessen pain. Conversely, anything that focuses the attention of the person on the pain tends to increase it. Hundreds of examples ranging from the trivial to the dramatic could be used to illustrate this point. The pain of minor burns and scratches in children is relieved by a kiss, a dab of colored antiseptic, or a tape bandage. A small child that has fallen and bumped his head may pick himself up and start to play again only to start crying when his mother, looking anxious, asks him where he hurt himself. Athletes, soldiers, and even ordinary laymen carry out a necessary activity, despite serious injuries. Mr. Allen, who was burned, is a good example. Despite serious burns, he returned to his apartment to rescue his son. Once his son was safe, he fainted. The pain-relieving effect of distraction and activity is quite often seen in patients. When the nurse enters the room, the patient complains of pain and general discomfort. By the time the nurse has bathed him, placed him in a comfortable position, and administered whatever care is required to improve his general comfort, he may be experiencing very little pain. A similar effect of distraction frequently is seen in elderly people who spend much of their time alone. When a visitor first arrives, Mrs. Cotton complains of the pain in her joints and other discomforts. By the time the visitor is ready to leave, her pain may be all but forgotten. The nurse frequently uses distraction to lessen a patient's pain or discomfort. She talks to him during a procedure or instructs him to do something such as to take a deep breath or to squeeze her hand.

Pain that is long continued reduces the capacity of the person to tolerate pain. Miss Smart illustrates this point very well. She was a middle-aged woman with a diagnosis of subacute bacterial endocarditis; the bacteria causing the infection showed a high degree of resistance to available antibiotics. To try to control the infection, Miss Smart was given one or another antibiotic by intramuscular injection every two hours around the clock. Before too long, Miss Smart's body was studded with painful spots. Her ability to tolerate pain and discomfort was reduced to the point that she screamed at the slightest touch or jarring of her bed. Fatigue, sickness, debility, and repeated painful procedures reduced her tolerance to pain to an exceedingly low level. Once the injections were discontinued and her condition improved, she was able to tolerate pain as well as most people.

When the pain experienced by the patient is mild or moderate, diversions such as music, reading, visiting, or crafts may serve to distract the attention of the patient from pain. This is not meant to be a universal prescription, however. In the patient who is suffering severe pain, attempts at diversion may increase the tension of the patient. Diversion should be employed when it is indicated, and avoided at other times. In general, patients who are acutely ill, including those who have recently undergone major surgery, should be protected from overstimulation and fatigue. What they need is a quiet, calm, and restful atmosphere combined with a feeling that they can trust those responsible for their care to meet their needs. Less acutely ill patients, and most particularly those with long-term illness, may be benefited by diversional activities that are suited to their state of health and personal interests. These patients should also be protected from overfatigue, as fatigue lowers the tolerance of the patient to pain.

The fact that the effectiveness of analgesic drugs is increased by telling the patient that the drug will relieve his pain has been demonstrated by experimental study. In some patients pain can be relieved by the assurance that the injection or pill he is receiving will relieve his pain. This is known as the placebo effect. This does not mean, as it is generally interpreted to mean, that the patient does not have pain. By reassuring the patient that something is being done for his pain, his attention is distracted from the pain and his apprehension is relieved. A nurse is appropriately utilizing the placebo effect when she says to the patient as she administers a pain-relieving medication, "I have something (a hypodermic or pill) that will relieve your pain." Occasionally, the physician prescribes an injection of water or saline for its placebo effect, but a nurse should never make the decision to give a patient a placebo without such an order. Psychological factors are of importance in all patients who have pain. They should be utilized to the benefit of the patient.

Another factor in the suffering caused by pain is the feeling of the patient that he has or does not have some degree of control over his pain. In order to provide the patient a feeling that he has some control over his pain, some physicians allow certain of their patients to keep analgesics, such as acetylsalicylic acid, at the bedside. When the patient is in pain and the nurse is responsible for the administration of an analgesic drug, she can add to the sense of security of the patient by administering it promptly.

When movement aggravates pain, as it is likely to do, every effort should be made to prevent unnecessary pain. Attention should be given to minimizing both the sensation of pain and the fear of pain. The first step is to prepare the patient for what to expect and for what is expected of him. For example, "We have come to turn you to your other side. We will use the turning sheet. You can help by holding your spine as 'stiff as a poker.'" Suggestions made by the patient should be treated with kindness and respect. Therefore, when the patient says, "I always keep my neck from moving by placing my hands on each side of my face," the nurse responds by saying, "Fine, we will tell you when we are ready and then you can help." The nurse should use discretion in following the suggestions of the patient; one that is harmful should not be followed. The patient should be told why his suggestion is rejected in such a way that his self-esteem is maintained. Courtesy and tact should be characteristics of the behavior of the nurse at all times.

The patient who has been, or is, in pain is frequently reluctant to move. Whether or not movement of the patient is essential at a particular time depends on the needs of the patient and of the situation. If harm is likely to result to the patient unless he is moved, then he should be encouraged to move or to permit himself to be moved. Often allowing a patient to wait for a short time in order to give him an opportunity to mobilize his resources will lessen his reluctance. He should be assured that enough competent assistance is available so that he will be moved with a minimum of discomfort. The number of persons required to move a patient is not always the deciding factor. One or two skillful nurses who are trying to do what must be done gently may be all that is required. Finally, the patient should know why he should move or be moved at this particular time. Sometimes the reluctance of the patient results not so much from his lack of acceptance of what has to be done, but from the fact that he is ill.

The patient's fear of pain can be minimized by providing his care in such a manner that he knows that those who are giving him care will do their best to protect him from unnecessary pain. All care should be characterized by gentleness, steadiness, and smoothness. Force, haste, or rough, jerky movements have no place in the care of the patient in pain. Noise, confusion, and ineptitude are disturbing to the patient in pain and should therefore be eliminated. In patients who have a painful illness, expressions of negative feelings are common. The nurse should try to accept these as part of his illness and continue to treat the patient with kindness and consideration. Undue levity and boisterousness should be avoided. Though the nurse does not help the patient by being as depressed by the pain as he is, neither is he aided by excessive cheerfulness. What is generally beneficial is a combination of acceptance of the fact of the suffering of the patient and an air that implies that something can and will be done to lessen it.

Attention to the physical aspects of pain is also important in its prevention and relief. All body structures should be maintained in anatomical alignment. Support should be provided as needed to achieve positions which will eliminate strain on parts. Basic to securing good alignment and to preventing strain on muscles is a firm mattress. When a patient is heavy, a board under the mattress may be required to achieve a firm surface. In some institutions a nurse may place a board under the mattress when it is required; in others a prescription from a physician must be secured. In the prevention of strain, the body and any of its parts should be moved as a unit. In moving the torso, the patient can assist by trying to keep his spine straight and stiff. The movements of all who participate in the turning should be synchronized, so that everyone moves together. Counting "one, two, three, go" is helpful. Devices such as casts, braces, and corsets may also be utilized to keep the spine and other joints immobile.

To move an extremity, the general principles already enunciated apply. The part should be supported so that strain is minimized and unnatural movements are avoided. Both hands may be used, supporting the part on the palms of the hands, or the extremity can be supported by placing the hand and arm under its length. Pressure should be avoided over painful areas. Here again, movement may be made less painful by the use of a splint, brace, cast, or even a pillow to support the painful part while it is moved.

In postoperative patients with incisions through the chest or abdominal wall, coughing causes more or less pain. The patient should, of course, be taught that coughing is part of his postoperative management and how to cough. He should also know that the discomfort in his incision can be decreased by supporting the wound when he coughs. Whether the nurse or the patient provides the support depends on the location of the incision and the wishes and the capability of the patient. In patients who cough in excess of that required to maintain the patency of the tracheobronchial tree, a binder may be required to provide continuing support for the incision.

When immobility of the trunk or thigh is required, or movement is accompanied by excessive pain, the desired result may be attained by placing the patient on a Foster, Stryker, or Bradford frame. They also facilitate the giving of patient care.

Swelling, particularly in a tissue surrounded by a bony wall or encased in a circular bandage or cast, is painful. The most effective treatment is to reduce the swelling by utilizing the force of gravity to remove the excess fluid. Mrs Erie offers a good example. She was admitted for the reduction of a fractured tibia which was followed by the application of a cast. Several hours after the cast was applied, she called and asked to have something for her pain. Her toes on the affected side were cyanotic, cold, and swollen. Instead of getting Mrs. Erie an analgesic, the nurse elevated her leg on pillows and told Mrs. Erie that, as soon as the swelling was relieved, her pain would disappear. An hour or so later Mrs. Erie said that she was free of pain and was able to eat breakfast.

Nurses also administer medications to relieve pain. The means by which different drugs relieve pain differ. They act by: (1) removing the cause of pain, (2) decreasing consciousness, (3) lessening the conduction of impulses over pain fibers, (4) raising the threshold for pain perception, and (5) lessening the awareness, or appreciation, of the significance of pain. To illustrate, pain in the patient with a peptic ulcer increases when the hydrochloric acid is undiluted by food or fluids. Relief of the pain is afforded by alkali or bland foods such as milk. These substances do not attack the basic cause of the ulcer, but they are effective in relieving the immediate cause of the pain.

The drugs most commonly used to suppress consciousness are the general anesthetics. Although they can be utilized to suppress pain of all types, their use is limited almost entirely to the operative period of surgical therapy. Local anesthetics are most frequently employed to prevent pain during a surgical procedure, but they may also be used to relieve pain that does not respond to the more usual methods of treatment. Alcohol or procaine, when injected into a nerve, interrupts the transmission of nerve impulses. The procedure is known as a nerve block and is employed to prevent pain incident to making a surgical incision or in the treatment of painful diseases. In the instance of Mr. Westwind, a surgeon injected alcohol into his gasserian ganglion about 18 months previous to the resection of his trigeminal nerve. He was free from pain for about a year.

Drugs commonly utilized to relieve pain are known as analgesics. Modell,[64] classifies analgesic drugs as the greater, or addictive, analgesics and the lesser, or nonaddictive, analgesics. The most important member of the first group is morphine. Its substitutes, such as meperidine hydrochloride and methadone hydrochloride, are also useful. The lesser, or nonaddictive, drugs fall into four groups. They are the salicylates, antipyrine, the coal tar derivatives, and cinchophen. Drugs that are not of themselves analgesics may contribute to the relief of pain when combined with an analgesic by decreasing the capacity of the patient to evaluate pain and the meaning of pain. Thus a patient may be given acetylsalicylic acid (aspirin) in combination with phenobarbital or one of the so-called tranquilizers, such as chlorpromazine. Acetylsalicylic acid is believed to raise the threshold to pain, or the point at which the patient experiences pain. As a result of the action of chlorpromazine or some other tranquilizing drug, the patient is less concerned with the significance of his pain. For specific information about various drugs, the

[64] Walter Modell, "Pain," in Relief of Symptoms, 2nd ed., C. V. Mosby, St. Louis, 1961, pp. 75-104.

reader is referred to a textbook on pharmacology. Morphine appears to have both effects, as it is effective in allaying the apprehension of the patient as well as in lessening his perception of pain. In fact, there is experimental evidence that morphine diminishes pain only when the level of anxiety is high.[65]

In the selection of an analgesic for a patient, the physician considers a number of factors—the nature and location of the pain, the elements contributing to the pain, the length of time that the patient can be expected to have pain, the probable outcome of the patient's illness, and the effects of the drug itself. For example, morphine or one of its substitutes is likely to be prescribed for the patient who has just had abdominal surgery and who can be expected to require pain relief for a period of not more than 48 hours. Under these circumstances the danger of addiction is minimal. In fact, in any condition in which pain is severe, addiction is not as likely to develop as when the pain is mild. By way of contrast, when pain is mild or moderate and/or the patient is expected to require relief for a long period of time, the physician usually prescribes the mildest drug in the smallest dosage that can be expected to afford relief. The selection of the medication and the interval at which it is given is the prerogative of the physician. The nurse administers the medication within the framework of the prescription of the physician. When the physician prescribes the medication at stated intervals, the drug must be given at the times prescribed unless the patient develops signs of depression of the respiratory or nervous system or other toxic effects. When the prescription left by the physician permits the nurse to use her discretion, then she may give the drug as often as required. Usually the prescription or the policy of the agency sets some limits on the maximum frequency with which a drug can be administered. This is usually every three to four hours. Generally, the patient gets more benefit from the drug if his pain is not allowed to become too severe. There is some evidence to support the observation that patients who can count on having their pain relieved promptly suffer less pain than those who cannot. Dickman made a study to determine the effect of knowing or not knowing on the quantity of drug required by postoperative patients for comfort. Patients who knew that they could have a pain-relieving medication required less medication than those who did not know.[66] Most patients tolerate painful or unpleasant procedures better if they have their medication before the procedure is performed. During the first 48 hours after surgery or immediately after the development of a painful disorder, such as a myocardial infarction, addiction is not very likely to develop.

To summarize, pain is a subjective experience. Since every person is different, each patient can be expected to behave in an individual manner when he is in pain or in a pain-provoking situation. There is abundant psychological and experimental evidence to indicate that psychological factors are of great

[65] Melzak, *Op. cit.*, p. 43.

[66] Helen Mae Dickman, *A Pilot Study of Pain in The Postoperative Patient*, unpublished Master's Essay. Detroit, 1959.

importance in the pain experience. To prevent and relieve his pain, the way the patient feels and thinks about his pain must be taken into account. The nurse cannot always know why one patient has more or less pain than does another, but she can assume that there is a reason. She can modify the care of the patient so that unnecessary pain is avoided. Pain cannot always be eliminated, but it can be made more bearable by kind and thoughtful care.

The nurse has another responsibility to the patient who is in pain, that is, to observe pain and its effects. Pain may originate in superficial or visceral structures or in the central nervous system. Superficial pain is initiated by the effect of an injurious agent on the skin. The points at which tissue damage and pain occur have been demonstrated to be very close. Sensitivity of the skin to painful stimuli varies from anesthesia, to hypesthesia, to hyperesthesia. In anesthesia, the skin is insensitive to painful stimuli. In hypesthesia, a greater-than-normal stimulus is required to evoke pain. In hyperesthesia, the skin is abnormally sensitive. Anesthetic and hypesthetic skin lacks the normal protective mechanisms against heat, cold, pressure, and trauma. Depending on the extent and location of these areas, protective measures may be required in the protection of the patient. Hyperesthesia is common in acute febrile diseases and in neuritis. In the latter condition the skin may be exquisitely painful over the affected area. Stimuli that would not ordinarily cause any discomfort may result in severe pain. The area may even have to be protected from the weight of bed coverings by a cradle. Hyperesthesia of the edges of a wound is common, and when it occurs, the patient can be assured that it is expected and will disappear in time.

With severe superficial pain the defense mechanisms of the body can be expected to be mobilized. There is an increase in the activity of the sympathetic nervous system and in the production of epinephrine, with tachycardia the peripheral vasoconstriction resulting. With the increase in the heart rate and vasoconstriction, the blood pressure can be expected to rise. In patients who do not express their discomfort either verbally or by a change in facial expression, the nurse may have to depend on evidences of increased sympathoadrenal activity, such as sweating, tachycardia, and a rise in blood pressure, to detect pain. A generalized increase in muscular tension may also indicate pain.

Pain can be deep, such as that occurring in bones or viscera. Pain in bones is often dull, aching, and localized. Pain in the viscera is usually dull and diffuse. Pain impulses arising in deep muscles and in the viscera are mediated by common sensory structures and can be projected to the skin. This contributes to difficulty in identifying the origin of the pain. For example, difficulty may be encountered in distinguishing between the pain of cholelithiasis, peptic ulcer, and myocardial infarction. Accompanying pain in the viscera is a type of pain called referred pain. Why referred pain occurs has not been completely explained. The pain occurs in the superficial structures supplied by the same sensory apparatus as the organ that has been injured. The explanation usually given is that the brain is unable to locate the specific origin of the pain and therefore projects it to the skin. The following are illustrations of disorders characterized by referred pain. In tuberculosis of the hip, pain is frequently referred to the knee. In myocardial infarction, pain may be referred to the precordium, the neck, the shoulder blades, and the left arm. The patient may have so much pain in his shoulder that he hesitates or refuses to move his arm and, as a result, develops a frozen shoulder.

Severe deep pain differs from superficial pain in that it is more likely to cause failure in homeostatic defense mechanisms. Weakness, hypotension, pallor, sweating, bradycardia, and nausea and vomiting are common. These signs and symptoms can be observed in patients with a variety of thoracic and abdominal conditions. Examples include myocardial infarction, perforations of abdominal viscera, and biliary or renal colic.

Central pain is a type of pain which is perceived in the mind of the individual and for which there is no peripheral cause at the time the pain is experienced. The classical example is phantom limb, a painful condition that has been known for many years. The patient has pain and other sensations in the amputated limb even when he can see that the limb has been removed. For example, one patient asked to have a pillow in his bed to support his amputated leg. He had the feeling that he had to hold his leg up off the bed. The sensation was relieved by placing a pillow in the bed where his leg would have normally rested. Many patients have sensations that appear to originate in the amputated extremity which in time disappear. Occasionally, however, these sensations persist for years, and they may be so severe that the person is incapacitated.

The manner in which pain is elicited differs with different types of tissues. The skin is sensitive to cutting, burning, pricking, and trauma. Severe pain is induced in skeletal muscles by ischemia. This is the basis for Mr. Elderly's pain during exercise. He has severe atherosclerosis which limits the ability of the arteries to increase the blood supply to his legs during exercise. When he walks for a block or so, he develops a severe cramplike pain in the calf of his leg which is known as intermittent claudication. Pain in the skeletal muscles can also be caused by prolonged contraction and by the injection of irritating substances into them. Ischemia is also the cause of pain in the heart muscle. The ischemia may be relative or absolute. In atherosclerosis or as a result of arterial spasm, the capacity of the coronary arteries to deliver blood to the heart muscle may be inadequate. When Mr. Plump increases his activity, he develops a cramplike pain in his chest. Essentially Mr. Elderly and Mr. Plump have a similar problem. Both of them have pain because their arteries are unable to deliver sufficient blood to maintain muscular activity. In both, pain is protective inasmuch as it acts as a warning. With the onset of pain they stop whatever they are doing; they rest and allow their muscles to recover. They also learn to avoid activities that precipitate the pain. When an artery supplying a muscle is obstructed, pain continues for some time. It is not relieved by rest or by drugs that dilate arteries and increase the blood supply.

Pain in the gastrointestinal tract is caused by trauma to engorged mucosa and by stretching or spasm of smooth muscle. The intestine and stomach can be cut or burned without giving rise to pain. Stretching or spasm of smooth muscle in the biliary and urinary tract also causes severe pain. Arteries also give rise to pain when they pulsate excessively as in migraine headaches or in arteritis.

Observation of the patient is necessary to the collection of information on which the nurse bases her judgment that the patient does or does not have pain of sufficient degree to require relief. From her observations of the patient, the nurse also decides on the course of action that she will take to treat the pain experienced by the patient. The first step is to determine whether or not the patient is in pain. When a patient is asleep or resting quietly, he is not likely to be in pain. When he is aroused he may complain of pain and then lapse back into sleep. The belief that all postoperative patients and patients with cancer have pain is erroneous. Keats[67] cites a study of another investigator who found that 44 per cent of 237 patients did not complain of pain after operation. In his own series he found that 21 per cent of 104 patients who had either a gastrectomy or colectomy received no more than one dose of a narcotic drug during the entire postoperative period. Some of these patients received none. Despite the above, it is invalid to conclude that a patient who does not complain of pain is comfortable.

When the patient complains of pain, he should be asked to indicate its location and to describe it. The patient may be asked to point to the painful area. Leading questions should be avoided as they may result in the patient giving misleading information. The question should be phrased so that the cause of the discomfort experienced by the patient can be determined. The resulting answer may indicate that the patient is in pain or that he is sleepless, is suffering from discomfort from a nasal or oxygen catheter, has a sore throat, headache, or backache, is in an uncomfortable position in bed, has an overdistended bladder, or has some other condition other than pain from an operative incision or relating directly to his disease. The selection of the method of treatment should be based on the cause of the discomfort. Information should be elicited about any situation or condition that provokes or relieves the pain. For example, Mrs. Robin continued to complain of pain five or six days after a gastroenterostomy. Her nurse noted that the pain was always precipitated by Mr. Robin's visit. About the same time, Mrs. Robin also made the comment that she always felt so good after she had a "hypo." Both facts were reported to her physician. As Mrs. Robin was showing early signs of addiction to morphine, the drug was discontinued and other therapy prescribed.

The quality of the pain and other characteristics of the pain should be noted and recorded preferably in the words used by the patient. The mode of onset of the pain, its duration, severity, and time of onset are all important.

[67] Arthur S. Keats, "Post Operative Pain: Research and Treatment," *Journal of Chronic Diseases*, IV, 1956, 72-83.

When the character of the pain experienced by the patient changes or pain appears in a new or unexpected area, this information should be reported to the physician. Whether this is done immediately or delayed until the next regular visit of the physician depends on the possible significance of the pain. Severe pain or pain and other symptoms and signs indicating involvement of the viscera should usually be reported before an analgesic drug is administered, as the drug may mask the patient's pain and thus eliminate an indispensable factor in helping the physician to identify the nature and location of visceral involvement.

In addition to the description of the pain by the patient, there is usually other evidence to indicate that a patient has pain. For example, restlessness, discomfort indicated by facial expression, hands pressed over the painful area, moaning or other sounds indicating pain, irritability, refusal to move or moving carefully, perspiration, and anorexia. When the pain is severe, the blood pressure may be elevated or depressed and the pulse and respiratory rate altered. Not all of these effects are unique to pain. Restlessness is also common in hypoxia, and it is important to identify its cause before treatment is instituted. Anorexia occurs in many types of illness. When pain is long continued, it contributes to the debility of the patient by decreasing his food intake. In just a few weeks, Mr. Westwind (trigeminal neuralgia) lost 25 lb. Each time he tried to eat, a paroxysm of pain was precipitated. Therefore he refused to eat. Pain, even when it is not induced by the suggestion of food, is so all-encompassing that everything else becomes unimportant.

Observation of the patient should continue after measures have been taken to relieve pain. Observation should be directed toward determining the success or failure of the treatment and any undesired effects. Some of the drugs used to relieve pain depress the respiratory and other centers in the brain. A patient may have an idiosyncrasy to any one of these drugs. When the patient exhibits unusual behavior shortly after a drug is administered and his behavior improves after a period of time, the probability is that there is a relationship between his behavior and his reaction to the drugs. Examples have been cited earlier in the chapter. Patients who have severe pain are often afraid that the pain will continue or return or that the pain indicates they have a serious illness from which they will die. They are afraid to allow themselves to relax and to go to sleep. When they are under the watchful eye of a nurse whom they trust to meet their needs, they have less need to remain alert. The external environment of the patient should also be controlled so that the therapy has an opportunity to be effective. A quiet, cool, but not cold environment is usually conducive to rest. For some patients the feeling of safety is increased by having a relative or good friend sit quietly at the bedside. The relative may require some instruction as to how he should behave and some recognition of the value of his contribution to the patient. Furthermore, the nurse should continue to assume the responsibility for the care and supervision of the patient. The relative should supplement, not replace, the nurse.

Pain and fear of pain are common to most illness. The extent to which each aspect predominates varies with the individual and with the cause of his illness. Pain is useful because it serves to warn the individual that something is wrong and spurs him into appropriate action. It is harmful when it frightens him so much that he avoids action or when it exhausts his physical and psychological resources.

The nurse's responsibilities in the care of the patient as they relate to pain are summarized in the following objectives:

1. To care for the patient so that preventable pain is avoided.
2. To evaluate the nature and cause of the patient's pain, so that appropriate measures may be instituted.
3. To convey to the patient that he can count on or trust the nurse (nurses) to meet his needs.
4. To continue to offer comfort and support to the patient whose pain persists despite the best efforts of all concerned.

As an addendum, at a number of points in the discussion of pain, reference was made to the necessity for the nurse to evaluate the degree of pain experienced by the patient. The writer is haunted by a patient who was selected by a student for the purpose of studying her nursing care requirements. The patient, who was approximately 40 years old, had been an actress as a child, but was now destitute. She was divorced and lived with her mother. She had developed a severe proctitis as a consequence of large doses of radiation in the treatment of cancer of the cervix. Because of her dependent behavior, she was seen by a psychiatrist who described her as being immature and childlike. Despite her pleas for relief of what is known to be an exquisitely painful condition, pain-relieving medications were withheld until she became mentally disorganized. She was punished for being an immature and incompetent person who whined and cried and was generally unpleasant. Although Mrs. Child Actress is an extreme example, the incident is uncommon only in degree. When a patient says he has pain, his complaint should be treated seriously. Insofar as is possible, the cause should be determined and appropriate treatment undertaken.

A symptom that is of some importance during the recovery of the patient is fever. For the first two or three days postoperatively some slight elevation of temperature and of leukocyte count is to be expected, as there is always some tissue damage. A marked increase in body temperature during the first 24 to 72 hours frequently indicates a developing atelectasis. Later elevations may denote phlebothrombosis, thrombophlebitis, and wound infection. See Chapter 11.

Hiccough, singultus, is an annoying, though not usually dangerous, symptom. It results from the paroxysmal and intermittent contraction of the diaphragm combined with a sudden closure of the glottis. It may be the result of chemical or mechanical irritation of the peritoneum or pleura that invests the diaphragm. Hiccoughs will often respond to simple measures—a drink of water, something that startles the person, a cough, a change in position. Other procedures that may be prescribed by the physician include rebreathing air in a paper bag, carbon dioxide inhalation, gastric lavage or suction, and sedatives. In extreme cases in which hiccoughs are prolonged and do not respond to other treatments, crushing the phrenic nerve may be required. Severe and continuous hiccoughing is exhausting because it interferes with rest and the ingestion of food and fluid.

How does surgical therapy threaten the self-concept of the patient?

In the discussion of the preoperative phase of surgical therapy, some mention was made of the psychological aspects of surgery as a threat to the survival of the individual. Many aspects of surgical therapy can provoke anxiety. This anxiety may be further augmented by the disease, or what the person perceives to be the disease, that makes surgery necessary. Many aspects of the total surgical experience threaten the self-concept of the individual. During the operative phase of his treatment, the patient loses complete control over what happens to him. He is utterly dependent on the surgeon, the anesthetist, and the assistants to the surgeon. The patient faces, and then experiences, pain and fear of pain. Throughout the entire experience, from the day he becomes aware that he is ill until he has completed his convalescence, the unknown plays a part in his reactions. Was surgery necessary? Was it successful? Was the cause of his illness cancer? Was it all removed? Has the doctor told him the truth?

The surgical treatment of disease frequently threatens his self-concept, by actual fact or by the perception of the individual. These are the persons who, though they make a full physiological recovery, have some change in their anatomy that threatens their self-concept. Full psychological recovery depends on their accepting the change in themselves as necessary and for their welfare. This involves a change in self-concept without a prolonged period of depression or other evidence of failure to accept reality.

Types of surgery that place the greatest strain on the adaptive capacity of the individual are those involving the loss of a part of the body: (1) that is obvious to others, such as an eye or an extremity, (2) in which the patient has an emotional investment, or (3) that involves an obvious change in function, such as a colostomy, ileostomy, or cystostomy. The patient can and should be expected to experience grief and anger. He may also feel shame or guilt. The psychosocial aspects of illness are discussed in some detail in Chapter 6, and the reader is referred to it for a more complete discussion of this very important aspect of the care of the surgical patient.

Summary

In the last century, surgical therapy has become a reality; diseases in all parts of the body are now treated by surgical methods. In its development, surgery was first made safe for the patient by the development of techniques of hemostasis, asepsis, anesthesia, and increased skill in incising and treating tissues. More recently, advances in knowledge have made it possible to extend the care, so that attention is given to making the patient safe for surgery. As a result, most patients are restored to health and vitality with a minimum of discomfort and disability. This is true of patients in all age groups and even those who have extensive surgery. Some of the complications which may delay recovery or cause death have been indicated.

Despite numerous possibilities for difficulty in the postoperative period, most patients make what is called an uneventful recovery. In those who do develop a complication, signs and symptoms are usually detected early so that procedures are promptly instituted to correct the problem. Much of the credit for the reduction in operative morbidity and mortality is given to the application of knowledge of physiology, microbiology, and psychology to the care of the patient in all phases of his operative experience. Credit is also given by surgeons to nurses who, in the care of patients, carry out, or assist patients in carrying out, procedures to protect and support bodily processes. Because of the amount of time nurses spend with patients, they also are in a position to observe and report early signs and symptoms that indicate a complication is developing. Despite the united efforts of the patient, nurse, and doctor, complications do occur. Many of the possibilities have been indicated in the preceding discussion. Surgery places stress on physiological and psychological functioning. Even in minor surgery, the combination of the effects of an anesthetic and a surgical procedure may result in the depression or disorganization of function. If continued, some disturbances in function are self-perpetuating or lead to more serious changes which are difficult to correct.

Complications that develop in the postoperative period can be summarized as having their origin in: (1) failure to restore the function of one or more systems—respiratory, gastrointestinal, urinary, or cardiovascular, (2) stress which exceeds the adaptive capacity of the individual—shock, hemorrhage, psychological disturbances, (3) failure to heal the wound, and (4) sepsis—wound infection or infection of other structures such as the urinary bladder, peritoneum, parotid gland, and abscess formation.

The complications that have their origin in the respiratory system have been discussed in Chapter 7. Because of their importance in the postoperative phase of surgery, they are emphasized here. They are believed to have their origin in obstruction or blocking of the tracheobronchial tree by its secretions or in aspiration of saliva and gastric secretions. They are prevented by the initiation of measures that have as their purpose the removal of respiratory- and gastrointestinal-tract secretions.

During the postoperative period the objective in the care of the patient is to provide the patient with the care that will enable him to return to optimal physiological and psychological functioning. The surgical procedure, including the route of approach, the anesthetic, the pain-relieving medications, and bed rest combine to depress and to disorganize bodily functions. An important part of the patient's care is to anticipate, protect, and maintain the functions that are disrupted. To do this effectively requires some understanding of physiology and how function can be maintained until the patient can carry on his own functions. In assessing the needs of the patient who is in the postoperative period, the nurse should try to determine the functions with which he requires assistance. Individual factors, such as age and personal habits, that may influence the prognosis of the patient should be given consideration. For example, the elderly patient can be expected to have a smaller reserve capacity with which to respond to stress. His respiratory reserve is less and he is more susceptible to respiratory complications than he was earlier in his life. The patient who has chronic bronchitis as a consequence of heavy smoking over a period of years also is predisposed to respiratory obstruction. In addition, the fact that he has a chronic cough renders him more liable to wound disruption. Both these patients, then, require more than usual attention to those procedures in their care that are directed toward keeping the tracheobronchial tree clear of secretions.

Only a small part of the patient's convalescence is spent in the hospital. As soon as the requirements of the patient can be met at home, he is likely to be dismissed from the hospital. Plans for the discharge of the patient should include instruction in the aspects of his care that require some modification in his patterns of daily living. He should know when he should visit his physician, how much rest and exercise he should take, any modifications of his diet that are required, and when he can anticipate returning to work. Even when the patient has made what is called an uneventful recovery, the nurse should ask herself the question, will this patient and his family be able to meet his needs after he leaves the hospital? If the answer is yes, as it will be in many instances, then nothing more needs to be done. If the answer is no, then the next question is, what kind of help does he or his family require? And then, what are the resources in the community that can be utilized to provide the help the patient and his family require? What steps should be taken to secure continuing care for the patient?

REFERENCES

Books

Brunner, Lillian Sholtis, et al., *Textbook of Medical-Surgical Nursing,* J. B. Lippincott Company, Philadelphia, 1964.
Cannon, Walter Bradford, *Bodily Changes in Pain, Hunger, Fear, and Rage,* Charles T. Branford Co., Boston, 1929.

Crowley, Dorothy M., *Pain and Its Alleviation,* University of California, Berkeley, California, 1962.

Davis, Harry A., *Principles of Surgical Physiology,* Paul B. Hoeber, Inc., New York, 1957.

Davis, Loyal (ed.), *Christopher's Textbook of Surgery,* 8th ed., W. B. Saunders Co., Philadelphia, 1964.

Dunbar, Helen Flanders, *Emotions and Bodily Changes,* 4th ed., Columbia University Press, New York, 1954.

Elman, Robert, *Surgical Care: A Practical Physiologic Guide,* Appleton-Century-Crofts, Inc., New York, 1951.

Franklin, Benjamin, *A Dissertation on Liberty and Necessity, Pleasure and Pain* (reproduced from the First Edition), The Facsimile Text Society, New York, 1930.

Fuerst, Elinor, and LuVerne Wolff, *Fundamentals of Nursing,* 3rd ed., J. B. Lippincott Co., Philadelphia, 1964, pp. 58-93.

Glenn, Frank and John M. Beal, Guest Editors, "Immediate Post Operative Complications," *The Surgical Clinics of North America,* XLIV, No. 2, April, 1964, W. B. Saunders Company, Philadelphia, pp. 303-564.

Goodman, Louis S., and Alfred Gilman, *The Pharmacological Basis of Therapeutics,* 2nd ed., The Macmillan Company, New York, 1955.

Gius, John Armes, *Fundamentals of General Surgery,* 2nd ed., The Yearbook Medical Publishers, Inc., Chicago, 1962.

Hardy, James D., *Pathophysiology in Surgery,* The Williams & Wilkins Co., Baltimore, 1958.

Harmer, Bertha, and Virginia Henderson, *Textbook of the Principles and Practice of Nursing,* 5th ed., The Macmillan Company, New York, 1955, pp. 989-1047.

Leithauser, D. J., *Early Ambulation and Related Procedures in Surgical Management,* Charles C Thomas, Springfield, Illinois, 1946.

Lewis, C. S., *The Problem of Pain,* The Macmillan Company, New York, 1944.

Livingston, W. K., *Pain Mechanisms,* The Macmillan Company, New York, 1943.

MacBryde, Cyril Mitchell, ed., *Signs and Symptoms: Applied Pathologic Physiology and Clinical Interpretation,* 3rd ed., J. B. Lippincott Co., Philadelphia, 1957.

Maingot, Rodney, *Abdominal Operations,* 4th ed., Appleton-Century-Crofts, Inc., New York, 1960.

Marshall, Henry Rutgers, *Pain, Pleasure, and Anesthetics,* The Macmillan Company, New York, 1894.

Montag, Mildred, and Ruth P. Stewart Swenson, *Fundamentals in Nursing Care,* 3rd ed., W. B. Saunders, Philadelphia, 1959, pp. 403-17.

Moore, Francis D., *Metabolic Care of the Surgical Patient,* W. B. Saunders Co., Philadelphia, 1959.

Sadove, Max, and James H. Cross, *The Recovery Room,* W. B. Saunders Co., Philadelphia, 1956.

Shafer, Kathleen Newton, *et al., Medical-Surgical Nursing,* 3rd ed., The C. V. Mosby Co., St. Louis, 1964.

Smith, Dorothy W., and Claudia D. Gips, *Care of the Adult Patient,* J. B. Lippincott Company, Philadelphia, 1963.

Tichener, James L., and Maurice Levine, *Surgery as a Human Experience,* Oxford University Press, New York, 1960.

White, James C., and William H. Sweet, *Pain: Its Mechanisms and Neurosurgical Control,* Charles C Thomas, Springfield, Illinois, 1955.

Wohlgemuth, A., *Pleasure-Unpleasure,* Cambridge University Press, Cambridge, 1919.

Wolff, Harold G., and Stewart Wolf, *Pain,* Charles C Thomas, Springfield, Illinois, 1948.

Wolff, Harold G., *Stress and Disease,* Charles C Thomas, Springfield, Illinois, 1953.

Zimmerman, Leo M., and Rachmiel Levine (eds.), *Physiologic Principles of Surgery,* 2nd ed., W. B. Saunders Co., Philadelphia, 1964.

Articles

Abdellah, Faye G., "Methods of Identifying Covert Aspects of Nursing Problems. A Key to Improved Clinical Teaching," *Nursing Research,* VI, June, 1957, pp. 4-23.

Adams, Ralph, Burke Fahlman, and Jacqueline Lord, "New Fashions in Surgical Attire," *American Journal of Nursing,* LIX, July, 1959, pp. 1102-7.

Adriani, John, "Some New Anesthetic Agents," *American Journal of Nursing,* LXI, May, 1961, pp. 60-62.

Adriani, John, "Local Anesthetics," *American Journal of Nursing,* LIX, January, 1959, pp. 86-88.

Alstead, Stanley, "Pain and Analgesia: The Philosophic Background," *Practitioner,* CLXXXIV, January, 1960, pp. 5-9.

Ansell, Julian S., "Nephrectomy and Nephrostomy," *American Journal of Nursing,* LVIII, October, 1958, pp. 1394-96.

Aring, Charles D., "The Nature and Significance of Chronic Pain," *Medical Clinics of North America,* XLII, November, 1958, pp. 1467-79.

Barber, Theodore X., "Hypnosis-Analgesia and Placebo Effect," *Journal of the American Medical Association,* CLXXII, February 13, 1960, pp. 680-83.

Beecher, Henry K., "Evidence for Increased Effectiveness of Placebos with Increased Stress," *American Journal of Physiology,* CLXXXVII, 1956, pp. 163-69.

Berblinger, Klaus W., "The Influence of Personalities on Drug Therapy," *American Journal of Nursing,* LIX, August, 1959, pp. 1130-32.

Bird, Brian, "Psychological Aspects of Pre-operative and Post-operative Care," *The American Journal of Nursing,* LV, June, 1955, pp. 685-87.

Bonsnes, R. W., "Postoperative Parenteral Nutrition," *Surgical Clinics of North America,* XXXVII, April, 1957, pp. 307-20.

Boyle, Rena E., "How Well Do We Know the Patients We Know Best?" *American Journal of Nursing,* LVIII, November, 1958, pp. 1540-43.

Brant, Charles S., Herbert Volk, and Bernard Kutner, "Psychological Preparation for Surgery," *Public Health Reports,* LXXIII, November, 1958, pp. 1001-7.

Brush, Brock E., John H. Wylie, and Joseph Beninson, "Some Devices for the Management of Lymphedema of the Extremities," *Surgical Clinics of North America,* XXXIX, December, 1959, pp. 1493-98.

Bulbulian, Arthur H., R. Quentin Rayer, and Charles J. Restall, "A New Nasal Anesthesia Mask Specially Designed for Oral Surgical Procedures," *Proceedings of the Staff Meetings of the Mayo Clinic,* XXXVI, March 1, 1961, pp. 105-12.

Council on Drugs, "Halothane," *Journal of the American Medical Association,* CLXX, August 8, 1959, pp. 1811-13.

Council on Drugs, "Hydroxydione Sodium Succinate," *Journal of the American Medical Association,* CLXVIII, September 20, 1958, pp. 285-87.

Dallenbach, Karl M., "Pain: History and Present Status," *American Journal of Psychology,* LII, No. 3, July, 1939, pp. 331-47.

Eckenhoff, James E., and Martin Helrich, "Study of Narcotics and Sedatives for Use in Preanesthetic Medication," *Journal of the American Medical Association,* CLXVII, May 24, 1958, pp. 415-22.

Edgar, Irving I., "Surgery and Lord Lister," *Journal of the History of Medicine,* XVI, April, 1961, pp. 145-60.

Engel, George L., "Psychogenic Pain," *Medical Clinics of North America,* XLII, 1958, pp. 1481-96.

Feldberg, W., "A Physiological Approach to the Problem of General Anesthesia and Loss of Consciousness," *British Medical Journal,* II, October 24, 1959, pp. 771-82.

Fisk, Jean E., "Nursing Care of the Patient with Surgery of the Biliary Tract," *American Journal of Nursing,* LX, January, 1960, pp. 53-55.

Fitzwater, Janet, "New Equipment of the Operating Room," *American Journal of Nursing,* LXI, August, 1961, pp. 54-55.

Frenay, Sister Mary Agnes Clare, "Balanced Anesthesia and Induced Hypothermia," *American Journal of Nursing,* LV, October, 1955, pp. 1245-47.

Gregg, Dorothy, "Anxiety—A Factor in Nursing Care," *American Journal of Nursing,* LII, November, 1952, pp. 1363-65.

Gregg, Dorothy, "Reassurance," *American Journal of Nursing,* LV, February, 1955, pp. 171-74.

Hardy, J. D., "The Nature of Pain," *Journal of Chronic Diseases,* IV, July, 1956, pp. 22-25.

Haugen, Frederick P., "Current Concepts of the Pain Process," *Journal of Chronic Diseases,* IV, July, 1956, pp. 4-10.

Hulse, Wilfred C., and Louis Lowinger, "The Psychological Management of the Pre and Post Operative Patient," *American Practitioner and Digest of Treatment,* VII, June, 1956, pp. 927-36.

Joergenson, Eugene J., and Richard Carter, "The Safe Conduct of the Patient Through Surgery," *Medical Clinics of North America,* XLIII, July, 1959, pp. 1223-42.

Karp, Mary, "Changing Concepts and Present Trends in Anesthesiology," *Surgical Clinics of North America,* XXXIX, No. 1, February, 1959, pp. 219-29.

Kaufmann, Margaret A., and Dorothy E. Brown, "Pain Wears Many Faces," *American Journal of Nursing,* LXI, January, 1961, pp. 48-51.

Keats, Arthur S., "Postoperative Pain: Research and Treatment," *Journal of Chronic Diseases,* IV, July, 1956, pp. 72-83.

Lundy, John S., "Amnesia-Analgesia for Management of Children Too Young to Cooperate," *Journal of the American Medical Association,* CLXVI, February, 1958, pp. 453-55.

Meyer, Bernard C., "Some Psychiatric Aspects of Surgical Practice," *Psychosomatic Medicine,* XX, March, 1958, p. 203.

Mikal, Stanley, "Surgical Physiology of the Colon," *American Journal of Proctology,* XII, April, 1961, pp. 93-98.

Molander, David W., and Richard D. Brasfield, "Liver Surgery," *American Journal of Nursing,* LXI, July, 1961, pp. 72-73.

Nourse, Myron H., "Management of the Patient Who Fails to Void After Surgery," *Journal of the American Medical Association,* CLXXI, November 28, 1959, pp. 1778-79.

Ostrow, Mortimer, "The Biological Basis of Human Behavior," *American Handbook of Psychiatry,* in Silvano Arieti (ed.), Basic Books, Inc., New York, 1960, pp. 58-85.

"Pre- and Post-operative Care," *Surgical Clinics of North America,* XXXIX, December, 1959, entire issue.

Quint, Jeanne C., "Nursing the Patient with Endarterectomy," *American Journal of Nursing,* LVIII, July, 1958, pp. 996-98.

Reams, Gerald B., and Elma J. Powell, "Postoperative Catheterization—Yes or No?" *American Journal of Nursing,* LX, March, 1960, p. 371.

Robertson, William H., "Post Operative Wound Disruption," *American Practitioner and Digest of Treatment,* IX, October, 1958, pp. 1615-20.

Rothenberg, Sanford F., "Post Operative Intractable Pain," *Medical Clinics of North America,* XLIII, July, 1959, pp. 1243-57.

Russell, E. S., "Hypothermia," *Canadian Nurse,* LVI, August, 1960, pp. 693-94.

Russell, Ritchie W., "Postgraduate Clinical Notes: Pain," *Postgraduate Medicine,* XXIII, February, 1958, p. 112.

Spaulding, Earle H., and Ellen K. Emmons, "Chemical Disinfection," *American Journal of Nursing,* LVIII, September, 1958, pp. 1238-42.

Taufic, Marjorie R., "Nursing the Patient After Nephrectomy," *American Journal of Nursing,* LVIII, October, 1958, pp. 1397-98.

Vandam, Leroy D., and Thomas K. Burnap, "Hypothermia," *New England Journal of Medicine,* CCLXI, September 10, 1959, 546-53, and September 17, 1959, pp. 595-603.

Virgadamo, Barbara T., "Care of the Patient with Liver Surgery," *American Journal of Nursing,* LXI, July, 1961, pp. 74-76.

Wallace, George, "Preanesthetic Medication Without Narcotics," *Journal of the American Medical Association,* CLXXIII, June 18, 1960, pp. 797-99.

Wolff, H. G., and J. D. Hardy, "On the Nature of Pain," *Physiological Reviews,* XXVII, April, 1947, pp. 167-99.

Woodbridge, Philip D., "Changing Concepts Concerning the Depth of Anesthesia," *Anesthesiology,* XVIII, July, 1957, p. 536.

Zborowski, Mark, "Cultural Components in Responses to Pain," in E. Gartley Jaco, ed., *Patients, Physicians and Illness,* The Free Press, Glencoe, Illinois, 1958, pp. 256-68.

Unpublished Material

Bobus, Helen, "Problems of Student Nurses in Caring for Surgical Patients," Unpublished Master's Thesis, University of Pennsylvania, 1955.

Little, Dolores E., "Identification of Principles and Concepts of Nursing Care in Relation to Expected Needs of Surgical Patients by Analysis of Selected Nursing Content," Unpublished Master's Thesis, University of Washington, 1957.

Walsh, Sister Margaret, "Quantitative Study of the Treatments and Medications Currently Employed in the Care of Intrapartum and Postpartum Patients," Unpublished Master's Thesis, The Catholic University of America, 1956.

16 : Nursing in Rehabilitation[1]

> An optimist is a person who sees a green light everywhere. The pessimist sees only the red light. But the truly wise person is colorblind.
>
> Albert Schweitzer

Rehabilitation.

Rehabilitation has become an often used and vital word. One is made constantly aware of objects, buildings, areas, and people being "rehabilitated." A few uses of the word, such as the rehabilitation of cemeteries, are too ridiculous to be credible. The rehabilitation of whole countries or cities, although overwhelming, does seem possible. Rehabilitating a beautiful old home in the city can be more of a status symbol than owning a sprawling modern home in surburbia. In considering the "rehabilitation" of criminals, one returns to the point of origin—the rehabilitation of human beings.

The word "rehabilitation" connotes many things to society. What was of value previously will be retained. The entity will be deleted of broken and unnecessary components. Emphasis is placed on totally eliminating those qualities that detract from beauty or function. The entity not only has new life, but is better able to justify its existence. Planning the rehabilitation of a permanently disabled person is done on the basis of his eventual return to this society.

Certainly everyone is free to use the word "rehabilitation" as he desires; however, those who work with the permanently disabled, as well as the disabled person himself, have as a result an even greater task presented them, for society has come to expect useless elements of rehabilitated entities to be replaced, but society does not always remember that a permanent disability of a human being cannot be removed. The difficulties of and pressures on a permanently disabled person become more clear to us when we realize it is not possible for him to be given those attributes necessary for coping with all aspects of society.

The physically disabled.

Persons who are physically disabled have malfunctioning of some part of their neuromuscular-skeletal system. These acquired or congenital conditions

---

[1] This chapter was contributed by Nancy Martin, Assistant Professor, College of Nursing, University of Illinois, Chicago, Illinois.

are considered to be either acutely, permanently, or progressively disabling. Although within each of these categories one finds disabilities that vary greatly in degree of severity, they must be differentiated in order to determine what type of rehabilitation is necessary. Each of the three areas presents unique problems.

Acute disabilities are those conditions that may or may not be severe initially. The function that was lost is expected to return. The disability is reversible. Even though the term "acute" is used, the length of time necessary for return may be months. Examples of such conditions are: fractures of long bones; severe infections that, in this case, leave no residual (poliomyelitis, Guillain-Barré syndrome); and cerebral vascular accident without organic brain damage and with complete return of function.

Return of function does not occur in a patient with a permanent disability. The lost function or part cannot be restored. Although in some cases it is possible to substitute for the loss in such a manner as to allow the person to lead a "normal" life, the disability remains. Such conditions as amputation; paraplegia and quadriplegia; cerebral vascular accident with organic brain damage, paresis, or paralysis; poliomyelitis with residual paralysis; and cerebral palsy fall into the category of permanent disabilities.

Muscular dystrophy, multiple sclerosis, and myasthenia gravis are often the only conditions considered to be progressively disabling. Certainly they may be the first to come to mind. In this group also are the following: recurring rheumatoid arthritis; chronic osteomyelitis; congenital bone deformities producing traumatic arthritis or osteoarthritis.

This chapter will consider rehabilitation of the permanently disabled. The nurse is advised to remember that although remaining physical abilities may be increased and strengthened, the patient must learn to accept and to live with his disability. Return of function does not occur, and all rehabilitation goals must be formulated with this as the basis.

Need for rehabilitation.

Interest in rehabilitation was fostered in this country because of the permanently disabled servicemen who received their injuries during World Wars I and II. From the expansion of the field of rehabilitation has come the physiatrist, or physician who practices rehabilitation and physical medicine. (The nursing student is urged to explore the writings of Rusk, Kessler, and Magnuson, who were involved in the evolution of this specialty.) That there is ever greater need for rehabilitation is obvious. The increasing population, as well as the increasing contact of more persons with high-powered machinery such as automobiles, cannot help but produce greater numbers of permanently disabled persons. In order to meet the total needs of the permanently disabled many specialties, or disciplines, have combined their services and function as a team. The team generally consists of physician, nurse, social worker, psychologist, psychiatrist, vocational counselor, and occupational, physical, and speech therapists. This team functions within an agency where care is given to either acutely or chronically ill persons. *Chronic* as used in this chapter does not connote custodial care, but rather the prolonged stage following the initial acute period of the disability.

Immediately following injury or illness the disabled person will receive care in a general hospital. The services of these institutions usually are not limited to care of the patient with a neuromuscular-skeletal condition. The type of care and how it is given are extremely important during the acute stage of the disability, as the foundation for future rehabilitation goals begins when the patient is admitted to this agency. Following the acute period of illness, the patient may be admitted to another institution or to another division of the hospital for more lengthy treatment. These agencies are the rehabilitation centers, and their philosophies are directed toward rehabilitation of the patient with a neuromuscular-skeletal disorder. It should be noted that initially emphasis was placed on private and separate rehabilitation centers; however, an increasing number of general hospitals are providing rehabilitation units within their own confines.

The combined services of these institutions alone cannot meet the total needs of permanently disabled persons. Other official and nonofficial agencies should be an integral part of the rehabilitation process. More often than not, a local, state, or federal agency will be involved: e.g., Visiting Nurse Association, Division of Services for Crippled Children, Office of Vocational Rehabilitation.

Rehabilitation nursing.

Many ask whether rehabilitation nursing is a specialty, and whether there is a body of knowledge peculiar to the rehabilitation nurse. It is true that some professional nurses have learned and practiced specific nursing care measures while working primarily with severely physically disabled persons. Only recently have the results of their pioneering efforts been recognized. Now the nursing care indicated for assisting severely disabled persons can become part of the basic knowledge of all professional nurses. While there will continue to be those who prefer practicing in an agency whose main purpose is the rehabilitation of disabled persons, all nurses should be prepared for the specific situations and problems associated with the care of the patient afflicted with a neuromuscular-skeletal condition, just as all nurses have a role in any patient's rehabilitation process. The agency in which the nurse is employed will determine only the degree of intensity of her rehabilitation activities.

First, the nurse in a general hospital must direct her attention toward keeping the newly admitted patient alive. She must be aware of the physiological reactions that occur as a result of a neuromuscular-skeletal disability. For example, she must know that the person who has sustained an injury resulting in a severed spinal cord will not perspire below his level of injury. The remaining innervated areas of the body must now assume the entire responsibility for the insensible water loss mechanism. If the injury to the spinal cord is in the region of the cervical vertebrae, all the body areas, including the head, neck and shoulders, may be affected. The nurse should anticipate an extremely high temperature elevation and be prepared to institute measures to assist the body in lowering the temperature. See Chapter 11.

The initial atmosphere in which the patient finds himself will have much bearing on his entire rehabilitation program. It is essential to remember the great physical and psychological shock these patients experience immediately following a neuromuscular-skeletal injury and address our efforts accordingly. An intelligent regimen must begin early or difficulty will be encountered in enlisting not only the patient's cooperation, but his consent. Attempts at instituting a regimen only several days after admission may be met with refusal by the patient. It is imperative that the patient have confidence in the nurse's ability. Unless the nurse is capable of meeting the patient's physical needs, and meeting them well, her efforts in other areas of concern (emotional, social) will be of little value. The complex of these problems, if not anticipated and met, hinders the patient's progress, and may result in no rehabilitation being possible. The great responsibility of helping to create this introductory atmosphere is that of the nurse in the general hospital.

The function of the nurse employed in a rehabilitation setting will be determined by the philosophy of that institution. She may be responsible for teaching the patient dressing techniques, or for communicating his dressing progress to the discipline responsible for the initial teaching. She may follow the teaching program outlined by a part-time speech therapist, or she may be primarily responsible for observing whether the patient utilizes the retraining the speech therapist feels he has accomplished. Above all, she must assist the patient in planning and reorganizing his time in order that the new goals he does achieve become a daily part of his life.

Possibly her most important responsibility will be to communicate and interpret the patient's progress, when on the patient unit, to the other disciplines. It is essential she observe not only his increased physical capabilities, but his interactions with staff, other patients, and his visitors. After a taxing day in the various therapies, the patient will be physically and emotionally exhausted. The patient unit is his "home," and the atmosphere must be conducive to relaxation. The nurse should be sensitive to his expressions of feelings of his progress. He should be told she realizes these days are exhausting. There could be no better time for well-chosen words of realistic encouragement. The rehabilitation process is a slow and difficult one, and its day-by-day progress only makes more apparent to the patient the full meaning of his disability.

To the visiting nurse or public health nurse goes the responsibility of observing the results of efforts accomplished during the acute and chronic periods of care. No amount of rehabilitation activities instituted in either of the two former agencies will be of any value if the patient is not prepared to function outside their protective environments. Besides determining his physical status and abilities, the visiting or public health nurse must be alert to the entire complex of the patient's reactions on returning to his home. Although his activities may not be so extensive as before his disability, she must ascertain if he is participating to his fullest potential. And if not, why not?

Hospitals of all kinds tend to protect patients, and the impact of coping again with the outside environment—now with a disability—is overwhelming. This pertains to the family as well as the patient. The nurse can help to resolve many of the problems faced by the patient. Many, such as inability to find employment, she cannot. Her only recourse then is to listen and give realistic support and encouragement. The public health nurse's role is to help the patient and family cope with the reality of the consequences of the disability.

The combined efforts of nurses in the two hospitals and in the public health agency have immeasurable value to the total rehabilitation of the person afflicted with a neuromuscular-skeletal disability. Their activities are of equal importance and carry equal responsibility. Each stage is a vital part of the whole. If in any of the three areas the nurse does not strive to assist the patient to reach his optimum potential, she is answerable to herself, the patient, and her colleagues.

The rehabilitation process.

Determination of Needs for Rehabilitation

A comprehensive approach to the patient's needs is essential. Permanent disability involves much more than physical limitations. Psychosocial, vocational-economic, and physical needs can best be determined by the team of specialists. The number of team members involved in an individual patient situation corresponds to the specific needs of that patient. For example, if, as a result of a cerebral vascular accident, a patient has sustained severe organic brain damage, there is little need for the services of a vocational counselor or speech therapist. On the other hand, if the patient can utilize the services of the entire team and benefits from spiritual guidance, his clergyman may become an active team participant.

It is the task of the rehabilitation team to determine how the needs of the patient may best be met. Their efforts are directed toward increasing his assets and substituting new methods for achieving old activities. Frequent team discussions, at which their observations are shared, inform them all of his progress. More often than not, a positive or negative sign will have been noticed by at least two disciplines. For example, John, a high school senior, sustained paraplegia as a result of a football injury. Three months after the accident he was admitted to a rehabilitation center. When the team first discussed possible goals for John, all departments reported he was greatly depressed and withdrawn. Further, he appeared to have no interest in increasing his abilities, and refused to do much of what he was then capable. This situation continued throughout the first month. At team conference one and a half months after admission it became apparent that his attitudes and desires were changing. The nurse reported that John was now a full participant in ward activities and was more concerned about his physical appearance. The physical therapist reported he had expressed beginning interest in transfer from bed to wheel chair. Two weeks later the vocational counselor told of John's asking if he now could continue his school work required for graduation. At the following team conference, all disciplines reported John appeared to be actively and positively involved in his rehabilitation program.

By combining their skills and knowledge of the patient's gains, necessary revisions in goal setting are made. At times this means arriving at the decision that the patient is not a candidate for extensive rehabilitation and other plans are necessary for him. This is always a difficult task, and one not arrived at without extensive consideration of the entire patient situation. It is extremely unfair to demand of the patient that of which he is incapable. Moreover, it is unfair to other patients if the team's time and energy are frustratingly exhausted.

The rehabilitation team must not only be positively involved in the patient's program, but all members must be working together and all at the same time. Each discipline, as needed by individual patients, is responsible for a unique area, and again, all of these areas are needed for the whole. Often, as in John's situation, the team must begin without the patient's cooperation as he may need to see the possibilities before becoming an active participant. Many complications arise and time is lost if a comprehensive program is not attempted. Further, the experienced team anticipates both physical and emotional delays. The complexities of a permanent disability demand the utmost patience of all concerned.

Viewing the Patient as an Individual

All persons, able-bodied or disabled, must be viewed as individuals. We cannot predetermine either the patient's physical or emotional capabilities by knowing only his disability. A person having sustained an injury resulting in quadriplegia may be completely self-sufficient and may provide valuable services to his employer and colleagues. Another, following traumatic amputations of both upper extremities, may refuse prosthetic devices and remain at home, providing no service to anyone.

We must not underestimate the capabilities of the disabled person. For example, seven-year-old Jimmy, diagnosed as having cerebral palsy, was admitted to a general hospital for an obturator neurectomy to relieve adduction contractures of his legs. He was unable to communicate verbally with the nursing staff. No information was available about his abilities, and, as his home was in another state, none was obtained from his parents. Complete custodial care was given this boy. Jimmy was fed, diapered, and allowed to remain totally inactive. Since he was unable to talk, no other means of communication were explored. When he was discharged to his parents, the nursing staff was shocked to learn that before admission Jimmy was completely toilet-trained and could communicate by using a word board. Many months of frustrating work by both the boy and his mother were undone by persons not attempting all possible means of communication with him, and not viewing Jimmy as the individual he was.

Successful Rehabilitation Program

If a patient can be described as being successfully rehabilitated, then one may assume all goals have been met. Only by determining and accomplishing short-term goals can the ultimate realistic goal be reached. Whether this ultimate long-term goal is partial self-care or returning to the community as a full participant does not alter the necessity for all concerned to strive for the possible—not probable—way of life for the patient. No excessive desire for unobtainable goals by any person involved can bring them about. Just as we must accept the patient's abilities, so too must we recognize his limitations. Achieving goals within the realm of possibility is difficult enough. Unrealistic goals and false encouragement can frustrate the patient to the point of rendering him incapable of achieving that which is possible. However, this is not to say that any patient's potential may not be greater than first believed. Caution and discretion are wise when initially informing the patient and his family of long-term goals. Changes in their lives caused by the disability are traumatic; having to tell them at a later date that the initially stated potential cannot be met is even more damaging.

Appropriate timing is inherent for a successful rehabilitation program. Positive patient and family motivation as well as the program outlined by the rehabilitation team is needed. Often these constituents are ready, but at differing times; and although it is possible to proceed for a period, total rehabilitation will not occur until the patient, his family, and the team are all working toward the same goal—and at the same time.

The problems of the rehabilitation process do not stop when the patient returns to the community. There are many reasons for the disappointments that often occur. The patient's former associates, both vocational and avocational, are rarely prepared for the role they must assume with him. Are the patient and his family capable of assisting friends and associates in this adjustment? There is no better test of the comprehensive guidance given by the team. When the visiting or public health nurse is a member of the team, at least in the final period of the patient's hospitalization, the knowledge and guidance of the team are carried into the home.

Although society is more aware that the permanently disabled person can participate in some manner, it is not told how this is possible. Moreover, society knows neither what nor how to assist—only that assistance is expected. All of this only compounds the final test of a successful rehabilitation program: does the patient increase his abilities after discharge? He should reach his highest potential at home, not while hospitalized.

The Patient Who Cannot Be Rehabilitated

If we state a patient cannot be rehabilitated because he lacks motivation, we are incorrect. Reaction and attitude are always a result of motivation. As far as the rehabilitation process is concerned, patient motivation may be positive or negative. It is important to remember he is motivated in some direction, and will respond accordingly. Herein lies one of the frustrations of rehabilitation.

The area of secondary gains from a disability is vast. The reader is urged to explore other works whose attention is directed to these considerations. In writing of "motivational consequences," Wright states:

A disability may serve many purposes. The person may wish to insure continuing financial compensation that his disability provides; he may welcome the dependency facilitated by his disability; his disability may satisfy a masochistic need for punishment; it may afford him social sanction for avoiding competitive striving, which he fears. . . . The point is a simple one. When a disability is satisfying for one reason or another, it becomes magnified through beliefs and expectations.[2]

Physical limitations may be the determining factors in the decision that a patient cannot be rehabilitated. Here again the situation is not an uncomplicated one. Often the determinant is a medical component. For example, if an elderly person has had bilateral lower extremity amputation as a result of arteriosclerosis with accompanying arteriosclerotic heart disease, the task of learning to walk with prosthetic devices may be considered too great a strain for the already weakened heart. Therefore, the best means of life for this patient would be from a wheel chair. It is necessary again to mention realistic goal setting. When the patient is unable to meet the stated potential because of lack of physical ability, then the original plans and subsequent program were in error. Too frequently we view a rehabilitated person in terms of ambulation—with or without braces. If, however, the early decision had been wheel chair existence, much physical and emotional energy would have been spared.

When thinking of future employment possibilities, the issue becomes more complicated in proportion to the extent of physical limitation. A unilateral lower entremity amputee faces a relatively uncomplicated situation. The problems of the severely afflicted rheumatoid arthritic, paraplegic, or multiextremity amputee are quite another matter. An employer hiring a person with

---

[2] Beatrice Wright, *Physical Disability: A Psychological Approach,* Harper & Brothers, New York, 1960, p. 173.

physical limitations understandably will choose the least afflicted. Employment environmental facilities must be negotiable for the wheel chair-bound. The practicality of the situation often provides insuperable obstacles. The greater the intelligence, the greater are future employment possibilities. For example, a person afflicted with quadriplegia must now depend almost completely on his mind. If he does not possess the necessary mental abilities, there can be no realistic thought of vocational goals.

It must be clearly understood that the patient may not accept a proposed vocational change. An area of great concern to the vocational counselor is helping the disabled person make the necessary adjustments. By using testing devices that determine the patient's mental and manual abilities, new vocational areas are made apparent. The possibilities can only be presented; here again the decision is the patient's.

Rehabilitation of persons with permanent disabilities is extremely expensive. The expense of time and physical and emotional energy can be greater than financial expense. The complete rehabilitation process of a patient will not be possible if any of these basic requirements cannot be met. The rehabilitation team can only work with what remains after the disability, and the emotional response of the patient is often more important than his retained physical abilities. However, even the patient who does not emotionally accept his disability can be upgraded physically, and will therefore be able to live better than before his partial rehabilitation. The most minor achievements rarely occur without great effort and understanding on the part of everyone involved in the rehabilitation program.

The Patient's Role

No matter how brilliantly conceived a rehabilitation program may be, it will be worthless unless the patient is involved. He must be motivated positively—and this is the essence of rehabilitation. Whereas the rehabilitation team is the body of the process, positive patient motivation is the soul. The driving force must come from within the patient, even though the team makes evident his potential and provides continued support and encouragement.

To become positively motivated demands a revision of self-concept. The patient is no longer the physical being he was. Until such time as he recognizes and comprehends this all-important fact, no changes in how he now views himself will occur. In too many instances we expect him to have had a secure and positive self-concept prior to his disability. The patient is what he was before his injury—only more so. If he was cognizant of his strengths and weaknesses, such an awareness will tend to continue. If, however, he had not found his role previous to his disability, it will be extremely difficult for him to do so now. The situation in which he now finds himself and his premorbid personality are essential factors in revising his self-concept. We cannot expect changes in self-concept or positive motivation to occur rapidly. This is a process which requires greatly differing lengths of time, and will depend on the individual. Determining whether or not a patient is positively motivated is a very difficult undertaking, and cannot and should not be done by one person.

Just as we must anticipate a delay in motivation, so too should we be alert to pseudomotivation. If the patient regularly attends his therapies and, in all other ways, is following (seemingly) the plan we have provided, we tend to assume he is a part of his rehabilitation process. This is not necessarily the true situation. There is no better way to be unaffected or overlooked by others than to perform in the manner expected. For example, Mary Simmons, a 30-year-old paraplegic, always seemed eager to attend the occupational and physical therapy appointments. She left the patient unit early enough to assure arriving early for therapy. The physical therapist presented a view of Miss Simmons quite different from what the nursing staff imagined. Although Miss Simmons was willing to exercise and increase the strength of her upper extremities, she would not agree to learn ways of compensating for the lost function of her lower extremities, e.g., transfer from bed to wheel chair.

Psychosocial Situations the Nurse Will Encounter

The stages of psychological shock, denial, depression, and anxiety usually precede acceptance of a permanent disability. Initially, the patient will be concerned with the loss of the body part or function. Psychological shock may be expected no matter what the disability. Even the person who has agreed to amputation of an extremity usually will experience a period of mourning for the lost body part.

It is impossible for the able-bodied to realize the full psychological impact on a person who is suddenly unable to move below his waist. In his eyes and in the eyes of many others he immediately loses the attributes making him the unique individual he was, and he becomes part of the nonspecific world of the crippled. Whether or not the full consequences are evident to him at once is of little import. He need only know he no longer can move, feel, or care for himself; and in ways he never knew existed, he is dependent on others. The shock is profound, and does not leave.

The patient may express denial in numerous ways: refusing to enter into or to allow planning for rehabilitation; refusing needed surgical procedures; outwardly accepting physical and occupational therapies, while inwardly believing the disability is not permanent. The patient's denial is not difficult to understand. If he believes the condition does not exist, the reality of the situation need not be faced. By assuming, as in Miss Simmon's case, the disability is temporary, the patient will see no need for rehabilitation.

As the full impact of the disability becomes obvious to the patient, he enters into a stage of depression. The disability has not gone away; physical sequelae further insult his disabled body; family savings are fast being exhausted; he can never return to his former vocation; previous life plans no longer are attainable. He is constantly reminded of his lost manhood. If he is of no value to himself, how can he possibly be to those who formerly depended on him? Society, with its pressures and emphasis on increasing production, offers no place for him. There seem to be no solutions to his problems, and he becomes further depressed and withdrawn. Again, he may exhibit various behavioral patterns, refusing all care, food, and fluids; refusing to talk; refusing to sleep, or sleeping all the time with the sheet pulled over his head.

Hopefully, throughout the stages of shock, denial, and depression, realistic potentials have been made apparent to the patient. Being so vitally concerned with self and his inability to meet former goals, he is easily overwhelmed by well-meant but indiscreet barrages of future possibilities. Therefore, making him aware of the positive aspects of his reality should be done carefully and appropriately.

Those around the patient should be alert to expressions of anxiety. As he is unsatisfied with his present state, if he believes there may be means of improving it, he will begin the adjustment of his self-concept. So much must be changed, and he realizes almost all can be done only by him. As he begins in his disability program, the slowness of his progress and inherent frustrations increase his anxiety. He may express overconcern about further physical harm to himself; he may be verbally abusive to those around him; he may suddenly take great interest in family affairs, and become dogmatic over seemingly trivial matters. One person, or everyone in his environment, may be the recipient of his expressions. If this is not understood and managed correctly, irreparable damage will occur. The value to the patient of progressing through these agonizing periods is the eventual acceptance of his disability. He cannot ignore or deny the lost function; it is part of him. And, viewing himself as a whole, he can now see his abilities and limitations. Ideally this is the point at which he joins the rehabilitation team in his program.

How much easier it would be for all concerned if we could predict the time needed for these stages. If only they could occur once—and in order! But this just does not happen. The length of time varies from days to months to years; the stages are mixed. There may be progression and regression. Only by observing his behavior and being sensitive to his expressions can we determine our approach. We cannot propel him through these areas as we wish. No matter how great our desire or efforts, he cannot and should not move forward in our predetermined way. And this is what is meant by seeing and accepting each person as an individual. We must remember he may stop and remain in any stage. As he belongs to himself and not to us, this is his right. However, he then cannot be viewed as a candidate for a successful rehabilitation program. When we perceive it otherwise, we fool only ourselves.

If we use one word to describe the nurse's approach, it should be adaptable. She must be alert to the patient's manner of expressing just where he is in his adjustment process. She must know when to move ahead with him and when to leave him alone. She must be aware of the time when he becomes an active participant. Or she must accept the decision that he is not a rehabilitation candidate. Only by being objectively observant can she appraise; only by being adaptable can she function; and only by functioning can she fulfill her role.

Psychosocial Situations Within Family

When viewing the family, again we are considering individuals. It is unrealistic and hazardous to assume all in the family group possess the same attributes and have the same relationship with the patient. For example, 20-year-old Tom sustained severe flaccid paralysis as a result of poliomyelitis. The father perceived his son's paralysis as destroying his plans for Tom joining him in business, while the mother viewed the disability as a means of keeping Tom dependent on her. Had Tom wanted independence, planned to live alone, and never wished to join his father in business, the situation would be even more complex. The nurse must be alert to the separate manifestations by individual family members, and their effects on the patient. The following discussion will be directed toward broad reactions and needs of family members.

If the patient-family relationship was positive prior to the disability, the manner in which each accepts the disability will affect the other. The family will go through the stages of adjusting as did the patient. Their eventual interpretation of the disability will also depend on how the disability meets or thwarts their desires—both for the patient and for themselves.

Untold benefits to the patient result from continued support, encouragement, and love given by the family. They are capable of sustaining him in ways not open to any outsider. He needs to feel he is still an integral family member. If he is led to believe his role is no longer essential, and, indeed, he is a burden, the effect can be devastating. We should remember he may well feel this under any circumstances, and even the slightest affirmation by a family member (or friend) can prohibit later attempts at bringing him into family matters.

It is usually a very sad state when a patient is rejected by one or more of the members of his family. Regression in his rehabilitation process is caused by such things as being ignored by his family; divorce proceedings; disposition of property; and the moving of his family to another area. The nurse may or may not know of these occurrences; it is difficult in either event. We must also realize that at times family rejection is understandable. When, for example, previous to his disability, the patient was a "ne'er-do-well" or a tyrant, creating and not solving family problems, the prospects of caring for him now may be more than the family can do or should be expected to do.

An ever-present problem that the nurse will encounter when working with the family is fear. The family may be able to express their fear, but more often than not, they will attempt to conceal it—for they think this is what is expected of them. The family may be incapable of localizing their apprehension or anxiety even if they wish to communicate; therefore, the nurse should anticipate their fear. The initial explanation of the disability will be given the family by the physician. It is the responsibility of the nurse to ascertain if they are aware of what to expect when first visiting the patient. They will be immediately concerned about his physical condition. Such things as whether he will live or die and what equipment is being used are of prime importance to them at this time. Trauma when first seeing the patient, even after being told what to expect, is great. The range of concern here is wide, depending on the condition: coma; stertorous breathing; hemiplegia; side rails; Stryker frame; water mattress. Families can be extremely frightened by assistive breathing devices such as an oxygen tent, tracheostomy, or positive pressure machine. Before and after this first visit, the nurse must provide time for explanation and questions.

The patient's physical appearance frightens the family. Following a cerebral vascular accident the patient may drool or be incontinent—the arm and leg appear glaringly lifeless. The patient who has sustained a cervical vertebral injury can move only his arms and head—but even "his arms do not move right," and "his fingers don't move at all." Their fear of physical contact with him can be twofold: either repulsion because of his appearance, or fear of causing further damage to him. They are frightened because they do not understand what has occurred, and yet they are afraid of knowing the truth. Their fear cannot be ignored.

When working with family members, no matter what the diagnosis, the nurse should approach them positively and realistically. The patient's progress and potential are to be made evident to them. Just as the patient needs support, so does the family. Care must be taken to avoid inappropriate reassurances, for this is equally as damaging to the family members as to the patient.

Sufficient time must be provided the family for questions. As the patient's condition changes, so too will the family's interests and concerns. Although the nurse should expect repetition in what the family states or asks, she must be alert to the family's asking the same question of many persons. This may mean no one has discovered what is really being asked. For example, Mr. Walker was admitted to a general hospital following a cerebral vascular accident. Mrs. Walker visited her husband daily, and several times during each visit, she would ask various members of the nursing staff if there were enough nurses on duty who knew how to give him the care he needed. When she continued to be concerned about this, the head nurse spoke at length with her. She found Mrs. Walker was really afraid of not being able to care for him at home, and was not at all worried about the care given Mr. Walker by the nursing staff.

When the family states their need for assistance that requires referral to another agency it is essential that the nurse know appropriate resources and method for the referral. The decision to seek assistance is not one easily made. What to the nurse may seem to be an obvious and a routinely met need can be extremely embarrassing and degrading to the family. When families ask for help, the referral should be swiftly and tactfully accomplished. They must be given specific and correct information and should not be left with the awareness that their need may or may not have been heard but was not answered. The nurse will be well acquainted with services available in her own institution. The task of determining the proper assistance agency will be greatly decreased if there is a social service department within her institution. When there is none, she must be familiar with official and nonofficial agencies in the community. Usually it will be the function of one agency to provide information on services offered by all agencies in the community, and the nurse should utilize this agency. Larger cities usually have an index or sourcebook of community agencies.

There are increasing numbers of groups formed by families of persons afflicted with the same disability. The value of families sharing problems and goals with each other is obvious. For example, nothing may be more comforting to parents who finally accept that their child has cerebral palsy than meeting other parents who have experienced and coped with the multitude of ever-present fears and discouragements.

The family may be provided reading materials that are written for the layman, e.g., *Care of the Patient with a Stroke,* by Genevieve Smith. By reading about the condition their family member has, they may more readily understand the entire situation. Even the most dedicated medical and paramedical personnel cannot hope to cover all necessary areas when talking with families. Furthermore, the family cannot quickly assimilate all information given to them verbally. More often than not, the family will return with new and important questions.

The family should be helped to understand the behavior patterns and personality manifestations of the patient. So often the patient does not behave as he did before the disability. Such things as hostility or silence of the paraplegic and drastic mood swings and cursing by the patient who has had a cerebral vascular accident must be explained. The family cannot and should not be expected to encounter and cope with these manifestations alone.

Preparing the Family for Home Care

The family is included in giving care gradually. Activities such as placing a pillow comfortably and correctly, and pouring the amount of water that will enable the patient to hold the glass himself, can begin when the family seems ready. Knowing when the family is ready is not always easy. Generally it is wise to begin when there no longer is grave concern for the patient's life. The frustrating feeling of utter uselessness can overcome the fear of physical contact. The physical care of a person afflicted with a neuromuscular-skeletal condition is complex. Besides the obvious weakness or loss of function of the body part or parts, many other physical problems occur. If professional persons become overwhelmed by the physical needs of these patients, they should be even more aware of their responsibilities to the family. Not only does the family need to know why and how activities of daily living are accomplished, but they must understand the even greater problem of how to allow the patient to do what he can for himself. How much easier it is to protect those we love by doing for them rather than seeing them struggle to do for themselves.

The nurse must carefully ascertain the effect on the patient caused by family members assisting him. If the assistance is gradual and matter of fact, and if the patient is allowed to do what he can, he will usually accept it. Although we often speak of promoting patient independence, we must not forget there will be times when the family will and should pamper the patient. The pressures of stressing independence, while seeing how terribly real the discouragements are, can become intolerable. Both family and patient can benefit and are supported by the occasional sharing of humor, tears, and overindulgence.

After a period of weeks many institutions allow patients to go home for week-end visits. With continuous teaching the family will know how all care for the patient is accomplished. Range of motion exercises, how to prevent further injury to the patient, transfer from bed to wheel chair—all should be comfortably understood. If the preparation of both patient and family has been comprehensive, the technicalities of Foley catheter irrigations, brace applications, and dressing techniques should present no problems. Having the family progress with the patient has several advantages: they are a part of his rehabilitation; his progress in the realistic program is apparent; and they are being prepared for his return home.

The following example is too frequently seen: Mrs. Hicks had suffered a cerebral vascular accident with subsequent right hemiplegia and severe expressive aphasia (inability to communicate verbally). Mr. Hicks visited his wife daily, and when he arrived, he usually found her in a wheel chair waiting for him. Not until the time he attempted to lift her into the car to take her home did he realize she had always been tied in the wheel chair to keep her from falling. It is imperative the family know what the patient can do for himself and the length of time required for completion of activities. If two hours and a quiet environment are required for the patient to dress himself, then this should be provided. In the event the family will be unable to keep the patient at home, this information is also required for selection of the proper nursing home.

When planning the physical environment for home care, the family should be discouraged from making early and expensive alterations in their home. The exact changes required can best be determined by occupational and physical therapists. Because of the financial strain disabilities bring about, their recommendations are geared to adapting what is presently in the home as opposed to purchasing expensive equipment. Further, only toward the end of hospitalization can the need for all necessary environmental changes and devices be determined. Often very little in the way of alteration is required.

Nursing Personnel

The nursing student cannot anticipate the personnel with whom she will eventually practice her profession. She knows there are full- and part-time professional nurses, nursing technicians, licensed and unlicensed practical nurses, aides and orderlies; and that they all have varying backgrounds and philosophies. The desired objective is for all to work together for the patient's benefit. The difficulties encountered and their solutions are not unique to caring for the patient with a permanent disability, but the need for team work and continuity of approach cannot be better demonstrated than by considering care of this type of patient.

Although the nonprofessional personnel may have had few educational experiences, it is not unusual to find them possessing great insight and enormous capabilities. Often they are the first to know that the patient is entering a new stage of adjusting to his disability. One must remember that the nonprofessional staff is subjected to as many, if not more, positive and negative experiences with patient and family as is the professional nurse. We cannot expect them to understand or accept manifestations such as hostility; those with specific preparation find it difficult. When the nurse becomes disappointed in the nonprofessional staff for not utilizing her instructions and demonstrations of proper positioning and prevention of deformities, she should address her attention to their total knowledge of the patient situation and to how they feel about it. Being able to work out feelings of fear, anger, or frustration about a severely disabled person alone is not to be expected of the nonprofessional person.

It is the view of the author that there is but one means of attempting an organized and comprehensive approach to the care of patients—and that is the nursing team conference. Pertinent information obtained from the conferences should be formulated into a nursing care plan. If a patient card index is used in the institution, this is the most practical method of transmitting the plan. As the plan must change with the patient's progress, so too should the information on the care plan. An outdated or redundant written care plan is as bad as no plan at all. Involving all nursing personnel in planning care means far more than exchanging observations and knowledge. When all are informed of the patient's progress or regressions, all become active participants in his rehabilitation. Nurses who employ this approach know of its value to all concerned, and are able to find the necessary time for conferences. The following situation occurred in a large respiratory center. All of the patients had a severe paralysis as a result of poliomyelitis, and required the assistance of either a respirator or a rocking bed. It came to the attention of the head nurse that when a patient wanted to know if he would move or walk again, often he would first ask the cleaning lady from the housekeeping department. Several days later the question would be put to aides or orderlies. Practical nurses were next in succession; eventually the question was put to the registered nurses. Length of time needed for this sequence ranged from days to weeks. Through team discussions the head nurse emphasized the importance of this question, and how it should best be attended to. Thereafter, when the first questions began, they were reported to the head nurse, who, in turn, relayed the information to the physician. Within a day the patient was visited by the ward physician and psychiatrist. At this time an explanation of the patient's future physical potential was given.

What the Nurse Can Do

When considering what the nurse can do for the patient, one may easily feel overwhelmed. So much must be understood about the disability and its aftermath. Specific nursing techniques are modified to meet the needs of the patient, and yet these things "are done to him" because of his loss. The more involved the physical condition, the greater in number are the procedures. Sequelae are as physically and emotionally damaging as the initial disability. When they have no meaning to the nurse in terms of her approach and activities, she may be assured she is giving little more than custodial care. For example, as was stated earlier, a person does not perspire in the areas that are not innervated. The consequent extreme perspiration from innervated areas may be frightening to the patient. The patient with a high vertebral injury may perspire so freely in the areas of head and neck that a bath towel will be saturated in five minutes. Not only must the patient be kept dry, but he obviously also must be told what is happening. It is essential that the nurse assist the patient in maintaining and modifying his identity. What she does is not so important as how and why she does it. An example is phantom pain and phantom sensation (the feeling of pain or sensation in a part that has been amputated). When, following surgery, the amputee is not told these phenomena usually occur, he may question not only his own sanity, but, indeed, that of the surgeon. If the patient has agreed to amputation of three toes and postoperatively he feels pain in these toes, he may be afraid the surgeon has amputated the wrong toes. Further, if he is unaware phantom pain is a common occurrence, he is unlikely to ask for medication to relieve pain in toes that supposedly no longer exist.

The problems of the patient with a severed spinal cord are more numerous and complex. Some of these complications are preventable; some are not. Most do not happen early in the disability and, therefore, are an excellent example of why diligent concern on the part of the nurse must continue—just as must the disability for the patient. All nurses, no matter in what area they practice, are responsible for the prevention of complications. Often nurses in both the general hospital and rehabilitation agency, and the public health or visiting nurse see the same patient with the same complication but in differing degrees of severity.

One such complication is that of spasms. Following the initial spinal cord injury, the patient enters a period known as spinal cord shock. During spinal cord shock the paralysis is flaccid. Spinal shock may last from weeks to months. Eventually, the lower motor neuron, or reflex arc, which has not been damaged, begins to function again. Since there is no longer central nervous system control or modulation of the reflex arcs below the level of injury, the paralysis becomes and remains spastic. Involuntary muscular contractions of the lower extremities will be observed. Very little stimulus is needed to set the reflex arc into action. Such things as jarring of the bed, pressure of a sheet on a leg, or merely touching of the leg can send the part into spasm. The patient will notice his leg "moves" or "jumps." It is not difficult to imagine the meaning of this event to the patient. Whereas his legs have been "dead," they now obviously have "come back to life."

The patient often is still in the general hospital, and the nurse in this setting should help him understand what is happening. It can be very difficult to assist the patient to accept the fact that this new event has nothing to do with regaining control of the paralyzed part. He may or may not ask what is happening; indeed, he may be too afraid to ask. Nevertheless, one can be quite assured he and his visitors are aware of the movement.

Spasms vary in severity from person to person. They may present no problem at all and, in fact, may be of physiological value. On the other hand, they may increase in severity to the point of producing permanent flexion contractures. Only as the months pass can their result be determined. The nurse in the rehabilitation setting will see the patient learning to live with his spasms. The constant tap-tap-tap of a shoe on a wheel chair footrest when the leg is in spasm is annoying at best. Spasms may increase to the point of preventing the patient from wearing long leg braces—thereby prohibiting ambulation. The accompanying discouragement is felt by all involved.

When the physiatrist feels that because of spasms no further rehabilitation can be accomplished, corrective surgery will be offered to the patient. Accepting or refusing rhizotomy (section of the posterior roots of the spinal nerves) is another decision that can be made only by the patient. Rhizotomy will result in a permanent flaccid paralysis as it destroys the reflex arc; but it will enable him to continue his rehabilitation process. Rhizotomy removes the little but obvious life remaining in his legs, and precludes the miracle of walking again. Few patients accept it immediately; some never agree to the procedure. Again, no amount of persuasion can or should speed the patient into making an affirmative decision. The rehabilitation team can only make apparent why rhizotomy is indicated. Theirs is not the final judgment. The patient may be discharged to his home to consider alternatives and make his decision.

This is the time the visiting or public health nurse will visit the patient. She may or may not know why he is home; he may or may not tell her voluntarily. Her success in assisting him in this adjustment will be greatly increased if this patient's referral contains information essential for his comprehensive care at home. She must determine at what stage he is, and remember what events led him to that stage. His attitudes, interests, and behavior are understandably related to the weight of his problem.

When the decision is in the affirmative, the patient returns to the general hospital for the surgery. It is not uncommon for the same nursing personnel who cared for him when his spasms first began, again to plan his care. He is the same person as before, but now with more problems. Additional disappointments have altered his behavior, and the nurse must adapt her approach accordingly. Above all, it is imperative he be supported in the decision he has made.

Skin breakdown is always a matter of grave concern to the paralyzed person. Able-bodied persons constantly shift their body weight to relieve and redistribute pressure. This is not possible for the paralyzed person. Due to lack of sensation, they are not aware when they have been in one position too long; and if they were aware, they could not move because of motor paralysis. Prolonged pressure, particularly over a bony prominence, causes a lack of circulation—which is the etiology of a decubitus ulcer. Ischemia is the first stage in the formation of a decubitus ulcer. This is noticed by a blanching of the skin. At this point strict measures to prevent formation of the ulcer should be instituted at once. The second stage is termed "hyperemia." The area will be red, raised, and warm to the touch. Cell destruction and hemorrhage have already occurred. This is the time most decubiti are observed, and one notes a general flurry of activity to prevent further skin breakdown. In the nonparalyzed these efforts often are of value; however, it is extremely difficult to halt this process in the paralyzed person. The final stage is a break in the skin. No matter how small the area, it is now a decubitus ulcer.

The anatomical areas most often affected are over bony pominences that receive the greatest degree of pressure. The sacrum, iliac crests, ischial tuberosities, greater femoral trochanters, and heels are common sites. Other sites are anterior tibial crests, knees, elbows, and scapulae. It will be noted that some of these areas normally are protected by fat pads. Both muscle and fat pad atrophy play an important part in the formation of decubiti. The necrotic process continues, and unless very carefully attended, the ulcer proceeds below the subcutaneous fat. There could be no better medium for bacteria.

Prevention is the best treatment for a decubitus. All areas of possible breakdown must be inspected frequently. This does not mean only during the morning bath or evening care, but every time the nurse is in the patient's room. These areas should be washed with copious amounts of soap and water solution, prepared by mixing equal quantities of liquid soap and water, and receive circulation-stimulating massage. Good results have been observed from placing patients on sheepskin or alternating pressure mattresses.

Nursing students are told of the importance of turning patients from the day they begin their education as nurses. It is repeated so often it at times assumes the character of the boy crying "wolf!" But there is no other effective way of preventing decubiti. For the paralyzed bed patient, turning is as essential to skin integrity as breathing is for life. All four sides are to be utilized, and the patient should be turned at least every two hours. If a turning schedule is not begun soon after the disability occurs, an ulcer will form, leaving only three sides for positioning—and so the process goes. An ulcer can occur in a matter of a few hours. Usually decubiti can be prevented by establishing and carrying out a regular schedule of turning. Maintenance of skin integrity is almost completely the responsibility of the nursing staff. There should be no reason for the physician to write orders for these patients to be turned. While decubiti will occur in some instances in spite of diligent nursing care, many occur as a direct result of negligence.

No matter whether in bed or in wheel chair, it is imperative the body weight be distributed evenly over as wide a surface as possible. The larger the area of weight distribution, the less the chance for ischemia to occur. It is important to remember the special problems of the paralyzed patient under 20 years of age. Like any paralyzed patient, they often lean to one side of the wheel chair. These young patients not only are prone to great skin problems, but tend to develop scoliosis due to incomplete bone ossification.

When a decubitus does form, treatment will be as ordered by the physician. It is fairly safe to say there are almost as many methods of treatment as there are physicians. Beyond agreeing that the area should be kept clean, any number of treatments are seen. If infection is present, antibiotics usually will be given. Negative nitrogen balance can be expected as a consequence of the metabolic response to injury. A greater amount of nitrogen is excreted by the body than can be ingested. Because of protein loss due to tissue breakdown, protein-sparing agents are sometimes given. Although it is not possible to reverse negative nitrogen balance in the period immediately following injury by a high dietary intake of protein, the patient must be encouraged to eat foods containing sufficient protein, vitamins, and minerals. After the catabolic phase is completed, protein foods are essential to an adequate anabolic response. Vitamins B and C (ascorbic acid) are also essential to wound healing.

A sterile dressing will usually be placed over the ulcer. Never, under any circumstances, are doughnuts to be used. They only serve to put increased pressure on the area juxtaposed to the ulcer. The desired objective is to reduce pressure. Desirably, no pressure will be placed on the ulcer. If there are decubiti in several areas, this may be impossible, and the sterile dressings over the decubiti should be covered with large, bulky pads.

When the ulcer penetrates the subcutaneous fat, plastic surgery usually is necessary. In addition to performing a full-thickness skin graft the surgeon will often shave the underlying bony prominence until it is paper-thin. As the full-thickness graft cannot compensate for the former fat pad, a protruding bony prominence can penetrate the flap graft.

As soon as possible the patient should become involved in daily observation of the condition of his skin. In order to examine all of his body surface a long-handled mirror should be used. He should be taught how to shift his weight to relieve pressure in both wheel chair and bed, and he should do this every 30 minutes. He is to be warned about the danger of pressure areas developing on his legs; since he has no sensation, injuries from ill-fitting braces and burns can occur without his awareness.

Psychological trauma caused by the formation of decubiti can be great. If the patient is with others who have decubiti, he soon learns what a decubitus would mean to his own rehabilitation program. They begin quickly and progress rapidly. This new body insult is but another cause for increased dependence on others. Decubiti are always unsightly, and often draining and foul-smelling. The nurse should never be more tactful than when giving care to a decubitus ulcer. Not infrequently, decubiti progress to the point of prohibiting any activity other than bed rest. The patient is "grounded." He can no longer be in a wheel chair; all therapies must be accomplished from his bed. Again the rehabilitation process is at a standstill and cannot be resumed until the decubitus heals. At this point the physical sequelae can complicate each other. For example, if a full-thickness flap skin graft is indicated, the plastic surgeon will probably not attempt the procedure if spasms are severe, since within a few hours extremity movement caused by spasms can destroy the graft. Therefore, rhizotomy may be essential before surgical repair of the decubitus is considered. Once more a major decision must be made by the patient. Months may elapse before additional goals can even be attempted.

Problems With Elimination

Bowel and bladder problems also plague the patient with paraplegia. A regimen must be established for each as soon as possible or physical and psychological trauma will occur. Consideration here will first be given to urinary complications.

Bladder sensation and control are lost following complete transection, or cross section, of the spinal cord. Immediately after the injury the bladder becomes atonic, or without tone, and remains so throughout the period of spinal shock. When reflexes again affect the detrusor muscle, the bladder will empty itself. The amount of urine the bladder is capable of holding varies. If the bladder can accommodate 250 to 350 ml and then expel this urine, the patient is said to have an automatic or reflex bladder. Initially an indwelling catheter will have been inserted. When attempts are made to "train" the bladder, the catheter will be clamped for one to four hours and then un-clamped for drainage. If, after a period of time, the bladder continues to empty itself, the catheter will be removed. Hopefully the bladder will continue to hold, then expel, its maximum amount of urine. When the reflex bladder is a reality, expulsion of urine will be mainly determined by the amount of fluid the patient drinks. He must carefully calculate his intake in order to know when to anticipate the expulsion of urine. Expulsion of urine may be facilitated by tactile stimulation of the areas innervated by the pudendal nerve, and by exertion of manual pressure over the bladder.

The length of time required for training the bladder varies greatly. Some patients are never able to achieve a reflex bladder, and therefore will need permanent indwelling catheters or cystostomies. The male patient may wear an external collecting device which will be attached to his leg. At this time there are no successful female collection devices; therefore, the female patient will usually wear sanitary pads as well as rubberized pants.

Urinary complications are a constant area of concern to the paralyzed. Disuse osteoporosis brings about abnormal calcium deposits. Although they can occur at any place in the body, these calculi are often seen in the genito-urinary tract. Oliguria, retention, and stasis of urine also precipitate stone formation and infection. Chills, temperature elevation, decreased urinary output, or hematuria may be the first sign of urinary complication.

It is imperative to keep in mind all the disorders that could occur, and watch for their signs other than the patient's complaint of pain, as these patients no longer feel any sensation. The absence of pain has significance not only for genitourinary complications, but indeed for all medical disorders. The nurse must remember these patients are as prone to develop internal disorders as are nonparalyzed persons, i.e., appendicitis, cholecystitis, peptic ulcer.

Autonomic dysreflexis (disturbed or abnormal reflexes) can occur when, due to a plugged catheter or bladder or urethral obstruction, tremendous back-up of urine greatly distends the bladder. This constitutes a medical emergency and must be corrected immediately. Again the patient cannot tell you his bladder is greatly distended. However, he will be extremely anxious, and may complain of a severe headache. The reflexes sent by the distended bladder may be carried via the internuncial neurons to all parts of the cord. Blood pressure will usually be elevated; it is not uncommon to observe a systolic reading of 300. Other signs are slow pulse, diaphoresis, pilomotor reflex, and temperature elevation. This complication will most often occur when an indwelling catheter is being utilized. The patient who has an automatic bladder should realize there is urinary retention at a time earlier than that required for such a urinary back-up to occur. The nurse should determine whether the catheter is patent. This situation must be reported to the patient's physician immediately.

Since most urinary bacteria thrive in alkaline media, attempts may be made to maintain an acid medium. Mandelamine, or mandelic acid, may be given. The patient should also be encouraged to drink fruit juices that assist in maintaining the acidity of urine. Such fruits are cranberries, plums, and prunes. The most important single measure will be an adequate fluid intake. At least 3,000 ml daily must be taken; the significance of this amount cannot be overemphasized. As soon as possible the patient should assume responsibility for drinking the sufficient amount, as it will be a daily activity for him for the rest of his life.

After discharge the patient will be followed very carefully by the physician. Intravenous pyelograms and X rays of the genitourinary tract will be done every three to six months. The patient must know the signs of urinary complications, such as oliguria and hematuria, and the importance of contacting his physician immediately when these signs occur. The physical, social, and psychological problems that arise as a result of loss of bladder control are as important to consider as any others encountered in the rehabilitation of the permanently disabled. Obviously, genitourinary surgery as well as rhizotomy and plastic surgery can halt the rehabilitation program. Not infrequently all three surgical procedures are seen in the same patient.

Problems with evacuation of feces occur generally with nonambulatory patients. The additional complication of paraplegia only compounds this ever-present concern for nurses. For one of many reasons, the diet is usually not conducive to facilitating normal bowel movements. Greatly diminished physical activity lessens the possibility of regular evacuation. Further, the patient no longer has sensory or motor functioning necessary for evacuation. Far too often constipation and subsequent impaction are the rule and not the exception for these patients. The necessary efforts of nurses in rehabilitation centers would be substantially assisted if the patient's bowel program were established prior to discharge from the general hospital. This is another area where early attention, planning, and action can prevent unnecessary waste of time and energy and alleviate emotional disturbances.

The usual hospital treatments for constipation are enemas. This approach to the problem of evacuation for the patient with paraplegia will never suffice as a desirable bowel program. Repeated enemas decrease normal bowel tone, and in the instance of the paralyzed patient, the highest degree of peristalsis possible must be maintained. Enemas should be utilized only as specific beginning steps in initiating a bowel program. They should never under any circumstances be considered the total solution to evacuation for the paralyzed person. Another often seen, but equally incorrect, method of approaching this problem is manual removal of feces. Again, this is indicated only when it is a component of a carefully prepared plan for setting up a bowel program. Overzealous attention to manual evacuation should be carefully avoided. Not infrequently the patient's poor food intake hinders evacuation. Until such time as the patient does eat a well-balanced diet, difficulties can be expected. Insufficient fluid intake also precludes formation of a bowel program.

The initial step when setting up a bowel program is to determine the time of day most convenient for evacuation after the patient returns to his home. If he will need the assistance of others, obviously it must be a time when there are persons in the home. Generally the time chosen will be early morning or evening. Regulating the bowel function is accomplished by using mineral oil, prune juice, and suppositories. Determining the amount needed is done by the trial-and-error method. If 6 A.M. is to be the time for evacuation, 1 oz of mineral oil and 200 ml of prune juice are taken at the hour of sleep on the previous night. At 5:30 A.M., a suppository is given. Or the patient may require only prune juice and a suppository, and action of the suppository may occur within five minutes. The important consideration here is to experiment with these three items until the most workable pattern is achieved. Once begun, the plan must be continuous; inattention of only one day can destroy weeks of effort.

The nurse may anticipate delay in establishing the program. During the period before the schedule is achieved, bowel movements can occur at any time, thereby causing embarrassment and discouragement to the patient. Psychological trauma caused by evacuation during meals, during visiting hours, or at occupational or physical therapy is obvious. Through continued efforts, patience, and support to the patient, a workable bowel program will evolve. The patient does need a definite program for the rest of his life, and only by working toward evacuation at a specific hour can he control this function; there is no reason to delay its establishment. Optimism is in order, as a plan can be achieved with time. The value to the patient of once again "controlling" evacuation of feces is immeasurable.

Prevention of Contractures and Deformities

When at rest or inactive for long periods of time, limbs tend to assume positions that, unless altered, produce deformity. Not only are flexors and adductors the stronger muscle groups, but assuming positions of flexion and adduction affords relief of pain. We can be assured deformities and contractures will occur in certain conditions, i.e., cerebral vascular accident and rheumatoid arthritis, unless preventive measures are begun early and are continuous. The nursing student is urged to examine her own position when supine. The importance of diligent attention may then be more apparent to her. She will observe that her feet are in plantar flexion and her legs are externally rotated. Not infrequently her arms will be adducted and flexed.

From the time of admission the body should be maintained in good physiological alignment. This is accomplished by the use of sandbags, pillows, trochanter rolls, and footboards. Far too often utilization of these devices is neglected by all concerned after the initial discussion in introductory nursing classes. Further, one often sees these devices in the patient's environment, but they are serving no useful purpose. One such example is the footboard. Indeed, it is on the bed; however, the feet of the patient are fully 4 in. from it, and are demonstrating plantar flexion. Due to the great inflexibility of footboards, and variances of patient's heights, some nurses have found it of value to fashion their own footboards. Sandbags, which provide stability, are placed in a cardboard box (such as the kind that contain intravenous solutions); the box is then covered with a small sheet. The position of this footboard may be altered according to the height of the patient. Nurses also are often faced with a lack of sandbags. This may be a suitable project for auxiliary groups working in or with the hospital. Five-, seven-, and ten-pound sandbags are relatively easy to make. The benefits to all are apparent.

Only at such time as the physician orders active or passive range of motion for the patient should the indicated exercises begin. The length of time following the disability until range-of-motion exercises can be started will be determined by the patient's condition. For example, if a cerebral vascular accident has occurred as a result of thrombus or embolus, these activities may be indicated within 48 hours after the accident. If, however, the stroke was caused by hemorrhage, the physician may not allow activity for six to eight weeks. When exercises are indicated and ordered, the necessity of their daily occurrence cannot be overemphasized. Talking with the physician about when he wishes exercises to begin is always in order.

In the event the nursing student has not taken an extremity through range of motion, and consequently does not know how it feels to move another person's limbs, she is urged to practice on a colleague. The "patient" should present her with two situations: first, she should make the limb as limp and lifeless as possible; second, her limb should assume and maintain positions of slight adduction and flexion.

The nurse may anticipate tightness and resistance when working with patients who have been inactive for a period of time. Inactivity of only a few days' duration produces limitations of motion and pain on movement. One such example is the "frozen shoulder" seen in patients who have suffered a cerebral vascular accident; the pain can be excruciating. For this reason sometimes these patients are encouraged to use their unaffected arm for taking the affected arm through range of motion, as they will know better than anyone else their own degree of pain tolerance. Daily range of motion should show some degree of increasing joint mobility.

The patient who has had a stroke should always have his affected arm supported by a sling when either sitting or walking. If the arm is not supported, subluxation or partial dislocation of that shoulder may ensue. When a sling is used, two considerations are important. First, the wrist must also be supported to prevent wrist drop. Second, the weight of the arm in the sling should not exert excess pressure on the cervical vertebrae. The knot should be lateral to the vertebrae, and a foam rubber or felt pad may be placed over the vertebrae to reduce the pressure.

The nurse must be alert to flexion contractures about the hip joint in addition to those at the knee and foot. The onset of hip flexion may be quite insidious. Elevation of the head of the bed, no matter to what degree, will have some effect on the hip joint. It is helpful for these patients to be in a flat position several times daily. The origin of external rotation of the leg is at the hip joint; therefore, the wise nurse places sandbags along the outer aspect of the upper leg as well as along the lower leg. Before placing sandbags, one should attempt to position the extremity in some degree of overcorrection (i.e., internal rotation of the leg), so that with the stronger opposite pull or external rotation, a neutral position may be achieved. The legs should be maintained in a neutral position, neither externally nor internally rotated. A small pillow may be placed under the lower legs to relieve pressure from the heels, thus preventing decubitus formation in these areas. Care must be taken that the pillow does not cause knee flexion, which in turn would produce contracture.

Respiratory Complications

Respiratory complications plague the disabled. The reasons are as numerous as are the basic diagnoses. The patient with paralysis due to poliomyelitis or traumatic quadriplegia may lack control of breathing and coughing mechanisms and therefore may require assistance with both. The patient who has suffered a cerebral vascular accident with resultant paralysis is also prone to hypostatic pneumonia. Nothing can be more frustrating to the nurse than telling such a patient to cough, and hear him repeat the word "cough," but no longer be able to comprehend what the word means.

These patients must be protected from possible respiratory infections. Every precaution must be taken to prevent contact with persons having upper respiratory infections. If the patient is at all capable of coughing, he should do so hourly. Turning is also essential in reducing the possibility of pulmonary congestion. The sooner the patient may be in an upright position, the less are chances for respiratory complications to occur. Never under any circumstances should oral fluids be given until it has been clearly ascertained that the patient can swallow. Aspiration pneumonia occurs when well-meaning but unthinking persons give fluids to the unconscious or dysarthric (paralysis or weakness of speech, swallowing or tongue musculatures) patient.

Additional Disorders of the Patient Who Has Suffered
Cerebral Vascular Accident With Organic Residual

Hemiplegia or hemiparesis is easily observable and presents definite indications for specific nursing care. However, equally important to the comprehensive care of the patient who has had a stroke is the area of communication, perception, and "inner thinking." Their individual meaning for each patient is inherent for good nursing care. Ascertaining the extent of brain damage is difficult and requires specific testing by highly skilled persons. Often these services are not available in general hospitals; therefore, the nurse will rarely have exact information about difficulties in these areas. By being aware of commonly seen sequelae, and reporting her observations, she can provide invaluable assistance to medical and paramedical disciplines. Moreover, nursing care will be planned around the capabilities and limitations of the patient.

Aphasia

Before discussing the various types of aphasia, it would be well to consider language per se. Language is a set of symbols by which we make our thoughts known to ourselves as well as others. Expressive language is that language used to reveal our needs and thinking to other persons. Receptive language is the language each of us uses to understand what others communicate to us. Inner language is that language individuals use to think or talk to themselves. The patient who has had a stroke may have had damage of varying degree to any or all of these three types of language. Therefore, if a patient is said to have expressive aphasia, it does not mean that he cannot hear and understand what is said to him or said in his presence. This fact must be clearly and completely understood by all persons (staff, visitors, and other patients) coming into contact with patients who are unable to speak. When attempting to communicate with such a patient, the nurse should talk with him as if he does understand her. Above all it should never be forgotten how devastating and frightening it would be to the patient to have others discuss within his hearing the hopelessness of his condition.

Verbal communication is the desired objective. Early and continued attempts to determine whether or not an aphasic patient can communicate in this manner are essential. If the patient does not demonstrate the ability to communicate verbally, it must be ascertained if he understands what is being said to him. The patient who appears to be expressively aphasic may be capable of responding nonverbally to questions asked him that require "yes" or "no" answers. When he does respond by shaking his head or blinking his eyes, he should use these devices appropriately. However, neither the patient nor those in his environment should be allowed to rely on nonverbal communication if verbal communication is possible for him.

Agraphia is the inability to write words on command or to formulate ideas in written expression, although copying may still be possible. The inability to solve mathematical problems is acalculia. Word blindness, or lack of reading comprehension, is alexia.

When the patient has total expressive and receptive aphasia he is said to be globally aphasic. Global aphasia results from severe organic brain damage; therefore, rehabilitation potential for these patients is quite limited.

Expressive or receptive aphasia does not mean the patient is incapable of producing word sounds. He may utter nonintellectual word forms in substitution for meaningful speech. Such an example is emotional utterance. This is demonstrated by such things as words of endearment or by cursing. Previous to his stroke, the patient may have controlled the desire for saying these words, but due to damage to the higher centers of the brain he is no longer capable of this control. The patient may demonstrate automatic speech. He may repeat an entire song or prayer, but have no awareness of its meaning. The patient may be capable of social speech, comprised in the main of common salutations. He may say "Good morning," or "How do you do." When social speech is uttered at an appropriate time one may easily overlook the presence of a basic aphasic problem. The nurse who makes daily morning rounds would do well to engage such a patient in other areas of conversation. Another example is serial content. Here the patient is capable of giving such things as the days of the week or months of the year in sequence, although he does not know the meaning of all or of individual words.

Perseveration is repetition with or without provocation on either a verbal or motor level. The word or act is meaningless, although initially it may have been appropriate for one response. If the patient demonstrates a "yes" or a "no" perseveration but is capable of other meaningful speech, he should be asked questions that cannot be answered with either of these words. Even though perseveration should be halted and a new activity begun, one must be discriminate, as this may be the patient's first attempts at communication.

Agnosia

Agnosia is the inability to comprehend sensations. A person with tactile agnosia cannot perceive an object by feel. Auditory agnosia is demonstrated by an inability to understand the meaning of environmental sounds such as the ringing of a telephone. Visual agnosia is the loss of comprehension of objects by sight. Patients demonstrating auditory agnosia will often also have visual agnosia.

Apraxia

Whereas agnosia is a sensory loss, apraxia is the inability to perform acts without motor loss. A nonverbal, or motor, apraxia is demonstrated by a patient picking up a comb but having no idea of its use. Although he may use the article automatically, he cannot do so on command. Persons with a verbal apraxia are unable to utilize the speech musculature.

Flexibility, again, is the basis of approach to the patient with aphasia. The nurse must have some idea of the language disorder demonstrated, but no issue should be made of the loss. Sentences should be simple and short. A soft, but easily understood voice should be used. An excessively loud voice is to be avoided. When assuming one is unable to hear, the speaker shows a tendency to speak far more loudly than necessary. It is essential not to bombard the patient with questions. If questions come too quickly, his answers may be behind by several questions. In such event even though his answers are correct, they may appear inappropriate and/or incorrect. It is wise to anticipate the word a patient is attempting to say. Although he should not be supplied the word immediately, he also should not be forced beyond his frustration point. After supplying the word for the patient, he should be encouraged to repeat it. Above all, his speech should not be interrupted or depreciated in any manner. Any speech the aphasic patient utters should be encouraged. If his speech is discouraged in any way he may make no further attempts at communicating.

Inner Thinking and Personality Disorders

When brain damage has occurred, it is not possible to determine the exact amount of "inner thinking" disturbance. We cannot completely know how the patient views himself or what he feels about his disability. His present state may be totally overwhelming, or because of severe inner thinking difficulty, he may be unaware of his condition. Accompanying personality disorders are often seen. Inappropriate behavior may be obvious to hospital personnel. Moreover, personality and behavioral changes will be observed and may be mentioned by the patient's family.

The patient is easily overwhelmed by excess environmental stimuli. He should be asked to concentrate on only one object or activity at a time. Overloading him with many requests, or even several areas of conversation, confuses him greatly. The patient who has suffered brain damage needs to have his environment controlled and structured for him whether or not aphasia is demonstrated. Unnecessary stimuli are to be eliminated, and the setting should be quiet and composed. All possible efforts at assisting him in adjusting to his present state must be made. These patients show tendencies toward rigidity and inflexibility. They cannot adjust to rapid and unfamiliar happenings. They may demand that their daily physical care be done in the same sequence. Such patients can become extremely agitated if objects in the room are not arranged in a specific order. By not following the pattern required by the patient, one may frustrate him to the point of making future adjustments impossible. Working with such a patient often is extremely trying, but the nurse must remember the patient is attempting not only to exhibit some control over his environment but to communicate with it as well. And this is the desired objective. Moreover, it must be kept in mind that the extreme anxiety demonstrated when making his desires known may be quickly followed by a complete reversal in the patient's manner. Just as they are easily exasperated, so, too, are they pleased.

The patient should not be confronted with daily changes. A routine should be established and continued. When at all possible, the same person on each shift should care for him until he is capable of communicating comfortably. Only when it is demonstrated to the patient that he and his needs are understood will he feel comfortable and supported, and he will not be at ease if he anticipates a changing atmosphere. No long-term goals can be attempted until the patient is secure with those caring for him.

These patients are usually withdrawn, as they are unable to express themselves or cope with their environment. It is not unusual for them to exhibit no interest in what is occurring around them. This may be seen even in the nonaphasic patient. Further, the patient may appear to be more alert at some times than at others. When these situations occur, the nurse should try to stimulate the patient in some way. The object is to assist the patient in communicating with someone or something other than himself. The areas the nurse may explore are limitless, and her efforts are to be continued until some means of reaching the patient is found. Often the family can be of assistance through either their presence or knowledge of his interests. Not infrequently an object that was dear to the patient may begin his interest. Bringing him such things as a picture of a family member or a family Bible can be of great value.

Since efforts are to be directed toward bringing him again in touch with reality, allowing him constantly to be absorbed in a nonparticipatory activity should be avoided. An example of this is looking at television or listening to the radio. It is quite possible to be in the presence of either of these media and to be completely uninvolved. This is not to say that under certain circumstances utilizing these media should not be attempted; i.e., the patient who was previously a baseball fan might benefit from watching a game on television. Indiscriminate use, however, may force the patient into further withdrawal.

When communicating with the patient, the nurse must be aware of another often seen complication. Persons who have suffered a stroke are prone to concretism. By this it is meant they are unable to think abstractly. Therefore, the nurse should refrain from statements such as, "Turn on your side closest to the window so that you can see the robins." None of these words may have any meaning for the patient now. He should be shown in some manner—possibly even turned toward the window—and then told to "see the birds."

Persons having sustained a cerebral vascular accident are highly prone to mood swings. Inappropriate laughing or crying is not necessarily provoked. For no apparent reason the patient may weep unconsolably and, just as strangely and suddenly, laugh uncontrollably. Even though this phenomenon is understood and accepted by family and personnel, it can be greatly disturbing. The important factor here is that those in contact with the patient (including other patients) know they are not responsible for the mood swings.

When the patient begins doing activities for himself, various other problems arise. Incoordination and confusion more often than not lead to unsuccessful attempts, no matter what the activity. It is imperative the patient be encouraged to continue these efforts. Often the nurse must demonstrate even the most rudimentary methods of self-care, and these demonstrations will have to be repeated. This is particularly true when dressing or other self-care activities are taught. In all things, it is important to remember these people tend to demonstrate past and not recent recall. For example, the patient may remember where a shirt is worn, but not recall the previous day's instructions of how to get his paralyzed arm through the sleeve.

Due to his awkward motions and inability to perform activities correctly, the patient may become more anxious and frustrated. Impulsivity is commonly seen as a result of frustration. The patient is unable to see the consequences of an act. An example is striking at and knocking over a pan of bath water into the bed because he is unable to wring out the washcloth. It is because of such impulsive acts and concretism that a decision may be made that the patient cannot safely be alone by himself for any period of time.

The patient should be encouraged to continue attempting an activity to his frustration point. Not uncommonly, he may at this point summon all of his energies and be successful. The nurse must not forget that the overt demonstrations of his great anxiety will be followed by a smile of satisfaction.

If the patient is provoked (by himself or others) beyond his frustration point, a catastrophic response may ensue. This is a psychobiological response of the entire organism when successful completion of an activity is not possible.[3] Expression of catastrophic response ranges from wild thrashing about to unconsciousness. The nurse must take great care not to frustrate the patient to this extreme. When it does occur, her action must be swift and sure. Observing this reaction is extremely upsetting, the nurse needs to think clearly and calmly. As casually as possible, whatever activity the patient is demonstrating must be stopped, even if it means being stopped physically.

Often as activities of daily living are begun, nursing personnel become aware of the patient's visual loss. For example, reaching for a glass but knocking it over may indicate the absence of complete visual acuity. Hemianopsia, or loss of one half of the visual field of one or both eyes, may be present without the patient's being aware of his loss. This may also account for his bumping into objects. Having the patient read aloud is one means of determining hemianopsia. If this is present, words or groups of words will be omitted from each line of print. Patients are taught to compensate for the loss of visual acuity or the effect of hemianopsia by scanning, or rotating the head, so that the object being scrutinized may be fully seen.

Activities of Daily Living

Daily self-care for permanently disabled persons is far too individualized to state a panacea. Although ingenuity of the nurse may be taxed to the point of exhaustion, it is her responsibility to determine the most feasible and safe manner self-care can be accomplished. And this is self-care for the patient after discharge—not for the convenience of the nursing staff. Inherent in self-care is the understanding by the patient and his family of how complications are prevented.

The problems involved are as basic as being certain all areas of the body will be washed. Simple though it may sound, such a goal is not without frustration. If the patient with paraplegia denies his legs are a part of him, he is not going to wash them—long-handled sponge or not! How does one ever teach a person to place a washcloth in a positioned paralyzed right hand for washing the left axilla, if this person is unaware he has a right side? The "body image" of the patient who has had a stroke will determine what he washes and what he ignores.

No matter in what areas she is responsible for patient teaching, regardless of the place of teaching, the needs of the patient will determine her plan. Teaching must be continuous and purposeful. Intensity and design of the

---

[3] Jon Eisenson, "Therapeutic Problems and Approaches with Aphasic Adults," in Lee Edward Travis (ed.), *Handbook of Speech Pathology*, Appleton-Century-Croft, Inc., New York, 1957, p. 473.

teaching plan are as important for the multiextremity amputee as for the quadriplegic. What is taught must be presented in a well-defined and vital manner. If it is not, the patient cannot be expected to recognize the significance of what he needs to know.

What the Nurse Cannot Do

The old and true saying that a nurse is not capable of being all things to all people cannot be better emphasized than when considering rehabilitation of the physically handicapped. One person cannot possibly accomplish the total rehabilitation of permanently disabled persons alone. Of necessity, the needs of the patient and difficulties encountered in meeting them demand the attention of several highly skilled disciplines. When, as still occurs, necessary team members are not available, goals for the patient must be set accordingly.

Too frequently in hospitals nurses assume overprotection of the patient. The patient "belongs" to the nursing personnel. He may spend most of a day in X ray or two hours in physical therapy, but he returns where he belongs— to the patient unit. Although this is not without some benefit, nurses can be quite perplexed by the all-too-obvious fact that the patient is not hers alone. To begin with, the patient belongs to himself. Moreover, it is shocking indeed to learn that the patient is as valuable to the occupational therapist and social service worker (and vice versa) as he is to nursing personnel.

This problem is particularly evident in a rehabilitation setting. The full complement of paramedical disciplines seems able to meet most if not all of the patient's needs. Many activities nurses have done for so long are now accomplished by disciplines educated expressly for those functions. Finding one's role where there seems so little role left is a common problem these nurses share. With diligence and patience the nurse can find her place on the team; but never will it be found if she attempts to duplicate the services of other disciplines. With the increasing numbers of services offered in general hospitals, this problem will be unique to the nurse in a rehabilitation setting for only a short period of time. As in so many other examples, the situations nurses encounter in care of the permanently disabled are not restricted to rehabilitation.

Impose Her Values on the Patient

Nurses must at all times refrain from imposing their own values on patients under their care. Assisting the patient in his rehabilitation program provides excellent opportunity for seeing in the patient that which the nurse desires to see. The particular situations encountered with the disabled patient are complex for more than one reason. First, this type of patient is usually hospitalized for far longer periods of time than the nondisabled patient. Therefore, her feelings of identification with the patient, or nonacceptance of his manner of adjusting to his disability, will have more time to develop. It is extremely difficult to change one's opinion of such a situation when the reasons for forming the opinion are constantly reinforced. With contact of many weeks the situation becomes increasingly trying for all. Her perception of the patient will determine what goals the nurse can visualize for him. The nurse who cannot accept a patient because his reaction is not what she imagines hers would be will possess neither the patience nor the interest necessary for planning and working with him. Moreover, efforts toward rehabilitation by such a nurse can only be considered for unrealistic goals, as they will be geared toward her incorrect perception of the situation.

Nonobjectivity

Occasionally the tragedy of the situation becomes the prime concern of the nurse. In allowing herself to see only the disastrous effects of the disability on one or more lives, she is utterly of no value to the patient or her colleagues. Patients and families deserve positive support and are quite without need for yet another weakness on the way back to a purposeful existence. It is the obligation of the nurse to maintain an objective approach, and this is to be accomplished by whatever means necessary.

Equally as damaging to all concerned is the nurse who becomes so emotionally involved with the patient that she feels no one else is capable of giving the care needed. Thereby she meets her own emotional needs and not those of the patient. This nurse misleads only herself.

Female nursing students must be alert to disabled male patients who attempt to form romantic relationships with them. Nothing could better prove the continued existence of his manhood than having a young female romantically interested in him. The young paraplegic who becomes (or remains) a Don Juan can provide an extremely difficult situation. Nurses who do become thus involved need help in determining their motivation for such attachments.

When for any reason the nurse realizes she is no longer capable of being objective in a patient situation, she should seek help and guidance. Maintaining a purposeful approach with patients is extremely difficult and not easily accomplished. Admitting to herself that she needs help and then seeking the necessary guidance are actions far more beneficial to the patient and herself than any others she could take.

Approach of the Nurse

As stated earlier, the nurse must be flexible and she will receive her clues for this flexibility from the patient. Listening to him and understanding what he says will tell her how best to formulate her approach. Having knowledge of the classical picture of the disability and how the patient's condition is similar to it is not enough.

The fear of saying the wrong thing to the patient is great. Wondering when she will inadvertently mention an activity no longer possible for the patient constantly plagues the nurse. The nursing student must understand that at some time she will err in her choice of words or topic of conversation. Only when she does make what she considers to be a gross error will the nurse realize how groundless were her fears. More often than not the understanding response of the patient will control the situation. He, too, has anticipated such an occurrence and will be prepared. There is no more astounding and rewarding facet of human capabilities than unexpected strength. Physical disability does not necessarily negate emotional resources. Further, after discharge the patient's associates cannot provide him the controlled environment found in hospitals; therefore, supposedly ill-chosen words could serve as a means of preparing him for what he will later encounter. The fact is, avoiding reference to his disability is often for the nurse's own benefit; and when this is the case, neither the patient nor the nurse is moving toward acceptance of his disability.

Efforts necessary for assisting the patient to reach his highest potential are thwarted for many reasons. The work is not glamorous or dramatic, and not infrequently it is totally unrewarding. Attempts at realizing well-conceived plans are often met with complete nonacceptance, and therefore will have been to no avail. It must be clearly understood that frustration is the rule and not the exception. How, then, should the nurse approach the patient with a permanent disability?

First and foremost, she must always remember she is responsible for neither the disability nor what eventually will be the fate of the patient and his family. What has happened to them *is not her fault*. There will be times when remembering this will be the only means of enabling the nurse to function as she must.

It is imperative she examine the motives for her actions and operate for the patient's benefit—not her own. She must carefully gear her thinking about the patient to his physical and emotional state; she must be aware of where he comes from, and to what environment he will return. Knowing all these factors separately is not sufficient; they must be combined and their effect on the patient—at that time—be determined.

The nursing student can be assured that when goals are accomplished, the meaning to all is immeasurable, for this cannot occur unless both patient and nurse work together to the extreme limits of their capabilities, and when it does, the rewards for both are great.

REFERENCES

Books

Brock, S. (ed.), *Injuries of the Brain and Spinal Cord and their Coverings,* 4th ed., Springer & Co., New York, 1960, Chaps. 19 and 20.
Cecil, R. L., and R. F. Loeb, (eds.), *Textbook of Medicine,* 11th ed., W. B. Saunders Co., Philadelphia, 1963, pp. 1611-19.
De Jong, R. V., *The Neurological Examination,* 2nd ed., Harper & Brothers, New York, 1958, Chaps. 44 and 53.
Garrett, J. F., *Psychological Aspects of Physical Disability,* U.S. Government Printing Office, Washington, D.C., 1952.

Garrett, J. F., and E. S. Levine, *Psychological Practices with the Physically Disabled,* Columbia University Press, New York, 1962.

Myklebust, H. E., *Auditory Disorders in Children,* Grune and Stratton, New York, 1954, Chap. 7.

Peplau, Hildegarde, *Interpersonal Relations in Nursing,* G. P. Putnam's Sons, New York, 1952.

Prather, G. C., and F. H. Mayfield, *Injuries of the Spinal Cord,* Charles C Thomas, Springfield, Illinois, 1953.

Rusk, H. A., and E. J. Taylor, *Living with a Disability,* Blakiston, Garden City, New York, 1953.

Smith, Genevieve, *Care of the Patient with a Stroke,* Springer Co., New York, 1959, p. 148.

Super, Donald, *Appraising Vocational Fitness,* Harper & Brothers, New York, 1949, Chaps. 1, 4, 6 (pp. 86-104), and 15.

Towel, Charlotte, *Common Human Needs,* National Association of Social Workers, New York, 1952, pp. 37-72.

Travis, Lee Edward (ed.), *Handbook of Speech Pathology,* Appleton-Century-Crofts, Inc., New York, 1957, Chaps. 12, 13, and 14.

Viscardi, Henry, *Give Us the Tools,* Eriksson-Taplinger Co., Inc., New York, 1959.

Wepman, Joseph, *Recovery from Aphasia,* The Ronald Press Co., New York, 1951, Chaps. 10 and 11.

Wright, Beatrice A., *Physical Disability—A Psychological Approach,* Harper & Brothers, New York, 1960.

Articles

Martin, M. A., "Nursing Care in Cervical Cord Injuries," *American Journal of Nursing,* LXIII, No. 3, pp. 60-66.

Visotsky, H. M., D. A. Hamburg, M. E. Goss, and B. Z. Lebovits, "Coping Behavior Under Extreme Stress," *Archives of General Psychiatry,* V, November, 1961, pp. 423-48.

Unpublished Material

Halper, Anita, "The Aphasic Patient," Unpublished lecture, given at The Rehabilitation Institute of Chicago, Chicago, Illinois, 1962.

Kir-Stimon, William, "Psychological Aspects of Physical Disability," Unpublished lecture given at the Rehabilitation Institute of Chicago, Chicago, Illinois, 1962.

Neal, Richard, "Medical Aspects of Physical Disability," Unpublished lecture given at the Rehabilitation Institute of Chicago, Chicago, Illinois, 1960.

Vultee, Fredrick, "Rehabilitation of the Physically Disabled," Unpublished lecture given at the Rehabilitation Institute of Chicago, Chicago, Illinois, 1960.

17 : Epilogue

PART A : Patients with Diabetes Mellitus

After saying that a good play does not require an epilogue, Shakespeare adds one to *As You Like It*. Though an epilogue may not be necessary, some of the content previously presented has been selected and applied to patients experiencing two different types of disorders. In the first part, six patients who have diabetes mellitus and who experienced a variety of complications are described. Information basic to understanding their needs has been selected and applied. In the second part, Mr. Allen, a patient who has been burned, is described. Information required to understand and meet his needs is presented. These patients illustrate many of the problems commonly experienced by persons who are ill.

In the not too distant past one of the critical tests of the skill of a nurse was her ability to meet the needs of a patient with an acute infectious disease such as typhoid fever or pneumonia. When the patient recovered, the nurse could rightly take credit for having made an important contribution to his recovery. As infectious diseases have been brought under control, the incidence of chronic illness has risen so that they now account for a significant portion of morbidity and mortality. The challenges presented by patients who are chronically ill are no less great than they are with patients with acute infectious diseases. Chronically ill patients are likely to have a wider range of problems than are patients whose illnesses are of short duration. Moreover, the welfare of persons with a chronic disorder often requires a greater variety of services than are needed to meet the needs of the acutely ill. Restoration of the patient to his optimum status and prevention of progress of his illness often demands the continued efforts of the patient, his family, the nurse, the physician, and other health and welfare personnel as well as the members of the community. With patients in whom progress toward recovery is slow and in whom control or prevention of the progression of disease is the goal rather than complete recovery, the nurse may not be able to see immediate results of her efforts. Instead of a relatively brief and intensive relationship in which the patient is dependent on the nurse, the nurse often has a more or less prolonged relationship with the patient. This relationship with the patient fluctuates from time to time, from dependence to independence to interdependence. To meet the needs of the patient, the nurse should be able to identify clues indicating the type of relationship best suited to the needs of the patient at a given time and to adapt her behavior accordingly. She must also be able to tolerate failure of the patient to make dramatic progress toward recovery.

Today the test of the skill of the nurse is her ability to meet the needs of the chronically ill patient. If a single disease were to be selected as the modern-day test of nursing knowledge and skill, diabetes mellitus would undoubtedly receive many votes. There are many reasons that this is true. Diabetes mellitus has a relatively high incidence. It affects all age groups. Its complications are many and serious. There are, however, effective means for its detection, diagnosis, and treatment. With modern methods of therapy, persons with diabetes mellitus can live almost as long as those who do not have diabetes. Even more important, they can have full and useful lives with few restrictions on their activities. Young men with diabetes mellitus have been Rhodes scholars, mountain climbers, and tennis champions. Young women with diabetes mellitus go to college, successfully complete programs in nursing or teaching, marry, bear and rear children, and otherwise lead successful lives.

Health programs, as they relate to diabetes mellitus, have two general objectives. The first is to prevent or, if this is not possible, to delay the onset of the disease. The second is to maintain the health and vigor of the individual throughout his life. In the achievement of these objectives the nurse has three general responsibilities. The first is to aid in the detection of persons who are predisposed to or in the early stages of diabetes mellitus. The second is to participate in the education of the patient, his family, and the community in the management of diabetes mellitus. The third is to meet the needs of the sick person for nursing. Frequently the nurse performs all these functions more or less simultaneously.

No nurse should accept the responsibility for the care of the patient with diabetes mellitus unless she knows as much as the well-educated patient is expected to learn about his disease. She should also be willing and able to recognize that the patient may well feel differently about having diabetes mellitus than she thinks he should. Not infrequently a patient is told that he is fortunate to have diabetes rather than cancer or tuberculosis. The advantages that diabetes mellitus has over diseases such as cancer are derived from comparing it with them, and they are expressed by physicians and nurses who do not have diabetes. In contrast, the patient compares diabetes with health. The feelings of the patient result from the implications diabetes mellitus has for him now and in the future. The nurse can be helpful to the patient by accepting his feelings as having a cause and by creating a climate in which he is free to express them. Eventually, most patients come to accept their diabetes with a reasonable degree of equanimity. A sound program of instruction adapted to the individuality of the patient can be expected to make a positive contribution to the acceptance by him of his therapeutic regimen.

As a basis for discussing the knowledge which the nurse needs if she is to meet the needs of patients with diabetes mellitus, the histories of six patients are summarized below. Some of the material was collected for other purposes so the details in all instances may not be complete. Selection of information is on the basis of what is most pertinent to this discussion. The material contained in the summary will be commented upon in the appropriate sections. Of the six patients it will be noted that five are female and one is male. They range in age from 15 to 73 years. Two of these six persons are college graduates and were diabetic at the time they entered college. One of them, Miss Arthur, lived in a dormitory and ate in a college cafeteria throughout her years in college; she had no problems in the selection of her diet. Both Miss Arthur and Mr. Benedict are self-supporting, and he has thus far been able to support his family. Although these patients do not present all the problems faced by patients with diabetes mellitus, they do evidence many of those that are common. Since they have all had their disorder for some time, they do not illustrate all the problems of the patient who has been recently found to have diabetes mellitus.

Had these six people lived 100 years ago, the probability is that only Mrs. Curry and Mrs. Delft would have survived more than a year or two after the onset of the disease. One hundred years ago the prognosis of the diabetic child was hopeless. His status was similar to, and probably no better than, that of the child who now has leukemia. Once the diagnosis was established, few children lived longer than a year. For the most part, the child led a miserable existence until he died in diabetic acidosis. Many persons now live as long as or longer than the life expectancy for nondiabetics of the same age. The average diabetic, however, lives about three-quarters of the life expectancy of the nondiabetic.

The changes having taken place in the length of life following a diagnosis of diabetes mellitus are illustrated by the following figures. From 1900 to 1914, the average patient lived 4.9 years. Child diabetics lived about a year, while adults lived somewhat longer. In the years 1956 to 1957, the average for Joslin's series was 18.2 years.[1] These statistics will probably be improved, for some of the persons on whom they are based are still alive. Of the six patients cited below, the average life span among those who developed diabetes as children is 13 years.

The factors contributing to the great improvement in the life expectancy of persons of all ages who have diabetes mellitus include: (1) greater understanding of the nature of normal as well as abnormal energy metabolism, (2) more appreciation of the value of diet in the control of hyperglycemia, (3) the discovery of insulin and its use in therapy, (4) the discovery of oral hypoglycemic agents, (5) the recognition that the control of diabetes mellitus is the responsibility of the patient and his family, and (6) the development of educational programs to prepare the patient to assume this responsibility. It now appears to be possible to identify persons who are predisposed to diabetes mellitus. Application of this knowledge may lead to the early indentifi-

[1] Elliot P. Joslin, Howard F. Root, Priscilla White, and Alexander Marble, *The Treatment of Diabetes Mellitus*, 10th ed., Lea & Febiger, Philadelphia, 1959, p. 228.

Summary of Six Patients' Histories

Factor	Bonnie	Miss Arthur	Mr. Benedict	Mrs. Curry	Mrs. Delft	Mrs. Keen
Age	15	22	29	62	71	73
Age at onset	4	13	8	60	62	55
Years of known diabetes	9	9	21	2	5	17
Sex	F	F	M	F	F	F
Severity	Severe	Severe	Severe	Mild	Mild	Severe
Reason for present hospitalization	Acidosis (numerous admissions in the past)	Hypoglycemia with unconsciousness	Evaluation of diabetes and investigation of complications	Myocardial infarction	Possible cerebro-vascular accident	Control of diabetes preparatory to operation
Present signs and symptoms	Nausea Vomiting Abdominal cramps Lips and tongue dry and parched Kussmaul breathing Glycosuria Ketonuria	Blood sugar on admission 55 mg/100 ml Unconscious	Weakness Easily fatigued Blurring of vision	Onset with diabetic retinopathy	Poor vision Blurring Severe frontal headaches Nausea and vomiting	Glycosuria Hyperglycemia Increased blood cholesterol
Adequacy of control	Poor	Generally excellent	Recent years generally satisfactory	Good with diet	Satisfactory with diet	Poor
Family history of diabetes	Grandmother diabetic	No family history known	Father and sister diabetic	Mother diabetic	None known	Sister diabetic
Weight at onset	Average	Average	Average	Obese	Obese	Obese

Summary of Six Patients' Histories—Continued

Factor	Bonnie	Miss Arthur	Mr. Benedict	Mrs. Curry	Mrs. Delft	Mrs. Keen
Therapy						
Diet	CHO 150 Protein 90 Fat 120	Diabetic	Low salt Diabetic	Diet 1,200 calories	Controlled by diet	CHO 175 Protein 80 Fat 80
Insulin	38U/NPH	Protamine	NPH	0		Lente insulin 10 U at time of discharge
Tolbutamide	—	—	—	Started with current hospitalization	—	Attempted, unsuccessfully
Exercise		Plays golf and tennis	Drives a car 90 miles a day			
Complications	Acidosis and cystitis	Hypoglycemia	Diabetic retinopathy	Myocardial infarction	Retinopathy Cerebrovascular accident	Cataracts Myocardial ischemia
			Early hypertension	Diabetic retinopathy		
			Nephrosclerosis			
Employment	School	Secretary	Office worker	Housewife	Housewife	Housewife
Responsibilities	Self	Self	2 young children	Husband	Lives with daughter	Lives with daughter

cation of individuals who are predisposed and to the prevention of or delay in the development of the disease.

According to available statistics, the incidence of diabetes mellitus is increasing. In 1900 diabetes mellitus ranked twenty-seventh as a cause of death. In 1957, it was eighth.[2] The total number of persons with diabetes mellitus, that is, the morbidity rate, is not known for certain. If, however, the findings of the study made in Oxford, Massachusetts, apply generally, there are about 3,000,000 persons in the United States with diabetes mellitus. About 2,000,000 are known diabetics, while approximately 1,000,000 are unaware of its presence. These figures are based on the Oxford study in which 70 persons were found to have diabetes. Of these, 40 were known and 30 were unknown diabetics.[3]

In a study reported by Lipkind,[4] screening tests were made on hospital outpatients and blood donors, and 7,164 persons were screened for diabetes. Of these, 1.3 per cent were diagnosed as diabetic. In another program 15,535 persons were screened and 210, or 1.35 per cent were found to be diabetic.[5]

Furthermore, the incidence of diabetes mellitus tends to rise with each decade through the fifth and sixth decades of life, the number of persons who have the disorder can be expected to rise as life expectancy increases. The fact that diabetic children are living to maturity increases the number of diabetics who are alive at one time. Moreover, when they marry and have children, the number of persons carrying the diabetic trait is increased. The incidence is highest in the parts of the world where food is most available and the need for exercise least. In parts of the world where there is little or no medical care and the collection of statistics is in a primitive state, little accurate information is available about the incidence of any disease.

Joslin[6] summarizes the factors contributing to the reported incidence of diabetes mellitus by saying that the frequency is highest where: (1) the average age is highest; (2) women predominate; (3) obesity is most frequent; (4) medical supervision is closest; (5) deaths are most accurately reported; and (6) the proportion of Jews is greatest. Some of these points will be discussed further later.

Despite the increase in the importance of diabetes mellitus as a cause of morbidity and mortality, it is not a modern disease. Nor is the disorder limited to human beings, for it appears in dogs, cats, and cows. The first recorded reference to diabetes mellitus is believed to be in the Papyrus Ebers,

[2] United States National Office of Vital Statistics, "Vital Statistics—Special Reports, National Summaries," L, No. 4, April 7, 1959, Table 1.

[3] H. L. C. Wilkerson and L. P. Krall, "Diabetes in a New England Town," *Journal of the American Medical Association*, CXXXV, September 27, 1947, pp. 209-16.

[4] Jason B. Lipkind, "Evaluation of Continuous Diabetes Screening in a Hospital Outpatient Department," *Public Health Reports*, LXXVIII, June, 1963, pp. 471-76.

[5] Glen W. McDonald, John B. Hozier, Gail F. Fisher, and Arvo B. Ederma, "Large Scale Diabetes Screening Program for Federal Employees," *Public Health Reports*, LXXVIII, July, 1963, pp. 553-60.

[6] *Op. cit.*, pp. 20-54.

which dates back to about 1500 B.C.[7] The first description of the clinical manifestations of diabetes mellitus was by Aertaeus, who described it as a melting of the flesh into the urine. Urine was described in the fifth century by Susruta as honey urine. Some 1,200 years later, Thomas Willis reported that the urine from a patient with diabetes mellitus tasted sweet.

In 1775, Dobson identified the material in urine as sugar. Almost a century later the first reasonably accurate determinations of the quantity of glucose in the blood were made by Claude Bernard. He also discovered glycogen as well as the function of the liver in its storage. In 1869 Langerhans described the islet cells in the pancreas that now bear his name. About 20 years later Von Mehring and Minkowskin demonstrated that diabetes mellitus was induced in a dog by pancreatectomy. Banting and Best, in 1921, isolated insulin from the islet cells in the pancreas, and in 1922 they made insulin available for patients. Because insulin usually corrects the disturbance in carbohydrate metabolism, scientists believed that the nature of diabetes mellitus was understood. This belief was shaken in 1930 when Houssay reported that the severity of diabetes mellitus following pancreatectomy in the dog could be ameliorated by the removal of the anterior pituitary gland. More recently Long and Lukens have demonstrated that the same effect can be produced in the cat by adrenalectomy. Recent studies in the metabolism of fat show that insulin is necessary for the synthesis and storage of fat in fat depots. These and other investigations indicate that the pathological physiology of diabetes mellitus is complex and probably not subject to a simple explanation. After more than ten years of study (1945 to 1955) Sanger and his associates finally clarified the structure of the insulin molecule. It is a polypeptide consisting of two chains joined by three -S-S- (disulfide) bridges. He was able to demonstrate the sequence of amino acids in the molecule, as well as the fact that the sequence of amino acids differs somewhat in different species. Human and whale insulin are most similar to each other, while beef and sheep insulins differ in certain respects. Although these differences do not appear to affect their action as insulin, they do affect the degree to which they are antigenic. Some patients who develop allergic responses to beef or sheep insulin are able to tolerate pig insulin.

How is diabetes mellitus defined?

The oldest definition of diabetes mellitus is based on the observation that certain persons have a disorder characterized by the excretion of an abnormally large volume of urine, that is, polyuria. The term "diabetes," which is derived from the Greek and means to pass through a siphon, was therefore applied to this condition. Mellitus—*mel* is Latin for honey—was added in the eighteenth century by Willis, who discovered that the urine from patients with diabetes mellitus tasted sweet. Based on the current state of knowledge dia-

[7] Ralph H. Major, *Classic Descriptions of Disease*, Charles C Thomas, Springfield, Illinois, 1948, p. 235.

betes mellitus can be defined as a chronic hereditary disorder not only of carbohydrate metabolism but of fat, protein, electrolyte, and water metabolism as well. Authorities generally agree that the metabolic defects result from a relative or absolute lack of insulin. Hypoinsulinism may result from (1) a failure of the beta cells in the islands of Langerhans to secrete sufficient insulin, (2) the reduced effectiveness of insulin, or (3) the increased destruction of insulin by the liver and possibly other tissue.

Historically, failure of the beta cells to secrete sufficient insulin has been given the most attention. Increased destruction is not prominently considered at this time. Considerable evidence is accumulating that in the adult type of diabetes particularly anti-insulin activity of the serum is a major factor. Specific insulin-binding activity may reside in the serum albumin-alpha, alpha$_2$, or gamma globulin fraction. Diabetes may be present while the insulinlike activity of splenic vein blood is normal.[8]

Since the liver and a number of endocrine glands—including the anterior pituitary, the adrenal, and the thyroid—participate in the homeostasis of glucose, they may play a role in the development of diabetes mellitus in some patients. In the past emphasis has been placed on the disturbance in carbohydrate metabolism in diabetes mellitus. There are, however, alterations in protein and fat metabolism as well. There is a possibility that had the disturbance in the capacity to utilize fat been as easily identified as the glucose factor, diabetes would be defined as a disorder of fat metabolism. In the acute form of the disease, the glycosuria and the products of increased protein and fat catabolism are all factors in polyuria. In severe, untreated diabetes mellitus, ketoacidosis, dehydration, coma, and death occur.

The consequences of a deficiency in the supply of insulin can be observed in all systems of the body. The functions of nervous, cardiovascular, respiratory, gastrointestinal, and renal excretory systems are all affected in one or more phases of the disease. In most patients the degree of severity can be modified by adequate treatment. In older obese adults the tendency to ketosis is usually absent, but vascular complications due to atherosclerosis is a common problem. In older patients vascular disorders may precede or follow its development. Juvenile diabetics have a tendency to develop atherosclerosis at an earlier age than nondiabetics. Four of our six patients present evidence of atherosclerosis and other arterial disease. Despite numerous admissions to the hospital for the regulation of her diabetes, Mrs. Keen never was in ketoacidosis. Young lean adults and children are, in contrast to the older obese diabetic, subject to ketoacidosis. Bonnie has been in the hospital on numerous occasions for the treatment of this complication. As a child, Mr. Benedict was in ketoacidosis on several occasions. Except for one episode associated with the clinical onset, Miss Arthur has not developed ketoacidosis. There is some question as to whether or not there are two different types of diabetes mellitus

[8] J. Vallance-Owen, "Insulin Antagonists," *British Medical Bulletin*, XVI, September, 1960, pp. 214-18.

or whether the differences in manifestations represent variations in degree of severity.

What kinds of evidence support the belief that a relative or absolute lack of insulin is responsible for the manifestations observed in diabetes mellitus?

Much of the evidence that diabetes mellitus is due to a deficiency in insulin supply is indirect. Until recently there has been no test by which the level of insulin in the blood could be identified. Much of the evidence has been obtained by experiments on animals and from the observation that severe diabetes mellitus cannot be controlled without insulin. Permanent diabetes mellitus in animals can be induced in a number of ways. These include: (1) the removal of nine tenths or more of the pancreas, (2) the destruction of the beta cells in the islands of Langerhans by a chemical such as Alloxan, (3) the prolonged administration of crude extracts of the anterior pituitary gland or of purified growth hormone, and (4) the prolonged parenteral administration of glucose.

The latter two experimental conditions appear to have a common element: they increase the demand for insulin by causing a persistent elevation in the blood sugar. Since the secretion of insulin is believed to be regulated by the level of glucose in the blood, a continued elevation in blood glucose places a strain on the beta cells in the pancreas. Eventually insulin-secreting cells are exhausted. After animals treated with the growth hormones or prolonged administrations of parenteral glucose die, their beta cells in the pancreas are usually found to have undergone degeneration. At autopsy, some, but not all, diabetics are found to have experienced destruction of the beta or islet cells. Hyperglycemia can be induced temporarily in some persons by the administration of adrenal cortical hormones and by excessive dosages of thyroid hormones. It disappears when these hormones are discontinued.

With what disorders or abnormalities is diabetes mellitus frequently associated?

Diabetes mellitus is induced in persons who are treated by pancreatectomy for the removal of a malignant neoplasm in the pancreas or who have chronic pancreatitis. It also occurs in a high percentage of patients who have hemochromatosis, a disorder of iron metabolism characterized by the deposit of iron in the pancreas and other tissues. Deposits in the skin lead to a characteristic coloring which gives the disorder its name, bronze diabetes. The deposits of iron in the tissues lead to irritation and fibrosis. With destruction of the beta cells in the pancreas, diabetes mellitus ensues. It commonly accompanies Cushing's disease, a disorder in which there is an increase in the secretion of adrenal cortical steroids.

What factors appear to be involved in the development of diabetes mellitus in man?

Two and possibly three factors appear to be important in the development of diabetes mellitus in man. They are heredity, obesity, and possibly hormonal disturbances (other than insulin). The relationship of heredity to diabetes mellitus has been observed since at least the seventh century A.D. Despite evidence that heredity is a factor in diabetes mellitus, it cannot be demonstrated in all persons. Statistics from different clinics indicate that from 20 to 50 per cent of diabetic individuals have a positive family history for diabetes. A number of possible reasons are offered to explain the difficulty in identifying the hereditary factor in some individuals. Since the onset of diabetes may occur at any time during the lifetime of an individual, but is usually after 40 years of age, a child may develop diabetes mellitus before it develops in one of his parents. A potential diabetic may also die from some other cause before diabetes develops. Further, whether or not some individuals develop diabetes appears to depend on the presence of some other predisposing factor, such as obesity. Knowledge of diseases suffered by earlier generations is often limited. Since most authorities state that diabetes is inherited as a mendelian recessive, to develop diabetes one must inherit the trait from both parents. Thus the trait may be carried for a number of generations before it is combined with a like trait in one individual. Some authorities also suggest that more than one gene may be involved. The reader will note that in four of our six patients there is a history of diabetes in the family.

In older individuals, heredity may be a predisposing rather than a direct cause of diabetes mellitus. For it to develop some other conditions placing a strain on the pancreas must be present; one such condition is obesity. The exact role of obesity in the development of diabetes is not understood. Seventy-five to eighty per cent of older diabetics are, however, obese at the time of the onset of the disease. It has recently been suggested that obesity in diabetes is a result of preferential utilization of insulin for fat synthesis and storage; that is, muscle tissue may be unable to utilize insulin owing to certain anti-insulin substances in the serum and its action is concentrated on adipose tissue. Therefore, the diabetic may be obese because he is diabetic, not diabetic because he is obese. Three of the patients in our group, and all of these over 50 years of age at the time of onset, were obese. Some persons gain weight just preceding the onset of diabetes mellitus. In many patients a loss of weight is accompanied by an amelioration of the condition. During periods in history when food is scarce, as in Europe during World War II, the incidence of diabetes tends to fall. In regions of the world where food is scarce, diabetes is infrequent.

Children differ from adults inasmuch as obesity is not a factor in the development of diabetes mellitus. The onset in children frequently occurs during periods of increased linear growth. Despite considerable evidence implicating obesity as a predisposing factor in diabetes mellitus, the nature of the relationship remains uncertain.

A deficiency in the supply of available insulin in relation to the quantity required to prevent hyperglycemia is conceded to be the principal endocrine factor in diabetes mellitus. The possibility exists that disturbances in the functioning of other endocrine glands may in some instances play a significant role in its genesis. To date, proof is lacking that abnormal function of glands such as the adrenal cortex or anterior pituitary causes diabetes mellitus unless the reserve capacity of the beta cells is inadequate. The hormones secreted by the adrenal cortex or anterior pituitary may precipitate diabetes mellitus in persons who have a pre-existing tendency to diabetes mellitus. Evidence to support a possible relationship of other hormones to the development of diabetes mellitus is derived from animal experiments and the observation that persons with acromegaly,[9] Cushing's syndrome,[10] and hyperthyroidism sometimes manifest hyperglycemia and glycosuria. Some persons under treatment with adrenal cortical hormones or adrenocorticotrophin also develop hyperglycemia. Because of their capacity to provoke hyperglycemia and glycosuria in persons who are predisposed to diabetes mellitus, hydrocortisone and cortisone may be employed to identify persons who are in the latent ("prediabetic") stage of the disease.

Animal experiments, such as those previously cited in the review of the development of knowledge of diabetes mellitus, also implicate the anterior pituitary and the adrenal cortex in the pathogenesis of diabetes mellitus. The injection of large dosages of anterior pituitary extracts injures islet cells. Houssay and his co-workers demonstrated that removal of the anterior pituitary decreases the severity of diabetes in the depancreatized animal.[11] Other investigators have demonstrated that the same effect can be produced by adrenalectomy.[12]

Studies such as the ones cited above cannot, of course, be made on human beings. Diseases in which hyperfunction of glands occurs can, however, provide information not otherwise available. With the developments in biochemistry, methods are becoming available whereby the various hormones appearing in blood, urine, and other body fluids can and will be identified.

There are two sources of information about the effects of hormones and glucose metabolism in the living human being. Hormonal changes occurring during pregnancy have a diabetogenic effect.[13] Women who are predisposed to, but have not yet developed, clinical diabetes mellitus may have an abnor-

---

[9] A disorder caused by an eosinophilic adenoma of the anterior pituitary which secretes an excess quantity of the growth hormone.

[10] A disorder characterized by hypersecretion of the glucocorticoids of the adrenal cortex.

[11] Charles H. Best, "Carbohydrate Metabolism," in Charles H. Best and Norman Burke Taylor, *The Physiological Basis of Medical Practice,* 7th ed., Williams & Wilkins Co., Baltimore, 1961, p. 830.

[12] *Ibid.,* p. 829.

[13] White, in Joslin, *Op. cit.,* p. 703.

mal glucose tolerance curve which returns to normal on the termination of the pregnancy. Women who have exceptionally large babies are more likely to develop diabetes at a later date than those whose babies are of average or small size. According to Joslin, 90 per cent of women whose babies weigh 13 lb at birth become diabetic.[14] Most authorities agree that giving birth to a infant weighing more than 9 lb is indicative of latent diabetes. Some believe that the large size of the infant is due to hypersecretion of the growth hormone.

In permanent diabetes the growth hormone can be shown to elevate the blood sugar. It is believed to inhibit the peripheral utilization of glucose and prevent the utilization of insulin by muscle and other tissues.[15] The adrenal steroids promote the formation of glucose (gluconeogenesis) by the liver and may decrease its peripheral utilization.

Other evidence supporting the hypothesis that hormonal imbalance influences the development of diabetes mellitus is that the incidence of the disease rises in women at the time of menopause and continues to be higher in women than in men after the menopause. Before the age of 45 years, the incidence is about equal in men and women.

The mechanisms of action by which hormones other than insulin predispose to the development of diabetes mellitus have not been proved. Several hypotheses have been proposed. They include: (1) the hormone or hormones act in some manner to decrease the secretion of insulin; (2) the hormone or hormones antagonize, inhibit, or block the peripheral action of insulin; and (3) the hormone or hormones act indirectly by producing conditions that increase the demand for insulin.

Although the primary endocrine defect in diabetes mellitus is believed to be a lack of available insulin, this does not preclude the possibility that other hormones play a role in its pathogenesis. As knowledge of the action of hormones is advanced, there is an increasing body of evidence indicating that hormones do not function independently of each other. Instead, the action of a hormone at a given time depends on the presence or absence of other hormones as well as other conditions within the organism. This does not mean that each hormone does not have a principal sphere of activity, but that the action of each hormone is dependent on existing conditions. For example, in animals the growth hormone does not injure islet cells when insulin is administered simultaneously with it.

From time to time reference is made in literature to the hormone glucagon, which has been extracted from the islet cell in the pancreas. When it is injected, it causes a transient elevation in the blood sugar similar to that caused by epinephrine. There is not convincing evidence at this time that it plays a role in the pathogenesis of diabetes mellitus.

Despite the frequency with which the onset of diabetes is coincident with an

14 *Ibid.*, p. 14.
15 Best and Taylor, *Op. cit.*, pp. 832-33.

infection, infection is believed to act as a precipitating rather than an etiological factor. The changes that occur during the infection serve to intensify the disorder so that the clinical manifestations become evident. Changes that increase the insulin requirement, during infection, include an increase in the secretion of adrenal cortical steroids in response to stress and an increase in the rate of metabolism as a result of fever. Fever also predisposes to dehydration and acidosis, which also tends to aggravate the diabetic state.

Vallance-Owen[16] of England has demonstrated an anti-insulin factor in the albumin-alpha 1 globulin fraction of the serum proteins which rises with acute infection and may be responsible for increased insulin resistance at this time. However, other studies indicate that this factor may be a degradation product of the insulin molecule itself, and the whole significance is not yet clear.

Diabetes mellitus also increases susceptibility to certain types of infections, particularly those of the skin. In preinsulin days carbuncles and furuncles were frequent and difficult to cure. Once they developed, the diabetic state was intensified and with it the resistance of the skin to infection was further diminished. As a student in nursing, the author once cared for an elderly man, Mr. Samuel, who had a huge carbuncle involving the entire back of his neck. Until his diabetes was brought under control, the infection continued to spread. After the adequate treatment of the diabetes mellitus was instituted, the area healed rapidly. The control of the infectious process also had a beneficial effect on his diabetes. As the carbuncle healed, his insulin requirement dropped. Another patient, Miss Murphy, was treated for furuncles (boils) for over a year. When her urine was finally tested for sugar, she was found to have glycosuria. With the control of her diabetes, her boils healed. The behavior of Mr. Samuel and Miss Murphy was in no way unusual. Infection has an adverse effect on diabetes mellitus, and diabetes mellitus increases the difficulty of controlling certain types of infections.

The fact that diabetes mellitus appears to be more common among certain groups of people than others merits some comment. The incidence is higher among those who live in urban areas than those who live in rural areas. This is probably due to the fact that, in the past at least, persons living in urban areas are more sedentary than those living in rural areas. It is recognized that exercise decreases the demand for insulin. The possibility also exists that persons living in urban areas are more likely to have adequate medical care available. The quality of medical care may also be better, and a higher *apparent* incidence of diabetes may be shown.

Most authorities emphasize that the incidence of diabetes mellitus is higher among Jews than among non-Jews. Joslin attributes this finding to the high incidence of obesity among Jewish people.[17] Cohen[18] challenges the belief

---

[16] *Op. cit.*, pp. 214-18.
[17] Joslin, *Op. cit.*, p. 67.
[18] A. M. Cohen, "Prevalence of Diabetes Among Different Ethnic Jewish Groups in Israel," *Metabolism, Clinical and Experimental*, X, 1961, pp. 50-57.

that the incidence is higher among Jews than non-Jews. He suggests that it is based on data collected in clinics patronized by a disproportionate number of Jewish people. In the study of the incidence of diabetes mellitus in Israel, Cohen found the incidence to be similar to that of people living in other countries. He also discovered that the Yemenites and Kurds, who traditionally have a very low incidence of diabetes mellitus, became diabetic at about the same rate as other Israelis when they adapted Western habits—food as well as habits of living and working.

To recapitulate, the manifestations of diabetes mellitus result from a relative or absolute lack of insulin. Some of the possible causes for this deficiency have been suggested. Heredity, obesity, and hormonal factors have been observed to be associated with the development of diabetes mellitus. What the role of each of these factors is in the genesis of diabetes mellitus is still in some doubt. The combination of optimum age, obesity, and hereditary tendency may be sufficient to induce diabetes mellitus. The tendency to develop the disease may be further increased by such factors as a strenuous life, dietary excesses, and too little exercise.

What theories have been advanced to explain the pathophysiology of diabetes mellitus?

Though progress has been made in understanding the nature of the metabolic disturbances in diabetes mellitus, much remains to be learned. A number of hypotheses have been proposed to explain the pathological physiology of the disorder. Two that are frequently mentioned in literature are the underutilization and the overproduction theories. The underutilization theory emphasizes that hyperglycemia results because of a suppression in the peripheral (muscle) use of glucose. According to the overproduction theory, hyperglycemia results from the excessive formation of glucose from nonglucose sources, that is, by gluconeogenesis. Recent evidence indicates that both factors probably are involved. Because the abnormal is presumably easier to understand when the normal is understood, the reader may wish to reexamine the features of energy metabolism in Chapter 10. A brief review of glucose metabolism is included here. As defined earlier, energy metabolism is a process whereby the energy stored in food is gradually liberated by a series of stepwise chemical reactions for use in cells or is converted to a form in which it can be stored for future use.

Since glucose is not chemically a very active substance, it must be activated before it can be used at body temperature. Glucose is converted into the chemically active glucose-6-phosphate. This reaction requires the presence of the enzyme hexokinase and is the first step in the utilization of glucose, regardless of whether the glucose is converted to glycogen, utilized as energy, or converted to fat and stored. The entrance of significant quantities of glucose into the cell also requires a transport mechanism. Once glucose enters the cell and is converted to glucose-6-phosphate, the cell is protected against too much energy at one time by the stepwise release of energy. Further different pathways are available in the utilization of glucose and many chemical reactions in the utilization of glucose are reversible. Not only is energy liberated and utilized, but it is fixed as chemically useful energy and stored in the form of high-energy bonds such as the high-energy phosphate bonds.

A number of conditions must be met for energy metabolism to proceed normally. In the first place appropriate metabolites in the proper form must be present. Some of these are supplied from exogenous as well as endogenous sources, and they must enter the cell at an appropriate rate, neither too slowly, nor too rapidly. For example, at least 100 gm of glucose must be metabolized daily to prevent the utilization of fat at an excessively rapid rate. Most of this comes from outside sources as the quantity of glycogen stored in the liver is sufficient to supply the glucose needed for about five hours. Some chemical reactions depend on the presence of certain metabolites which are formed during metabolism to provide the energy required for the reaction. For example, the transfer of glucose into cells and its conversion into glucose-6-phosphate requires the presence of high-energy adenosinetriphosphate. In some chemical reactions a metabolite necessary to spark the reaction is released or regenerated at the end of the reaction so that it is again available. For example, oxaloacetic acid is required at the beginning of the Krebs cycle to start the oxidation of acetic acid. It is regenerated at the end of the reaction.

In addition to the availability of appropriate metabolites at varying stages of metabolism, enzymes and coenzymes are required to catalyze the various chemical reactions involved in the release or storage of energy. Some of these are synthesized by the cells while others, such as thiamine, must be ingested in the diet.

A third factor in metabolism in multicellular organisms is the regulation of various phases of metabolism by hormones. There is a considerable body of knowledge of the effects of the action of hormones. This has been derived from observation of persons suffering from a deficiency or excess of one or more hormones and from animal and tissue culture experiments. Little is known of their mode of action. One or more of the following are possible: (1) enhancing the rate at which metabolites are transported through the cell membrane; (2) accelerating the speed of a chemical reaction—one step; and (3) influencing the direction or pathway taken in the metabolism of a metabolite. Whatever the mechanism of action of hormones, tissue culture studies demonstrate that hormones are not required for energy metabolism within cells. Moreover, animals from whom endocrine glands have been removed continue to survive provided they are carefully protected from changes in their environment. Hormones apparently act to enable the organism to adapt to its environment, but how they do this awaits further understanding of cellular activity.

Although the metabolism of glucose is discussed in some detail in Chapter 10, some of the factors that play a role in the homeostasis of glucose are presented below. An understanding of the pathophysiology of diabetes mellitus as well as of metabolic acidosis depends on this knowledge.

The fact that the regulation of the level of glucose in the blood is complex should not be surprising. Some tissues such as the brain utilize only glucose in metabolism and they are as dependent on glucose as they are on oxygen. As in other homeostatic conditions, the level of glucose in the blood depends on the relationship of supply to use, excretion, and storage. These factors can be summarized briefly as those tending to elevate the level of glucose in the blood balanced against those tending to lower its level. If equilibrium is to be maintained, any disturbance in the level of glucose in the blood must be counteracted by one or more mechanisms tending to restore the level of glucose to predisturbance levels.

What are the factors tending to elevate the level of glucose in the blood?

In the regulation of the level of glucose in the blood, certain cells recognize the need of the organism for glucose. When this need is sufficiently great, it is translated into the sensation hunger. Hunger motivates the individual to search for, find, and ingest food. There are three sources or routes by which glucose enters into the blood. The usual route of entry is by absorption from the alimentary canal. A second and much less common route is by parenteral injection as by intravenous infusion. Parental injection is usually reserved for patients who are unable to ingest food into or absorb it from the alimentary tract. A third route of entry is the secretion of glucose by the liver. In time of need, the liver can maintain the level of glucose in the blood within normal limits, despite the absence of food intake. Although the liver is able to do this in the absence of hormonal factors, the rate at which glucose is secreted into the hepatic vein by the liver is modified by hormones.

The process by which the liver converts glycogen to glucose and secretes it into the hepatic vein is known as glycogenolysis. This is a rapid reaction occurring in a matter of minutes. The rapid conversion of glycogen to glucose is adapted to protect the individual in emergency situations against a drop in blood glucose. Since the total quantity of glycogen in the liver is limited (a 1,500-gm liver probably contains no more than 60 gm of glucose), glycogen cannot be expected to protect the level of glucose in the blood for more than a brief period of time.[19] The process is regulated by epinephrine and possibly glucagon.

Glucose is also formed in the liver by a process known as gluconeogenesis. As the term implies, new glucose is created or formed from noncarbohydrate sources. In gluconeogenesis the liver converts amino acids after they have

[19] Jay Tepperman, *Metabolic and Endocrine Physiology,* Yearbook Medical Publishers, Inc., Chicago, 1962, p. 151.

been deaminized (NH_2 removed) to glucose. The source of the amino acids is the muscles of the body. Gluconeogenesis differs from glycogenolysis in two respects. Rather than being a rapid and brief source of glucose to the blood, it is a slow and sustained reaction. It protects the level of glucose in the blood in disorders in which the supply of glucose is deficient or loss is excessive. Thus the level of glucose in the blood is maintained in starvation, despite a failure in the supply from exogenous sources. It is also maintained in disorders of the kidney in which excessive quantities of glucose are lost in the urine.

Whereas the rate of glycogenolysis is regulated by epinephrine and glucagon, the rate of gluconeogenesis is regulated by the adrenal glucocorticoids (Cortisol or hydrocortisone). The exact mechanism by which the adrenal steroids regulate the conversion of amino acids to glucose is not known. According to Tepperman,[20] the adrenal steroids are believed to "permit" the anabolism-catabolism equilibrium to be tipped in the direction of protein breakdown. The adrenal steroids may also facilitate the conversion of amino acids to glycogen in the liver.

In addition to protecting the level of glucose in the blood by making more glucose available to the blood, reduction in the utilization of glucose by peripheral tissues may also be a factor in the maintenance of the blood glucose. In starvation, tissues adapt in such a manner that they utilize less glucose than when the glucose supply is adequate. One factor in adaptation to starvation is a drop in total metabolism. On the basis of tissue culture experiments it is postulated that the muscles of starving animals utilize relatively more fatty acids than glucose.[21]

Similar to other aspects of glucose metabolism, hormones are believed to regulate the processes involved in blocking the peripheral use of glucose. These hormones, which are often called insulin antagonists, are the growth hormone (anterior pituitary) and the adrenal glucocorticoids. The nature of the action of these hormones in blocking peripheral glucose oxidation is not known.

One factor that may possibly contribute to the elevation of glucose in the blood is an increase in the rate of destruction of insulin. A number of tissues, especially the liver, have been demonstrated to inactivate insulin. The insulin-destroying mechanism in the liver has been referred to as insulinase, but the nature of the system has not been firmly established.

Another factor influencing the level of glucose in the blood is the state of hydration of the patient. In severe dehydration, the level of glucose in the blood tends to rise. Dehydration is one factor in the marked rise in the level of glucose in the blood of acidotic patients.

What forces act to lower the level of glucose in the blood?

A variety of factors contribute to the lowering of glucose in the blood. Just as the sensation hunger motivates food-seeking behavior, satiety (satisfac-

[20] *Ibid.,* p. 151.
[21] *Ibid.,* p. 152.

tion) tends to depress it. The normal response to satiety is to cease ingesting food or to decrease the supply of exogenous glucose. After absorption, glucose is distributed through the body water, thereby reducing its concentration in any compartment, including that of the blood. A third mechanism for lowering the blood glucose is exercise. Exactly how exercise affects the level of glucose in the blood is not well known. It is valuable in the treatment of diabetes mellitus, because it lowers the blood sugar independently of the effect of insulin.

Although a number of hormones regulate the mechanisms involved in elevating the level of glucose in the blood, the only hormone known to lower the blood glucose is insulin. The secretion of insulin is believed to be regulated by the level of glucose in the blood. A rise in the blood glucose acts as a stimulus to secretion of insulin, while a fall inhibits it. Similar to other regulatory mechanisms when the amount of glucose ingested at one time is in great excess, the quantity of insulin secreted may be greater than that required to lower the blood glucose to an appropriate degree. As a consequence the blood glucose may fall below the base line established earlier.

How does insulin act to remove glucose from the blood?

Insulin promotes the removal of glucose from the blood by three principal effects. It facilitates the conversion of glucose to fat (lipogenesis) in adipose tissue and the liver. It speeds the conversion of glucose to glycogen, especially in the muscles, and the oxidation of glucose in insulin-sensitive tissues. In the absence of insulin all these processes are depressed to some extent. Some of the theories advanced to explain the actions of insulin follow. Though the mechanism(s) by which insulin acts are not known, three modes of action have been suggested. The most generally accepted mechanism of action at this time is that insulin facilitates the transport of glucose across the cell membrane. How this is accomplished is not known. Whether insulin increases the permeability of the cell membrane to glucose or acts on the chemical or enzymatic mechanisms for the transfer of glucose into the cells remains to be proved. The rate at which a metabolite enters cells is important, as too rapid a rate of entry may cause the cell to be overloaded with it. The too slow entry of the metabolite will cause the cell to be "starved" for it.

The second and older theory for which there is some support is that insulin acts in some way to promote the phosphorylation of glucose. One theory proposed to explain the action of insulin on phosphorylation is that insulin antagonizes the inhibiting effect of the growth hormone on hexokinase, and the adrenal glucocorticoid hormones intensify the effect of the anterior pituitary hormones. Some authorities have suggested that the pituitary and adrenal cortical hormones antagonize the action of insulin by increasing glucose formation from fat and protein, that is, by gluconeogenesis.

A third theory suggests that insulin acts by increasing the efficiency with which the cell forms adenosinetriphosphate. An adequate supply of this high-energy substance is necessary for glucose to be entered into the metabolic pathway. It should be clear that these and other theories are not mutually exclusive. Some authorities suggest that insulin may act at more than one point in the transport and utilization of glucose.

The maintenance of the level of glucose in the blood results from a balance between the forces tending to raise and to lower it. As with other homeostatic conditions, the forces influencing blood glucose in health are in dynamic equilibrium. When there is a shift in one direction, mechanisms are initiated to counteract the change and to restore the blood glucose to normal. If the disturbance has been great, the correcting mechanism tends to overshoot the mark before equilibrium is attained. From the above, it should be clear that the regulation of the blood glucose is highly complex. Disorders resulting in an elevation in the level of glucose in the blood may result from a disproportionate increase in the activity of mechanisms for elevating the blood glucose or from a failure in the mechanisms regulating the lowering of it.

Explain the pathophysiology of diabetes mellitus.

In light of present-day knowledge, diabetes mellitus appears to be due to an absolute or relative lack of insulin and the effects of insulin deficiency on carbohydrate and fat metabolism. As in other disorders of function, some of the manifestations in diabetes mellitus are due to the effects of the disorder and some are due to the response of the organism to biochemical and physiological changes.

In what respects is the adaptation of metabolism in the cells in starvation similar to the pathophysiological changes in diabetes mellitus?

Some understanding of the pathophysiological changes in diabetes mellitus can be gained by reviewing the adaptation of the cells to starvation. Among the important differences, however, is the fact that the alterations occurring in starvation have survival value, inasmuch as they protect the cells against a deficient food supply. In contrast, in diabetes mellitus, because these changes are too intense, they predispose to harm the individual rather than to protect. In starvation as well as in diabetes, the individual cells substitute fat for glucose as fuel. The first change initiating acidosis is a decrease in the utilization of glucose by the peripheral tissues, accompanied by a mobilization of stored (depot) fat in the form of free fatty acids. They are also known as non- or unesterfied fatty acids.[22]

Besides the mobilization of fatty acids, the rate of breakdown of tissue proteins is intensified. The resulting amino acids are deaminated in the liver

[22] An ester is formed by the combination of an alcohol with an acid. In the process, water as well as the ester is formed.

and converted into glucose (gluconeogenesis). In starvation there is usually some ketonemia (elevation of ketone bodies in the blood) and ketonuria (excretion of ketone bodies in the urine). When the supply of food is inadequate, the shift from glucose to fat metabolism has survival value. It enables the individual to adapt to an insufficient supply of exogenous glucose. Adaptation is further supported by a lessening in the rate at which cells utilize glucose.

In the instance of Bonnie as well as among other diabetics, the failure in glucose utilization stems not from a lack of supply of glucose, but from a relative or absolute lack of insulin required for the utilization of glucose. Many older diabetics who were obese at the onset of their disease presumably utilize sufficient glucose, so that there is not an excessively rapid mobilization of fat. They are not predisposed to acidosis. In young and lean adults with a severe form of the disease, metabolic acidosis is a continuing possibility. Acidosis occurs when some event upsets the balance between the quantity of insulin required and that available. Although we do not know what the precipitating event was in the instance of Bonnie, she may have omitted her insulin. If this was the case, acidosis may have been precipitated by an absolute lack of insulin. If, as is more likely, some sudden and unexpected stress increased her insulin requirement, her insulin deficiency was relative rather than absolute. She had enough insulin to meet her usual requirements, but not enough to cover the emergency. Among the common precipitating causes of acidosis are infection, physical trauma, and emotional stress. A not infrequent event associated with the onset of acidosis in Bonnie was nausea and vomiting. It was not known whether the nausea and vomiting were associated with an acute gastrointestinal disorder or with the onset of acidosis. With their advent, she failed to ingest either food or fluids. Thus Bonnie was deprived of a supply of exogenous glucose.

Although the factors contributing to the development of acidosis in Bonnie are not known with certainty, they include the possibility of one or more of the above, that is, (1) failure to take her insulin, (2) some disturbance increasing her insulin requirements, and (3) abstinence from food and fluids as a consequence of nausea and vomiting. From Bonnie's history, her diabetes can be presumed not to have been maintained under very good control. As a 15-year-old, emotional stress arising from her relationships with her parents, teachers, or peers as well as how she felt about herself and the fact of having diabetes mellitus may have contributed to an increased need for insulin.

As a consequence of insulin deficiency, utilization of glucose by the cells is diminished, as in starvation, and the conversion of glycogen in the liver to glucose (glycogenolysis) is increased. Since the quantity of glycogen stored in the liver is small, it serves only as a temporary source of glucose. Though slower to be effected, a more sustained source of glucose is the formation in the liver of glucose from deaminated amino acids (gluconeogenesis). Since there is an imbalance between the factors tending to elevate the blood glucose and those tending to lower it in favor of those tending to elevate it, the blood glucose rises. The elevation in the blood glucose partly compensates for the lack of insulin inasmuch as it makes more glucose available to the cell.[23] With an elevation in the concentration of glucose in the blood, more glucose is available to, and is presumed to enter, the cell. Theoretically, a sufficient elevation in the blood glucose should make enough glucose available to supply required energy. Elevation of the blood sugar is in part limited by the renal threshold.[24]

Loss of glucose in the urine has several undesirable effects. First, it is wasteful, and unless food intake is increased in proportion to loss, it will be associated with a loss in body weight and strength. Second, glucose is osmotically active. It holds water in the urine and thereby causes polyuria. With polyuria, not only water but electrolytes such as potassium and sodium are lost. Thirst and an increase in fluid intake prevent dehydration, unless and until the individual develops nausea and vomiting. With dehydration, the blood becomes concentrated and blood volume falls; blood pressure drops and circulation to the tissues fails. In the kidney, failure of blood flow results in anuria and eventually leads to coma and death. As circulation to the tissues fails, generalized tissue anoxia causes a shift to anaerobic metabolism. Lactic acid appears in increasing concentrations in the blood and reflects an elevation of the hydrogen ions in the cell. Unless the condition is corrected by improving the supply of oxygen to the cells, death ensues. The sequence of events resulting from the effects of a lack of insulin on carbohydrate metabolism is diagrammed in Figure 17-1-A.

Early presenting signs of diabetes mellitus are hyperglycemia and glycosuria. Symptoms, in some instances also signs, are thirst (polydipsia), increased urine output (polyuria), and increased appetite (polyphagia), often with weight loss and weakness. The effects of a decrease in the use of glucose are due to (1) loss of calories and (2) the effects of the loss of water and electrolytes on the capacity of the individual to maintain the circulation.

The deficiency of insulin and diminution in the use of glucose have important effects on the capacity of the individual to synthesize, store, and maintain storage depots of fat. With a lack of insulin and failure to utilize normal amounts of glucose, large quantities of fat are mobilized from fat stores and are poured into the blood in the form of fatty acids. In the severely ill patient, such as Bonnie and Miss Arthur, fat may be mobilized from fat tissue.

The liver is inundated with fat, most of which it metabolizes only to the acetyl CoA stage. The two carbon atom fragments unite to form acetoacetic acid (diacetic acid and beta hydroxybutyric acid), and an accumulation of

---

[23] The effects of the raising of the blood glucose are an example in a living system of the law of mass action; that is, the speed of a chemical reaction is proportional to the molecular concentration of the reacting substances in a solution.

[24] The normal renal threshold is about 160 to 180 mg of glucose per 100 ml of blood. In patients who have longstanding diabetes mellitus the renal threshold is usually elevated, occasionally markedly.

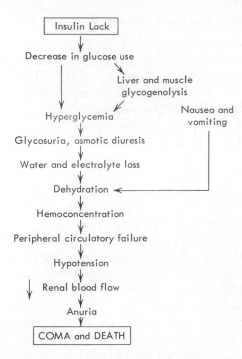

Insulin Lack

Decrease in glucose use

Liver and muscle
glycogenolysis

Hyperglycemia

Nausea and
vomiting

Glycosuria, asmotic diuresis

Water and electrolyte loss

Dehydration

Hemoconcentration

Peripheral circulatory failure

Hypotension

Renal blood flow

Anuria

COMA and DEATH

FIGURE 17—1-A. The effect of insulin lack on carbohydrate metabolism. (Adapted, with permission, from Jay Tepperman, *Metabolic and Endocrine Physiology*, Year Book Medical Publishers Inc., Chicago, 1962, Fig. 47, p. 154.)

these acids in the blood results in metabolic acidosis, one of the characteristic features of which is Kussmaul breathing (deep and rapid breathing). In addition, as the production of ketoacids exceeds the capacity of the kidney to reabsorb them, they are excreted in the urine, and in the process of excretion they take cations such as sodium and potassium with them. Since electrolytes are osmotically active, they also require water for their excretion. With the loss of sodium ions, the total quantity of sodium in the body is diminished, and with the decrease, the water-holding power of extracellular fluid is also reduced. With a loss of sodium, the total volume of water in the extracellular

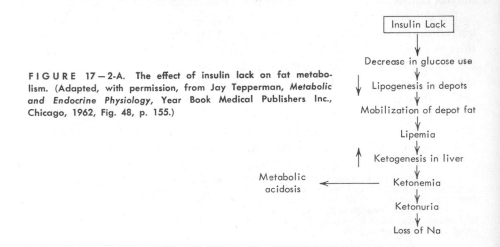

FIGURE 17—2-A. The effect of insulin lack on fat metabolism. (Adapted, with permission, from Jay Tepperman, *Metabolic and Endocrine Physiology*, Year Book Medical Publishers Inc., Chicago, 1962, Fig. 48, p. 155.)

Insulin Lack

Decrease in glucose use

Lipogenesis in depots

Mobilization of depot fat

Lipemia

Ketogenesis in liver

Metabolic
acidosis

Ketonemia

Ketonuria

Loss of Na

fluid falls. Blood volume drops and predisposes to peripheral circulatory failure. The effects of a deficiency of insulin on fat metabolism are summarized in Figure 17-2-A.

Not only does a lack of insulin impair the use of glucose and fat, but it also affects protein metabolism. With a deficiency in the supply of insulin, protein synthesis, especially in muscles, is lessened and protein catabolism exceeds

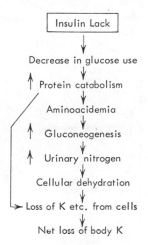

Insulin Lack

↓

Decrease in glucose use

↓

↑ Protein catabolism

↓

Aminoacidemia

↓

↑ Gluconeogenesis

↓

↑ Urinary nitrogen

↓

Cellular dehydration

↓

→ Loss of K etc. from cells

↓

Net loss of body K

FIGURE 17—3-A. The effect of insulin lack on protein. (Adapted, with permission, from Jay Tepperman, *Metabolic and Endocrine Physiology*, Year Book Medical Publishers Inc., Chicago, 1962.)

protein anabolism. The amino acids released as a result are deaminated in the liver, the NH_2 fragment is removed, and the carbon-containing residues are converted to glucose or fatty acid. Protein catabolism results in a loss of nitrogen and potassium from the body and thereby contributes to dehydration and its associated effects.

From the foregoing discussion, it should be obvious that despite the direct relationship of insulin to carbohydrate metabolism, insulin also influences the manner in which fat and protein are metabolized. Adequate supplies of insulin facilitate the use of glucose and favor synthesis and storage of fat. Inadequate insulin is accompanied by impaired use of glucose and, as a result, mobilization of fatty acids, in some instances triglycerides, and amino acids. As a consequence, nutrition of the cells is reduced, water and electrolytes are lost, and, unless these deficits are corrected, circulation to the tissues is threatened.

How is the presence of diabetes mellitus established?

Because hyperglycemia is accompanied by glycosuria, diabetes mellitus is one of the easiest of diseases to detect. The finding of glucose in the urine is presumptive but not conclusive evidence that a person has diabetes mellitus as glycosuria can be present in a person who is nondiabetic. Glycosuria occurring after the excessive ingestion of carbohydrates is known as alimentary glycosuria. The person who has this form of glycosuria may well be prediabetic. Glycosuria also occurs in persons who have a low renal threshold for

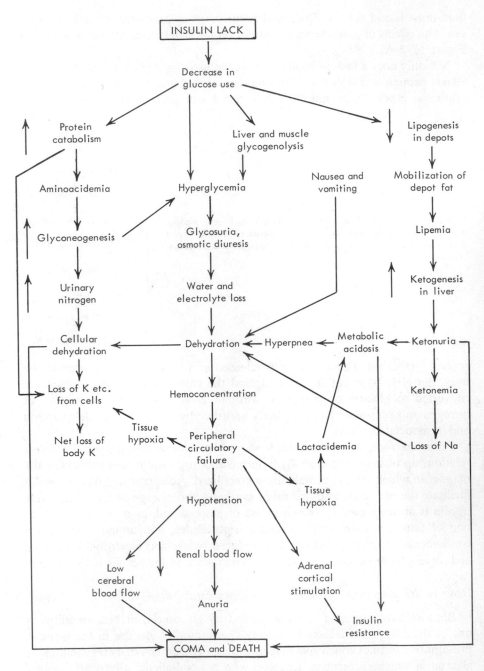

FIGURE 17—4-A. Composite summary of the pathophysiology of diabetic acidosis. Note particularly connections among the three general areas of metabolism. (Adapted, with permission, from Jay Tepperman, *Metabolic and Endocrine Physiology,* Year Book Medical Publishers Inc., Chicago, 1962.)

glucose. The most frequent cause is, however, diabetes mellitus. The presence of reducing substances in the urine (mellituria) can also be associated with lactation (lactose lactosuria) and rare "metabolic errors" (pentosuria, fructosuria, etc.). These substances will give a positive reaction with Benedict's solution and commonly used testing agents (Clinitest®), but can be differentiated by test strips containing glucose oxidase (Testape®, Clinistix®). Glycosuria plus ketonuria is almost pathognomonic of diabetes mellitus. The diagnosis of diabetes mellitus is established by the presence of hyperglycemia in a person who is fasting or who cannot adapt at a normal rate to the stress produced by the ingestion of 100 gm of glucose.

In many patients the diagnosis of diabetes mellitus is not established until the patient develops a complication. In some persons the disorder is discovered when they visit their physician for a medical examination. Other cases are discovered because an alert nurse encourages a patient with symptoms suggesting diabetes mellitus to seek medical attention. Still others are identified during community screening programs. These programs are usually sponsored by the American Diabetes Association through its local branches and the county medical society. Each fall these groups sponsor a Diabetic Detection Week. During the week materials are made available through the local pharmacies so that individuals can test their urine for glucose. An educational program is carried on at the same time to encourage individuals to avail themselves of this opportunity. The program is publicized by the various communication media. On specified days materials for testing urine are made available by the local pharmacies. Persons found to have glycosuria are referred to their physicians for diagnosis and, if need be, treatment.

Nurses have a number of opportunities to assist in the identification of persons who have diabetes mellitus. The suspicion of the school nurse should be aroused when a child develops polyuria and polydipsia. The public health nurse who visits in the home should be alert to the possibility of diabetes in family members. Recently a visiting nurse who was making a call to a mother with a new baby inquired about other members of the family. She learned that five-year-old Suzie was unusually irritable and that she was constantly "passing water," that she drank an unusual amount of water and was constantly hungry. The nurse obtained and tested a sample of urine. When she found that it was highly positive for glucose and acetone, she informed the mother that the child should see a physician as soon as possible. An appointment was made with the family physician, who examined Suzie and confirmed the fact that she had diabetes mellitus.

Some patients are discovered to have diabetes after they are admitted to the hospital. Most hospitals have a rule that before a patient can undergo any type of surgical procedure, his urine must be checked for glucose. In two instances known to the author, a nurse noted on the morning of surgery that the urine of a patient had not been checked for sugar. On testing the urine, it was found to contain glucose. In both instances surgery was delayed until the patient's diabetes was brought under control.

In addition to opportunities for the nurse to participate in programs for the identification of persons who have diabetes mellitus, nurses have a role in the prevention of the disease. Because of the hereditary predisposition to diabetes mellitus, persons with diabetes are advised not to marry other diabetics or into families with a known history of the disease. Because of the frequency with which diabetes in the middle-aged person is associated with obesity, individuals are encouraged to avoid overweight by diet and exercise. About 10 per cent under the average weight is usually advocated for those over 30 years of age.

What are some of the factors influencing the nature of the onset of diabetes mellitus?

In the young, the onset of diabetes mellitus is likely to be rapid and acute, while in the middle-aged, obese adult, it is often slow. Among the latter, diabetes may be present for some time before the individual becomes aware of its manifestations. One estimate is that the middle-aged, obese adult is diabetic for about as many years before the disease is discovered as he survives after the diagnosis is made. Often, though not invariably, onset is precipitated by some physical or emotional stress.

The six patients whose histories are summarized on pages 1278-79 illustrate the classical types of onset. In Bonnie, Miss Arthur, and Mr. Benedict, all of whom developed diabetes mellitus as children, onset was rapid. Although each of them had manifested polyuria, polydipsia, and polyphagia for an indefinite period, diagnosis was not established until they developed ketoacidosis. In retrospect Mrs. Arthur remembered that Miss Arthur had been eating very well, but she attributed Miss Arthur's appetite to the fact that her daughter was growing.

Among the three older diabetics, Mrs. Delft and Mrs. Curry were discovered to be diabetic when they sought medical attention for complications of diabetes mellitus. Mrs. Curry had blurring of vision from retinopathy. Mrs. Delft also had blurring of vision as well as dizziness, and weakness on one side of her body. Mrs. Keen sought medical attention after observing that some urine which she had spilled left a shiny residue on drying.

In summary, in the young the onset is often more rapid and acute than in the mature, obese adult. Unless signs and symptoms are discovered early, acidosis is precipitated by some stress such as a respiratory infection which intervenes and the individual becomes acutely ill. In the middle-aged, obese adult onset is likely to be less acute. Diagnosis follows the discovery of glucose in the urine on a routine physical examination, or in association with an infection, or after a person seeks medical attention for the diagnosis and treatment of a related or unrelated disorder.

From the nature of the onset, the signs and symptoms manifested by patients at the time of diagnosis vary greatly. Not all adult patients are aware of any symptoms characteristic of diabetes mellitus. Discovery of glycosuria leads to an examination of the blood and the finding of hyperglycemia. Glycosuria is often, but not always, accompanied by polyuria, polydipsia, and polyphagia.

In women patients, glycosuria is frequently associated with pruritus—itching—of the vulva. The glucose in the urine may irritate the skin as it dries. It also serves as an excellent medium for the growth of *Monilia*. Excoriation of the skin from scratching provides sites for the entrance of microorganisms. Prevention and relief of pruritus depend on the elimination of glucose from the urine by controlling the diabetes. Scrupulous cleanliness is also imperative.

Another result of glycosuria and the other metabolic disturbances in diabetes is loss of weight and strength. In some patients, polyphagia is sufficient to compensate for the glucose lost in the urine. In severe forms of the disease, as much as a pound of glucose may be lost each day into the urine. In terms of calories the person loses 4 calories with each gram of glucose excreted in the urine and as many as 2,000 calories may be lost each day by a person with severe diabetes. Mrs. Keen had enough glucose in her urine for it to be seen after the water evaporated. In the severe diabetic, weight loss is inevitable unless the disease is brought under control. When weight loss is accompanied by a loss of tissue proteins, weakness is to be expected. In the preinsulin days, loss of weight in the severe diabetic was often extreme and patients experienced marked weakness. Young emaciated diabetics are pictured as supporting themselves by leaning on a wall as they walk. According to Duncan,[25] weakness is the most common complaint presented by his patients. Weakness and weight loss are not specific to diabetes mellitus, as they occur in any debilitating disease. Impotence is not infrequent in males.

To reiterate, not all adult patients have symptoms when they are found on medical examination to have diabetes mellitus. The chemical changes that are pathognomonic of the disease are hyperglycemia and glycosuria. With glycosuria, osmotic diuresis occurs and the patient becomes aware of voiding frequently in large amounts. Polyuria is followed by polydipsia and polyphagia. In women pruritus of the vulva is also associated with glycosuria. When the hyperglycemia is insufficient to compensate for the inefficient glucose metabolism, fat and protein catabolism are increased which leads to an increase in the ketone bodies in the blood serum and urine. Despite increased appetite, loss of weight and strength occurs. Unless the diabetic condition is corrected, the individual with severe diabetes will go on to dehydration and possibly to peripheral vascular failure and death.

As stated earlier, patients frequently do not seek medical attention until

[25] Garfield G. Duncan, *Diseases of Metabolism*, 4th ed., W. B. Saunders Company, Philadelphia, 1959, p. 780.

they develop a complication. Mrs. Curry was not aware of any symptoms of diabetes until she developed blurring of vision resulting from diabetic retinopathy. In contrast, Mrs. Keen sought medical attention because she had marked glycosuria. Infection, by intensifying the diabetes, is sometimes the event that brings the patient to the physician.

Most of the complications resulting from diabetes mellitus were present in one or more of our six patients. They include hypoglycemia and acidosis, both of which require prompt and intensive treatment, and many of the disorders associated with longstanding diabetes mellitus. These include nephrosclerosis, diabetic retinopathy, cataracts, and atherosclerosis. None of our patients had tuberculosis, which occurs more frequently among diabetics than among nondiabetics.

Although not all patients experience it, hypoglycemia is an ever-present possibility in the patient who takes insulin. Situations which predispose to hypoglycemia, or, as it is commonly called, insulin reaction, include a delay in or omission of a meal, an increase in the amount of exercise taken, or an improvement in the patient's glucose tolerance. An error in the measurement of insulin, resulting in excess dosage, can also be responsible. The manifestations of hypoglycemia have been listed and discussed in Chapter 10. Hypoglycemia, particularly when severe or repeated, is generally regarded as a serious condition. Many of the signs and symptoms are the result of the effect on the brain of lowering of the blood sugar. A marked fall in the blood sugar may be accompanied by unconsciousness. Severe and repeated periods of hypoglycemia may cause permanent damage to the brain. Miss Arthur was unconscious at the time of her admission. She could not explain why she had developed hypoglycemia as she said that she had neither delayed eating nor taken more than her usual amount of exercise. The principal change in her life was that she had taken a new position a week previously. Emotional stress may be reflected in a change in the blood glucose, usually in the direction of an elevation. Possibly Miss Arthur experienced an elevation in the level of glucose and she increased her insulin dosage. She was embarrassed by her condition as she took pride in keeping her diabetes under control; she was also worried lest she lose her new position.

Bonnie had two mild attacks of hypoglycemia as her diabetes was brought under control. She felt nervous and perspired profusely. Both patients recovered promptly following the administration of glucose. Because Miss Arthur was unconscious, she was given 100 ml of 10 per cent glucose by intravenous infusion. Patients who are unconscious should never be given fluids by mouth. Bonnie was given 2 teaspoonfuls of corn syrup dissolved in half a glass of water. Suitable substitutes include 100 ml of orange juice or a lump or two of sugar. Patients should be instructed to treat the first indications of hypoglycemia without delay. When patients are hospitalized, they should be encouraged to report suspicious symptoms. There should be no delay in treatment. In some hospitals the method to be used in the treatment of hypoglycemia is included in the standing orders. In others individual physicians leave a prescription or ask to be called. Whatever the practice, there should be no unnecessary delay in instituting effective therapy. Furthermore, should the nurse be in a position where there is some doubt as to whether the patient is hypoglycemic or acidotic, and the physician is not readily available, she should treat the patient for hypoglycemia. Delay in its correction can result in harm to the patient. Five or ten grams of glucose will not affect the course of acidosis appreciably.

As will be emphasized when the various types of insulin are presented, the patient who is taking regular insulin is always aware that he is hypoglycemic. He can, therefore, protect himself from a severe reaction. In contrast, the patient who is taking long-acting insulin may not have warning and can pass directly into an unconscious state. If he happens to be driving an automobile, or is in a position involving danger, the possible consequences to himself and others are obvious.

The prevention of hypoglycemia is preferable to its cure. Patients should be instructed to maintain an inflexible meal schedule, insofar as possible. The distribution of carbohydrate through the day should take into account the time of maximum action of the type of insulin the patient is using. When a meal is delayed, 5 to 10 gm of glucose should be taken, and this glucose can be subtracted from the next meal. Exercise should be regular rather than sporadic, and when it is increased, the patient may take 5 to 10 gm of glucose to prevent hypoglycemia. During a period in which a patient is recovering from an acute illness or his diabetes is being brought under control, as in the instance of Mrs. Keen and Bonnie, nurses should be alert to the possibility that the tolerance of the patient for glucose is likely to be improving and hypoglycemia may occur. Changes in the behavior of the patient should be interpreted in this light.

Though the urine may provide information about the level of glucose in the blood, the results may also be misleading. When urine accumulated in the bladder over a period of time is tested, it can contain glucose despite the presence of hypoglycemia at the time. For example, Mr. Rugge, a known diabetic, was admitted to the emergency room of City Hospital in an unconscious state. A catheterized specimen of urine was examined for glucose and produced a maximum color change, that is, it was 4+ for glucose. He was transferred to an inpatient ward, where another sample of urine was obtained and tested for glucose. This time glucose was absent. Mr. Rugge was given 10 gm of glucose by intravenous infusion. In a matter of seconds, consciousness returned, and in less time than it takes to tell, he was sitting up in bed demanding, "What happened? Why am I here? I'm hungry. Can't somebody get me something to eat?" Prompt and effective treatment of hypoglycemia quickly restores the individual to well-being. Untreated, it may cause irreparable harm.

The second complication of diabetes mellitus that is in the nature of an emergency is acidosis or ketoacidosis. Dr. Edward Rynearson, in his lectures to student nurses, emphasizes this point by saying that the patient in diabetic acidosis is to the physician what acute perforation of a viscus is to the surgeon. The point he is emphasizing is that the patient requires prompt and energetic treatment, if he is to survive. Joslin[26] states that the first three hours after therapy is started are most important to the recovery of the patient.

Before insulin became available, acidosis accounted for about two thirds of the deaths among young diabetics. Since the introduction of insulin, acidosis is generally less frequent and the prognosis of the patient is good, provided the patient is promptly and adequately treated. Acidosis is seen most commonly in the young at the onset of diabetes mellitus and among those who cannot or do not keep their diabetes under control.

Our teen-ager, Bonnie, presented a typical picture of the onset and course of acidosis. She was found to have diabetes mellitus at the age of four and has been admitted for the treatment of acidosis on numerous occasions. On one occasion she was comatose; that is, she could not be aroused. Details of each period of acidosis differed somewhat, but her present attack is reasonably representative. The day before she was admitted to the hospital she vomited throughout the day. During the night she developed abdominal cramps and her lips were dry and parched. When her mother brought her to the hospital, she walked into the emergency room, but required a great deal of assistance from her mother. She was described by the admitting physician as lethargic. She had Kussmaul respirations; her skin and tongue were dry and her eyeballs were slightly soft.

Constituents in her urine and blood were compatible with acidosis. Her blood sugar was elevated to 312 mg per 100 ml of blood plasma. Acetone was present at a dilution of 1 to 20, but not at 1 to 40, and was indicative of a severe degree of acidosis. Carbon dioxide content was 15.2 mEq per liter. It was 20.8 mEq per liter when the test was repeated four hours after treatment was initiated. Three tests revealed increased concentration of her blood as a result of dehydration. Her leukocyte count was elevated to 19,500, her hemoglobin was 17.6 gm per 100 ml of blood, and her hematocrit was 53 volumes per cent. Electrolytes, sodium, potassium, and chlorides were within normal limits. Normal values may, however, have been the result of some degree of dehydration. Had the normal volume of water in the blood been present, the levels of the electrolytes would probably have been depressed. At the time of admission Bonnie's urine was 4+ for both glucose and acetone.

The clinical picture presented by Bonnie is fairly typical of patients in acidosis. The effects were due to the acidosis and the accompanying dehydration. The degree of hyperglycemia she experienced was not as great as sometimes occurs. Though not common, blood glucose levels of as high as 1,000 mg have been observed. Moreover, acidosis does not always accompany a moderate elevation of the blood sugar. Despite a blood glucose of 276 mg and poor control of her diabetes, Mrs. Keen has presented no evidence of acidosis.

[26] *Op. cit.*, pp. 371-72.

Though all the reasons are not known, diabetes is generally more severe in children and in lean young adults than it is in older obese adults. They invariably require insulin. Control is made more difficult by a number of elements. Infections are both more common and more severe in children then they are in adults. Exercise tends to be erratic. The emotional pattern, particularly during adolescence, tends to be unpredictable. Both the parents and the child want the child to grow and develop normally. Despite some exceptions, the child wants to be like others of his age and sex and to do what they do. Any abnormality can be a cause of stress. Child-parent relationships may be such as to be a cause of stress. During the period of adolescence, the child is also striving to separate himself from his parents and to become a separate and unique individual.

At the time Bonnie was admitted, she presented characteristic signs and symptoms of the patient experiencing metabolic acidosis. She was nauseated, had been vomiting, and she had abdominal cramps. Her breathing was of the Kussmaul type. Her urine contained both glucose and ketone bodies. She was markedly dehydrated; her skin was dry and her lips dry and parched. Her eyeballs were soft from the loss of fluid. Her tongue was furry and furrowed. Her hematocrit was slightly elevated (53 per cent), as was her hemoglobin (17.6 gm per 100 ml). The elevation in her leukocyte count was also due to dehydration. Dehydration is due to loss of water by vomiting and by hyperventilation. Another important source of loss of water was through the kidney. For a time the kidney is able to protect a nonacidotic individual against water loss by way of other avenues, such as vomiting, by excreting concentrated urine. Two factors prevented Bonnie's kidney from conserving water. Her renal threshold for sugar was exceeded, so that water was used to excrete sugar. Second, the kidney plays an important role in the maintenance of acid-base balance by conserving or eliminating excess anions or cations. Elimination of either anions or cations requires water. In acidosis, cations are required to excrete the anions of the ketoacids. The mechanisms by which the kidney conserves cations, other than the hydrogen ions, also fail. (See Chapter 8.) Acidosis, therefore, contributes to the depletion of water and electrolytes. With the loss of water the concentration of the blood increases and the blood volume decreases. These changes, if severe and continued, predispose to peripheral vascular collapse.

To accommodate the increase in anions of the ketoacids, the concentration of bicarbonate anions is lowered by hyperventilation (Kussmaul breathing, see Chapter 8), and sodium cations are made available to maintain electroneutrality. One result is a reduction in the carbon dioxide content as well as in the carbon dioxide-combining power of the blood plasma. The latter is the result of the sodium ion being unavailable to combine with the bicarbonate ion. On admission the carbon dioxide content of Bonnie's blood had been lowered to 15.2 mEq per liter. The normal range is from 21 to 30 mEq per liter.

Though the skin of the patient in acidosis is often florid, Bonnie was pale.

She was less alert than usual, but she was not stuporous. Drowsiness followed by stupor, coma, and death can be expected unless the acidosis is corrected.[27] Some patients in acidosis are restless and thrash about and moan in bed. Until the patient is fully recovered, he should not be held responsible for his own safety. Side bars should be raised or placed on the bed. When the patient is excessively restless, they may need to be padded to protect him from injury. In some hospitals, a nurse or physician remains with the patient until he is well on his way to recovery. It is essential that the patient be under intelligent and continuous observation.

Eventually, if the acidosis continues, the circulation fails. The pulse becomes weak and thready, and the blood pressure falls; anuria develops, and the patient dies. When adequate therapy is instituted early enough, recovery is the rule.

When Bonnie was admitted to the hospital, the immediate problem in her care was to correct the acidosis and its effects. The therapeutic plan that was initiated had three objectives. They were (1) to restore normal carbohydrate metabolism, (2) to replace water, minerals, and other substances lost in the urine and vomitus, and (3) to protect Bonnie from injury. All these objectives were carried out more or less simultaneously.

To restore the normal rate of carbohydrate metabolism, Bonnie was given insulin. Patients whose diabetes is of long standing are frequently resistant to insulin, and they are likely to require more insulin when they develop acidosis than do newly discovered diabetics. The longer the acidosis is allowed to persist, the more resistant the patient is likely to be to insulin. Some patients may require 1,000 or more units before there is a drop in the level of glucose in their blood, but Bonnie did not require such a large amount. In the first four hours after she was admitted to the hospital, she received 330 units of insulin. To ensure a prompt effect, unmodified or regular insulin was placed in the intravenous fluids as well as injected subcutaneously. Only unmodified, regular, or crystalline insulin is administered in intravenous fluids. Later isophane (N.P.H.) insulin was also prescribed for Bonnie. During the first 24 hours the total amount administered was 400 units. A fall in the level of glucose and the disappearance of ketone bodies from Bonnie's blood and urine indicated that glucose metabolism was sufficient to suppress the excess metabolism of fat. Particularly in patients who are treated aggressively, glucose may be administered by intravenous infusion to prevent or treat hypoglycemia. As soon as patients retain fluids taken by mouth, fluids containing glucose, such as orange juice, are often prescribed by the physician.

Simultaneously with the measures instituted to restore carbohydrate metabolism, Bonnie was given intravenous fluids to correct dehydration and the electrolyte deficits. Solutions are usually selected on the basis of the extent of

[27] Drowsiness is defined as a pathological state of sleepiness. Stupor is a state of unconsciousness from which the individual can be aroused. He lapses back into unconsciousness after stimulation ceases. In coma, the patient cannot be aroused. All are different degrees of depression of mental alertness.

electrolyte deficits and the availability of laboratory facilities to check the level of the electrolytes in the blood plasma. Bonnie received 500 ml of Ringer's lactate solution, 1,000 ml of physiological saline with 5 per cent bicarbonate of soda, and 4,000 ml of physiological saline by intravenous infusion. In addition, she ingested about 2,200 ml of fluids by mouth. Oral fluids consisted of 600 ml of beef broth, 600 ml of orange juice, and approximately 1,000 ml of water. Her total fluid intake was therefore 9,900 ml. Her urine output during the first 24 hours following hospitalization was 1,850 ml. The relatively small output of urine in relation to the intake of fluid provides some clue to the extent of her dehydration. Although the 9,900 ml of fluid administered intravenously to Bonnie may appear large, it is probably the average amount required by patients in diabetic acidosis. Patients treated aggressively sometimes receive as much as 10,000 ml over a period of a few hours.

Bonnie was placed on bed rest as soon as she was admitted. Patients with diabetes are usually advised to go to bed immediately when they are unwell. Reduction in activity reduces metabolism and should thereby decrease the catabolism of fat and protein.

To reduce the fluid lost by vomiting and to prevent gastric dilatation, fluids were withheld for two hours after Bonnie was admitted. Gastric lavage, which is frequently performed at the time of the admission of the patient to the hospital, was not performed. Gastric aspiration with or without lavage removes fluids accumulated in the stomach and relieves gastric dilatation. It may shorten the length of time the patient is unable to retain fluids. Usually, fluids are withheld for one hour after the completion of the gastric aspiration. After fluids were started and until Bonnie received her usual diet, she was given 100 ml each of broth and orange juice. Broth is a good source of sodium and potassium salts as well as of water and is usually well tolerated when served hot. Orange juice is also a good source of potassium as well as of glucose and water. Other fluids, such as ginger ale, serve the same purposes.

The therapeutic plan for Bonnie is similar to that utilized in the medical treatment of most patients in acidosis. Since every patient is an individual, the details of the treatment required by each patient will differ. Physicians differ in their beliefs about how patients should be treated and this will be a modifying factor. Knowledge changes as a result of observation, study, and research. Practices vary because the assumptions on which practice is based vary.

Although all persons who care for the patient have a responsibility for the safety of the patient, perhaps much of the burden for his protection falls on the nurse. During the period when the patient is less than normally responsive, he must be protected from falling and from the effects of pressure. As stated earlier, side rails should be raised or placed on the bed. Bed covering over the lower extremities should be elevated with a cradle. Should the patient be in shock, care should be taken to prevent injury by burning or pressure. If hot-water bottles are used, the temperature should not be greater than 105°

F, and the bottle should not rest against the patient. Insofar as is possible, patients should be moved and turned regularly unless they are so restless that this is unnecessary. When the patient is restless precautions must be taken to prevent falling or injury from unprotected side rails. He should, of course, be also protected from overheating and chilling. Extra heat should not be applied to patients in a state of vascular collapse, as heat increases vasodilatation and intensifies the failure of the circulation. Albeit all patients should be protected from sources of infection, in no patient is this more important.

As emphasized earlier, the response of the patient to therapy, and often whether or not he recovers, depend on the promptness with which therapy is initiated. Depending on the situation, the nurse may be called upon to prepare, administer, and supervise the therapeutic regime prescribed by the physician. In addition, the nurse is responsible for observing the patient and his reaction to therapy. She may be required to modify the therapy in relation to its effects on the patient and report to the physician only when the patient fails to respond in the desired manner to the prescribed therapeutic regime.

As stated earlier, the medical therapy of the patient, including Bonnie, consists of insulin and fluids. The nurse is responsible for administering these promptly and accurately. The nurse usually collects the urine and sometimes tests it for glucose and acetone. Since insulin dosage is usually in relation to the quantity of glucose and acetone in the urine, accurate and regular testing is important. The length of the interval at which testing is performed varies from one-half to two hours. When voided specimens are used, all urine may be checked. In some clinics the collection of urine specimens is facilitated by the introduction of an indwelling catheter. In others, this is not done because of the increased possibility of infection of the urinary tract.[28] When urine is used as an index of the level of glucose in the blood at a specific time, a freshly secreted specimen must be obtained for testing. The blood may also be tested in place of or to supplement urine testing.

Patients receiving insulin without adequate amounts of glucose may continue to have ketone bodies in the urine in the absence of glycosuria. One patient stands out in the memory of the author. She was a young woman who had an appendectomy in the morning. Since she was a known diabetic, she was given insulin. During the first night after surgery she was found to have ketone bodies but no glucose in her urine. She also had Kussmaul respirations. Her physician was called, and both glucose and insulin were administered. Evidence of developing acidosis was rapidly corrected.

Patients being treated for acidosis may also become hypoglycemic. Although hypoglycemia does not usually occur suddenly, it may. Bonnie developed a mild hypoglycemic reaction after she had been under treatment for acidosis for about six hours.

Any patient who receives a large volume of fluid by intravenous infusion should be subject to careful observation. Patients may be anuric at the time of

[28] Diabetics are predisposed to urinary-tract infection.

admission or may develop anuria later. The reasons for the occurrence of anuria have been presented. Observation of the urine output, including quantity and frequency of voiding, is highly important. As dehydration is corrected, urine output should increase. In general, the capacity of the patient to tolerate a large volume of fluid will depend on the severity of his dehydration, his general health status, and the adequacy of his cardiovascular and renal systems. Any patient receiving a large volume of fluid should have the rate of infusion and its general effects closely observed by a person who is well informed.

Because the recovery of the patient depends on the restoration of homeostasis, the related factors have been emphasized. Although physiological homeostasis is given priority, this does not mean that the patient as a human being should be neglected. Care should be taken to avoid making unwarranted statements in the presence of the patient or talking about other patients in his presence. Conversation should include the patient, but should not make unnecessary demands on him. He should be informed about the care he is receiving and, as he is able, the progress he is making. Attention should be paid to his physical comfort as well. Until the survival of the patient is assured, attention is, however, directed toward three principal objectives—to restore normal carbohydrate metabolism as promptly as possible, to replace the water and electrolyte balance, and to protect the patient from harm. If the recovery of the patient is to be ensured, time is of the essence. Consequently, when a patient is admitted, therapy should be started promptly.

By the evening of the day Bonnie was admitted to the hospital, her dehydration had been corrected. Although several days elapsed before her blood glucose became relatively stable, ketonemia had been largely corrected. She was able to eat the food prescribed on her diet. About seven o'clock in the evening following her admission, she passed 425 ml of urine and was more alert than she had been. From thence forward, she made rapid progress. A week later she was dismissed from the hospital.

How can Bonnie and others who have severe diabetes mellitus prevent diabetic acidosis?

Another question that may be raised is why did Bonnie and her parents allow her to become seriously ill before medical attention was sought? Some of the answers sound easy, but in actual practice they may not be. Acidosis ought to be prevented by continuous and conscientious control of diabetes mellitus. All patients, particularly those who have a tendency to ketosis, should go to bed and call a physician at the first indication of an infection. Bonnie has never been a very well-controlled diabetic. Whether the instability of her diabetes is due to neglect or to an exceptionally severe form of the disease or both is not really known. Her mother is a nurse. She assures the physician that his instructions are carefully followed, and they may well be.

Treatment was not sought until Bonnie was seriously ill. Why not? Were Bonnie and her family ashamed of their failure, or did they not recognize what was happening? Had other members of the family had a similar illness and recovered promptly? Perhaps neither Bonnie nor her parents really understood the nature of diabetes mellitus. Patients and the members of their families may appear to be more knowledgeable than they really are. Since the answers to the questions about why Bonnie develops acidosis frequently are not known, only guesses can be made about them.

Recently a youngster whose medical history parallels that of Bonnie came to the attention of the author. The child, Bobby, was in and out of the hospital at frequent intervals. On a recent admission to the hospital the nurse who cared for him decided to investigate the reasons for his repeated attacks of acidosis. In this instance, the nurse learned that neither Bobby nor his parents had any real understanding of the nature of diabetes mellitus or why certain procedures were important. The nurse made a detailed teaching plan, checked it with the physician to be sure that what she was planning to present to the patient was not in conflict with his instructions, and proceeded to instruct the patient and family. The mother was delighted. Best of all, six months later Bobby was well and active; he had not missed a day of school nor had he been unwell. This had never happened before. Not all problems in the control of diabetes mellitus are as easily solved as were Bobby's. From his previous history, however, Bobby probably would have continued to be in and out of the hospital if a nurse had not tried to identify the reason for his failure to remain well and initiated an appropriate teaching plan.

In the instance of Bonnie, the answer is not known. Multiple factors including a lack of knowledge, physical and emotional problems of adolescence, and relationship problems with parents, peers, teachers, and others may be involved, as well as the fact that the disease is difficult to control.

In addition to acidosis, tuberculosis is another complication that has decreased in frequency. In preinsulin days, it was one of the frequent causes of death among diabetics. Since insulin has become available and the nutritional status of patients can be maintained at reasonable levels, the incidence of tuberculosis has dropped. Tuberculosis continues to be from two to four times more prevalent among diabetics than among nondiabetics, however.

With the increase in the life expectancy of patients with diabetes mellitus, chronic complications involving the vascular and nervous systems and the kidney have become increasingly important. Reference to the patients presented on pages 1278-79 shows that four of the six patients have vascular complications; one of the four has a renal disorder as well. Studies such as the one cited by Duncan[29] indicate that a high percentage of persons who develop diabetes in childhood and live into adult life develop vascular complications. Ninety-two per cent of 200 patients who had had diabetes mellitus from childhood and whose diabetes was of 20 or more years' duration presented

---

[29] Garfield C. Duncan, *Op. cit.*, p. 858.

evidence of vascular disease. Vascular complications also are frequent among persons who are middle-aged or older at the time of onset. Vascular complications occur earlier and to a more severe degree in diabetics than in nondiabetics.[30] They are more rapidly progressive in young persons who have longstanding diabetes that has been inadequately treated. More than 50 per cent of the deaths in patients who have had diabetes for more than 15 years are due to vascular lesions.[31] All types of arteriosclerosis occur alone or in combination. The arteries most commonly involved are those supplying the lower extremities, the heart muscle (coronary arteries), the brain, the eye, and the kidney.[32]

Vascular complications are important because they have a high incidence and their incidence among persons with diabetes is rising. Once established, they tend to be progressive. They differ from acute complications as they do not cause the diabetes to become more severe. Though most authorities state that vascular disorders are likely to develop earlier and progress more rapidly in those in whom therapy is inadequate, vascular complications also develop in those with mild diabetes. Sometimes, as in the instance of Mrs. Curry, the diabetes is discovered when the patient seeks treatment for a complication. Since the problems presented by patients with vascular complications are similar, these are discussed in Chapter 10.

Complications involving the kidney are very common among patients with longstanding diabetes mellitus. Renal complications include those resulting from arteriolarsclerosis, intercapillary glomerulosclerosis, and pyelonephritis. All these conditions can and do occur in nondiabetics. They are, however, likely to be more severe and more rapidly progressive in diabetics than in nondiabetics. When they are progressive, they lead to a loss of renal reserve and with it to azotemia (the accumulation of the wastes of protein metabolism in the blood).

Of the renal disorders the one most commonly associated with diabetes mellitus is pyelonephritis, but the most characteristic is intercapillary sclerosis or Kimmelsteil-Wilson's disease. This disorder is frequent and its incidence is rising. Though its diagnosis requires renal biopsy, it is presumed to be present when edema, hypertension, azotemia, and proteinuria are present. Other pathology frequently associated with intercapillary sclerosis is diabetic retinopathy and anemia. Although it may remain stable for long periods of time, once severe edema and albuminuria occur the life expectancy of the patient can be measured only in months. The reader may remember that Mr. Benedict has edema and hypertension. Though he is not aware of the seriousness of his condition, his prognosis is guarded. He has had known diabetes for 21 years.

Complications arising from the effects of diabetes on the various structures of the eyes are frequent. Arteriosclerosis of the retinal arteries, as well as

[30] *Ibid.*, p. 858.
[31] *Ibid.*, p. 788.
[32] *Ibid.*, p. 782.

hemorrhages and exudates into the retina, lead to loss of vision. In three of our patients retinitis is present. A fourth patient has cataracts. Although the type of cataract occurring most frequently in diabetic patients does not differ from the ordinary senile cataract, they do occur somewhat more frequently among diabetic patients than among nondiabetics. The problems of the patient are those of any individual who is losing or loses his vision. About 18 per cent of blindness is associated with diabetes mellitus.

Not much is known about the pathological changes responsible for the neurological complications. Neuropathies occur in the peripheral nerves as well as elsewhere in the nervous system. When the spinal cord is involved, the changes in the posterior and lateral columns are identical with those found in pernicious anemia. Patients with peripheral neuritis often suffer numbness, tingling, and pain which is sometimes very severe.

Among the complications involving the skin are furuncles (boils) and carbuncles (multiple boils adjacent to each other). In health, the skin serves as a storehouse for glycogen. In uncontrolled diabetes, the glycogen in the skin is depleted and the glucose content of the skin rises with the hyperglycemia. When diabetes is poorly controlled, the skin is predisposed to infections by the *Staphylococcus aureus*. There is also evidence that function of the polymorphonuclear leukocytes is impaired. Two requirements, that is, control of diabetes and cleanliness of the skin and clothing, are important to the prevention of skin complications.

Vascular, renal, and neurological complications usually develop over an extended period of time. Their increasing incidence is related to the fact that diabetics as well as nondiabetics have an improved life expectancy. All these complications occur earlier and are more rapidly progressive than in the nondiabetic.

What are the measures that are available for the control of diabetes mellitus? On what principles are they based? What are the objectives of therapy? What are the responsibilities of the nurse to the patient with diabetes mellitus?

As stressed earlier, successful control of diabetes mellitus depends on the intelligent cooperation of the patient and his family. Unlike recovery from an acute infectious disease, recovery does not follow a period of acute illness. Diabetes mellitus is permanent. Remissions can and do occur when the disease is discovered early and treated aggressively, but even these patients should not think of themselves as cured.

The days and weeks that immediately follow the diagnosis of diabetes mellitus are important in the life of the patient. During this time he learns what it means to be diabetic and, hopefully, how he can control his disease. The general objectives of his medical therapy include: (1) to individualize his regime so that he can live as full and useful a life as is possible within the limitations of his disorder; (2) to correct the underlying metabolic abnormalities or, to state it in positive terms, to restore homeostasis; (3) to attain and maintain ideal body weight; and (4) to prevent or delay the onset and progression of complications of the disease.

The fundamental methods used in the treatment are insulin or hypoglycemic agents, diet, exercise, and education. In the prevention of complications good hygiene is also important. The continued management and control of diabetes mellitus depends on the patient. Education as to the nature and behavior of his disease is required so that he understands the reasons for what he must do and develops the skills required for it.

At the time the patient learns that diabetes is incurable, he should learn that it is controllable. Whether or not it is kept under control depends to a large extent on himself and his family. In the past, physicians have tended to assume the primary responsibility for the regulation of diabetes. The trend is toward placing the responsibility for control on the patient and his family. Doctors and nurses are available and willing to help him assume this responsibility, however. Furthermore, the measures that are required are for his well-being. The patient learns to control his disease because this is the way to good health. He does not take insulin or other medications and regulate his food intake to please the doctor or the nurse or someone else, but to promote health. The control of diabetes mellitus is a way of life, but it should not be all of life.

When a person learns that he has diabetes mellitus, even when he has suspected its presence, he suffers some degree of emotional shock. The degree of shock will depend on the individual and what the diagnosis and treatment mean to him. Any pre-existing problem can be expected to be intensified. The patient and his family can be expected to react to knowledge of the diagnosis as they do to other crisis situations in life. Authorities frequently emphasize the advantages of diabetes over disorders such as cancer. In time the patient may come to a similar conclusion, but at the time the diagnosis is established he is thinking of what he has lost and not of other more serious possibilities. He compares diabetes with health and he prefers health. Furthermore, diabetes does not render an individual less susceptible to other chronic illnesses. The nurse can usually be of more help to the patient if she can help him to identify and express his feelings rather than telling him how lucky he is.

When diabetes is diagnosed in a young child, the parents are the ones who experience the negative feelings. Their child is less than perfect. If the disease is to be controlled, the child must have special care and attention. Questions arise. Will other children in the family develop the disease? Is the fact that the child is ill the result of something the parent did or thought he did not do? Of our six patients, Bonnie, at four, probably had few, if any, preconceived ideas about diabetes mellitus. Try, however, to imagine the feelings of an eight-year-old boy or a 13-year-old girl who learns that he or she has diabetes. Are they likely to be consoled by the fact they they do not have leukemia?

In addition to the fact of diabetes itself, negative emotions are usually engendered by the measures required in treatment. Although children of five or younger learn to inject their own insulin, older adults find this procedure particularly frightening. Men and women who are employed may be concerned about whether they will be able to continue in their current jobs. Those who are not yet gainfully employed face the possibility that diabetes will limit their choice of vocation as well as their chances of getting and holding a position. Will others know and if they do will the diabetic be accepted? Will he be able to do what his friends do? Will he be able to marry and to have children? Boys who have dreamed of being athletes find their ambitions threatened. Restrictions real and imagined are likely to appear to be insurmountable to the patient and to his family as well.

A danger common to any patient with a disease requiring long-term therapy is that when the person feels well, he will decide that he is cured and discontinue his regime. Or when he finally realizes that he is not going to get well in the usual interpretation of the term, he may decide to try some quick cure such as a special food or a cure-all. Deviations from the prescribed regime will result in a loss of, at best, the control of his diabetes mellitus and, at worst, his life.

Although much has been accomplished to reduce the cost of insulin, diet, and medical supervision, diabetes mellitus does place an economic burden on families whose incomes are limited. For this reason, patients with diabetes mellitus may be declared medically indigent at a higher level of income than nondiabetics. Enough problems have been raised to suggest that the psychological stresses arising in relation to a diagnosis of diabetes mellitus are many and highly individualized.

During the period immediately following diagnosis the patient and his family require psychological support. This should start with the patient's admission to the office of the physician, to the clinic, or to the hospital. The type and amount of support will vary with each individual. Both the patient and his family have a right to expect that professional personnel try to understand their feelings and to accept their behavior as having meaning. An important objective in the care of the patient should be to provide a climate in which he feels accepted, so that he will feel free to express his feelings and be supported in his attempts to accept his diagnosis and what it entails. The nurse should try to convey to the patient that, while she understands or is trying to understand his feelings, he will be able to learn to do what he must do and will be provided with the necessary assistance.

The objectives of the therapy of diabetes are achieved by diet, insulin, exercise, and education. Physicians differ about the degree to which chemical control is necessary. Some advocate strict chemical control so that glycosuria is prevented and the level of glucose in the blood is maintained at normal or nearly normal levels. Both hypo- and hyperglycemia are to be avoided. Those who support strict chemical control state that it reduces the severity of diabetes and lessens the likelihood of degenerative changes developing and that when they develop, their rate of progress is slowed. A further argument is that insulin requirements are less when blood glucose is maintained at normal or near normal levels. For example, at the time Mrs. Keen was admitted, she was taking 35 units of isophane insulin and 24 units of regular insulin each day. At the time she was discharged, she was taking 10 units of Lente insulin daily. For a person on a limited budget, as Mrs. Keen was, the reduction in insulin dosage reduced the cost of treatment, a not unimportant consideration.

Those who disagree with the strict chemical control approach say that this method neglects the individuality of the patient, because the therapy is directed against the disease rather than toward the person. This argument does not necessarily apply, however. Not all physicians believe that chemical control is either necessary or desirable. Some physicians believe that hyperglycemia and glycosuria can be disregarded as long as ketosis is avoided and normal weight and strength are maintained. For example, they would not be concerned because Mrs. Keen's blood glucose was elevated most of the time or because she had marked glycosuria more or less continuously. She would be given enough insulin to keep her feeling well and to keep her urine free of ketone bodies. Some physicians who support this approach place no restrictions on the diet. Others encourage the patient to restrict his intake of concentrated carbohydrates, especially those lacking other nutrients. Physicians who favor clinical control believe that the incidence of degenerative complications is not high enough to warrant the restrictions required to achieve chemical control. Moreover, they say that the patient feels better.

Many physicians and, if the truth were known, patients adopt a regime between the two. The physician tries to prescribe a diet that is acceptable to the patient and takes into account the severity of his disease. Some patients prefer a strict regime, while others do better when the approach is more flexible. Since insulin has become available, a nutritious and satisfying diet can usually be achieved.

Root and Bailey[33] state that diet planned for long-continued use should meet the following criteria:

1. Its caloric content should be sufficient to meet the patient's needs as determined by his age, sex, activity, and growth requirements. For example, because Bonnie is still growing and is presumably more active, she requires a higher caloric intake per unit of body surface than Mrs. Curry. Because Mr. Benedict is a man, he utilizes more calories than women do.

2. The distribution of calories and the proportions of carbohydrate, protein, and fat should remain about the same from day to day. The specific foods eaten may vary greatly. Some authorities make this point

[33] Howard F. Root and C. Cabell Bailey, "Diet in the Treatment of Diabetes Mellitus," in Michael G. Wohl and Robert S. Goodhart (eds.), *Modern Nutrition, In Health and Disease,* 2nd ed., Lea & Febiger, Philadelphia, 1960, pp. 680-81.

by saying that the proportions of the various nutrients as well as the meal schedule should be inflexible. Great flexibility can, however, be exercised in the selection of specific foods.

3. Most diabetic diets contain less carbohydrate than the normal diet. The quantity of protein and fat is usually a little higher. The reduction in carbohydrate is accompanied by the elimination of concentrated sweets and pastries.

4. The calories should be planned to support the ideal rather than the actual weight. The obese patient can be expected to lose weight. The underweight person should gain weight.

5. The diet should be planned so that it provides for an adequate intake of all nutrients, including minerals and vitamins.

The physician makes the decision as to the content and distribution of carbohydrates, proteins, and fat in the diet of the patient. The nurse and the dietitian translate the prescription into terms of food and methods of food preparation. In the hospital, the dietitian often is responsible for the formal dietary instruction. In small hospitals and in public health agencies nurses must often assume the responsibility for the basic instruction of the patient. In some public health agencies dietary consultants are available to give guidance and other help to the nurse. Unless the patient receives detailed instruction and the diet is planned to take into account his usual food pattern, he is quite likely to return to his previous dietary or to unnecessarily restrict his food intake.

Proudfit and Robinson[34] list nine points that should be kept in mind when the diet is planned. Some of the points are included above and will not be further reviewed. In the achievement of the first one, that is, the planning of the diet in terms of the individual pattern of living of the patient, the nurse, wherever she is employed, is in a particularly advantageous position to be helpful. The nurse should obtain information about the economic status of the patient, what foods are available to him as well as their cost, his religion, national origin, social status, occupation, idiosyncrasies, misconceptions, and beliefs about food, facilities for preparing food, and where and with whom he eats. Unless the family dietary is inadequate, the family food pattern is used as a base. One of the objectives is to disrupt the family as little as possible. The food pattern of the patient is kept as nearly like the rest of the family's as is possible. The visiting nurse can often be of great service to the person who prepares the meals for the person with diabetes. For the most part special foods are not required. Water-packed canned fruits and vegetables are now available at most grocery stores. They can be substituted for fresh fruits and vegetables when these are not available or are expensive.

The patient and the person who prepares his meals should learn to identify the carbohydrate, protein, and fat content of foods. They should know why

[34] Fairfax T. Proudfit and Corinne H. Robinson, *Normal and Therapeutic Nutrition*, 12th ed., The Macmillan Company, New York, 1961, pp. 467-68.

the carbohydrate content is restricted. When a patient is in ketosis, the carbohydrate content may be restricted to 100 gm per day, as was done when Bonnie was first admitted. At the time she was dismissed, her diet prescription was for 150 gm of carbohydrate, which is well within the usual range.

Whether patients are taught to weigh, measure, or approximate the size of servings depends on the views of the physician. Patients with compulsive personalities may be more comfortable when they weigh their food while others may reject the idea entirely. The patient and the person who prepares his food should be well acquainted with food exchange lists and know how to use them.

In many patients, diabetes mellitus cannot be controlled by dietary measures alone. In only two of our six patients was this possible. In young persons and those with moderate or severe diabetes insulin is required. Two general types of insulin, unmodified and modified, are available. Unmodified insulin, commonly known as regular insulin, was the first type to be available. It is promptly absorbed after subcutaneous injection and its effect is begun within one-half hour after it is injected. It reaches its maximum effect in from two to three hours. Because it may be injected intravenously as well as subcutaneously and it acts quickly, it is used in the treatment of diabetic acidosis. It is also used to supplement the effect of the types of insulin with prolonged actions.

Modified insulins differ from regular insulin in that something is added to make the insulin relatively insoluble and thereby delay the rate at which it is absorbed with the result that the period over which the insulin acts is prolonged. Classified according to the length of the period over which they act, modified insulins are of two types—long-acting and intermediate-acting. Protamine zinc insulin, the first of the modified insulins to be developed, has a prolonged action. It was developed by Hagedorn of Denmark, who added a basic protein, protamine—a substance obtained from the sperm of a certain fish—to insulin. Protamine absorbs insulin and delays the rate at which it is absorbed as the protamine must be broken down before the insulin is released. Because of its prolonged action, hyperglycemia in patients requiring more than 40 units of insulin is difficult to control with protamine zinc insulin. Although the period of maximum action is from 12 to 24 hours, action may continue for from 48 to 72 hours. There is, therefore, an overlapping of dosages, making it difficult to secure a uniform depression of the blood glucose. Hypoglycemic reactions are frequent.

A more nearly physiological effect can be achieved by administering part of the insulin dosage as unmodified and part as protamine zinc insulin, either as two separate injections or by mixing the two and giving one injection. The success of this method depends on the ability of the patient to assume responsibility for measuring and mixing the two types of insulin. A commercially prepared mixture of protamine zinc insulin and regular insulin is now available.

Following the introduction of protamine zinc insulin, other modifications were introduced that more nearly met all the following criteria. They require only one injection, have a sufficiently rapid onset of action, and are absorbed over an appropriate period of time. The three most successful preparations are isophane or N.P.H. insulin, globin insulin, and Lente insulin. Isophane insulin is a modified protamine zinc insulin. It behaves essentially like a mixture of 2 parts regular to 1 part protamine insulin. As the two types are mixed, the problems in administration are simplified. The essential difference between globin and isophane insulin is that globin rather than protamine is used to prolong the period of absorption.

The Lente insulins are the newest preparations. They differ from other slow-acting insulins in that they do not contain a foreign protein. They are made by precipitating insulin with zinc and then resuspending it in an acetate buffer solution. By altering the conditions under which the preparations are made, particles of different sizes can be made. Ultra Lente contains particles of large size and has the duration of action of over 30 hours; its duration of action is similar to that of protamine zinc insulin. Lente insulin contains particles of small size. Insulin is released more rapidly from small than from large particles, and duration of the action of Lente insulin is approximately 24 hours. Semi-lente insulin is composed of amorphous particles, and the duration of its action is from 12 to 18 hours. The two preparations of insulin in most common use today are isophane and Lente insulin. The types of insulin along with the time of onset, period of maximum action, and duration of action are summarized in Figure 17-5-A.

FIGURE 17 – 5-A
Time of Action of Various Insulin Preparations

Type of Insulin	Time of Onset, Hours	Period of Maximum Action	Duration of Action
Insulin injection U.S.P.	½	3	6
Crystalline zinc insulin	1	3	8
Globin zinc insulin	2–4	8–16	16–24
Isophane insulin injection (N.P.H.)	2	10–20	28–30
Protamine zinc injection	6–8	12–24	48–72
Lente insulin (insulin zinc suspension)	4–5	12–16	20–24

The objective of insulin therapy is to enable the individual to utilize sufficient food to meet his nutritional needs and, within limits, his desire for food. For many patients this objective can be achieved by a single injection of protamine zinc insulin or one of the intermediate-acting insulins, either alone or in combination with crystalline insulin. The ideal preparation of insulin would be one in which the insulin is released in response to hyperglycemia. At this time there is no such preparation. A reasonably good approximation can, however, be achieved in many patients. This is done by planning the distribution of carbohydrate in the diet of the patient and his pattern of exercise in relation to the duration of action of the type of insulin used. Since individuals differ from each other and the same individual differs from time to time, the details of the therapeutic plan will be different for each person. Persons who require less than 40 units of insulin a day often do very well on a single injection of protamine zinc insulin. Miss Arthur had been able to control her diabetes with 35 units of protamine zinc injected each morning. Those who require more than 40 units of protamine zinc insulin to control their diabetes usually respond better to one of the intermediate insulins either singly or in combination with crystalline insulin. There are some persons whose diabetes is very difficult to control, that is, to prevent rapid shifts in the level of glucose in their blood, despite attention to the therapeutic regime.

Application of knowledge of the duration of the action of each of the various insulins enables the physician, nurse, or patient to predict when hyperglycemia and hypoglycemia are most likely to occur. The physician prescribes the distribution of carbohydrate in the diet of the patient in relation to the type of insulin used. To protect patients who are receiving protamine zinc insulin from nocturnal hypoglycemia, some of the carbohydrate from the evening meal is saved for a lunch at bedtime. Milk and crackers or toast and butter are satisfactory. Patients taking intermediate-acting insulin are frequently advised to save some of the carbohydrate from their lunch as a mid- or late-afternoon snack. By distribution of the intake of carbohydrate over the time when insulin absorption is at its height, the patient is protected from attacks of hypoglycemia. The importance of the mid-afternoon and prebedtime lunch should be emphasized to the patient. Although regular and crystalline insulins do not induce hypoglycemic reactions without warning, modified insulins do. A hypoglycemic reaction may not be too serious when the person is in the protected environment of his home, but a sudden loss of consciousness when out in public can endanger his life. If he is driving a car, not only the person's life but the lives of others are in danger. Some physicians recommend that patients who are planning to drive a car in the later afternoon take 5 to 10 gm of glucose before starting out. A fourth to one-half glass of orange juice or a Life Saver or two contain enough glucose to protect the patient from hypoglycemia. As pointed out earlier, the patient requires less insulin when his diabetes is under control than when he is hyperglycemic. During periods when control is being established, he should, therefore, be observed for signs of hypoglycemia. He should also be asked to report any changes in the way he feels. The patient should learn the common manifestations of hypoglycemia.

Although hypoglycemic attacks may occur at any time, patients on Isophane, globin, or Lente insulin are most likely to have them in the late afternoon. Bonnie had an attack of hypoglycemia about four o'clock on two successive afternoons. As a result, her physician prescribed that one slice of toast be saved from her lunch to be eaten at three-thirty in the afternoon. Patients receiving protamine zinc insulin may be hypoglycemic during the early morning hours when they are asleep. Mrs. Arthur discovered her daughter to be unconscious when she tried to waken her in the morning. Nurses should observe patients for unusual behavior. If a patient who is asleep cannot be aroused, the doctor should be notified immediately. Patients presenting evidence of hypoglycemia should be treated promptly with 5 to 10 gm of glucose. This may be in the form of a lump of sugar, a half-cup of orange juice, or Karo syrup in water. Following treatment the patient should be under continued surveillance as there is a tendency for patients who are taking modified insulin to have one or more recurrent attacks. Milk, with or without crackers, provides more continuous protection than orange juice or other sugar solutions. When the hypoglycemia is accompanied by unconsciousness, glucose administered by intravenous injection results in a prompt recovery.

Another factor that predisposes to hypoglycemia is exercise. Exercise is a valuable part of the therapeutic regime, because working muscle does not require insulin to utilize glucose. As a result, the patient with diabetes is encouraged to exercise regularly. The type, amount, and degree of activity should be about the same from day to day. Sudden increases, particularly in the patient who is taking insulin, are to be avoided. The beneficial effect of exercise sometimes creates problems for the patient who has been hospitalized. Hospital space and policy often make it difficult for the patient to duplicate the amount of exercise he takes outside the hospital. After his discharge, he may have a series of hypoglycemic attacks. To prevent this, some physicians encourage patients who are able to leave the hospital for an afternoon, or several afternoons, to try to duplicate their usual activity. When patients must for some reason exercise more than is usual, they should protect themselves by taking 5 to 10 gm of glucose (1 to 2 lumps of sugar).

Because patients have to buy insulin they should know that there are different types but that they should not substitute one type or strength for another without discussing this with their physician. They should also learn that insulin dosage is expressed in units and that a unit has the same power to lower the blood sugar whatever the number per milliliter of solution or the type of insulin. A unit of insulin is determined by its blood sugar-lowering effect when it is injected into a rabbit. Preparations are concentrated so that 1 ml of solution contains 10, 20, 40, 80, or 100 units. Because of the differences in potency, care should be exercised in the identification of the number of units per milliliter. To lessen the chance of error, some hospitals require that two nurses check the label on the bottle against the order and the label against the quantity of insulin in the syringe. Textbooks used in courses of introduction to nursing cover the details of subcutaneous injections, so they will not be repeated here. The physician prescribes the type, dosage, and time insulin is to be administered to the patient as well as when to instruct and who is to be instructed. Ideally, instruction should begin as soon as the diagnosis is established. Joslin says that, when at all possible, the patient should inject his first dose of insulin.[35]

This practice has the advantage of not allowing the patient time to worry about whether or not he will be able to do it. Joslin is of the opinion that delay only increases the difficulty for the patient. Patients should be taught that since insulin is a protein, it is advisable to keep it in a cool place, but that it should not be allowed to freeze. With the exception of the Lente insulins, the supply in current use need not be refrigerated. Lente insulins should be refrigerated.

Syringe and needle should be sterilized by boiling before each injection. Boiling is simplified by placing the separated barrel and plunger of the syringe and the needle in a metal strainer. The strainer is placed in a saucepan of cold water and boiled for five minutes. When the syringe is removed from the water, care should be taken not to contaminate any part of the needle or syringe that comes in contact with the insulin or is introduced into the patient. When the syringe and needle are kept in alcohol, the alcohol container should be emptied, washed, and boiled at the time the syringe is sterilized. Before the syringe is filled with insulin, alcohol should be removed from the barrel by moving the plunger in and out of the barrel a number of times. The skin over the site of injection should be clean, and just before the injection is made, it should be cleansed with alcohol.

The hour at which the patient takes his insulin will depend on the type of insulin, the severity of his diabetes, when his blood sugar is highest, and the practices of his physician. The most common time is 20 to 30 minutes before breakfast for patients receiving one injection a day. Modified insulins containing a precipitate should be gently rotated until the sediment is thoroughly mixed with the clear solution. Vigorous shaking should be avoided to prevent bubble formation.

Insulin, though usually called a protein, is a polypeptide and is digested in the alimentary canal. It must, therefore, be administered parenterally. The usual method is by subcutaneous injection into loose subcutaneous tissues. Because daily, or more frequent, injections are required over the lifetime of the individual, care should be taken to rotate the sites, so that one area is not used more often than once each month. When a patient injects his own insulin, the anterior aspects of the thigh and the abdomen are usually the most convenient sites. For those patients who have automatic syringes, the lateral aspect of the upper arm may also be used.

Local reactions may occur at the site of injection. Local allergic reactions are common when patients are taking protamine zinc insulin and are unusual when other types of insulin are used. The reaction is manifested by redness, swelling, itching, and discomfort at the site of injection. The first symptoms

[35] *Op. cit.,* p. 283.

appear in from 2 to 12 hours after the injection and reach their height in from 18 to 24 hours. In from three to four weeks this type of reaction subsides. Fortunately, patients rarely are allergic to the protein of insulin itself. When they are, they are more likely to be allergic to beef or sheep insulins than to pork insulin.

Other local reactions may result from repeated injections of insulin into the same site over a long period of time. In some patients, adipose tissue hypertrophies and causes local areas of swelling. In other patients, adipose tissue atrophies leaving concave depressions in the skin. Children of both sexes and adult females seem to be predisposed to this condition. The cause is not known. The rotation of the sites of injection is encouraged to prevent either hypertrophy or atrophy of adipose tissue. Fat atrophy is also less likely to occur if insulin is administered at room temperature.

A considerable number of persons whose diabetes is rapidly brought under control with insulin develop a temporary presbyopia, a condition in which the individual can see at a distance, but has difficulty in accommodating to near vision. Particularly to the young patient, presbyopia may be quite disturbing. He should be reassured that the condition will clear up in from three to four weeks and delay having his eyes examined for glasses as any prescription obtained during this period will not be suitable later.

The patient with diabetes mellitus should carry with him some form of identification which includes not only personal data, but the fact that he is diabetic, his insulin dosage, and the name of his physician. Carrying a card is of greatest importance to those who are taking insulin or who are subject to ketosis. A number of types of identification tags and cards are available. A coin-size tag on a chain or bracelet has the advantage of being less likely to be separated from the individual. Additional information can be placed on a card and carried in a billfold.

When a patient requires insulin, he will usually require at least one injection every day for the remainder of his life. There are exceptions, but this is the general rule. He, or a member of his family must learn to measure and to inject the insulin. The instruction of the patient including the injection of his own insulin should be begun immediately. Judgment should be exercised so that the patient is not overwhelmed by too much information offered at one time. Instructions should be repeated as often as necessary.

Besides insulin, what drugs are useful in the control of the level of glucose in the blood?

Valuable as insulin is in the control of diabetes mellitus, to be effective it must be administered either by subcutaneous injection or by intravenous infusion. Consequently, when the sulfonylureas were found to have a hypoglycemic effect, hope was aroused that an effective oral substitute had been discovered. Subsequent experience with the sulfonylureas has demonstrated that, like other drugs, they have limitations as well as uses. They are effective in newly discovered diabetics who are (1) over 40 years of age, (2) not susceptible to ketosis, (3) not overly obese, but (4) in whom hyperglycemia is not controlled by diet alone. They are not effective in young diabetics or in older diabetics whose disease is severe. For example, tolbutamide, a sulfonylurea, was not successful in controlling hyperglycemia in Mrs. Keen. Patients subject to ketosis or with severe diabetes require insulin. Tolbutamide is sometimes used by patients who require large dosages of insulin to reduce the amount of insulin required. Sulfonylureas may become ineffective, and insulin is then required when diabetes worsens or during an infection or other stress. The sulfonylureas are believed to stimulate the beta cells in the pancreas to secrete insulin. They are not insulin but act on the beta cells to increase the output of endogenous insulin.

One of the most widely used of the sulfonylureas is tolbutamide, or Orinase. It is short-acting as its effect lasts only about four hours. It is safe and effective as about 35 per cent of patients who are resistant to ketosis respond favorably to it.

Duncan[36] emphasizes that each patient receiving tolbutamide should have individual instructions. They should know that: (1) although tolbutamide is effective in many older diabetics, it rarely is in the young, (2) it is not a form of insulin, (3) it does not act like insulin, and (4) it is not effective during infections or other forms of stress as insulin is required at these times. In some patients the favorable effect of the sulfonylureas lasts only from four to six months. Other measures—diet and exercise—are still important and should not be neglected. The only real change in the regime of the patient is that he can take tolbutamide by mouth rather than taking insulin by subcutaneous injection. When, as is not at all uncommon, the patient is taking several different drugs, some system should be devised that helps him to remember which of these drugs controls his blood sugar.

As repeatedly emphasized, diet, exercise, and, when required, insulin or an insulin substitute, form the framework in the treatment and control of diabetes mellitus. Since diabetes mellitus is an incurable disease characterized by failure in the homeostasis of glucose, fats, and proteins, good health depends on conforming to the therapeutic regime. As stated earlier, successful control of diabetes mellitus depends on the patient and his family assuming responsibility for the management of his condition. Consequently, education assumes a significant role in therapy.

Unlike many chronic diseases, in diabetes relatively simple methods are available to check the effectiveness of the measures used to control hyperglycemia. The concentration of glucose and of acetone in the blood or urine can be determined by relatively simple tests. Examinations of the urine for glucose and acetone are so simple that lay-men easily learn to perform them. Determinations of the level of glucose in the blood are somewhat more com-

[36] Duncan, *Op. cit.*, p. 856.

plicated. To secure accurate information about the degree to which the homeostasis of glucose is being achieved, food and insulin should be delayed until after the blood has been withdrawn. A newly admitted patient should be instructed about the days when blood is taken to be tested for glucose. He may, sometimes, need to be reminded about why he has not received his breakfast. The nonhospitalized patient who has blood drawn in the office of his physician or in the outpatient clinic should be informed of what is expected of him. He should know whether or not he should omit his breakfast and insulin and whether or not he should bring his insulin and breakfast with him. The latter practice may be encouraged particularly for patients who have a limited income. In the preparation of the patient for some of the newer screening and diagnostic tests, the patient may be instructed to eat his regular or a special meal.

Although the concentration of glucose in the blood of a fasting person provides accurate information about the adequacy of control of diabetes mellitus, the frequency with which the test is performed is limited by the fact that blood must be withdrawn before it can be examined. Under most circumstances, the quantity of glucose in the urine provides a reasonably accurate estimate of the degree to which the homeostasis of glucose is being achieved. Because urine is easily obtained and glucose and acetone are excreted in the urine when the renal threshold is exceeded, and the qualitative test for glucose and acetone are relatively simple, urine is widely used to evaluate the control of diabetes mellitus. Depending on the severity of the diabetes and, whether or not the patient takes insulin, as well as the views of the physician, the patient may be instructed to test his urine as frequently as four times a day or as infrequently as once or twice a month. For most individuals who work, two testings a day are a practical maximum. During a period in which a diabetes mellitus is under regulation or is changing, more frequent testing may be desired to determine when hyperglycemia and/or hypoglycemia occurs.

Whereas blood to be tested for glucose is usually taken when the patient is fasting, no simple statement applies to the kinds of samples of urine examined for glucose. All urine may be saved for 24 hours, so that the total quantity of glucose excreted per day can be determined. Each and every voiding may be checked as a means of evaluating fluctuations in the blood glucose. The patient may be instructed to void at specific times of the day and the urine is added to previous voidings and mixed. A sample of the mixture is then tested for sugar and acetone. In another method the patient voids and discards the voiding unless a 24-hour specimen is being collected, when the urine is added to previous voidings. He drinks a glass or two of water and then one hour later collects a sample of urine (a fresh specimen) for testing. Since the urine is secreted over a known and relatively short period of time, it more accurately reflects the level of glucose in the blood at the time of testing than is likely to be true of the other methods. Whatever method is used, however, the patient should be instructed in its use. He should have practice not only in performing the method he will use at home but in evaluating the results. If he is to adjust his insulin dosage in relation to the quantity of glucose in his urine, he should also be given explicit written as well as verbal instructions and should practice adjusting his insulin dosage while he is still being instructed.

The standard method for determining the quantity of glucose in the urine is the Benedict test. Benedict's solution is an alkaline solution of cupric hydroxide. When it is heated in the presence of an aldehyde group $H—\overset{\overset{\textstyle H}{|}}{C}=O$, the blue cupric ions are reduced to brick-red cuprous ions. Since the glucose molecule contains an aldehyde group, when urine containing glucose is added to Benedict's solution and the mixture is heated, this reaction occurs. Cuprous hydroxide forms a precipitate which settles out on standing. To perform the test 1 teaspoon of Benedict's solution is measured and placed in a clean test tube. Eight drops of urine are added. The test tube is placed upright in a pan of boiling water and boiled for five minutes. The color changes vary from the clear blue of cupric hydroxide to the brick red of cuprous hydroxide. Scales for comparison are found in various textbooks. An effective method for teaching nurses and patients to estimate the amount of glucose in the urine is to prepare a series of test tubes containing varying amounts of glucose and then, after heating the solution, to seal the open end of the tube by heating it in an oxhydrogen flame.

Since the introduction of the Benedict test, procedures have been developed that make it possible to test the urine both easily and quickly. These include the following:

1. Clinitest method, a modification of the Benedict test. The reagent tablet is dropped into a measured amount of urine. The results are similar to those of the Benedict test. Since the tablets lose their potency when they are exposed to moisture, bottles containing Clinitest tablets should be tightly stoppered.

2. Galatest. In this test the active agent is bismuth. A drop or two of urine is placed on a small mound of powder. When glucose is present, the bismuth is reduced and the powder changes to gray or black.

3. Glucose oxidase tests. These tests are based on the fact that an enzyme, glucose oxidase, converts glucose to glyconic acid. Unlike other tests for identifying glucose in the urine, these tests are specific for glucose.

   Two commercial tests are available that make use of glucose oxidase reaction. *Tes-Tape* not only identifies the presence of glucose in the urine, but gives a rough approximation of the quantity of glucose present. The test is simple to perform, since a strip of impregnated paper is dipped into the urine. Color changes take place in about a minute. When glucose is present, the color changes to varying shades of green or blue.

Clinistik, the second glucose oxidase test, is similar to the *Tes-Tape*. A specially prepared tip of a stick is placed in urine. These tests have the advantage of being easy and quick to perform. *Tes-Tape* or Clinistik is used in community detection drives.

When glucose is present in appreciable quantities, the urine is also tested for ketone bodies. To test for diacetic acid, a 10 per cent water solution of ferric chloride is added, drop by drop, to 5 ml of freshly voided urine. A wine-red color indicates the presence of diacetic acid.

Acetest is a simple test for acetone. A drop of freshly voided urine is placed on a tablet which contains aminoacetic acid, disodium phosphate, and sodium nitroprusside. A positive test is indicated by a purple tint, from lavender to a deep purple. The more intense the color, the greater the amount of acetone.

The tests for glucose and for ketone bodies are useful in evaluating the success of the control of diabetes mellitus. The patient should be instructed to seek medical attention immediately when the quantity of glucose in the urine increases over 1+ or 2+ as well as when ketone bodies appear in the urine. An experienced and intelligent diabetic patient may be able to evaluate why glucose appears in his urine and to make the appropriate adjustment. When these adjustments are not successful, he, too, should see his physician.

Diet, insulin, and exercise have as their objective the maintenance of the homeostasis of glucose. Analysis of the blood and urine for glucose and urine enables the patient and his physician to evaluate success in achieving and maintaining homeostasis. Although not specifically related to the control of diabetes mellitus, certain hygienic habits lessen the danger of skin infections such as boils and also help to protect tissues with a limited blood supply. For convenience, the habits which should be developed by the diabetic are divided into general hygiene, care of special areas, and care of the feet. If the patient is hospitalized, all these measures should be observed in the care of the patient. When the nurse is sufficiently aware of the importance of these measures and encourages the patient to practice what he is taught, the patient is more likely to be impressed with their importance than if they are neglected. Converscly, if the nurse does not carry out the necessary procedures in the care of the patient and does not help the patient to follow them, their importance is likely to be minimized to the patient.

What should the patient be taught concerning general hygiene?

The diabetic patient should be the cleanest person "on the block." Personal cleanliness, as well as clean clothing, is very important. Diabetic patients are more susceptible to "athlete's foot" and to pyogenic infections of the skin than nondiabetics. Cleanliness reduces the number of bacteria and other micro-organisms on the skin. The removal of the secretions from between the toes and from the skin makes conditions less favorable for the growth and multiplication of bacteria.

Instruction must be practical. This means that it should be adapted to the situation of the patient, including his customs, his habits, and his living conditions. For example, although a daily bath is frequently recommended as a desirable practice, some modifications are often necessary. For the patient with very dry skin frequent bathing intensifies the dryness and predisposes to itching. A patient living in a cold-water flat or in a farmhouse where water has to be carried in and out and where only one room is heated may find the effort and lack of privacy great obstacles to seriously considering a daily bath. Habits and customs also differ from one group to another. The elderly man who has always bathed once or twice a week is not likely to take kindly to a daily bath. When frequent bathing is rejected or is impractical, the nurse should stress the daily washing of the feet, the neck, and the pubic region.

In the diabetic patient the care of the feet cannot be overemphasized. Arteriosclerosis develops earlier and progresses more rapidly than it does in the nondiabetic. An injury to the toes that would pass unnoticed in the non-diabetic can, if neglected, lead to gangrene of the toe, foot, and leg. The feet of the diabetic patient require special care.

Today, with increased life expectancy and the availability of insulin for the control of severe diabetes, diabetic patients are living longer than at any other period in history. Diabetic coma, although still a serious complication, is no longer responsible for a high proportion of deaths, especially among young diabetics. Complications associated with diabetes mellitus usually result from arteriosclerosis. The thickening of the walls of the small arteries in particular results in a lessening of the blood supply to the tissues, which in turn reduces the ability of the tissues to respond favorably to injury. Consequently, when an older diabetic is admitted to the hospital, he should not only receive the care given to the nondiabetic patient, but special attention should be given to protect his lower extremities from injury. One of the most common causes of injury to the lower extremities is heat. Diabetics are remarkably sensitive to heat and may be burned by hot-water bottles, electric pads, and hot, moist packs. Therefore, heat in any of the above forms should not be applied below the knees. If moist dressings are applied, they should be just warm (100° to 105° F.).

Extremities of the diabetic patient should be protected not only from heat, but from the effects of pressure. A cradle placed under the covering at the foot of the bed prevents pressure from above and allows for freedom of movement. If the patient lies in one position more or less continuously, or if his blood supply is especially poor, a soft pillow under the ankle or heel will help lessen the pressure. Nurses caring for diabetic patients cannot exercise too much care in the protection of the patient's feet from injury. Cleanliness, protection of the feet, well-fitting shoes and hose, proper cutting of the nails, and prompt treatment of injuries when they occur are imperative. See Chapter 9 for more detailed instruction.

The diabetic patient should be taught to treat minor infections such as a common cold or an acute gastrointestinal infection by going to bed. He should avoid the use of sweetened cough mixtures and other agents which are sometimes taken during acute respiratory infections. He should test his urine at three-hour intervals during the day and at six-hour intervals during the night. Since any infection in the diabetic patient is an emergency, he should call his doctor and follow his advice.

The period during which the severity of diabetes is being evaluated and regulation is effected should be utilized to prepare the patient and the members of his family to assume the responsibility for controlling his diabetes. During this period he should learn what he needs to know to understand the nature of his disease and develop the skills needed to maintain his control. The objective should be for him to be the master of diabetes mellitus, rather than for it to be his master. The reward of mastery is a more nearly normal life. He should learn to avoid all excesses. Idleness is to be avoided as well as excess strain, tension, anxiety, emotional upsets, and overfatigue. Eight to ten hours' sleep at night and, if convenient, an hour of rest at midday is beneficial.

Some hospitals have well-organized plans for the instruction of patients with diabetes mellitus. Both group and individual instruction are arranged. More recently, some of the content has been programmed and placed on a teaching machine. Each method has its advantages and disadvantages. One of the advantages of group instruction is that the patient may be encouraged when he learns that other people's problems are not unlike his own. Patients may have an opportunity to share experiences and solutions to problems. Individual instruction allows for modification of the plan for the needs and problems of the patient. Programmed instruction permits the patient to progress in learning at his own rate. Theoretically, he does not progress until he has mastered each step. This form of instruction also insures that each patient receives a minimum of instruction. A well-planned program should cover all aspects required by the patient.

Whether patients are taught in groups or individually, instruction should be carefully planned and adapted to the needs of each individual patient. A variety of factors may interfere with the ability of the patient to learn. Sometimes, a patient is of low intellectual level. Other factors are more frequently responsible, however. The fact that the patient is adjusting to a new and anxiety-provoking diagnosis may decrease his learning capacity for the time being, because he is unable to give his attention to learning. His ability to learn may be lessened because he is not feeling well. Frequently the time that he is in the hospital is too short to master the necessary knowledge and skill. As soon as he begins to feel well, he is discharged. His ability or willingness to reveal significant factors in his home and work situation may be lacking. He may interpret instructions too literally. For example, Mr. Simon ate hamburgers every day for lunch because his doctor told him to eat what he had been eating in the hospital. This was all he could remember having been served for lunch while he was in the hospital. Also, the patient may not follow through with his prescribed treatment. This may be due to the stress involved in his adjustment at home or because he fails to understand the importance of continued treatment. The adjustment of the patient and his family is usually facilitated by a visit from a friendly professional nurse. When the patient's instruction has been inadequate, the services of the visiting nurse as a teacher are practically indispensable.

If the patient is to successfully assume the long-term management of diabetes mellitus, he needs to understand its nature and the measures that are used in its control. He also requires practice in a supportive environment until he develops skill and confidence in his ability to carry out the necessary procedures. For the nurse to provide the patient with the assistance that he needs, she should have a body of knowledge and have developed skills in teaching as well as in the performance of necessary procedures. In these programs nurses are usually responsible for certain aspects of the instruction of the patient. They should, therefore, be familiar with the total program. In hospitals and other agencies that do not have an organized instructional plan, the nurse should discuss the content of her plan for teaching with the physician so that the patient is protected from conflicting instructions, as this can be a source of psychological stress to the patient. Further, the nurse may be able to secure the cooperation of the physician and the dietitian in initiating a program of instruction.

If the patient is to be prepared to assume the management of his condition, he should receive the maximum rather than the minimum of instruction. To accomplish this, teaching should begin as soon as the diagnosis is established. When the physician's prescription is required before teaching can be started, it should be sought early. Most of the objections of physicians to nurses teaching patients are based on an experience in which a nurse used poor judgment in what she told a patient. In the experience of the author, these fears usually can be laid to rest by adequate preparation and discussion with the physician before the teaching is started.

Most, though by no means all, patients are motivated to learn. When the patient is unable for one reason or another to learn, members of the family or a neighbor may be enlisted to give the necessary assistance. Mrs. Delft never learned to administer her own insulin. Her son came each morning on his way to work to inject it. Certainly it would have been more convenient had Mrs. Delft learned to administer her own insulin. She refused, however, saying, "I just can't stick myself." Some patients such as Mrs. Curry do not see well enough to measure insulin and to carry out the details of the procedure.

In addition to making the most of the patient's interest in learning and being sure that he knows what he is to learn, the teaching should provide for thoughtful or understanding learning. Time should be taken to learn what the patient already knows or thinks he knows, as well as what he wants to know about diabetes. In the opinion of the author, there is a tendency to overestimate what persons who have had diabetes for some time know about their disease and its control. Although the average patient may not benefit from knowing the chemical reactions involved in the testing of urine, he is much more likely to test his urine regularly if he understands why he tests it and if he knows how to use the results. Sometimes the physician may ask the patient to keep a record of the results of urine testing. The patient should know that the information will help guide the physician in regulating his diabetes. As in other learning, the program should provide for sufficient repetition to make certain that the patient has had sufficient knowledge and practice to care for himself with confidence. Some of the factors that influence the amount of practice that a given patient needs are: the ability of the patient to learn, his interest in learning, and his confidence in himself. A great deal of encouragement is sometimes necessary. Emphasis should be on accomplishment rather than on failure.

As in other types of learning, the situation should provide the patient with an opportunity to perform procedures as nearly as possible as they will be carried out at home. For example, when Bonnie learns to administer her own insulin, she should learn the various parts of the procedure separately, but she should practice the procedure as a whole; that is, she should measure the dosage of insulin, make the injection, and care for the syringe following its use.

Practice periods should be distributed over a period of time rather than be limited to a single intensive practice. Unless the instruction of the diabetic patient is carefully planned, this factor in learning is likely to be disregarded. Instruction may include little more than a hasty demonstration and inadequate practice. The patient is then dismissed with the vain hope that he has mastered a set of complicated instructions and that he will be able to manage his diabetes. The worried patient goes home hoping for the best. Often, as a result of failure to appreciate the importance of the control of diabetes plus a lack of confidence in his ability to care for himself, the patient lapses into his old habits and sooner or later is readmitted to the hospital where the same procedure is repeated.

It follows that if the instruction of every diabetic patient is to be adequate, this instruction must be planned. The plan for the patient's instruction must suit the individual patient and his situation if it is to work. However, whether the instruction of the diabetic patient is given by a special instructor or is shared by a number of people, each person should know what his responsibilities are and every provision should be made to see that these functions are accomplished.

A not unimportant, but frequently little appreciated, part of teaching the patient is the teaching given by the nurse in her care and supervision of the patient. The nurse is in a favorable position to encourage the patient to express and examine his feelings about diabetes mellitus, to learn his misconceptions and doubts, and to answer or obtain answers to his questions. Some instruction she gives directly as instruction. Other teaching is done by example, for if she carries out and supervises his care conscientiously she does much to impress him with its importance. For example, if she collects the urine specimens promptly and correctly, she does much to impress the patient with the importance of regular and frequent testing of the urine. If she uses care in washing the feet of the patient and dries them well with a soft cloth, the patient is more certain to follow the example set. If the nurse insists that the patient who starts barefooted for the bathroom stop and put on his slippers, she is not only emphasizing what he has been taught, but she is giving him actual practice in it. The patient who is provided with a footstool and encouraged to elevate his feet is learning by doing.

Throughout the discussion of the needs of the patient with diabetes mellitus, emphasis has been placed on the importance of preparing the patient to manage himself, so that his diabetes is kept under control. Diet, exercise, and, when necessary, insulin or an insulin substitute are the principal measures used in the control of diabetes mellitus. Education is an essential aspect of therapy.

Because the patient and his family must eventually assume the responsibility for the management of the diabetes mellitus, the nurse must not do for the patient what he is able to do for himself. She should, however, interpret her actions so that he understands the reason for encouraging him to care for himself. She should also give recognition to progress made by the patient. The nurse must exercise a high degree of judgment in making the decision that the patient is or is not ready to assume more responsibility for his own care. In some instances, the patient is unable to assume full responsibility for his care and a member of his family must be taught to assist him. Insofar as the patient is able to participate, he should be included in any instruction. Whenever possible, one or more members of the family should also be included in the instructional plan, as family members can be helpful to the patient.

Even when instructions given in the physician's office or in the hospital are well planned and carried out, the patient and/or his family still may have some problems. When a visiting nurse service or public health nurse is available in the community, the patient can be helped to make the adjustment to full responsibility by a few visits from a nurse. Even when a patient is well taught in the hospital, problems are likely to arise in his adjustment at home or to his work situation. In addition to the usual sources of stress in hospitalized patients, he is adapting to diabetes and all that is entailed in its control.

Since anesthesia and surgery lessen the patient's glucose tolerance, the diabetic who has surgery must be diligently observed for signs of both diabetic coma and insulin reaction. Signs of either should be promptly reported. The patient's fluid intake and output should be promptly and carefully measured and recorded. On the day of surgery and for several days thereafter, all urine voided should be tested for sugar. Orders for parenteral fluids and insulin should be carried out promptly and as ordered. Frequently and regularly turning the patient, encouraging deep breathing, keeping the patient warm without overheating him, maintaining his fluid intake after food is allowed, seeing that his diet promptly follows his insulin injection are all important, as is encouraging him to eat all the food on his tray. If he does not, the amount of food left should be reported to the dietitian.

Summary

The nurse has two major responsibilities to the diabetic patient. They are the instruction of the patient in the management of his condition and his care during illness. The sick diabetic patient has all the problems of any person who is ill plus special ones which must be recognized and met. The nurse who assists in the care of diabetic patients has the satisfaction of knowing that the well-instructed diabetic patient has a good chance of living almost as long and as well as if he were not a diabetic.

PART B : Mr. Allen, A Patient Who Was Burned[37]

On the bright, crisp morning of October 15, Mr. Marshall Allen arose as usual at five o'clock. He dressed and started for the kitchen. A spark of static electricity, generated by his hob-nailed boots as he passed over the living-room rug, ignited gas that had escaped from a leaky gas stove. The force of the explosion that followed knocked him to the floor. He was slightly burned by the fire which was started by the explosion. He recovered quickly and went into the bedroom to get his son, seven-year-old Bobby, whom he carried to the head of the stairs outside their apartment. At this point, he fainted. Bobby in panic ran back into the apartment to get his overalls. As Mr. Allen revived, he heard Bobby's screams for help. He crawled back into the apartment, threw a coat over Bobby, and crawled back to the head of the stairs. Having extinguished the flames on himself and his son by beating them out with his hands, he then fainted again. This time he did not regain consciousness until he was in the admitting room at Emergency Hospital. After he had fainted, Bobby's screams aroused the neighbors, who called the fire department and the police.

Since Mr. Allen lived near the hospital, and was unconscious, he was placed on a stretcher between two clean sheets and transported to the hospital without treatment. Had he been having pain he would have been given an analgesic, probably morphine. Had the distance over which he would have had to travel been great, he might well have been given saline solution intravenously.

On their arrival in the admitting room of Emergency Hospital, it was determined that Bobby was much less seriously burned than his father. Bobby's total burned area was limited to about 4 per cent of his body surface. He had some second-degree burns on his left arm and a small area of first-degree burn on his face.

Mr. Allen, however, was hospitalized for the treatment of second- and third-degree burns over about 30 per cent of his body; most of them were second degree. From Figure 17-1-B the reader can see that his burns were distributed over his face, neck, both arms and hands, and the upper two thirds of his posterior chest. Because he had facial burns and some respiratory distress, tracheal burns were considered to be a possibility, and a tracheostomy was considered, but was determined to be unnecessary. Continued observation for indication of respiratory distress was necessary. To arrive at the percentage of body surface burned, his physician used the rule of nines. In Figure 17-2-B

---

[37] This part was contributed by Joyce Passos, Assistant Professor of Nursing, College of Nursing, Wayne State University, Detroit, Michigan.

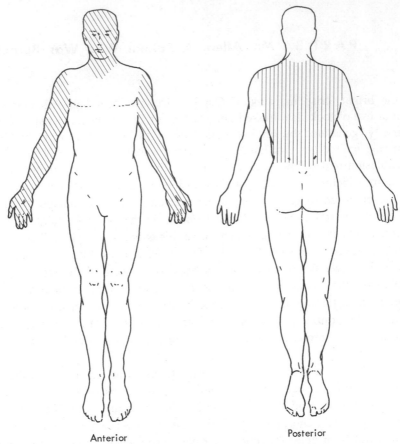

Anterior   Posterior

FIGURE 17—1-B. Distribution of burns on Mr. Allen's body surface. Anterior. Posterior.

the body is divided so that each area is equivalent to approximately 9 per cent of the total body surface.[38]

The history, taken from relatives, and the physical examination of Mr. Allen revealed the following information:

Personal data

 Age, 45 years; born in South Carolina.

 Migrated to big industrial city at age 29.

 Married and divorced twice; first wife was the mother of his two children.

 Children: Matthew, aged 18—lived with his mother; Bobby, aged 7—lived with Mr. Allen.

 Income—$100.00 per week.

 Occupation—welder.

 Living accommodations—second floor, three-room apartment in a lower-middle-class neighborhood (one bedroom).

[38] C. P. Artz and E. Reiss, *The Treatment of Burns*, W. B. Saunders Co., Philadelphia, 1957, p. 11.

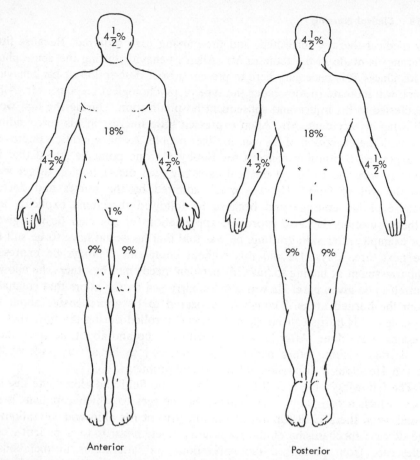

$4\frac{1}{2}\%$ $4\frac{1}{2}\%$

18%   18%

$4\frac{1}{2}\%$ $4\frac{1}{2}\%$ $4\frac{1}{2}\%$ $4\frac{1}{2}\%$

1%

9%   9%   9%   9%

Anterior   Posterior

FIGURE 17—2-B. Rule of nines. A rapid method of estimating percentage of body surface involved. Anterior. Posterior. (Adapted. Courtesy of C. P. Artz and E. Reiss, *The Treatment of Burns*, W. B. Saunders Co., Philadelphia, 1957, p. 11.)

Hospital insurance—none.

Income insurance—$49.00 per week.

Religion—no preference. Believed in God, thought what happened was God's will and that God would help him to recover.

Physical status

Slender, well-built man who had always been healthy. He appeared to be in good state of nutrition. His weight at the time of admission was about 165 lb (75 Kg).

Personal habits—smoked, and drank three to four bottles of beer a day.

Education—grade school.

Family—in addition to his children, he was one of six children. He appeared to have a close relationship with one brother and his wife.

The extensive table on the following pages summarizes, and emphasizes the pathophysiological changes that occurred in Mr. Allen because of his burns, the medical therapy instituted, and the nursing care required. Because little reference is made in the table to Mr. Allen's behavior during the acute phase of his illness, it is necessary here to present a brief description of his behavior, which will indicate to the reader the type of psychological response Mr. Allen manifested to his injury and subsequent hospitalization. During the first week following his accident, Mr. Allen expressed little interest in his surroundings and, with the exception of his son, in other people. As his condition improved, he expressed continuing concern for Bobby. At one point he stated that his recovery was due to "good medical care, my own determination to get well, and the will of God." He was much admired by the nurses and doctors because of his courage and because he followed directions explicitly and without question. He also expressed appreciation for the care he was given. For example, after skin grafting, he was told that he would have to lie still for the next three days. He did this without complaint. Though he expressed embarrassment at having to have his personal needs met by others, he allowed himself to be given care. He was also embarrassed by the odors that emanated from the burned areas. Though he appeared to be apprehensive about the dressing of his burns causing pain, he was controlled during the time that the dressings were done. After he was allowed to be up and about, he spent much of his time visiting other patients. He appeared to be a very independent person. He avoided discussion of his personal problems.

The following table includes discussion of the fluid and electrolyte disturbances which accompany severe burns; the dangers to which a patient is exposed when there is disruption of the integrity of the skin and alterations in the defense mechanisms of the respiratory tract; hazards to a patient's convalescence from prolonged immobilization; and alterations in metabolism, especially of proteins, in the immediate and long-term postburn period. In each case, the medical therapy instituted for Mr. Allen is presented, and there is detailed elaboration of action indicated for, and taken by, the nurse.

At the time Mr. Allen was admitted to Emergency Hospital, there was no doubt that he had been subject to severe psychological and physiological stress. Both his survival and that of his son had been threatened. He had reacted to this threat not just once, but twice. He was thrown to the floor with sufficient force that he lost consciousness, and he was burned. His burns were of a critical nature, as he had second- and third-degree burns over 30 per cent of his body and his burns were complicated by possible injury to the respiratory tract. These burns involved his face, arms, and hands.

Undoubtedly, when Mr. Allen recovered consciousness following the explosion, his impulse was to flee. However, as a parent he had to control this impulse and rescue his son. His son, on being released by the father, panicked as he found himself outside the apartment in his night clothes. Because his father was unable to restrain him, Bobby returned to the apartment to get his overalls. The father's and son's reactions represent two types of reactions to stress. In one, action is appropriate and thereby contributes to survival. The other is inappropriate and in this instance not only was ineffective, but increased the chance of injury or death. Despite differences in their behavior, similar psychological and physiological changes were undoubtedly taking place. By the mechanisms of repression or suppression the father was able to block out his pain on being burned, so that he could save his son. That he had pain is evidenced by the fact that he fainted each time after he rescued his son.

From the previous descriptive material, the reader will recognize that Mr. Allen fulfilled the role of a patient as is expected in our culture. As a result, he was accorded the approval of those who were responsible for his care. He showed great bravery in rescuing his son. Though he was very ill, he cooperated by making progress toward recovery. As he improved physically, he accepted the care that was necessary. He expressed his appreciation to those who cared for him and followed the instructions (orders) of the professional staff explicitly and without question. As a cooperative patient he merited and received their approval. He was able to be dependent when his condition required him to be. As his condition improved, he resumed his independent status. His expressed goal, to make a quick recovery so that he could resume the care of his son and return to work, was socially acceptable. Although he was not in a position to assume the entire financial burden for his care, he was not held to be responsible. Those who cared for him also expressed respect for the fact that he did not discuss his personal problems or complain that his wife had left him with the responsibility for rearing a young boy. His brother and his sister-in-law also behaved as relatives are expected to behave. They expressed appropriate concern for the welfare of the patient and were satisfied with a minimum of explanation. When the time came for Bobby to be discharged, they took him into their home. They visited Mr. Allen regularly and appeared to be interested in his welfare. The patient frequently expressed his appreciation for their kindness. Both Mr. Allen and his son recovered. Mr. Allen expressed his appreciation for the efforts of all who assisted in caring for him and his son.

Some of the ways in which Mr. Allen responded psychologically have been indicated in the description of how he came to be burned and in his general behavior during his recovery. He was reluctant to talk about how he came to be burned and what happened immediately following the accident. Artz and Reiss[39] say that this is a common reaction. Apparently the patient who has been severely burned wants to forget the suffering that he has experienced. Mr. Allen was unusual; despite the serious nature of his burns, he was able almost from the beginning to cooperate with the doctors and nurses. Patients who have been burned are frightened. They are frequently demoralized, and not infrequently whining, depressed, and demanding, easily discouraged, and certain they will not recover. These behaviors may continue for days or weeks. Mr. Allen, probably by sheer force of will, presented a calm and

[39] *Ibid.,* p. 209.

composed exterior to all who dealt with him throughout his period of hospitalization. The energy required to effect this composure might well have been directed to the healing of his injured body; it is impossible to say to what extent his progress was affected by his directing so considerable an effort into maintaining his composure. There is no doubt, however, that the fact that he was so cooperative and composed made ministering to him considerably easier and more pleasant for all concerned with his care and recovery.

Changes	Observations and Medical Therapy	Nurse Should
Inhalation of carbon particles (smoke) and superheated air which accompanied Mr. A.'s burn resulted in some depression, and possible destruction, of the defense mechanisms which contribute to the cleansing action of the respiratory tract:	Watch closely for any signs of respiratory distress.	On admission, observe for: Singed nasal hairs, Blackened rim of nares, especially when adjacent skin is not burned, Rapid, noisy respirations—as wind passing over a dry reed, Hoarseness, Dry, wracking cough, Cyanosis of unburned skin and toenail beds, Râles, Black particles and/or blood in sputum coughed up.
Extreme temperature and absence of any moisture in inhaled air leads to: drying of protective mucin, cessation of flagellation of cilia, and sustained contact of debris with mucosa.		
High temperature and presence of foreign bodies in prolonged contact with tracheobronchial mucosa leads to: vasodilatation, increased capillary permeability, and edema possibly leading to laryngeal obstruction.		
Skin surfaces involved by burn included: Right side of face, all of anterior neck surface, both arms and hands, and upper two thirds of posterior chest.	Check vital signs every 30 minutes.	Know location and operation of: Oxygen equipment Laryngoscope Endotracheal tube Tracheostomy set Aspirator Check vital signs frequently: Blood pressure: Place cuff around left thigh, stethoscope over popliteal space with leg extended. After intravenous injection is started in left saphenous vein, speed up rate before insufflating cuff and deflate quickly. Pulse: Count with stethoscope during blood pressure reading; after intravenous injection, take pulse in left temporal or left femoral, popliteals, or if possible, in pedal pressure points. Respirations. Temperature: Take rectally.
Although blood pressure and pulse are not as sensitive indices of circulatory status and adequacy of therapy as they are in circulatory collapse due to hemorrhage, they should be recorded every 30 minutes in the early phase of therapy, since serious difficulty is certain when the pulse suddenly increases or blood pressure suddenly falls.[1]		

[1] C. P. Artz and E. Reiss, *The Treatment of Burns*, W. B. Saunders Co., Philadelphia, 1957, p. 36.

Changes	Observations and Medical Therapy	Nurse Should
Mr. A. was considered to be critically burned according to the starred items in the following criteria: A. Critical burns *1. Burns complicated by respiratory tract injury. 2. Partial-thickness burns of more than 30% of body surface. *3. Full-thickness burns of face, hands, feet, genitalia, or, more than 10% of body surface. 4. Burns complicated by fractures or major soft-tissue injury. 5. Electrical burns. 6. Deep acid burns. B. Moderate burns 1. Partial-thickness burns of 15 to 30% of body surface. 2. Full-thickness burns less than 10% of body surface, provided the hands, face, or genitalia are not involved. C. Minor burns 1. Partial thickness of less than 15% of body surface. 2. Full thickness of less than 2% of body surface. Extent of Mr. A.'s burn was estimated by the rule of nines (as shown in Fig. 17-2-B). The initial estimate of the type and amount of fluids to be administered to Mr. A. in the first 48 hours was calculated by the Brooke formula, according to the severity of the burn:[2] A. 0.5 ml. colloid per Kg of body weight for each 1% of body surface burned. B. 1.5 ml. electrolyte solution per Kg of body weight for each 1% of body surface burned (0.9% solution of saline widely used). C. 2,000 ml glucose in water.	Keep femoral vein cutdown open at all times. *Intravenous injection fluids for first 12 hours (see Chapter 8).*	

[2] *Ibid.*, pp. 41-42.

Changes	Observations and Medical Therapy	Nurse Should
Clinical shock is a preventable syndrome, provided adequate therapy can be instituted soon after injury.		Prepare patient for a cutdown in right femoral vein. In clear, unexcited, low tones explain to Mr. A.—whether or not he asks or seems frightened—that he will have:
Mr. A. arrived at Emergency Hospital 45 minutes after he rescued his son. To ensure that Mr. A. would receive uninterrupted fluid and electrolyte therapy essential to the early management of his burns, an intravenous cannula was inserted by cutdown into the right femoral vein, and tied securely; in addition, an intracatheter was inserted in his left saphenous vein, on the medial aspect of the ankle.	Set up: 1,000 ml dextrose 5% in water. 1,000 ml isotonic saline Femoral vein cut down.	1. Two tubes into his veins by which to feed him for a while. 2. A tube into his bladder to be sure of how his kidneys are working. 3. An immediate trip to the operating room, so his burns can be cleansed in the shortest time and with the best protection and minimal pain for him.
One ml of aqueous heparin solution, 1%, was to be injected every 4 to 6 hours into the cutdown tubing, to help prevent thrombosis at the tip of the catheter. (This does not significantly affect the coagulation mechanism.) Therapy with fluids and electrolytes is the most important aspect of the early management of burns. Among the alterations in fluid and electrolytes is a decrease in the circulating plasma volume due to the passage of water, electrolytes, and proteins into the interstitial space around the burned area. Since more water than protein is lost into this space an increase in the concentration of circulating plasma protein occurs. With the increase in the plasma proteins osmotic pressure rises and fluid moves from the cells to the interstitial fluid to restore osmotic pressure relationships. Thus the rest of the body is dehydrated by the fluid loss. Some degree of anemia occurs because erythrocytes are destroyed by hemolysis and loss by bleeding into the burned area.	Foley catheter to gravity drainage stat. Urine volume and specific gravity every hour.	4. Medication to ease the pain and help him relax. Assemble two independent intravenous injection setups with prescribed solutions, placing one on each side of Mr. A. Set up male catheterization tray for physician, or if he is occupied with intravenous injections, use qualified male attendant.
Free hemoglobin released from hemolyzed cells may be filtered in the glomeruli and may produce renal damage. Although early hemoconcentration may be present, the diminished number of erythrocytes becomes apparent after the volume of water in the body is restored to normal.		

Changes	Observations and Medical Therapy	Nurse Should
The sodium content of the extracellular fluid is depleted by a large amounts of sodium entering the edema fluid in the burned area. When sodium continues to be lost in edema fluid and by diuresis, the patient may remain in negative sodium balance for several weeks. Loss of bicarbonate (HCO₃) accompanies that of sodium. The loss of bicarbonate may be aggravated by starvation, ketosis and retention of acid metabolic products by the kidneys. Consequently, acidosis often develops.	*On admission* Hematocrit—60 mm % (N = 40-50 mm %) Hemoglobin—14.2 gm % (N = 12-18 gm %) Total protein—5.2 gm % (N = 7.2 gm %) Albumin—3.4 gm % (N = 5.2 gm %) Globulin—2.0 gm % (N = 1.8 gm %) Blood sugar—148 mg % (N = 70-120 mg %) Type and cross-match for 1 unit of blood. Set up two additional units.	Connect indwelling catheter to sterile drainage set and a sterile, stable, *calibrated* collecting reservoir. Be sure connecting drainage tubing is free of any obstruction which will interfere with free gravity flow and that collection unit is protected against being turned over or broken. (E.g., if a bottle is used, suspend from bed frame.) Be sure measurement is done in a receptacle with calibrations at least as fine as 5 ml.
When plasma is administered by intravenous infusion protein levels are usually increased early in treatment. Later, however, the patient is likely to lose more protein than is assimilated and to continue to do so until healing occurs.[3]		Be sure volumes are measured and recorded every hour and that volumes less than 30 ml or greater than 50 ml per hour are reported immediately to the physician. Urinary volumes in excess of 100 ml every hour indicate overloading, while urinary volumes below 10 to 20 ml every hour for two or more hours indicate need for more energetic therapy.
The increased capillary permeability to protein is limited to the burned areas and does not occur at sites away from the wound. A rapid loss of extracellular fluid from the uninjured parts of the body is first manifested by a reduction in extracellular fluid, which is mainly a mixture of NaCl and NaHCO₃. Thus the shift of extracellular fluid into the burned areas represents a loss of Na salts and water by the unburned parts (dehydration).		Measure and record specific gravity every one hour or as often as cumulative hourly volumes enable the urinometer to float. A concentration in excess of 1.020 to 1.030 may indicate progressive hemoconcentration and should be reported stat.

[3] *Fluid and Electrolytes*, Abbott Laboratories, No. Chicago, Illinois, April, 1961, p. 46.

Changes	Observations and Medical Therapy	Nurse Should
Thus the tremendous accumulation of Na in injured tissues plays a primary role in the reduction of plasma volume, and provides the rationale for use of isotonic Na solution in the treatment of burn shock. The greatest fluid losses occur deep in the wound. Third-degree burns are misleading, as they are characterized by a dry surface (eschar) and a small amount of visible swelling. Large quantities of fluid may accumulate in deep tissue without any evidence of swelling. Relatively small changes in a measurable parameter, such as the circumference of a limb, may be associated with a surprisingly large fluid accumulation. In third-degree burns, the entire thickness of the skin is destroyed. Capillaries are thrombosed close to the surface of the wound, with the result that: 1. Erythrocytes are removed from circulation (contributes to anemia). 2. Fluid exchange ceases (explains why fluid losses do not originate in the most severely burned tissues). Water and electrolytes do not exchange in the eschar of a third-degree burn. The extensive fluid loss appears to be due to injury of a large volume of tissue beneath and surrounding the area of full-thickness skin destruction; the deeper the wound, the greater the fluid loss. Pulmonary edema may develop in the severely burned patient owing to: 1. Excessive fluid therapy. 2. Damage to respiratory tract due to inhalation of noxious gases. 3. Invasive pulmonary infection. However, with improvements in fluid therapy this is becoming rare in a patient such as Mr. A., who has far less than 60% of his body surface burned, and whose age and general health favor his recovery.		Note character of urine for: Deepening of amber color. Pink tinge (indicating presence of blood). Casts, sediment (indicating albumin or cells). Odor. Observe him for changes in C.N.S. function which will reflect hypoxia (indicating need to intensify fluid replacement and/or to administer O_2), and report stat.: Restlessness. Disorientation. What is your name? Where are you? What day, time, year? Irrational, maniacal behavior. Observe for nausea, vomiting, report stat. (May indicate: circulatory collapse, stress response, acute gastric dilatation, paralytic ileus, increasing intensity of pain, or nonspecific effect of injury.) Observe for thirst (usually first sign of fluid deficit). Observe for signs and symptoms of pulmonary edema: Increased restlessness; Cyanosis of toenail beds, feet, ears, conjunctival sac; Increase in moist, labored respirations; Complaints of feeling of chest constriction, desire to sit up; Marked increase in pulse; Alteration (possible decrease) in B.P.; Hemoptysis. Observe burned areas for amount, kind of drainage. Observe unburned areas for contour, size, resistance of tissues to palpation, to estimate accumulation of fluid in tissues. With Mr. A, this may be most evident in: feet, ankles, calves, thighs, presacral area, genitalia.

Changes	Observations and Medical Therapy	Nurse Should
Mr. A.'s burns were débrided in the operating room without a general anesthetic. The recency of his injury (1½ hours postburn he was in the operating room), his stoical cooperation, and the administration of morphine, 10 mg, on admission, made it possible to complete débridement with only a small amount of local anesthesia.		
On his admission to the surgical ward, the doctors decided to supplement his intravenous fluid therapy with oral salt solution, which is considerably the best form if the patient can tolerate it. (8 hours after injury, Mr. A. had had no nausea or vomiting.)	Give Haldane's solution, 30 to 60 ml, every one hour as tolerated. Intravenous cutdown set: 1,000 ml dextrose 5% in saline. Run in by 12 midnight.	Mix: 4 Gm of NaCl = 1 tsp; 2 Gm of bicarbonate of soda = ½ tsp; in 1 qt. of water, keep chilled for optimum tolerance, and offer Mr. A. about 15 ml every 15-20 minutes, increasing volume and decreasing frequency as tolerated. (May flavor with lemon if physician has no objection.) Observe for evidence of gastric retention. Keep minutely accurate record of all intake, by every route.
The lymphatic system apparently plays a major role in picking up the leaking plasma proteins, thus increasing its ability to draw fluids from the tissues and convey them back to the depleted vascular compartment.[4] In uncomplicated burns of minor extent, the rate at which edema fluid is withdrawn from the wound approximates the rate of its accumulation. In more extensive burns, and particularly those complicated by infection, the wound edema may persist for 2 to 3 weeks.	Intravenous injection to follow: 500 ml dextrose 5% in water.	Be sure intravenous solutions are numbered, administered, and recorded in sequence. Observe cutdown site for evidence of phlebitis: Palpate thigh and low abdomen for increased tension, induration; Note any streaks of red around site; Note any increase in warmth of area compared with other extremity; Check rectal temperature at least every 4 hours; Enlargement of part;
Within 48 hours after his injury, Mr. A.'s extremities and genitalia demonstrated evidence of retained fluid, his urinary output had ranged from 30 to 60 ml in one hour, and he had demonstrated no signs or symptoms of overloading. On the third postburn day, diuresis began, with hourly volumes ranging from 80 to 120 ml per hour; there was a decrease in his lower extremity circumferential measurements, and a weight loss of 3 lb. By the fourth postburn day, Mr. A.'s intravenous fluid therapy was discontinued, and he was able to maintain an adequate intake of food and fluids by mouth.		Observe, estimate or measure, record, and report output from all sources: Stools, especially important if Mr. A. should develop diarrhea; Sweating, and drainage from exposed areas: Note number of times linen must be changed; estimate...

[4] Arthur Grollman, *Clinical Physiology*, McGraw-Hill Book Co., Blakiston Div., New York, 1957, p. 135.

Changes	Observations and Medical Therapy	Nurse Should
		mate degree of saturation. Vomiting Sputum Urine (as ordered above)
With extensive destruction of his body's first barrier against infection, invasion of microorganisms, and covered with charred clothing and dirt as the burned areas were, Mr. A. was subject to infection by anaerobic microbes, especially *Clostridium tetani*.	Tetanus toxoid, 0.5 ml S.C. stat.	Explain that the injection is to protect him against infection (lockjaw?). Because this induces active immunity, observe for signs and symptoms of anaphylaxis (see Chapter 5).
Infection is always a hazard in burn cases, and may delay the reabsorption of edema fluid at the site of the burn.[5] It was therefore imperative to promote as clean and rapid a closure of Mr. A.'s wounds as possible.	N.P.O Prepare for O.R. stat. Prepare morphine, 10 mg, for intravenous injection stat.	In admitting room, have generous supply of masks, gowns, gloves, with provision for clean storage and discard areas. Be responsible for seeing that all personnel who come in contact with Mr. A. don all three.
Immediately on his arrival in the admitting room, Mr. A. had all of the burned areas scrubbed by one physician using a phisohex solution, while the second physician initiated intravenous fluids. Phisohex (diphenol in a detergent base, with G.-11) is particularly effective against gram-positive bacteria, and has the added advantage that it leaves a protective film on the area to discourage establishment of secondary infection. This cleansing procedure was done with surgical aseptic technique. All debris and detached epidermis were then removed, blisters were broken, and the skin was trimmed in preparation for grafting in the operating room.		Explain to Mr. A. that all personnel are in special dress to protect him from infection of his burns. Check with physician about whether he has requested brother to sign operative permit after physician has explained need for grafting to Mr. A. If necessary, have operative permit signed.
General agreement exists that full-thickness burns should be excised and the defect grafted as soon as possible to: 1. shorten the period of protein loss, 2. diminish infection and toxic absorption, 3. reduce scar formation.	Débridement of second- and third-degree burns of both arms and hands, right side of face, all of anterior neck, and of second-degree burns of upper ⅔ of posterior trunk.	Assure Mr. A. and family about security of his valuables, reassure them that his appearance at this time is not necessarily indicative of a poor prognosis, and inform family of the unit to which he will be transferred after leaving the O.R. Call the ward to allow time for preparation of a room to receive Mr. A. after he is grafted.

[5] *Fluid and Electrolytes, Op. cit.*, p. 46.

Changes	Observations and Medical Therapy	Nurse Should
	Postage-stamp grafts from left anterior thigh were applied to anterior surface of both forearms. Occlusive dressings applied to both hands, with fingertips exposed. Fine-mesh gauze applied to donor site. All but hands to be treated by exposure. Have Circo-Electric bed to receive patient from O.R. table.	Be sure entire bed is washed down with a bactericidal solution and sterile sheets are used to make up anterior and posterior frame mattresses. Be sure mattresses and any pillows to be used in positioning are protected with soft plastic covers.
Partial-thickness burns treated by the exposure method heal uneventfully beneath the protective covering of the crust. If kept dry, the dead skin of a full-thickness burn seems to serve as an excellent cover for the wound to protect it from bacterial invasion.[6]		
During the first 48 hours after exposure, patients have pain and complain of chilling, but they are quite comfortable after the crust has formed.	Demerol, 75 mg I.M. every 3 hours prn.	
Treatment by exposure eliminates need for frequent dressing changes; it is well established that frequent anesthesia of a severely injured patient is detrimental to his prognosis.[7] It is not known how crust formation occurs without infection. However, when bacteria are transplanted to a new environment, there is a preliminary period in which certain bacteria die off		

[6] Artz and Reiss, *Op. cit.*, p. 74.
[7] *Ibid.*, p. 76.

Changes	Observations and Medical Therapy	Nurse Should

and others fail to multiply. In their effort to adjust metabolically to a new environment, bacteria are thwarted by what happens on the exposed burned surface; the exudate dries and the bacteria are subjected to an environment that is cooler than body temperature. Drying is a deterrent to bacterial reproduction. Proliferation of contaminating microorganisms is hindered, and the dried cover prevents invasive infection.

Antibiotics are given prophylactically. Penicillin diffuses freely into the exudate of recent burns. As drying proceeds, concentration of penicillin on the burned surface actually increases, and it is likely that the fully formed crust has a considerable quantity of penicillin incorporated in it.

The eschar of a full-thickness burn is composed of dehydrated dead skin. As long as it remains dry, it appears to be an effective barrier against invading microorganisms. Since bacteria around the hair follicles and in the sweat glands remain viable in many full-thickness burns, a certain amount of infection always occurs beneath the eschar, which is dead skin and must ultimately be removed.[8]

The following microorganisms are the most common contaminants of unhealed burn wounds:
Gram-negative: *B. proteus, E. coli; Pseudomonas*
Gram-positive: *Staphylococcus albus* and *aureus, Streptococcus* —alpha, beta, and gamma.

Partial thickness burns should show crust formation within 48 to 72 hours, with epithelial regeneration under the crust producing a healed surface in 14 to 21 days.

Chloromycetin, 250 mg p.o. every 6 hours.
Penicillin, 1.2 million units, intramuscularly every 12 hrs.
Streptomycin, 0.5 gm every 12 hours, intramuscularly.

Request chloromycetin suspension to limit amount of water. Mr. A. would otherwise be required to take pills every 6 hours.
Rotate injection sites among upper outer quandrants of glutei, anterior superior glutei as they attach to crest of each ileum, and right quadriceps.

Select a single room or cubicle, prepare the unit, and assign personnel to care for Mr. A. in a way which will promote the priority need to prevent infection and promote epithelization:

I. Reverse precautions
A. All materials coming in contact with Mr. A. must be sterile until crust and eschar have formed; then strict medical asepsis must be maintained until his wounds are covered by epithelium.

---

[8] *Ibid.*, pp. 74-75.

1347

Changes	Observations and Medical Therapy	Nurse Should

Full-thickness burns should develop eschar within 48 to 72 hours after exposure, with liquefaction occurring beneath it within 12 to 21 days.[9]
 	
In treating the burns of Mr. A.'s hands, it was most important to achieve a good functional result. Occlusive dressings are preferred because:
1. Position of function is better maintained.
2. Demarcation between areas of second and third degree can be detected earlier.
3. Separation of the eschar is more rapid.[10]
 	
Success of the exposure method depends almost entirely on how adequately complete exposure and immobilization of all burned areas can be achieved so that crust and eschar can form. The protective cover must be managed in such a way as to prevent softening and maceration or cracking.
 	
Elevation of burned areas hastens fluid absorption (edema) and should be used unless it causes undue discomfort. Infection may originate from bacteria which survive deep within the wound or from outside contaminants. Two types of infection may develop:
1. Local invasive—cellulitis, lymphangitis, regional lymphangitis.
2. Generally invasive—septicemia: a positive blood culture in combination with the signs and symptoms of invasion of the blood stream.
	I. Protective isolation.
	II. Change position every 2 hours.
	III. Turn 30 degrees side to side, and front to back.
	IV. Prevent:
	  A. Flexion of arms.
	  B. Turning of head.
	  C. Disturbance of fine-mesh gauze covering donor site.
	  D. Friction over posterior trunk when turning.
	V. Cough and deep-breathe every hour.
	VI. Check pulse, respiration, and temperature every hour, and blood pressure every 4 hours.
	VII. Do not allow patient to use bandaged hands.
		1. All personal care equipment must be sterilized before placing it in his unit.
		2. Individual thermometer and, if possible, sphygmomanometer and stethoscope, should be separated for his use.
		3. All personnel must be instructed and expected to wear gloves, gown, mask.
		4. All linen must be sterile.
		B. Clean and dirty areas for storage and discard of equipment should be clearly labeled and all personnel instructed in their use.
		C. All visitors should be assured that Mr. A.'s isolation is to protect him from them, and be properly dressed and instructed before being allowed to enter Mr. A.'s unit. (They should be prepared to expect rather extensive facial edema within the early postburn period, so that they—and consequently the patient—are not frightened and repulsed by the inevitable change in his appearance.)
		D. Room should include a sink with running water. If this is not available, modifications requiring use of hand-wash basins should be carefully thought out and their use made clear to all who enter the unit before they are allowed in to see or work with Mr. A.
		E. Floor and furniture in unit should be damp-dusted at least once a day by person assigned to care for Mr. A., unless housekeeping staff can be instructed in, and carry out, satisfactory isolation precaution procedures.

[9] *Ibid.*, pp. 66-69.
[10] *Ibid.*, p. 77.

Changes	Observations and Medical Therapy	Nurse Should

Principal therapeutic problem is to prevent septicemia prior to the time when a granulating barrier is established. Septicemia is probably the most serious complication in burns, causing—directly or indirectly—about 50% of the deaths.

Patients who develop septicemia after three weeks either fail to grow granulation tissue or experience destruction of this previously formed barrier. The sudden disappearance of apparently healthy granulations within a period of a few days is one of the most discouraging occurrences in treatment of a severe burn. Since the disappearance of granulation and the onset of septicemia are almost simultaneous, it is impossible to identify which is cause and which effect.

However, it is reasonable to suppose that impairment of the granulating barrier against infection creates a condition that facilitates invasion of the blood stream.

Onset of septicemia may be insidious or acute. A blood culture is indicated in any burned patient whose rectal temperature is 103° F. or higher.

Clinical features of septicemia may include:

1. High temperature (104° to 107° F. rectally)
2. Rapid and regular pulse
3. Hypotension and oliguria
4. Paralytic ileus
5. Disorientation
6. Increased bleeding tendency
7. Mild jaundice

It is to prevent this dreaded complication that therapy includes:

1. Removal of eschar

Nurse Should

II. Place bed in a position in relation to door and windows that will prevent drafts over the patient as people leave and enter his room.

III. Assignment of staff

  A. Case method, not functional, to reduce numbers of persons having to enter room.

  B. Use best qualified person available, a registered nurse if possible, to enable the most to be done by the fewest hands.

  C. Allow nobody in the unit who has any signs of an upper respiratory infection, or evidence of any other impending illness.

IV. Temperature and humidity control

  A. Have room at least 75°-80° F., with high humidity. (To decrease Mr. A.'s feeling cold and to promote crust and eschar formation.)

  B. Add moisture to air by placing a protected water source over heater or by using a cold-steam humidifier.

    1. During immediate postburn period, a "tent" of sterile sheets may need to be made over Circo-Electric bed frame and cold steam directed into his immediate environment to promote hydration of oropharyngeal-tracheal mucosa.

    2. After reaction of mucosa of respiratory tract has subsided, and normal defense mechanisms are again operating (48-72 hours), "tent" may be removed and humidifier directed into entire unit. Door must be kept closed at all times.

Schedule Mr. A.'s plan of care so that he is not left isolated behind a closed door for prolonged periods of time. Extensive physical care should be consolidated to conserve his energy and minimize pain, but frequent visits to check

Changes	Observations and Medical Therapy	Nurse Should
		his output, offer fluids, and bring his mail, should be provided.
2. Systemic antibiotics 3. Grafting[11]		Bathe any unburned skin with phisohex when giving personal hygiene care. Instruct Mr. A. to deep-breathe and cough:
Many factors contribute to the acute need to ensure that Mr. A. is vigorously encouraged to maintain pulmonary function:		1. Inspire against pressure of nurse's hands on anterior-lateral surface of his thorax.
1. He will have some degree of tracheobronchial edema due to inhalation of superheated air.		2. Expire forcibly, with assistance of nurse's hands, to compress thorax as completely as possible.
2. He may have some degree of bronchitis due to his history of being a cigarette smoker.		3. After a sequence of exchanges, cough at the onset of the expiratory phase.
3. He must be immobilized for many days to promote healing of his wounds.		4. Have tissue over Mr. A.'s nose and mouth before he coughs.
Positioning which will best promote function following the prolonged immobilization necessary for patients with burns includes:		Position, turn, and exercise him to provide optimal exposure of all burned areas, redistribution of pressure, and immobilization of arms and head:
1. Extension of neck.		1. Head must be in neutral position with sandbags placed to prevent rotation (to protect grafts on neck) when Mr. A. is on posterior frame.
2. Anatomical position of trunk and hips.		
3. Almost complete extension of the knees.		On anterior frame, forehead support and body weight promote immobilization.
4. Dorsiflexion of ankles to prevent shortening of Achilles tendon.		Do not address Mr. A. until you are standing directly in his vision.
5. Anatomical position of shoulders, except in burns of the axilla where the shoulders should be abducted to 90 degrees.		Place bed so he can see those entering his room without having to turn his head.
6. Extension of the elbow to 140 degrees unless there is a burn in the antecubital fossa.		2. As soon as cutdown is discontinued, and crust has formed on donor site, Mr. A. can be encouraged to move both legs freely, being careful not to strike
7. Extension of the wrist and flexion of the fingers.		

[11] Ibid., pp. 147-55.

Changes	Observations and Medical Therapy	Nurse Should
		donor site against anything. Teach, supervise, and encourage:
		Quadriceps setting exercises,
		Gluteal setting exercises,
		Flexion extension exercises of legs and feet,
		Wiggling toes, and pressing on footboard (see Chapter 9.)
		3. Keep elbow joint as nearly straight as possible, support arms (under elbow to produce extension) with rolled towels, bath blankets, or small pillows to elevate hands just above shoulder (to promote venous return and decrease edema of wrapped hands) when Mr. A. is on posterior frame.
		On anterior frame, support to arms should be placed under wrists with arms extended, so that weight of arms will keep elbow joint straight.
		4. As long as hands are wrapped, provide only for elevation of extremities and observe for signs of impaired circulation.
		When dressings are removed, and granulation has become established, Mr. A. should begin simple gross movements (probably holding a glass with both hands, squeezing a gauze pad, flexion-extension of arm and fingers) under direction of physiotherapist.
After three days, when intravenous fluid therapy was no longer necessary, Mr. A. was allowed to "stand" with Circo-Electric bed in the perpendicular position. When he was able to tolerate this for more than 15 minutes, he was assisted to stand on the floor, take a few steps, and return, ensuring that his head and arms remained immobile. Ambulation then progressed in frequency and duration, but he remained on the frame until the fourteenth postburn day, when his posterior chest wounds exhibited a healed surface.		5. To provide for regular frequent exposure of his posterior chest burn, Mr. A. should be turned prone and his back exposed for one hour every two hours, at least until he is able to be out of bed with his back exposed. Whenever Mr. A.'s posterior chest or arms are in contact with any surface—frame or supportive devices—the burned areas must be covered with sterile, fine-mesh, gauze absorptive dress-

Changes	Observations and Medical Therapy	Nurse Should
		ing to protect the exposed and granulating surfaces. A good protective covering will usually form in 72 to 96 hours.
		6. As soon as facial burns have granulated, Mr. A. should be encouraged to chew gum and blow up balloons.

In Protein Metabolism

Proteins are the basic components of cellular protoplasm, composed of carbon, hydrogen, oxygen, nitrogen, and often sulfur. With complete hydrolysis, proteins yield various crystalline amino acids, which may be:

1. Synthesized into protein,
2. Metabolized to H_2O and CO_2 for energy production, or
3. Converted to glucose or fat.

Of the 23 known amino acids, 10 are essential in the diet because they cannot be synthesized in the body; foods containing these are called complete proteins. Incomplete protein can be synthesized from products of glucose and fat metabolism and also occurs in vegetable proteins.

Amino acids absorbed in the intestine go directly to the liver via the portal vein, where some are stored and others are sent on to body tissues.

In the absence of food, protein will be deprived of its nitrogen and converted into glucose to keep up the blood sugar level and to provide the glucose essential to the burning of body fat for fuel. As much as 58% of protein, by weight, may thus be turned to glucose to be burned along with fat for fuel, or serve as the sole source of fuel when body fat is exhausted. The nitrogen output of the fasting man is thus

Changes	Observations and Medical Therapy	Nurse Should
raised because he uses protein for fuel as well as for building purposes.		
To minimize this extravagant use of protein in a patient unable to ingest (or digest) food by the oral route, carbohydrate should be given to supply the glucose necessary to provide energy and spare protein.	1,000 ml dextrose 10% in water intravenous daily × two.	Execute observation and precautions previously indicated in Chapter 8 in relation to intravenous therapy instituted in admitting room at time of arrival.
The normal adult is in nitrogen equilibrium; intake equals excretion, and the total quantity of protein stores remains essentially stable. Positive nitrogen balance implies that the rate of anabolism exceeds the rate of catabolism. Negative nitrogen balance exists when catabolism exceeds anabolism.		
In the early postburn period, Mr. A. was in negative nitrogen balance (excessive catabolism) due to imbalance created by excessive losses in wound exudate and increased excretion of urinary nitrogen, mostly as urea, resulting from hydrolysis of proteins for energy and extensive destruction of tissue protein by burn injury. When amino acids are burned for fuel, they are deprived of their nitrogen and reduced to compounds containing only carbon-hydrogen-oxygen, which burns like sugar and fat. The nitrogen, being of no use as fuel, is converted into a relatively harmless soluble substance, urea, and excreted in the urine.		
An adult ingesting a normal diet excretes from 10 to 15 gm of urinary nitrogen a day; the same adult, following an extensive burn, may excrete as much as 30 gm of urinary nitrogen a day. During the first few days postburn, increased excretion of urinary nitrogen is not evident because of impaired renal function. High excretion becomes evident within 3 to 5 days postburn, reaching a maximum in the first and		

1353

Changes	Observations and Medical Therapy	Nurse Should
second postburn week. Magnitude of urinary nitrogen loss varies with the following factors: 1. There is a rough correlation between the severity of the burn and the amount of nitrogen excreted; the more extensive the burn, the larger the nitrogen excretion. 2. Preburn body weight is positively correlated with nitrogen excretion. 3. Men generally excrete more than women. 4. Usually increased nitrogen excretion does not occur in patients malnourished before injury. Excellent healing has been known to occur in the presence of marked negative nitrogen balance; however, persistent negative nitrogen balance, such as occurs following extensive burns, results in serious debilitation, increased susceptibility to infection, poor granulation tissue, and poor graft takes and often is responsible for the death of the patient. Force-feeding programs to offset nitrogen losses are contraindicated. Although it is theoretically possible to achieve nitrogen equilibrium in the early postburn period, the seriously burned patient during the first 5 to 10 postburn days is unable to tolerate oral intake required to increase protein ingestion. He often suffers nausea, vomiting, and gastrointestinal atony manifested by abdominal distention and decreased peristalsis. Forced feeding may be followed by unusually severe gastric dilatation, which may then persist for several days. A crucial element in improving the patient's nutrition is proper timing. Mr. A. tolerated chilled Haldane's solution well, and it was decided on the fourth postburn day to offer him additional oral intake.	Offer full liquids up to 90 ml per hour as tolerated.	Offer liquids up to 90 ml per hour as tolerated. Assess Mr. A.'s tolerance for, and encourage: cream soups,

Changes	Observations and Medical Therapy	Nurse Should
		eggnogs, flavored if necessary, and meat stock broth
		Identify Mr. A.'s favorite drinks:
		1. Disliked plain milk, but took large amounts on cereal and in coffee.
		2. Liked 2 cups of coffee, took 2 tablespoons of sugar in each cup.
		3. Liked ice cream.
		4. Tolerated high-protein powdered-milk preparation for supplementary feedings if flavored heavily with coffee or strawberry and served cold.
		Refrain from forcing more than Mr. A. takes willingly, to avoid his developing a strong aversion to food early in his convalescence.
		Allow 10 to 15 minutes for offering liquids, as Mr. A. is unable to hold container, and his willingness to drink may be in direct proportion to the relaxation and encouragement of nurse's attitude.
		Observe closely for:
		1. Eructation
		2. Nausea
		3. Abdominal distention
		4. Complaints of cramps, abdominal pain.
		Discontinue feedings if any of above signs or symptoms develop, and report to M.D. immediately.
		Estimate exudate lost in dressings and on linen.
		Weigh patient daily after he is allowed out of bed. Keep accurate record of all intake and output.
Plasma proteins serve as a reservoir of protein during the catabolic phase following severe injury.		
A loss of 30 gm of tissue protein represents an accompanying loss of approximately 1 gm of total protein per 100 ml of serum.		

Changes	Observations and Medical Therapy	Nurse Should
Loss of protein, especially albumin (smaller molecule), but also globulin (larger molecule), tends to persist until wound healing is complete. Albumin levels do not rise above normal except in the presence of hemoconcentration or dehydration. A decline in serum albumin levels follows prolonged malnutrition or loss of protein, either in the urine or by extravasation, as in burns. In third-degree burns with extensive granulating wounds, the exudate nitrogen is closely correlated with the amount of suppuration. A loss of 5 to 7 gm of nitrogen into the exudate per day is not uncommon in such burns; thus, early wound closure is of paramount importance. In this same postburn period, a low nitrogen intake contributes further to the negative nitrogen balance.	Have one unit of albumin ready to add to intravenous in A.M.	Observe for anaphylactic reaction: Mild: slight elevation of temperature; skin—red, itching, urticaria. Severe: dyspnea, violent cough, cyanosis, marked elevation of temperature, skin eruptions, pulse variations, feeling of chest constriction.
An energetic nutritional regimen of a high-protein, high-caloric diet, instituted 7 to 10 days after burning, may reduce substantially the duration of negative nitrogen balance. Unless special efforts are made to achieve ingestion of such a diet, negative nitrogen balance can be expected to last more than a month. The well-treated burned patient returns to nitrogen equilibrium, or more likely to positive balance, after a month.	3,500-calorie high-protein, high-vitamin diet. Offer in no less than 6 equal feedings.	Encourage complete proteins: milk eggs cheese and cottage cheese fish fowl liver, kidneys veal pork lamb lean meat
In a high-calorie, high-protein diet, the ratio of calories to nitrogen in the intake is important because protein synthesis will not occur in the absence of adequate caloric intake. The calorie : nitrogen ratio is the ratio of nonprotein calories to protein nitrogen in the diet. 1 gm of carbohydrate equals 4 calories 1 gm of fat equals 9 calories		Encourage proportional intake of incomplete proteins: legumes—3 to 4 servings per day cereals cereal products: bread, whole-wheat crackers Encourage low alkaline ash juices (to minimize renal cal-

Changes	Observations and Medical Therapy	Nurse Should
1 gm of protein equals 4 calories.		culus formation while increasing vitamin, mineral, and fluid intake): cranberry juice raspberry juice plum juice
About 40 to 50% of the chemical energy of carbohydrate and fat, and 80 to 85% of the chemical energy of protein, is converted to heat in the process of metabolism. A lack of caloric intake from the first two food sources will result in gradual combustion of body tissue. The burned patient loses weight as he loses muscle mass and fat. His depletion syndrome includes low levels of total body protein, potassium, magnesium, sulfate, and other intracellular ions. Water and extracellular salts tend to remain in excess until the patient approaches nitrogen equilibrium.		
B complex vitamins, especially thiamine, are essential to the enzyme systems responsible for facilitating use of glucose by the cell.	Vitamin B complex capsules II p.o. bid.	
Ascorbic acid is essential for growth, cell activity, maintenance of strength of blood vessels, and formation of supporting tissues. Plasma ascorbic acid concentration is low after severe burns; ascorbic acid is one of the precursors of the adrenocortical steroids and thus is depleted during the body's response to stress. This, in combination with increased tissue demands for vitamin C for healing the extensive areas of injury, requires administration of large doses of ascorbic acid.	Ascorbic acid, 500 mg p.o t.i.d.	Encourage foods rich in vitamin C. Ask family to contribute some of the following, if not available in quantity from the kitchen: citrus fruits melons berries tomatoes raw vegetables
Anemia develops rapidly in severely burned patients who survive the initial period of shock. Amount of destruction of red blood cells (RBC's) following thermal injury is variable, and in general is a significant problem only with deep burns. Mechanism of early RBC losses includes:	FeSO₄ 0.6 gm p.o. b.i.d.	Encourage foods high in iron: beans soybeans green leafy vegetables: kale

Changes	Observations and Medical Therapy	Nurse Should

1. RBC's trapped in the burned area at the time of injury are hemolyzed.		turnip
		lean meats—liver
		dried fruits:
		  prunes
		  apricots

2. Delayed hemolysis is observed for 24 to 48 hours after injury, resulting from lysis of RBC's that are partly damaged by heat.		Observe stools for black color. Instruct patient that this is not harmful.

3. Thrombosis of blood occurs in the capillaries of burned tissues and contributes to the RBC mass decrease.		Note any changes in consistency of stool:
		  diarrhea
		  constipation

4. The phenomenon of sludging is well demonstrated in burns.		Give pills with meals to minimize nausea.

Although thermal injury to erythrocytes in the dermal blood vessels results in anemia, this effect may not be evident at first because of hemoconcentration present before fluid replacement. An elevated bilirubin may indicate anemia in the early postburn stage. Jaundice—the yellow color of skin, sclerae, and mucous membranes—is due to an increase in bilirubin in the plasma. Hemolytic jaundice is due to an overproduction of bilirubin, due to increased breakdown of erythrocytes, in excess of the amount of bile pigment that the liver can excrete. Normally, 0.1 ot 1.5 mg of bilirubin loosely associated with protein is present in 100 ml of human serum.

Mr. A.'s bilirubin was 1.2% mg on his fourth postburn day; however, he never manifested jaundice.

With the re-establishment of his fluid and electrolyte balance, nitrogen equilibrium, and integrity of skin, Mr. A.'s care was designed to increase his mobility and improve his nutritional state. The nursing staff worked closely with Mr. A.: his physiotherapist, the dietitian, and Mr. A.'s family throughout the duration of his hospitalization to achieve those objectives.

REFERENCES

Part A

Books

Ellenberg, Max, and Harold Rifkin (eds.), *Clinical Diabetes Mellitus,* The Blakiston Division, McGraw-Hill Book Company, Inc., New York, 1962.
Joslin, Elliot P., *Diabetic Manual,* 10th ed., Lea & Febiger, Philadelphia, 1959.
Joslin, Elliot P., *The Treatment of Diabetes Mellitus,* 10th ed., Lea & Febiger, Philadelphia, 1959.
Lindberg, Ann Morrow, *Gift from the Sea,* Pantheon, New York, 1955.
Williams, Robert H. (ed.), *Diabetes,* Paul B. Hoeber, Inc., New York, 1960.

Articles

A.D.A. Forecast, American Diabetes Association, Inc., published bi-monthly for patient education.
Allan, Frank, "Current Concepts in Therapy—Education of the Diabetic Patient," *New England Journal of Medicine,* CCLXVIII, January 10, 1963, p. 93, 1963.
Babcock, Charlotte, "Attitudes and the Use of Food," *Journal of the American Dietetic Association,* XXXVIII, June, 1961, pp. 546-51.
Beaser, Samuel B., "Diabetes Mellitus," *New England Journal of Medicine,* CCLIX, No. 11, September 11, 1958, pp. 525-32; CCLIX, No. 12, September 18, 1958, pp. 573-81.
Bergen, Stanley S., and Theodore B. Van Wallie, "The Glucagon Problem," *New York State Journal of Medicine,* LXI, March 1, 1961, pp. 779-83.
Best, Charles .H., "Diabetes Since Nineteen Hundred and Twenty," *Canadian Medical Association Journal,* LXXXII, May 21, 1960, pp. 1061-66.
Bouton, Malcom A., and Joseph B. Cortisin, "A Diabetes Case Finding Program," *American Journal of Public Health,* L, April, 1960, pp. 524-30.
Caso, Elizabeth K., "Diabetic Meal Planning—A Good Guide Is Not Enough," *American Journal of Nursing,* LXII, November, 1962, pp. 76-78.
Clarke, C. A., "The Genetics of Diabetes Mellitus," *Diabetes,* X, No. 3, May-June, 1961, pp. 175-77.
Collens, William S., and Morris M. Banowitch, "Use of Oral Hypoglycemic Agents in Treatment of Diabetes Mellitus," *New York State Journal of Medicine,* LX, September 1, 1960, pp. 2689-2701.
Crossman, Ruth, "Nursing Care," *American Journal of Nursing,* LVIII, January, 1958, pp. 101-28.
Danowski, T. S., "Some Principles of Diabetes Care," *Diabetes,* IX, No. 4, July-August, 1960, pp. 292-95.
Daughaday, William H., "Hydrogen Ion Metabolism in Diabetic Acidosis," *Archives of Internal Medicine,* CVII, January, 1961, pp. 63-68.
DeLawter, DeWitt E., and James M. Moss, "Tolbutamide," *American Journal of Nursing,* LVIII, August, 1958, pp. 1106-8.
Ellenberg, Max, "Diabetic Neuropathy," *Annals of Internal Medicine,* LII, May, 1960, pp. 1067-75.
Fabrykant, Maximilian, "Laboratory Aids in Diagnosis," *New York State Journal of Medicine,* LX, December 1, 1960, pp. 3846-56.
Fajans, Stefan, and Jerome W. Conn, "Comments on the Cortisone-Glucose Tolerance Test," *Diabetes,* X, January-February, 1961, pp. 63-67.
Fineberg, S. K., "Obesity and Diabetes: A Reevaluation," *Annals of Internal Medicine,* LII, April, 1960, pp. 750-60.
Fischer, Alfred E., "Management of the Newborn Infant of the Diabetic Mother," *New York States Journal of Medicine,* LXI, January 15, 1961, pp. 292-96.
Fitzgerald, M. G., *et al.,* "The Effect of Sex and Parity on the Incidence of Diabetes Mellitus," *Quarterly Journal of Medicine,* XXX, January, 1961, pp. 57-70.
Glover, Virginia M., "Working with the Patient—A Case Study," *Nursing Outlook,* VIII, May, 1960, pp. 278-79.

Gould, Gertrude, and Jean Golden, "Teaching the Diabetic at Home," *American Journal of Nursing,* LVII, No. 9, September, 1957, pp. 1170-71.

Hardinge, Mervyn, and Hulda Crooks, "Lesser Known Vitamins in Foods," *Journal of the American Dietetic Association,* XXXVIII, March, 1961, pp. 240-45.

Hauns, E. A., "The Current Role of Insulin in the Era of Hypoglycemic Agents," *American Practitioner,* XIII, January, 1962, pp. 3-15.

Hinkle, L. E., Jr., "The Influence of the Patient's Behavior and His Reaction to His Life Situation upon the Course of Diabetes," *Diabetes,* V, September-October, 1956, pp. 406-7.

Hooker, Ann D., "Camping and the Diabetic Child," *Journal of The American Dietetic Association,* XXXVII, August, 1960, pp. 143-45.

Jay, Arthur N., "Hypoglycemia," *American Journal of Nursing,* LXII, January, 1962, p. 77.

Joslin, Elliott, "Diabetes in the Future," *Diabetes,* X, No. 2, March-April, 1961, pp. 148-51.

Krall, Leo P., "The Management of Diabetes with the Aid of Oral Hypoglycemic Agents," *Medical Clinics of North America,* XLV, July, 1961, pp. 823-38.

Levine, Rachmiel, and M. S. Goldstein, "Action of Insulin," *Scientific American,* CXCVIII, June, 1958, pp. 99-109.

MacNeil, Ann, "Urine Testing—When the Diagnosis Is Diabetes," *American Journal of Nursing,* LXI, No. 11, November, 1961, pp. 67-69.

Martin, Marguerite M., "The Diabetic at Home," *American Journal of Nursing,* LVI, October, 1956, pp. 1294-98.

Martin, Marguerite M., "Detection Is Your Protection," *American Journal of Nursing,* LX, No. 11, November, 1960, pp. 1608-9.

Martin, Marguerite M., "A Teaching Center for Diabetics," *American Journal of Nursing,* LVIII, No. 3, March, 1958, pp. 390-91.

Martin, Marguerite M., "The Unconscious Diabetic Patient," *American Journal of Nursing,* LXI, November, 1961, pp. 92-94.

Meyer, William J., "Continuous Diabetes Screening in a Rural Area," *Public Health Reports,* LXXV, No. 9, September, 1960, pp. 784-90.

Miller, Emery C., and William J. Reeves, "Severe 'Juvenile' Diabetes of Thirty-nine Years' Duration," *Diabetes,* IX, March-April, 1960, pp. 104-5.

Moss, James M., and DeWitt E. DeLawter, "Oral Agents in the Management of Diabetes Mellitus," *American Journal of Nursing,* LX, No. 11, November, 1960, pp. 1610-13.

Mulholland, H. B., John A. Owen, and J. Brookins Taylor, "Complications of Diabetes," *Disease a Month,* June, 1960.

Pollack, Herbert, "Nutritional Aspects of Therapy for Diabetes," *Postgraduate Medicine,* XXX, December, 1961, pp. 598-603.

Rouse, George P., Jr., "Pregnancy and Diabetes," *American Journal of Nursing,* LVIII, No. 1, January, 1958, pp. 100-1.

Shlevin, Edmund L., and Paul Pedowitz, "Pregnancy and Diabetes," *New York State Journal of Medicine,* LXI, January 1, 1961, pp. 130-35.

Sister M. Maureen, and Irene Beland, "The Nurse and the Diabetic Patient," *American Journal of Nursing,* XLVI, No. 9, September, 1946, pp. 606-9.

Smith, Kendrick, "Diabetic Neuropathy," *Postgraduate Medicine,* XXX, September, 1961, pp. 223-28.

Special papers from the Joslin Clinic, *Geriatrics,* XVII, May, 1962, pp. 317-44.

Tomhave, Wesley G., "Treatment of Diabetes Mellitus with Oral Hypoglycemic Compounds," *The Medical Clinics of North America,* XLVII, No. 1, January, 1963, p. 53.

Tulloch, J. A., and R. C. Lambert, "Latent Diabetes," *Diabetes,* X, No. 3, May-June, 1961, pp. 207-10.

Unger, Robert, "Medical Emergencies in Diabetes," *Medical Clinics of North America,* XLVI, March, 1962, pp. 487-93.

Wilson, Shirley M., and Roselia L. Dumm, "Tolbutamide on Trial," *American Journal of Nursing,* LVIII, No. 8, August, 1958, pp. 1108-9.

Winter, Frank C., "Diabetic Retinopathy," *Journal of the American Medical Association,* CLXXIV, September 10, 1960, pp. 143-46.
Zarowitz, Harold, "The Prediabetic State," *New York State Journal of Medicine,* LX, December 15, 1960, pp. 4056-60.

Part B

Books

Artz, Curtis P. (ed.), *Research in Burns,* F. A. Davis Company and the American Institute of Biological Sciences, Philadelphia, 1962.
Artz, Curtis P., and Eric Reiss, *The Treatment of Burns,* W. B. Saunders Company, Philadelphia, 1957.
Bland, John H., *Clinical Recognition and Management of Disturbances of Fluid Balance,* W. B. Saunders Company, Philadelphia, 1956.
Brown, James Barrett, and Frank McDowell, *Skin Grafting,* 3rd ed., J. B. Lippincott Company, Philadelphia, 1958.
Colbeck, J. C., *Control of Infections in Hospitals,* American Hospital Association, Chicago, 1962.
Corrigan, Marjorie J., and Lucille E. Corcoran, *Epidemiology in Nursing,* The Catholic University of America Press, Washington, D.C., 1961.
Fuerst, Elinor V., and LuVerne Wolff, *Fundamentals of Nursing,* 3rd ed., J. B. Lippincott Company, Philadelphia, 1964.
Hardy, James D., *Pathophysiology in Surgery,* Williams & Wilkins Company, Baltimore, 1958.
Harkins, Henry N., ed., *Surgery: Principles and Practices,* 2nd ed., J. B. Lippincott Company, Philadelphia, 1961.
Williams, R. E. O., ed., *Infections in Hospitals,* F. A. Davis Company, Philadelphia, 1963.

Articles

Artz, Curtis P., and John K. Hoopes, "Current Knowledge of Fluid Balance in Burns," *American Journal of Surgery,* CIII, March, 1962, pp. 316-19.
Balch, Henry H., "Resistance of Infection in Burned Patients," *Annals of Surgery,* CLVII, January, 1963, pp. 1-19.
Colebrook, Leonard, John M. Duncan, and W. P. Dallas Ross, "The Control of Infection in Burns," *The Lancet,* CCLIV, June 12, 1948, pp. 893-99.
Cope, Oliver, and Francis D. Moore, "A Study of Capillary Permeability in Experimental Burns and Burn Shock Using Radioactive Dyes in Blood and Lymph," *Journal of Clinical Investigation,* XXIII, March, 1944, pp. 241-57.
Cope, Oliver, *et al.,* "The Nature of the Shift of Plasma Protein to the Extravascular Space Following Thermal Trauma," *Annals of Surgery,* CXXVIII, December, 1948, pp. 1041-55.
Evans, Everett, *et al.,* "Fluid and Electrolyte Requirements in Severe Burns," *Annals of Surgery,* CXXXV, June, 1952, pp. 804-15.
Kriegel, Julia, "A Coordinated Infection Control Program," *Nursing Outlook,* IX, March, 1961, pp. 152-54.
Krumanocker, Josephine, "A Master Nursing Care Plan for the Burn Patient," *Tomorrow's Nurse,* III, June-July, 1962, pp. 20-25.
Lawrence, C. A., "The Effects of Disinfectants on Antibiotic Resistant and Antibiotic Sensitive Strains of Micrococcus Pyogenes, Var. Aureus," *Surgery, Gynecology and Obstetrics,* CVII, December, 1958, pp. 679-84.
Lowbury, E. J. L., "Infection of Burns," *British Medical Journal,* I, April 2, 1960, pp. 994-1001.
Lund, C. C., and N. C. Browder, "The Estimation of Areas of Burns," *Surgery, Gynecology and Obstetrics,* LXXIX, October, 1944, No. 4, pp. 352-58.
Lyons, Champ, "Problems of Infection and Chemotherapy," *Annals of Surgery,* CXVII, June, 1943, pp. 894-902.
Markley, Kehl, *et al.,* "Fatal Pseudomonas Septicemias in Burned Patients," *Annals of Surgery,* CXLV, February, 1957, pp. 175-81.

Moncrief, J. A., "Complications of Burns," *Annals of Surgery,* CXLVII, April, 1958, pp. 443-75.

Mortimer, Edward A., Jr., "Hospital Staphylococcal Infections: Interruption of Transmission as a Means of Control," *Medical Clinics of North America,* XLVII, No. 5, September, 1963, pp. 1247-56.

Nahmias, Andre J., "Infections Associated with Hospitals," *Nursing Outlook,* XI, No. 6, June, 1963, pp. 450-53.

Price, Philip B., *et al.,* "Bacterial Invasion in Experimental Burns," *Surgical Forum,* VI, March, 1955, pp. 64-67.

Rabin, Captain Erwin W., *et al.,* "Fatal Pseudomonas Infection in Burned Patients," *The New England Journal of Medicine,* CCLXV, December 21, 1961, pp. 1225-31.

Schumer, William, "Recent Advances in the Management of Burns," *Surgical Clinics of North America,* XLIII, No. 1, February, 1963, pp. 229-44.

Weller, Charles, "Oral Hypoglycemic Agents," *American Journal of Nursing,* LXIV, No. 3, March 1964, pp. 90-92.

Wilson, Ben. J., and Jerry A. Stirman, "Initial Treatment of Burns," *Journal of American Medical Association,* CLXXIII, June 4, 1960, pp. 509-16.

Index

Aorta, coarctation of (continued)
defined, 588n
hypertension and, 680–81
occlusions of, 490–91
sclerosis of, 650
structure of, 649–50
Aortic bodies, receptors in, 425
Aortic insufficiency, 588, 627
Aortic valve, 570
Aphasia, 1265–67
global, 1266
motor, 1095
sensory, 1095
Aplasia, defined, 114
and hypoplasia in bone marrow, 706–709
Apnea, defined, 453
Appendicitis, 116, 299, 703, 892, 1138–39
enemas contraindicated in, 1155
Appetite, defined, 743–44
Apraxia, 1267
Arachnoid, 1066
Aramine (metaraminal), 640
Aramine bitartrate (metaraminal bitartrate), 515–16, 1179
Arborviruses, 207
Areolar connective tissues, 53
Ariboflavinosis, 743
Arm-lift–back-pressure artificial respiration, 431
Arsenic, 151
Arsphenemine, 278
Arteries: see also Arteriosclerosis; Atherosclerosis; Circulatory system; specific arteries
aneurysms of: see Aneurysms
described, 561–62, 649
ischemia and, 116–21
movement of blood and, 562
tests of blood flow in, 668
thrombosis of, 667–68
Arteriography, 669
Arterioles
action of, 501
constricted, 428
degeneration of, 140
described, 650
peripheral resistance and, 674
Arteriosclerosis
age at onset of, 650
aneurysms from, 313n
coronary, heart block and, 618–19
death rate from, 80
heat sensitivity with, 308
obliterans, 563
Arteriovenous fistulae, 656
Arteriovenous shunts, defined, 588n
Arthralgia, 267

Arthritis
disability from, 85
prevention of residual injury in, 310
prolonged, 49
in rheumatic fever, 244, 259, 575–76
scar tissue in healing from, 314
as symptom, 267
Arthus reaction, 273, 275
Artificial kidney: see Kidney
Artificial respiration, 430–36
objectives of, 430–31
methods of, 430–36
oxygen administered as, 430
Arteriovenous fistulae, 656
Ascariasis, 881
Aschoff bodies, 573
Ascites
defined, 523
fluid shifts with, 506
in liver disease, 824
treatment of, 145
Ascorbic acid: see Vitamin C
Asepsis, 72, 232, 1166–68
development of, 218, 1132, 1133–36
slackness in, 220
Asphyxia
causes of, 399
fast development of, 402
from lung cancer, 950
from obstruction of trachea, 394
from openings in thoracic cavity, 422
Aspiration, 395, 1163
Aspirin (acetylsalicylic acid), 153–54
as antigenic agent, 274
for pain relief, 276, 954, 1226
as poison, 153–54
use during fever, 912
Astereognosis, 1097
Asthma, 472–73
allergic, 277–78, 282–83
breathing with, 273
bronchial, 416
cardiac, 458–59, 596–97
disability from, 86
injury in, 49
morphine and, 1158
obstruction with, 400
secretions increased by, 406
severe, 285
treatment for, 288
Asynergia, 1091
A.T. 10: see Dihydrotachysterol
Atabrine hydrochloride, 75
Ataxia, 1079, 1091
Atelectasis, 477
causes of, 420, 424
defined, 394
effects of, 399

predisposition to, 308, 407
prevention of, 399
Atherosclerosis, 88, 633
as cause of disease, 118–19
coronary, 627–33
diet and, 630
generalized, 564
harmful effects of, 440
heart block and, 619
hypertension and, 678, 681
as intrinsic disease, 292
obesity and, 72
predisposition to, 846
tissue repairs and, 314
Athetosis, 1087
Athlete's foot, 280
Atmospheric pressure, 383–89
Atomic bomb, 136–37
Atopy, defined, 266
ATP (adenosine triphosphate), 863, 849
Atria, 567
Atropine sulfate, 393–94, 620, 682, 1158
anticholinergic effects of, 394
for colic, 160
Atrophy, 108–11
causes of, 109
classifications of, 109–11
defined, 108
disuse, 109–11
Auditory agnosia (word deafness), 1095, 1267
Auditory nerve, 1092
Auerbach's plexus, 760
Aureomycin, 180
Auricular fibrillation: see Fibrillation, auricular
Auriculoventricular node, 617
Autoimmune diseases
defense mechanisms in, 269
defined, 270
Autonomic nervous system, 1080
activation of, 249–54
affecting alimentary canal, 760–62
heart and, 44
imbalance in, 363
Axillary temperature, 901
Axons, 1071–73
Azotemia, 1311
defined, 555
rapidly developing, 545
Azure A, in test for stomach cancer, 968

B

Babinski reflex, 1099
Bacillary dysentery, 882
Backache
cause of, 244
prevention of, 245
Bacteremia, defined 301

Blood pressure (*continued*)
in preoperative evaluation, 1147
maintenance despite blood loss, 44
movement of, 562
ranges of, 671–73
regulation of, 40, 44–45, 673–97
capillary fluid shift mechanism, 673–74
drugs to lower, 692–97
kidney, 677–78
sympathetic nervous system, 675–77
in shock, 512–13
Blood sludge, formation of, 294
Blood sugar: *see* Glucose
Blood transfusions, 523, 1185–94
dangers of, 268, 509, 716, 1189–93
Blood urea nitrogen, 550
Blood vessels: *see also* Arteries; Capillaries; Circulatory system; Hemorrhage; Veins
activation of, 250
blood escaping from, 160
collapse of, 519
degeneration of, 140
diseases of, 653
in inflammation, 292–95
occlusion of, 118
as point of exit, 40
structure of, 649–51
tone of: *see* Vascular tone
Blue babies, 566
BMR: *see* Basal metabolic rate
Body defenses, 42–43
Body fluids: *see also* Fluid and electrolyte balance; *specific fluids*
as cause of injury, 160–61
composition of, 485–87, 496
loss of, 488
with burns, 292–93, 506
containing proteins, 503
in irradiation, 137
in metabolic acidosis, 538
obstructive, 391
physiological changes, 507–508
supply of, 487–88
transportation of, 500–506
Body structure, heat loss and, 905
Body temperature: *see also* Fever; Hypothermia
alteration in, 900–19
acclimatization to cold, 915–16
adaptation to extremes in temperature, 908–10

elements in heat production, 903
factors in heat loss, 903–908
maintenance of, 40
regulation of, 42
as symptom, 63, 305
Body walls as protection, 42
Boils
evacuation of, 310
manipulation of, 300
Bone: *see also specific bone diseases*
as calcium source, 158
cancer of, 953
demineralization of, 110
formation of, 1059–60
infections of, 224, 313
preoperative preparation for, 1157
injury to, 262
necrosis of, 145
osteitis fibrosa cystica, 1061
oxygen lack in, 382
parathormone acting on, 530
as protective structures, 240
water content of, 488
Bone marrow, 135, 721
aplasia and hypoplasia of, 706–707, 717
depression of, 278, 296
destruction in leukemia of, 950
erythrocyte formation in, 52, 389, 705–707
hyperplasia in, 113
injury to, 114
macrophages in, 297
Botulism, 185–86
Bowel
cancer, 970
cleansing of, 811
gangrene of, 116
preoperative preparation of, 1155
regulation of, 800, 806
ulceration of, 160
Bowman's capsule, 491
Boyle's law, 383–84
Bradford frame, 1225
Bradycardia, 765
Bradypnea, defined, 453
Brain: *see also* Cerebellum; Cerebral cortex; Cerebrospinal fluid; Neural regulation; Reticular formation
atherosclerosis and, 633
atrophy of, 110
blood-brain barrier, 1068
blood supply of, 1069
breathing affected by, 454
cerebral metabolism, 1069
cranial nerves, 395, 1091–93
disturbance of function of, 518
edema of, 294, 408

respiratory failure and, 428
as response to injury, 783
hypertension and, 682
inadequate blood supply to, 306, 381–82, 512
increased intracranial pressure, 765, 783, 1100–1101
integration of function of, 1081–83
lumbar puncture and 1103–1104
microscopic structure of, 1071
prefrontal lobes, 1095
protection of, 1065
response to frustration in injury to, 348, 1007
seizures, 1101–1103
solvents and, 150
tracheostomy and, 407–408
tumors of, 428
vestibular nuclei, 1087
weight of, 109
Brain concussion, 124, 428
Brain contusion, 124
Breasts: *see also* Mastectomy
abscesses of, 217
cancer of, 927, 965
effect of hormones on, 937–38, 955, 977
Breath sounds, 401
Breathing: *see* Respiration
Bretylium, 693, 694
Bromides, poisoning by, 528
Bromsulfalein (BSP) excretion test, 820–21
Bronchi
activation of, 250
aid in removal of foreign bodies, 393
muscular contraction of, 273
obstructed, 394, 399
perforation of, 403–404
Bronchial aspiration, 402
Bronchiectasis, 404, 416, 469–70, 540
cleaning mechanisms and, 404
Bronchioles, 399–400
emphysema in, 416–17
muscle fibers in, 437
muscle spasms of, 406
Bronchitis: *see also* Tracheobronchitis
chronic, 416, 468
disability from, 86
Bronchogenic carcinoma, 154–55, 935–36
Bronchographs, 469
Bronchopneumonia, 407
in concentration camps, 191
Bronchoscopy, 402–405
care of patient during, 403
complications from, 403–404

Bronze diabetes, 1283
Brucellosis, leukopenia in, 298
Bruises, 124
  pain with, 302
Brunner's glands, 789
Bubonic plague: see Plague
Buccal mucosa, spots on, 63
Buerger-Allen exercises, 666
Buerger's disease, 658–70
Buffer systems
  defined, 484
  function of, 531–32, 536
Buffers
  defined, 484, 531
  in respiratory acidosis, 540
Bullas, rupture of, 420
Bundle of His, 616
  blocking, 618–19
Burn scars, cancer of, 939, 940
Burns, 1333–58
  as acute inflammations, 305
  of aged people, 1144
  anemia in, 717
  classification of, 128–29
  food intake after, 261
  healing of third-degree, 314
  loss of fluids with, 292–93
  response to, 238, 262
  rule of nines, 1333, 1335
  severe, 253
  thermal, 127–28
  tissue restoration in, 49
Burrows' solution, 288
Buttocks, edema of, 522–23, 598

C

Cachexia, 952
Caffeine (coffee, tea), 622
  in hypertensive headaches, 682
Caisson disease, 384–86
Calamine lotions, 276
Calciferol, 158, 159
Calcium, 1058–62
  in blood coagulation, 725–26
  in fluid balance, 493
  functions of, 530–31, 1059–62
  lost during rest, 1207–1208
  neuromuscular irritability from decrease in, 504
  regulation of, 157–60
Calcium gluconate, administration of, 531
Calculi, 110, 159–60
  biliary, 161
Calories, 828–44
  for diets, 842–44
  required, 828–31
  sources of, 831–32
Cancer: see also Carcinoma; Tumors; specific types of cancer

among ancient animals and people, 924–25
benign vs. malignant neoplasms, 931–35
cancer quacks, 999–1000
carcinogenic agents, 939, 941–43, 961–62
care of patient with, 960–62
  resuming normal activities, 977–82
  role of nurse, 923–24
  widespread and progressive disease, 982–93
as cause of diarrhea, 802
as cause of pleurisy, 303
chemotherapy in, 975–77
compared to other types of disease, 944–46
death rate from, 80, 81, 85
detection
  in men, 967
  in women, 965–66
diagnosis, 969
discovery of suspicious lesions, 968–72
etiology of, 935–36
hormones as factor in, 937–38
host susceptibility to, 936–37, 938–39
incidence of and trends, 925–26
from ionizing radiation, 130–31, 138, 145–46, 941–42
ionizing radiation to treat, 974–75
of larynx, 408–409
leukocytosis in, 298
mechanical effects of, 947–50
naming of, 929–30
of nasal sinuses, 130
normal cell growth and, 135–36, 922–23, 928–30
pain in, 952–55, 1165, 1230
patients' reaction to diagnosis and treatment of, 87, 149, 958–60, 983–96
phases in, 960
prevention of, 962–67
psychological effects of, 955–58, 978–81
recent increase of, 925–28
rectal examination for, 967–68
research on, 946
seven danger signals, 970–71
in situ, 945
smoking and, 56, 154–55, 940
of stomach, 789
surgery in, 972–73
  history of, 972–73
  objectives of, 973

as palliative measure, 973–75
symptoms of, 946
systemic effects of, 950–52
types of therapy, 971
typing and grading of, 970
viruses and, 205
Cannon, W. B., 38, 249
Capillaries
  buds of, 316
  described, 650–51
  erythrocytes concentrated in, 126
  function of, 500–503
  importance of, 649
  increased permeability of, 137, 140, 521
    caused by physical and chemical agents, 501
    in allergies, 272–73
  interstitial fluid returned to, 503
  membrane, 500
  pulmonary, 437–38
Capillary fluid shift mechanism, 673–74
Capillary fragility test, 721
Carbohydrates
  in diabetes mellitus, 1281, 1282, 1296, 1306
  diet low in, 787
  dumping syndrome and large amounts of, 786
  energy extracted from 848–60
  in stomach, 785
Carbon dioxide
  in acidosis, 417, 538
  capillary permeability increased by, 501
  combining power, 544
  content, 452, 544
  function of, 459, 531
    anion level determined by, 532–34
  level of
    decreased, 438
    in plasma, 454
  narcosis, 417, 474
  respiratory centers and, 455
  solubility of, 383–85
  as stimulant to respiration, 426
Carbon monoxide
  hemoglobin and, 149–50; see also Carboxyhemoglobin
  poisoning from, 439–40
Carbon tetrachloride, 150, 312
Carbonic acid
  in alkalosis, 540–42
  in buffer systems, 532
  decomposition of, 533
  ratio of, 536–38
  in respiratory acidosis, 539–40
Carbonic anhydrase, 533, 1017

Degenerative diseases, chronic, 56, 1124
Dehydration, 507–508
  cellular, 507–508
  from drinking sea water, 46
  from irradiation, 142
  from mouth breathing, 392
Dehydrocholic acid (Decholin), 601
Demerol (meperidine hydrochloride), 660, 987, 1158, 1226
  for colic, 160
  depression of respiratory system from, 540
Dendrites, 1071
Dentures during surgery, 1159
Dermatitis: see also Contact dermatitis
  as delayed reaction to allergy, 279
  exfoliative, 278
  treatment for, 288
Dermatomyositis, 49, 568n
Desoxycorticosterone, 680, 1020, 1032, 1036
  in scar tissue experiments, 316
Desoxyribonucleic acid: see DNA
Desquamation from irradiation, 140
Diabetes insipidus, 1028–29
Diabetes mellitus, 1027, 1275–1332
  abnormalities associated with, 1283
  acidosis in, 525, 769, 1294–98, 1304–1308
  atherosclerosis and, 629
  care of feet in, 661, 1327
  cause of mortality in, 80
  control of, 1312–23, 1326–32
  definition of, 1281–82
  diagnosis of, 1297–1300
  factors affecting blood glucose level, 1290–92
  glucose tolerance test for, 861
  heredity in, 50
  history of, 1277–81
  hospital therapy, 1306–1309
  hygiene in, 1326–28
  incidence of, 1280, 1287–88
  injury and, 260–61
  insulin in, 1025, 1282–83, 1292–97, 1302–1308
  specific types of insulin and therapy, 1317–22
  intensified severity of, 856
  life expectancy in, 1277
  obesity and, 72, 846
  onset of, 1295–1302

other drugs, 1322–23
  patient instruction, 1328–31
  prevention of acidosis, 1309–10
  similarity to starvation, 1293–97
  tests for effective control of, 1323–26
  uncontrolled, 314, 538, 832
  urine testing in, 1324–26
Diacetic acid, 538
Diagnosis, making of, 809–12
Dialysis, 528–30
Diamox (Acetazolamide), 524, 826, 853, 1017
Diaphoresis: see Perspiration
Diaphragm, 425
  pressure on, 405
Diarrhea, 63, 771, 1127–28
  with allergies, 273
  causes of, 804
  in chronic alcoholism, 156–57
  described, 800–806
  infantile, 81
  neurogenic origin of, 801
  as protection, 189
  severe, 538
  as symptom of irradiation sickness, 137
  water loss in, 506
Diathermy, 128, 244
Dichlordiphenyl-trichlorethane: see DDT
Diets
  in anemia, 708, 712, 719
  in atherosclerosis, 630
  defined, 737–38
  in diabetes mellitus, 739, 1315–17
  elimination, 283–84
  in hypertension, 691–92
  low-sodium
    in heart failure, 606–607, 647
    in hypertension, 692
    possible salt depletion, 692
  in myocardial infarction, 647
  nursing responsibilities regarding, 739–40
  for obesity, 842–45
Diffusion, defined, 485
Digestive juices as cause of injury, 160–61
Digitalis, 526, 602–605, 618
  ECG and, 626
  effect of calcium on, 1060
  premature beats and, 622–23
  toxic symptoms, 604
Digitalization, defined, 604
Digitoxin, 524, 603–604
Dihydrotachysterol, 1062
Dihydroxyphenalaline, 695
Dilantin Sodium (diphenyl-

hydantoin sodium), toxic effects of, 713
Diphtheria
  airway obstructed in, 396
  antibodies for, 197
  antitoxin for, 87, 186, 201
    administration of, 265
    allergy to, 276
    development of, 173
  carriers of, 182
  complications of, 157
  control of, 202
  death rate from, 80, 175
  exotoxin in, 185–87
  heart block and, 618
  recurrence of, 75
  susceptibility to, 203
Diphtheritic myocarditis, 588
Disease: see also Illness, "benign" vs. "malignant"
  compared with health, 54
  defined, 53–54
  etiology of
    adaptive responses, 48–50
    general beliefs of cause of, 167–74
    germ theory, 168, 172–74, 1134
    immunological defense, 269
    molecular theory, 53–54
    multiple factors theory, 57, 61
    natural phenomenon, 54
    "necessary and sufficient" concept, 56
    respiratory, 463–71
  factors influencing specific cause of, 59
  major causes of, 79–80
  manifestations of, 61–62
  prevention of
    application of, 74–79
    defined, 67–68
    knowledge of, 72–74
    measurement of, 68
  rate of: see Morbidity
  signs and symptoms of, 62–64
  study of, 58–61
  transmitted by blood transfusions, 1190–91
  wasting, 49
Disodium calcium versenate, 151
Disodium phosphate, 532
Diuresis, 43, 151
  fluid intake and, 527
Diuretics
  in congestive heart failure, 600, 605–608
    digitalis and, 603, 605
  enzyme system and, 1017
  in hypertension, 693
  mercurial, 526
  overuse of, 519
Diuril (chlorothiazide), 606

Hypothermia (*continued*)
metabolic rate and, 452
methods of induction of, 916
tissue requirements reduced in, 832
ventricular fibrillation in, 625
Hypothermia blankets, 916–18, 1055
Hypothyroidism (myxedema), 588–89, 1021, 1041, 1042, 1044–47, 1056–58
anemia in, 714
atherosclerosis and, 629
complication of thyroidectomy, 1055
obesity and, 831
tachycardia and, 621
tissue requirements reduced in, 832
Hypovolemic shock, 786
Hypoxia, 381, 386–88, 701
anxiety with, 414
cyanosis and, 387–88
development of, 388–89, 417, 429–30, 440
disorders causing, 273, 428, 437, 552
erythropoiesis and, 48, 714, 722
intensified by catheters, 413
metabolic rate lowered in, 452
respiratory centers affected by, 426
signs and symptoms of, 439
as stimulus to dyspnea, 455
tracheostomy for, 407–408

I

Icterus index, 720
Idiocy, hypothyroidism and, 1041
Ileostomy, 161, 519, 759
Ileus, paralytic, 1196
Illness: *see also* Disease
acceptance of, 358–59
"benign" vs. "malignant," 685, 924
expense of, 351
disability from, 85
objectives of therapy in, 87–93
period of, 195–96
psychosocial aspects of: *see* Psychosocial aspects of illness
Immunity, 174, 264–68
defined, 264, 266
Immunization: *see* Vaccination
Impetigo, 217, 218, 224
Increased intracranial pressure
care of patient with, 1100–1101

Incubation periods, 195
for food poisoning, 221–22
Infants: *see* Children
Infarct, defined, 117–18
Infarctions, 116, 117–18; *see also specific infarctions*
healing of, 313
Infections, 117–26; *see also specific organs*
acute fulminating, 49
chronic, 157–60
defense mechanisms against, 188–89
diabetes mellitus and, 1287, 1312, 1327–28
dormant, 181
face mask to control, 230–32
food intake after, 261
house cleaning to control, 232–33
inapparent (missed, abortive cases), 183
inflammation from, 290–307
leukocytes in, 703
predisposition to, 278, 394
prevention of wound infection, 1166–68
as response to injury, 262
staphylococcal, 47, 191, 209–11, 216–34
characteristics of, 221–24
diagnosis of, 204
spread of, 225–33
types of, 223–24
streptococcal, 50
diagnosis of, 204
of heart valves, 572
hemolytic, 217, 219
in rheumatic fever, 573–75
in trauma, 123–26
vehicle of transmission of, 184
Infectious diseases, 164–234; *see also specific diseases*
acute, 196–202
in childhood, 176
care of patients with, 208–16
control of, 199–202
nurse's responsibilities, 165–67
as cause of death, 36, 73, 81, 174–76
as cause of respiratory failure, 428
causes of, 175–95
chronic, 157–60
course of, 195–96
diagnosis of, 203–205
disability from, 85
elements in development of, 193–95
fever with, 196–97
general characteristics of, 164–65

history of, 165–74
identifying persons susceptible to, 202–203
immunity to, 264–68
inflammation from, 290–307
prevention of, 74–75
respiratory, summary of, 463–77
staphylococcic: *see* Infections, staphylococcic
theories of cause of, 167–77
Infectious hepatitis: *see* Hepatitis
Infectious mononucleosis: *see* Mononucleosis, infectious
Infiltration
defined, 115
fatty, 155–57
Inflammations, 48, 116, 291–307
acute, 305
as allergic response from drugs, 275
chronic, 305
classified, 301–305
definition, 291–92
described, 291–92
exudate of: *see* Inflammatory exudate
hemorrhagic, 304
inhibited, 259
lymphocytes in, 297
neutrophils in, 296–97
to prevent infection, 189
products of, 501
response to, 301
role of blood vessels, 292
of serous membranes, 506
signs and symptoms in, 305–307
treatment of, 307–11
vascular congestion from, 396
Inflammatory exudate, 295–98
movement of, 292
reduction of, 310
removed by coughing, 300, 310, 401
types of, 303–304
Influenza
convalescence from, 197
death rate from, 80, 171
epidemics of, 206
exposure to, 56
fever and, 911
frequency, 176
as predisposition to pneumonia, 228
among smokers, 56–57
vaccine for, 202
virus for, 207, 467
Injurious agents
kinds of effects, 107–108
objectives of nursing care derived from knowledge of, 106

Kidneys, functions of (*continued*)
failure in, 518–19, 520, 527–28
hydrogen ion concentration, 534–37, 540
insufficiency in, 519
sodium regulation as, 499
waste removed by, 485
heart failure and, 592, 593, 598
hydrostatic pressure and, 438
hypertension and, 679, 680, 681–82, 687
increase in size of, 112
injury to, 514
ischemia of, 514
in glomerular nephritis, 552
prolonged, 545
mercury and, 151
microscopic structure, 491
oxygen lack in, 381–82
parathormone acting on, 530
preoperative evaluation of, 1148–49
in regulation of blood pressure. 677–78
renal colic, 159
scar tissue in, 313
single, 114
solvents and, 150
structure of, 489–94
summary of disorders of, 545–57
transplantation of, 271
tuberculosis in, 199
water retained by, 257
Kimmelsteil-Wilson's disease, 1311
Kline tests, 214, 1190
Klinefelter's syndrome, 1014
Koch's postulates, 173
Kohlmer test, 214
Koplik spots, 63
Krebs cycle, 156. 849–51
Küpffer cells, 296, 812
Kussmaul breathing, 538
defined, 459
development of. 556
in diabetes mellitus, 1296, 1305
Kwashiorkor, 157, 438
Kyphosis, 418

L

Laceration, 125
Lactic acid
presence of, 439
reoxidation of, 382
Lactodehydrogenase (LDH), 63, 1016
Lanatoside C (Cedilanid), 603
Laryngeal nerves
injury during thyroidectomy, 1054
severance of, 397-98

Laryngeal stridor, 401–402
Laryngectomy, 408–409, 957, 982
Laryngitis, 465–66
Laryngoscope, 810
Larynx, 390–91
artificial, 957–58
cancer of, 408–409
diphtheria and, 186
edema of, 273, 276, 404
mucous membrane of, 186
obstructed, 399, 408
opening into, 395
rendered insensitive, 398
spasm of, 407
Law of partial pressures, 383–84
Law of solubility of gases, 383
LDH, 63
Lead, 151, 716
Lecithin, 816
Lecithinase, 187
Legs: *see also* Extremities, lower
gangrene of, 116
exercises of, 1209–10
ulcers of, 716
Leiomyofibroma of uterus, 929, 949–50
Leithauser, D., 1207
Leprosy, 177
Leptomeninges, 1066
Lesions: *see* Injury; *specific lesions*
Leukemia, 935, 938, 942, 955
chronic lymphatic, 267
destruction of bone marrow in, 950
drugs for, 976, 977
fever in, 913
increase in incidence of, 927
from irradiation, 146
leukocytes in, 703
lymphocytic, 716
virus as cause of, 943
Leukocidins, 187, 223, 229
Leukocyte count, 720, 914, 922
Leukocytes (white blood cells), 702, 720
abnormalities of, 703
change in level of, 63
count in rheumatic fever, 575
destroyed: *see* Leukocidins
disappearance of, 137, 316
effect of hemolysins and leukocidins on, 187
granular (polymorphonuclear), 278, 702
in infections, 703
in inflammation, 296–99, 303
pavementing of, 294
as wandering cells, 297
Leukocytosis, 123

in acute conditions, 306
in myocardial infarction, 642
occurrence of, 298
with sunburn, 129
Leukopenia, 135, 141, 298
Leukoplakia, 939, 942, 966
Lavarterenol Bitartrate (Levophed, norepinephrine), 515–16, 639–40, 1179
Levin tube, 1149–52
Levophed: *see* Levarterenol Bitartrate
Lichenification, defined, 280
Life expectancy, 68–71, 78–79, 82–83
Linens, care of contaminated, 232–33
Linkage of chromosomes, 1012
Lipase, 1016
Lipemia, 550, 863
Lipids
accumulation of, 292
as antigens. 267, 270
in fatty infiltration, 156–57
as phospholipids, 158
regulation of level of, 863
Lips
chancres on, 212
dehydrated condition of, 507
swelling. 273
Lithiasis, 159–60
Liver
amyloid degeneration in, 157
atrophy of, 110
bilirubin in, 715
cancer, 942
cirrhosis of, 889–91
anemias with, 823
frequency of, 80
sodium excess with, 520
as defense, 189
disease of
blood changes in, 823
edema with, 824
water and electrolyte imbalance in, 824
estrogen and. 772
fatty infiltration of, 156–57
functions of, 812–16
tests for, 820–21
glycogenesis in, 250, 260–61, 1290–91, 1294–96
heart failure and, 592
hepatomegaly, 112
hypertrophy of, 112
in hemolytic anemia, 716
increased hemolysis in, 716
in metabolic acidosis, 538
obstruction of, 760

Mental retardation, 1013
Meperidine hydrochloride
  (Demerol), 660, 987,
  1158, 1226
  for colic, 160
  depression of respiratory
    system from, 540
Meprobamate, in congestive
  heart failure, 608
Mercaptopurine (6-mercap-
  topurine), toxic ef-
  fects of, 713
Mercurial diuretics, 526, 693
  enzyme system and, 1017
Mercury, 150–51
Mercury chloride, 222
Mesantoin (methyl-phenyl-
  ethyl hydantoin),
  717
Mesenchymal tissues, regeneration of, 312
Metabolic acidosis, 126
  causes of, 537–40
  development of, 556
  hyperventilation in, 459
  nursing care during, 539
Metabolism: see also Basal
    metabolic rate;
    Homeostasis
  acids produced by, 531
  adjustment of, 43
  in diabetes mellitus, 1288–
    92
  disorders of
    hypermetabolism, 38,
      127, 307
    myocardium and, 588–
      89
    tachycardia and, 621
  intermediary
    described, 827–28
    disturbances in, 155–57
  of protein, 852
  in response to injury, 256–
    63
  waste products of, 40–41
    excreted by kidney, 488
Metabolites
  pH of, 531
  from proteins, 492
  toxic, 305
Metaplasia, 113–14
Metaraminal (Aramine),
  640
Metaraminal bitartrate (Aramine Bitartrate),
  515–16, 1179
Metastasis, 932–34, 950,
  951
Metastatic abscesses, 224
Methacholine chloride, 1031
Methadone hydrochloride,
  1226
Methemoglobin, cyanosis
  and, 387
Methenamine mandalate
  (Mandelamine),
  1202
  for urine sterilization,
  547

Methotrexate (Amethop-
  terin)
  toxic effects of, 713
  in treatment of cancer,
  976
Methyl alcohol, as poison,
  152
Methyl-phenyl-ethyl hydantoin (mesantoin),
  717
Miasmic influences, 169–72
Microglia, replacement with,
  312
Microorganisms, 175–95
  as cause of disease, 185–
  89
  characteristics of, 194–95
  in current theory, 175–77
  discharged, 400
  hosts and, 175–93
    brought together, 191–
    93
    effects of disturbance on
      balance between,
      178–81
    relationship between,
      175–78
    susceptible, 182–85,
      190–91
  localized, 301
Microphages: see Phago-
  cytes
Midbrain, 1081, 1088
Middle ear infections, 461
Migraine headaches, 269,
  276
Milieu intérieur, 39
Milk
  calcium in, 530
  constipating faculty, ef-
    fect of, 748
Milliequivalent, defined, 484
Mineralocorticoids, 680,
  1032; see also Aldos-
  terone
Minerals, deficiency in, 707–
  709
Minute ventilation, defined,
  449
"Missed cases," defined,
  183
Mitochondria, 1020
Mitosis, 921, 1014
  of malignant neoplasm,
  932
Mitral valve disease, 438,
  579, 587
Moisture, heat loss and,
  905–906
Molybdenum, 828, 868
Mongolism, 1014
Monilia, 217
Monocyte, 911
Mononucleosis, infectious,
  298, 588
  tests for, 204
Monosodium phosphate
  from bisodium phosphate,
  535
  in buffer systems, 532
  excreted, 537

Morbidity
  acute, 205
  causes of, 86
    digestive disturbances,
    800
    infectious diseases,
    174–77
    major, 79–87
    peptic ulcers, 790–91
    respiratory disease, 459–
    62
    staphylococcic infections,
    216–17
Morphine sulfate, 393, 1226
  administration of, 245
  allergy to, 286
  in anxiety and dyspnea,
    458, 596, 597, 608
  for colic, 160
  depression by, 540
  in myocardial infarction,
    637
  patient's response to,
    1158, 1227
  as poison, 517
Mortality: see Death
Motion sickness
  drugs for, 769
  vomiting with, 765
Motor aphasia, 1095
Motor cortex, 1096–99
Mountain sickness, signs,
  and symptoms of,
  388–89
Mouth
  as air passageway, 392
  in anemia, 719
  dehydrated condition of,
  507
  functions of, 777–79
  suctioning of, 406–407
Mouth-to-mouth respiration,
  430–32
Mucous colitis, 764
Mucous membrane: see also
  Skin
  acid in contact with, 531
  alimentary canal, 789–90
  allergies affecting, 276,
  396
  bleeding in, 727
  buccal, 63
  catarrhal inflammation of,
  304
  drying of, 410
    in dehydration, 507
    in oxygen therapy, 447–
    48
  edema of, 400
  exposure of, 114
  as external environment,
  38
  of gastrointestinal tract,
    160, 764, 774–76
  intestinal, 760
  minimized trauma to,
  413–15
  nasal, 392, 396
  as protection, 42, 123–24
  pseudomembrane, 396
  response to irritation, 401

Mucous membrane
(continued)
superficial ulceration of,
186
swelling of, 461
two characteristics of,
392–93
virus infection of, 208
warming action of, 392
Mucous patches, 213
Multiple factors, in causation
of disease, 57, 61
Multiple myeloma, 267
Multiple sclerosis, 270
Mumps
frequency of, 176
glands affected by, 778
swelling with, 204
Murmurs, heart, 571
Muscles
atrophy of, 108, 110–11
cells of, 108
ciliary, 250
contraction of smooth,
272, 273, 762
in alimentary canal,
762–63
hyperresponsive, 400
treatment of, 288
effect of potassium on,
504–505, 526
heavy, 47
hypertrophy of, 112–13
ischemia of, 122–23, 309
paralyzed, limitation
from, 418
skeletal
contraction of, 382
for respiration, 425
as venous pump, 652
spasms of, 159, 244, 305
in influenza, 467
relief from, 531
at ulcer site, 793
storage in, 53
tension of
in illness, 243–47
as indication of emo-
tional state, 363–64
in tracheobronchial tree,
399–400, 405, 406
twitching of, 554
water content of, 448
Muscular dystrophy, 425
Myalgia, with influenza, 467
Myasthenia gravis
defined, 425, 778n
fatigue with, 778
respirators for, 434
swallowing with, 783
Mycobacteria, 583
Myelin, 1071–73
Myenteric plexus (Auer-
bach's), 760
Myocardial infarction, 63,
588, 635–48, 681
angina pectoris differentiated from, 635
defined, 568n
effect of, 253
fever after, 306

healing from, 313
incidence of, 628
later effects of, 644–48
leukocytosis in, 298
patient study of, 636–38
scar formation in, 643
shock with, 515
therapy in, 442–43, 639–
48
rest, 308, 609–10, 641–
42, 647
Myocarditis, defined, 304
Myocardium
antigen of, 271
diseases of, 588–89; see
also Myocardial in-
farction
angina pectoris, 634–35
Aschoff bodies, 573
classification of, 588
heart failure and, 587–
89
pericardial disease and,
583
enlargement of, 47
failure of, 516
function and structure of,
583–86
automaticity and rhyth-
micity, 615–18
hypertrophy of, 112, 113
irritability of, 530
oxygen lack in, 381–82
sensitivity to digitalis, 526
Myoglobin, 707, 715
Myoneural junction, 504
Myositis, defined, 304
Myxedema: see Hypothy-
roidism
Myxoviruses, 207, 463

N

Narcosis, carbon dioxide,
417, 474
Narcotics: see Drugs; specific drugs
Nares, 392
Nasal polyps
with allergic rhinitis, 282,
396
illustrated, 397
Nasal tubes for stomach intubation, 780–81,
1149–55
Nasopharynx, diphtheria
and, 186
Nausea, 63
from falling oxygen ten-
sion, 389
from hypoxia, 388
as protection, 764–65
as symptom of irradiation,
137
before vomiting, 768
Neck
collapsed veins in, 519
staphylococci on, 226
Necrosis, 116–18; see also
specific sites
Nembutal (Pentobarbital),
1157

Neoplasms: see Cancer;
Tumors
Neostriatum, 1086
Neo-Synephrine (phenyl-
ephrine hydrochlo-
ride), 1031
caution in use of, 396
Nephritis: see also Glo-
merular nephritis
chronic, 80
defined, 304
healing of, 313
hemorrhagic, 224, 305
injury in, 49
Nephrons, 491–92
Nephrosclerosis, 549, 1020
Nephrosis, protein lost in,
545
Nephrotic syndrome, 549
Nerves: see Neural regulation; Nervous system;
specific nerves
degeneration of, 1073
Nervous system, 1018; see
also Autonomic nerv-
ous system; Neural
regulation; Sympa-
thetic nervous system
anemia and, 718–19
central nervous system
organization of, 1064–
66
controls of
respiratory, 405, 425,
427
swallowing, 395
in diabetes mellitus, 1312
glomerular nephritis and,
556
hypertension and, 679
hypoxia and, 386–87
pain and, 1216–21
in regulation of blood vessels, 652
relationship between en-
docrine system and,
1024
in serum sickness, 276
in shock, 1177
stimulation of
by cocaine, 403
dyspnea from, 455
syphilis and, 214
surgery on, to relieve
spasm or pain, 1165
virus infections, 208
Nervous tissue, water content of, 488
Neural regulation, 1064–
1110; see also Brain
blood-brain barrier and,
1068
blood supply of brain,
1069
cerebral cortex, 1082
absence of, 1085
function of, 1093–99
cerebral metabolism, 1069
cerebrospinal fluid, 1066–
68
cranial nerves, 1091–93

1385

Osmotic pressure (*continued*)
   of extracellular fluids, 488
   increase in, 506
   reduced, 518
   increased, 507
Osteitis fibrosa cystica, 1061
Osteomalacia, in adults, 556
Osteomyelitis
   described, 224
   healing of, 313
   protein loss from, 866
Osteoporosis, defined, 110
OT, 203
Otitis media, 461
Outpatient clinics for syphilis
   treatment, 212
Ovarian cysts, 931, 948
Ovulation, temperature during, 908
Oxidation-reduction reac-
   tions, 379–80
   end products of
      heat as, 494
      water as, 488
   enzymes required for, 440
   stages of, 849
Oxygen, 379–478
   administration of, 442–49
      for acidosis, 417–18
      for artificial respiration,
         430–36
      for asthma, 472
      for carbon monoxide
         poisoning, 150, 440
      for emphysema, 473–74
      observation of patient
         receiving, 448
      for pneumonia, 470
      prescribed, 442–43
      for shock, 515
      safety and, 445–46, 448
   in blood
      failure in blood trans-
         portation and, 563–
         64
      hemorrhage and, 1181–
         82
      high altitudes and, 389
      number of erythrocytes,
         703
   decrease in blood's power
      to carry, 52
   described, 445
   failure in transporting,
      439–49
   in heart disease, 615, 625,
      634
      congestive heart failure,
         607
      myocardial infarction,
         641
   tension, 381*n*
   poisoning, 448
   preparation of patient for,
      447
   as stimulant to respiration,
      426
   supply of, 379–438
      deficit in, 16, 386; *see
         also* Hypoxia
      obstructed, 393–415

   regulation of, 425–36
   source of, 383
   tests determining, 449
   threatened, 379–80
   to tissues, 381–82
Oxygen tents, 444–45, 909,
   1048
Oxyhemoglobin
   as buffer systems, 484,
      532
   carrying of, 439
   formation of, 438
   temperature and, 902
Oxytocin, 1019, 1022, 1024

P

Pacemakers, artificial, 619
Pain, 1216–32
   abdominal, 776–77
   with breathing, 405–406
   with bruises, 302
   in cancer, 952–55, 1165,
      1230
   changes in breathing due
      to, 426
   drugs for, 1223, 1226–27
   expressions of, 343–44
   in joints, 275, 276
   observation and recording
      of, 1228–32
   from peptic ulcers, 793–
      94
   phantom, 1256
   psychic component of,
      351, 1221–25
   as reaction to injury, 260,
      262
   as sign of inflammation,
      305
Paleostriatum, 1086
Palliative surgery, 1164
Palpitation, heart, 600
   in anemia, 600, 718
Pancreas
   cancer of, 1164
   digestion of, 161
Pancreatectomy, 1016
   diabetes mellitus and, 1283
Pancreatic juice
   escaped, 302
   as example of interstitial
      fluid, 486
Pancreatitis, acute, 515,
   891–92
Pandemic, defined, 165
Panhypopituitarism, 1027–
   28
Pantothenic acid, in en-
   zymes, 853
Pantopium hydrochloride,
   608
Papanicolaou smear exami-
   nation, 966, 1163
Papaverine hydrochloride
   administration of, 245,
      667
   for colic, 160
Papilledema, 682
Papillomas, 942
Para-aminosalicylic acid
   (PAS), 200

Paracentesis, performance
   of, 825–26
Paradoxical breathing, defined, 420–22
Paraffin section, 1163
Paralysis
   of ciliary action, 405
   disability rate from, 86
   flaccid, 110
   obstructive, 391
   overstimulation as cause
      of, 108
   respiratory, 540, 1265
   of soft palate, 398, 779
   of vocal cords, 397–98
Paralytic ileus, 253, 1195,
   1196
Paraplegia, 1244–45
   elimination problems in,
      1260–63
   prevention of contractures
      in, 1263–65
   prevention of decubiti in,
      1258–60
Parasites, 176–78
   facultative, 178
   malarial, 176–77
   obligatory, 178
   obstructing lymph chan-
      nels, 503
Parasympathetic nervous
   system
   activities of, 41, 250–54
   increased, 399–400
   epinephrine and, 287
   inhibited, 249, 255
   relation to gastrointestinal
      tract, 761–62
Parathyroid glands
   hormone from, 42, 530,
      1058–62
   removal of, 530
Paratyphoid fever, 183
Parenchyma of the liver,
   726, 821–23
Parenteral injections, 510–11
Paresthesias, 718, 1072
Parkinson's disease, 1087
Paronychia, 224, 224*n*
Parotitis, 224, 885
   described, 778–79
   predisposition to, 392
Paroxysmal dyspnea, 458–
   59, 596–97
PAS, 200
Pasteur, L., 172–73
Patent ductus arteriosus, defined, 588*n*
Pathogenicity, defined, 184–
   85
Pathogens, 55–56, 164
Patients, 7–30, 198, 366
   conversations with, 372–
      75, 552–53
   dependence of, 358–59
   dying, 89–97, 333–34
   home care of, 100–101,
      333
   increasing security of,
      369–75
   isolated, 198

Proctitis, 145, 874–75
Proctosigmoidoscopy, 967–68
Prodromal period, 196
Prolactin, 1026
Properidin system, 193
Proprioceptive pathway, 1077
Propylthiouracil, 1052
Prostate
bleeding after surgery on, 727, 1181
cancer of, 948–49
hyperplasia of, 112
Prostration, acute, 222
Protein-bound iodine (PBI) test, 1041
Protein shells, function of, 206
Proteins
deficiency of
effects of, 866
predisposition to, 866–67
diet high in, 787
energy extracted from, 848–60
enzymes, 1014–18
in fluid balance, 493
loss of, 502–503, 550, 832, 911
permeability to, 500–501
in plasma, 502
return of escaped, 500
specific dynamic action of, 903
synthesis of, 1010, 1013
utilization of, 864–65
water for storage of, 495
Prothrombin, 725–29, 816
Prothrombin time, 644–46
Protons, defined, 131
Protoveratrine, 698
Pruritus, 556–57
Psittacosis, 183
Psoriasis, 49
Psychological effects of illness
cancer, 955–58
hypertension, 686–87, 688–91
myocardial infarction, 643–44
palpitation, 600
permanent disability, 1249–53
regression, 360
tachycardia, 621–22
Psychological response to injury, 318, 320, 322
Psychological stress, 57–58
causes of, 350–57
defined, 348–50
discomfort from, 362
from disparity in beliefs, 346
due to lack of speech, 410
due to expense of illness, 351
from dyspnea, 456–57

hypertension and, 684, 688–91
mild, 257
minimizing, 368–69
pain and, 1221–25
from radiation treatment, 141
role definitions as source of, 350–57
surgery and, 1233
preoperative phase, 1137, 1139–43
Psychology defined, 326–27
Psychosocial aspects of illness, 326–76
cultural: see Cultures
emotional homeostasis, 347–48
emotional reactions, 357–75
inner thinking and personality disorders, 1267–70
intellectual responses, 346–47
place of residence, 337–38
professional education, 345
socioeconomic status, 338
time orientation, 334–38
value systems, 338–43
Ptyalin, 778
Pubic hair, preoperative shaving of, 1156
Pulmonary embolism, 1202–1207; see also Thrombosis
Pulmonary function: see Lungs
Pulmonary hypertension, 699–702
Pulse
changes in, 63
in children, 622
digitalis and, 603–605
in heart block, 619
pulsus bigeminus, 603
thready, 519
water-hammer (Corrigan's), 588
Pulse deficit, defined, 603
Pump oxygenator, 916
Punch, 1163
Purified protein derivative (PPD), 203
Purkinje cell, 1088, 1089
Purkinje system, 617
Purpura, 556, 727, 731
Pus (purulent exudate)
contents of, 300
described, 303
obstructive, 391
removal of, 310, 424
in wounds, 316
Push-pull artificial respiration, 430–31
Putamen, 1086
Pyelonephritis, 224, 548, 677, 679, 687, 1311
described, 547–50

Pyemia, 224
Pyloric muscle, hypertrophy of, 112–13
Pyoderma, 224
Pyogenic infections, 267, 703
Pyothorax, 424
Pyramidal tracts, 1097–99
Pyridoxine, 853
Pyrogen, 910–11
Pyrosis (heartburn), 784
Pyruvic acid, 382

Q

Quadriplegia, 1248
Quinidine, 717
Quinidine sulfate, 624
Quinine, 75, 716
poisoning, 624
dermatitis from, 278

R

Rad, defined, 132
Radial nerve, injury to, 1072–74
Radiation, 129–49
heat in, 904
injury from, 114, 129–41
ionizing, 130–49, 706
as cause of cancer, 130–31, 138, 145–46, 941–42
defined, 131
effects of, 130–32, 132–33, 136–39
emotional psychological stress in patients, 141
hazards to person handling, 145–46
sensitivity to, 133–35
sources of, 132
in treatment, 139–48
in treatment of cancer, 974–75
related nursing care, 140, 143
sickness from, 141–42
and staphylococcic infections, 228
Radical neck resection, 408
Radioactive gold
in treatment of cancer, 974
in treatment of ascites and pleural effusion, 145
Radioactive iodine
to test thyroid gland, 1042
in treatment of cancer, 974
in treatment of hyperthyroidism, 1053
Radioactive isotopes, 132, 143–45, 921
Radioautography, 928
Radiomimetic drugs, 148–49
Radium therapy, 130
theory, 132–33
nursing care, 143–44, 147–48
salts, ingested, 144
Rales, defined, 401

Thrills, defined, 657
Throat, sore, 207
  following bronchoscopy, 404
  with syphilis, 213
  from tonsilitis, 464
Thrombectomy, 659
Thrombin, 725–26, 729
Thromboangiitis obliterans, 658–70; *see also* Buerger's disease
Thrombocytes (blood platelets), 702, 720
  abnormalities of, 135, 278, 703
  bleeding and, 727, 728
  level of, 137, 273
Thrombophlebitis, 655, 725, 1204–1205
Thromboplastin, 725–26
Thrombosis: *see also* Anticoagulant drugs
  arterial occlusion and, 490–91, 667–68
  atherosclerosis and, 632–33
  cerebral, hypertension and, 682
  fibrous connective tissues in healing of, 313
  with homografts, 268
  intracardiac, 568–69, 572, 614–15
  mural, 624, 667
    defined, 568n
  in small vessels, 294
  in peripheral vascular disease, 659
  in postoperative patients, 1202–1207, 1210
  surgical removal, 659
Thymus, 156
Thyroid crises, 910, 913, 1055
Thyroid gland, 111
  hormones of, 1019–21, 1041–58; *see also* Thyroxin
  neoplasms in, 929, 950, 974
  surgical removal of, 397, 408, 1054–56, 1137–38
Thyroid-stimulating hormone, 111n, 1026, 1042
Thyrotoxicosis, 678, 1044–56
Thyrotrophic hormones (TSH): *see* Thyroid-stimulating hormone
Thyroxin, 42, 111, 856, 1019–21, 1042
  caloric intake and, 831
  in injury, 256–57
  as regulator of cellular metabolism, 42
  as regulator of heat production, 907–908, 1041
Tidal volume, defined, 449

Timed vital capacity, 449–50
Tissues
  anatomic barriers within, 194
  crepitus of, 403–404
  excess of, 43
  lack of oxygen supply to, 381–82
  necrosis of, 116–18, 642–44
  reduced requirements of, 832
  repair of, 314–17
  replacement of: *see* Fibrous connective tissue; Scar tissue
  transplantation of foreign, 268–69
Tobacco: *see* Smoking
Toenails, cutting of, 660–61, 662
Tolazoline hydrochloride (Priscoline hydrochloride), 667
Tolbutamide, 1323
Tongue
  dehydrated, 507
  in lack of sodium, 519
Tonsillectomy, bleeding after, 727, 1180–81
Tonsillitis, 464
Total lung capacity, 450
Tourniquets in pulmonary congestion, 607
Toxin, 106, 186
Trachea
  mucous membrane, 114
  obstructed, 399, 408
    by encrustrations, 410
  perforation of, 403–404
Tracheal suctioning, 413–15
Trancheobronchial tree, 393–415
  increased secretion, 272
  obstructions of, 393–415
    air passing through fluids, 401
    bronchoscopy performed, 402–405
    removal of mucus from, 393
    stab wounds, 423
    tracheostomy performed, 407–15
  patency of, 390
  suctioning of. 430
Tracheobronchitis, 304, 407, 1146
Tracheostomy, 407–15
  for bronchiectasis, 469
  care of, 413–15
  care of tubes, 412
  in emphysema, 415, 450
  for laryngeal edema, 276, 1054
  tray for, 398
Trachoma, 177
Traction for muscular tension, 244
Tranquilizers, 797–98, 1226

Transitional cells, 921
Transplantation of foreign tissue, 268–69
Transportation
  causes of failure, 563
  related nursing care, 564–65
  symptoms and signs of failure, 563–64
Transudates, 438, 486
Trauma, 49
  degree and type of, 262
  effects of, 119, 123–26, 506, 790
  food intake after, 261
  to mucosa, 413–15
Tremor, 826, 1087
Trenchfoot, 126
Trendelenburg position, 406
Trends in health care, 99–101
Trephining, 168, 1131–32
Trichinosis, 882
Triethylenemelamine (TEM), 706
Trigeminal nerve, 1092
Trigeminal neuralgia, 1219–20
Tri-iodothyronine, 1041, 1042
Trochlear nerve, 1092
Trophic hormones, 111n
TSH, 111n
Tube feedings, 781
Tuberculosis, 209–11, 416
  advanced, 306
  allergies of, 279–80
  avian, 264
  bovine, 200–201
  calcification following, 158
  as cause of adrenal insufficiency, 1034
  as cause of pleurisy, 303, 424
  death rate from, 71, 80, 81
  destruction of lung in, 418
  development of, 56, 175–76
  diagnosis of, 203–204
  diarrhea with, 802
  disability from, 86, 174
    benefits for, 461
  drugs for, 73, 75
  effects of, 157, 179
  fever in, 910–11
  frequency of, 175, 191
  incubation period for, 195
  obesity and, 831
  pericardial infection in, 583
  pulmonary, 191, 199
  reaction in, 297
  recurrence of, 181
  susceptibility to, 190, 738
  treatment of, 199–200
Tularemia, 183
Tumors, 923; *see also* Cancer
  in alimentary canal, 774, 807
  brain, 428